Mosby's®
PHARMACY
TECHNICIAN
Principles and Practice

Mosby's® PHARMACY TECHNICIAN

Principles and Practice

Seventh Edition

Karen **Davis**
AAHCA, BHS, CPhT
Pharmacy Technician Education Consultant
Society for the Education
of Pharmacy Technicians (SEPhT)
Lyons, Georgia;
Pharmacy Technician Program Instructor
Florence Darlington Community College
Florence, South Carolina

Tony **Guerra**
PharmD, RPh
Professor
Des Moines Area Community College
Ankeny, Iowa

ELSEVIER

Elsevier
3251 Riverport Lane
St. Louis, Missouri 63043

Publishing Director: Kristin Wilhelm
Senior Content Strategist: Luke E. Held
Director, Content Development: Ellen Wurm-Cutter
Content Development Specialist: Elizabeth McCormac/Dominque McPherson
Senior Project Manager: Beula Christopher
Senior Book Designer: Amy L. Buxton

Printed in India

Last digit is the print number: 9 8 7 6 5 4 3 2 1

Working together
to grow libraries in
developing countries

www.elsevier.com • www.bookaid.org

Reviewers

Melissa Ballard, CPhT, BA
Director, Pharmacy Technician Program
Mountwest CTC
Huntington, West Virginia

Lacey Crawford, CPhT, PhTR
Pharmacy Technician Instructor
Science and Health Sciences
Kilgore College
Kilgore, Texas

James Graves, PharmD
Clinical Pharmacist
University of Missouri Inpatient Pharmacy
Columbia, Missouri

Chelsea Jones, RN, CPhT, CSPT
Pharmacy Education Manager
University Hospitals
Cleveland, Ohio

Lisa Jones, EdS, MH A, CPhT
Pharmacy Technician Academic Coordinator
Aiken Technical College
Graniteville, South Carolina

Genevieve Lamarre, BSc Pharm
Pharmacist,
Chair of Pharmacy Technology
John Abbot College
Montreal, Quebec, Canada

Simon Majeur, PharmD, MSc
Pharmacist
Jon Abbott College
Montreal, Quebec, Canada

Preface

You are about to embark on an exciting journey into one of today's fastest-growing fields in health care. Whether you work in a hospital pharmacy, community pharmacy, mail-order pharmacy, Internet pharmacy, or another location, the knowledge you will gain from this textbook and its supplements will prepare you well for your new career. The authors and publisher have tried to equip you with all the background knowledge and tools you need to succeed on the job. *Mosby's Pharmacy Technician: Principles and Practice* was designed as a fundamental yet comprehensive resource representing the latest information for preparing pharmacy technician students for today's challenging job environment.

Who Will Benefit From This Book?

Pharmacy technicians are increasingly called on to perform duties traditionally fulfilled by pharmacists. This development occurred because federal regulations now require pharmacists to spend more time with patients to provide patient education. As the number of pharmacy technicians in the United States and Canada continues to grow, the need to outline a scope of practice for the pharmacy technician profession has become more urgent. *Mosby's Pharmacy Technician: Principles and Practice* provides students with solid coverage of the information they need to succeed while giving the instructor the tools to present the information effectively and efficiently.

Why Is This Book Important to the Profession?

This textbook maps directly to the Pharmacy Technician Certification Examination (PTCE) and the American Society of Health-System Pharmacists (ASHP) Curriculum. The Pharmacy Technician Certification Board (PTCB) set its blueprint for the PTCE, most recently updated in 2020. The blueprint divides the information into four Knowledge Domains and Areas: Medications, Federal Requirements, Patient Safety and Quality Assurance, and Order Entry and Processing. ASHP's current Model Curriculum, most recently revised in 2018 and implemented in 2019, provides details on how to meet the goals defined in the *ASHP Accreditation Standards for Pharmacy Technician Education and Training Programs.* It includes objectives and instructional objectives for each goal and examples of learning activities for each portion of the program, including the didactic, simulated (laboratory), and experiential program components. The most recent revision allows programs to seek accreditation as entry-level or advanced programs. This text is designed to cover all entry-level standards as well as many of the advanced standards. The criteria defined in the PTCB Blueprint (the foundation of the PTCE) and the ASHP Model Curriculum are designed to help pharmacy technicians work more effectively with pharmacists, provide more excellent patient care and services, and create a minimum standard of knowledge across all 50 states in the United States and the provinces throughout Canada to help employers determine a knowledge base for employment.

Organization

For this edition, *Mosby's Pharmacy Technician: Principles and Practice* has been completely reworked to relate to the PTCB Blueprint (the foundation of the PTCE) and ASHP Model Curriculum. This textbook remains a reliable and understandable resource, written specifically for pharmacy technician students and technicians already on the job, including those preparing for the certification examinations. The writing style, content, and organization guide today's pharmacy technician students to better understand anatomy and physiology, diseases, and, most importantly, the drugs and agents used to treat those diseases. The textbook is divided into two parts, **Pharmacy Practice** and **Pharmacology and Medications,** and includes two appendices and a glossary.

Part One, Pharmacy Practice, provides an in-depth overview of pharmacy practice as it relates to pharmacy technicians. Highlights of Part One include the history of medicine and pharmacy; law and ethics (and regulatory agencies); competencies, associations, and settings for pharmacy technicians; communication; dosage forms (and routes of administration); conversions and calculations; drug information references; community pharmacy practice (including prescription interpretation); institutional pharmacy practice (including long-term care and medication order interpretation); additional pharmacy practice settings (including managed care, mail-order pharmacy, and pharmaceutical industry); bulk repackaging and non–sterile compounding; aseptic technique and sterile compounding; pharmacy stock and billing; medication safety and error prevention; and pharmacy operations management. This part gives the pharmacy technician student a comprehensive look at the vast world of pharmacy practice today.

Part Two, Pharmacology and Medications, provides an overview of each body system and the medications used to treat common conditions that afflict these systems. Highlights of Part Two include drug classifications; therapeutic agents for all the body systems (i.e., nervous; endocrine; musculoskeletal; cardiovascular; respiratory; gastrointestinal;

renal; reproductive; immune; eyes, ears, nose, and throat; dermatological; and hematological), in addition to over-the-counter (OTC) medications. It also covers the emerging world of complementary and alternative medicine (CAM). Unique to this part are detailed discussions of anatomy and physiology and photographs of several drugs used to treat various conditions of each body system.

This edition includes two appendices. Appendix A, Top 200 Prescription Drugs, lists the 200 most commonly prescribed legend drugs, their classifications, and the indications for their use. Appendix B, Top 30 Herbal Remedies, lists some more popular herbal remedies and their commonly reported uses. The Glossary contains all key terms and definitions listed in the textbook.

Distinctive Features

Learning Objectives

The organizational format of this textbook facilitates the learning process by providing students and educators with detailed learning objectives that address the cognitive knowledge required to master each chapter's content. These learning objectives are listed at the beginning of each chapter, giving students and instructors definitive evaluation tools to use as each chapter's content is covered.

Key Terms

Key terms are identified and defined at the beginning of each chapter, providing students with a valuable terminology overview. These key terms are included in the Glossary at the back of the book and are supplied in flashcard form on the Evolve site to allow students to test their knowledge of the chapter's terms and definitions.

Scenario

In Part One (Pharmacy Practice), pharmacy technician scenarios are provided at the beginning of each chapter, and scenario checkups appear throughout the chapter. These scenarios offer practical applications for pharmacy technician students and allow them to "connect" with their future beyond the classroom. The scenarios in the chapters often involve authentic pharmacy technicians sharing their fears, likes, hopes, and aspirations, providing a "real-world" feel to the book and inspiration for the student.

Tech Notes

Helpful pharmacy technician notes are interspersed throughout the chapters, providing interesting historical facts, drug cautions, hints, and safety information. These notes enhance students' acquisition of the practical information they need in a pharmacy setting.

Tech Alerts

Tech Alert boxes highlight essential information the pharmacy technician needs to remember when in the pharmacy. The Tech Alert often functions as a medication safety reminder or presents proper drug names.

Technician Profile

In Part One (Pharmacy Practice), technician profiles are shared to help pharmacy technician students "connect" with their future beyond the classroom. These profiles provide insight into life after graduation and often show students the different types of jobs and responsibilities they may take on once they enter the real-life profession of pharmacy technician.

Mini Drug Monographs

Drug monographs with pill photographs are provided in Part Two (Pharmacology and Medications), where each body system is discussed. In addition to a photo of the drug, these monographs include the drug class, generic and trade names, indication, route of administration, common adult dosage, mechanism of action, side effects, and required auxiliary labels. The monographs provide students with quick, easy-to-understand information about specific drugs. Clinical Pharmacology powered by ClinicalKey provides all pill photo images used in the Mini Drug Monographs.

Do You Remember These Key Points?

These chapter summaries are placed at the end of every chapter to recap the highlights and most important topics covered. These summaries of each chapter's key points can serve as a study tool, reminding students of the subject areas they may need to review before taking an examination on the chapter's content.

Review Questions

Multiple-choice review questions are included at the end of every chapter (and in interactive form on the Evolve site). This section provides students with a unique review tool as they prepare both for classroom and certification examinations once they are ready to begin their professional lives as pharmacy technicians. Just as the key points serve as a study tool and chapter summary, these review questions allow students to quiz themselves on the chapter content, assess their knowledge of essential chapter topics, and evaluate which topics need follow-up review.

Technician's Corner

The Technician's Corner, which appears at the end of every chapter, provides critical thinking questions to help students prepare for on-the-job experiences.

Ancillaries

Considering the broad range of students, instructors, programs, and institutions for which this textbook was designed, an extensive package of supplements has been designed to complement this seventh edition of *Mosby's Pharmacy Technician: Principles and Practice*. Each of these comprehensive supplements has been thoughtfully developed with the shared goals of students and instructors: to produce students who are well-equipped for a career in pharmacy and well-prepared to earn their certification. All of these supplements and their inventive features (with the exception of the Workbook/Lab

Manual) can be found on the Evolve site (see inside front cover for access information). They include the following materials.

For the Instructor

TEACH Instructor Resource

TEACH for *Mosby's Pharmacy Technician* is designed to help the pharmacy technician instructor prepare for class by reducing preparation time, providing new and innovative ideas to promote student learning, and helping to make full use of the rich array of resources available. This wholly revised manual includes the following:

- Detailed Lesson Plans that map to the chapter objectives (as well as the ASHP Standards)
- PowerPoint presentations
- Student Handouts
- Answer Keys for the Chapter Review Questions as well as Workbook/Lab Manual exercises

Additional Instructor Ancillaries

- ASHP Mapping Guide
- Image Collection

- Test Bank
- Competency Skills Checklists

For the Student

Ancillaries Available on the Evolve Site

- Review Questions
- Practice Exam
- Appendices from the textbook

Student Workbook/Lab Manual

The student Workbook/Lab Manual is a unique blend of a traditional workbook combined with lab exercises that enhance the student's ability to perform in class. This valuable product includes:

- Exercises to reinforce key concepts taught in this textbook
- Skill Check-off Sheets to correspond to textbook procedures
- Opportunities for students to reflect critically on topics as they develop critical thinking and decision-making skills
- Complete lab activities that will relate to practice

Contents

SECTION ONE Pharmacy Practice

Karen Davis

1 History of Medicine and Pharmacy, 3

History of Medicine, 4
Advances in Drug Therapy and Vaccinations, 10
History of Pharmacy, 12

2 Pharmacy Law, Ethics, and Regulatory Agencies, 19

US Food and Drug Administration History, 21
Description of Laws, 23
Controlled Substances, 31
Drug Monographs, 43
Prescription Regulation, 47
Special Prescribing Programs, 50
Pharmacy Sites, 51
Occupational Safety and Health Administration, 52
The Joint Commission, 52
Legal Standards, 53

3 Competencies, Associations, and Settings for Technicians, 57

Historical Data, 59
Competencies, 60
Nondiscretionary Duties, 61
National Certification for Technicians, 70
Professionalism in the Workplace, 78
The Future of Pharmacy Technicians Is Bright!, 81

4 Communication and Role of the Technician With the Customer/Patient, 83

Communication, 84
Conclusion, 91

5 Dosage Forms and Routes of Administration, 94

Where Did Pharmacy Abbreviations Originate?, 96
"Do Not Use" List, 96

Dosing Instructions, 102
Classifications of Medications, 102
Classifications of Drug Sales, 102
Dosage Forms, 103
Routes of Administration, 112
Other Considerations: Form and Function, 116
The Use of Excipients, 118
Manufactured Products, 119
Packaging and Storage Requirements, 119
Medical Terminology, 119

6 Conversions and Calculations, 125

History of Pharmacy Calculations, 126
Roman Numerals, 127
International Time (Military Time), 128
Temperature Conversion Between Fahrenheit and Celsius, 129
Basic Math Skills, 129
Measurement Systems, 132
Calculations With Liquid Medication, 137
Business Calculations, 145

7 Drug Information References, 149

Researching a Drug, 150
References Used in Pharmacy, 151
Pocket-Sized Reference Books, 156
Electronic Referencing, 156
The Internet, 158
Journals and News Magazines, 159
Additional Types of Information, 159
Considerations When Choosing a Reference, 161

8 Community Pharmacy Practice, 163

Role of the Pharmacy Technician, 165
Prescription, 166
Prescription Processing, 170
Prescription Preparation, 173
Other Pharmacy Technician Duties, 176
Pharmacy Layout, 177
Communication, 181
Elderly Patients, 182
Other Pharmacy Services, 185

9 Institutional Pharmacy Practice, 190

Types of Hospitals, 192
Hospital Pharmacy Standards and Procedures, 194

Pharmacy and Nursing Staff Relationship, 194
Hospital Orders, 195
Institutional Pharmacy Technicians, 199
The Future of the US Health Care System, 210

10 Additional Pharmacy Practice Settings and Advanced Roles for Technicians, 213

Advanced or Specialized Pharmacy Technician
   Opportunities, 214

11 Bulk Repackaging and Nonsterile Compounding, 222

Bulk Repackaging, 224
Nonsterile Compounding, 228
Packaging, 247
Documentation, 247
Safety, 250
Compounding Professionalism, 250
Regulatory and Quality Control, 250
Veterinary Medications, 250
Personnel Training, 251
Compounding Calculations, 251

12 Aseptic Technique and Sterile Compounding, 255

Terminology Used in Pharmacy, 257
Standard Precautions for a Health Care Worker, 257
Supplies, 258
Routes of Administration, 262
Medication Delivery Systems, 262
United States Pharmacopeia <797>, 263
Aseptic Technique, 271
Hand Placement, 273
Use of Ampules to Prepare Medications, 274
Education and Training, 282

13 Pharmacy Billing and Inventory Management, 286

Formulary and Drug Utilization, 288
Generic Versus Trade Name Drugs, 289
Types of Private and Group Medical Insurance
   Plans, 290
Government-Managed Insurance Programs, 291
Current Use of Medicare and Medicaid Insurance, 292
Third-Party Billing, 297
Other Methods of Payment, 303
Inventory Management, 303

14 Medication Safety and Error Prevention, 314

Overview, 315
Five Rights of Medication Safety, 315
What Constitutes an Error?, 316
Types of Medication Errors, 316
Responsibility for Errors, 318
Where Errors Are Made, 318
Why Errors Occur, 319
Risk Evaluation and Mitigation Strategies, 320
Drug Interactions as a Source of Error, 321
Errors in the Pharmacy, 322
Errors Related to Patient Care, 323
Age-Related Errors, 323
Necessity of Reporting Errors, 325
Common Pharmacy Technology, 328
Patient Dose-Specific Orders, 330
United States Pharmacopeia <797> Regulations, 330
Medication Reconciliation, 331
Quality Assurance Practices and Risk Management, 333
Other Considerations, 333
Training and Education, 334
Conclusion, 334

15 Pharmacy Operations Management and Workflow, 337

Overview, 338
Community Pharmacy, 338
Institutional Pharmacy, 343
Improving Efficiency Techniques, 345
Getting Started, 345

SECTION TWO Pharmacology and Medications

Tony Guerra

16 Drug Classifications, 351

Classifying Drugs, 352
Brand Versus Generic Versus Chemical Names, 352
Tall Man Lettering in Brand and Generic Medications
   Versus the Use of Generic Prefixes, Suffixes, and
   Infixes, 352
Medication Characteristics, 353
Drug Trials, 353
Four Phases of Drug Testing, 353
Anatomy, Physiology, Pharmacology,
   Pharmacodynamics, and Pharmacokinetics, 353
Pharmacokinetics: ADME, 354
Pharmacodynamics, 354
Drugs and Receptors, 355
Agonists and Antagonists, 355

Therapeutic Index, 355
Drug Interactions, 356
Other Drug Effects, 356
Drug Classifications by Drug Enforcement
    Administration Schedules I, II, III, IV, and V, 360

17 Therapeutic Agents for the Nervous System, 363

Nervous System Introduction, 366
Central Nervous System, 369
Peripheral Nervous System, 371
Conditions of the Nervous System and Their
    Treatments, 372

18 Therapeutic Agents for the Endocrine System, 397

Anatomy of the Endocrine System, 400
Description of Hormones and Glands, 401
Functions of the Endocrine Glands, 403
Conditions of the Endocrine System and Their
    Treatments, 409

19 Therapeutic Agents for the Musculoskeletal System, 425

Anatomy and Physiology of the Skeletal System, 427
Anatomy and Physiology of Skeletal Muscle, 427
Common Conditions Affecting the Musculoskeletal
    System, 427
Other Select Medication Classes That Affect the
    Musculoskeletal System, 441

20 Therapeutic Agents for the Cardiovascular System, 447

Anatomy of the Heart and Vasculature System, 451
Regulation of the Heart and Vasculature, 453
Common Medication Classes Used to Treat Cardiac
    Conditions, 453
Conditions Affecting the Cardiovascular System, 457

21 Therapeutic Agents for the Respiratory System, 478

Structure and Function of the Respiratory System, 480
Disorders and Conditions of the Respiratory System, 485

22 Therapeutic Agents for the Gastrointestinal System, 503

Form and Role of the Gastrointestinal System, 505
Anatomy and Physiology of the Gastrointestinal
    System, 505
Conditions Affecting the Gastrointestinal System, 508

23 Therapeutic Agents for the Renal System, 525

Anatomy and Physiology of the Renal and Urologic
    Systems, 527
Conditions Affecting the Renal and Urologic
    Systems, 531

24 Therapeutic Agents for the Reproductive System, 545

Female Reproductive System, 547
Conditions Affecting the Female Reproductive
    System, 550
Male Reproductive System, 560
Conditions Affecting the Male Reproductive
    System, 562
Sexually Transmitted Diseases, 568
Hepatitis C, 572

25 Therapeutic Agents for the Immune System, 575

Anatomy and Physiology of the Immune System, 577
Autoimmune Disorders, 584
Transplant Rejection, 591
Immunizations, 592

26 Therapeutic Agents for Eyes, Ears, Nose, and Throat, 598

The Eyes (Ophthalmic System), 601
Conditions That Affect the Eye, 602
The Ears (Auditory System), 613
Nose and Sinuses, 616
The Throat, 618

27 Therapeutic Agents for the Dermatologic System, 622

Anatomy and Physiology of the Dermatologic
    System, 624
Common Conditions Affecting the Dermatologic
    System, 625

28 Therapeutic Agents for the Hematologic System, 643

Anatomy and Physiology of the Hematologic
    System, 645
Conditions Affecting the Hematologic System, 646

29 Over-the-Counter Medications, 661

US Food and Drug Administration Regulations, 662
How a Prescription Drug Becomes an Over-the-Counter
    Drug, 662
Patient Perceptions and Safety of OTC Medications and
    Herbal Supplements, 663
Common Routes of Administration for Over-the-Counter
    Drugs, 663
Considerations for Special Populations, 669
Restricted Over-the-Counter Products, 669
Urinary Incontinence (Overactive Bladder), 670

30 Complementary and Alternative Medicine, 672

What Is Complementary and Alternative Medicine?, 673
FDA Regulation of Dietary Supplements, 673
Medical Food, 674
Types of Complementary and Alternative Medicine, 675

APPENDIX A   Top 200 Prescription Drugs, 685

APPENDIX B   Top Herbal Remedies, 690

Glossary, 691

Index, 705

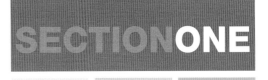
Pharmacy Practice

1   History of Medicine and Pharmacy, 3

2   Pharmacy Law, Ethics, and Regulatory Agencies, 19

3   Competencies, Associations, and Settings for Technicians, 57

4   Communication and Role of the Technician with the Customer/Patient, 83

5   Dosage Forms and Routes of Administration, 94

6   Conversions and Calculations, 125

7   Drug Information References, 149

8   Community Pharmacy Practice, 163

9   Institutional Pharmacy Practice, 190

10   Additional Pharmacy Practice Settings and Advanced Roles for Technicians, 213

11   Bulk Repackaging and Nonsterile Compounding, 222

12   Aseptic Technique and Sterile Compounding, 255

13   Pharmacy Billing and Inventory Management, 286

14   Medication Safety and Error Prevention, 314

15   Pharmacy Operations Management and Workflow, 337

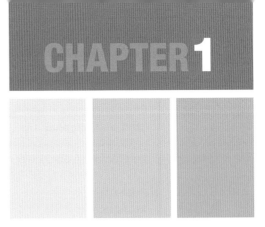

CHAPTER 1

History of Medicine and Pharmacy

Karen Davis

OBJECTIVES

1. Discuss the following related to the history of medicine: (a) discuss ancient beliefs of illness and medicine from 440 BCE through 1600 CE, (b) list common ancient treatments that prevailed in Western civilization, (c) describe 18th- and 19th-century medicine and identify influences that major wars had on medicine, (d) describe the wide use of opium and the problems surrounding opium use and differentiate between opiates and opioids.
2. Discuss advances in drug therapy and vaccinations.
3. Discuss the following related to the history of pharmacy: (a) identify the role that early pharmacists played in society; (b) describe how the first pharmacies began in the United States; (c) describe the first technicians in pharmacy; (d) list major ways pharmacy has changed over the past 100 years; (e) list important current trends in pharmacy in relation to pharmacy technicians.

TERMS AND DEFINITIONS

Apothecary Latin term for pharmacist; also, a place where drugs are sold

Bloodletting The practice of draining blood; believed to release illness

Caduceus Often confused as the symbol of the medical field; it is a staff with two entwined snakes and two wings at the top

Dogma A principle or set of principles laid down by an authority as incontrovertibly true

Hippocratic oath An oath taken by physicians concerning the ethics and practice of medicine

Inpatient pharmacies Pharmacies in a hospital or institutional setting

Laudanum A mixture of opium and alcohol used to treat dozens of illnesses through the 1800s

Leech A type of segmented worm with suckers that attaches to the skin of a host and engorges itself on the host's blood

Maggots Fly larvae that feed on dead tissue; used in medicine to clean wounds not responding to routine antibiotics

Medicine The science and art dealing with the maintenance of health and the prevention, alleviation, or cure of disease

Opioid Any agent that binds to opioid receptors

Opium An analgesic that is made from the poppy plant

Pharmacist Person who dispenses drugs and counsels patients on medication use and any interactions it may have with food or other drugs

Pharmacy A place where drugs are sold

Pharmacy technician Professional who works under the pharmacist's supervision to provide medications and health care services safely to patients

Pharmacy Technician Certification Board (PTCB) Issues a national examination for pharmacy technicians

Shaman A person who holds a high place of honor in a tribe as a healer and spiritual mediator

Staff of Asclepius The symbol of the medical profession; it is a wingless staff with one snake wrapped around it

Trephining A practice of making an opening in the head to allow disease to leave the body

IMPORTANT PEOPLE

Aristotle	Greek scientist, philosopher
Asclepius	Greek god of healing and medicine
Bacon, Roger	English scientist responsible for scientific methods
Crick, Francis	Co-discoverer of the molecular structure of DNA, the double helix
Domagk, Gerhard	Developed sulfonamides and synthetic antibiotics
Fleming, Alexander	Discovered penicillin, the first antibiotic
Galen, Claudius	Greek physician
Hippocrates	Greek physician and philosopher, considered to be the father of medicine
Mendel, Gregor	Scientist and monk, known as the father of genetics
Nightingale, Florence	Nurse who was responsible for improving the unsanitary conditions at a British base hospital during the Crimean War, reducing the death count
Paracelsus	Swiss physician, philosopher, and scientist
Pasteur, Louis	French scientist, discovered several vaccines and invented pasteurization
Watson, James	Co-discoverer of the molecular structure of DNA, the double helix

Scenario

Kelly is a new pharmacy technician student at a local career college. She begins her course of study by learning about the history of pharmacy. Why is this an important part of Kelly's education?

History of Medicine

Ancient Beliefs and Treatments

Medicine has been practiced for thousands of years. Archaeological discoveries have unearthed civilizations that have documented the use of minerals, animals, and plant parts to heal the sick. Certain remedies, such as herbs, have been used consistently throughout history. For example, herbs have been used for centuries for minor ailments such as intestinal problems, arthritis, and gout.

Many ancient treatments for illness were based on the dreams or visions of the believers. A **dogma**, such as gods being able to both cause and cure illnesses, is based on a set of principles (eg, religious or ideological doctrines) proposed by authoritarians. These principles are based on writings from respected spiritual authorities rather than scientific evidence. One belief about healing the sick was that severe illness was caused by evil spirits. To rid a person of an evil spirit, a cut was made into the skull to give the spirit a portal through which to leave. This type of treatment was called **trephining** and often was performed by a tribal **shaman** (a spiritual person in a tribe who cares for the spiritual, medicinal, and physical health of the tribe). Tribal shamans were believed to have the gift of being able to communicate with spirits. Other shamans believed that they were connected with a special spirit who helped them render the evil spirits harmless through the use of prayer, herbs, or potions. Shamans were prevalent throughout societies in ancient times. Some still exist in various societies throughout the world. In North America, various Inuit and Native American tribes held shamans in high esteem. However, many popular beliefs of the past have mostly disappeared.

The Medical Staff

The **staff of Asclepius** is the formal symbol of medicine and is associated with **Asclepius**, the Greek god associated with healing. The staff of Asclepius is a wingless walking stick with a single serpent wrapped around it. Because snakes shed their skin, the snake was believed to signify renewal of youth. The **caduceus** is often mistakenly used as a symbol of medicine. The caduceus is the staff of Hermes, a Greek god; the staff represented magic and had two serpents wrapped around it, usually with two wings at the top (Fig. 1.1). For example, in 1902 the US Army erroneously adopted the caduceus as an emblem of the Medical Corps, leading to its mistaken use as a symbol of medicine. Although many organizations still use the caduceus to represent medicine, the true staff of Asclepius has been adopted as a symbol by authoritative health organizations, such as the World Health Organization and the American Medical Association.

The Evolution of Medicine

The early path of medicine was not a smooth road. Throughout the ages, many plagues killed thousands of people. The existence of microbes, unseen by the eye, was not known to be responsible for many of the diseases that caused death and

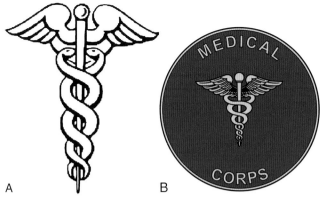

FIG. 1.1 (A) Caduceus. (B) Army Medical Corps emblem.

despair. Despite advances made through early history, most remedies for physical ailments tended to be extreme. Other ancient remedies have been used for hundreds of years. Prevalent thoughts included the belief that sickness was an entity within the body that needed a means to leave the body. Another widely held belief was that spirits were responsible for illness. In many cultures, the most common form of treatment, prayer, has remained the only way to cure illness.

Hippocrates (460–357 BCE), born on the small island of Cos near Greece, was a third-generation physician. He taught at a school of medicine on Cos, which was one of the first medical schools established. He believed in the prevailing concept of that era: life consisted of a balance of four elements that were linked to the qualities of good health. These four qualities were wet, dry, hot, and cold. In addition, he believed that illness resulted from an imbalance of the four humors of the body system: blood, phlegm, yellow bile, and black bile. These four humors were linked to the four basic elements: blood is air, phlegm is water, yellow bile is fire, and black bile is earth. Methods used to treat imbalance of the humors included bloodletting and natural laxatives.

Hippocrates was responsible for many advances in the world of medicine. Some of his observations included the effects of food, climate, and other influences on illness. He was one of the first physicians to record his patients' medical illnesses. This new way of viewing the causes of illnesses eventually led to the belief that sickness originated from something other than the supernatural. Hippocrates believed that the spirit of the patient was just as important as the condition being treated, and he promoted kindness to the sick. He also believed in letting nature do the healing and promoted resting and eating light foods. He taught that doctors needed to rebalance the four humors. Most of his teachings have been documented in a collection of books called the *Corpus Hippocraticum*. Although many of the writings are now thought to be from different authors, they still reflect the teachings of Hippocrates.

Today's medical schools still use the **Hippocratic oath** as part of their graduation ceremony. Box 1.1 presents the revised version of the Hippocratic oath used today. The Hippocratic oath outlines the physician's responsibility to the patient. Hippocrates practiced what he preached with respect to exercise, rest, diet, and overall moderation in

---

BOX 1.1   The Hippocratic Oath[a]

I swear to fulfill, to the best of my ability and judgment, this covenant:

I will respect the hard-won scientific gains of those physicians in whose steps I walk, and gladly share such knowledge as is mine with those who are to follow.

I will apply, for the benefit of the sick, all measures which are required, avoiding those twin traps of overtreatment and therapeutic nihilism.

I will remember that there is art to medicine as well as science, and that warmth, sympathy, and understanding may outweigh the surgeon's knife or the chemist's drug.

I will not be ashamed to say "I know not," nor will I fail to call in my colleague when the skills of another are needed for a patient's recovery.

I will respect the privacy of my patients, for their problems are not disclosed to me that the world may know. Most especially must I tread with care in matters of life and death. If it is given me to save a life, all thanks. But it may also be within my power to take a life; this awesome responsibility must be faced with great humbleness and awareness of my own frailty. Above all, I must not play at God.

I will remember that I do not treat a fever, chart a cancerous growth, but a sick human being, whose illness may affect the person's family and economic stability. My responsibility includes these related problems, if I am to care adequately for the sick.

I will prevent disease whenever I can, for prevention is preferable to cure.

I will remember that I remain a member of society, with special obligations to all my fellow human beings, those sound of mind and body as well as the infirm.

If I do not violate this oath, may I enjoy life and art, respected while I live and remembered with affection thereafter. May I always act so as to preserve the finest traditions of my calling and may I long experience the joy of healing those who seek my help.

[a]Written in 1964 by Louis Lasagna, Academic Dean of the School of Medicine at Tufts University, and used in many medical schools today.
From *https://www.medicinenet.com/hippocratic_oath/definition.htm*

---

lifestyle. Various records have documented his death as occurring in 377 BCE, whereas others record his death as having occurred in 357 BCE. Because of the advances he promoted in the world of medicine, it is not surprising that Hippocrates is known as the father of medicine. Before the existence of Hippocrates and other innovative scientists, people believed that they were at the mercy of the gods or supernatural forces.

Tech Note!

The origin of the term *black humor* stems from the belief that too much of the black bile humor resulted in a person showing signs of melancholy.

Later in history, the Greek philosopher and scientist **Aristotle** (384–322 BCE) was responsible for many advances in the areas of biology and medicine. His main area of interest was biology and the study and classification of various organisms. He classified human beings as animals. Because the Grecian belief system in those times did not allow dissection of the dead, he described much of human anatomy from observations he made from dissections of other animals. This included in-depth descriptions of the brain, heart, lungs, and blood vessels.

Claudius Galen (129–210) began to study medicine at the age of 16. He attended medical schools in Greece and the famous Alexandria School of Medicine in Egypt. He later resided in Rome and was the personal physician of the Roman imperial family. Although he was born nearly 600 years after Hippocrates, he followed many of the same beliefs, such as eating a balanced diet, exercising, and practicing good hygiene. He contributed greatly to the study of medicine, writing more than 100 books on topics such as physiology, anatomy, pathology, diagnosis, and pharmacology. Many of his books were used in medical schools for 1500 years. He proved that blood, rather than air, flowed through arteries.

Philosopher and alchemist **Roger Bacon** (1214–1294) further refined and explained the importance of experimental methods, which focused on observation, hypothesis, experimentation, and verification. During Bacon's time, most explanations were based on tradition, not fact. He preferred to rely on mathematics and measurement to prove his theories. He is considered an important contributor to what is now known as the scientific method.

Paracelsus (1493–1541), a Swiss physician and alchemist, believed that it was important to treat illness with one medication at a time. At the end of the Middle Ages, it was a common practice to give multiple remedies or large quantities of agents that had not been tested previously. Through experimentation and documentation of the effectiveness and dosage of each individual agent, Paracelsus was able to produce many medications. He introduced one of the most popular tonics of that time—laudanum, which was used to deaden pain. Table 1.1 lists major figures and their influences throughout medical history.

TABLE 1.1
Advances in Medicine

Name	Year	Medical Advance
William Harvey	1628	Writes first book on blood circulation through the heart
James Lind	1747	Discovers that citrus fruits prevent scurvy
Rene Laennec	1816	Invents stethoscope
James Blundell	1818	Performs first blood transfusion
Crawford W. Long	1842	Uses ether as a general anesthetic
Joseph Lister	1867	Publishes *Antiseptic Principle of the Practice of Surgery*
Louis Pasteur	1870s	Establishes germ theory of disease
Wilhelm Roentgen	1895	Discovers x-rays
Ronald Ross	1897	Demonstrates that malaria is transmitted by mosquitoes
Felix Hoffman	1899	Develops aspirin
Karl Landsteiner	1901	First describes A, B, AB, and O blood groups
Sir Frederick Gowland Hopkins	1906	Suggests existence of vitamins and concludes they are essential to health
Dr. Paul Dudley White	1913	One of the first cardiologists; pioneers use of electrocardiograph
Edward Mellanby	1921	Discovers that lack of vitamin D causes rickets
	1922	Is the first to use insulin to treat diabetes
Sir Alexander Fleming	1928	Discovers penicillin[a]
Gerhard Domagk	1932	Discovers sulfonamides
Dr. John H. Gibbon, Jr.	1935	Successfully uses heart-lung machine (on cat) to continue circulating blood while patient was in surgery
Selman A. Waksman	1943	Discovers streptomycin
Paul Zoll	1952	Develops first cardiac pacemaker
James Watson, Francis Crick	1953	Describe double-helical structure of DNA
Dr. Joseph E. Murray	1954	Performs first kidney transplant
Dr. Luc Montagnier, Dr. Anthony Galo	1983	Discover the human immunodeficiency virus (HIV), the virus that causes acquired immunodeficiency syndrome (AIDS)
James Thomson	2007	Discovers how to use human skin cells to create embryonic stem cells; performs study in laboratory at University of Wisconsin

TABLE 1.1
Advances in Medicine—cont'd

Name	Year	Medical Advance
Laurent Lantieri	2008	Performs the first full face transplant
Deborah Persaud	2013	Becomes the first to cure baby of HIV in the United States
Researchers at Massachusetts General Hospital in Boston	2013	Produce first kidney grown in vitro in the United States
Organovo	2014	Develops 3D organ printing through tissue engineering
KardiaMobile	2019	Launche the AliveCor mobile app for personal electrocardiography monitor
Researchers at Washington University School	2020	Develop first blood test for Alzheimer disease

aAlthough discovered in 1928, it was not isolated and used as an antibiotic until 1938.

Ancient Herbal Remedies

Over the millennia, some prevalent treatments consisted of multiple mixtures of plants, roots, and other concoctions. Digestion of the type of plant that resembled the organ affected by disease also was believed to cure illnesses. For example, those with liver problems ingested a plant called *liverwort* (named because the leaves were shaped like a liver). Other popular treatments included using garlic for inflammation of the bronchial tubes, wine and pepper for various stomach ailments, onions for worms, and tiger fat for joint pain. It was difficult to detect which, if any, of the ingredients administered actually worked, because many concoctions contained a multitude of ingredients. As strange as many of these archaic remedies seem, there were many people who were "cured" because of their strong belief in the treatment given or their belief in the person treating them.

Throughout history, popular religious beliefs revolved around the idea that evil spirits were the cause of illness in a person who had sinned. This belief may have persisted partly because no one had the slightest idea about germs or genetics. Many times, through trial and error (error sometimes causing death), certain treatments were found to be fairly effective.

Anytime new theories are proposed, they can be met with some skepticism and disbelief. Eventually, medicine and science discovered methods to answer this need for corroboration, leading to modern approaches and effective treatments for disease. A new hypothesis should be treated as a possible answer that has not been disproved. As new sciences emerge and new methods are devised to test hypotheses, the results can lead to medical advances. This was especially evident throughout the golden age of microbiology.

◎ Scenario Checkup 1.1

Kelly is assigned to create a poster board showing the advances of medicine throughout ancient history. What should she focus on when creating her poster? What important pieces of information from ancient history relate to today's pharmacy practice that Kelly could show on her poster?

Eighteenth- and Nineteenth-Century Medicine

From the time of Galen, it was widely believed that the four humors could be rebalanced through the use of cathartics to clean out the bowels; diuretics to lessen the imbalance of body fluids; emetics to empty the stomach; and bloodletting to lessen body fluids, heart rate, and temperature. Physicians brought this theory to America, where such techniques were widely used, especially **bloodletting**.

Bloodletting had its origins in Egypt more than 3000 years ago and later spread into all areas of Europe through the Middle Ages. Just as trephination of the skull was believed to release evil spirits, bloodletting was thought to be an effective way of lessening excess body fluids that were believed to cause illness. Artifacts such as sharp bones, sharks' teeth, thorns, and sharpened sticks were thought to be the earliest instruments used in bloodletting. During the 19th century, some even used bloodletting as preventive medicine to ensure good health. A well-known victim of bloodletting in the United States during the 18th century was George Washington, who suffered from an infection and died of complications from bloodletting. At that time, it was wrongly believed that the body contained 12 quarts of blood; however, it contains only 6 quarts, and President Washington was bled of 4 quarts over a 24-hour period.

One bloodletting treatment involved using **leeches**. These bloodsucking worms were gathered, stored, and used to remove blood from patients. The leech has the ability to latch onto the skin with sharp, teethlike appendages and engorge itself to nearly twice its size on a person's blood. Leeches also emit a natural anticoagulant, hirudin, that allows the blood to flow freely. Leeches were used in specific places, such as the vagina to treat menorrhea. Once the leeches were finished eating, they would normally detach themselves; if not, they were encouraged to detach with the use of salt. Bleeding would continue until it was necessary to manually stop the flow of blood with bandages. Today, leeches are used in microsurgery and plastic surgery to prevent blood clots.

TABLE 1.2
Examples of Prescription Compounds From the 1900s

Infusion of Dandelion, &c.	Interpretation of Formula
Infusi Taraxaci, fℨiv	4 fluid ounces of infusion of dandelion
Extracti Taraxaci, fℨij	2 fluid drachms of extract of dandelion
Sodæ Carbonatis, ℨβ	½ drachm of sodium carbonate
Potasse Tartratis, ℨiij	3 drachms of potassium tartrate
Tincturæ Rhei, fℨiij	3 fluid drachms of tincture of rhubarb
Hyoscyami, gtt. xx	20 drops [19] of henbane tincture
Signa.—One-third part to be taken 3 times a day. In dropsical and visceral affections.	

Another form of bloodletting, venesection (phlebotomy, or drawing blood), was widely used in the 1700s and 1800s for those who did not want leeches applied. The physician would heat the air inside a small cup and place it on the skin, which would draw up the skin tissue, along with its blood flow (called *wet cupping*). At this point, a lancet would be used to cut into the skin, the cup would be removed, and 1 to 4 ounces of blood would be collected. Many patients succumbed to this procedure until the early 1900s, when this type of treatment was declared quackery.

Fortunately, medicine did advance through the 19th century in many ways. Medical schools arose throughout Europe, specifically in France and Germany. Many of the doctors trained in these schools came to the United States and brought with them this European influence in medicine. Medicinal recipes were written in Latin until the 1900s. Table 1.2 presents an example of a commonly compounded prescription. Because Latin was used in medicine and **apothecary** products, this order could be interpreted by most practitioners. Although there have been many changes in the accepted abbreviations and weights in medicine, the fluid ounce can still be seen on pharmacy bottles. Several important medical advances that have changed medical treatments and lengthened the human life span are listed in Table 1.1.

Throughout the 19th century, the church became active in scientific research as well. A monk named **Gregor Mendel** experimented on plants and noticed the changes from generation to generation with respect to color, size, and appearance. He used pea plants to determine how traits were transferred from one to another and in doing so determined the basics of genetics. In 1822, he determined how stronger plants could be propagated through heredity. It was not until the 1900s, however, that other scientists were able to continue his work and enlighten the scientific world with the theory of genetics. As a result of his work, Mendel became known as the father of genetics.

Florence Nightingale was born in Florence, Italy, in 1820 and is best known as a nurse who spent her career caring for the wounded. She believed in cleanliness and its benefits to the medical field. She started a hospital and founded a school for nurses. Her writings sparked worldwide health care reform.

North American Medicine

In early North America, as new immigrants brought their families from Europe and other parts of the world, disease followed. At that time, doctors were responsible not only for diagnosing conditions but also for preparing the necessary remedies to cure patients. Disease was widespread in the colonies, and many people did not survive the voyage across the sea from Europe, succumbing to diseases such as scurvy and severe intestinal infection. Patients were at a disadvantage throughout the colonies because there were few doctors and even fewer hospitals. The first pharmacists, known as druggists at the time, were doctors until pharmacy became a specialty. The term *druggist* was widely used from the 1700s until the mid-1800s to describe the practitioners of pharmacy, eventually leading to the title *pharmacist.*

Remedies used in early American history included cinchona bark (quinine) for the treatment of malaria. More unconventional and dangerous treatments also were used; for example, mercury was used to treat syphilis. Many people died of mercury poisoning because of its toxicity. Many people also died of typhoid fever, malaria, diphtheria, and dysentery. The need for doctors and treatments increased dramatically. The average life expectancy was approximately 40 years, and many families lost several children to childhood diseases, such as smallpox, for which no vaccines were available. Most treatments were concoctions handed down through family tradition. If a person were to use a doctor, he or she most likely would be treated at home or in the doctor's office, with treatments ranging from minor procedures to surgery. Table 1.3 presents some typical remedies used in the 1800s in the United States.

Tech Note!

Vaccines were not developed until 1796, with the first immunization against smallpox in England. Smallpox vaccination was stopped in 1971 because the disease had been eradicated worldwide. Polio is another serious illness that has been eradicated in developed countries through the use of an effective vaccination strategy. However, childhood immunization remains important to prevent the spread of wild-type polio infection worldwide. Countries such as Nigeria, India, Pakistan, and Afghanistan have been experiencing a resurgence of polio, which makes all countries that no longer immunize for this disease vulnerable to infection.

TABLE 1.3
Typical Remedies During the 1800s in America

To stop earaches	Blow tobacco smoke into the ear.
To treat a cold	Combine a mixture of sugar, mineral oil, sulfur, ginger, lemon, and whisky in 8 oz of water; drink this and go to bed.
For baldness	Rub the head with an onion in the morning and at night before bed until the skin becomes red, and then rub it with honey.
For worms	Take a tablespoon of molasses and mix it with tin rust and ingest.
For stomach aches	Mix strychnine and other alkaline additives into an oral solution.
For cough and cold	Mix terpin of hydrate with codeine or heroin into an oral solution.
For eye infections	Add mercury to other ingredients such as eye drops.

Opium and Alcohol One of the most popular tonics made for medicinal use in the early United States contained opium and alcohol. Its effectiveness was surpassed only by its addictiveness. This tonic was given as a sedative and to dull the sensation of pain. Paracelsus (as mentioned earlier in this chapter) introduced the opium-alcohol mixture called **laudanum** in the 16th century, and laudanum was used as a medicinal remedy. Laudanum was used widely throughout Europe in the Victorian era. During the Civil War, laudanum not only was used to treat painful wounds from the battlefield (Box 1.2) but also found its way into households throughout the United States for less severe problems. Laudanum was used mostly by white middle-class to upper-class women for

BOX 1.2   The Civil War

From 1861 through 1865, the US Civil War claimed more lives than any other war in American history. More than 1 million soldiers died on the battlefield. Soldiers who did not die of their wounds succumbed to tuberculosis, typhoid fever, dysentery, and a host of other diseases, including measles, mumps, and chickenpox. Diseases spread rapidly as a result of the overcrowded and close quarters of men who had never been exposed to these diseases. Field hospitals were unsanitary and over-crowded. Many men died of infections caused by amputations and gunshot wounds. Medication was not available most of the time, and anesthesia was limited to chloroform, from which many men died as a result of an overdose of the drug. Those who were hurt on the battlefield received care from undertrained medical staff with less than adequate equipment in nonsterile conditions. Most of the doctors (in the states) had minimal training; usually they completed an apprenticeship in lieu of formal training.

BOX 1.3   Laudanum Recipe From 1669

16 ounces of sherry wine
2 ounces of opium
1 ounce of saffron
1 ounce powder of cinnamon
1 ounce powder of cloves

a host of problems, including nervousness, diabetes, diarrhea, gastric problems, menstrual pain, and even morning sickness. Laudanum was also used to calm screaming babies. Individuals became addicted at an alarming rate. Many mortalities and miscarriages were attributed to this agent. Even though it was well known by the 18th century that opium and alcohol were addictive, alternative remedies were hard to find. Box 1.3 presents an example of a laudanum recipe from 1669 that was used as a remedy for dysentery. Another alcohol-based liquid was absinthe. The herb *Artemisia absinthium* was mixed with alcohol and other additives. Absinthe was served with water and sugar and was purported to rid a person of tapeworms, among other ailments.

Tech Note!

Alcohol use has been dated back to 3500 BCE in Egypt. Opium has long been a part of human history; opium plants have been found as part of Neolithic burial sites. Cultivated opium made its appearance in Egypt about 1300 BCE; from Egypt, opium was traded to Greece and eventually other parts of Europe.

Origin of opium (opiates). **Opium** has a long history for medicinal relief of pain and recreational use. Opium is a by-product of the plant *Papaver somniferum*, commonly known as the opium poppy. The sap is taken from the head of the poppy. The raw opium is then precipitated from the sap. The result of this process is a potent drug that causes an analgesic effect. Although *opiate* was a term used for a drug derived from opium, the more common term is **opioid**, which refers to both synthetic and semisynthetic medications. Opiates and opioids react on the same opioid receptor sites, which are located in the central nervous system and gastrointestinal tract (see Chapter 22). The effects associated with the opioid receptors include analgesia, respiratory depression, pupil constriction, reduced gastrointestinal motility, euphoria, dysphoria, sedation, and physical dependence. Opioids and opiates have many of the same side effects, including nausea and vomiting. When used properly, the opioid drugs are effective and help many patients who otherwise would suffer extreme pain. Not until 1909, under the Opium Exclusion Act, did the prohibition of opium importation (except for medicinal purposes) begin in the United States (see Chapter 2).

Twentieth-Century Medicine

In the 1900s many new medicines were discovered; some of the earlier, groundbreaking discoveries were for medicines that were useful in treating infections. The Scottish physician and bacteriologist **Alexander Fleming** accidentally contaminated a plate of bacteria with mold while working in his laboratory in 1928; the mold inhibited the growth of the bacteria, and he named the mold *penicillin*. Many years of failed and successful experimentation by many scientists followed before penicillin was recognized as a useful medicine. It was not until after 1938 that penicillin would undergo mass production and be used worldwide as a helpful antibiotic. Penicillin was the first antibiotic discovered and is still in use today. The first synthetic drug, a sulfonamide, was discovered by **Gerhard Domagk** in 1938 and was derived from a chemical dye found to inhibit bacterial growth. This sulfonamide was used extensively during World War II to treat infections that were a result of battle wounds. Today, sulfonamides are primarily used to treat urinary tract infections. Many antibiotics were discovered in the years after penicillin and sulfa.

In the 20th century, Rosalind Franklin, a British scientist, discovered the density and helical shape of DNA. Her work would lay the foundation for another particularly important discovery made by **James Watson** and **Francis Crick**. In April 1953, they published a scientific paper presenting the structure of the DNA double-helix, the molecule that carries genetic information from one generation to another. In 1962, Watson and Crick received the Nobel Prize in Physiology or Medicine, along with Maurice Wilkins, for their important contributions to science.

Advances in Drug Therapy and Vaccinations

Many of the most famous chemists, biologists, and doctors who contributed to science were from European countries such as Germany, England, France, and Poland. **Louis Pasteur** (France), who is best known for the pasteurization process, was also responsible for discovering vaccines, such as the anthrax vaccine. Most recently, because of the coronavirus disease 2019 (COVID-19) pandemic, research has introduced new technology, such as mRNA, when creating vaccines. These do not affect the DNA but rather teach cells to make a protein that affects the immune response. Table 1.4 provides a list of pathogens and diseases that were discovered, along with the vaccines administered to prevent these diseases.

TABLE 1.4
Examples of Important Vaccine Advances in Medicine[a]

Scientist	Year of Discovery	Organism/Disease Identified	Vaccine
Edward Jenner (England)	1796 (acknowledged in 1800)	Smallpox	Smallpox vaccine
Robert Koch (Germany)	1876	Anthrax, tuberculosis	BioThrax vaccine[b,c]
Louis Pasteur (France)	1877–1887	*Staphylococcus, Streptococcus, Pneumococcus*	Rabies, chickenpox, cholera, anthrax vaccines
Emil von Behring (Germany)	1890	Antitoxins	Tetanus/diphtheria/typhoid fever vaccine (DPT)
	1896	Typhoid fever	
	1926	Whooping cough	Pertussis vaccine
	1945	Influenza	Various vaccines used currently: Fluarix, Fluvirin, Fluzone, FluLaval intranasal, FluMist
Jonas Salk (United States)	1955	Polio	First polio vaccine
Albert Sabin (United States)	1962	Polio[d]	First oral polio vaccine
	1964	Measles	Vaccine combo (measles, mumps, rubella [MMR])
	1967	Mumps	Vaccine combo (MMR)
	1970	Rubella	Vaccine combo (MMR)
	1974	Chickenpox[e]	Varicella (Varivax) vaccine
	1977	Pneumonia	Pneumovax vaccine
	1978	Meningitis	Menactra, Menomune vaccines
	1981	Hepatitis B	HepB (Engerix-B, Recombivax HB)
	1992	Hepatitis A	HepA (Havrix, Vaqta) HepA/HepB combo (Twinrix)
	1998	Lyme disease	Vaccine removed from US market in 2002 because of low demand

TABLE 1.4
Examples of Important Vaccine Advances in Medicine—cont'd

Scientist	Year of Discovery	Organism/Disease Identified	Vaccine
	2003	Influenza	FluMist (first nasal vaccine for influenza approved in the United States)
	2006	Human papillomavirus	HPV (Gardasil)
	2006	Varicella-zoster virus (shingles)	Zostavax vaccine
	2009	Swine flu	H1N1 vaccine
	2010–2011	Influenza	H3N2 vaccine
	2010	*Streptococcus pneumoniae*	Prevnar 13 vaccine
	2013	Hand-foot-mouth disease vaccine	Enterovirus 71
	2014	HPV, meningococcal influenza	Gardasil 9, Trumenba, Rapivab, Fluzone
	2015	Meningitis	Yellow fever booster, Bexsero
	2016	Cholera	Vaxchora
	2019	Ebola	ERVEBO vaccine
	2020	COVID-19, coronavirus	Spikevax, Comirnaty, Novavax

[a]For more information on vaccines, refer to Chapter 25.
[b]For military use only.
[c]Not used in the United States.
[d]Oral polio vaccine is no longer used for routine vaccination in United States because the disease has been eradicated in that country.
[e]Given to individuals born after 1956.

Are Old Remedies Making a Comeback?

Many archaic treatments fell out of favor during the middle to late 19th century, yet certain ones prevail. For instance, patients are bled daily in all types of medical settings. For example, if a physician orders a blood test to be done on a patient, up to 30 mL of blood will be taken from the patient's vein. This, of course, is used to diagnose an illness rather than as a curative measure, yet these techniques originated in the distant past, and today no one would question such a technique. The disorder hemochromatosis is a hereditary condition in which the body absorbs too much iron, which is stored in organs and can cause serious damage. The current treatment for this disorder is to remove blood (phlebotomy) on a regular basis.

The US Food and Drug Administration (FDA) approved the use of both leeches and maggots in the medical setting in 1976. This may seem strange and not much of an advance in medicine. The origins of this type of treatment stem from research in the repair of tissue that has been severely damaged, such as that found in patients who have undergone reconstructive surgery or skin grafts or patients with infections. Surgical reattachment of veins can result in coagulation before blood flow is reestablished to the affected part, thus killing the affected tissues. Leeches are used to siphon excess blood from the area and prevent coagulation from taking place too soon. They are applied one at a time over 20 minutes for up to 2 days as necessary. Leeches are cared for and stored in the refrigerator in the pharmacy. They may not be the first choice of a physician, but they have been used successfully in many cases as a means of avoiding amputation.

Because dead skin is the main dietary intake of **maggots**, they can be used to remove dead skin. Antibiotics are normally used as the first course of treatment; however, when they are ineffective, physicians have used maggots to do the manual work of restoring the wound to a recoverable stage. Maggots not only eat the dead tissue; they also have the ability to kill the bacteria that are the cause of the infection. Treatments involving both leeches and maggots are very inexpensive compared with other treatments.

Other remedies are being studied, such as the honey produced by some bees (manuka honey). The medicinal attributes of this type of honey include the ability to heal wounds. Manuka honey keeps the wound moist, is bacteria free, and has a high sugar content, along with minerals, vitamins, and amino acids that may promote healing. In 2007, the FDA and Health Canada approved its use for wounds and burns. In 2010, it was approved to treat leg ulcers and diabetic foot ulcers. In 2012, the FDA approved manuka honey wound dressings to be sold over the counter to treat abrasions, lacerations, and minor cuts. As medicine advances, it is wise not to forget the past, because many historical treatments and remedies may be the answer for future cures. Pharmacy plays a part in both the historical and future advances in medicine and treatments because the roots of medicinal knowledge run deep.

History of Pharmacy

Early Pharmacists

The expanding population and the subsequent increasing need for trained medical personnel influenced the need for specialists such as veterinarians, eye doctors, and **pharmacists**. In addition, the shipping of medicines to America from England was becoming difficult as the colonies separated from England. After the Civil War, apothecaries (pharmacies) began to emerge in towns across America. Manufacturing plants were built, and people were trained to prepare medications accurately. As the physician's role changed from distributing drugs to diagnosing disease and performing surgery, the role of the pharmacist emerged. The first pharmacy school opened in 1821 at the College of Pharmacy and Sciences in Philadelphia. The school is now called the University of the Sciences in Philadelphia. Through the 1800s, pharmacists compounded nearly every drug ordered by physicians. Various sizes of ornate apothecary jars were used to store herbs and ingredients (Fig. 1.2). The instructions for preparing remedies were contained in medical recipe books. Ingredients such as chalk for heartburn, rose petals for headaches, and oils, herbs, and spices filled containers in the apothecary. Although many of the ingredients in early compounded remedies are no longer used, several are still in use today, such as aspirin, digoxin, and others.

Another type of interesting container associated with the pharmacy was the show globe. Show globes have been the beacons for pharmacies dating back as far as the early 1600s. It is thought that they were placed in the apothecary stores of the town to let visitors know the status of the health of the town. Red meant there was illness or that the town was in quarantine because of disease, whereas green meant the town was healthy and thus it was safe to come into the town. It is also said that signs were posted on the doors of contagious individuals, rather than relying only on the globes. Decorative globes (Fig. 1.3) showed patrons the pharmacist's competencies in chemical mixtures. More ornate globes were layered in various colors, resulting in a striped appearance. This was done by using various liquids of differing densities,

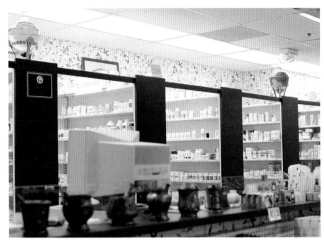

FIG. 1.3 Large show globes (seen on top of shelf). An assortment of different mortars and pestles (seen on countertop).

causing a layered effect. These types of jars are now displayed in many pharmacies, along with other artifacts from the past.

Early Pharmacy in America

The first **pharmacy** managed by a registered pharmacist opened in New Orleans in 1823. Starting in the mid-1800s and early 1900s, the soda fountain became an extension of the town drugstore. The first soda fountain pharmacy opened in the mid-1800s, and they gained popularity in the early 1900s. Prohibition in 1919 also helped with the proliferation of soda fountains. With the invention by a pharmacist, Jacob Baur (1921), of a soda fountain that dispensed carbon dioxide, soda fountain units could easily prepare all types of carbonated drinks.

Pharmacists would make and market their own recipes to be used for various treatments. It was common to find drugs mixed with flavorings, along with effervescent soda water, to treat ailments or provide a boost of energy. Both caffeine and cocaine were also often used in sodas. Some of the many conditions mineral water was supposed to cure were obesity, upset stomach, depression, and nervous disorders. Pharmacists sold phosphate sodas and ice cream favorites, worked the lunch counter, and filled the prescriptions for the day. The first 7-Up drink was made with lithium and was sold from soda fountains for conditions such as gout, uremia, and rheumatism. In 1886, Coca-Cola was invented by John Pemberton, a pharmacist in Georgia. The soft drink was marketed as a tonic and contained extracts of cocaine and caffeine until 1905, when cocaine was removed from the recipe because of changing public opinion regarding its use. It was not until later, after the Harrison Narcotic Drug Act of 1914 (see Chapter 2), that pharmacists were prohibited from making cocaine-containing preparations and began to sell plain soda drinks.

Table 1.5 presents a list of pharmacists and inventors. By the late 1800s, the soda shop/pharmacy was so popular that people came to drink the sweet concoctions whether they were ailing or not. This type of pharmacy setting undoubtedly added to the image of the friendly neighborhood pharmacist as a person who could be trusted. The stereotypic local neighborhood pharmacist who wore a white jacket,

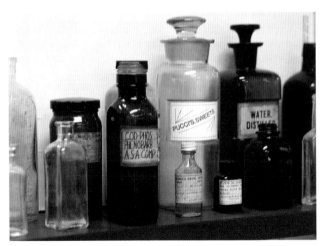

FIG. 1.2 Many ingredients (compounds) were combined to make medications.

TABLE 1.5
Famous Pharmacists

Charles Alderton	Invented Dr. Pepper
Caleb Bradham	Invented Pepsi-Cola
Susan Hayhurst	First woman to graduate from the Philadelphia School of Pharmacy
Charles Elmer Hires	Invented Hires Root Beer
John Pemberton	Invented Coca-Cola
William Proctor, Jr.	Father of American Pharmacy; founded American Pharmaceutical Association in 1852
Ella Phillips Stewart	One of the first African American female pharmacists in the United States
James Vernor	Invented Vernors ginger ale
Harvey A.K. Whitney	Founder and first president of the American Society of Hospital Pharmacists in 1942

packaged medications, and sometimes worked the soda machine has all but disappeared, except in a few shops where a person may still purchase an old-fashioned malt or milkshake while waiting for a prescription to be filled.

Early Pharmacy Technicians

The first **pharmacy technicians** were those enlisted in the military because of the high demand for medications to treat injuries and illness. These individuals were trained on the job not only to fill prescriptions but also to perform many of the functions of a pharmacist. To this day, military technicians have a broader scope of training than civilian technicians. Technicians also were employed by pharmacists who owned drugstores. Family members helped behind the counters, filled stock, and waited on customers. These early pharmacy clerks then moved on to become what we now call **pharmacy technicians**.

An urgent need for standardized training arose in the 1960s as pharmacist organizations, such as the American Society of Health-System Pharmacists (ASHP), the Michigan Pharmacists Association (MPA), and the American Pharmacists Association (APhA), realized that technicians would be able to better serve the patient with additional training. Technicians play such an important role in the health care of patients that it is important for them to understand all aspects of their required tasks in the pharmacy. At the first conference on pharmacy technicians held by the ASHP in 1988, many of the topics involved pharmacy technician training, although other important aspects of the pharmacy setting, such as the lack of technician involvement in the workplace, were also discussed. In 1995 the **Pharmacy Technician Certification Board (PTCB)** was formed, which was responsible for creating a national examination for technicians (see Chapter 3).

Although the transition from clerk to technician is fairly recent in history, forecasts indicate that the pharmacy technician will play a critical role in the future pharmacy setting. New job positions are constantly being created for technicians who have the necessary skills and knowledge to fill them. Clinical technicians now assist the pharmacist with a variety of tasks such as anticoagulation monitoring. They may also manage the automation and pharmacy coordination systems in certain pharmacies. Table 1.6 presents an outline of the important chronological events that have transformed the position of pharmacy technician into its current role.

TABLE 1.6
Advances in the Field of Pharmacy Technology

Year	Description of Change in Pharmacy
1940s	The origins of a training program for technicians are established in the military (US Army).
1969	American Society of Health-System Pharmacists (ASHP) begins to establish national guidelines for pharmacy technicians to improve standards.
1973	National Association of Chain Drug Stores (NACDS) begins support of technicians and on-the-job training programs.
1975	ASHP creates a set of guidelines for the hospital pharmacy technician.
1977	ASHP creates competencies for technicians in organized health care settings and qualifications for entry-level technicians in hospitals.
1979	Massachusetts College of Pharmacy starts a pharmacy technician training program.
1979	American Association of Pharmacy Technicians (AAPT) is formed.
1981	Michigan Pharmacists Association (MPA) starts the first examination program for certifying pharmacy technicians. ASHP creates a bulletin for technical assistance on guidelines for pharmacy technician training programs.
1982	ASHP creates accreditation standards for training programs.
1987	Illinois Council of Hospital Pharmacists (ICHP) begins an examination program to certify technicians.
1988	ASHP Research and Education Foundation holds a conference on the use of technicians in pharmacy. The conference addresses on-the-job training, quality care, voluntary certification of technicians, and the roles and responsibilities of a pharmacy technician in the hospital setting.
1991	Pharmacy Technician Education Council (PTEC) is formed.

Continued

TABLE 1.6
Advances in the Field of Pharmacy Technology—cont'd

Year	Description of Change in Pharmacy
1994	The Scope of Pharmacy Practice Project addressing task analysis of pharmacy technicians is completed.
1995	Pharmacy Technician Certification Board (PTCB) is created by the ASHP, American Pharmacists Association (APhA), ICHP, and MPA.
1996	ASHP and APhA publish the first *White Paper on Pharmacy Technicians.* It addresses the need for national standards in training pharmacy technicians.
1997	ASHP, APhA, American Association of Colleges of Pharmacy (AACP), AAPT, and PTEC collaborate on a model curriculum for training courses for pharmacy technicians.
2000	PTCB updates the task analysis of pharmacy technicians.
2002	The second *White Paper on Pharmacy Technicians: Needed Changes Can No Longer Wait* is published.
2004	Major online search engines select PharmacyChecker.com to verify the validity of online pharmacies.
2008	Congress passes the Ryan Haight Online Consumer Protection Act banning online pharmacies from selling controlled substances based on online patient consultations.
2009	Task Force on Pharmacy Technician Education and Training Programs meets in Rosemont, Illinois. It was established by the National Association of Boards of Pharmacy (NABP) to review the existing state requirements for technician education and training and to recommend national standards.
2010	At its 106th Annual Meeting in Anaheim, California, the NABP passes resolution No. 106-7-10, resolving to continue to encourage states to adopt uniform standards for pharmacy technician education and training programs.
2010	Google removes PharmacyChecker.com as a certifying authority for online pharmacies. Currently, online pharmacies can be verified by Verified Internet Pharmacy Practice Sites (VIPPS).
2011	The CPE Monitor is launched as a collaborative effort by the NABP and the Accreditation Council for Pharmacy Education (ACPE).
2011	PTCB launches the CREST Initiative by hosting a summit focused on the areas of consumer awareness, resources, education, state policy, and testing as they relate to pharmacy technicians.
2013	PTCB announces certification program changes.
2014	All sterile compounders must be licensed by July 1 Drug Enforcement Administration reschedule of hydrocodone combinations to CII.
2015	ASHP and ACPE join to form the Pharmacy Technician Accreditation Commission (PTAC), a pharmacy technician training accrediting organization.
2019	ASHP/ACPE standards revision of training programs for advanced and entry level technicians.
2019	PTCB begins a new program for advanced certified technicians (CPhT-ADV) that requires completion of new speciality certificate programs.
2020	PTCB begins new eligibility requirements and offers an updated PTCE examination.
2021	The PREP Act allows for qualified pharmacy technicians to administer COVID-19 vaccines, tests, and childhood vaccines, regardless of state requirements.
2022	PTCB acquires the educator's organization PTEC.
2023	The PTCB removes the age requirements for CPhT testing.

As of January 2023, the PTCB had certified more than 788,000 technicians nationwide. In addition, there are 1250 CPhT-Adv or certified advanced pharmacy technicians. Beginning in 2019, PTCB began to offer specialty certificate programs in various areas. Completing these allows a CPhT to earn the designation as CPhT-Adv. Currently there are 21 states that require CPhT certification. This demonstrates the seriousness of this profession and the need for standardized competencies in the workplace. Up until the PTCB examination was established, most technicians had a high school diploma, although it was not mandatory; also, background checks were not done in every state. After the PTCB was established, not only were educational standards instituted but salaries were increased for many certified technicians. Attitudes have changed over time as well. Technicians once were viewed as incompetent in many areas of pharmacy but nonetheless a threat to replace pharmacists with cheap labor. Views now have changed because even with the increase in technicians in the workplace, pharmacists still are in high demand. Technicians are now a part of the health care team, and most pharmacists are confident that they can delegate tasks to technicians, knowing that the job will be done correctly. It is no coincidence that as higher standards and educational requirements have been set for the pharmacy technician, pharmacists' trust in technicians has increased.

Changing Pharmacy Requirements

Times have changed and so have the requirements of today's pharmacist. The educational requirements for a pharmacist include successful completion of a GPhC-accredited master of pharmacy school (MPharm). This is a full-time 4-year degree. In addition, there is a period of working as a trainee, where work is observed. To work, all states require licensure and a passing score on the Pharmacy College Admissions Test. Coursework usually includes biology, chemistry, anatomy, and physics.

Pharmacists who received a bachelor of science in pharmacy before this change have been allowed to work in pharmacy without obtaining a doctor of pharmacy degree. Pharmacist licensure also requires examination through the National Association of Boards of Pharmacy (NABP), in addition to examination according to the state's pharmacy laws; candidates for licensure must demonstrate competency by passing these examinations. Today's pharmacist also needs in-depth and broad communication skills to communicate effectively with doctors, other health care team members, and patients.

Today's typical pharmacy technician is required to do an array of tasks, all of which require competencies in many areas. Therefore, in some states, technicians are required to complete additional education and national certification. Currently, there are no nationally standardized requirements for pharmacy technicians. Technicians assist the pharmacist in community settings by entering and maintaining patient medications and history, preparing prescriptions, managing inventory and third-party billing, and compounding specialized medications (Fig. 1.4).

In an institutional setting, which includes hospital and other types of **inpatient pharmacies**, tasks include supplying floor stock, preparing parenteral medications, transcribing physicians' orders, and managing inventory for automated dispensing cabinets. Other practice areas, such as long-term care, nuclear medicine facilities, and insurance or call centers, require technicians to be trained in specialty areas. In all pharmacy settings, technicians require strong communication and organizational skills (see Chapter 4).

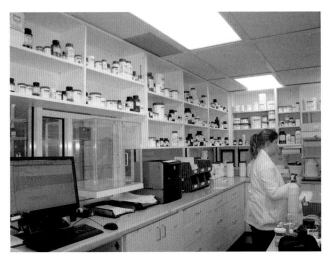

FIG. 1.4 Pharmacy technician working in the pharmacy.

Entry-level pharmacy technicians must possess skills in pharmacology, laws and regulations, compounding, medication safety, inventory and billing, and technology. They can also obtain specialty certifications and may participate in providing specialty services. In some cases, participation may be governed by state law, professional licensing boards, and certifying bodies. For example, some pharmacy technicians assist in anticoagulation or pharmacokinetics services, working under the supervision of a pharmacist to review patients' laboratory results and determine the drug concentration and its relation to the therapeutic response of the patient. Pharmacists will then write the necessary change in medication strength based on the laboratory results. Other specialty duties include, but are not limited to, oncology, pediatrics, geriatrics, and compounding services.

New specialty certifications and opportunities for technicians also are available. In 2019, PTCB began offering an advanced credential (Advanced Certified Pharmacy Technician [CPhT-Adv]) and some specialty certificates. Critical Point offers specialized training in sterile products and hazardous drug compounding. Many hospitals allow technicians to prepare chemotherapy drugs and offer advanced positions as medication reconciliation technicians (see Chapter 10 for more information on the advanced practice setting for pharmacy technicians).

Trust in Pharmacists and Technicians

Over the decades the pharmacist has become known as a person who can be trusted to provide truthful information, someone in whom a person can be comfortable confiding. Although some traditions continue, times have changed concerning the role of the pharmacist. The most prevalent change can be seen in the inpatient setting of the hospital. As the competency of a pharmacist has become more "clinical" and involved in the patient's overall well-being and health, pharmacists are becoming more involved, alongside physicians, in the appropriate prescribing of medications and their dosages. These clinical pharmacists are found in the community pharmacy and in hospital settings.

Another important change in pharmacy concerns the laws governing patient consultation. The Omnibus Budget Reconciliation Act of 1990 (OBRA '90; see Chapter 2) addressed several issues concerning patient education and monitoring of medications. Although initially consultation was required to be offered only to Medicaid patients, most states have developed statutes that require pharmacists to provide written and/or oral consultation to all patients who are prescribed new or changed medications. Consultation is meant to inform and educate the patient about the medication he or she is taking. Because of these changes in the way pharmacies function, virtually every pharmacy employs pharmacy technicians. Thousands of technicians help lighten the load of filling prescriptions and performing other nondiscretionary tasks. Therefore it is important for the patient to be able to trust a technician to provide the best care by filling the correct medication and referring the patient to the pharmacist for appropriate counseling. Most pharmacists agree that it is important for pharmacy technicians to maintain a standard of knowledge about pharmacy practice. Thus far, national certification is one of the best markers for ensuring a minimum level of competency in pharmacy.

Pharmacists have earned the trust of their patients over many decades, and it will take time for technicians to earn the same trust. This requires a true commitment to the profession of pharmacy on the part of the pharmacy technician. Through education, training, and good communication skills, technicians can gain the trust of the patients whom they serve.

◉ Technician Profile

As a pharmacy technician for 3 years at a community hospital, Julia has learned how to build trust with her colleagues in and out of the pharmacy. She is required to fill orders in a fast-paced but exciting environment. She works alongside a pharmacist, Dr. Ellen, to whom Julia has proven that she can do her job competently. Dr. Ellen hired Julia after she finished her pharmacy technician training at a local college and received her national certification. Julia has gained Dr. Ellen's trust and the trust of the nurses and physicians who rely on her to fill the medication orders in the busy hospital setting. She is careful, efficient, and friendly and thoroughly enjoys her career.

Technicians of the Twenty-First Century and Beyond

In the new millennium, with the roles of pharmacists and technicians becoming more clearly defined, new concerns arise. We must be aware that just as the advances of medicine through the ages met with much resistance, so has the profession of pharmacy. Changes in the roles of pharmacists, technicians, and even clerks have met their share of obstacles, mostly from within the medical community. Some physicians are not eager to have pharmacists writing orders, even if the medications are simple. Likewise, technicians have been perceived as posing a threat to pharmacy. Some pharmacists think that technicians may take jobs away from pharmacists or may increase the pharmacist's liability if someone who is not properly trained makes a mistake. Therefore there is disparity across the United States regarding the duties of a pharmacy technician. In some states, pharmacies limit technicians' duties to a clerical level. In other states, technicians are required to have training and/or be certified as pharmacy technicians before they are employed. All technicians must be aware of the laws in their state. (To find out more about the laws in your state pertaining to pharmacy technicians, visit the website *http://nabp.pharmacy*.) Each year more pharmacies are requiring a certain level of education from their technicians. This in turn allows for the expansion of job duties and possibly higher pay for the technicians.

Technicians' duties continue to expand and change. In some pharmacies, technicians regularly enter new prescription orders into the computer. This task previously was done exclusively by a pharmacist. The pharmacist is moving into a more highly clinical role, not only counseling patients but also working with the medical staff. To a degree, the technician now does what the traditional pharmacist did: a health professional who transcribed orders, pulled medications, and filled prescriptions. Advanced pharmacy technicians who have additional education may perform tasks that require more responsibility, and some organizations and colleges are offering specialized training programs for pharmacy technicians. Education in medication history, inventory management, quality improvement, immunization, speciality compounding, and analysis are just a few of the specialty roles being offered for technicians.

◉ Scenario Checkup 1.2

As Kelly reads this chapter, she wonders what her role will be like in the pharmacy as a pharmacy technician. What would you tell her? How would you tell her about the role of the pharmacy technician and how it has evolved over time? What would you tell her about how to maintain a professional image?

Do You Remember These Key Points?

- Terms and definitions used in this chapter
- Common ancient beliefs, including the dogmas of those eras
- Common treatments used for conditions in earlier times
- Early American medical practices and challenges during the Civil War
- The use of opium in the 19th century
- Advances in medicine over the centuries
- Major figures who influenced the changes in the dogmas of medicine
- The use of leeches and maggots throughout history
- The beginnings of the roles of pharmacists and pharmacy technicians
- How the roles have changed for pharmacists and pharmacy technicians
- Some of the specialty roles that are available for advanced technicians

◉ Scenario Follow-Up

Kelly has learned that the history of medicine and pharmacy has provided a strong foundation for the career field she is pursuing. There have been clear medical advances throughout history that have had an important impact on the pharmacy profession of today. Kelly will be better prepared to enter the workplace as a result of her knowledge of the evolution of the pharmacy technician's duties and responsibilities.

Review Questions

Multiple Choice Questions

1. During the Civil War, many soldiers died as a result of:
   A. Unsanitary conditions
   B. Postsurgical infections
   C. Gunshot wounds
   D. All of the above

2. Which of the following choices best describes sources of materials for remedies in ancient times?
   A. Chemicals, minerals, vitamins
   B. Minerals, animals, prayer
   C. Minerals, animals, plants
   D. Plants, seeds, minerals
3. Which of the following statements is *not* true?
   A. Sulfonamides are synthetic antibiotics.
   B. Sulfonamides are used for urinary tract infections.
   C. Gerhard Domagk discovered sulfonamide.
   D. Sulfonamide was one of many new antibiotic classes discovered in the 1800s.
4. Taking new prescriptions over the phone and entering them into the computer are tasks a _____ can do.
   A. Pharmacist
   B. Pharmacy technician
   C. CPhT
   D. All of the above
5. The PTCB was founded by which of the following entities?
   A. ASHP, MPA, CPhA, PTEC
   B. MPA, ICHP, APhA, ASHP
   C. NAPB, ASHP, MPA, ICHP
   D. APhA, ASHP, NABP, PTEC
6. Opium and alcohol were once used to:
   A. Desensitize a person to pain
   B. Help ease depression
   C. Treat anxiety
   D. All of the above
7. The word *apothecary* means:
   A. Pharmacist
   B. Store
   C. Drug
   D. Both A and B
8. The first pharmacy technicians were:
   A. Family members
   B. Clerks
   C. Military technicians
   D. All of the above
9. Pharmacy technicians perform the following functions *except:*
   A. Filling prescriptions
   B. Compounding medications
   C. Counseling patients
   D. Ordering medications
10. The PTCB is an organization that:
    A. Regulates all pharmacy technicians
    B. Gives a national examination for pharmacy technicians
    C. Was founded by several pharmacist associations
    D. Both B and C

■ Technician's Corner

Discuss why pharmacists consistently rank among the most trusted professionals. Research the 2013 annual poll conducted by Gallup to find out what percentage of respondents rated pharmacists "very high" on honesty and ethical standards. Do technicians benefit from these statistics?

Bibliography

Anderson MJ, Stephenson KF. *Scientists of the Ancient World*. Springfield, NJ: Enslow; 1999.

Ballington DA. *Pharmacy Practice for Technicians*. 3rd ed. St Paul, MN: EMC/Paradigm; 2006.

Moulton C, ed. *Ancient Greece and Rome*. Vol 3. New York: Simon & Schuster; 1998.

Narcto D. *The Complete History of Ancient Greece*. San Diego: Greenhaven; 2001.

Suplee C. *Milestones of Science*. Washington, DC: National Geographic; 2000.

Websites Referenced

CDC Recommendations for Shingles Prevention. SHINGRIX (Zoster Vaccine Recombinant, Adjuvanted) for HCPs Available at: shingrixhcp.com.

Centers for Disease Control and Prevention. List of vaccines used in United States. Available at: https://www.cdc.gov/vaccines/vpd/vaccines-list.html.

Centers for Disease Control and Prevention. Vaccine preventable deaths and the global immunization vision and strategy, 2006–2015. *MMWR Morb Mortal Weekly Rep.* 2006;55(18):511-515. Available at: http://www.cdc.gov/mmwr/preview/mmwrhtml/mm5518a4.htm.

Ella Phillips Stewart. Available at: Wikipedia.

Encyclopedia Mythica. Asclepius. Encyclopedia Mythica Online. Available at: http://www.pantheon.org/articles/a/asclepius.html.

Florence Nightingale. Biography, Facts & Nursing | HISTORY.

Gallagher J. Hand, foot and mouth disease: first vaccine. *BBC News.* Available at: http://www.bbc.co.uk/news/health-22689593.

Gardasil 9. Available at: https://www.gardasil9.com/.

Greek Mythology.com. Asclepius. Available at: https://www.greekmythology.com/Other_Gods/Asclepius/asclepius.html.

Hayhurst S. Available at: http://explorepahistory.com/displayimage.php?imgId51-2-189F.

Mayo Foundation for Medical Education and Research, Mayo Clinic staff. Hemochromatosis. Available at: http://www.mayoclinic.com/health/hemochromatosis/DS00455/.

Greek Medicine: The Four Humors. Available at: http://www.greekmedicine.net/pathology/Pathologies_of_Black_Bile.html.

National Alliance of Advocates for Buprenorphine Treatment. Opiates/opioids. Available at: http://www.naabt.org/education/opiates_opioids.cfm.

Pharmacy Technician Certification Board. New certificate offerings. Available at: Credentials - Credentials - PTCB.

Pharmacy Technician Certification Board. PTCB certifications granted statistics. Available at: State Regulations and Map (ptcb.org).

Prevnar vaccine. Available at: http://www.fda.gov/Biologics BloodVaccines/Vaccines/ApprovedProducts/ucm201667.htm.

Roger Bacon, The Medieval 'Wizard' Who Pioneered Modern Science Available at: allthatsinteresting.com.

Shultz S. *Epidemics in Colonial Philadelphia From 1699–1799 and the Risk of Dying*. Archiving Early America. Available at: http://www.earlyamerica.com/review/2007_winter_spring/epidemics.html.

The discovery of the molecular structure of DNA: the double helix. Available at: https://www.nobelprize.org/educational/medicine/dna_double_helix/readmore.html.

Timeline of medicine and medical technology. Available at: http://en.wikipedia.org/wiki/Timeline_of_medicine_and_medical_technology.

University of Wisconsin–Madison. Scientists guide human skin cells to embryonic state. *ScienceDaily*. Available at: http://www.sciencedaily.com/releases/2007/11/071120092709.htm.

Vivian J, Fink J. OBRA '90 at sweet sixteen: a retrospective review. *US Pharm*. 2008;33(3):59-65. Available at: http://www.uspharmacist.com/content/t/pain_management,miscellaneous/c/10126/.

Pharmacy Law, Ethics, and Regulatory Agencies

Karen Davis

<table>
<tbody>
<tr>
<td>

OBJECTIVES

</td>
<td>

1. List the history of federal drug laws in chronological order.
2. Describe the implications of the Health Insurance Portability and Accountability Act (HIPAA).
3. Explain how the Patient Protection and Affordable Care Act (ACA) and the Drug Quality and Security Act (DQSA) have changed health care.
4. Discuss the following related to the US Food and Drug Administration (FDA) and Drug Enforcement Administration (DEA): (a) define the functions of the FDA and DEA, (b) describe the process for reporting any problems with a drug or any adverse reactions to the FDA, and (c) explain the three classes of drug recalls defined by the FDA.
5. Describe the proper handling of controlled substances and explain the necessary forms and regulations used for controlled substances.
6. Discuss the following related to drug monographs: (a) list the basic information contained in a drug monograph, (b) explain the purpose of boxed warnings and MedGuides, and (c) list and explain the five pregnancy categories established by the FDA.
7. Discuss the following related to prescription guidelines: (a) list who can prescribe medications and medical devices, (b) describe prescription orders and prescription labels, and (c) perform the function of verifying a DEA number.
8. Describe special prescribing programs and explain the purpose of risk management programs for prescription drugs.
9. Explain the verification process for Internet pharmacies.
10. Explain the Occupational Safety and Health Administration (OSHA) guidelines as they pertain to pharmacy.
11. Explain the purpose of The Joint Commission.
12. Explain why pharmacy technicians must be knowledgeable about the law when performing nondiscretionary duties and discuss the differences between morals and ethics.

</td>
</tr>
</tbody>
</table>

TERMS AND DEFINITIONS

Act A statutory plan passed by Congress or any legislature that is a bill until it is enacted and becomes law

Adulteration The mishandling of medication that can lead to contamination or impurity, falsification of contents, or loss of drug quality or potency. Adulteration may cause injury or illness to the consumer

Amendment A change in an original act or law

Barbiturate A drug derived from barbituric acid; a barbiturate acts as a central nervous system depressant. Barbiturates are often used in the treatment of seizures and as sedative and hypnotic agents

Board of Pharmacy (BOP) State board that regulates the practice of pharmacy within the state

Boxed warning Drug warning that is placed in the prescribing information or package insert of the product and indicates a significant risk for potentially dangerous side effects. It is the strongest warning

19

the US Food and Drug Administration (FDA) can give. It is common in the pharmacy profession to call these warnings "Black Box Warnings" because of their appearance in a drug label; the warning is often enclosed in a black outlined box to draw attention to the content

Controlled substance Any drug or other substance that is scheduled I through V and regulated by the US Drug Enforcement Administration (DEA)

Drug diversion The intentional misuse of a drug intended for medical purposes; the DEA usually defines diversion as the recreational use of a prescription or scheduled drug. Diversion also can refer to the channeling of the prescription drug supply away from legal distribution and to the illegal street market

Drug Enforcement Administration (DEA) Federal agency within the US Department of Justice that enforces US laws and regulations related to controlled substances

Drug utilization evaluation (DUE) A process that ensures that prescribed drugs are used appropriately. The main desired outcome of any DUE program is an increase in medication-related efficacy and safety

Ethics The values and morals used within a profession

Health Insurance Portability and Accountability Act of 1996 (HIPAA) Federal act that protects patients' rights, establishes national standards for electronic health care communication, and ensures the security and privacy of health data

Legend drug Drug that requires a prescription for dispensing; these drugs carry the federal legend: "Federal law prohibits the dispensing of this medication without a prescription"

Medicaid Federal- and state-operated insurance program that covers health care costs and prescription drugs for low-income children, adults, and elderly and those with disabilities

Medicare Federal- and state-managed insurance program that covers health care costs and prescription drugs for individuals older than 65, persons younger than 65 with long-term disabilities, and individuals with end-stage renal disease

Misbranding Labeling of a product that is false or misleading; label information must include directions for use; safe and/or unsafe dosages; manufacturer, packer, or distributor; quantity; and weight

Monograph Comprehensive information on a medication's actions within that class of drugs. Also lists generic and trade names, ingredients, dosages, side effects, adverse effects, how the patient should take the medication, and foods or other drugs (eg, over-the-counter [OTC] medications, herbals) to avoid while taking the medication

Morals Standards concerning or relating to what is right or wrong in human behavior

Narcotic A nonspecific term used to describe a drug (such as opium) that in moderate doses dulls the senses, relieves pain, and induces profound sleep but in excessive doses causes stupor, coma, or convulsions and may lead to addiction. From the standpoint of US law, opium, opiates (derivatives of opium), and opioids, in addition to cocaine and coca leaves, are "narcotics"

National Drug Code (NDC) A 10-digit number that indicates specifics of a prescription drug or an insulin product. The NDC specifies the drug manufacturer, the drug product (drug strength, dosage form, and formulation), and the package size

National Formulary (NF) A book of standards for certain pharmaceuticals and preparations not included in the USP; revised every 5 years and recognized as a book of official standards by the Pure Food and Drug Act of 1906

Negligence A legal concept that describes an action taken without the forethought that should have been taken by a reasonable person of similar competency

Occupational Safety and Health Administration (OSHA) US government–managed agency that oversees safety in the workplace; created Safety Data Sheet (SDS) requirements

Omnibus Budget Reconciliation Act of 1990 (OBRA '90) Congressional act that changed reimbursement limits and mandated drug use evaluation, pharmacy patient consultation, and educational outreach programs

Over the counter (OTC) Describes medication that can be purchased without a prescription; nonlegend medications

Physicians' Desk Reference **(PDR)** One of the many reference books on medications; it compiles and publishes select manufacturer-provided package inserts and prescribing information useful for health professionals

Pregnancy categories A system used by the FDA to describe five levels of assessment of fetal effects caused by a drug; a required section of current prescription drug labeling. First introduced in 1979, the system is being reevaluated for usefulness and inclusion in the prescription label

Protected health information (PHI) A term used to describe a patient's personal health data. Under HIPAA, this information is protected from being shared or distributed without permission

Pure Food and Drug Act of 1906 Act that led to the creation of the FDA and was enacted to prevent mislabeling or misbranding of medicines

Safety Data Sheet (SDS) (formerly known as MSDS sheets) A document providing chemical product information. An SDS includes the product name, composition (chemicals in the product), hazards, toxicology, and other information about the proper steps to take with spills, accidental exposure, handling, and storage of the product. Filing of an SDS in the pharmacy or workplace is usually a requirement for meeting Occupational Safety and Health Administration (OSHA) standards

The Joint Commission (TJC) An independent, nonprofit organization that accredits hospitals and other health care organizations in the United States. Accreditation is required to be eligible for Medicare and Medicaid payments

Tort An act that causes harm or injury to a person intentionally or because of negligence

United States Pharmacopeia (USP) An independent, nonprofit organization that establishes documentation on product quality standards, drug quality and information, and health care information on medications, OTC products, dietary supplements, and food ingredients to ensure that they have the appropriate purity, quality, and strength

United States Pharmacopeia–National Formulary **(USP-NF)** A publication of the USP that contains standards for medications, dosage forms, drug substances, excipients, medical devices, and dietary supplements

US Drug Enforcement Administration (DEA) Federal agency within the US Department of Justice that enforces US laws and regulations related to controlled substances

US Food and Drug Administration (FDA) The agency within the US Department of Health and Human Services that is responsible for ensuring the safety, efficacy, and security of human and veterinary drugs, biological products, medical devices, the national food supply, cosmetics, and radioactive products

Scenario

Laura is a new technician at a local chain pharmacy. She graduated from an accredited technician training program in which she learned about her roles and responsibilities as a pharmacy professional. As she begins her career, she thinks about her legal liabilities. Does she need malpractice insurance in case she makes a medication error? What if she unknowingly violates a Health Insurance Portability and Accountability Act (HIPAA) regulation?

The practice of pharmacy is governed by a series of laws, regulations, and rules enforced by federal, state, and local governments. The practice of pharmacy is also subject to policies and procedures established by institutions and/or pharmacy management at each pharmacy site. The number of rules and regulations is staggering, and most of us cannot easily decipher the legal tangle of words; however, we are required to follow these rules and regulations. This chapter presents the most basic laws and regulations that pertain to pharmacy, pharmacists, and especially the technician. A good understanding of these laws is necessary to pass the Pharmacy Technician Certification Board (PTCB) examination; more important, it is necessary to know your responsibilities when working in pharmacy. An overview of the history of the **US Food and Drug Administration (FDA)** is given, and its present-day functions are described. The laws are listed in chronological order, along with a short description of how and why each was enacted. Common record-keeping practices are covered. The legal liabilities of pharmacists and technicians are explained. Morals and ethics are discussed at the end of this chapter because they play a vital role in the decisions technicians make in pharmacy practice.

US Food and Drug Administration History

The FDA was established in 1862, along with the US Department of Agriculture (USDA). The FDA is the oldest consumer protection agency in the US federal government. The FDA's Division of Chemistry consists of a staff from several disciplines, including chemists, physicians, veterinarians, pharmacists, microbiologists, and lawyers. Until 1901, the Division of Chemistry evaluated applications for new drugs for use in humans or animals, food and color additives, medical devices, and infant formulas. The chief chemist in the Division of Chemistry at that time, Harvey Wiley, changed the direction of the division, establishing scientific authority by researching the effects of chemical preservatives used in the production of foods and drugs, exposing potential hazards in products, focusing on consumer safety, and eventually paving the way for government regulation. Inspectors in the department visited thousands of food and other manufacturing facilities each year. In 1901, the Division of Chemistry was renamed the Bureau of Chemistry. Wiley's efforts led to the first passage of major legislation, the **Pure Food and Drug Act of 1906.** The new agency was to make many more changes in its authority and scope as it grew. In 1927, the agency's name was changed to the Food, Drug, and Insecticide Administration, and in 1930 the name was shortened to the FDA. The FDA remained under the authority of the USDA until 1940, when the agency became part of the Federal Security Agency. As the FDA continued to regulate new applications for drugs, devices, and other products, the agency was transferred to the Department of Health, Education, and Welfare (HEW) in 1953 and eventually was placed under the authority of the US Public Health Service within HEW in 1968. In 1980, the FDA was moved from HEW to the newly created US Department of Health and Human Services (DHHS).

Early Activity of the US Food and Drug Administration

Since the FDA's founding, the agency has investigated the **adulteration** and **misbranding** of agricultural goods used for food and drugs. Hundreds of bills were introduced in Congress to establish standards to protect the health of consumers, yet the FDA's ability to regulate and enforce these standards remained limited, leaving the primary control of domestically produced food and drugs to the individual states. The laws varied widely from state to state. Meanwhile, horrible incidents continued to occur, such as the deaths of 13 children and 9 babies in 1902 after they were injected with a tainted batch of tetanus diphtheria antitoxins. In June 1906 President Theodore Roosevelt signed the Pure Food and Drug Act of 1906, also known as the Wiley Act. This important act gave the government the power to administer and prohibit the interstate transport of unlawful food and drugs. Drugs had to meet the standards of strength, quality, and purity established by the **United States Pharmacopeia (USP)** and the **National Formulary (NF)** guidelines; any variations from the guidelines had to be plainly listed on the product label. The label could not mislead the consumer, and all ingredients had to be listed on the label. The law also prohibited the addition of any ingredients to a food that would substitute for the food, conceal damage, pose a health hazard, or constitute a filthy or decomposed substance.

Wiley's authority was challenged and undercut many times by the Supreme Court as attempts were made to form standards affecting food and drug manufacturers. The FDA suffered a severe setback in 1912 when the Supreme Court determined that the law enforcing the regulation of drugs did not apply to false therapeutic claims. The controversy lay in the attempt to prove that the drug companies intended to defraud the consumer. This Supreme Court ruling undermined the Wiley Act, and many manufacturers won court cases, allowing their products to be sold to consumers. In 1912, Wiley resigned from the FDA, and at this point the bureau focused more closely on drug regulation because this was a great concern.

With a new presidential administration taking over in 1933 under Franklin D. Roosevelt, the FDA was able to change its authority to include both quality and identity standards for food and drugs, prohibition of false therapeutic claims for drugs, and coverage of cosmetics and medical devices. The FDA had the right to inspect factories and control the advertising of products. The FDA countered advertisements of drug claims by exposing the horrible but true results of certain drugs. For example, an eyelash dye that blinded some women as a result of dangerous additives had been widely advertised to consumers. A medication tonic made with radium as an additive was found to cause a slow and painful death for the user. All products were protected under the previous laws. For the next 5 years, a bill that would replace the 1906 revised law was stalled in Congress. It took tremendous effort to pass new standards enforceable by the FDA. In 1937, a Tennessee drug company advertised a new sulfanilamide elixir specifically intended for children. The toxic solvent was untested (per then current laws), and more than 100 people died—mostly children. It was later determined that the solvent was similar to antifreeze, which is fatal to humans and animals. Unfortunately, this type of deadly scenario was repeated several times before the necessary changes in the laws of that time were made. As a result of public

pressure, Congress finally passed the 1938 Federal Food, Drug, and Cosmetic Act. The act required manufacturers to prove to the FDA that a drug was safe for use before marketing it, and the manufacturers had to provide directions on the drug's label for its safe use. The act also mandated standards for foods, set tolerances for certain poisonous substances, and authorized factory inspections. The FDA was given authority to enforce the standards. Just a few months after passage of the act, the FDA determined that sulfa and other drugs required a prescription from physicians before they could be purchased. Clarification of what constituted a prescription drug versus an **over-the-counter (OTC)** drug was established in 1951 with the enactment of the Durham-Humphrey Amendment (Fig. 2.1). Other laws passed in the 1950s banned carcinogenic additives to foods.

Another potential tragedy was averted in the United States in the 1960s when the drug thalidomide, a sedative used in Europe, was found to cause severe birth defects, including grossly deformed limbs, when administered during pregnancy. The drug was never approved for use in the United States. The Kefauver-Harris Drug Amendments of 1962 were revolutionary in their scope for ensuring the safety and effectiveness of medications in the US market. Another growing concern was the use and abuse of amphetamines, **barbiturates,** and other potentially addictive agents. The FDA was given more control over these agents with the enactment of the Drug Abuse Control Amendments of 1965. This control was eventually delegated to the **Drug Enforcement Administration (DEA)** in 1968. In 1973, some of the responsibilities of the FDA were given to the Consumer Product Safety Commission (CPSC). These included oversight of hazardous toys, flammable fabrics, and potential poisons in consumer products. Other provisions in the 1960s allowed for greater FDA oversight to ensure the safety and effectiveness of veterinary drugs and additives to animal feed.

Before 1938 the US Post Office Department and Federal Trade Commission were in charge of ensuring the safety of cosmetics and medical devices; after 1938, regulating cosmetics and medical devices became the responsibility of the FDA. The advertising of various quack products was widespread throughout the country; claims such as increasing the

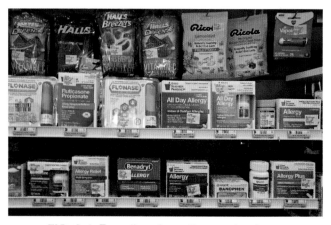

FIG. 2.1 Examples of over-the-counter drugs.

life span, curing conditions, and protecting one's health were unfounded in many cases. However, in 1976, another disaster occurred when an intrauterine device that claimed to prevent pregnancy caused serious injury to thousands of women. Only then did the 1976 Medical Device Amendments allow the FDA to regulate and approve these types of devices and recall ineffective or dangerous devices.

With continued consumer and political pressure, the FDA has influenced new laws such as the Orphan Drug Act (ODA), which was passed in 1983 and targeted all rare diseases. The ODA influenced expanded research and availability of new treatments for acquired immunodeficiency syndrome (AIDS), cancer, and genetic diseases. (An overview of several acts and **amendments** is presented in the following section.) The FDA has continued its mission to ensure public safety, including the oversight of dietary supplements that present safety problems, make false or misleading claims, or are otherwise adulterated or misbranded.

Description of Laws

What is an **act?** An act is a statutory plan passed by Congress or any legislature that is called a *bill* until it is enacted, at which point it becomes a law. An amendment is a change in the original act or law. The following examples are brief because the various acts and amendments encompass broader descriptions. Further reading is suggested to gain a deeper insight into the laws that pertain to pharmacy and patient rights. Table 2.1 presents a list of well-known federal laws, in chronological order, that are discussed in this chapter.

1906 Pure Food and Drug Act

The 1906 Pure Food and Drug Act was one of the first laws enacted to stop the sale of inaccurately labeled drugs. All manufacturers were required to have truthful information on the label before selling their drugs. Although this act was well intentioned, many drugs still made their way onto the market because of continued false claims regarding their effectiveness. Additional changes were made to this act that ultimately required manufacturers to prove the effectiveness of the drugs through methods such as scientific studies.

1914 Harrison Narcotics Act

By 1912 international meetings were being held to curb the increase in trafficking of highly addictive substances. The International Opium Convention of 1912 was one of these meetings. Limitations on opium transport and recreational use were attempted. The Harrison Narcotics Act of 1914 was enacted in the United States in parallel with international treaties to curb the recreational use of opium. Individuals could no longer purchase opium without a prescription, and it became harder to obtain opium for nonmedical purposes. The Harrison Narcotics Act required practitioner registration, documentation regarding prescriptions and dispensing, and implementation of restrictions regarding the importation, sale, and distribution of opium, coca leaves, and any derivative products.

TABLE 2.1
Well-Known Federal Food and Drug Laws

Year	Law
1906	Pure Food and Drug Act
1912	International Opium Convention
1914	Harrison Narcotics Act
1938	Federal Food, Drug, and Cosmetic Act
1951	Durham-Humphrey Amendment
1962	Kefauver-Harris Amendments (thalidomide disaster)
1970	Comprehensive Drug Abuse Prevention and Control Act
1970	Poison Prevention Packaging Act
1972	Drug Listing Act
1983	Orphan Drug Act
1987	Prescription Drug Marketing Act
1990	Anabolic Steroids Control Act
1990	Omnibus Budget Reconciliation Act of 1990 (OBRA '90)
1994	Dietary Supplement Health and Education Act (DSHEA)
1996	Health Insurance Portability and Accountability Act of 1996 (HIPAA)
2000	Drug Addiction Treatment Act (DATA 2000)
2003	Medicare Modernization Act (MMA)
2005	Combat Methamphetamine Epidemic Act (CMEA)
2006	Dietary Supplement and Nonprescription Drug Consumer Protection Act
2010	The Patient Protection and Affordable Care Act (ACA)
2013	The Drug Quality and Security Act (DQSA)

1938 Federal Food, Drug, and Cosmetic Act

The 1938 Federal Food, Drug, and Cosmetic Act was enacted because the earlier Pure Food and Drug Act of 1906 was not worded strictly enough and did not include cosmetics. Two important concepts introduced in this new act were adulteration and misbranding. For example, false or exaggerated claims commonly were placed on new drug labels and often misled the consumer. This was considered misbranding. All addictive substances were required to be labeled "Warning: May be habit forming." This act also provided the legal status for the FDA. Adulteration deals with the preparation and/or storage of a medication. Mishandling of the food or drug may cause injury or even death to a consumer. This act described the exact labeling for products and defined misbranding and adulteration as illegal. The new law also required drug companies to include package inserts and directions to the consumer regarding safe use (see Food and Drug Administration and Drug Enforcement Administration, later in the chapter).

1951 Durham-Humphrey Amendment

The 1951 Durham-Humphrey Amendment added more instructions for drug companies and required the labeling "Caution: Federal law prohibits dispensing without a prescription." Under this amendment, certain drugs require a physician's order and supervision. This amendment also made the initial distinction between **legend drugs** (by prescription only) and OTC medications that do not require a physician's order (also known as *nonprescription drugs*).

1962 Kefauver-Harris Amendments

The Kefauver-Harris Amendments enacted in 1962 were groundbreaking in their attempts to ensure the safety and effectiveness of all new drugs on the US market. The amendments gave the FDA specific authority to approve a manufacturer's marketing application before a drug could be made available for commercial use. Firms now had to prove safety and provide substantial evidence of effectiveness for the drug's intended use. The required evidence had to consist of adequate and well-controlled studies. The amendments helped establish rules of clinical drug investigation and required the informed consent of study subjects. The amendments also required that drug-related adverse events be reported to the FDA. The regulation of prescription drug advertising was transferred from the Federal Trade Commission to the FDA, and the burden was put on the drug manufacturing companies to ensure quality as "good manufacturing practice" (GMP) standards were established. One example of the effectiveness of the FDA is illustrated by its role in preventing the sale of thalidomide in the United States. In Europe, people were taking this new medication to help them sleep. In the early 1960s, European women who had taken thalidomide while pregnant gave birth to children with severe defects, including the absence of limbs. The FDA postponed approving thalidomide until just before the birth defects across Europe were reported. Very few cases were reported in the United States; those reported were due to women obtaining thalidomide from outside the United States. Consumers became aware that drug companies were not doing enough to test the drugs they were marketing. More laws ensued after the thalidomide tragedy to better safeguard the public; this also greatly increased the time and money spent on testing a drug for safety and effectiveness.

1970 Comprehensive Drug Abuse Prevention and Control Act (Also Known as the Controlled Substances Act)

The DEA was formed to enforce the laws concerning controlled substances and their distribution. A stair-step schedule of controlled substances was introduced, based on the drug's intended medical use, the propensity of a drug to be abused, and safety and dependency concerns. The five-level stair-step schedule of controlled substances requires stricter rules for low-numbered classifications and less strict rules for higher numbered categories. Schedule I is the most restrictive and is defined as drugs with no medically accepted use in the United States. The prescription of a schedule V drug is less restricted and requires less documentation than that for a schedule II drug.

1970 Poison Prevention Packaging Act

The Poison Prevention Packaging Act (PPPA) of 1970 required manufacturers and pharmacies to place all medications in containers with childproof caps or packaging. This includes both OTC and legend drugs. The standard specifies that medication should not be able to be opened by at least 80% of children under the age of 5 and that at least 90% of adults should be able to open the medication within 5 minutes. Exceptions to this act include physician requests for non-childproof caps for their patients, certain legend medications, hospitalized patients, or a specific request by the patient.

Before the implementation of this act, there were hundreds of unintentional deaths of children under the age of 5 years as a result of ingestion of either drugs or household chemicals. The first attempt to prevent these tragedies was the Hazardous Substances Labeling Act of 1960. Pharmacist Homer George of Mississippi was the driving force behind the first National Poison Prevention Week (occurring yearly in March). Individual states followed by implementing poison control centers. It was not until 1970 that the PPPA was enacted; it is now under the authority of the CPSC. It is estimated that more than 1.4 million childhood deaths have been prevented annually because of childproof caps (for more information, see the CPSC website at *https://www. cpsc.gov/Business–Manufacturing/Business-Education/Business-Guidance/PPPA*). Box 2.1 presents PPPA guidelines for exempt drugs.

1972 Drug Listing Act: National Drug Code

In 1972 the Drug Listing Act (**National Drug Code [NDC]**) was implemented under the authority of the FDA. Every drug has a unique 10-digit number divided into three segments. The numbers identify the labeler, product, and trade package size (Fig. 2.2). The first set of numbers (labeler code) is assigned by the FDA. The second set (product code) identifies the specifics of the product. The third set of numbers (package code) identifies the specifics of the package size and types. Both product and package codes are set by the drug company. The example in Box 2.2 presents a specific overview of each part of the code.

1983 Orphan Drug Act

The 1983 Orphan Drug Act (ODA) encouraged drug companies to develop drugs for rare diseases by providing research assistance, grants, and cost incentives to manufacturers. Before this act, companies had no incentive to develop medications and spend millions of dollars and many years of trials to treat a disease that affected a small portion of the population. Therefore several regulatory restrictions were waived for diseases that affected fewer than 200,000 people in the United States. The act also covered diseases that affected more than 200,000 people if it could be proved that the cost of developing and testing a drug could not be recovered by the eventual sales. In addition, the act encouraged manufacturers to develop drugs for rare diseases by providing marketing exclusivity for orphan drugs for a period of 7 years after FDA approval.

BOX 2.1 Poison Prevention Packaging Act Guidelines (Exempt Drugs)[a]

All medications must be dispensed with a childproof cap, with the exception of the following:
- Anhydrous cholestyramine powder
- Betamethasone tablets, 12.6 mg or less contained in dispenser packages
- Colestipol, no more than 5 g
- Conjugated estrogens containing no more than 32 mg
- Contraceptives in daily dispensing sets
- Erythromycin ethylsuccinate tablet packages not containing more than 16 g
- Erythromycin granules, no more than 8 g in suspension
- Hormone replacement therapy products that contain one or more progestin or estrogen substances
- Mebendazole containing no more than 600 mg in dispenser packages
- Medroxyprogesterone tablets
- Methylprednisolone tablets containing no more than 84 mg
- Norethindrone mnemonic (memory-aid) packages containing no more than 50 mg
- Pancrelipase powder, capsule, or tablet forms
- Prednisone package containing no more than 105 mg
- Sacrosidase preparations in glycerin and water
- Sodium fluoride containing no more than 264 mg per package
- Sublingual forms of isosorbide dinitrate 10 mg or less
- Sublingual forms of nitroglycerin
  or
- All medications dispensed in a hospital or nursing home do not require childproof packaging
  or
- Customer requests medication not be dispensed with childproof cap; may be a "blanket" request for all prescription medications
  or
- Physician requests medication not be dispensed with a childproof cap; may be a blanket request for all prescription medications

[a]The National Capital Poison Control Center can be contacted at 1-800-222-1222 or at the website *http://www.poison.org*.
US Consumer Product Safety Commission. Poison prevention packaging: a text for healthcare professionals. *http://www.cpsc.gov/*.

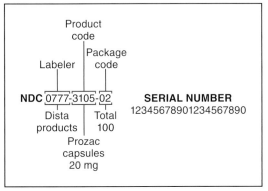

FIG. 2.2 Example of a National Drug Code (NDC), broken down by section.

BOX 2.2 National Drug Code Number Specifics

NDC 50580-449-05

50580: First five positions indicate the **labeler code;** this identifies any firm that manufactures or distributes (under its own name) the drug (includes **repackers** or **relabelers**).

449: Second set of numbers indicates the **product code;** this identifies a specific strength, dosage form, and formulation for a particular drug. Examples include active ingredients and size, shape, color, or imprinted code on drug, in addition to any other distinguishing markings on the drug.

05: Third set of numbers indicates the **package code** and identifies package types and sizes. For example, drug is in a bottle, vial, or box; drug's quantity or amount, such as in milliliters, ounces, or pints for liquids.

If the NDC number contains **two asterisks** at the end, this identifies the product as a bulk, raw, nonformulated controlled substance.

Because the NDC directory is limited to prescription and insulin drugs, certain products may not be listed. Reasons include the following:
- The product is not a prescription drug or insulin.
- The manufacturer has notified the US Food and Drug Administration (FDA) that the drug is no longer being produced.
- The manufacturer has not complied with all requirements; the drug is not included until all information has been provided to the FDA.

1987 Prescription Drug Marketing Act

The 1987 Prescription Drug Marketing Act (PDMA) addressed issues related to the distribution and wholesale pedigree of human prescription drugs. The intent of the act was to solidify the legal supply channel of prescription drugs from manufacturers to authorized distributors and wholesalers. The act helps prevent counterfeit drugs and ingredients in the supply chain and limits the diversion of pharmaceutical samples and prescription drugs.

1990 Omnibus Budget Reconciliation Act

The origins of the **Omnibus Budget Reconciliation Act** date to 1987, when Congress addressed the problems regarding health care quality for the elderly. With increasing numbers of elderly entering nursing homes, great concern arose over the substandard care being provided, the high nursing personnel-to-patient ratios, and the unhealthy conditions present. OBRA '87 set requirements for facilities participating in Medicare and Medicaid programs and addressed enforcement mechanisms. A minimum standard of care was required, and a change began to take place, transitioning nursing homes from uncomfortable institutions to comfortable, homelike environments providing higher quality care. However, the provisions of OBRA '87 did not address individual privacy rights. The **Omnibus Budget Reconciliation Act of 1990 (OBRA '90)** affected the responsibilities of practicing pharmacists and health care personnel in general. The act outlines specifics for pharmacies to participate in the Medicaid Drug Rebate Program. Medicaid is a state and federal government–managed program that provides medical coverage for low-income individuals. OBRA '90 has profoundly affected pharmacy responsibilities. This act states that a pharmacist must offer to counsel (at the time of purchase) all Medicaid patients who receive new prescriptions. OBRA '90 also requires **drug utilization evaluation (DUE).** The intent of DUE under OBRA '90 is to ensure that all medications being prescribed to patients would be reviewed for appropriateness. Three important provisions of OBRA '90 include:

1. *Evaluation of drug therapy:* This must be completed before a prescription is filled (prospectively). Pharmacists must review drugs for appropriateness, possible drug interactions, contraindications, correctness of drug dosage, and duration of therapy to ensure the patient's safety.
2. *Review of drug therapy:* This is a long-term review of provision 1 through the use of software programs and includes educational interventions intended to ensure the quality of prescribing by physicians.
3. *DUE board review:* The board reviews, evaluates, and develops strategies to improve patient care and reduce costs for those covered by the Medicaid program.

In addition, the DUE must include systems such as computer programs that alert the pharmacist to possible drug interactions, precautions, and other pertinent information that the patient should know. Pharmacies must document and maintain records to track consultations and outcomes. Although OBRA '90 is specific to **Medicaid** coverage, pharmacies usually now counsel all patients on medications that have been prescribed. If these provisions are not met, the pharmacy cannot receive federal reimbursement for medication and may face civil liability proceedings. The Board of Pharmacy (BOP) in each state oversees OBRA '90 compliance. It can also impose fines on both pharmacies and pharmacists for noncompliance, although a patient may refuse counseling.

1996 Health Insurance Portability and Accountability Act

The **Health Insurance Portability and Accountability Act of 1996 (HIPAA)** established the principle of **protected health information (PHI).** HIPAA's privacy rules are meant to protect certain health information. Standards of PHI address the use and disclosure of an individual's health information. Entities that are covered by PHI are obligated to comply with all requirements in the rules of HIPAA, which became effective in 2003. A HIPAA-covered entity is a health care provider, a health plan, or a health care clearinghouse. This includes entities that process nonstandard health information they receive from another entity into a standard format (eg, standard electronic format or data content or vice versa).

All covered physicians were required to update their HIPAA policies and procedures and otherwise implement the changes required by these regulations no later than the September 23, 2013, compliance date. These new rules

meant physicians needed to update their business associate agreements and their notices of privacy practices. The rules also required them to understand the importance of encryption of electronic PHI.

◉ Scenario Checkup 2.1

Laura continues to work at the local chain pharmacy. She is able to put into practice the skills she learned in school. One day she finds herself filling a prescription for her daughter's fiancé. She recognizes the drug as a maintenance medication for individuals infected with the human immunodeficiency virus. Should she share this information with her daughter? Why or why not? Is this a legal or an ethical dilemma?

Patient Confidentiality

Confidentiality is another aspect of ethical work. The definition of confidentiality is to keep privileged information about a customer from being disclosed without his or her consent. This includes information that may cause the patient embarrassment or harm. Under federal law, patients have the right to privacy concerning their medications, treatment, or any aspect of their health care. These laws affect all areas of medicine, including pharmacy, concerning issues of obtaining, transferring, and accessing patient information. Changes have been made throughout all medical facilities and medical information centers that limit access to patient information in charts and computer databases. A patient's approval is required for the release of any information about the patient to any third party, including insurance companies, physicians, and pharmacies. Because pharmacy technicians and other health care professionals have access to information about a patient's condition, medications, and other personal information, they are responsible for keeping the patient's information confidential.

What Information Is Protected?

The HIPAA Privacy Rule protects all "individually identifiable health information" held or transmitted by a covered entity or its business associate, in any form or media, whether electronic, paper, or oral.

What Does This Mean for the Pharmacy?

Patient information must be communicated on a need-to-know basis, with the provision that the entity is covered under the HIPAA health information rules and regulations. This means that the physician can call and request information about his or her patient. The patient's health insurance company can request information on the participant. The pharmacist can share information with the patient about his or her own coverage or medications.

How Is Information Protected on the Computer?

Several safeguards help protect electronically transmitted patient information. The sender of electronic PHI is required to use encryption to convert the information into a nonreadable format. Decryption is the reverse process. The encryption technology must be approved by the National

Institute of Standards and Technologies to ensure its effectiveness in protecting patients' rights.

What Are the Rights of the Patient?

Under HIPAA, patients have the following rights:
- The right to ask to see and obtain a copy of their health records.
- The right to have corrections added to their health information.
- The right to receive a notice that tells them how their health information may be used and shared.
- The right to decide whether they want to give their permission before their health information can be used or shared for certain purposes, such as for marketing.
- The right to obtain a report on when and why their health information was shared for certain purposes.
- If patients think that their rights are being denied or their health information is not being protected, they can:
  - File a complaint with their provider or health insurer
  - File a complaint with the US government
  - Either authorize or not authorize any sharing of their personal or medical information
  - Change or rescind this permission any time they desire

The HIPAA Privacy Rule specifically permits certain persons identified by the patient, such as a spouse, family members, or friends, to receive information that is directly relevant to the patient's care or the patient's payment for health care. If the patient is present or is otherwise available before the disclosure and has the capacity to make health care decisions, the covered entity may discuss this information with the family and these other individuals if the patient agrees or, when given the opportunity, does not object.

For example, when a person comes to a pharmacy and requests to pick up a prescription on behalf of an individual he or she identifies by name, a pharmacist, based on professional judgment and experience with common practice, may allow the person to do so.

Examples of What the Technician Cannot Do

As a pharmacy technician, you may not do the following:
- Offer any personal or medical information pertaining to the patient to any entity not covered under HIPAA rules and regulations
- Share any information with any family member or friend, co-worker, manager, or any entity not covered under the HIPAA rules and regulations

Box 2.3 presents additional examples.

Examples of What is Not Covered Under Health Insurance Portability and Accountability Act Patients' Rights

If you work as a pharmacy technician for a health plan or covered health care provider:
- The HIPAA Privacy Rule does not apply to your employment records.
- The rule does protect your medical or health plan records if you are a patient of the provider or a member of the health plan.

BOX 2.3 Examples of Breaching Confidentiality

Explain why the following examples are in violation of HIPAA regulations.

Example 1: Ms. K has cancer. Two pharmacy technicians discuss her condition and the medications she is taking. A co-worker of Ms. K overhears this information and tells her employer.

Example 2: A computer screen is left on that shows a patient's health information and can be seen by other patients.

Example 3: A regular customer of the pharmacy asks the technician for another patient's phone number; the customer knows that patient.

Example 4: A technician looks up personal patient information because the technician is curious about the patient.

Example 5: A technician gives drug information over the phone to a family member of the patient.

Public Health Activities

Covered entities may disclose PHI to the following:
1. Public health authorities authorized by law to collect or receive such information for preventing or controlling disease, injury, or disability and to public health or other government authorities authorized to receive reports of child abuse and neglect
2. Entities subject to FDA regulation regarding FDA-regulated products or activities for purposes such as adverse event reporting, tracking of products, product recalls, and postmarketing surveillance
3. Individuals who may have contracted or been exposed to a communicable disease when notification is authorized by law
4. Employers, regarding employees, for information concerning a work-related illness or injury or workplace-related medical surveillance to comply with the Occupational Safety and Health Administration (OHSA) or similar state law

Law Enforcement Purposes

Covered entities may disclose PHI to law enforcement officials for law enforcement purposes under the following six circumstances, subject to specified conditions:
1. As required by law, such as court orders
2. To identify or locate a suspect, fugitive, material witness, or missing person
3. In response to a law enforcement official's request for information about a victim or suspected victim of a crime
4. To alert law enforcement of a person's death, if the covered entity suspects that criminal activity caused the death
5. When a covered entity thinks that PHI is evidence of a crime that occurred on its premises
6. By a covered health care provider in a medical emergency not occurring on its premises, when necessary to inform law enforcement about the nature of a crime, the location of the crime or crime victims, and the perpetrator of the crime

Examples

1. Can I have a friend pick up my medications and medical supplies for me?

   Yes; under HIPAA, pharmacists are allowed to give prescription medications and supplies to a family member, friend, or any person you send to pick up the medications or supplies.

2. If my daughter calls the pharmacy to ask about whether my medications are ready, can they tell her?

   Yes; but no other information can be given out.

3. If I cannot speak the language and a stranger offers to interpret the exchange between myself and the pharmacist, is this okay?

   Yes; as long as you do not object.

4. Is a pharmacist permitted to have the customer acknowledge receipt of the notice by signing or initialing the log book when picking up prescriptions?

   Yes; provided the individual is clearly informed on the log book of what he or she is acknowledging and the acknowledgment is not also used as a waiver or permission for something else that also appears on the log book (such as a waiver to consult with the pharmacist). The HIPAA Privacy Rule provides covered health care providers with discretion to design an acknowledgment process that works best for their businesses (see the website https://www.hhs.gov/hipaa/for-professionals/privacy/laws-regulations/index.html).

2000 Drug Addiction Treatment Act. The Drug Addiction Treatment Act of 2000 (DATA 2000) permits physicians to prescribe controlled substances (preapproved by the DEA) in schedules C-III, C-IV, or C-V to individuals with opioid addiction for the purpose of maintenance or detoxification treatments. This act is different from the regulations that oversee methadone maintenance treatments for opioid addiction. Certain controlled substances have been found to effectively attenuate the craving for opioids and also prevent withdrawal symptoms. Patients must be in a treatment program that provides additional support services. Physicians must complete a training course and must be registered with and certified by the DEA to prescribe these agents. If the physician is in private practice, he or she may treat only up to 30 patients at one time. After 1 year the physician may apply to treat up to 100 patients.

2003 Medicare Modernization Act. Medicare is a government-managed insurance program that provides assistance to people older than age 65. In addition, those who are younger than age 65 with disabilities and individuals with end-stage renal failure are covered under this program. Medicare has a long history, starting in 1965. In 2003, a major change took place for millions of Americans with the passage of the Medicare Modernization Act (MMA). This revision provided a drug discount card to beneficiaries with low incomes who require pharmacy company assistance for obtaining medications. The new program is administered under the Medicare Advantage program, which began in 2006. This allows Medicare participants to offset high drug costs, which should also reduce preventable hospitalizations resulting from lack of medication treatment.

◉ Scenario Checkup 2.2

Laura is assigned to cover the register in addition to performing her regular prescription-filling duties at a local chain pharmacy. It is a particularly busy day, and two technicians have called in sick during her shift. A customer comes to the register and asks to purchase two boxes of Sudafed. Laura has the person sign the log book but does not ask for identification. What are the possible negative implications for Laura in this transaction? What are the laws regarding the purchase of pseudoephedrine in your state?

2005 Combat Methamphetamine Epidemic Act. Until 2004, the drug pseudoephedrine (PSE) was sold OTC as a decongestant and was not limited in quantity for purchase by the consumer. Several different manufacturers produce this drug, and it was stocked outside the pharmacy on the shelves of every store that carried cold remedies. The OTC status of PSE was changed when the US government became aware of its diversion and use as an ingredient in the preparation of methamphetamine (Fig. 2.3).

In 2005, Congress passed the Combat Methamphetamine Epidemic Act (CMEA) in response to this problem. The bill addressed all areas of the manufacturing, law enforcement regulations, and sale of this drug. Although PSE is still labeled as a "noncontrolled substance" in over 30 states, the manufacture, distribution, and sale of this drug must follow several strict guidelines. According to these guidelines, only a licensed pharmacist or technician may dispense, sell, or distribute this drug (Box 2.4). According to the National Association of State Controlled Substances Authorities (NASCSA) 2016 report, approximately 32 states have implemented electronic reporting to track PSE sales using the National Precursor Log Exchange (NPLEx). Arkansas, which originally utilized MethMonitor, was the most recent state to move to the NPLEx platform. Two states, Oregon and Mississippi, along with 63 Missouri counties and cities, now require a prescription for PSE products. At least 100 bills in 27 states have been introduced that would require a prescription for obtaining PSE. Mexico has actually banned the drug completely.

According to the United States Government Accountability Office (GAO) 2013 report, the nationwide meth lab count dropped to a low of 6951 in 2007 as a result of the passage of the CMEA and state laws restricting the sales of precursors. Unfortunately, that number then rose to more than double that figure by 2010, reaching a total of 15,314 reported labs. Experts attribute this spike to technology advances and working around the system through coordinated group buys. Since 2010, more states have implemented the use of NPLEx to track PSE sales and several states have further restricted PSE purchase quantities. Since the GAO publication, the nationwide meth lab count is again decreasing every year, with the National Drug Threat Assessment (NDTA) 2020 reporting a meth lab count below 1000 in 2019. However, a decrease in meth lab numbers does not mean that the threat of meth is fading. In fact, meth availability and usage are on the rise. One example of that rise can be seen in the 1600% jump in meth seized by the 23 drug task forces (including Northern Kentucky's) that are funded through the Ohio High-Intensity Drug Trafficking Area agency from 2015 to 2019 (and the 2019 numbers are

U.S. Department of Justice
Drug Enforcement Administration
Office of Diversion Control

Problem
Pseudoephedrine and ephedrine, both List 1 chemicals, are highly coveted by drug traffickers who use them to manufacture methamphetamine, a Schedule II controlled substance, for the illicit market. The diversion of over-the-counter, pseudoephedrine-containing products is one of the major contributing factors to the methamphetamine problem in the United States. Inappropriate retail level purchases by individuals attempting to procure pseudoephedrine for the illicit manufacture of methamphetamine have been documented as a source of much of the pseudoephedrine found in clandestine methamphetamine laboratories. These purchases, which are accomplished by methods such as "*smurfing*" and *shelf sweeping*, violate Federal law and may expose the seller to criminal and civil penalties.

Common Pseudoephedrine Products
Common cold products including, but not limited to Sudafed®, Tylenol®Cold, Advil®Cold, Drixoral®, Benadryl® Allergy & Cold Tablets, Robitussin®Cold Sinus & Congestion, as well as many generic brands.

Retail Thresholds
The Methamphetamine Anti-Proliferation Act (MAPA) limits the thresholds of pseudoephedrine drug products to 9-gram single transactions with the package size not to exceed 3 grams.

Nine (9) Gram Single Transactions--Three (3) Grams per Package
- 120 mg pseudoephedrine HCl = 92 tablets
- 120 mg pseudoephedrine HCl = 31 tablets
- 60 mg pseudoephedrine HCl = 184 tablets
- 60 mg pseudoephedrine HCl = 62 tablets
- 30 mg pseudoephedrine HCl = 367 tablets
- 30 mg pseudoephedrine HCl = 123 tablets

Common Methods of Diversion
- *Smurfing* involves the retail purchase of sub-threshold amounts by organized groups of individuals that either send in multiple purchasers into the same location or visit a large number of different locations.
- *Shelf sweeping* occurs when individuals or groups remove all the shelf stock and exit the store, similar to a "smash and grab" shoplifting technique.
- *Shoplifting* occurs when individuals remove stock from the shelves and exit the store without paying.

All of the above methods can be prevented by limiting access to products or by utilizing mirrors or other surveillance equipment such as cameras.

Suspicious Purchase Items
Camping fuel, lithium batteries, large quantities of matches, iodine, coffee filters, rock salt, battery acid, swimming pool acid (when purchased in unusual quantities or under unusual circumstances).

Theft or Loss of List I Chemicals
The DEA reminds List I chemical handlers of the regulatory requirement: "A regulated chemical handler must immediately report thefts or losses to the nearest DEA office and should notify state/local law enforcement and regulatory agencies. A written report must be submitted to the DEA within 15 days of discovery of the theft or loss". (CFR 21 §1310.05)

Improper Sales
"Any person who possesses or distributes a listed chemical knowing or having reasonable cause to believe that the listed chemical will be used to manufacture a controlled substance, except as authorized by this title, shall be fined in accordance with Title 18, or imprisoned not more than 20 years, or both". (Title 21 U.S.C. 841 (c)(2))

FIG. 2.3 Drug Enforcement Administration poster on the misuse of pseudoephedrine. (Courtesy Drug Enforcement Administration, Washington, DC.)

incomplete). The 2020 NDTA noted a 55% increase in DEA methamphetamine seizures from 2018 to 2019 and a 75% increase in overall meth-related reports since 2014.

Table 2.2 presents an overview of other pharmacy-related acts.

BOX 2.4 Combat Methamphetamine Epidemic Act 2005

- Pseudoephedrine storage: Behind the counter or locked in a cabinet.
- The maximum amount sold may not exceed 3.6 g in a calendar day or 9 g per 30 days retail, and 7.5 g per 30 days by mail order.
- Purchaser's identification must be provided.
- Documentation may be done electronically or by log book. If a log book is used, it must be a bound book.
- Records of all information must be kept for at least 2 years.
- Documentation required:
  - Drug name
  - Drug strength
  - Drug amount
  - Date/time of sale
  - Customer's name
  - Customer's address
  - Customer's signature

▮ Tech Note!

In Oregon and Mississippi, pseudoephedrine is a schedule III controlled substance, whereas in Illinois, Iowa, and Kansas, it is a schedule IV.

2010 Patient Protection and Affordable Care Act. In March 2010, President Obama signed into law the Patient Protection and Affordable Care Act (ACA). This comprehensive health care reform makes preventive care more accessible and affordable for many Americans. The ACA has a number of provisions that were phased in over a period of years, beginning in 2010 and continuing through 2020. The law requires insurance companies to cover all applicants with new minimum standards, including individuals with preexisting conditions. Many components of the ACA involve pharmacy professionals, such as the following:

- Electronic health record incentives and e-prescribing
- Medication therapy management
- Accountable care organizations
- The Independence at Home Demonstration Project

Pharmacy technicians need to be knowledgeable about the ACA and the changes dealing with medication management and Medicare Part D. Well-informed technicians build credibility for the profession and for themselves as an important part of the pharmacy team. More information on the

TABLE 2.2
Additional Pharmacy-Related Laws

Year	Act	Abbreviation	Description
1967	Fair Packaging and Labeling Act	FPLA	Label must show net contents; name and place of business of manufacturer, packer, or distributor; and net quantity of contents in terms of weight, measure, or numerical count. Measurement must be in metric and US units.
1972	Drug Listing Act	DLA	Provides the FDA with an accurate list of all drugs manufactured, prepared, propagated, compounded, or processed by a drug establishment regulated under the FDA. This act amends the Federal Food, Drug, and Cosmetic Act and prevents unfair or deceptive packaging and labeling.
1990	Anabolic Steroids Control Act	ASCA	Because of anabolic steroid misuse by athletes, this act helps enforce regulations on abuse.
1990	The Humanitarian Device Exemption— Safe Medical Devices Act	SMDA	This act encourages discovery and use of devices intended to benefit patients in treatment and diagnosis of diseases or conditions that affect fewer than 4000 individuals in the United States.
1990	Nutrition Labeling and Education Act	NLEA	This act covers food items and their labeling; vitamins, minerals, or other nutrients are on the label and in some cases are highlighted.
1994	Dietary Supplement Health and Education Act	DSHEA	This act better defines the term *dietary supplements* to include herbs such as ginseng, garlic, fish oil, psyllium, enzymes, glandulars, and mixtures of these. Consumers must be informed of health-related benefits. Manufacturers of these supplements are held to the same regulations. Labels cannot mislead consumers. Labels must include nutritional values.
1997	Food and Drug Administration Modernization Act	FDAMA	New drugs are being reviewed and released into the public faster. Millions of persons have a wider and more timely access to information on new medications.
2005	Combat Methamphetamine Enhancement Act of 2010	CMEA	This act amended the Controlled Substances Act to increase the compliance of retailers and distributors of pseudoephedrine products. All persons engaged in the sale of pseudoephedrine must self-certify that they have trained personnel to comply with the Combat Methamphetamine Epidemic Act. Also, distributors can sell only to retailers who are registered with the DEA.
2006	Physician's Labeling Rule	PLR	Drug manufacturers classify drug information into five pregnancy categories: A, B, C, D, and X
2009	Family Smoking and Tobacco Control Act	Tobacco Control Act	Gives FDA authority to regulate the manufacture, distribution, and marketing of tobacco products
2016	21st Century Cures Act	Cures Act	Helps to accelerate medical products innovation and provision to patients faster and efficiently
2023	Mainstreaming Addiction Act	MAT Act	All health care providers with a standard control license can prescribe buprenorphine for opioid use disorders

ACA can be obtained at the website *https://www.healthcare.gov/glossary/affordable-care-act/*.

2013 Drug Quality and Security Act. In November 2013, President Obama signed into law a bill that gives the FDA greater oversight of bulk pharmaceutical compounding and enhances the agency's ability to track drugs through the distribution process. This legislation was prompted by the deadly fungal meningitis outbreak in the fall of 2012 that resulted from unsanitary conditions at a compounding facility in Massachusetts. The Drug Quality and Security Act (DQSA) comprises two separate acts: the Compounding Quality Act and the Drug Supply Chain Security Act.

The Compounding Quality Act creates a new class of compounding manufacturers that voluntarily register with the FDA as an "outsourcing facility." These manufacturers will be regulated similar to traditional pharmaceutical manufacturers and will be able to sell to hospitals in bulk.

The Drug Supply Chain Security Act addresses concerns relating to counterfeit, falsified, and substandard prescription medication. This act requires the FDA to create and implement a national tracking system to be used by manufacturers. Bar coding technology will be used to introduce pharmaceutical products into the supply chain. This new track-and-trace pedigree system for drugs will be phased in over 10 years.

In 2012, counterfeit vials of bevacizumab (Avastin), a cancer medication, were found in the United States. They were introduced from Britain and traced back to a Turkish wholesaler. The vials had no active ingredient.

Food and Drug Administration and Drug Enforcement Administration

Two government agencies that are important in the practice of pharmacy are the FDA and the DEA. The FDA now is an agency of the DHHS (see the discussion of the history of the FDA presented earlier in this chapter). The main function of the FDA is to enforce the guidelines for manufacturers to ensure the safety and effectiveness of medications. The Federal Food, Drug, and Cosmetic Act established standards that prohibit misbranding, adulteration, and misleading labeling of any products before they are provided to consumers. Any food, drug, or product that contains any avoidable, added, poisonous, or harmful substance is unsafe and is considered adulterated. To prevent misbranding, manufacturers must meet the following packaging standards under the Federal Food, Drug, and Cosmetic Act:

1. Mandatory drug labeling (see Drug Monographs, later in the chapter)
2. Standards of identity
3. Imitation foods
4. Nutritional information for special dietary foods
5. Manufacturers may not advertise false or misleading statements about their product

Examples of misleading information on product labeling include the following:

1. Incorrect, inadequate, or incomplete identification
2. Unsubstantiated claims of therapeutic value
3. Inaccuracies concerning condition, state, treatment size, shape, or style
4. Substitution of parts or material
5. Ambiguity, half-truths, and trade puffery
6. Failure to reveal material facts, consequences that may result from use, or existence of difference of opinion

The other enforcement department is the DEA. This agency was created later under the Department of Justice. The function of the DEA is to prevent illegal distribution and misuse of controlled substances. The DEA also issues licenses to practitioners, pharmacies, and manufacturers of controlled substances. The DEA's primary role is to enforce the nation's federal drug laws.

Food and Drug Administration Reporting Process and Adverse Reactions

The FDA has a toll-free number (1-800-FDA-1088) for reporting any defect found in OTC medications or any drug problem noted by a person. A technician or pharmacist also may use this number to report any problems with a drug, whether it is OTC or legend (prescription). A product that looks different from its normal package should be reported. Adverse reactions also should be reported to the FDA's MedWatch program. Any medication reaction that may cause disability, hospitalization, or death should be reported, along with any less disabling type of reaction such as fainting or other types of reactions that

may not have been listed in the drug monograph. MedWatch is the program under the FDA that allows consumers and health care professionals to report discrepancies or adverse reactions to medications. The MedWatch form for such reports can be found in many drug reference publications and drug compendia databases or online at the website *https://www.fda.gov/safety/medwatch-fda-safety-information-and-adverse-event-reporting-program*. The patient and reporting person's identities are kept confidential (Fig. 2.4).

> ### ■ Tech Note!
>
> Follow MedWatch on Twitter to keep up with the latest drug safety information and adverse event reporting! US FDA MedWatch@FDAMedWatch or the website *https://www.fda.gov/safety/medwatch-fda-safety-information-and-adverse-event-reporting-program*.

Recalled Drugs

The FDA does not typically order recalls but instead may request (in writing) a recall by the manufacturer. Only if the manufacturer refuses and there is clear evidence of a risk to human health may the FDA enforce such a request. The manufacturer can voluntarily recall items that have been found to be defective or somehow tainted. This is done by several means, such as television news or newspapers, and recall notifications can be downloaded from the FDA website. In addition, the manufacturer must notify by e-mail, phone, or fax all entities that may have dispensed the product and must include instructions on how to handle each type of recall (Box 2.5). Once the product has been recalled, it is destroyed, and an investigation is conducted to determine why the product was defective.

All stock must be pulled from the shelves according to the guidelines of the manufacturer. The manufacturer supplies a return form with instructions for reimbursement. The three classes of recalls are as follows:

Class 1: The highest level of recall; it deals with products that could cause serious harm or prove fatal. This includes life-saving drugs. This level also includes foods that contain toxins or labels that do not list ingredients that may cause allergies.

Class 2: The next level, which deals with products found to cause a temporary health problem or to pose a slight threat of serious harm. This level includes drugs that are dispensed at less than the strength labeled on the container; it does not include drugs used in life-threatening events.

Class 3: The lowest level, which is used for products that may have a minor defect or other condition that would not harm the patient but that prevents the drugs from being resold. This level includes a drug container defect (eg, a faulty cap), a product with a strange color or taste, or the lack of English labeling on retail food items.

Controlled Substances

Controlled substances, such as barbiturates, opioids, benzodiazepines, and central nervous system stimulants, are

DEPARTMENT OF HEALTH AND HUMAN SERVICES
Food and Drug Administration

Form Approved: OMB No. 0910-0291
Expiration Date: 6/30/2015
(See PRA Statement on preceding general information page)

MEDWATCH Consumer Voluntary Reporting
(FORM FDA 3500B)

Section A – About the Problem

What kind of problem was it? *(Check all that apply)*

☐ Were hurt or had a bad side effect *(including new or worsening symptoms)*

☐ Used a product incorrectly which could have or led to a problem

☐ Noticed a problem with the quality of the product

☐ Had problems after switching from one product maker to another maker

Did any of the following happen? *(Check all that apply)*

☐ Hospitalization – admitted or stayed longer

☐ Required help to prevent permanent harm *(for medical devices only)*

☐ Disability or health problem

☐ Birth defect

☐ Life-threatening

☐ Death *(Include date)*: _____

☐ Other serious/important medical incident *(Please describe below)*

_____

_____

_____

Date the problem occurred *(mm/dd/yyyy)*

Tell us what happened and how it happened. *(Include as many details as possible)*

_____

_____

_____ | Continue Page |

List any relevant tests or laboratory data if you know them. *(Include dates)*

_____

_____

_____ | Continue Page |

For a problem with a product, including

- prescription or over-the-counter medicine
- biologics, such as human cells and tissues used for transplantation (for example, tendons, ligaments, and bone) and gene therapies
- nutrition products, such as vitamins and minerals, herbal remedies, infant formulas, and medical foods
- cosmetics or make-up products
- foods (including beverages and ingredients added to foods)

⇨ **Go to Section B**

For a problem with a medical device, including

- any health-related test, tool, or piece of equipment
- health-related kits, such as glucose monitoring kits or blood pressure cuffs
- implants, such as breast implants, pacemakers, or catheters
- other consumer health products, such as contact lenses, hearing aids, and breast pumps

⇨ **Go to Section C (Skip Section B)**

For more information, visit *http://www.fda.gov/MedWatch*

Submission of a report does not constitute an admission that medical personnel or the product caused or contributed to the event.

FIG. 2.4 Food and Drug Administration MedWatch form. (Courtesy Drug Enforcement Administration, Washington, DC.)

Section B – About the Products

Name of the product as it appears on the box, bottle, or package (Include as many names as you see)

Name of the company that makes the product

Expiration date (mm/dd/yyyy)	Lot number	NDC number

Strength (for example, 250 mg per 500 mL or 1 g)	Quantity (for example, 2 pills, 2 puffs, or 1 teaspoon, etc.)	Frequency (for example, twice daily or at bedtime)	How was it taken or used (for example, by mouth, by injection, or on the skin)?

Date the person first started taking or using the product (mm/dd/yyyy): _____

Date the person stopped taking or using the product (mm/dd/yyyy): _____

Why was the person using the product (such as, what condition was it supposed to treat?)

_____

_____

_____

Did the problem stop after the person reduced the dose or stopped taking or using the product?   ☐ Yes   ☐ No

Did the problem return if the person started taking or using the product again?

☐ Yes   ☐ No   ☐ Didn't restart

Do you still have the product in case we need to evaluate it? (Do not send the product to FDA. We will contact you directly if we need it.)

☐ Yes   ☐ No

⇨ **Go to Section D (Skip Section C)**

Section C – About the Medical Device

Name of medical device

Name of the company that makes the medical device

Other identifying information (The model, catalog, lot, serial, or UDI number, and the expiration date, if you can locate them)

_____

_____

Was someone operating the medical device when the problem occurred?

☐ Yes

☐ No

If yes, who was using it?

☐ The person who had the problem

☐ A health professional (such as a doctor, nurse, or aide)

☐ Someone else (Please explain who)

_____

For implanted medical devices ONLY (such as pacemakers, breast implants, etc.)

Date the implant was put in (mm/dd/yyyy)	Date the implant was taken out (If relevant) (mm/dd/yyyy)

⇨ **Go to Section D**

For more information, visit *http://www.fda.gov/MedWatch*

Submission of a report does not constitute an admission that medical personnel or the product caused or contributed to the event.

FORM FDA 3500B (4/13)   **MedWatch** Consumer Voluntary Reporting   Page 2 of 3

FIG. 2.4, cont'd

Continued

Section D – About the Person Who Had the Problem

Person's Initials	Sex ☐ Female ☐ Male	Age *(at time the problem occurred)* or Birth Date	Weight *(Specify lbs or kg)*	Race

List known medical conditions *(such as diabetes, high blood pressure, cancer, heart disease, or others)*

_____

_____

Please list all allergies *(such as to drugs, foods, pollen, or others)*

List any other important information about the person *(such as smoking, pregnancy, alcohol use, etc.)*

List all current prescription medications and medical devices being used.

_____

| | Continue Page |

List all over-the-counter medications and any vitamins, minerals, supplements, and herbal remedies being used.

| | Continue Page |

⇨ **Go to Section E**

Section E – About the Person Filling Out This Form

We will contact you only if we need additional information. Your name will not be given out to the public.

Last name	First name

Number/Street	City and State/Province

Country	ZIP or Postal code

Telephone number	Email address	Today's date *(mm/dd/yyyy)*

Did you report this problem to the company that makes the product (the manufacturer)? ☐ Yes ☐ No	May we give your name and contact information to the company that makes the product (manufacturer) to help them evaluate the product? ☐ Yes ☐ No

Send This Report by Mail or Fax

Keep the product in case the FDA wants to contact you for more information. Please do not send products to the FDA. Mail or fax the form to:

Mail: MedWatch Food and Drug Administration 5600 Fishers Lane Rockville, MD 20857	**Fax:** 1-800-332-0178 (toll-free)

Thank you for helping us protect the public health.

For more information, visit *http://www.fda.gov/MedWatch*

Submission of a report does not constitute an admission that medical personnel or the product caused or contributed to the event.

FORM FDA 3500B (4/13)   **MedWatch** Consumer Voluntary Reporting   Page 3 of 3

FIG. 2.4, cont'd

BOX 2.5   Sample Recall Notification

The US Food and Drug Administration (FDA) posts press releases and other notices of recalls and market withdrawals by the firms involved as a service to consumers, the media, and other interested parties. The FDA does not endorse either the product or the company.

Recall—Firm Press Release

Company Announcement

Fresenius Kabi Issues Voluntary Nationwide Recall of 13 Lots of Ketorolac Tromethamine Injection, USP Because of the Presence of Particulate Matter in Reserve Samples

Summary

Company Announcement Date:
April 20, 2020
FDA Publish Date:
April 20, 2020
Product Type:
Drugs
Reason for Announcement:
Presence of Particulate Matter
Company Name:
Fresenius Kabi USA, LLC
Brand Name:
Toradol

Product Description:

Ketorolac tromethamine injection, USP, 30 mg/mL, and ketorolac tromethamine injection, USP, 60 mg/2 mL

Fresenius Kabi USA, LLC is voluntarily recalling 13 lots of ketorolac tromethamine injection, USP, 30 mg/mL, 1-mL fill in a 2-mL amber vial and ketorolac tromethamine injection, USP, 60 mg/2 mL (30 mg/mL), 2-mL fill in a 2-mL amber vial to the user level because of the presence of particulate matter composed of the following elements: carbon, silicon, oxygen; and polyamides. Particulate matter was found in eight reserve sample vials.

Administration of products containing particulate matter could obstruct blood vessels and result in local irritation of blood vessels, swelling at the site of injection, a mass of tissue that could become inflamed and infected, blood clots traveling to the lung, scarring of the lung tissues, and allergic reactions that could lead to life-threatening consequences.

Ketorolac tromethamine, a nonsteroidal antiinflammatory drug, is indicated for the short-term (up to 5 days in adults) management of moderately severe acute pain that requires analgesia at the opioid level. The total combined duration of use of oral ketorolac tromethamine and ketorolac tromethamine injection should not exceed 5 days.

Listed is a table of the recalled lots distributed nationwide to wholesalers, distributors, hospitals, and pharmacies between May 5, 2018, and December 16, 2019, and a copy of the label:

Product Name/ Product Size	NDC Number	Product Code	Batch Number	Expiration Date	First Ship Date	Last Ship Date
Ketorolac tromethamine injection, USP, 30 mg/mL, 1-mL fill in a 2-mL amber vial	63323-162-01	160201	6118737	04/2020	05/30/2018	06/27/2018
			6118902	04/2020	08/01/2018	08/15/2018
			6119052	05/2020	06/25/2018	07/25/2018
			6119752	08/2020	09/28/2018	12/06/2018
			6122349	07/2021	09/16/2019	11/04/2019
			6122538	09/2021	11/01/2019	12/16/2019
Ketorolac tromethamine injection, USP, 60 mg/2 mL (30 mg/mL), 2-mL fill in a 2-mL amber vial	63323-162-02	160202	6119229	06/2020	08/09/2018	10/30/2018
			6119273	06/2020	09/26/2018	03/30/2019
			6119843	09/2020	11/11/2019	01/07/2020
			6121115	02/2021	03/30/2019	04/22/2019
			6121451	03/2021	04/29/2019	08/05/2019
			6121452	03/2021	07/12/2019	10/22/2019
			6121496	03/2021	06/21/2019	12/10/2019

Fresenius Kabi is notifying its distributors and customers by letter and asking customers and distributors to check their stock immediately and to quarantine and discontinue the use and distribution of any affected product. Distributors should notify their customers and direct them to quarantine and discontinue distributing or dispensing any affected lots and to return the product to Fresenius Kabi. The recall letter and response form are available at *https://www.fresenius-kabi.com/us/pharmaceutical-product-updates*.

Customers with questions regarding this recall may contact Fresenius Kabi at 1-866-716-2459 Monday through Friday, during the hours of 8:00 am to 5:00 pm Central Time. Consumers should contact their physician or health

care provider if they have experienced any problems that may be related to taking or using this drug product.

Adverse reactions or quality problems experienced with the use of this product may be reported to the FDA's MedWatch Adverse Event Reporting program either online, by regular mail, or by fax.

- Complete and submit the report online.
- Regular mail or fax: Download form or call 1-800-332-1088 to request a reporting form, then complete and return to the address on the preaddressed form or submit by fax to 1-800-FDA-0178.
- Or contact Fresenius Kabi at 1-800-551-7176, Monday through Friday, during the hours of 8:00 am to 5:00 pm

Continued

BOX 2.5 Sample Recall Notification—cont'd

or by e-mail at *http://productcomplaint.USA@fresenius-kabi.com* or *adverse.events.USA@fresenius-kabi.com*.

This recall is being conducted with the knowledge of the US Food and Drug Administration.

About Fresenius Kabi

Fresenius Kabi *(http://www.fresenius-kabi.com/us)* is a global health care company that specializes in medicines and technologies for infusion, transfusion, and clinical nutrition. The company's products and services are used to help care for critically and chronically ill patients. The company's US headquarters is in Lake Zurich, Illinois. The company's global headquarters is in Bad Homburg, Germany. For more information about Fresenius Kabi worldwide, please visit *http://www.fresenius-kabi.com*.

Company Contact Information

Consumers

Fresenius Kabi
1-866-716-2459

Media

Matt Kuhn
847-550-5751
matt.kuhn@fresenius-kabi.com

US Food and Drug Administration. Safety alerts; Fresenius Kabi USA, LLC initiates nationwide voluntary recall of 13 lots of ketorolac tromethamine injection, USP, 30 mg/mL, and ketorolac tromethamine injection, USP, 60 mg/2 mL. *https://www.fda.gov/safety/recalls-market-withdrawals-safety-alerts/fresenius-kabi-issues-voluntary-nationwide-recall-13-lots-ketorolac-tromethamine-injection-usp-due*.

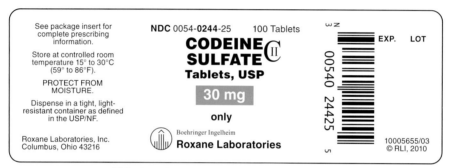

FIG. 2.5 Codeine label showing C-II imprint.

substances that are addictive and have the potential to be abused. Opioids, such as codeine and morphine, are substances created from opium and are addictive. When they are consumed over time, a person can build up a tolerance to their effects and require increased doses. Each type of controlled substance is assigned a rating that depends on its addictive and abuse potential. Fig. 2.5 presents an example of a labeled **narcotic**.

Ratings of Scheduled (Controlled) Substances

The letter C (meaning controlled substance) is used in addition to Roman numerals to indicate the addictiveness and abuse potential of controlled substances. In 1970, Congress established five levels of control based on the potential for abuse. The strongest level in terms of abuse potential are C-I drugs. These drugs have been determined to have a high potential for abuse and to have no acceptable medical purpose; they also are deemed unsafe for use under medical supervision. This category includes such drugs as D-lysergic acid diethylamide (LSD) and heroin. Pharmacies do not stock drugs in the C-I class because they do not have any medicinal use in the United States. Therefore physicians cannot prescribe C-I drugs for their patients. All medicinal controlled substances are placed in the following four categories: C-II, C-III, C-IV, and C-V. Table 2.3 shows the schedule, types of medications, and abuse potential for each level of controlled substances.

▽ **Tech Alert!**

Effective October 6, 2014, hydrocodone combination products are considered schedule II under the Controlled Substances Act. This change by the DEA (from schedule III) means that stricter schedule II controls and sanctions now apply to these products. For more information, see the *Federal Register.*

Individual states establish rules concerning controlled substances, such as storage and record-keeping. Schedule C-V medications (referred to as *exempt controlled substances*) may be kept OTC in some states because of their low potential for abuse. However, even for exempt controlled substances, specific rules govern the quantity kept on hand and the records that must be retained by the pharmacy when these substances are purchased by consumers. Many states require C-II drugs to be kept (before filling) in locked storage areas because of their high potential for abuse.

The US Attorney General has the authority to decide under which schedule a drug should be placed. The decision is made after careful consideration of the scientific findings and recommendations from various authorities on the dependency potential for each agent. Some drugs may be labeled under two different schedules because the dose may alter the dependency of the drug. Sometimes controlled substances can be reevaluated. For example, dronabinol (Marinol) previously

TABLE 2.3
Typical Controlled Substances

Drug Level	Type of Medication		Potential for Abuse
	Generic Name	**Trade Name**	
C-I	LSD cocaine (crack or street) peyote heroin marijuana (cannabis)		Drugs that have no accepted medical use in the United States and have very high abuse potential
C-II	meperidine oxycodone/APAP oxycodone/ASA hydromorphone methylphenidate fentanyl codeine morphine amphetamines methadone opium hydrocodone/acetaminophen hydrocodone/APAP hydrocodone/ibuprofen	Demerol Percocet Percodan Dilaudid Ritalin Duragesic[a] Vicodin[a] Norco Vicoprofen[a]	High potential for abuse; used for medicinal purposes; abuse may lead to severe psychological or physical dependence
C-III	acetaminophen/codeine #2, #3, #4 testosterone	Tylenol/codeine[a] Depo-Testosterone	Potential for abuse under this schedule is less than that of controlled substances under C-II; abuse may lead to moderate or low physical dependence or high psychological dependence; most schedule III drugs are combination narcotics
C-IV	diazepam lorazepam pentazocine chlordiazepoxide flurazepam phenobarbital quazepam	Valium Ativan Talwin[a] Librium[a] Dalmane[a] Dormalin[a]	Potential for abuse is low compared with C-III drugs; abuse may lead to limited physical or psychological dependence
C-V	diphenoxylate/atropine- codeine/guaifenesin promethazine/codeine	Lomotil Cheratussin AC Phenergan/codeine[a]	Low potential for abuse compared with C-IV drugs; abuse may lead to limited physical or psychological dependence

[a]Brand discontinued; now available only as generic.

APAP, Acetyl-*p*-aminophenol (acetaminophen); *ASA,* acetylsalicylic acid (aspirin).

was classified as a C-II drug but now is a C-III drug. In contrast, certain illegal street drugs are used primarily for procedures in hospitals; for example, topical cocaine is used locally to stop bleeding and provide anesthesia before suturing.

Cannabis Legality

Under the Controlled Substances Act (CSA) of 1970, the possession of cannabis is illegal and is categorized as a schedule I substance. Each state, however, can determine recreational or medical use policies individually. This is very controversial and varies widely from state to state. The medical use of cannabis is legal in 39 states and approved recreationally in 21.

Cannabidiol

Pharmacies now sell cannabidiol (CBD), which is an oil derived from the cannabis plant. It is available in oils, creams, and even gummies. The uses vary for treatment of pain, asthma, epilepsy, migraines, and lung diseases.

Tamper-Proof Prescriptions

Many states have changed to a new type of prescription for controlled substances. These new prescriptions have up to eight different tamper-proof security marks on them. These features were designed to protect a prescriber's intended order from forgery and fraud. Several features eliminate the usefulness of photocopying the prescription order. The prescription forms can be ordered with any or all of the features. The DEA must approve the printer company that prints the new prescriptions, but no specific format has been established because each state may adopt its own features, colors, or size (check with your individual state board of pharmacy for more information). The individual features of these tamper-proof forms are listed in Box 2.6, and Fig. 2.6 shows a sample prescription form.

- Tamper-resistant background ink shows attempts to alter script by patient.
- Thermochromatic ink box shows "SECURE" when rubbed or heated.
- Each prescription sheet has an individual numerical identifier so that lost or stolen prescription pads can be invalidated.
- Each sheet is sequentially numbered for internal and state-mandated record-keeping.
- Security feature warning bands are on the front of each script to detail security features.
- Penetrating magnetic ink is used to print the prescriber's information on the script, preventing chemical "lifting" of information during forgery.
- Secure prescriptions have "coin reactive" ink; message appears when the back of the pad is rubbed with a coin.
- Photocopied features:
  - Hidden security "VOID" appears when photocopied on most high-end photocopiers.
  - Reverse-printed RX (lighter colored) notations in upper corners of pad drop out when photocopied to appear white.
  - All secure prescriptions have a high-security watermark on the reverse side that cannot be copied and can be seen only when held to a light source at an angle.
  - MicroPrint security borders are present, which are tiny printings of a security message along the edges of a pad that combine to form a solid line when digitally scanned or copied.

Registration Requirements for Maintaining Narcotics

The DEA uses three main registration forms in the regulation of controlled substances. Only Form 224 is needed by the pharmacy to dispense controlled substances. The following is a list of form numbers issued by the DEA, along with additional requirements:

- To manufacture or distribute controlled substances: Form 225.
- To manage a controlled substances treatment program or compound controlled substances: Form 363.
- To dispense controlled substances: Form 224 (must be renewed every 3 years using Form 224a).
- To order or transfer schedule II substances: Form 222. This must be done by the receiving registrant to the registrant transferring the drugs. A final count of the drugs must be completed on the day of transfer. No copy needs to be sent to the DEA, but a copy should be kept on file for 2 years for DEA inspection.
- Authorization to destroy damaged, outdated, or unwanted controlled substances: Form 41. Retail pharmacies can request this form from the DEA only once a year. (Hospitals may request a "blanket destruction" permission form, which allows them to destroy a controlled substance multiple times throughout the year.) For retail pharmacies, a letter must be sent to the DEA for approval, along with the completed Form 41, at least 2 weeks before destruction. The request letter must contain the names of at least two people who will witness the destruction and the proposed date and method of destruction. The disposal of the scheduled drug or drugs must be witnessed by a licensed

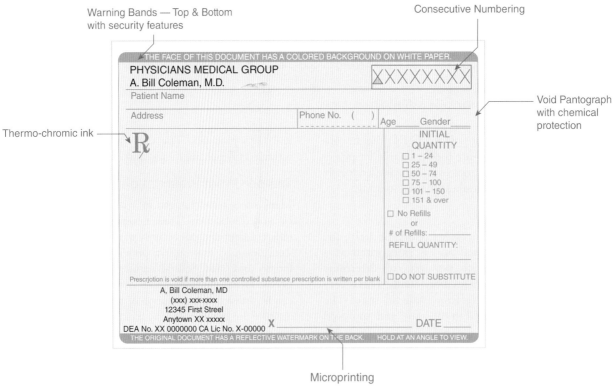

FIG. 2.6 Example of a tamper-proof prescription.

physician, pharmacist, registered nurse (RN), or law enforcement officer. Signed copies of Form 41 must then be forwarded to the DEA.

- Retail pharmacies that want to engage in wholesale distribution of bulk quantities of drugs containing PSE, phenylpropanolamine, or ephedrine must register with the DEA: Form 510.
- For loss or theft of a controlled substance: Form 106. Required information includes the name and address of the pharmacy, DEA registration number, date of loss or theft, police department notified, type of loss or theft, drug name, and symbols or cost codes used by the pharmacy in marking containers (if applicable).

Refilling Controlled Substances

The DEA guidelines for C-II substances allow physicians to write up to three separate prescriptions at one time for multiple drugs, to be filled sequentially over 90 days. The date of each subsequent prescription must be written on the order, and the prescription cannot be filled before that date. Each state's **Board of Pharmacy (BOP)** may implement additional guidelines that control the amount of controlled substances that can be refilled.

Most states limit refills of schedule C-III through C-V drugs to a maximum of five times or within 6 months from the original order, whichever comes first. In addition, the amount ordered on the refills may not exceed the original order. The length of time for keeping records may also vary by state, but a record must be kept of controlled substance refills showing the pharmacist's initials and the date the refill was dispensed. (A list showing each state's BOP can be found at the website *https://nabp.pharmacy/*.)

Ordering Controlled Substances

A pharmacy has two ways to obtain schedule II controlled substances from a distributor: electronic or paper filing of DEA Form 222. Form 222 (Fig. 2.7) *must be signed* by the pharmacist who signed Form 224 or a person who has been *legally assigned* power of attorney by that pharmacist. This triplicate form must be completed only with a pen, a typewriter, or an indelible pencil. The top copy, or Copy 1, and the middle (DEA) copy, or Copy 2, with the carbon paper, are sent to the supplier or manufacturer by the pharmacy *receiving/ordering* the drugs.

The pharmacy retains the bottom copy (Copy 3). When the medication is shipped to the pharmacy, the middle (DEA) copy is forwarded to the DEA to prove that the medication has been properly received. When the pharmacy receives the controlled substances, the pharmacist compares the pharmacy's copy of Form 222 with the invoice and signs and dates both. The invoice and the form are stapled together and retained for 2 years. If any error is made, the form becomes invalid but must be

Sample DEA Form 222							
See Reverse of PURCHASER'S Copy for Instructions	No order form may be issued for Schedule I and II substance unless completed application form has been received (21 CRF 1305.04)					OMB APPROVAL NO. 1117-0010	
TO:	STREET ADDRESS						
CITY AND STATE		DATE	TO BE FILLED IN BY SUPPLIER				
			SUPPLIER DEA REGISTRATION NO.				
	TO BE FILLED IN BY PURCHASER						
	No. of Packages	Size of Package	Name of Item	National Drug Code		Packaging Shipped	Date Shipped
1							
2							
3							
4							
5							
6							
7							
8							
9							
10							
◄ LAST LINE COMPLETED *(MUST BE 10 OR LESS)*		SIGNATURE OF PURCHASER OR ATTORNEY OR AGENT					
Date Issued	DEA Registration No.	Name and Address of Registrant					
Schedules							
Registered as a	No. of this Order Form						
DEA Form 222 (Oct. 1992)	US OFFICIAL ORDER FORMS - SCHEDULES I & II DRUG ENFORCEMENT ADMINISTRATION SUPPLIER'S Copy 1						

FIG. 2.7 Drug Enforcement Administration Form 222. (Courtesy Drug Enforcement Administration, Washington, DC.)

retained for reference; therefore the pharmacy cannot erase mistakes or throw away the form. When returning any C-II drugs, the pharmacy must have the manufacturer or wholesaler fill out the same form (Form 222) to request the controlled substance; the pharmacy then is the provider who retains the top copy and sends the middle copy to the DEA. Other controlled substances (C-III, C-IV, and C-V) are ordered on normal invoice forms, but invoices must be filed and retained for possible DEA or state BOP inspection. These should be kept separate from other nonscheduled drugs for easy retrieval. Once the scheduled drugs have been received, the invoice forms for schedules III through V must be kept for no less than 2 years.

> ### ▇ Tech Note!
>
> Under the authority of the Controlled Substances Act of 1970, the Controlled Substances Ordering Systems (CSOS) now allows electronic filing of DEA Form 222. This allows more stock to be ordered than is possible using the paper form. A smaller amount of controlled stock usually must be kept in the pharmacy because ordering is quicker and stock can be ordered more often.

Record-Keeping

A pharmacy has three methods of filing controlled substances and legend drugs (Table 2.4). Although federal law allows any one of these three methods to be used, a state's BOP may require a specific method. Each time a controlled substance is issued to a patient or nursing station, it must be logged out of the pharmacy stock (Fig. 2.8) as required under state law. Levels are first counted; the amount of each drug must be correct. Then the technician or pharmacist subtracts the amount taken. The remaining stock is double-checked for accuracy. This same standard holds for returning items or adding new stock to the inventory.

Narcotic Inventory

Narcotics are at high risk for **drug diversion** and must be inventoried differently from normal nonscheduled drugs. The pharmacy maintains a perpetual inventory of these medications. This means that once the inventory is started, it does not end; instead, it continues until the drug is no longer stocked. The basic principle is to identify an initial count of all controlled substances and to monitor the count as drugs are dispensed by subtracting the amount taken out of stock; this also involves adding to the count all drugs received by the pharmacy and placed into stock. This can be done either in pen in a ledger or through the use of software. The type of ledger or software used differs between community and institutional pharmacies, although basic information is required. Although the technician may be responsible for keeping track of all transactions, a pharmacist must validate all counts. In addition, overall periodic counts are done weekly or monthly by pharmacists. The DEA requires an inventory to be taken every 2 years; the DEA does not require a copy of the inventory taken. Any discrepancies that are identified must be investigated and explained.

Reverse Distributor

The term *reverse distributor* indicates all controlled substances that are unwanted, unusable, or outdated are returned to the distributor. These must be dealt with in accordance with DEA regulations. All transactions must be under the control of a person authorized by the DEA to handle controlled substances; this process is meant to deter the loss or misuse of drugs, also known as *drug diversion*. If a controlled substance becomes outdated or damaged, the pharmacy must return the substance to the manufacturer or return the substance to a company that collects controlled substances and then either returns them to the manufacturer or arranges for their disposal. These authorized companies may call themselves reverse distributors or returns processors. If nurses or pharmacy personnel use a partial dose of a controlled substance, two parties are required to witness and sign off on the destruction or waste of the drug. All liquid and solid medications must have proper documentation, which is kept for 2 years. To destroy medication, DEA Form 41 must be filed. This is determined by an agent of the DEA, which instructs the applicant how to proceed. The completed form must include the following:

- Date
- Name of substance
- Dosage form
- Number of units
- Reason for destruction
- Manner of destruction
- Applicant's signature

▇ TABLE 2.4
Three Methods of Filing Controlled Substances and Legend Drugs

System	Drawer I	Drawer II	Drawer III
1	C-II separate	C-III, C-IV, C-V	All other prescriptions
2	C-II separate	C-III, C-IV, C-V,[a] and all legend drugs	
3	C-II, C-III, C-IV, C-V[b]		All other prescriptions

[a]If any C-III, C-IV, or C-V controlled drugs are kept with noncontrolled drugs (system 2) or mixed with C-II drugs (system 3), they must be stamped with a red C for easy identification. All records must be kept on site for no less than 2 years. Many states, however, have requirements for keeping records longer; remember that the strictest law is the one that must be followed. When taking inventory, the technician must have exact counts of C-II substances at all times. The final count can be inventoried only by a licensed pharmacist.
[b]Technicians should consult the regulations of the individual state.

Oxycodone/APAP 5/325 mg Tablets

Date	Prescription/Invoice#	Quantity	Patient/Supplier	Balance	Initials	Current Inventory Count	Discrepancy
4/8/18	Rx#12345	25	10	15	JJ	15	0
4/9/18	Invoice#9876	100	Glaxo	115	KB	115	0

A

Previous Days Count			20	15	35	2	12	9	21	25	5	19	4	16	
Date	Patient	Dispensed	Oral						Inj						SIGNATURE
			Codeine 30 mg	Diazepam 5 mg	Hydrocodone/APAP 5/325 mg	Lorazepam 5 mg	Oxazepam 15 mg	Oxycodone ER 10 mg	Meperidine 25 mg /mL	Meperidine 75 mg /mL	Diazepam 5 mg/mL	Hydromorphone 5 mg/5 mL	Morphine 1 mg/mL	Morphine 10 mg/mL	
9/21/18	*Jane Smith*	*10 mg Meperidine*							*20*						*Paul James RN*
9/21/18	*Add to stock*	*John Whey CPhT*		*25*		*27*		*24*			*25*		*29*		*Sean Ray RN*

B

FIG. 2.8 (A) Pharmacy log sheet. (B) Nursing floor log sheet.

Records must be kept on all drugs destroyed as determined by state law.

Tech Note!

Because opioids in general are widely used to treat patients for pain, technicians, pharmacists, and nurses come in contact with these drugs daily. This has led to many cases of addiction in health care workers. All narcotics such as opioids and other controlled medications must be accounted for and must not be left out in the open, where they could be misused. All controlled substances must be signed into and out of stock in pen to create a permanent record.

Scenario Checkup 2.3

Laura is a dedicated employee who has demonstrated honesty and ethical behavior on a consistent basis. She is trusted by the pharmacists she works with and acts in a professional manner with all customers. Ms. Smith, a regular customer, has her child's Adderall prescription faxed in so that the medication will be ready to pick up when she arrives. Laura prepares the prescription, double counts it, and has the pharmacist complete the final check. When Ms. Smith arrives, Laura asks for the original prescription. Ms. Smith tells her she forgot to get it on the way out of the physician's office. She promises Laura she will bring it in tomorrow. What should Laura do?

Filling, Refilling, and Transferring Prescriptions for Controlled Drugs

Original Filling of C-II Through C-V Drugs Schedule II through V drug prescriptions can be accepted by the pharmacy in written, oral, or fax form according to certain DEA provisions and/or circumstances. A schedule C-II order may be called or faxed ahead of time, but the original prescription, signed by the prescriber, must be presented before it is actually dispensed. Although the following regulations are outlined according to the DEA, each state normally has additional restrictions that must be followed. For information on your specific state's guidelines, visit your state's BOP website, which can be found at the National Association of Boards of Pharmacy website (*http://www.nabp.net*).

Emergency Filling of C-II Drugs An oral order in place of a written prescription is permitted only in emergency situations. The guidelines are as follows:

1. The physician determines that the patient needs the C-II drug and considers it to be an emergency, with no alternative treatment possible.
2. The physician cannot give a written prescription to the pharmacist. This may be because the physician is away from the office.
3. The pharmacist must obtain all information from the physician, including the drug name, strength, dosage form, and route of administration. The physician's name,

address, phone number, and DEA number are required. All information must be recorded in written form.

4. The amount of the drug can be only enough to sustain the patient through the emergency period. The pharmacist should indicate on the prescription that it is being filled because of an emergency.

5. The pharmacist must make every effort to verify the physician's authority unless he or she knows the physician personally.

6. The prescriber has 7 days to produce the written and signed prescription to the pharmacist. Each state may impose shorter time limits. In addition, the prescription must have written on its face "Authorization for Emergency Dispensing." If this is not done, the pharmacist must notify the DEA. The written prescription must be attached to the oral record of the prescription.

7. There is no time limit when a C-II drug must be filled after being signed by the prescriber; however, the pharmacist must determine whether the patient still needs the medication (eg, a drug filled several weeks after the order was written).

8. No limits are placed on the quantity of C-II drugs.

9. There may be additional provisions established by state BOP regulations.

Schedule C-III, C-IV, and C-V drugs may be reduced to written form if called into the pharmacy. All required prescription information must be obtained by the pharmacist, including the prescriber's DEA number.

Refilling of C-II Through C-V Drugs For refilling prescriptions according to DEA regulations, controlled substances are placed into three categories: C-II, C-III and C-IV, and C-V.

1. Schedule C-II drugs may not be refilled.

2. Schedule C-III and C-IV drugs may be refilled only up to five times or within 6 months after the date the prescription was written, whichever occurs first. Patients are allowed to request refills by e-mail or by phone.

3. Schedule C-V drugs can be refilled as often as prescribed on the prescription.

When C-III, C-IV, and C-V drugs are refilled, the following required information must be provided on the back of the prescription: pharmacist's initials, refill date, and the amount of drug that is refilled. In addition, a pharmacy may use a data-processing system to store and retrieve C-III, C-IV, and C-V prescription refill information. To meet DEA regulations, the following criteria must be met:

1. Pharmacies must use one of two methods: manual or computerized log for refills.

2. A daily hard copy is printed, and pharmacists verify all refills they have authorized.

3. A log book is kept in which all controlled refills are verified by the pharmacist.

4. A computer system is used to print a refill-by-refill audit for any specific strength, dosage, or form, retrievable by either generic or trade name.

5. In case the computer system is not functioning, the pharmacy must have an alternative procedure for authorizing

documentation. These data are entered into the computer system as soon as possible.

Partial Filling of C-II Through C-V Drugs Schedule III, IV, and V drugs may be partially filled if the pharmacist does not have enough in stock. The pharmacist must note on the prescription the amount filled, and the remaining amount must be dispensed within 6 months.

Schedule II drugs may be partially filled if the pharmacist does not have the full quantity in stock. The pharmacist must note on the prescription the amount filled, and the remaining amount may be dispensed within 72 hours of the first fill. If the amount cannot be filled within 72 hours, the pharmacist must notify the prescribing physician because no further quantity may be supplied after this time.

Transferring Controlled Drug Prescriptions (C-II Through C-V Drugs) Schedule III, IV, and V prescriptions may be transferred to another pharmacy one time only. The receiving pharmacy must have all of the information required on an original prescription, including the prescriber's DEA number, and the information must be transcribed into written form. Schedule II prescriptions are not transferrable because they can be filled only once.

Dispensing Without a Prescription Schedule V drugs that are sold over the counter in some states are required to be dispensed by the pharmacist. The pharmacist must determine whether the medication is necessary and must follow these guidelines:

1. The purchaser must be at least 18 years of age.

2. The purchaser must show identification, including proof of age.

3. No more than 240 mL or 48 solid doses of opium can be sold.

4. No more than 120 mL or 24 solid doses of any other controlled substance can be sold.

5. No more than a 48-hour supply may be sold without a prescription to any one purchaser.

6. A schedule V log book is kept with the purchaser's name and address, name and quantity of medication sold, date dispensed, and pharmacist's initials.

7. The log book must be kept for 2 years.

8. If there are no federal or state laws that require a prescription to dispense schedule V drugs, dispensing without a prescription is permitted.

Lending or Transferring C-II Through C-V Drugs to Another Pharmacy A pharmacy may lend scheduled drugs to another pharmacy as long as the following guidelines are met:

1. The pharmacy to be lent the medication is registered with the DEA to dispense controlled substances.

2. The lending pharmacy must record that it lent the medication, and the receiving pharmacy must record that it obtained the medication.

3. If a schedule II drug is lent, it must be documented on a DEA Form 222 by the pharmacy lending the C-II drug. The form must indicate the name, dosage form, and quantity of the drug, and the name, address, and DEA registration number of the pharmacy receiving the drug.

4. No more than 5% of the total number of dosage units of controlled substances can be dispensed by a pharmacy within a calendar year unless the pharmacy is registered as a distributor.

Mailing Controlled Substances (C-II Through C-V Drugs) A pharmacy is allowed to mail any controlled substance, as long as it is mailed in a container that is not marked with the contents' information. The inner container must be labeled to indicate the name and address of the dispensing pharmacy.

Drug Monographs

Under the FDA labeling regulations, the following information must be available in **monographs,** also known as package inserts or official prescribing information, because of the lack of space on most drug containers. Physicians often refer to this information as published in the *Physicians' Desk Reference (PDR).* It also is available from free online resources, such as the National Library of Medicine *(https://www.nlm.nih.gov/),* which provides files from the FDA database. The information in the package labeling is also found in the monographs published in many print and online nationally recognized drug compendia. All official label information is required to give the date of the most recent revision. As new information emerges or is reported, new monographs are written or revised. Therefore it is important to have an updated copy of the required information in the pharmacy's referencing materials. If an updated copy is not available, the package insert from the medication container can be consulted for the most recent information. The following is the type of information contained in a package insert.

- FDA monograph information
- FDA prescription drug labeling, containing a summary of the essential scientific information for the safe and effective use of the drug; it should meet the following specific requirements:
  - Be informative and accurate
  - Use language that is not promotional in tone, false, or misleading
  - Not make claims or suggested uses for drugs when there is insufficient evidence of safety and unsubstantiated evidence of effectiveness
  - Contain information based whenever possible on data derived from human experience
- The information on prescription drug labeling is also referred to as:
  - Prescribing information
  - Package insert
  - Professional labeling

The Highlights section of the official prescribing information is approximately half a page in length and provides a quick reference summary of the most important information about the prescription drug. The drug manufacturer is required to include a list of all changes made within the past year to ensure that the most updated information is available for the prescriber. The Highlights of the label cover the following topics and are cross-referenced to the corresponding full prescribing information section for additional details:

1. Indications and Usage
2. Dosage and Administration
3. Dosage Forms and Strengths
4. Contraindications
5. Warnings and Precautions
6. Adverse Reactions
7. Drug Interactions
8. Use in Specific Populations
9. Drug Abuse and Dependence
10. Overdosage
11. Description
12. Clinical Pharmacology
13. Nonclinical Toxicology
14. Clinical Studies
15. References
16. How Supplied/Storage and Handling
17. Patient Counseling Information

Full prescribing information now includes the following:
- Table of contents section (recent change). This easy-to-use reference helps practitioners quickly locate specific information rather than having to scan the whole document.
- Generic and trade names and date of initial US approval.
- Boxed Warning section: Each drug may or may not have one.
- The use of bullets is limited to 20 lines for ease of reading.
- Complete prescribing information can be accessed using a cross-referencing number or the hyperlink given (see Boxed Warning, later in the chapter).

1. Indications and Usage

The following information may be found in this section:
- The conditions the drug is approved to treat, listed in bulleted form for ease of reading
- Pharmacological class of the drug (to remind the prescriber of the drug's mechanism of action)
- All limitations, such as patients who should not use the drug

2. Dosage and Administration

This section includes the recommended dosage regimen, dosage range, the manner in which the medication should be administered, and pharmacological information.

3. Dosage Forms and Strengths

This section lists all the dosage forms and their strengths. Product identification information such as color and scoring is also listed in the How Supplied section.

4. Contraindications

This bulleted section lists clear situations in which the drug should absolutely not be used. It describes specific conditions in which the risk from taking the medication clearly outweighs any possible therapeutic benefit, in addition to known hazards of the drug. The order in which contraindications are listed is based on the likelihood of occurrence and the size of the population studied.

5. Warnings and Precautions

This section is an abbreviated summary of the most clinically adverse reactions and actions to take when such reactions occur. In addition, information is given on the monitoring parameters of these side effects.

6. Adverse Reactions

This section lists the most commonly occurring adverse reactions and the incidence of these effects. Separate listings are required for adverse reactions reported from clinical trials or from postmarketing experience. Additional details are given on the nature, severity, and frequency of adverse reactions and the relationship to dosage and demographics. This section also provides advice on how to report adverse reactions to manufacturers by telephone or electronically (or both) by using MedWatch to record reactions.

7. Drug Interactions

Both food and drug interactions are listed, as are instructions on how to prevent or lessen the interaction. Also included in this section are conditions in which the drug interaction necessitates a dosage adjustment (also found under Clinical Pharmacology).

8. Use in Specific Populations

This section is a bulleted summary of the use of the medication in various patient populations, including pregnant patients (see Pregnancy Categories, later in the chapter), patients in labor and delivery units, pediatric patients, geriatric patients, patients with renal impairment, and patients with hepatic impairment. Also included are cross-references to sections that can be reviewed to determine necessary prescribing adjustments.

9. Drug Abuse and Dependence

If patients have shown any tendency to become addicted to the medication or if the medication has been found to be abused by patients, the information is listed in this section.

10. Overdosage

Information on toxicity and the use of antidotes is provided in this section.

11. Description

This section lists specifics about chemical agents and ingredients, such as the drug's chemical formula.

12. Clinical Pharmacology

This section describes how other drugs can interact with the medication and alerts the prescriber to adverse reactions. Also included is a "Microbiology" data subsection for the drug, if applicable. Drug interaction data also may be found in the section Drug Interactions.

13. Nonclinical Toxicology

This section contains information on studies conducted during the development of the drug, including in vitro studies (ie, performed in test tubes), drug formulation, and in vivo efficacy studies (eg, performed in live animals).

14. Clinical Studies

This section summarizes the most important studies that establish the effectiveness and safety of the drug in humans. Not all studies are included.

15. References

A list of reference materials that may be accessed for further information specific to the drug is presented in this section.

16. How Supplied/Storage and Handling

Information about how the medication is supplied often is given in chart format because it lists the varying strengths, amount of drug per container, dosage form, and whether the medication has any special requirements, such as protection from light or storage in a refrigerator.

17. Patient Counseling Information

This section contains suggested pertinent information about the drug that professionals should convey to their patients. The FDA-approved patient labeling is written for a lay audience. Even drugs given in the hospital by a health care professional may have patient counseling information.

Hyperlinks can be used to access specific information. The FDA requires structured product labeling in a standardized electronic file format and the use of embedded computer tags to help health professionals improve patient care.

The FDA and the National Library of Medicine created the DailyMed labeling resource; it can easily be downloaded and is available to professionals and patients electronically free of charge (see *https://www.nlm.nih.gov/*). Fig. 2.9 shows a sample of important information found in a drug monograph.

Boxed Warning

A **boxed warning** is encased in a bold border in the manufacturer's insert; health care professionals often refer to the boxed warning as a *Black Box Warning*, even though this is not the official labeling term for the warning. This type of warning is required on medications and other products that carry a high risk potential for the consumer. The label indicates the proper use of a drug to avoid or decrease the possibility of serious or life-threatening side effects. Warnings can be very specific or may include an entire class of drugs, such as antidepressants. Antidepressants have been found to cause an increase in suicidal behavior in adolescents, especially those with prior psychiatric disorders. Box 2.7, Part A, presents an example of a boxed warning; Part B presents a sample list of agents with boxed warnings.

MedGuides

MedGuides are paper handouts that are available with many prescription medicines. Many medications with boxed warnings also come with MedGuides. The guides address issues specific to particular drugs and drug classes, and they contain FDA-approved information that can help patients avoid serious adverse events. A MedGuide is distributed by the pharmacy with each prescription and each prescription refill because the information for the patient may change frequently.

HIGHLIGHTS OF PRESCRIBING INFORMATION

These highlights do not include all the information needed to use Imdicon safely and effectively. See full prescribing information for Imdicon.

IMDICON ® (cholinasol) CAPSULES
Initial U.S. Approval: 2000

WARNING: LIFE-THREATENING HEMATOLOGICAL ADVERSE REACTIONS

See full prescribing information for complete boxed warning.

Monitor for hematological adverse reactions every 2 weeks for first 3 months of treatment (5.2). Discontinue Imdicon immediately if any of the following occur:
- Neutropenia/agranulocytosis (5.1)
- Thrombotic thrombocytopenic purpura (5.1)
- Aplastic anemia (5.1)

―――――――――――――――――RECENT MAJOR CHANGES―――――――――――――――――

Indications and Usage, Coronary Stenting (1.2) 2/200X
Dosage and Administration, Coronary Stenting (2.2) 2/200X

―――――――――――――――――INDICATIONS AND USAGE―――――――――――――――――

Imdicon is an adenosine diphosphate (ADP) antagonist platelet aggregation inhibitor indicated for:
- Reducing the risk of thrombotic stroke in patients who have experienced stroke precursors or who have had a completed thrombotic stroke (1.1)
- Reducing the incidence of subacute coronary stent thrombosis, when used with aspirin (1.2)
  Important limitations:
- For stroke, Imdicon should be reserved for patients who are intolerant of or allergic to aspirin or who have failed aspirin therapy (1.1)

―――――――――――――――――DOSAGE AND ADMINISTRATION―――――――――――――――――

- Stroke: 50 mg once daily with food (2.1)
- Coronary Stenting: 50 mg once daily with food, with antiplatelet doses of aspirin, for up to 30 days following stent implantation (2.2)
Discontinue in renally impaired patients if hemorrhagic or hematopoietic problems are encountered (2.3, 8.6, 12.3)

―――――――――――――――――DOSAGE FORMS AND STRENGTHS―――――――――――――――――

Capsules: 50 mg (3)

―――――――――――――――――CONTRAINDICATIONS―――――――――――――――――

- Hematopoietic disorders or a history of TTP or aplastic anemia (4)
- Hemostatic disorder or active bleeding (4)
- Severe hepatic impairment (4, 8.7)

―――――――――――――――――WARNINGS AND PRECAUTIONS―――――――――――――――――

- Neutropenia (2.4% incidence; may occur suddenly; typically resolves within 1-2 weeks of discontinuation), thrombotic thrombocytopenic purpura (TTP), aplastic anemia, agranulocytosis, pancytopenia, leukemia, and thrombocytopenia can occur (5.1)
- Monitor for hematological adverse reactions every 2 weeks through the third month of treatment (5.2)

―――――――――――――――――ADVERSE REACTIONS―――――――――――――――――

Most common adverse reactions (incidence 2%) are diarrhea, nausea, dyspepsia, rash, gastrointestinal pain, neutropenia, and purpura (6.1).

To report SUSPECTED ADVERSE REACTIONS, contact (manufacturer) at (phone # and Web address) or FDA at 1-800-FDA-1088 or ***http://www.fda.gov/medwatch***

―――――――――――――――――DRUG INTERACTIONS―――――――――――――――――

- Anticoagulants: Discontinue prior to switching to Imdicon (5.3, 7.1)
- Phenytoin: Elevated phenytoin levels have been reported. Monitor levels (7.2)

―――――――――――――――――USE IN SPECIFIC POPULATIONS―――――――――――――――――

- Hepatic impairment: Dose may need adjustment. Contraindicated in severe hepatic disease (4, 8.7, 12.3)
- Renal impairment: Dose may need adjustment (2.3, 8.6, 12.3)

See 17 for PATIENT COUNSELING INFORMATION and FDA-approved patient labeling
Revised: 5/200X

FIG. 2.9 Highlights of a drug monograph. *Continued*

FULL PRESCRIBING INFORMATION: CONTENTS*
WARNING–LIFE-THREATENING HEMATOLOGICAL ADVERSE REACTIONS

1 INDICATIONS AND USAGE
    1.1 Thrombotic Stroke
    1.2 Coronary Stenting
2 DOSAGE AND ADMINISTRATION
    2.1 Thrombotic Stroke
    2.2 Coronary Stenting
    2.3 Renally Impaired Patients
3 DOSAGE FORMS AND STRENGTHS
4 CONTRAINDICATIONS
5 WARNINGS AND PRECAUTIONS
    5.1 Hematological Adverse Reactions
    5.2 Monitoring for Hematological Adverse Reactions
    5.3 Anticoagulant Drugs
    5.4 Bleeding Precautions
    5.5 Monitoring: Liver Function Tests
6 ADVERSE REACTIONS
    6.1 Clinical Studies Experience
    6.2 Postmarketing Experience
7 DRUG INTERACTIONS
    7.1 Anticoagulant Drugs
    7.2 Phenytoin
    7.3 Antipyrine and Other Drugs Metabolized Hepatically
    7.4 Aspirin and Other Non-Steroidal Anti-Inflammatory Drugs
    7.5 Cimetidine
    7.6 Theophylline
    7.7 Propranolol
    7.8 Antacids
    7.9 Digoxin
    7.10 Phenobarbital
    7.11 Other Concomitant Drug Therapy
    7.12 Food Interaction

8 USE IN SPECIFIC POPULATIONS
    8.1 Pregnancy
    8.3 Nursing Mothers
    8.4 Pediatric Use
    8.5 Geriatric Use
    8.6 Renal Impairment
    8.7 Hepatic Impairment
10 OVERDOSAGE
11 DESCRIPTION
12 CLINICAL PHARMACOLOGY
    12.1 Mechanism of Action
    12.2 Pharmacodynamics
    12.3 Pharmacokinetics
13 NONCLINICAL TOXICOLOGY
    13.1 Carcinogenesis, Mutagenesis, Impairment of Fertility
14 CLINICAL STUDIES
    14.1 Thrombotic Stroke
    14.2 Coronary Stenting
16 HOW SUPPLIED/STORAGE AND HANDLING
17 PATIENT COUNSELING INFORMATION
    17.1 Importance of Monitoring
    17.2 Bleeding
    17.3 Hematological Adverse Reactions
    17.4 FDA-Approved Patient Labeling

*Sections or subsections omitted from the full prescribing information are not listed.
Retrieved from http://www.fda.gov/ohrms/dockets/ac/06/briefing/2006-4210b_13_01_physician%20labeling%20rule.pdf

FIG. 2.9, cont'd

BOX 2.7   Boxed Warnings

Special Warnings and Information

- Explanation of the types of serious side effects that may occur
- Monitoring recommendations, such as blood tests and pregnancy tests before and while using the medication; signs and symptoms that may occur during treatment
- Indication of other medications that cannot be taken at the same time
- Instructions to the prescriber regarding information that must be given to the patient before dosing
- The steps to be taken if an adverse reaction may have occurred (MedWatch: 1-800-FDA-1088)

Example of Drugs Requiring Boxed Warning

- Seroquel
- risperidone
- Zyprexa
- Brilinta
- Linzess
- Tygacil
- Lamictal
- levofloxacin
- ciprofloxacin
- pioglitazone
- rosiglitazone

The FDA requires that MedGuides be issued with certain prescribed drugs and biological products when the agency has determined the following:

- Certain information is necessary to prevent serious adverse effects.
- The patient should be informed about a known serious side effect of a product.
- Patient adherence to directions for the use of a product is essential to the product's effectiveness.

Pregnancy Categories

A pregnant woman's fetus is susceptible to the effects of drugs taken by the mother. The drug may be transmitted to the fetus during its developmental stages, causing birth defects. The FDA established five **pregnancy categories** that indicate the potential of a drug to cause fetal defects; the categories are based on the ratio of risks to benefits (Box 2.8). These categories are set for each drug based on extensive clinical trials by the manufacturer. Both the prescriber and the pharmacist must counsel the patient to make sure the patient understands the risks involved before taking the agent.

BOX 2.8 Pregnancy Categories

Category A

Adequate and well-controlled studies have failed to demonstrate a risk to the fetus in the first trimester of pregnancy (and there is no evidence of risk in later trimesters).

Category B

Animal reproduction studies have failed to demonstrate a risk to the fetus, and there are no adequate and well-controlled studies in pregnant women.

Category C

Animal reproduction studies have shown an adverse effect on the fetus, and there are no adequate and well-controlled studies in humans, but potential benefits may warrant use of the drug in pregnant women despite potential risks.

Category D

There is positive evidence of human fetal risk based on adverse reaction data from investigational or marketing experience or studies in humans, but potential benefits may warrant use of the drug in pregnant women despite potential risks.

Category X

Studies in animals or humans have demonstrated fetal abnormalities and/or there is positive evidence of human fetal risk based on adverse reaction data from investigational or marketing experience and the risks involved in use of the drug in pregnant women clearly outweigh potential benefits.

Prescription Regulation

Who Can Prescribe?

The FDA and DEA have no authority in determining prescribers. Physicians and other medical prescribers are licensed by their individual state boards. The scope of practice is determined by the person's degree. For example, a podiatrist, a physician who treats conditions of the feet, can prescribe medications and devices that are used in treating foot conditions; a podiatrist would not and should not prescribe heart medication. The same is true for dentists, veterinarians, and optometrists because each is an expert in their specialty and not in others. Prescribers can vary from state to state; therefore the specific laws governing them are not covered. However, more states allow professionals such as nurse practitioners and physician assistants to prescribe a limited number of medications and/or devices. These practitioners are regulated at the state level; some are required to be supervised by a physician, who assumes responsibility for their prescribing methods and scope of knowledge. In all 50 states, nurse practitioners are allowed to prescribe medications independently. Florida, however, does not allow nurse practitioners or physician assistants to prescribe controlled substances, and optometrists cannot prescribe controlled

substances in five states. Each state also regulates whether it will accept out-of-state prescriptions written by practitioners who are not licensed in the state. Individuals who can prescribe controlled drugs must be registered as a midlevel practitioner with DEA Form 224. In some states, pharmacists are granted prescribing privileges under a collaborative drug therapy management agreement. This agreement is between a physician and a pharmacist and entails allowing the pharmacist to initiate, modify, and continue medication regimens; order laboratory tests; and perform patient assessments under a defined protocol. Montana, New Mexico, and North Carolina give pharmacists extended authority. Five other states (California, Massachusetts, Minnesota, North Dakota, and Washington) allow pharmacists to obtain a DEA number.

Who Can Receive a Prescription?

Clearly, a pharmacy technician takes in prescriptions, enters them, and fills them; the pharmacist is responsible for interpreting and reviewing the prescription before dispensing the medication. Many states prohibit pharmacy technicians from taking phone orders for legend drugs. All states require a pharmacist to authorize a phoned-in prescription for a controlled substance per DEA regulations. Often prescriptions are called in, faxed, or transmitted by computer from the physician's office by the physician or nurse. A pharmacist must translate any verbal orders into written form. In addition, if a patient wants a prescription transferred to another pharmacy, this transaction must be done between licensed pharmacists or pharmacy interns under the supervision of a pharmacist. A pharmacy intern also can receive prescriptions by phone.

Tech Note!

As of 2017, 17 states allow qualified technicians to accept verbal prescriptions called in by physicians or their representative.

Prescription Labels and Prescription Orders

The information on a prescription label is different from that required on a prescription order, although both must have patient and medication information (Fig. 2.10). The components of a prescription order and a prescription label are as follows:

Prescriber's prescription order
1. Name of prescriber
2. Address and phone number of prescriber
3. License number of prescriber (DEA number if applicable)
4. Date prescription was written
5. Prescriber's signature

Prescription label
1. Name of pharmacy
2. Address and phone number of pharmacy
3. Name of prescriber
4. Date prescription was filled
5. Prescription number
6. Any cautions described or provided on auxiliary labels

A

```
Dr. Tracy Crum                                          11287 E Villanova Drive
DEA#AC1243170                                           Aurora, CO 30358
LIC#44550                                               Phone: 303-555-1212


Date: 12/12/18


Patient's name:  Billie Jones          Age: 83 yrs
Address: 125 Grand Canyon Drive, Tucson, Arizona  85707



Rx:
                    Potassium chloride 20mEq tab
                    1 daily        #90

Substitution permitted Y N
Refills 1 2 3 4 5 6 7 8 9                    Signature____Tracy L Crum, MD
```

B

```
                        Thomas Pharmacy
                        519 Barney Lane
                      Clarksville, TN 03542
                      Phone: 931-555-1122


Patient: Christopher Gilbert
RX # G03011984


Dosage:   Clonazepam 1-mg tablets         Quantity #30


Take 1 tablet by mouth at bedtime


Refills 0
Filled: 12/12/18                          Expiration date: 09/25/18
Dr. Ronald Belham
```

FIG. 2.10 (A) Sample of the information required on a physician's prescription order. (B) Sample of the information on a medication label.

Special Labeling and Record-Keeping Considerations

Certain drugs require that additional, manufacturer-provided information be given to a patient because of the possibility of adverse effects from the medication; interactions between food, drugs, or supplements; and teratogenicity (genetic harm) to an unborn fetus. These instructions are known as *patient package inserts* and are distributed by the prescriber or the pharmacy dispensing the medication or device (Box 2.9).

Veterinary Medications

The FDA Food, Drug, and Cosmetic Act defines an animal drug as "any drug intended for animals other than man *(https://www.fda.gov/animal-veterinary/resources-you/fda-regulation-animal-drugs#overview)*. Special labeling is also required for animal medications. Prescribers must be a licensed veterinarian under federal law and include the statement: "Caution: Federal law restricts this drug to use by or on the order of a licensed veterinarian." In addition, written treatment records are maintained for 2 years for each animal treated.

■ Tech Note!

There are continuing education lessons specially for technicians regarding veterinary medication dispensing. This is a field in which technicians are increasingly being used.

BOX 2.9 Drugs Requiring Additional Information

- Estrogens
- Fertility drugs
- Injectable contraceptives
- Oral contraceptives
- Retinoids

Hospitals and community pharmacies differ in the length of time patient records must be kept. Record-keeping is regulated by state law. Both hospitals and community pharmacies are required to keep complete and accurate records of patients. For the purpose of simplicity, Table 2.5 lists community patient information separately from institutional requirements.

Repackaging

Unit dose medication that is prepared in the pharmacy requires the following record-keeping rules. Technicians traditionally prepare most of the unit dose medications in a pharmacy setting; the pharmacist verifies the preparations (except in states that allow tech-check-tech). Any medication taken from bulk packages and placed in blister packs or unit-dosing devices (eg, oral syringes) must have the following information on each individual label (Fig. 2.10):

1. Drug name (trade/generic)
2. Strength

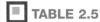 **TABLE 2.5**
Required Prescription Information[a]

Type of Facility	Patient's Full Name	Pre-scriber's Name	Name and Strength of Drug	Date of Issue	Pre-scription Number	Expiration Date	Lot and Control Number of Drug	Manu-facturer	Name of Drug Dispensed
Hospital	X	X	X	X	—[b]	X	—[b]	—[b]	X
Community	X	X	X	X	X	X	X	X	X
Home health	X	X	X	X	X	X	X	X	X

[a]Each medication sent to the floor has the manufacturer's name, the lot number, and the expiration date on each unit dose of medication. Hospital patients are not given prescription numbers; instead, orders are listed in the computer under a patient's medical record number, and a hard copy, often called the medication administration record (MAR), of all medications is made daily for the patient's chart.
[b]This information is not transcribed into the patient's electronic medical record.

3. Dosage form
4. Manufacturer
5. Lot number
6. Expiration date

All information must be logged into a binder or a system in which such information can be retrieved easily. More information on repackaging is presented in Chapter 11.

Drug Enforcement Administration Verification

All prescribers must be registered with the DEA to write prescriptions for controlled substances. When approved, the prescribers are given a nine-character identification code. This code is different for each prescriber. There is a method of verifying DEA numbers. The first two characters are composed of letters. The first letter is an A, B, F, M, or X, followed by the first letter of the prescriber's last name. Prescribers who are qualified to order medications to treat opioid addiction are assigned an X. The letter M is assigned to Medical Legal Partnerships (MLPs), such as nurse practitioners. For example, for Dr. D. Wong, MD, the DEA number could begin with AW or BW. The next seven digits are composed of numbers that form an equation. Procedure 2.1 presents the steps for verifying a DEA number.

 Tech Alert!

Hospital physicians are assigned an internal code number that is attached to their DEA registration number. This information must be kept by the institution for verification purposes (eg, AB1234567-045).

Procedure 2.1

Verification Process for Prescriber's Drug Enforcement Administration Number

Goal

To be able to determine whether a DEA number on a prescription is valid or a forgery.

Equipment and Supplies

• Paper, pencil, and a calculator may be used.

Example

Dr. Tom Johnston writes an order for Tylenol #3. The physician's DEA number is AJ1234892.

Procedural Steps

1. Verify that the first letter of the DEA number is A, B, F, or M (for nurse practitioners).
   PURPOSE: To confirm that the doctor or nurse practitioner has the authority to prescribe controlled substances.
2. Determine whether the second letter is the first letter of the prescriber's last name (in this case, J for Johnston).
   PURPOSE: To make certain that the letters match to prevent possible forgeries.

3. Use the formula: First, add the first, third, and fifth numbers in the DEA set (1 + 3 + 8 = 12).
   PURPOSE: To make certain the DEA number is valid.
4. Continue the formula: Second, add the second, fourth, and sixth numbers and then multiply by 2 (2 + 4 + 9 = 15; 15 × 2 = 30).
   PURPOSE: To verify that the DEA number is authentic.
5. Complete the formula: Finally, add the two sums together (12 + 30 = 42).
   PURPOSE: To complete the process and determine whether the DEA number is valid or a forgery.
6. Compare the results. If the last digit from your total (ie, 2) matches the last number in the DEA set, the number is valid. In this case all steps match; therefore the number is valid. If any of the key elements do not match, alert your pharmacist; the DEA number is invalid.
   PURPOSE: To continually be on the lookout for forged prescriptions and to use your skill in determining whether DEA numbers are valid or invalid.

Child-Resistant Packaging

Most medications are required to be packaged in containers that are exceptionally difficult for children to open. Hence, childproof caps were created. Unfortunately, the caps also can be difficult for some adults to open. There are some products which require childproof packaging (eg, aspirin, acetaminophen, ibuprofen, elemental iron, naproxen).

There are some exceptions to this regulation because of patients' need to access their medications easily (Table 2.6). In addition to these exceptions, medications can be packaged in non–child-resistant containers if certain requirements

■ TABLE 2.6
Prescription Drugs That Can Be Packaged in Non–Child-Resistant Bottles

Drug	Dosage Form
Betamethasone	Tablet
Cholestyramine	Powder
Colestipol	Powder
Erythromycin	Tablet, granules
Isosorbide dinitrate ($<$10 mg)	Sublingual, chewable tablets
Mebendazole	Tablet
Methylprednisolone	Tablet
Nitroglycerin[a]	Sublingual
Prednisone	Tablet
Sodium fluoride	Package

[a]Nitroglycerin is the only medication that does not have a dosage limit for filling the prescription without a childproof cap.

have been met: either the prescriber, such as a physician, orders the medication to be filled without a childproof cap or the patient requests that the medication be filled without a childproof cap. Usually this information is entered into the patient's medical record for future reference. Some pharmacies may require the patient to sign a release form that is kept in the patient record.

Special Prescribing Programs

Programs for Opioid Maintenance
Methadone Maintenance Treatment

Methadone is a schedule II controlled substance and is used to treat individuals addicted to opiates. Patients are to receive specialized treatment while taking this medication. No more than 1 day's supply may be filled by a pharmacy, and the medication must be taken in a physician's office or drug treatment center. Other brand names for methadone include Dolophine and Methadose. Although methadone is more commonly used to treat opioid addiction, it also can be prescribed by physicians (with appropriate DEA registration) as an analgesic to treat chronic pain and alleviate pain in cancer patients.

Suboxone and Buprenorphine

Suboxone and buprenorphine, which are sublingual tablets, are schedule III controlled substances that require special consent forms to be completed by the patient. Although most treatments are supervised either in a physician's office or in a clinical setting, a pharmacy may receive orders for small amounts to be delivered to a physician's office or to be picked up by a family member of the patient. Under federal law, prescribers must meet certain criteria. When the prescriber has met all conditions, the DEA issues him or her a special number with an X, identifying the individual as a qualified prescriber.

Opioid Use Addiction

To protect the public from overdose deaths of opioids, the Mainstreaming Addiction Treatment (MAT) Act was passed in 2023. This provides that all health care providers that have a standard controlled substance license can prescribe buprenorphine (Naloxone) for opioid use disorders. Naloxone is an antidote to opioid overdose and, given within 15 minutes, can restore normal breathing and consciousness to a patient. See Fig. 2.11 for a kit example.

Synthetic Opioid Fentanyl

According to the Centers for Disease Control and Prevention, synthetic opioid fentanyl is now the leading cause of deaths among US adults ages 18 to 45 *(https://www.globenewswire. com/news-release/2022/09/16/2517859/0/en/Fentanyl-is-Now-the-Leading-Cause-of-Death-for-American-Adults-The-Detox-Center-of-Los-Angeles-is-on-the-Front-Lines.html)*. Pharmacy technicians should be cautious to look for counterfeit pills that are being distributed in many forms or potential signs of opioid abuse.

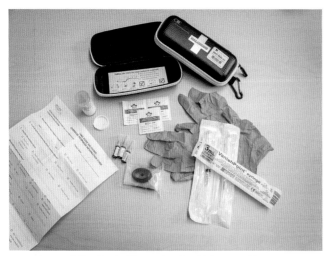

FIG. 2.11 Example of a Naloxone kit.

Risk Management Programs for Prescription Drugs

The Food and Drug Administration Amendments Act of 2007 gave the FDA the authority to require a Risk Evaluation and Mitigation Strategy (REMS) from manufacturers to ensure that the benefits of a drug or biological product outweigh its risks. Certain drugs are placed in a restricted status for use.

iPledge Program Under the Food and Drug Administration

The FDA regulates isotretinoin (formerly branded as Accutane and marketed now as Amnesteem, Claravis, and Absorica) under a special program called iPledge because of the severe adverse effects of the drug. It causes birth defects; therefore it is important that female users understand that they must take precautions to avoid becoming pregnant. In addition, possible side effects of suicidal thoughts and signs of depression are now associated with this drug. This agent requires a boxed warning. iPledge is a computer-based risk management program designed to increase awareness of the dangers of isotretinoin in an effort to eliminate fetal exposure to the drug. There are restricted distribution guidelines that must be followed before a patient can receive a prescription for isotretinoin.

Restricted drugs have different levels of restrictions based on REMS. Previously, the restriction for dispensing rosiglitazone-containing drugs consisted only of ensuring that the patient received a copy of the medication guide. The new restrictions require health care providers and patients to enroll in a special program for those prescribing and those receiving rosiglitazone-containing medicines.

Additional information about REMS and restricted drugs can be found on the FDA website at *https://www.accessdata.fda.gov/scripts/cder/rems/index.cfm*.

Drug Abuse and Monitoring Programs

In 2010, the National Drug Control Strategy was implemented because of the surge of prescription drug abuse and heroin addiction among adults. The National Institute on Drug Abuse (NIDA) lists more than 23 million persons over age 12 with an addiction to some type of illicit drug or alcohol. Yearly strategies are added such as the 2015 integration of substance abuse awareness and combating domestic drug trafficking and production. Partnerships through agencies such as the DEA and National Association of Boards of Pharmacies (NABP) have also created National Take-Back Initiative programs and electronic reporting systems such as the Prescription Drug Monitoring Program (PDMP) Inter-Connect Program.

The NABP PDMP InterConnect, developed by the National Boards of Pharmacy, is an interstate data system used to share prescription information and provides a more efficient means of combating drug diversion and drug abuse nationwide. To date, there are more than 49 states and territories participating in the program. For a complete listing of those participating and more information, see *http://www.nascsa.org/*.

The National Take-Back Initiative, established by the DEA, allows a safe, responsible, and convenient way for the public to dispose of unwanted drugs.

> ▽ **Tech Alert!**
>
> As a technician, it is important to be aware of any signs of abuse, fraud, or discrepancies when processing a prescription and report any suspicious activity to the pharmacist. The special programs listed previously are not all-inclusive. These are examples of the most common programs found in either the hospital or retail setting.

Pharmacy Sites

Brick-and-Mortar and Mail-Order Pharmacies

The term *brick and mortar* refers to a building, such as a retail pharmacy. A common practice is to mail medications through the post office or other authorized mailing system. This option has become even more accessible to patients because of the introduction of online pharmacies and mail-order pharmacies. Rules govern the way in which drugs are mailed. Prescription drugs can be mailed only by DEA-registered entities.

Online Pharmacies (e-Pharmacies)

In the 1990s, e-pharmacies began to appear on the Internet, which led to the opportunity for drugs to be ordered illegally. In addition, consumers could be defrauded because some e-pharmacies charged credit cards but did not mail the drugs ordered. The NABP began to accredit sites in 1999 to allow consumers to distinguish between legal and illegal sites. The label Verified Internet Pharmacy Practice Sites (VIPPS) indicates to the public that the website from which they are ordering drugs is both legitimate and licensed (more information is available at the website *https://safemedsonline.org/resource/find-a-certified-vipps-online-pharmacy/*). When linking to a pharmacy

Internet site, the customer should click on the label for authentication. At this time, VIPPS is a voluntary accreditation. Although verification is done by the NABP, the organization does not regulate the sites; instead, the websites are regulated by the state in which the pharmacy is physically located, along with federal guidelines. E-pharmacies have the same regulations as retail and mail-order pharmacies with regard to dispensing to out-of-state pharmacy locations, and they are also required to adhere to HIPAA regulations.

Ordering medications by the Internet has many advantages, including ease of ordering, lower prices, and easy accessibility to online information, which lessens the wait time when trying to ask a pharmacist for information. However, identifying illegal pharmacies is a constant struggle for both state and federal agencies. If a suspicious e-pharmacy is found, it should be reported to the NABP. If the wrong medication or label is dispensed, this should be reported to the state's BOP.

Signs that a pharmacy site probably is illegal include the following:

- Dispensing medications without having the customer mail in the prescription
- Faxing a prescription that cannot be confirmed as a valid prescription
- Dispensing medications on completion of a questionnaire
- Not having a preexisting examination or patient-prescriber relationship
- Inability to contact a pharmacist at the website for consultation

Occupational Safety and Health Administration

The purpose of the **Occupational Safety and Health Administration (OSHA)** is to make the workplace safe for employees. Box 2.10 presents an outline of common safety and health topics. A safe workplace involves having safe equipment and materials, being able to safely perform tasks, and ensuring that the policies and procedures of a company (including pharmacies) are safe. OSHA requires **Safety Data Sheet (SDS)** information on all potentially dangerous chemicals used in the workplace.

Safety Data Sheets

Almost all chemicals can be dangerous if ingested or spilled. In all workplaces, including pharmacies, all chemicals must

---

BOX 2.10   Common Safety and Health Topics

- Disposal of hazardous drugs
- Ergonomics
- Handling practices
- Hazard communication standards
- Hazardous drugs during administration
- Hazardous drugs during caregiving
- Hazardous drugs during preparation
- Hazardous drugs during storage
- Latex allergy
- Workplace violence

---

have an SDS on file in an SDS binder, or the SDS must be available electronically through a database. The binders are normally bright yellow and black. The information on these sheets includes the storage requirements, handling procedures, and actions to take if the chemical is spilled, sprayed into the eyes, or comes in contact with the skin. It is important to know where the binder or database is kept and to ensure that every chemical has a sheet on file. For example, phenol is a dangerous antiseptic agent often used in nerve blocks; it is stored in many institutional pharmacies. If it is spilled, it is important not to breathe in the fumes but to contain the spill as quickly as possible and call the appropriate department for cleanup. Normally, environmental services in a hospital will respond and handle the cleanup. It is extremely easy to get SDS information to protect the employees who will handle the agent. The phone number is always given by the manufacturer, which is required by law to distribute the information to the requesting party within 24 hours. Usually the manufacturer faxes the SDS directly to the business (more information can be obtained on OSHA's website at *http://www.osha.gov*). The SDS information not only is important but also is required by law.

The Joint Commission

In 1951 several medical associations created the Joint Commission on Accreditation of Healthcare Organizations (JCAHO) as an independent, nonprofit organization that voluntarily accredited hospitals. In 1959 Canada withdrew from JCAHO to form its own accrediting organization. It was not until 1964 that JCAHO began to charge for its surveys. The following year, hospitals were required to be accredited to participate in the Medicare and Medicaid programs. Over the following years, JCAHO expanded its range of compliances over hospitals and institutions. In 2007 JCAHO changed its branding to **The Joint Commission (TJC)**. TJC meets three times annually and has 32 voting board members, consisting of physicians, administrators, nurses, employers, a labor representative, health plan leaders, quality experts, ethicists, educators, and a consumer advocate. TJC accredits more than 20,000 health care organizations and programs throughout the United States, including 9500 hospitals and home care facilities. Organizations must be surveyed at least every 3 years. Once accredited, the organization may display TJC's seal of approval. Ratings of all institutions can be found on the organization's website at *http://www.jointcommission.org*. The benefits of accreditation and certification include the following:

- It provides the community with confidence in the quality and safety of care, treatment, and other institutional services.
- It identifies and addresses risk management and reduction.
- It provides professional advice and staff education to improve services.
- It is recognized by many health care insurers and other third parties (Medicare and Medicaid).
- It meets regulatory requirements in specific states.

TJC surveys all aspects of hospital services, including pharmacy services. Areas of concern in the pharmacy include how look-alike, sound-alike drugs are identified; communication; allergy notification; conflicting prescriptions; verbal orders; and other areas that may create an avenue for errors. All employees should be knowledgeable about the pharmacy's policies and procedures so they can answer any questions asked by TJC representatives. If a technician is asked a question to which he or she does not know the answer, the technician should answer honestly and should not try to make up an answer. TJC representatives may collect pharmacy data to monitor the pharmacy's performance, identify adverse drug reactions, and determine how the pharmacy identifies and has attempted to improve problems in these areas. In 2004, TJC created the "Do Not Use" list of abbreviations as a requirement. However, this requirement has met with resistance because surveys reveal that as of 2006, 22% of accredited organizations were still noncompliant with this standard. In 2010, the "Do Not Use" list was integrated into the National Patient Safety Goal as a part of the Information Management standards.

Legal Standards

State Laws

Each state has its own set of laws that pharmacists, interns, pharmacy technicians, and clerks must follow when working in the pharmacy. You must know the regulations of your state. All pharmacy personnel should become familiar with the laws by obtaining the regulations booklet from their state BOP. You will notice that many states have laws that differ from federal law. Remember that the strictest law is the one you follow. Therefore if the FDA states that you must keep records for no less than 2 years but your state regulations require 7 years for inpatient records, you would follow the strictest regulation, in this case your state regulation. To learn more about your specific state regulations and laws, go to your state's BOP website, which can be found at *http://www.napb.net*.

Liabilities

You also should be aware of federal and state liability laws pertaining to pharmacy technicians. A patient can make various charges against a pharmacy technician if the pharmacy technician caused damage because of **negligence** or intentional action in the workplace. A **tort** is defined as an act causing injury to a person intentionally or because of negligence. The word *negligence* may describe an action taken without the forethought that should have been applied by a reasonable person of similar competency; a mistake was made. For an intentional mistake, the penalty can range from criminal charges to the awarding of damages, which usually means that money is paid to the person or persons who were wrongly affected. A negligent mistake can affect a person's ability to continue to work as a technician and also may result in punitive damages (ie, monetary payment).

Mistakes occur for many reasons. Some happen because of an excessive workload or possibly staffing shortages, which can lead to a mishap and could be classified as a negligent tort. Criminal behavior, such as false insurance claims or diverting drugs, could be called an intentional tort and could

result in imprisonment. One of the questions you should ask your employer is whether you are covered under the company's legal department. If a lawsuit were to be filed with you as the plaintiff, do you know who would represent you? Many companies have lawyers who represent the company, although you should not assume that they would represent you. If you are not covered by your employer, you may want to purchase malpractice insurance. Most technicians do not have such insurance; it is a personal preference. At the very least, be aware of what your rights and responsibilities are, including legal considerations, before entering a workplace. Depending on the state in which the technician works, laws vary as they pertain to the liability of the technician. Therefore you must check your state laws as they pertain to you. If you are involved in or witness any incidents in the workplace, you should follow these guidelines:

1. Review your state's regulations.
2. Understand your employer's rules and practices.
3. Define your scope of employment.

If an "event" occurs in the pharmacy, you should be prepared in the following ways:

1. Know the name of your attorney.
2. Always be careful of what you say and to whom you say it if you are ever questioned by state or federal investigators pertaining to an incident.
3. Write down in-depth notes on the facts of the event (as soon as possible) and keep them for reference.

Both federal and state laws change frequently; it is your responsibility to keep up with the current regulations. Pharmacy departments keep close track of these changes and notify employees of changes, but you are the one who carries out these laws on a daily basis. Be sure to learn the specifics of a new rule or regulation and obtain clarification if necessary because not understanding a new rule or regulation and not seeking further guidance are unacceptable excuses. Because pharmacy technicians can be held accountable for their actions, this is a fundamental competency of all pharmacy technicians. In addition, the PTCB requires at least one continuing education (CE) unit in current law to be taken for recertification within a 2-year period.

⊙ Scenario Checkup 2.4

Laura continues her work as a trusted technician at a local independent pharmacy. She is busy serving customers in a caring and efficient manner.

One morning a young man comes to the counter and asks to buy the medication Plan B. Laura is morally against selling this "morning after" pill. She asks for identification, and the young man freely presents it. He is 20 years old. What are Laura's legal and ethical options in this situation?

Ethics and Morals in the Workplace

Ethics are the values and morals that are used within a profession. **Morals** are a person's beliefs concerning what is right or wrong in human behavior. Work ethics are a set of standards that should be followed by anyone working in a field. Work ethics are often outlined in the pharmacy protocol. One important factor that the pharmacy technician must remember is that he or she has a clear responsibility to the patient on many levels. Patients are consumers, and as consumers they have the right to receive goods that have been handled properly and are in good condition. They also trust the pharmacy personnel with their personal information, expecting that their information will be treated as confidential. Many times in a pharmacy, or any work setting, employees express their opinions concerning various medical procedures such as abortion, surgery, or a type of treatment. These are controversial topics, and the opinions that each person has are a part of personal morals or beliefs. Although each person has his or her own set of morals, many morals tend to coincide with the beliefs of others (eg, stealing is wrong).

In the workplace, however, technicians, pharmacists, and other health care workers are faced with patients who might have different morals. In these situations, ethics include the professional behavior of a technician regardless of a patient's morals. Ethics tend to overlap many morals and need to be separated in the workplace and in the public domain. When you assume the responsibility of serving the public in a setting such as the pharmacy, you accept work ethics that guide your behavior. For instance, in a hospital, there may be a need for medication that is used for the termination of pregnancy, emergency contraception, or other controversial treatments. The responsibility of the pharmacy staff is to provide services for all patients. If providing the service conflicts with your morals or your beliefs prohibit you from participating in servicing patients, you must communicate this to your supervisor.

For many decisions, just keeping small matters in perspective can help you make the right choice. Keeping patients' information confidential and working within the pharmacy's rules and guidelines, including policies and procedures, ensure that patients receive the best service possible. The technician should always remember that pharmacists, technicians, and clerks are present to serve patients and customers in a professional manner at all times, as outlined in the pharmacy technician's code of ethics (Box 2.11).

Professional Ethics

Professional ethics are systematic rules or principles governing right conduct. Each practitioner has the duty to adhere to the standards of ethical practice and conduct set by the profession. Pharmacy technicians have a responsibility to make informed decisions based on their specialized training. Professional codes of conduct must be followed. Respect is a

BOX 2.11 Pharmacy Technicians' Code of Ethics

Preamble

Pharmacy technicians are health care professionals who assist pharmacists in providing the best possible care for patients. The principles of this code, which apply to pharmacy technicians working in any and all settings, are based on the application and support of the moral obligations that guide the pharmacy profession in relationships with patients, health care professionals, and society.

Principles

- A pharmacy technician's first consideration is to ensure the health and safety of the patient and to use knowledge and skills to the best of his or her ability in serving patients.
- A pharmacy technician supports and promotes honesty and integrity in the profession, which includes a duty to observe the law, maintain the highest moral and ethical conduct at all times, and uphold the ethical principles of the profession.
- A pharmacy technician assists and supports the pharmacist in the safe, efficacious, and cost-effective distribution of health services and health care resources.
- A pharmacy technician respects and values the abilities of pharmacists, colleagues, and other health care professionals.
- A pharmacy technician maintains competency in his/her practice and continually enhances his/her professional knowledge and expertise.
- A pharmacy technician respects and supports the patient's individuality, dignity, and confidentiality.
- A pharmacy technician respects the confidentiality of a patient's records and discloses pertinent information only with proper authorization.
- A pharmacy technician never assists in dispensing, promoting, or distribution of medication or medical devices that are not of good quality or do not meet the standards required by law.
- A pharmacy technician does not engage in any activity that will discredit the profession, and will expose, without fear or favor, illegal or unethical conduct in the profession.
- A pharmacy technician associates with and engages in the support of organizations that promote the profession of pharmacy through the utilization and enhancement of pharmacy technicians.

The Institute for the Certification of Pharmacy Technicians (2007); Code of Ethics for Pharmacy Technicians—adapted from the American Association of Pharmacy Technicians Code of Ethics, published. *Am J Health-Syst Pharm* 60:37-51, 2003. *https://www.pharmacytimes.com/view/10-black-box-warnings-every-pharmacist-should-know.*

key component of professional behavior in the pharmacy. Technicians should always display a sincere respect for the pharmacist, the patient, and their health care colleagues. Being honest, trustworthy, and an all-around team player demonstrates professional ethics.

- Terms and definitions covered in this chapter
- Major federal laws affecting pharmacists and pharmacy
- The differences between the functions of the DEA and FDA
- The process for reporting any problems with a drug or any adverse reactions to the FDA
- The three classes of drug recalls defined by the FDA
- The proper handling of controlled substances, including the necessary forms and regulations
- The basic information contained in a drug monograph
- The purpose of boxed warnings and MedGuides
- The five pregnancy categories established by the FDA
- Who can prescribe medications and medical devices
- How to decipher a DEA number
- Risk management and drug abuse monitoring programs and their purpose
- Regulation and authentication of Internet pharmacies
- OSHA guidelines as they pertain to pharmacy
- The purpose of The Joint Commission
- The legal limitations of pharmacy technicians
- The difference between morals and ethics

◎ Scenario Follow-Up

As Laura continues in her retail pharmacy career, she has learned that it is imperative to keep abreast of the state and federal laws and regulations affecting her position. She understands that she can be held accountable for HIPAA violations and any medication errors in which she may be involved. Laura uses her continuing education courses to stay up to date on changes in the pharmacy profession. She also regularly checks websites maintained by the FDA, the DEA, and her state BOP for changes or legislation related to pharmacy law.

Review Questions

Multiple Choice Questions

1. The amendment that required the labeling "Caution: Federal law prohibits dispensing without a prescription" was the:
   A. Durham-Humphrey Amendment
   B. Kefauver-Harris Amendments
   C. OBRA '90
   D. None of the above
2. What is the purpose of the Orphan Drug Act?
   A. It enacts stricter rules concerning sales and distribution of controlled substances.
   B. It allows drug companies to bypass lengthy testing to treat persons who have a rare disease.
   C. It stops the use of drug testing in animals.
   D. It ensures the safety and effectiveness of manufacturing practices.
3. The law that requires pharmacists to counsel patients on new medications is:
   A. OBRA '90
   B. Comprehensive Drug Abuse Prevention and Control Act
   C. Prescription Drug Marketing Act
   D. Durham-Humphrey Amendment

4. The primary purpose of the FDA is to:
   A. Make arrests
   B. Ensure that safety and effectiveness standards for medications are met by manufacturers
   C. Prevent the distribution and illegal use of controlled substances
   D. Make sure all laws pertaining to physicians and pharmacists are followed
5. A pharmacy that will be dispensing controlled drugs must have which one of the following forms on file with the DEA?
   A. Form 222
   B. Form 224
   C. Form 363
   D. Form 225
6. The five categories of controlled substances are rated on the basis of:
   A. Cost
   B. Strength
   C. Conditions that they treat
   D. Potential for abuse
7. Which of the following health care providers is *not* one of the standard practitioners that all states accept?
   A. Doctor of podiatry
   B. Dentists
   C. Chiropractors
   D. Veterinarians
8. Safety Data Sheets (SDS) contain information on:
   A. Storage of a chemical
   B. Actions to take in case of a spill
   C. The combustion and stability of a chemical
   D. All of the above
9. Which classification of drug recall could cause a temporary health problem or a slight threat of serious harm?
   A. Class I
   B. Class II
   C. Class III
   D. Class IV
10. What is the maximum legal amount of pseudoephedrine that can be purchased per day?
    A. 7.5 g
    B. 3.6 g
    C. 9 g
    D. 62 tablets

■ Technician's Corner

Dr. Beth Golden writes an order for the following prescription:
- DEA#AG1958366
- Disp: hydrocodone/acetaminophen tablets #50
- Sig: Take 1 tablet q8h prn severe pain
- 0 refills

Determine whether this DEA number is correct and explain each step of the checking process.

Bibliography

Andrews S. The Affordable Care Act. *Todays Tech*. 2012;13:17.

Ballington DA. *Pharmacy Practice for Technicians*. 2nd ed. St. Paul, MN: EMC/Paradigm; 2002.

George T. Role of the advanced practice nurse in palliative care. *Int J Palliat Nurs*. 2016;22(3):137-140.

Gieringer DH. The safety and efficacy of new drug approval. *Cato J*. 1985;5(1):177-201.

Gray Morris D. *Calculate With Confidence*. 6th ed. St. Louis: Elsevier; 2013.

National Association of Boards of Pharmacy. *Survey of Pharmacy Law*. Mount Prospect, IL: The Association; 2005.

Nielsen JR, James JD. *Handbook of Federal Drug Law*. 2nd ed. Philadelphia: Williams & Wilkins; 1992.

Outterson K. The Drug Quality and Security Act—mind the gaps. *N Engl J Med*. 2014;370(2):97-99.

Potter PA, Perry AG. *Fundamentals of Nursing*. 8th ed. St. Louis: Elsevier; 2013.

Shargel L, Mutnick A, Souney P, et al. *Comprehensive Pharmacy Review*. 8th ed. Baltimore: Lippincott Williams & Wilkins; 2012.

Websites Referenced

American Veterinary Medical Association. *Prescriptions and pharmacies: FAQs for veterinarians*. Available at: https://avma.org.

Coffa D, Snyder H. Opioid Use Disorder: Medical Treatment Options. *Am Fam Physician*. 2019;100(7):416-425.

Diversion Control Division. CMEA (The Combat Methamphetamine Epidemic Act of 2005). Available at: https://usdoj.gov.

DeMio T. Meth is back and flooding the streets of Ohio and Kentucky, and it's uglier than ever. *The Enquirer*. February 20, 2020. Available at: https://www.cincinnati.com/story/news/2020/02/13/meth-opioids-new-epidemic-of-addiction/4551991002/.

Drug Enforcement Administration. DEA Releases annual National Drug Threat Assessment. March 2021. Available at: https://www.dea.gov/sites/default/files/2021-02/DIR-008-21%202020%20National%20Drug%20Threat%20Assessment_WEB.pdf.

Encyclopedia of Surgery. Barbiturates. Available at: http://www.surgeryencyclopedia.com/A-Ce/Barbiturates.html.

Food and Drug Administration. Drug recalls. Available at: https://www.fda.gov/drugs/drug-safety-and-availability/drug-recalls.

Food and Drug Administration Website. FluMist quadrivalent vaccine information. February 01, 2023. Archive of FDA. Available at: https://pagefreezer.com.

Food and Drug Administration. Legal requirements for the sale and purchase of drug products containing pseudoephedrine, ephedrine, and phenylpropanolamine. Available at: https://www.fda.gov/drugs/information-drug-class/legal-requirements-sale-and-purchase-drug-products-containing-pseudoephedrine-ephedrine-and.

Food and Drug Administration. National drug code directory. Available at: https://www.fda.gov/drugs/drug-approvals-and-databases/national-drug-code-directory.

Food and Drug Administration. Physician labeling rule requirements. Available at: https://www.fda.gov/drugs/laws-acts-and-rules/prescription-drug-labeling-resources.

HealthCare.gov. Affordable Care Act (ACA). Available at: https://www.healthcare.gov/glossary/affordable-care-act/.

Houck LK. The FDA law blog; GAO report assesses state approaches to control pseudoephedrine. February 26, 2013. Available at: http://www.fdalawblog.net/fda_law_blog_hyman_phelps/2013/02/gao-report-assesses-state-approaches-to-control-pseudoephedrine.html.

Legal Requirements for the Sale and Purchase of Drug Products Containing Pseudoephedrine, Ephedrine, and Phenylpropanolamine | FDA.

Murawski M, Villa KR, Dole EJ, et al. Advanced-practice pharmacists: practice characteristics and reimbursement of pharmacists certified for collaborative clinical practice in New Mexico and North Carolina. *Am J Health Syst Pharm*. 2011;68(24):2341-2350. Available at: https://www.medscape.com/viewarticle/754690.

National Association of State Controlled Substances Authorities. Impact of state laws regulating pseudoephedrine on methamphetamine production and abuse. April 18, 2016. Available at: https://nabp.pharmacy/members/programs-services/industry-information-networks/pmp-interconnect/.

National Boards of Pharmacy. NABP PMP InterConnect. Available at: https://nabp.pharmacy/members/pmp-interconnect/.

Perrone M. New restrictions on hydrocodone to take effect. *USA Today*. Available at: http://www.usatoday.com.

Safety Emporium. Sample SDS for benzoic acid. Available at: http://www.ilpi.com/msds/benzoic.html.

Schedules of controlled substances. Rescheduling of hydrocodone combination products from Schedule III to Schedule II (2014, August 22). 79 *Fed Regist*. No. 163, 49661 (to be codified at 21 CFR Part 1308). Available at: https://www.federalregister.gov/articles/2014/08/22/2014-19922/schedules-of-controlled-substances-rescheduling-of-hydrocodone-combination-products-from-schedule.

The Joint Commission. Standards. Available at: https://www.jointcommission.org/standards/.

USP information. Available at: http://www.usp.org/aboutUSP/.

USP–NF. Available at: http://www.usp.org/USPNF/.

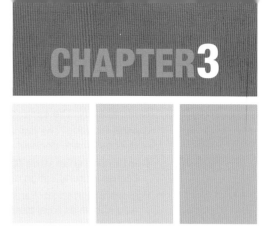

Competencies, Associations, and Settings for Technicians

Karen Davis

OBJECTIVES

1. Describe the competencies needed for technicians to be successful in various pharmacy settings.
2. Explain the term nondiscretionary duties and describe different nondiscretionary duties in inpatient, outpatient, and closed-door pharmacy settings.
3. Discuss the American Society of Health-System Pharmacists (ASHP) Model Curriculum and how it relates to pharmacy technician training programs and certification.
4. Discuss the following related to national certification for technicians: (a) state the differences among certification, licensure, and registration; (b) explain the benefits of obtaining technician certification; (c) explain the process by which a person can become a nationally certified pharmacy technician; (d) describe the various national certification examinations and their requirements; (e) list ways in which the Pharmacy Technician Certification Board (PTCB) national examination differs from the National Healthcareer Association (NHA) national examination; (f) describe the requirements that technicians must meet to maintain their national certification.
5. List specialty certifications available for technicians and explore the various websites that can be used to obtain continuing education credits.
6. List various opportunities available for technicians and discuss incentive programs.
7. List the various professional associations pharmacy technicians can join.
8. Explain the importance of professionalism in the workplace and the importance of networking as it relates to the job search.

TERMS AND DEFINITIONS

Accreditation Council for Pharmacy Education (ACPE) National agency for the accreditation of professional degree programs in pharmacy and providers of continuing pharmacy education

American Association of Pharmacy Technicians (AAPT) First pharmacy technician association; founded in 1979

American Pharmacists Association (APhA) Oldest pharmacy association; founded in 1852

American Society of Health-System Pharmacists (ASHP) Pharmacy association founded in 1942

American Society of Health-System Pharmacists (ASHP) Model Curriculum for Pharmacy Technician Education and Training A program that provides details on how to meet the ASHP goals for pharmacy technician training curricula

Board of pharmacy (BOP) A state-managed agency that licenses pharmacists and may either register or license pharmacy technicians to work in pharmacy

Certified pharmacy technician (CPhT) A technician who has passed the national certification examination; the technician can use the abbreviation CPhT after his or her name

Closed-door pharmacy A pharmacy in which medications are called in from institutions, such as long-term care facilities, and are then delivered; closed-door pharmacies are not open to the public

57

Communication The ability to express oneself in such a way that one is readily and clearly understood

Community pharmacy Also known as an outpatient or a retail pharmacy; these pharmacies serve patients in their communities; consumers can walk in and purchase a prescription or over-the-counter (OTC) drug

Competency The capability or proficiency to perform a function

Confidentiality The practice of keeping privileged customer information from being disclosed without the customer's consent

Continuing education (CE) Education beyond the basic technical education, usually required for license or certification renewal

Hyperalimentation Parenteral (intravenous) nutrition for patients who are unable to eat solids or liquids; also known as total parenteral nutrition (TPN)

Inpatient pharmacy A pharmacy in a hospital or institutional setting

Licensed pharmacy technician A pharmacy technician who is licensed by the state board; licensing ensures that an individual has at least the minimum level of competency required by the profession, unlike a registered pharmacy technician

National Association of Boards of Pharmacy (NABP) National organization for members of state boards of pharmacy

National Health Career Association (NHA) Certification organization for a variety of health care careers, including the Institute for the Certification of Pharmacy Technicians (ICPT)

National Pharmacy Technician Association (NPTA) Pharmacy association primarily for technicians; founded in 1999

Nondiscretionary duties Tasks that do not require professional judgment such as repackaging medications, managing inventory, filling automated dispensing machines, and billing

Outpatient pharmacy A pharmacy that serves patients in community or ambulatory settings

Parenteral medications A term most commonly used to describe medications administered by injection, such as intravenously, intramuscularly, or subcutaneously

Pharmacy Technician Accreditation Commission (PTAC) Agency-formed partnership between ASHP and ACPE for review and accreditation of pharmacy technician education and training programs

Pharmacy Technician Certification Board (PTCB) National board for the certification of pharmacy technicians

Professionalism Conforming to the right principles of conduct (work ethics) as accepted by others in the profession

Registered pharmacy technician A pharmacy technician who is registered through the state board of pharmacy; the registration process helps maintain a list of those working in pharmacies and may require a background check through the legal system; the registration process does not guarantee the level of the registrant's knowledge or skills

The Society for the Education of Pharmacy Technicians (SEPhT) SEPhT is a national technician organization that offers tools and useful information used in training and education of students and current practicing pharmacy technicians

Total parenteral nutrition (TPN) Large-volume intravenous nutrition administered through the central vein (subclavian vein), which allows for a higher concentration of solutions

◉ Scenario

Olivia is a newly hired technician at an independently owned pharmacy. She is required to register with the state board of pharmacy, but certification is not mandated. She is a graduate of a technical career college and remembers her instructor discussing the benefits of association membership. What are Olivia's membership options, and how can she find more information on this subject?

Technician qualifications and job descriptions vary from state to state. There are no mandatory national standards or requirements pertaining to technician duties or training needed. Therefore each state **board of pharmacy (BOP)** determines the standards required and how they are to be met by technicians.

Because of the rapidly changing health care system, the job descriptions and educational requirements of pharmacy technicians are quickly changing. Among the changes are increased responsibilities, the need for higher education, more legal responsibility, and certification mandates. This trend can be seen across the United States. Many BOPs now require completion of a program accredited by the **American Society of Health-System Pharmacists (ASHP)** for a person to become a registered technician. Currently many states require **Pharmacy Technician Certification Board (PTCB)** or **National Healthcareer Association (NHA)** certification and have accepted it as their measure of the knowledge base of pharmacy technicians. Positive aspects of these changes include a wider range of jobs available, bonuses, salary increases, and better benefits for technicians.

This chapter begins with an overview of the history of pharmacy technicians' duties and then explores important attributes for a successful career in pharmacy. Necessary job qualifications, expectations, and trends in pharmacy are explored, along with the importance of national pharmacy organizations and the benefits of pharmacy technician certification. This chapter also provides information about the preparation necessary to conduct a successful job search and explores the exciting advanced roles now available to the pharmacy technician. This information can help the student technician determine the best career path to follow, understand the various positions available, and attain the ultimate goals and benefits of this profession.

Historical Data

Historically technicians have answered to a variety of titles. These include pharmacy clerk, pharmacist assistant, and pharmacy aide. Technicians have held a variety of positions. Some of the job responsibilities have been billing, ordering, stocking medications, typing, answering the phone, greeting customers, troubleshooting, cashiering, and running errands. Technicians have been a part of the pharmacy field since the beginning of pharmacy (see Chapter 1). However, more recently, pharmacy managers and their respective state BOPs have been attempting to classify and clearly define the role of the pharmacy technician as the needs of pharmacy change.

Technicians' duties focus on tasks that do not require professional judgment but rather concentrate on their technical skills and training. Pharmacists' duties have moved from filling prescriptions and compounding simple agents to counseling patients and interacting with other medical professionals, such as physicians and nurses. This change can especially be seen in the hospital setting, where pharmacists are responsible for managing dosing of medications and participating on committees. The change in responsibility has been addressed many times over the course of pharmacy technician history by the ASHP, the **American Pharmacists Association (APhA),** and other pharmacy associations. The need for skilled personnel has never been greater.

One significant contribution to the improvement of the pharmacy technician profession was the development of the white paper. In 2002 the *American Journal of Health-System Pharmacists* addressed many of the challenges pharmacy faces by publishing the *White Paper on Pharmacy Technicians 2002: Needed Changes Can No Longer Wait*. A white paper argues a specific position or solution to a problem. The paper explores the diversity of pharmacy technicians' qualifications, knowledge, and responsibilities (Box 3.1). The white paper was endorsed by a panel of pharmacy organizations and comprehensively discussed issues pertinent to the promotion and growth of a competent pharmacy technician workforce.

In 2009 the Task Force on Pharmacy Technician Education and Training Programs met in Rosemont, Illinois. It was established by the **National Association of Boards of**

BOX 3.1 White Paper on Pharmacy Technicians 2002

1. *Education and training:* Encompasses the history of training techniques and programs. Explores the need for adjusting the length of the training program based on the functions of the technician. Course curriculum adjustments and adequacy are discussed.
2. *Accreditation of training programs and institutions:* Describes the types of training programs and the need for institutional accreditation. Explains why it is important to oversee these programs because there are no nationally recognized ones.
3. *Certification:* Covers the history and growth of the national certification process; describes the importance of certification, both for the establishment of minimum levels of competency and for the recognition of pharmacy technicians as paraprofessionals.

American Society of Health-System Pharmacists (ASHP). Available at: *http://www.pharmacycredentialing.org/Files/Technicians%20White%20Paper%20Jan%202003.pdf.*

Pharmacy (**NABP**) and was charged with the following mission:

1. Review the existing state requirements for technician education and training requirements for national technician training program accrediting organizations, such as the ASHP and the **Accreditation Council for Pharmacy Education (ACPE)** Core Competencies.
2. Recommend national standards for technician education and training programs and encourage BOPs to recognize them.

The NABP executive committee accepted the following recommendations from the task force:

- NABP should encourage BOPs to require as an element of pharmacy technician certification completion of an education and training program that meets minimum standardized guidelines.
- NABP should encourage BOPs to require as an element of pharmacy technician certification completion of an accredited education and training program.
- NABP should assist in developing a national accreditation system for pharmacy technician education and training programs that is based within the profession of pharmacy and uses a single accrediting agency.
- NABP should encourage ACPE and ASHP to work collaboratively to develop an accreditation system for pharmacy technician education and training programs that reflects all pharmacy practice settings and, if feasible, to consolidate the activities into one accrediting body, preferably the ACPE.
- NABP should encourage PTCB to change the process by which it determines who is qualified to sit for its examination to include completion of an accredited pharmacy technician education and training program and high school diploma or general education diploma (GED) verification.

- NABP should encourage the PTCB to provide the NABP with information on its certified pharmacy technicians (CPhTs), so that the NABP may enhance the pharmacy technician data contained in the NABP clearinghouse to provide the information necessary for the state BOPs to protect the public health.
- NABP should encourage the ASHP to revise its current accreditation standards for pharmacy technician education and training programs to require accredited providers to inform potential program applicants of applicable state requirements for registration or licensure.

In 2010, at its 106th Annual Meeting in Anaheim, California, the NABP passed resolution No. 106-7-10, resolving to continue to encourage states to adopt uniform standards for pharmacy technician education and training programs.

The PTCB launched the CREST Initiative by hosting a summit focused on the areas of consumer awareness, resources, education, state policy, and testing as they relate to pharmacy technicians. Summit participants made recommendations during the meeting pertaining to additional requirements for a candidate to sit for the Pharmacy Technician Certification Exam (PTCE). The following recommendations were proposed:

- The PTCB should require a minimum period of practical experience to be eligible for the PTCE.
- Mandatory criminal background checks should be required for all PTCE candidates. ASHP and ACPE joined to form the **Pharmacy Technician Accreditation Commission** and became known as ASHP/ACPE. In some references, this is also referred to as **PTAC**.
- All PTCE candidates should be required to complete a training program accredited by the ASHP.

Additional recommendations were made related to requirements for recertification. It is recommended that PTCB change the current requirements for CPhT recertification to:

- Accept only pharmacy technician–targeted and/or ACPE "T" and/or "P/T" designated continuing pharmacy education (CPE) credits for a total of 20 hours every 2 years.
- Require at least 15 of the 20 hours of CPE to be provided through the state BOPs, NABP, employer-accredited programs, or programs accredited by ACPE. The allowable continuing education (CE) hours from college courses have been reduced from 15 to 10, and allowable in-service hours have been phased out.
- Five hours of practical/employer-based CPE may be allowed as part of the 20-hour CPE requirement every 2 years.
- Maintain the requirement that 1 of the 20 required CPE credits be in pharmacy law.
- Require 1 of the 20 required CPE credits to be in medication/patient safety (effective in 2014).

In March 2012 the CREST Initiative steering committee, composed of 10 leaders in pharmacy, developed and launched a profession-wide survey on these recommendations. The survey was completed by more than 17,000 pharmacy technicians and pharmacists nationwide. Results from the survey will provide the PTCB Board of Governors and Certification Council with important input from the profession on advancing the work of pharmacy technicians and the future of the PTCB certification program.

In February 2013 the PTCB announced that these changes will be phased in over the next 7 years. The board of governors conducted a 90-day open online comment period to allow members of the pharmacy community to share their best practices for implementing the new requirements. The PTCB began releasing the policies and procedures on the implementation of these decisions in late 2013.

In February 2017 the Pharmacy Technician Stakeholders Consensus held a 3-day conference. Over 100 individuals attended on site, and access was available by webinars. Discussions revolved around current practice standards and qualifications for entry-level and advanced practice pharmacy technicians, with outcomes and recommendations to be published later in the year. More information can be found at *http://www.ptcb.org/about-ptcb/news-room/news-landing/2017/03/08/national-conference-of-pharmacy-stakeholders-seeks-consensus-on-pharmacy-technician-qualifications#.WcUs_oWcFYc*.

The Pharmacy Technician Career

Pharmacy technician is one of the hottest careers for individuals interested in working in the health care industry. Pharmacies all over the country need technicians. According to Yahoo Education, pharmacy technician was one of the top five growing health care careers in the United States in 2019. More than 417,000 technicians were employed as of May 2019 nationally. The occupation is expected to grow by 7% by year 2028. See the Bureau of Labor Statistics *Occupational Outlook Handbook* for more information *(https://www.bls.gov/ooh/healthcare/pharmacy-technicians.htm?view_full#tab-6)*.

Competencies

Competency can be defined as the capability or proficiency to perform a function. The practice of pharmacy includes a wide variety of settings. Technicians must have many different technical skills to function in each area. Box 3.2 lists chapters that cover common responsibilities and competencies. These competencies outline the roles and responsibilities that pharmacy technicians perform, which include the specific job-related knowledge and skills needed to ensure patient safety.

State and National Boards of Pharmacy

Each state in the United States has its own BOP, which is overseen by the NABP *(http://www.nabp.net)*. Each state's BOP serves many functions, including registering technicians and licensing pharmacists. The BOP also provides consumers with a way to file a complaint or report any problems or illegal actions they have experienced in a pharmacy. BOPs also review and update current rules and regulations pertaining to pharmacy practice. When new standards are implemented, BOP inspectors may visit any pharmacy to

BOX 3.2 Chapter References Citing Common Responsibilities and Competencies of a Pharmacy Technician

Pharmacy Law, Ethics, and Regulatory Agencies	Chapter 2
Dosage Forms and Routes of Administration	Chapter 5
Conversions and Calculations	Chapter 6
Drug Information References	Chapter 7
Community Pharmacy Practice	Chapter 8
Institutional Pharmacy Practice	Chapter 9
Bulk Repackaging and Nonsterile Compounding	Chapter 11
Aseptic Technique and Sterile Compounding	Chapter 12
Pharmacy Billing and Inventory Management	Chapter 13
Medication Safety and Error Prevention	Chapter 14

BOX 3.3 Examples of Federal Laws Governing Pharmacy

Prescription Records

A record of all prescriptions dispensed should be maintained for 2 years after the last refill. All systems used for maintaining records of any prescriptions must include the following:
- Prescription number
- Date of issuance
- Patient's identification (name, address)
- Name, strength, and dosage form of medication
- Quantity dispensed
- Practitioner's identification (Drug Enforcement Agency registration, if applicable)
- Pharmacist's identification

Patient Consultation (OBRA '90)

Pharmacists must screen the entire drug profile of all Medicaid recipients before their prescriptions are filled. Each patient must be given counseling on the medication that has been prescribed, including topics such as how to take the drug, storage of the drug, and side effects of the medication. Most states have passed regulations that require counseling of all patients according to the same processes, although the requirements for the provision of written and/or oral consultation may be different among the states.

For more information on pharmacy law, refer to Chapter 2.

determine its compliance with these new standards. If the pharmacy is found to be in noncompliance, the BOP has the authority not only to impose fines but also to close the pharmacy until compliance is attained. If a pharmacy technician is found guilty of a violation of pharmacy law, the BOP can revoke his or her registration or license, depending on the state regulations.

The NABP and state BOPs are currently studying the expanded use of technicians in the pharmacy field. For example, technicians in California who have achieved a specific level of competency are granted the additional job duty of monitoring other pharmacy technicians. In Tennessee, technicians can take physicians' verbal orders over the phone. More states are requiring technicians to be registered, certified, and/or licensed. This examination of the current uses of technicians no doubt will reveal the skill level necessary for various types of pharmacy tasks, and ultimately changes will be made by each state BOP. BOPs also may change technician-to-pharmacist ratios in pharmacy settings. A knowledge of pharmacy law (Box 3.3) is essential before a person can work in a pharmacy environment. Federal laws govern all 50 states. In addition, each state's BOP has specific laws, regulations, and guidelines that pertain to pharmacy practice in that state (Box 3.4). When state laws differ from federal laws, the strictest law should be enforced. (For more information on the legal requirements of pharmacy technicians, see Chapter 2.)

⊙ Scenario Checkup 3.1

Olivia is enjoying her new position at the family-owned pharmacy. She is counting pills, reconstituting medications, and checking out customers at the register. She is allowed to answer the phone and take refill orders. Olivia has been on the job for approximately 3 months. She wonders why she has not been allowed to input prescriptions on the computer yet. Her typing speed is 28 words per minute. Why do you think the pharmacist has not put her on the computer yet? What steps can she take to gain this additional responsibility?

Nondiscretionary Duties

Technicians perform many **nondiscretionary duties** in the pharmacy setting. These are tasks that do not require professional judgment. Examples include repackaging medications, managing inventory, filling automated dispensing machines, and billing. All of these tasks are clearly defined and should be easy to follow. This does not mean that anyone can do the job, however, because prior knowledge of pharmacy terms, drugs, and procedures is required. As job classifications in pharmacy expand, so will the level of pharmacological knowledge required for pharmacy technicians. Historically, the pharmacist was responsible for the final approval of any task completed in a pharmacy setting, although this is also changing. Some states now permit "tech-check-tech" approval procedures; this allows a certified technician, rather than a pharmacist, to check another technician's order-filling accuracy. Nondiscretionary duties prohibit technicians from interpreting scientific studies, counseling patients about medications, and conferring with other medical personnel about proper treatments.

BOX 3.4 Pharmacy Technician State Requirements

Alabama: Must complete a board-approved program and be registered with the state board.

Alaska: Complete an on-the-job training program directed by a pharmacist in charge and registered with the state board.

Arizona: Pharmacy Technician Certification Board (PTCB) certification required.

Arkansas: Must pass a board-approved training program or become nationally certified through PTCB.

California: The choices are as follows:
Earn an associate's degree in pharmacy technology
Finish a course that provides a minimum of 240 training hours or complete the American Society of Health-System Pharmacists (ASHP) training course
Graduate from a pharmacy school accredited by the ASHP
Complete training through the US armed services
Become PTCB certified

Colorado: New must reg as CPhT.

Connecticut: Must be trained by a pharmacy manager, and the training must be documented; then apply for state certification or obtain PTCB certification or another certification approved by Connecticut's Department of Certification of Pharmacy.

Delaware: No current licensure requirements for pharmacy technicians.

Florida: Must complete a board-approved training program.

Georgia: Must register with the state board of pharmacy.

Hawaii: No current license requirements for pharmacy technicians.

Idaho: Must pass the PTCE or another board-approved program and register with the board.

Illinois: Must complete pharmacy technician training program and become certified through PTCB.

Indiana: Must complete a board-approved training program or obtain the PTCB certification.

Iowa: Must register with the state board of pharmacy and obtain either NHA or PTCB certification within a year.

Kansas: Must be currently employed as a technician and pass a test provided by the state board.

Kentucky: Must be 16 or older, have a HS diploma or GED, and crim B/G ck.

Louisiana: Candidates must complete a board approved OR earn at least 600 hours of practical experience in a LA pharmacy.

Maine: Must have on-the-job training and register with the state board.

Maryland: Must obtain PTCB certification or complete a board-approved training program involving at least 160 hours of work experience but no longer than 6 months' duration.

Massachusetts: Say this candidates must be at least 18 yrs old and have a HS diploma or GED.

Michigan: Complete an employer-based training program or become nationally certified.

Minnesota: Complete an ASHP program, or board-approved program with a minimum of 240 hours, or a program offered through a military branch or board-approved institution, and then register with the state board of pharmacy.

Mississippi: Must apply for certification with the state board; then take either the NHA or the PTCB examination.

Missouri: Must register with board, but must be a CPhT to perform additional activities.

Montana: Must register with the state board and obtain NHA or PTCB certification.

Nebraska: Must register with the state board.

Nevada: Perform 1500 hours of on-the-job training as a pharmacy technician-in-training; or become nationally certified through the PTCB or another approved certifying agency and perform 500 hours of on-the-job training as a pharmacy technician-in-training; or complete a pharmacy technician training program accredited by the ASHP and perform 350 hours of on-the-job training as a pharmacy technician-in-training; or complete a pharmacy technician training program conducted by the Indian Health Service or a branch of the military and become nationally certified through the PTCB or another approved certifying agency.

New Hampshire: Must register with the state board.

New Jersey: Must register with the New Jersey Division of Consumer Affairs.

New Mexico: Must register with the state board as / noncertified, complete documented on-the-job training with a pharmacist, apply for certification, and obtain NHA or PTCB certification.

New York: Register with board and become CPhT through board approved course.

North Carolina: Do one of the following and register with the North Carolina Board of Pharmacy: Complete an employer-based on-the-job training program within 180 days of beginning employment in a pharmacy; or complete a board-approved pharmacy technician training program conducted by an accredited institution or college; or become nationally certified through the PTCB or another approved certifying agency.

North Dakota: Must complete a program accredited by the ASHP or complete training on the job under the supervision of a licensed pharmacist.

Ohio: Must register as a CPhT, registered tech, or trainee per board requirements.

Oklahoma: Must obtain a job in a pharmacy and complete on-the-job training provided by the pharmacist in charge or a staff pharmacist.

Oregon: Register with board an complete a on the job program apporved by board, OR obtain CPhT through PTCB.

Pennsylvania: register with board, complete a board approved program, and be a CPhT.

Rhode Island: Must complete a training program accredited by the AHSP; or finish a training program offered by the US armed services; or complete a program offered at a community college or earn NHA or PTCB certification.

South Carolina: Must register with the state board.

South Dakota: Either register with the South Dakota Board of Pharmacy as a pharmacy technician-in-training, complete a board-approved pharmacy technician training program, and pass the PTCE or become nationally certified through the PTCB or another approved certifying

BOX 3.4 **Pharmacy Technician State Requirements—cont'd**

agency and register with the state board as a certified pharmacy technician.

Tennessee: Must obtain a job in a pharmacy and then register with the state board.

Texas: Must register as a technician still in training and then complete a board-approved training program and obtain PTCB certification.

Utah: Must earn NHA or PTCB certification and complete a board-approved training program involving 180 hours of practical experience.

Vermont: Must register with the state board.

Virginia: Must complete a board-approved training program and sit for the state examination to obtain registration or earn PTCB certification and register with the state board of pharmacy.

Washington: Must pass a national certification examination on completion of a board-approved program for training.

Washington, DC: Complete a board-approved training program or complete a national certification.

West Virginia: must register as a trainee, complete board approved on the job training program and complete test, obtain a CPhT through PTCB OR ...CPhTs can complete 20 hours of on the job training and register as a technician.

Wisconsin: No current licensure requirements for pharmacy technicians.

Wyoming: Must earn PTCB certification and register with the state board.

Basic Nondiscretionary Skills

Typing

The number of prescriptions processed per day in a pharmacy directly relates to the speed and accuracy of the typist. This makes a fast and accurate pharmacy technician with a good working knowledge of medications a great asset.

Computers

Pharmacies use computers for many jobs, including dispensing medications and maintaining inventory. Dispensing systems accurately count and dispense medications, which reduces the rate of errors. Although these systems increase accurate dosing, human error still occurs. A knowledge of automation used in dispensing and computer programs such as Microsoft Word and Excel is essential to creating various reports, ordering, filling prescriptions, and maintaining inventory. Nothing replaces the knowledge of a skilled pharmacy technician to reduce error rates.

Reports and Documentation

Many pharmacies expect technicians to prepare various reports. A knowledge of computers and programs such as Microsoft Word and Excel can make a technician a valuable asset to the pharmacy. Because all pharmacies have integrated computers into their ordering, filling, and documentation procedures, technicians must be computer savvy.

Inventory Management

The task of ordering stock is the responsibility of a specific person in the pharmacy, although everyone should know how to order stock when necessary. Ordering stock, returning expired or damaged stock, and handling recalled items are duties in which pharmacy technicians should be competent. This skill is normally taught on the job because each pharmacy has its own way of handling stock inventory. An important aspect of an inventory technician is the storage requirements of the medications that arrive in the pharmacy. For more information on this topic, refer to Chapter 13.

Tech Note!

Technology is constantly changing! A technician must continually update and improve his or her computer skills to remain a valuable pharmacy team member.

Inpatient Setting Requirements

Inpatient pharmacy usually refers to pharmacies located in hospitals or institutions in which patients stay overnight or longer, depending on the procedures they require. Most departments in a hospital have medications and supplies that are specific to their department. These are supplied by the inpatient pharmacy. Therefore inpatient pharmacies traditionally have a wider range of stock than outpatient pharmacies, so that they can provide all the supplies required by each department. For example, the labor and delivery unit stocks a large amount of the drug oxytocin (which induces labor), whereas the intensive care unit and coronary care unit require a wide variety of cardiac medications in their stock areas. The cancer units may stock large amounts of morphine and other analgesics, and the pediatrics department stocks many drugs in liquid form for children. Inventory control of these areas is just one of the responsibilities of an inpatient pharmacy technician.

Other important tasks include preparing intravenous (IV) medications and **hyperalimentation** products (ie, total parenteral nutrition [TPN]) and performing nonsterile compounding of ointments and creams. The pharmacy loads patient medication drawers and/or automated dispensing systems that allow nurses to access medications. Various individuals in the health care institution are responsible for proper documentation of controlled substances and floor stock disposition; however, the inpatient pharmacy oversees the process. (For more information on hospital job descriptions and competency requirements, see Chapter 9.)

In addition to knowing the various drugs, strengths, and dosage forms, the technician must be able to immediately and appropriately react when emergency (stat) orders are received by the pharmacy. The dynamics of an inpatient pharmacy can fluctuate minute to minute, depending on the flow of patients into and out of the hospital. "Stat" doses are to be delivered within 15 minutes or less to the area requesting them, such as the emergency department, operating room, intensive care unit, or cardiac care unit. This duty often includes preparing IV solutions (Fig. 3.1).

> ### ■ Tech Note!
>
> The bottom line when working in any area of pharmacy is this: always make sure the pharmacist has checked all drugs and/or devices before they leave the pharmacy. If this step is taken, the technician is working within his or her scope of practice and fewer mistakes will occur.

Another aspect of the inpatient pharmacy is the preparation of unit dose medications (see Chapter 11), which are widely used in many hospital settings. Medications need to be repackaged because either (1) the drug companies do not have the medication available in unit dose or (2) the hospital has chosen to prepare its own unit dose medication for cost-saving reasons.

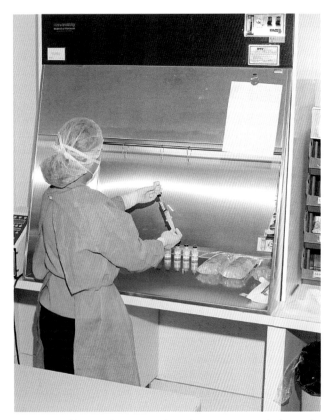

FIG. 3.1 Room for preparing intravenous solutions for inpatients.

◉ Scenario Checkup 3.2

Olivia joins the National Pharmacy Technician Association (NPTA). She visits the organization's website regularly. She notices many job opportunities in the hospital setting. Olivia finds that the beginning pay scale is often higher for the hospital pharmacy technician. She wonders whether she should explore this career avenue. What information and advice would you give her about this possible career move?

The following are common duties, roles, and responsibilities of technicians working in a hospital, nursing home, or other inpatient facility. Most inpatient pharmacy technicians who are interested in the following areas in pharmacy receive additional on-the-job training to prepare them for these additional tasks.

- *Inventory technician:* Orders all stock, handles billing, talks to drug representatives, and may be responsible for ordering lowest cost items.
- *Robot filler:* Many pharmacies are installing robots to fill patient medication drawers each day. Technicians must be trained to load these million-dollar mechanical robots and to keep them running smoothly.
- *IV technician:* Interprets orders and prepares all **parenteral medications**, in both large and small volumes, including controlled substance drips, **total parenteral nutrition (TPN)**, products, insulin drips, and any other special-order intravenous or intramuscular drugs.
- *Chemotherapy technician:* Receives orders and prepares all chemotherapeutic agents and their adjunct medications, such as antiemetics.
- *Anticoagulant technician:* Assists the anticoagulant pharmacist in contacting patients when patient follow-up is necessary or the patient's anticoagulation medication (eg, warfarin) or dosage needs to be changed.
- *Technician verifiers:* As a part of the tech-check-tech program, this specially trained technician checks the work of other technicians, including filling patient cassettes (plastic containers) and preparing floor stock. He or she performs the final verification of medication orders and identifies orders on a routine basis that need the pharmacist's intervention to improve the administrative experience.
- *Clinical technician:* Assists the clinical pharmacist with tracking patients' medications. The clinical technician may compile important data (eg, patient demographics, medication records, laboratory results) that the pharmacist needs to monitor and evaluate patient outcomes or the appropriateness of drug therapies or to monitor formulary compliance.
- *Pharmacy informatics analyst:* This specially trained technician works with the clinical applications specialists to maintain pharmacy software and computers, coordinate hardware and software updates, and work with the pharmacy informatics team (see the Sample Job Description box).
- *Supervisory technician:* Schedules other technicians and may even hire prospective technicians by reviewing their skills and backgrounds.

Pharmacy Informatics Analyst: Pharmacy Technician

If You Are a Pharmacy Informatics Analyst With 3+ Years of Experience, Please Skip!

What You Need for This Position:

- Pharmacy technician licensed in the State of South Carolina
- Experience with Cerner software!
- At least 3 years of experience in electronic medical record (EMR) pharmacy and clinical computer applications, including upgrading and implementing new systems and providing staff education
- Experience with Microsoft Office and project management software
- Knowledge of clinical pharmacy workflow and how computer applications would assist the pharmacy in these workflows

What You'll Be Doing:

- Supporting implementation, integration, and maintenance of technology to optimize medication use process
- Organizing and completing the validation of changes to the pharmacy modules, including testing, coordinating training, functional support, auditing, and documentation
- Identifying computer applications and needs of the pharmacy and clinical departments
- Ensuring that the objectives and goals of the clinicians are communicated and supported by the system and processing improvements that are implemented
- Communicating and coordinating with other clinical systems, applications analysts, and customers about changes and issues that have an impact on pharmacy systems
- Documenting general functional requirements and detailed technical specifications for pharmacy applications and test scripts
- Interacting with customers through various phases of implementation and maintenance
- Monitoring industry trends and technology advancements as they apply to the pharmacy and medication processes
- Coordinating problem resolution with support services and vendors
- Working closely with financial areas to modify and update charges
- Assisting with investigating and responding to billing and charge audits
- Producing reports as requested
- Maintaining **confidentiality** of records

What's In It for You:

- Competitive salary with a comprehensive benefits package
- Solid paid time off package, including personal time, sick time, and vacation time
- Offers extended illness bank, education and training, tuition reimbursement
- Great work environment!

Tech Note!

Did you know that technicians can work in the oncology field? Oncology pharmacy technicians assist pharmacists in caring for patients with various types of cancer. Typical duties include preparing chemotherapy IV admixtures, maintaining safety data sheet (SDS) information, calculating correct dosage volumes, and making sure that all guidelines for the handling of hazardous materials are followed. Oncology technicians work closely with patients and the pharmacist to provide optimal care. Job requirements include a high school diploma with a minimum of 2 years of experience in a pharmacy and also IV skills. IV certification is preferred, along with PTCB or NHA certification. In addition, many facilities have specific levels for technicians' responsibilities. The lowest level is tech I, followed by tech II, and then tech III. Each level requires a minimum amount of time spent working in the previous level. This type of structure allows for career advancement and salary increases based on responsibilities. In the community pharmacy, the structure of responsibilities is quite different.

Community (Outpatient) Setting Requirements

Working in an **outpatient pharmacy** or a **community pharmacy** setting can be one of the most difficult tasks in pharmacy because of the close interaction with patients.

This job tests the **communication** skills and stress levels of the technicians who work with the public. The job has a high volume of interaction on the telephone; these technicians register refill prescriptions and answer questions pertaining to various types of insurance coverage. Computer skills are often necessary to find specific patient information and to assist the customer over the phone or in person. Many neighborhood pharmacies fill a high volume of prescriptions daily (Fig. 3.2). It is not uncommon for a midsize pharmacy to fill 300 or more prescriptions a day, answer phone calls, and address patients' problems. In addition to filling prescriptions, the outpatient technician must be able to order stock in a timely manner. Smaller community pharmacies may keep minimal stock because of limited space and the limited variety of drugs prescribed by physicians in the area. The billing of various insurance companies is another skill the outpatient technician must master. This includes understanding the various rules, regulations, and special codes that may accompany each type of prescription claim.

The following list includes descriptions of the jobs performed by outpatient pharmacy technicians, in addition to descriptions of some of the new positions being filled by technicians in community pharmacies. Larger drug companies that are community based also have recognized the positive aspects of hiring technicians to fill certain positions.

- *Insurance billing technician:* This person must know the guidelines of Medicare, Blue Cross, Medicaid, and other

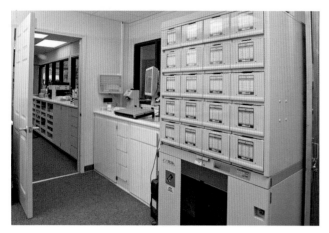

FIG. 3.2 Strip packaging machine.

insurance companies (see sample job description in the following box).

- *Retail technician:* This person must have excellent communication skills, phone skills, and prescription-filling abilities.
- *Inventory/stock technician:* This person must know contacts for fast service, be able to obtain products and drugs as soon as possible, and perform proper billing functions for the pharmacy, including processing returns, recalled drugs, and controlled substances.
- *Technician recruiter:* Some outpatient pharmacies and/or temporary agencies employ these technicians to recruit other technicians into their company.
- *Technician trainer:* Various outpatient pharmacies employ technicians to train newly hired technicians on computer programs and to master other necessary skills relevant to their specific pharmacy.
- *Technician manager:* Many retail pharmacies promote technicians to managerial positions. Their job is to supervise the pharmacy technician staff. The technician manager is responsible for interviewing possible new employees, developing and maintaining work schedules, making sure registrations and certifications are current, and working with the pharmacists to continually train and update the skills of the pharmacy technician employees.

Closed-Door Pharmacy Requirements

A **closed-door pharmacy** is exactly what its name implies. These pharmacies are not open to the public, and they are normally based away from institutional sites (Fig. 3.3). Depending on the types of service the closed-door pharmacy provides, couriers deliver the medications to home health clients, inpatient hospital pharmacies, specialty clinics, and assisted living or long-term care facilities. The job descriptions of home health pharmacy technicians incorporate some of the duties of both inpatient and outpatient pharmacy technicians. The technicians usually are processing prescription medications for patients weekly or monthly, which is similar to an outpatient setting. However, there are no patients, physicians, nurses, or other health care providers in the facility. Closed-door pharmacies are different in that the oral prescriptions usually are packaged differently. Flat cardboard blister packs are prepared by

technicians for use by nurses, who administer the drugs in the assisted living, long-term care, and home health settings (see Chapter 11).

Other technician responsibilities include preparing parenteral medications. Usually a few days' to a 1-month supply is filled each time, instead of only a 24-hour dose of medication. A licensed pharmacist checks all medications filled for a home care patient before they are delivered. Home health nurses may receive supplies from the pharmacy clinic, or the patient's family may pick up or have the supplies delivered. Examples of patients who may receive care at home include patients with kidney failure undergoing peritoneal dialysis and patients in hospice. Nuclear pharmacies are considered closed-door pharmacies and offer a unique work environment for pharmacy technicians. A nuclear pharmacy technician (NPT) is a highly specialized type of pharmacy technician

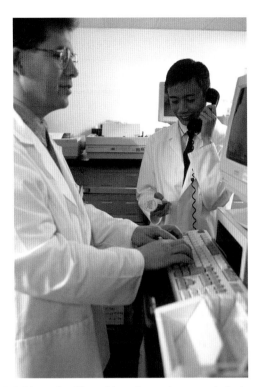

FIG. 3.3 Home health and long-term pharmacy industry setting.

who has specialized training and education in a clinical setting for nuclear pharmacy. An NPT works under the direct supervision of a licensed nuclear pharmacist.

Mail-Order Pharmacy and E-Pharmacy

Mail-order pharmacies and e-pharmacies are growing as the "baby boomers" reach maturity. The need to fill prescriptions expeditiously has increased as more medications have become available to treat commonly acquired illnesses specific to older persons. Large distribution centers process new prescriptions and refills. Technicians are also used in these settings. This is a relatively new area of pharmacy that is growing steadily. This growth is occurring partially because many aging Americans are living longer and are taking multiple medications that can be costly. By using mail order, they often can receive drugs at a lower cost.

In 2004, because of Congress's concern about counterfeit drugs, the major online search engines selected Pharmacy-Checker.com to verify the validity of online pharmacies. In 2005 an investigation by the US Food and Drug Administration (FDA) revealed that many drugs promoted online as "Canadian" were counterfeit and actually originated from other countries. In 2008 Congress passed the Ryan Haight Online Consumer Protection Act, banning online pharmacies from selling controlled substances based on online patient consultations. In 2009 a report from LegitScrip found that 80% to 90% of search engine–sponsored advertisements of online drug pharmacies (verified by PharmacyChecker.com) violated federal and state laws. In 2010 Google removed PharmacyChecker.com as a certifying authority for online pharmacies. Currently online pharmacies can be verified by Verified Internet Pharmacy Practice Sites (VIPPS).

Sample Job Description

Pharmacy Technician (Closed-Door Facility)

Employee type	Full time
Location	Main facility
Job type	Pharmaceutical, science, health care
Experience	1 to 2 years
Date posted	1/22/2018

Certified Pharmacy Technician
Job Details:

We have an opening for a certified pharmacy technician (CPhT) within a closed-door pharmacy. As a member of our team, you'll enjoy a customized approach to your career needs and comprehensive benefits! Join our dynamic team—apply today!

Certified Pharmacy Technician (Closed-Door Facility)
Job Details:

As a CPhT, you will be responsible for maintaining productivity and quality standards and legal and company compliance as you enter new prescriptions and assist in the preparation of prescriptions. Your responsibilities will include:
- Item entry
- Establishing or maintaining patient profiles, including lists of medications taken by individual patients
- Answering telephones, responding to questions or requests
- Assisting customers by answering simple questions, locating items, or referring them to the pharmacist for medication information

Job Requirements:
- 1 to 2 years of recent pharmacy experience
- Must have PTCB certification
- Must have excellent data entry skills
- Able to successfully complete background check and drug screen
- Pay, depending on experience
- Schedule to be determined

Benefits:
- Health insurance with prescription coverage
- Vision/dental plans
- 401(k) and deferred compensation programs
- Cafeteria plans
- Free continuing education (CE)
- Low-cost group health benefits for part-time associates

⊙ Scenario Checkup 3.3

Olivia's pharmacist, Karen, invites her to attend the local pharmacy association meeting as a guest. This group meets once a month, and its membership consists of pharmacists and certified pharmacy technicians. Olivia is so impressed that she joins the group that very night. She enjoys participating in various continuing education sessions and networking with other professionals. What do you see as the benefits Olivia might gain from her association with this group?

Training Programs for the Pharmacy Technician Student

Since 1982, when pharmacy technician accreditation programs were first established, the ASHP has been the leader in providing course curriculum and standards and offering students the best foundation for becoming technicians. Before the formation of technician schools, the ASHP/ACPE's training guidelines and standards were used in hospitals for training pharmacy interns. Accreditation continues to be a voluntary process under the Pharmacy Technician Accreditation Commission, a partnership formed in 2015 between ASHP and ACPE. Program accreditation is given to colleges and technical schools that apply and meet the requirements set by the ASHP/ACPE. An outline of topics for the **ASHP Model Curriculum for Pharmacy Technician Education and Training** is provided in Box 3.5. The ASHP

BOX 3.5 ASHP Model Curriculum for Pharmacy Technician Education and Training

The Key Elements are listed by Standard Categories as they pertain to the Model Curriculum (Standards 1–5).

Standard 1: Personal/Interpersonal Knowledge and Skills

Entry Level

1.1 Demonstrate ethical conduct.
1.2 Present an image appropriate for the profession of pharmacy in appearance and behavior.
1.3 Demonstrate active and engaged listening skills.
1.4 Communicate clearly and effectively, both verbally and in writing.
1.5 Demonstrate a respectful and professional attitude when interacting with diverse patient populations, colleagues, and professionals.
1.6 Apply self-management skills, including time, stress, and change management.
1.7 Apply interpersonal skills, including negotiation skills, conflict resolution, customer service, and teamwork.
1.8 Demonstrate problem-solving skills.

Advanced Level

1.9 Demonstrate capability to manage or supervise pharmacy technicians in matters such as conflict resolution, teamwork, and customer service.
1.10 Apply critical thinking skills, creativity, and innovation.
1.11 Apply supervisory skills related to human resource policies and procedures.
1.12 Demonstrate the ability to effectively and professionally communicate with other health care professionals, payors, and other individuals necessary to serve the needs of patients and practice.

Standard 2: Foundational Professional Knowledge and Skills

Entry Level

2.1 Explain the importance of maintaining competency through continuing education and continuing professional development.
2.2 Demonstrate ability to maintain confidentiality of patient information and understand applicable state and federal laws.
2.3 Describe the pharmacy technician's role, pharmacist's role, and other occupations in the health care environment.

2.4 Describe wellness promotion and disease prevention concepts.
2.5 Demonstrate basic knowledge of anatomy, physiology and pharmacology, and medical terminology relevant to the pharmacy technician's role.
2.6 Perform mathematical calculations essential to the duties of pharmacy technicians in a variety of settings.
2.7 Explain the pharmacy technician's role in the medication-use process.
2.8 Practice and adhere to effective infection control procedures.

Advanced Level

2.9 Describe investigational drug process, medications being used in off-label indications, and emerging drug therapies.
2.10 Describe further knowledge and skills required for achieving advanced competencies.
2.11 Support wellness promotion and disease prevention programs.

Standard 3: Processing and Handling of Medications and Medication Orders

Entry Level

3.1 Assist pharmacists in collecting, organizing, and recording demographic and clinical information for the pharmacists' patient care process.
3.2 Receive, process, and prepare prescriptions/medication orders for completeness, accuracy, and authenticity to ensure safety.
3.3 Assist pharmacists in the identification of patients who desire/require counseling to optimize the use of medications, equipment, and devices.
3.4 Prepare patient-specific medications for distribution.
3.5 Prepare non–patient-specific medications for distribution.
3.6 Assist pharmacists in preparing, storing, and distributing medication products, including those requiring special handling and documentation.
3.7 Assist pharmacists in the monitoring of medication therapy.
3.8 Maintain pharmacy facilities and equipment.
3.9 Use information from safety data sheets (SDS), National Institute of Occupational Safety and Health (NIOSH) Hazardous Drug List, and the United

---

States Pharmacopeia (USP) to identify, handle, dispense, and safely dispose of hazardous medications and materials.

3.10 Describe US Food and Drug Administration product tracking, tracing, and handling requirements.

3.11 Apply quality assurance practices to pharmaceuticals, durable and nondurable medical equipment, devices, and supplies.

3.12 Explain procedures and communication channels to use in the event of a product recall or shortage, a medication error, or identification of another problem.

3.13 Use current technology to ensure the safety and accuracy of medication dispensing.

3.14 Collect payment for medications, pharmacy services, and devices.

3.15 Describe basic concepts related to preparation for sterile and nonsterile compounding.

3.16 Prepare simple nonsterile medications per applicable USP chapters (eg, reconstitution, basic ointments and creams).

3.17 Assist pharmacists in preparing medications requiring compounding of nonsterile products.

3.18 Explain accepted procedures in purchasing pharmaceuticals, devices, and supplies.

3.19 Explain accepted procedures in inventory control of medications, equipment, and devices.

3.20 Explain accepted procedures used in identifying and disposing of expired medications.

3.21 Explain accepted procedures in delivery and documentation of immunizations.

3.22 Prepare, store, and deliver medication products requiring special handling and documentation.

Advanced Level

3.23 Prepare compounded sterile preparations per applicable, current USP chapters.

3.24 Prepare medications requiring moderate- and high-level nonsterile compounding as defined by USP (eg, suppositories, tablets, complex creams).

3.25 Prepare or simulate chemotherapy/hazardous drug preparations per applicable, current USP chapters.

3.26 Initiate, verify, and manage the adjudication of billing for complex and/or specialized pharmacy services and goods.

3.27 Apply accepted procedures in purchasing pharmaceuticals, devices, and supplies.

3.28 Apply accepted procedures in inventory control of medications, equipment, and devices.

3.29 Process, handle, and demonstrate administration techniques and document administration of immunizations and other injectable medications.

3.30 Apply the appropriate medication use process to investigational drugs, medications being used in off-label indications, and emerging drug therapies as required.

3.31 Manage drug product inventory stored in equipment or devices used to ensure the safety and accuracy of medication dispensing.

Standard 4: Patient Care, Quality, and Safety Knowledge and Skills

Entry Level

4.1 Explain the pharmacists' patient care process and describe the role of the pharmacy technician in the patient care process.

4.2 Apply patient and medication safety practices in aspects of the pharmacy technician's roles.

4.3 Explain how pharmacy technicians assist pharmacists in responding to emergent patient situations safely and legally.

4.4 Explain basic safety and emergency preparedness procedures applicable to pharmacy services.

4.5 Assist pharmacist in the medication reconciliation process.

4.6 Explain point-of-care testing.

4.7 Explain pharmacist and pharmacy technician roles in medication management services.

4.8 Describe best practices regarding quality assurance measures according to leading quality organizations.

Advanced Level

4.9 Verify measurements, preparation, and/or packaging of medications produced by other health care professionals.

4.10 Perform point-of-care testing to assist pharmacist in assessing patient's clinical status.

4.11 Participate in the operations of medication management services.

4.12 Participate in technical and operational activities to support the pharmacists' patient care process as assigned.

4.13 Obtain certification as a basic life support healthcare provider.

Standard 5: Regulatory and Compliance Knowledge and Skills

Entry Level

5.1 Describe and apply state and federal laws pertaining to processing, handling, and dispensing of medications, including controlled substances.

5.2 Describe state and federal laws and regulations pertaining to pharmacy technicians.

5.3 Explain that differences exist between states regarding state regulations pertaining to pharmacy technicians and the processing, handling, and dispensing of medications.

5.4 Describe the process and responsibilities required to obtain and maintain registration and/or licensure to work as a pharmacy technician.

5.5 Describe pharmacy compliance with professional standards and relevant legal, regulatory, formulary, contractual, and safety requirements.

5.6 Describe Occupational Safety and Health Administration (OSHA), National Institute of Occupational Safety and Health (NIOSH), and United States Pharmacopeia (USP) requirements for prevention and treatment of exposure to hazardous substances (eg, risk assessment, personal protective equipment, eyewash, spill kit).

Continued

5.7 Describe OSHA requirements for prevention and response to blood-borne pathogen exposure (eg, accidental needle stick, postexposure prophylaxis).

5.8 Describe OSHA Hazard Communication Standard (ie, "Employee Right to Know").

Advanced Level

5.9 Participate in pharmacy compliance with professional standards and relevant legal, regulatory, formulary, contractual, and safety requirements.

5.10 Describe major trends, issues, goals, and initiatives taking place in the pharmacy profession.

See *https://www.ashp.org/_/media/assets/professional-development/technician-program-accreditation/docs/model-curriculum-for-pharmacy-technician-education-training-programs-final-2018.ashx?la=en&hash=1613697B83DEEF83FE59C893985AFD7975A2764.*

designed this model to aid programs that are just starting up, in addition to current programs that are reviewing their curriculum. The ASHP/ACPE used the PTCB's scope of practice analysis data to determine the required outcomes for the programs. There are five new standards defining competencies as entry level and advanced level.

1. Personal/Interpersonal Knowledge and Skills
2. Foundational Professional Knowledge and Skills
3. Processing and Handling of Medications and Medication Orders
4. Patient Care, Quality, and Safety Knowledge and Skills
5. Regulatory and Compliance Knowledge and Skills

According to the current standards revised in 2019, a program can prepare students for entry level in 400 hours or advanced level in 600 hours.

The PTCB's CREST Initiative in 2011 and the NABP task force proposed new pharmacy technician roles and responsibilities. These new roles included medication safety positions, tech-check-tech, providing operational support for clinics, participating in medication reconciliation, and maintaining and optimizing technology. Based on the CREST initiatives and changes in practice, and to help prepare technicians for these expanded roles, beginning 2020, the PTCB requires that all PTCE candidates complete a training program accredited by the ASHP/ACPE. Currently, 47 states regulate technicians and, of those, 21 require PTCE in their requirements. There are also some states that require technicians pass a state-approved certification examination.

Different Levels of Pharmacy Technicians

There are four levels of pharmacy technicians: pharmacy technicians who have no specialized training or credentials and licensed, registered, and certified technicians. Each level has different qualifications, which may differ from state to state.

Pharmacy Technician

The first level of pharmacy technician requires no specialized training. Some states require pharmacy technicians to attain minimum standards such as a high school diploma and others do not.

Licensed Pharmacy Technician

A **licensed pharmacy technician** is licensed by the state BOP. *Licensing* is the process by which an agency of the government grants permission to an individual to engage in a given occupation based on the findings that the applicant has attained the minimum degree of competency necessary to ensure that the public health, safety, and welfare will be reasonably well protected.

Registered Pharmacy Technician

A **registered pharmacy technician** is a pharmacy technician who is registered with the state BOP. *Registration* is the process of making a list or being enrolled in an existing list; registration should be used to help safeguard the public through tracking of the technician workforce and preventing individuals with documented problems from serving as pharmacy technicians. Registration carries no indication or guarantee of the registrant's knowledge or skills. Each state determines whether CE is required of technicians to renew their registration.

Certified Pharmacy Technician

A **certified pharmacy technician** (CPhT) is one who has earned national recognition by a nongovernmental testing agency or association; *certification* indicates that the person has met predetermined qualifications specified by that agency or association (PTCB or NHA). CPhT currently is the main credential available to pharmacy technicians. Certification is an indication of the mastery of a specific core of knowledge. Certified technicians must renew their certification every 2 years and complete at least 20 hours of pharmacy-related CE, which must include 1 hour of pharmacy law and 1 hour of medication safety.

National Certification for Technicians

It should be the goal of every pharmacy technician student to become nationally certified. Certification means that you have passed a national examination demonstrating your knowledge of the skills needed to enter the pharmacy technician profession. Many employers prefer certified technicians and often offer them a higher pay scale. Certification, along with education, leads to better job security and additional employment opportunities.

During the infancy of any profession, there is a lack of regular guidelines and standards, or continuity. Currently five types of verification may be required or pursued by technicians: registration, licensing, certification, associate of science (AS) degree in pharmacy technology, or certificate in pharmacy technology. As outlined previously, registration is regulated by the state and requires that the applicant pass a standard background check, in addition to meeting BOP standards. Licensing also may be required by the state, but it is not currently required in all states. A CPhT earns a certificate that acknowledges that the technician has a basic understanding of all areas of pharmacy, including federal law. Maintaining certification requires CE to keep skills at a minimum level.

Pharmacy technicians work throughout the United States and in all types of pharmacy settings under different rules determined by the individual states, which makes this profession challenging. At some point in the near future, a national minimum standard for the profession must be agreed on across the United States. Although some variations will always exist from state to state, the overall skill level of a pharmacy technician should be a well-known standard. Currently technicians represent a wide range of skill levels, experience, pay, and belief systems. One of the most basic aspects is the lack of a common title. Pharmacy technicians also are known as pharmacy clerks and pharmacy assistants.

Two national groups certify technicians and are recognized by various states: the PTCB and the NHA. The PTCB was founded in 1995 by four organizations with the intent of implementing an examination that would certify that a technician has met a basic skill level (Box 3.6). The four organizations that founded the PTCB are the ASHP, the APhA, the Illinois Council of Health-System Pharmacists (ICHP), and the Michigan Pharmacists Association (MPA).

Table 3.1 presents a comparison of two examinations, the PTCE, offered by the PTCB, and the Examination for the Certification of Pharmacy Technicians (ExCPT), offered by the NHA.

As of December 5, 2013, the PTCB began offering one sample examination consisting of 90 multiple-choice questions to be taken within 110 minutes. The new Practice Test is designed to familiarize candidates with the PTCE. The Practice Test is built according to the same content specifications as the PTCE (updated in January 2020, although the Practice Test questions never appear on an actual examination. The cost for this official practice examination is $29. The PTCB expects to add more practice tests in the future. The actual certification examination, administered by the PTCB, is given at a professional testing center and is computerized. Testing can take place once an appointment is made. The PTCE is a computer-based examination administered at PearsonVue test centers nationwide. The PTCE is also offered online now as a proctored test. It is a 2-hour multiple-choice examination that contains 90 questions (80 scored questions and 10 unscored questions). Each question is shown with four possible answers, only one of which is the correct or best answer. Unscored questions are not identified and are randomly distributed throughout the examination. A candidate's examination score is based on the responses to the 80 scored questions. One hour and 50 minutes is allotted for answering the examination questions and 10 minutes for a tutorial and postexamination

---

BOX 3.6   Goals of the Pharmacy Technician Certification Examination and Eligibility Requirements

Goals

- To work more effectively with pharmacists
- To provide better patient care and service
- To create a minimum standard of knowledge for pharmacy technicians
- To help employers determine the knowledge base of pharmacy technicians

Eligibility Requirements to Take the Examination

- Full disclosure of all criminal and state board of pharmacy registration or licensure actions
- Compliance with all applicable PTCB certification policies
- Passing score on the Pharmacy Technician Certification Exam (PTCE)
- A candidate may be disqualified for PTCB certification on the disclosure or discovery of:
  - Criminal conduct involving the candidate
  - State board of pharmacy registration or licensure action involving the candidate
  - Violation of a PTCB certification policy, including but not limited to the Code of Conduct

The PTCB reserves the right to investigate criminal background, verify candidate eligibility, and deny certification to any individual.

Eligibility Requirements

To be eligible to apply for PTCB CPhT Certification, an applicant must complete one of the following requirements:

Pathway 1: A PTCB-recognized education/training program (or completion within 60 days)

Pathway 2: Equivalent work experience as a pharmacy technician (minimum 500 hours). This alternative path will serve experienced pharmacy technicians who were not in a position to attend a PTCB-recognized education/training program.

In addition to completing a PTCB-recognized education/training program or equivalent work experience, applicants must satisfy the following:

- Full disclosure of all criminal and state board of pharmacy registration or licensure actions
- Compliance with all applicable PTCB certification policies
- Passing score on the Pharmacy Technician Certification Exam (PTCE)

Once certified, certified pharmacy technicians (CPhTs) must report to the PTCB for review any felony conviction, drug- or pharmacy-related violations, or state board of pharmacy action taken against their license or registration at the occurrence and at the time of recertification. Disqualification determinations are made on a case-by-case basis.

Pharmacy Technician Certification Board. Available at: *http://www.ptcb.org* and National Association of Boards of Pharmacy. Available at: *https://www.ptcb.org/ guidebook/ptcb-certified-pharmacy-technician-cpht-program#cpht-eligibility-requirements*.

TABLE 3.1
Comparison of Technician Certification Exams

	ExCPT	PTCE
Organization name	National Healthcareer Association (NHA)	Pharmacy Technician Certification Board (PTCB)
Cost	$117	$129
Length of test	2 hours, 10 minutes 120 multiple-choice questions (100 scored, 20 pretest)	2 hours (5 minutes for tutorial, 1 hour 50 minutes for examination, 5 minutes for postexamination survey) 90 multiple-choice questions (80 scored, 10 unscored)
Frequency of testing	Continuous	Continuous
Testing providers/sites	PSI/Lasergrade	PearsonVue
Results available	Preliminary pass/fail results immediately on examination completion	Pass/fail results immediately on examination completion
Testing requirements	Be at least 18 years of age Have a high school diploma or GED equivalent Have successfully completed an approved pharmacy technician training program within the last 5 years *or* provide evidence of 1200 supervised pharmacy-related work experience in any 1 of the last 3 years Have not been convicted of or pled guilty to a felony Have not had any registration or license revoked, suspended, or subject to any disciplinary action by a state health regulatory board	Completion of a PTCB-recognized education/training program or equivalent work experience Full disclosure of all criminal and state board of pharmacy registration or licensure action Compliance with all applicable PTCB certification policies
Examination content	*Overview and Laws (25%):* Role, scope of practice, general duties, laws and regulations, and controlled substances *Drugs and Drug Products (15%):* Drug classifications, dosage forms, routes of administration, commonly prescribed brand and generic drugs *Dispensing Process (45%):* Prescription and medication order intake and entry, preparation and dispensation of prescriptions, calculations, sterile and nonsterile products, compounding, unit dose, and repackaging *Medication Safety and Quality Assurance (15%):* Best practices, safety strategies for error prevention, medication adherence, safe work environment, analysis of floor stock	Medications (40%) Federal requirements (12.5%) Patient safety and quality assurance (26.25%) Order entry and processing (21.25%)
Accredited by the National Commission for Certifying Agencies (NCCA)	Yes	Yes
Website	*https://www.nhanow.com/certifications/ pharmacy-technician*	*http://www.ptcb.org*
Recertification requirements	Every 2 years, 20 hours CE required, including 1 hour each of pharmacy law and patient safety Cost: $55	Every 2 years (no grace period), 20 hours CE requiring 1 hour each of pharmacy law and patient safety Cost: $49
Reinstatement requirements	Within 12 months of expiration date Cost: $55 for recertification, plus a reinstatement fee	Within 1 year of expiration date Cost: $89

▣ TABLE 3.1
Comparison of Technician Certification Exams—cont'd

	ExCPT	PTCE
Revocation	For false statements, cheating, conviction of a drug-related felony, revocation of registration/licensure by a state, documented violation of the NHA Pharmacy Technician Code of Ethics	For false statements, cheating, conviction of a crime or felony of moral turpitude (including but not limited to drug-related crimes), documented gross negligence, intentional misconduct, or deficiency in knowledge base
Number of technicians certified	N/A	More than 706,500 (as of December 2019)
States that have formally approved test for certification	All states that require certification. All states that either expand the number of permitted pharmacy technicians or the scope of pharmacy technician practice based on certification	50 states

ASHP, American Society of Health-System Pharmacists; *CE,* continuing education; *ExCPT,* Examination for the Certification of Pharmacy Technicians; *PTCE,* Pharmacy Technician Certification Examination.

survey. Calculators and scratch pads are provided by the test center. Scoring is done by an independent group that grades the various areas of pharmacy knowledge. The results are immediately calculated at the end of the examination.

The PTCE content was developed by experts in pharmacy technician practice, based on a nationwide Job Analysis Study completed in February 2012. The PTCB's Certification Council and Board of Governors reviewed the 2012 Job Analysis Study and approved a new blueprint for an updated PTCE, which launched on January 2020.

The PTCE assesses knowledge critical to pharmacy technician practice organized into nine knowledge domains, each with a number of knowledge areas (Box 3.7). It is currently the only pharmacy technician certification examination accepted in all 50 states. For more information, visit the PTCB's website at *http://www.ptcb.org.*

BOX 3.7 Pharmacy Technician Certification Exam Blueprint

Pharmacy Technician Certification Examination (PTCE) Content Outline

Effective January 1, 2020

1. Medication 40%
1.1 Generic names, brand names, and classifications of medications
1.2 Therapeutic equivalence
1.3 Common and life-threatening drug interactions and contraindications (eg, drug-disease, drug-drug, drug-dietary supplement, drug-laboratory, drug-nutrient)
1.4 Strengths/dose, dosage forms, routes of administration, special handling and administration instructions, and duration of drug therapy[a]
1.5 Common and severe medication side effects, adverse effects, and allergies
1.6 Indications of medications and dietary supplements
1.7 Drug stability (eg, oral suspensions, insulin, reconstitutables, injectables, vaccinations)[a]
1.8 Narrow therapeutic index (NTI) medications
1.9 Physical and chemical incompatibilities related to nonsterile compounding and reconstitution
1.10 Proper storage of medications (eg, temperature ranges, light sensitivity, restricted access)
2. Federal requirements 12.5%
2.1 Federal requirements for handling and disposal of nonhazardous, hazardous, and pharmaceutical substances and waste

2.2 Federal requirements for controlled substance prescriptions (ie, new, refill, transfer) and DEA controlled substance schedules[a]
2.3 Federal requirements (eg, DEA, FDA) for controlled substances (ie, receiving, storing, ordering, labeling, dispensing, reverse distribution, take-back programs, and loss or theft of)
2.4 Federal requirements for restricted drug programs and related medication processing (eg, pseudoephedrine, risk evaluation and mitigation strategies [REMS])[a]
2.5 FDA recall requirements (eg, medications, devices, supplies, supplements, classifications)
3. Patient safety and quality assurance 26.25%
3.1 High-alert/risk medications and look-alike/sound-alike [LASA] medications
3.2 Error prevention strategies (eg, prescription or medication order to correct patient, Tall Man lettering, separating inventory, leading and trailing zeros, bar code usage, limit use of error-prone abbreviations)
3.3 Issues that require pharmacist intervention (eg, drug utilization review [DUR], adverse drug event [ADE], OTC recommendation, therapeutic substitution, misuse, adherence, postimmunization follow-up, allergies, drug interactions)[a]
3.4 Event reporting procedures (eg, medication errors, adverse effects, and product integrity, MedWatch, near miss, root-cause analysis [RCA])

Continued

BOX 3.7   Pharmacy Technician Certification Exam Blueprint—cont'd

3.5   Types of prescription errors (eg, abnormal doses, early refill, incorrect quantity, incorrect patient, incorrect drug)[a]

3.6   Hygiene and cleaning standards (eg, handwashing, personal protective equipment [PPE], cleaning counting trays, countertop, and equipment)

4.   Order entry and processing 21.25%

4.1   Procedures to compound nonsterile products (eg, ointments, mixtures, liquids, emulsions, suppositories, enemas)[a]

4.2   Formulas, calculations, ratios, proportions, allegations, conversions, Sig codes (eg, b.i.d., t.i.d.,

roman numerals), abbreviations, medical terminology, and symbols for days supplied, quantity, dose, concentration, dilutions[a]

4.3   Equipment/supplies required for drug administration (eg, package size, unit dose, diabetes supplies, spacers, oral and injectable syringes)[a]

4.4   Lot numbers, expiration dates, and National Drug Code (NDC) numbers[a]

4.5   Procedures for identifying and returning dispensable, nondispensable, and expired medications and supplies (eg, credit return, return to stock, reverse distribution)

[a]Some or all of this statement reflects calculation-based knowledge.
DEA, US Drug Enforcement Agency.
PTCE Content Outline Effective January 1, 2020, v1.3, November 2018. *https://www.ptcb.org/lib24watch/files/pdf/168.*

The National Healthcareer Association

The NHA is accredited by boards of the National Commission for Certifying Agencies (NCCA) and the National Association of Chain Drug Stores (NACDS). (For more information about the NHA, visit *http://www.nhanow.com.*) The examination administered by the NHA is called ExCPT and is given throughout the country at various proctored testing sites. The NHA offers two 50-question sample examinations to practice online, at $25 each. One covers just math, and the other covers various areas of pharmacy. Currently ExCPT certification is not recognized in all 50 states. Technicians should check with their individual state BOPs and employers to determine which certifications are accepted.

Specialty Certifications

One of the recommendations of the 2011 CREST summit involved the creation of specialty pharmacy technician certifications. The PTCB Board of Governors is focused on ensuring that the PTCB program prepares CPhTs for the integral roles they play in supporting pharmacists in all practice settings. Currently the **National Pharmacy Technician Association (NPTA)** offers three specialty certification programs for technicians who want to enhance their skills and marketability: Sterile Products IV certification, Compounding certification, and Chemotherapy certification. To learn more about the PTCB, visit the website at *http://www.ptcb.org.*

⊙ Technician Profile

Avery is a lead controlled substance pharmacy technician at a Veterans Health Administration hospital. He has worked in the pharmacy for 5 years. Controlled substance distribution is a highly visible and sensitive area for the facility. Avery's position requires an individual who is willing to accept increased responsibility and at the same time pay close attention to details. Most of Avery's duties are performed in the pharmacy vault, setting up controlled substances for dispensing, making appropriate record entries, and reviewing controlled substance administration records. Avery is expected to maintain a high degree of accurate productivity and performance while being extremely sensitive to the contribution to total patient care. He checks in shipments of drugs and supplies, verifies the accuracy of those shipments, and ensures the proper storage of all items. All of Avery's activities are supervised by the pharmacy operations manager and the controlled substance pharmacist on duty.

Continuing Education

Technicians who meet the requirements of national certification may use the initials *CPhT* on their identification tag, indicating that they are a CPhT. To maintain their certification, they must earn CE credits. All valid CE credits must be approved by the ACPE, which is indicated on each CE course. ACPE accredits CE courses for both pharmacists and pharmacy technicians. Although technicians can currently take CE courses meant for pharmacists, the PTCB requires that all 20 hours needed for recertification must be pharmacy technician–specific CE credits. The letter P indicates that the CE course is designed for pharmacists, whereas a T indicates that the course is for technicians. In addition to the two levels of CE courses (ie, P and T), current courses may have 05 added to their name; this indicates that the CE course covers a patient safety topic. CE credits can be obtained through pharmacy organizations that offer free CE to members, journals that include CE units, and online webinars or traditional seminars. CE is less expensive for association members, and many drug companies offer free CE units to pharmacists and technicians. Independent pharmacists and other small businesses offer low-cost CE credit courses on the Internet (Table 3.2).

Currently more than one-third of jurisdictions have CE requirements for technicians to maintain their licensing, certification, or registration. In late 2011 the CPE Monitor was launched as a collaborative effort by the NABP and the ACPE. It provides an electronic system for pharmacists and pharmacy technicians to track their CPE credits. It also

TABLE 3.2
Examples of Continuing Education Websites for Technicians

CE Websites	Online CE	Live/Live Webinar CE	Cost[a]
http://www.uspharmacist.com	X		Free CE courses available
http://www.rxschool.com	X	X	Free CE courses available
http://www.powerpak.com	X		Free CE courses available
http://www.freece.com	X	X	Free CE courses available
http://www.pharmacytechnician.org	X	X	Free CE courses available for members
http://www.pharmacytechce.org	X	X	Free CE courses available for members

[a]Many programs are available at no charge; occasionally, fee-based programs also may be available, depending on the session provider.

CE, Continuing education.

offers state BOPs the opportunity to electronically authenticate the CPE units completed by their licensees, rather than requiring pharmacists and technicians to submit their proof of completion statements on request or for random audits. Requirements for each state vary; technicians should contact their state BOPs for information on CPE reporting requirements. In the future, this information may flow from CPE Monitor to the PTCB. The NABP e-profile can be completed by the pharmacist and/or technician at that organization's website *(http://www.nabp.net)*. Once the e-profile has been established, an NABP ID is issued, which is used to register with the CPE Monitor. The pharmacist and/or technician gives the ID to the provider when completing a CPE activity.

Tech Note!

Many employers may encourage certification and formally recognize achievement. Some pharmacy technicians may receive a raise in pay or expanded career responsibilities after completion of the Pharmacy Technician Certification Exam.

Box 3.8 lists both the qualifications and common duties of pharmacy technicians as established by the PTCB.

According to current statistics, there are more than 484,039 PTCB-certified technicians nationwide. Many states are beginning to recognize the importance of certification to guarantee that the technicians hired are competent in all

BOX 3.8 Common Job Duties and Requirements for Pharmacy Technicians

Job Duties

The following list represents the responsibilities expected of pharmacy technicians, depending on the pharmacy setting and the technician's scope of practice.
- Assist in inpatient dispensing
- Assist in outpatient dispensing
- Assist in purchasing and billing
- Assist patients in dropping off and picking up prescriptions
- Assist pharmacist in labeling and filling prescriptions
- Compound large volumes of intravenous mixtures
- Compound oral solutions, ointments, and creams
- Compound total parenteral nutrition (TPN) solutions
- Enter prescriptions into the computer
- Order medications
- Prepackage bulk medications
- Prepare chemotherapeutic agents
- Prepare intravenous mixtures
- Prepare medication inventories
- Schedule and maintain workflow
- Screen calls for pharmacists
- Verify that customer receives the correct prescription or prescriptions
- Work with insurance carriers to obtain payment and refilling authority

Knowledge, Skills, Training, and Education

State practice acts and employer policies determine training and education requirements. The following are some commonly desired characteristics.
- Ability to type 35 words per minute
- Ability to work in teams
- Attention to detail
- Hard-working
- Outgoing
- Pharmacy Technician Certification Board (PTCB) certification (may be desired or mandatory)
- Previous customer service experience
- Professional attitude
- Quick learner
- Strong communication skills
- Understanding of medical terminology and calculations

From Pharmacy Technician Certification Board. Career outlook. Available at: *http://www.ptcb.org/resources/career-outlook#.U7zFiPldVoM.*

areas of pharmacy (see Chapter 14, Discussion of Emily's Act). Employers increasingly are using these credentials as a requirement for hiring technicians.

Opportunities for Technicians

Pharmacies use computers daily; therefore software must be developed for pharmacy personnel. Some pharmacy-related fields require more education in specific areas, such as computers. With the proper educational training (eg, an AS degree or a bachelor of science [BS] degree in computer science), the pharmacy technician is well equipped to write software or provide support. In addition, because many technicians are given the responsibility of training technicians, their expertise may help them write curriculums, articles, and even books for pharmacy technicians. Many vocational schools hire experienced CPhTs to teach students the requirements for becoming competent pharmacy technicians. Completion of such training programs offers different degrees, such as certificates, an associate's degree (associate of arts [AA] or AS), or a bachelor's degree (bachelor of arts [BA] or BS).

Pharmacy technicians also can fill many other, less well-known positions, such as the following nontraditional jobs:

- *Pharmacy business management operators:* Pharmacy business management companies are beginning to realize the importance of knowing not only the trade and generic names of drugs but also their classifications. They are hiring technicians, rather than registered pharmacists, to help pharmacy customers over the phone, which is a cost savings for the company.
- *Computer support technician (Pyxis, SureMed):* Large companies that supply hospitals, community pharmacies, and other facilities with automated medication dispensing systems are employing technicians as support personnel.
- *Software writer:* Some pharmacy software writers are using technicians with additional computer background and/or training to prepare software services. Technicians use their terminology and drug knowledge to create new software programs.
- *Poison control call center operator:* Some poison control centers are using technicians to triage calls coming in to the 911 stations. If the call concerns something life-threatening, technicians transfer it to a pharmacist or poison specialist. If the call is less serious, technicians are authorized to take the call.
- *Nuclear pharmacy technician:* The technician may assist the pharmacist with handling of and preparing physicians' orders for radioactive medications used in diagnosis and treatment.
- *Director/instructor:* CPhTs can oversee technician training programs and/or serve as instructors in schools around the country. Some programs require a BS degree or vocational education teaching credentials.
- *Corporate pharmacy analyst:* Working through an independent management service, a technician surveys the efficiency in all areas of the pharmacy and recommends changes to help the pharmacy operate more productively

and efficiently. The analyst may travel and even work on The Joint Commission standards to prepare pharmacies for inspection.
- *Technician coordinator:* Coordinators oversee as many as 50 to 100 technicians in a large hospital pharmacy. They are responsible for training, regulation compliance, and scheduling of all pharmacy technician personnel.
- *Home infusion pharmacy technician:* Home infusion technicians assist the pharmacist in the preparation of IV solutions, injectable drugs, and enteral nutrition therapy. These medications are dispensed to the patient at home. Technicians process equipment and supply orders and must be knowledgeable about vascular access and infusion devices.

In addition to the positions listed, technicians may continue their education and apply for pharmacy school. Many pharmacists were once technicians. New positions are being developed by different types of pharmacies specifically for technicians. For instance, some hospitals are using pharmacy technicians in the anticoagulant clinic setting to assist the pharmacist in obtaining and assessing information on patient compliance, medication dosages, bleeding symptoms, and a patient's general state of health. Other hospitals are employing pharmacy technicians specializing in pharmacy informatics to provide support for their information and automation systems. Although these positions currently may be nontraditional, their numbers are growing. It would not be surprising if these jobs became commonly held positions for future technicians.

EXAMPLES	SETTING
Clinical pharmacy technician	Hospital
Anticoagulant pharmacy technician	Hospital
Program director—pharmacy technician	Vocational/ technical school
Medical billing specialist—pharmacy technician	Health care services
Certified pharmacy technician— loader, driver	Long-term care facility
Implementation pharmacy technician	Pharmacy benefits service
Data entry pharmacy technician	Institutional pharmacy

Incentive Programs

Pharmacies sometimes have an incentive program for employees who want to further their careers in pharmacy. Many pharmacists who began their careers as technicians have used this company benefit to their advantage. Many pharmacy employers provide incentives to their technicians for returning to school and becoming a pharmacist. They may reimburse tuition costs or give pay incentives for agreeing to be employed by the pharmacy a certain number of years on graduation from pharmacy school. Whether a company supports and partly funds a school program is something a prospective employee should consider when inquiring about a pharmacy position.

As the geriatric age group increases over the next decades, so will the need for qualified medical personnel. Pharmacy technicians are very knowledgeable about the challenges and benefits that pharmacy has to offer. The future of technicians still is being determined, but judging from the advances currently being made by technicians, the only limitations for pharmacy technicians are self-imposed. Many pharmacy companies reimburse their technicians after they pass the PTCB examination. This is more likely to take place in states in which certification is not mandatory but preferred. Attaining higher level skills, including becoming a CPhT, opens more doors for technicians in pharmacy.

Professional Technician Associations

There are many pharmacy associations that technicians can join (Table 3.3). Each association has requisite yearly dues, and each has different benefits. These organizations offer CE programs and regular conferences or seminars. The following sections give a brief history of each of the national associations. Throughout history it has become clear that professions that form associations provide their participants with an avenue to make changes and advance their careers.

It is important that pharmacy technicians not only join pharmacy associations to keep abreast of new information but also that they become active participants. Benefits of association membership include perks such as free CE courses and access to journals; opportunities to attend local, state, and national conventions; and numerous networking possibilities. Association membership is an excellent way for a technician to advance his or her career and form lifelong friendships with pharmacy colleagues.

American Pharmacists Association

The APhA, the oldest and largest pharmacist association, was founded in 1852. Members, including pharmacists, technicians, pharmacy students, scientists, and other interested parties, participate in conferences and discussions on pharmacy issues around the world. The association holds annual meetings, which offer opportunities for CE courses and networking. The APhA also participates in the formation of several important government policies, such as Medicare Part D. Technicians can join their local state pharmacists' association in addition to this national organization.

TABLE 3.3

Organizations and Associations for Pharmacy Technicians[a]

Technicians	Pharmacists	Educators	Annual Fees	Special Category/ Technician Student Fees	Journal or Magazine Included	Website
ASHP (has state chapters)						
Yes	Yes	N/A	$69 with journal[b]	No/state chapters vary	AJHP Journal[c]	http://www.ashp.org
APhA (has state chapters)						
Yes	Yes	N/A	$67 with journal[b]	No	JAPhA Journal[c]	http://www.pharmacist. com
AAPT						
Yes	Yes	N/A	$40	$10	None	http://www.pharmacytechnician. com
NPTA						
Yes	No	N/A	$69	No	Today's Technician	http://www.pharmacytechnician. org
NCPA						
Yes	Yes	N/A	$75	No	None	http://www.ncpanet.org
SEPhT						
Yes	Yes	Yes	FREE	N/A	N/A	http://www.thesepht.org

[a]Updated August 2016.

[b]Fees may vary based on state.

[c]Included for fee.

AAPT, American Association of Pharmacy Technicians; *APhA,* American Pharmacists Association; *ASHP,* American Society of Health-System Pharmacists; *N/A,* not applicable; *NCPA,* National Community Pharmacists Association; *NPTA,* National Pharmacy Technician Association; *PTEC,* Pharmacy Technician Education Council; *SEPhT,* The Society for the Education of Pharmacy Technicians.

American Society of Health-System Pharmacists

In 1942, 154 members of the (AphA) separated to form the American Society of Hospital Pharmacists. In 1945 this group established focus areas on minimum standards of pharmaceutical services in the hospital and education about new techniques and medications. The group expanded over time and in 1950 published its journal, *Mirror of Hospital Pharmacy*. After the group received feedback from more than 3000 hospitals, the journal began to publish recommendations to enhance the development of hospital pharmacy. In 1995 it expanded its outreach to areas other than hospital pharmacists. Under its new name, the ASHP, the association now includes other pharmacy settings, such as home care and ambulatory care; however, most of its members are pharmacists based in hospital settings. Since 2015 PTAC, a collaboration of ASHP and ACPE, has been responsible for the accreditation of pharmacy technician education and training programs. A new accreditation standard for pharmacy technician education and training programs took effect on January 15, 2015. The new standard was updated with 46 goals and objectives, to meet the future needs of practice, to protect the public, to serve as a guide for the development of pharmacy technician education and training programs, and to provide criteria for evaluation of new and established programs. The ASHP allows technicians to join, and local state chapters also are available.

American Association of Pharmacy Technicians

The **American Association of Pharmacy Technicians (AAPT),** the first pharmacy technician association, was established in 1979. It has always been managed by volunteer pharmacy technicians and participates in the advancement of pharmacy technicians. Its membership includes pharmacy technicians, pharmacists, and pharmacy students. The AAPT is a not-for-profit association that serves technicians' interests through the work of the executive board, committees, national office, and local chapters. The AAPT is very involved with the changes occurring in the pharmacy technician field. It offers CE programs and a career center to help technicians with their job searches.

National Community Pharmacists Association

The NCPA was founded in 1898 under the National Association of Retail Druggists. Members include pharmacists, pharmacy owners, managers, pharmacy students, and pharmacy technicians. The NCPA represents the professional and proprietary interests of independent community pharmacists. The association is dedicated to the continued growth and prosperity of the independent pharmacies in the United States. The NCPA is governed by elected officers, a chief executive officer, and a board of directors. NCPA committees include technology and communications, compounding, long-term care, national legislation and government affairs, and pharmacy payment programs. The NCPA works on many issues affecting the independent community pharmacy, including health care reform, Medicare Part D, pharmacy benefits manager transparency, and stopping legislation promoting mandatory mail-order prescription filling.

National Pharmacy Technician Association

The NPTA was started in 1999 in Houston. The next year, the association published its magazine, *Today's Technician,* and had its first convention. In 2004 the NPTA gained the approval of the ACPE and began offering its own CE courses. In 2005 the NPTA joined the Committee of European Pharmacy Technicians (CEPT), a European technicians' association. The NPTA also is part of an advocacy group that works to advance education and acknowledgment for technicians. The association's strategic vision includes the following:

- ACPE-accredited CE requirements
- Mandatory competency-based examinations
- Mandatory registration
- A pharmacy technician representative on each state BOP
- Standardized formal education and training requirements

The association is composed of pharmacy technicians from a variety of practice settings, such as retail, nuclear, hospital, independent, formal education, long-term care, and mail-order pharmacies. The NPTA is dedicated to advancing the value of pharmacy technicians in pharmaceutical care.

The Society for the Education of Pharmacy Technicians

The Society for the Education of Pharmacy Technicians (SEPhT) was formed by technician educators in 2011. Membership is free for educators and students. A comprehensive website offers a host of technician information such as safety, current drug information, success stories and articles, and links to other pharmacy and training-related information and educational simulation products. The mission includes a focus on enhancing the knowledge base of technicians and providing the professional development tools and simulated supplies for those educating and those practicing in the field of pharmacy.

Professionalism in the Workplace

Pharmacy is an important profession, and pharmacy technician is a great career. As with many things in life, you get out of it what you put into it. If you put 100% effort into your career as a technician, you can achieve a great deal of satisfaction.

A *profession* is a job, occupation, or line of work that becomes a career; a profession is founded on specialized training. **Professionalism** is conforming to the right principles of conduct (work ethics) as accepted by others in the profession. It takes time, hard work, and consistency to be respected as a professional. Because of the increasing depth of education and training that a pharmacy technician needs, today's technicians are the first generation of pharmacy technicians who have been considered professionals. If they do not meet certain responsibilities, they will remain

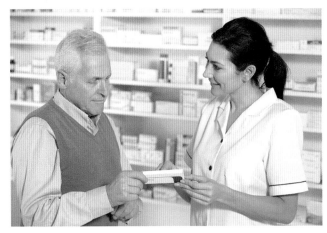
FIG. 3.4 Technician helping a customer.

pharmacy assistants and not professionals in the eyes of other health care professionals.

One of the measures of professionalism is projecting the correct behavior; this includes your attitude and interpersonal skills, in addition to your level of competence. Pharmacy technicians work daily with patients, pharmacists, physicians, and nurses (Fig. 3.4). How technicians conduct themselves in various situations reveals their professionalism and their personal maturity.

In a 2008 survey of more than 2000 businesses in the state of Washington, employers said entry-level workers in a variety of professions were lacking in several areas, including problem solving, conflict resolution, and critical observation. These employers came up with a list of six soft skills that every employee needs.

1. *Communication skills:* These skills include the ability to write a coherent memo, persuade others with a presentation, or simply be able to explain to a co-worker what one needs.
2. *Teamwork and collaboration:* Employers need people who can work together toward a common goal, who can easily transition from leader to follower, and who can meet assigned deadlines.
3. *Adaptability:* This skill focuses on the employee's ability to embrace learning and adapt to the changing needs of the organization.
4. *Problem solving:* Employers expect workers to face problems with a positive attitude. They want people who can explain a dilemma and how it should be approached, involving team members in devising a solution that provides measurable results.
5. *Critical observation:* This skill involves going beyond the ability to collect and manipulate data; it includes the ability to analyze and interpret it.
6. *Conflict resolution:* This skill entails being able to negotiate win-win solutions to serve the best interests of the company and the individuals involved.

According to the 2013 Professionalism in the Workplace Study, conducted by the Center for Professional Excellence (CPE) at York College of Pennsylvania, a large portion of the study's participants thought that the professionalism of new employees had decreased over the previous 5 years. Research points to the generation gap between hiring managers and human resources (HR) professionals and the younger entry-level employees as a possible cause. This gap seems to center around the definition of professional standards, which business leaders and managers do not think should change over time. They think that younger workers should conform to the current standards instead of changing them to match larger societal norms.

The results of the study showed that to be professional in the workplace, an employee should demonstrate the following qualities:
- Ability to remain focused and attentive
- Appropriate appearance
- Communication skills
- Honesty
- Interpersonal skills, including civility
- Punctuality and regular attendance
- Task completion

An unprofessional employee displays the following characteristics:
- A sense of entitlement
- Disrespectful or rude behavior
- Inappropriate appearance
- Poor time management
- Poor work ethic

Based on the research from the CPE study, the following can give a job candidate an edge in getting hired:
- Be committed to doing quality work
- Be prepared for the interview
- Control your on-the-job use of technology
- Learn what it means to be professional
- Remember, appearance matters

Professional Dress

Statistics from the 2013 Professionalism in the Workplace Study show that 80.6% of the respondents thought that appearance has a considerable impact on the probability of a candidate being hired. Appearance and attire were also linked with the public's confidence in an employee's ability to perform his or her job requirements. Pharmacy is predominantly a conservative profession. Dressing professionally includes proper clothing, shoes, and hairstyle. Unnatural hair color, facial jewelry, visible tattoos, or any other feature that draws attention away from your personality should be avoided. Medical personnel should appear to be professional, knowledgeable, and competent. It is important that the pharmacy technician show the public that he or she is professional and does not view the vocation as just a job (Fig. 3.5).

Pharmacy technicians must strive to maintain professional behavior when dealing with customers, pharmacists, and fellow health care workers. A professional is honest and dependable and displays integrity in all situations. Job candidates who understand professionalism have a distinct advantage over those who do not.

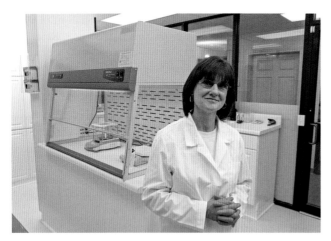

FIG. 3.5 Example of professional dress.

Tech Note!

Each year pharmacy technicians celebrate their profession. National Pharmacy Technician Day is observed on the Tuesday of National Pharmacy Week, which is always the third week of October.

The Resume

One of the first encounters you will have with your future employer is through your resume. Recruiters spend only about 10 seconds reviewing each resume. That is why yours should be concise, structured, and specific. Each resume objective should be tailored to the position for which you are applying. Update it regularly to include recent information pertinent to the current job application. Resumes should be approximately one page long. If possible, list jobs in which you have had customer service experience or those in which you managed yourself or others. These are highly valuable skills that will get you noticed. Because HR managers may not always be familiar with your former employers, it is a good idea to include a hyperlink to the company in the Experience section of your resume. Make sure you can obtain references from your employers at those jobs. Always have references ready on a separate page for your future employer. If you have little or no employment history, focus on your academic qualifications and related skills. Align your achievements with the qualities desired by the hiring organization. Demonstrate your goals and how you will add value to the organization. Seek help in writing your resume and have others look at it to see whether it looks professional (Box 3.9). Larger pharmacy companies may have a standardized format to automate the filing of your resume online. In such cases, it may be helpful to familiarize yourself with the information they request before submitting your application. Do not forget that many hiring managers use social media to search for employees. It is a good idea to include a hyperlink to your LinkedIn profile in the Contact section of your resume.

The Job Search

Job searching has changed drastically over the past several years. Applicants can no longer rely on a generic resume and

cover letter to get the job. Now it is about customization and standing out from the crowd. The following are a few suggestions to help you in today's competitive job market.

1. Search for specific jobs.
   - Online job listings can be difficult to decipher. Try to stick with sites, such as *US.jobs*, that will take you directly to the employer website, and apply for the position in which you are most interested.
2. Be prepared for multiple interviews, including some by Skype or webcam.
   - According to a 2017 *Forbes* article, 6 of 10 recruiters use video interviewing.
3. Contact the hiring manager directly.
   - Use sites such as LinkedIn to find specific contact information.
4. Create and maintain social media profiles.
   - LinkedIn, Twitter, and Facebook can serve as platforms to showcase your accomplishments. Employers are constantly scanning profiles on social media, so be careful what you post. Double-check your spelling and grammar.
5. Apply for numerous positions.
   - Interviewing keeps your skills sharp.
6. Stay positive.
   - A job search can be stressful, with setbacks and rejections. Remember, you have desirable skills to offer, and you will be an asset to any employer. Hiring managers prefer to hire happy people!

Box 3.10 presents websites that can be helpful in the job search.

Why not start your career while in school? Many student technicians are employed as pharmacy clerks. The benefits are endless; working as a pharmacy clerk not only can strengthen and expand the student's knowledge base about drugs but also can provide insight into the business of pharmacy and even a possible future job as a technician.

The Future of Pharmacy Technicians Is Bright!

The role of the pharmacy technician is changing! Technicians of the past focused on task-oriented jobs and could be trained by the employer. Today's technician positions are specialized and highly technical. The demand for educated, certified, and skilled pharmacy technicians is great. According to the Bureau of Labor Statistics *Occupational Outlook Handbook*, the pharmacy technician job market is expected to grow at a rate of 9% between 2014 and 2024, which is much faster than the average for all occupations. A technician who has graduated from an accredited program and is nationally certified will be the preferred hire. Traditional settings, such as the retail or hospital pharmacy, are not the only places you will find technicians working today. There are many other options for those who do not want to work in the traditional roles. For example, pharmacy technicians can be employed by the federal government (eg, Veterans Administration hospitals, prisons, and military pharmacies), quality control offices (repackaging facilities), software companies (pharmacy system software development), and insurance companies (medication consultants). These changes can be positive but challenging as pharmacy technicians take on new and expanded roles. Technicians should be excited about the possibilities the future holds. Advanced roles and certifications provide technicians with specialty roles and higher positions. The outlook for the pharmacy technician is bright!

Do You Remember These Key Points?

- The common responsibilities and competencies technicians need to function in various pharmacy settings
- Nondiscretionary duties and skills pharmacy technicians can perform
- The ASHP model curriculum and how it relates to technician training
- The levels of pharmacy technician status and the requirements of each
- The process involved in obtaining national certification and the benefits for technicians
- The requirements for maintaining national certification after passing the examination
- The advanced pharmacy positions and certifications available to pharmacy technicians
- The types of associations available for pharmacy technicians to join
- The importance of professionalism and networking and how they relate to the job search

⦿ Scenario Follow-Up

As Olivia continues in her independent pharmacy career, she gradually is gaining more responsibilities. She is now able to process prescriptions on the computer. She has learned the inventory ordering system and is involved in processing out-of-date medications. Her communication skills continue to improve, and she is beginning to recognize the customers by name. The pharmacists she works with are very pleased with her progress and professionalism and expect her to continue to excel.

Review Questions

Multiple Choice Questions

1. The pharmacy organization that accredits pharmacy technician education programs is the:
   A. National Pharmacy Technician Association
   B. American Association of Pharmacy Technicians
   C. Pharmacy Technician Accreditation Commission
   D. American Pharmacists Association
2. How often does a nationally certified pharmacy technician (CPhT) have to renew his or her certification?
   A. Yearly
   B. Biannually
   C. Biennially
   D. Every 3 years
3. Which of the following is considered a nondiscretionary duty a pharmacy technician can perform?
   A. Returning expired or damaged stock
   B. Recommending an OTC cold medication
   C. Advising patients about current medications
   D. Changing an order for an IV base
4. Which of the following organizations could revoke a technician's registration?
   A. BOP
   B. ASHP
   C. ACPE
   D. All of the above
5. All pharmacies in their respective states are overseen by:
   A. The National Association of Boards of Pharmacy
   B. Each state's board of pharmacy
   C. Pharmacy managers
   D. Consumer advocacy groups
6. Which of the following would *not* be performed by an inpatient pharmacy technician?
   A. Ordering stock
   B. Accepting payments from patients
   C. Filling medication orders
   D. All of the above would be performed by an inpatient pharmacy technician
7. Which quality is considered a soft skill preferred by employers?
   A. Honesty
   B. Experience
   C. Personality
   D. Adaptability

8. Once nationally certified by the PTCB, a technician must attain _____ CE units in medication safety every 2 years.
   A. 1
   B. 2
   C. 3
   D. 20
9. Which of the following is an example of a closed-door pharmacy?
   A. Children's hospital pharmacy
   B. Nuclear pharmacy
   C. Independent pharmacy
   D. Community pharmacy
10. When preparing a resume, you should:
    A. Have two or three pages to show all of your accomplishments
    B. Add your LinkedIn profile information to the Contact section
    C. Add your references to the bottom of your resume
    D. All of the above

◼ Technician's Corner

Julie is a recent graduate of an accredited pharmacy technician program. She just passed her national certification examination. She has been selected for an interview with a local community pharmacy. Julie has been asked to arrive for the interview with the pharmacist at 1 pm and to bring her resume. Discuss which steps Julie should take to prepare for this interview. How can she demonstrate professionalism and confidence? Julie has a small nose piercing. Should she remove this for the interview? Why or why not?

Bibliography

Academy of Managed Care Pharmacy. White paper on pharmacy technicians 2002: needed changes can no longer wait. *Am J Health Syst Pharm*. 2003;60:37. Available at: PTC-White-paper-2023_06142023.pdf (visanteinc.com).

American Society of Health-System Pharmacists. *Manual for Pharmacy Technicians*. 3rd ed. Bethesda, MD: The Society; 2004.

Gaunt MJ. *Medication safety: Cases of Name Confusion*. Pharmacy Times: June 15, 2010. Available at: pharmacytimes.com.

Harteker LR. *The Pharmacy Technician Companion*. Washington, DC: American Pharmacists Association; 1998.

Institute of Medicine (US) Committee on Quality of Health Care in America. In: Kohn LT, Corrigan JM, Donaldson MS, eds. *To Err is Human: Building a Safer Health System*. Washington, DC: National Academies Press (US); 2000.

Nordenberg T. Make no mistake: medical errors can be deadly serious. *FDA Consumer Magazine*. 2000:1-8.

US Food and Drug Administration. Laws. Available at: http://www.fda.gov.

Western Career College curriculum. Sacramento, Calif: Western Career College. Available at: https://westerncommunitycollege.ca/programs/health-care/pharmacy-assistant/.

Websites Referenced

A brief history of online pharmacy regulations. Available at: http://www.safemedicines.org/online-pharmacy-regulation.html.

Accreditation Council for Pharmacy Education. Available at: http://www.acpe-accredit.org/.

American Society of Healthcare Pharmacists. Model curriculum for pharmacy technician training. Available at: http://www.ashp.org.

Available at: http://jobsearch.about.com/od/resumetips/fl/best-resume-tips-2014.htm.

Available at: http://ptcb.org/docs/get-certified/new_ptce_blueprint.pdf?sfvrsn=6.

Available at: https://www.aacp.org/resource/council-credentialing-pharmacy-ccp.

Available at: http://www.jobs.net/jobs/rx-relief/en-us/job/united-states/pharmacy-technician-closed-door-facility/J3F45879MSBRMNFVYHP/.

Available at: http://www.linkedin.com/jobs2/view/9132852.

Available at: https://nabp.pharmacy/programs/cpe-monitor/.

Available at: http://www.ycp.edu/media/york-website/cpe/York-College-Professionalism-in-the-Workplace-Study-2013.pdf.

Center for Drug Evaluation and Research. Available at: http://www.fda.gov/cder.

Live Remote Proctoring Now Available for the ExCPT Pharmacy Tech Certification Exam. Available at: https://www.pharmacy-times.com/.

Pharmacy Technician Code of Ethics. Available at: https://www.pharmacytechnician.com/.

Pharmacy Technician Career Guide. Available at: http://V-TECS.org.

PTCB announces certification program changes by PTCB staff. Available at: https://www.ptcb.org/news/ptcb-to-change-cpht-program-eligibility-requirements-and-update-exam-in-2020.

CHAPTER 4

Communication and Role of the Technician With the Customer/Patient

Karen Davis

OBJECTIVES

1. Describe the communication skills needed in the delivery of direct patient care in the pharmacy setting.
2. Explain the communication cycle.
3. Identify various nonverbal and verbal communication skills.
4. Describe ways to improve vocal and verbal communication skills.
5. Use proper telephone and cell phone etiquette and describe its guidelines.
6. Describe the importance of written communication skills in today's workplace.
7. Identify communication skills needed to work with special groups of people, such as the terminally ill, non–English-speaking individuals, and hearing-impaired patients.
8. Explain the significance of working as an effective member of a team.
9. Identify ways to eliminate barriers to effective communication.

TERMS AND DEFINITIONS

Attitude A mental disposition or feeling a technician adopts toward customers, co-workers, or duties at work

Channel A means of communication that can be a written message, spoken words, or body language

Communication The ability to express oneself in such a way that one is understood readily and clearly

Compassion A feeling of wanting to help someone who is sick or in trouble

Diplomacy The skill of dealing with others without causing bad feelings

Etiquette An unwritten guideline or rule of behavior

Nonverbal communication Communication using messages or signals and no spoken language

Perception The way a person thinks about or understands someone or something

Tact The ability to do or say things without offending or upsetting other people

Verbal communication The sharing of information by individuals through the use of speech

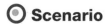

Scenario

Catherine is a lead technician at a local grocery store pharmacy. She is in charge of training newly hired technicians. Catherine and her supervising pharmacist have developed a 4-week program to help the new trainees integrate successfully into the pharmacy workplace. Currently, Catherine is working with Jackson, preparing for his first day on the job. Module one of the 4-week program is titled "Communication." What topics do you expect Catherine to cover with Jackson in this first section?

Communication

Probably one of the most prevalent concerns of pharmacy managers and pharmacists is the need for pharmacy technicians who are competent in the area of communication. **Communication** is the ability to express oneself in such a way that one is understood readily and clearly. Pharmacy technicians communicate daily with co-workers, health care professionals, and customers (Fig. 4.1).

Effective communication skills are critical in achieving optimal patient satisfaction and trust. Virtually all employers consider basic communication abilities a prerequisite to hiring. A competent technician has excellent written and verbal communication skills. In addition, technicians are expected to use skills such as **diplomacy, compassion,** sensitivity, responsibility, **tact,** and patience. Good communication is also important for patient safety. A technician who knows exactly what the patient needs and understands how to communicate is able to assist the person with confidence and accuracy.

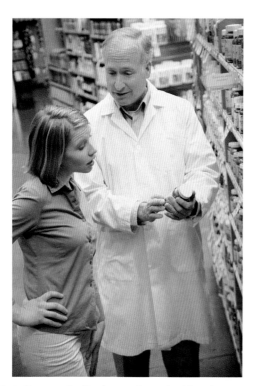

FIG. 4.1 Communication is very important for pharmacy technicians, especially in daily interactions with customers.

The Communication Cycle

The communication cycle involves two or more individuals exchanging information. The cycle consists of a sender, a receiver, a message, various channels of communication, and feedback (Fig. 4.2). The sender is the person who initiates the communication and sends the message across a **channel.** A channel can be written messages, spoken words, or body language. The receiver decodes the message and provides feedback according to his or her understanding of what is being communicated. To provide optimal patient care, pharmacy technicians must have a clear understanding of the communication cycle.

Listening Skills

Active listening is a communication technique in which listeners confirm understanding by restating or summarizing what they have heard in their own words. This helps both parties make sure the same thing is being discussed. Active listening helps keep the focus on the patient. Always remember the **perception** of the communicators when trying to convey a message. Showing empathy and listening are key components of ensuring the person that you are listening and are concerned about what they are saying.

Sometimes just listening to a person is all that is required.

If a customer is angry about a medication, regardless of the problem, just listening can ease the person's frustration. Instead of talking over the person or telling the person that he or she is wrong, try to listen until the person is finished and empathize with the dilemma. Most customers know a problem with a medication is not the fault of the pharmacy technician, but they want to be heard. A professional does not allow himself or herself to be directed by another person's inappropriate behavior. Pharmacy technicians must remember to always behave professionally.

Nonverbal Communications

Nonverbal communication, or body language, is the act of giving or exchanging information without using spoken words.

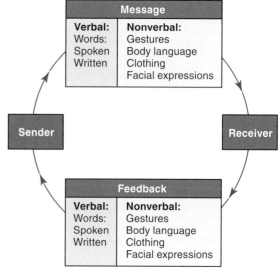

FIG. 4.2 Communication cycle.

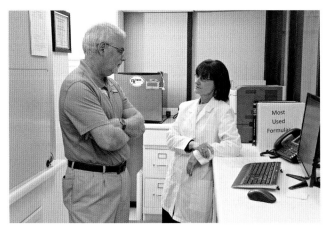

FIG. 4.3 Negative messages are too easily conveyed through nonverbal communication.

BOX 4.1 Example of Negative Body Language

Ms. Lehman walks up to the counter to have her prescription filled and asks whether it can be done within 5 minutes because her bus will be leaving. John, the pharmacy technician, rolls his eyes and shakes his head in disbelief, wondering why patients think they should never have to wait. He turns and walks away without saying a word.

Alternative response: John shows concern for Ms. Lehman and tells her that her prescription will be filled as soon as possible. John can ask the pharmacist to please fill the prescription as quickly as possible.

Procedure 4.1

Recognizing and Responding to Nonverbal Communications

Goal

To be able to recognize nonverbal communication and respond to it in a professional manner.

Equipment and Supplies

- Various statements that can be communicated in a nonverbal manner

Procedural Steps

1. Select a classmate as a partner who will play the role of a patient for this procedure. Use patients of varying cultural backgrounds and ability to communicate in English while practicing the procedure.
   PURPOSE: To practice nonverbal communication with a patient whose responses will not be predictable.
2. Take turns role-playing each nonverbal cue provided.
3. Use appropriate body language and other nonverbal skills in communicating with patients, family, and staff.
   PURPOSE: To make certain that the nonverbal communication sends the same message as the verbal communication.
4. Determine whether the receiver understood the message correctly.
   PURPOSE: To send a nonverbal message that is understood by the receiver.
5. Analyze communications in providing appropriate responses and feedback.
   PURPOSE: To continually improve the communications process among health care professionals, other staff members, and patients.

Everyone communicates on a daily basis; however, rarely do we take a step back and evaluate how effectively we are communicating. One important aspect of communication is facial expressions. The old phrase "actions speak louder than words" is true. When technicians are working closely with customers in the pharmacy setting or with co-workers, it is important that they maintain a caring but professional attitude at all times.

Most people make a judgment of others within the first 30 seconds of meeting. This is also true in the pharmacy setting. A professional should not bring his or her outside personal problems to work. Stress manifests in various ways, such as frowning, tensing the shoulders, biting one's lip, raising the eyebrows, folding the arms, placing the hands on hips, or other idiosyncrasies. Rolling your eyes or sighing loudly shows impatience and a lack of respect for the customer. If you are counting pills and scowling, the patient may assume you are frustrated. This could keep the person from asking questions or sharing important information (Fig. 4.3). If and when stress begins to transform into this type of body language, it is time to take a step back and maybe a deep breath to help regain focus. If your facial expression is pleasant, the patient will most likely respond in a positive manner. Exhibiting positive body language makes your communication with the patient more effective. The primary goal of pharmacy personnel is to help others, which can be accomplished by being friendly and remaining calm. Facial expressions can show many different emotions, thoughts, and biases. Because you are a pharmacy professional, it is imperative that the only body language you convey is that of a helpful and concerned pharmacy technician.

Box 4.1 presents an example of negative body language. Procedure 4.1 provides an exercise in practicing nonverbal communication.

Verbal Communication

Verbal communication is the sharing of information by individuals through the use of speech.

Verbal communication is an important tool in pharmacy. It is a skill that must be learned and practiced. To be an effective communicator, you must remember that your words and your voice are not always in agreement. Each is a separate entity and can be used to work for or against you. Remember, verbal communication skills have two parts: vocal and verbal.

Vocal Skills: How You Sound

Your voice is a powerful tool that affects the customer or person to whom you are talking. Words alone do not necessarily convey your meaning or feelings; the inflection (pitch), tone, speed, and volume add multitudes of information that is being picked up by the listener. As an example of the use of inflection, in the following statements, stress the capped word while you say each sentence to a partner, and notice your partner's response to each statement.

- IF you'll wait a moment, I'll get the information you need.
- If you'll WAIT a moment, I'll get the information you need.
- If you'll wait a moment, I'll get the information you need.

As you can see, or hear in this case, the way in which you emphasize a word in a sentence makes a big difference in how it is perceived.

How to improve your vocal communication skills

- Try not to talk using the same tone all the time (monotone voice) because it can lose the listener's interest and attention.
- Do not talk too rapidly to a customer; the customer may not be able to follow what you are saying.
- Talking very slowly indicates you do not know the answer; if the latter is the case, contact the pharmacist.
- People prefer a lower pitched voice; high, squeaky tones can annoy the listener, and they can result in the listener taking you less seriously.
- A loud or extremely soft voice can annoy and irritate people; speak in a medium tone of voice so you can be heard.
- Articulation is extremely important; mumbling, mispronouncing words, or using slang is one of the fastest ways of sounding unprofessional. Speak in clear, crisp words and sentences.

Verbal Skills: What You Say

Words are also a strong tool that can calm or escalate a situation between you and a customer or patient. Using intimidating words, belittling a person's opinion, or leaving the customer feeling embarrassed, angry, or sad may alienate the patient and result in a loss of business.

Tech Note!

Remember, customers can choose where they want to fill their prescriptions. Many choices are available to today's consumer. If patients can essentially get the same medication at numerous pharmacies, what is the deciding factor in where they take their business? When all things are equal, such as price and availability, the pharmacy staff is what makes the difference. People want to shop where they receive warm, friendly service and where the staff knows their name. Technicians can be that difference! As author and motivational speaker John C. Maxwell said, "People don't care how much you know, until they know how much you care!"

Be careful of the words you use while addressing a customer. If the customer is definitely wrong, do not tell the person that he or she is wrong. Instead, after carefully listening to the customer, point out the misconception to let the customer know that you understand how this point could be easily confused. Determine which of the scenarios in the following boxes is most appropriate.

Option 1

Customer: When I called earlier, they said the prescriptions would be done by noon; now you tell me they aren't ready. Why do you guys lie like that?
Technician: We don't lie; you probably called in late.
Customer: Oh no; I think I called it in around 10 am.
Technician: Well, either way, you'll have to wait.
Customer: Let me talk to your manager.

Option 2

Customer: When I called earlier, they said the prescriptions would be done by noon; now you tell me they aren't ready. Why do you guys lie like that?
Technician: I'm sorry; I know the automated system said they would be done by noon, but that's for prescriptions that were called in by a certain time. Did you call in your prescription before 9 am?
Customer: Oh no; I think I called it in around 10 am.
Technician: That's okay; let me go take a look to see whether we can get your prescription ready for you as soon as possible.
Customer: Thanks.

How to improve your verbal skills

- Reading increases your vocabulary.
- Take a course in communication.
- Several types of communication aids are available that you can use to increase your vocabulary, such as workshops, websites, and pharmacy technician organizational resources.
- Always try to put yourself in the customer's position when talking to him or her. Often the customer is sick or in pain and cannot control his or her emotions; however, you can control yours. Even if the customer is wrong, arguing will not help the situation; instead, it will energize the discussion with negativity. However, if a customer is abusive, the technician should not engage in this type of communication and should notify the pharmacist in charge immediately. If the pharmacist cannot rectify the problem, security is normally called, and the patient is escorted from the premises. Procedure 4.2 provides an exercise for practicing verbal communication skills.

Optimize Your Communication

The following are a few tips to optimize your communication abilities:

1. *Use open-ended questions.* This gets you more than just a "yes" or "no" answer. It shows the patient that the conversation is not just one way and that you care about his or her perspective. If you can get a dialogue going with

Procedure 4.2

Recognizing and Responding to Verbal Communications

Goal

To be able to recognize verbal communication and respond to it in a professional manner.

Equipment and Supplies

• Various patient scenarios

Procedural Steps

1. Select a classmate as a partner who will play the role of a patient for this procedure. Use patients of varying cultural backgrounds and ability to communicate in English while practicing the procedure.
   PURPOSE: To practice communication with a patient whose responses will not be predictable.
2. Take turns role-playing each scenario provided.
3. Demonstrate sensitivity appropriate to the message being delivered.
   PURPOSE: To send a clearly communicated message.
4. Demonstrate empathy.
   PURPOSE: To treat each person fairly and with dignity.
5. Apply active listening skills.
   PURPOSE: To make sure your patient understood your message and to allow him or her to communicate a response.
6. Restate the patient's response.
   PURPOSE: To ensure that you understood what the patient said.
7. Analyze communications in providing appropriate responses and feedback.
   PURPOSE: To continually improve the communications process between health care professionals, other staff members, and patients.

your customer, you may be able to avoid potential errors. For example, if you ask, "Do you have any allergies?" the customer may just say "No" or shake his head. However, if you say, "What type of medications are you allergic to?" the customer will give you a more detailed answer.

2. *Provide empathetic responses.* This shows the customer that you can see the situation from her point of view. When a patient thinks you understand how she feels, she is more inclined to share information that could assist with her care. For example, you might have a patient who had a long wait to see the physician with her sick infant. She is clearly stressed and is now waiting to pick up the baby's medication. She asks you why it is taking so long to get one bottle of medicine. An empathetic response might be, "I know you must be exhausted from all of this waiting. I assure you we are working diligently to get your child's medication ready. Helping her get well is our goal."

3. *Minimize distractions.* The goal for every conversation you have with a patient should be to communicate clearly and make sure your message is understood. If needed, take the patient to a quieter space, such as a designated counseling area, to answer any questions or clarify instructions. For example, you may have a patient who has received a prescription for tadalafil (Cialis). You ask if he would like to speak with the pharmacist about this new medication. He is hesitant because there are several customers within hearing distance. You should suggest that the patient speak with the pharmacist in the counseling area, which is private and away from the other customers.

Tech Note!

Always treat customers as you would want to be treated. Remember to be kind, courteous, and respectful at all times.

⊙ Scenario Checkup 4.1

Catherine has reviewed module one with Jackson, and he is ready to begin interacting with the customers. He will be answering the phone for the first part of his shift. She explains to him that the proper way to greet the customer on the phone is by saying, "Thank you for calling BG pharmacy. This is Jackson, a pharmacy technician. How may I help you?" Is it okay for Jackson to put his own touch on the greeting and change the format, as long as he is friendly? Why is it important for him to identify himself each time he answers the phone?

Telephone Etiquette

Another key area of communication in the pharmacy workplace is telephone interactions. A knowledge of proper phone etiquette is important when dealing with patients. **Etiquette** is an unwritten guideline or rule of behavior. Both traditional phone and cell phone guidelines are discussed.

Answering the phone in a busy pharmacy is traditionally the technician's job. Technicians conduct a great deal of daily business over the telephone. The manner in which they answer the phone can set the tone for the remainder of the conversation. A professional attitude and good judgment should be used at all times. With each call, the technician must decide either to direct the call to the pharmacist or to handle it himself or herself (Fig. 4.4).

Sometimes it is necessary to place a customer on hold. If the call must be placed on hold, the technician should check back with the caller at 1- to 2-minute intervals to reassure the patient that he or she has not been forgotten and to verify that the call has not been accidentally disconnected. If the customer raises his or her voice, the technician should let the complaint be aired without reacting negatively. The tone of voice used by the technician can either help resolve the problem or escalate a problem into a long, drawn-out argument. It is best to talk in an even tone and always be pleasant and professional. Arguing with the customer can fuel the fire, and the situation may get out of hand, with no resolution (Box 4.2).

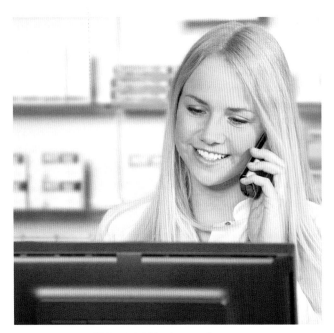

FIG. 4.4 Telephone etiquette.

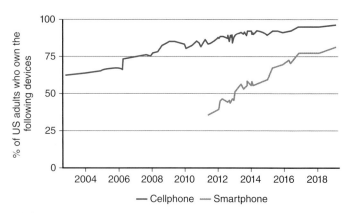

FIG. 4.5 Adult gadget ownership timeline. (Mobile technology fact sheet. Pew Research Center, Washington, DC; June 2019. Retrieved from *https://www.pewresearch.org/internet/fact-sheet/mobile/*.)

BOX 4.2   Example of Unacceptable Phone Etiquette

Patient: Hello, I'm calling because my medication looks different from before, and I need to know if it's the same drug or not.
Pharmacy technician: Would you please hold?
Patient: No, I need to know now because …
Pharmacy technician: [Places the patient on hold and forgets to get back to the patient.]
Alternate response: The technician waits to hear the patient's response to the question. When the patient says she cannot wait, the technician waits to hear why and then proceeds to help her.

Remember the following guidelines when interacting with patients and medical personnel over the phone:
1. Always clearly identify the place of business, your name, and your title when you answer the phone.
2. Carefully listen to the caller to determine the nature of the call.
3. Determine whether the task is within your scope of practice as a technician or whether the call should be forwarded to the pharmacist.
4. If the call can be handled by the technician, make an offer of assistance and restate the purpose of the call before placing the customer on hold or ending the conversation.

▽ **Tech Alert!**

Currently, there are 17 states where it is legal for a pharmacy technician to take an oral prescription from a prescriber and 4 states where they can administer immunizations. As the technician field evolves and more states require formal education, there is reason to think that technician responsibilities will continue to increase.

Cell Phone Etiquette

The Pew Internet Project's research, as of June 2019, demonstrated the following:
- 96% of American adults have a cell phone
- 81% of American adults have a smartphone
- Nearly 75% of American adults own a tablet computer
- Nearly 50% of all American adults own an e-reader

Adult gadget ownership has increased significantly over the past few years; these devices have become a fixture in our daily lives (Fig. 4.5). Mobile health apps are also popular, and patients are using these for lifestyle monitoring, testing, and information gathering. Examples include the following:
- Diabetes management apps to record glucose levels
- Pain management apps to aid with chronic pain management
- Cardiovascular (electrocardiograph [ECG]) testing app
- Maintaining up-to-date electronic health records information
- Using devices to assist with lifestyle and health management is ever increasing, and technicians are often the first contact for information or obtaining the information for a pharmacist to use in a patient interview.

Good cell phone etiquette is a must for today's pharmacy technicians. There are many ways that cell phones can distract them from delivering excellent customer care. Technicians must be careful not to talk or text on their cell phone while working. Even if you are looking up a drug or medication on your smartphone, it may give the patient the perception that you are focusing on something other than the task at hand. Resist the urge to check your messages or return calls until your break. Technicians have been terminated for inappropriate cell phone use while on the clock. If you have an emergency or an urgent message, ask your supervisor if you can step out for a moment to check on the call. Excellent patient care should always be your main focus. You cannot afford to be distracted when filling a prescription.

■ **Tech Note!**

Be sure to check with your supervisor about cell phone policies in your workplace. Always err on the side of caution and stay off your phone during work!

Here are a few guidelines for cell phone use in the pharmacy workplace:

1. Always give 100% focus to the customer in front of you. If you are on your phone, your attention is diverted.
2. Keep cell phones out of sight. This could mean in your locker, pocket, handbag, or briefcase.
3. Keep your cell phone on silent or vibrate.
4. Never text or talk on your cell phone while filling a prescription or dealing with a customer.
5. Keep personal calls to a minimum so you do not appear unfocused to the customers or the pharmacy team.

Virtual Communication Etiquette

In today's fast-paced world, communication is often offered through virtual meetings. This involves a group of people communicating over the internet in a host of locations. Good verbal skills are key as well as the ability to carry on discussions without seeing the person in some cases.

Remember these guidelines when participating in a virtual meeting:

1. Find a quiet place to take the call. Background noises, such as pets, children, radios, phones, fans, or even traffic, can be extremely distracting. Be aware of the sounds in your area and use the MUTE button unless you are the HOST and actively talking.
2. If you are a HOST, this means you are conducting the meeting. Keep the participants to a minimum, as the more there are, the harder it is to not talk over each other. Without verbal cues to indicate someone wants to speak, it is difficult to have one person talk at a time.
3. Be conscious of time and create an agenda. This is key to a successful meeting. If the meeting is set for a limit, it is imperative to stay on track to accomplish the goal of the meeting. Participants may have other obligations often called "hard stops" and will need to leave the meeting at the end time.
4. Keep it professional. Today there are a host of backgrounds and memes that can be used. Be aware of what you are using or where you are conducting the call from, and if on camera, dress as you would for an in-person meeting. A virtual meeting is just as important as an in-person meeting and should be treated as professionally as possible.
5. Test your equipment, camera, and software prior to the meeting. Make sure you don't have pop-up "notifications" showing if you are the host sharing your screen because they see this and it is distracting.
6. If you are recording the meeting, notify the participants ahead.
7. Use introductions and take notes.
   Overall, remember that a virtual meeting does not allow for verbal communication, and if conducted with a group, extra time must be included to allow for individual speakers. Respect everyone's time and be professional.
8. Join the meeting on time.

Written Communication Skills

In today's workplace, pharmacy technicians must be proficient in written communication. They must be able to document information, procedures, and actions accurately and clearly. The ability to coordinate written, oral, and electronic communications is vital to a successful pharmacy team. If the technician's writing is inaccurate or illegible, mistakes can be made and poor patient care can result. Technicians are responsible for written communications such as memos, e-mails, and ordering supplies. Employees with good writing abilities come across as more capable and more credible than their co-workers who make spelling or grammatical errors. In the workplace, remember to proofread all written communications, from e-mails to social media posts to company memos.

Message-taking is also especially important. Often technicians take multiple messages for refills or other tasks during a busy pharmacy shift. Sometimes there may be a delay between the time the message was taken and the time the message is relayed or acted upon. If the message was not written accurately and legibly, it may be misinterpreted. If a system is not in place on how to record and maintain incoming messages, some may be lost or simply forgotten. The more detailed the message, the less likely the technician is to make a mistake. Illegible handwriting by prescribers can also lead to interpretation problems. Many of the drug errors that have been reported in the news and in medical journals are due to poor handwriting (Box 4.3).

BOX 4.3 Example of Poor Written Communication Skills

Nurse Johnson calls the pharmacist to ask whether the two drugs she is about to administer are compatible. She is in a hurry. Joe North, certified pharmacy technician (CPhT), scribbles down the question but does not get the nurse's name or telephone extension. By the time the nurse calls back to contact the pharmacist, the dose is late and the patient has been in pain while waiting for a response.

Alternative response: The technician, Joe North, tells the nurse he will ask the pharmacist to return her call. Joe then asks for the nurse's name, station, and extension, in addition to the patient's name and medical record number.

Information That Should Be Obtained and Written Down in the Message

- Nurse's or caller's name
- Floor location and extension (hospital setting), the physician's callback number (community pharmacy), or the patient's preferred callback number
- The purpose of the call
- The time of the call
- The initials of the technician who took the call
- How soon the information is needed

Only then can a pharmacist quickly and easily relay the correct information to the appropriate person. If your handwriting is illegible, it can cost time and possibly result in a preventable error. There is no excuse for poor handwriting. Poor handwriting is one of the reasons physicians now are transitioning to electronic medication ordering. Thousands of preventable errors can be overcome through the use of computer ordering.

◉ Technician Profile

Shelia is an oncology pharmacy technician. She works for a large hospital. Under the direct supervision of the oncology pharmacist, Shelia prepares medication orders for cancer patients. Her duties include compounding or admixing intravenous (IV) drugs, calculating correct dosage volumes by converting between metric and apothecary equivalents, and checking all orders for completeness of information. Record-keeping is extremely important. Shelia checks all orders for insurance approval before admixing. This step is crucial because many of these medications are extremely expensive. She maintains current drug inventory and Safety Data Sheets (SDSs). All interoffice guidelines and those established by the Occupational Safety and Health Administration (OSHA) must be followed. Shelia's other duties include proper disposal of all materials, both chemotherapy and nonchemotherapy IVs. She must clean the hoods daily or more often as needed. Controlled substances are counted, and weekly logs must be accurate. The requirements for Shelia's position are 2 to 5 years of pharmacy experience in an IV setting, active state registration, certified pharmacy technician (CPhT) certification, and a clean background check and drug screen. Shelia loves her job because she is able to assist the pharmacist in providing quality medication and care to patients experiencing very difficult challenges. She thinks she makes a difference each and every day she goes to work.

Communications With Special Patient Groups

The goal of communication should be to understand and to be clearly understood. The technician should be sensitive to each customer and alert to any special needs the patient might have. This role begins when the technician greets the patient and accepts the prescription.

Terminally Ill Patients

Special consideration should be given to patients who are terminally ill. Remember that they may be feeling overwhelmed. Although each person copes with his or her own mortality differently, there are "normal" progressive steps that people experience. The five stages that terminally ill patients experience are as follows:

STAGE	EXAMPLE
Denial	"This can't be happening …"
Anger	"It isn't fair. I don't deserve this …"
Bargaining	"Please make me better, and I promise …"
Depression	"I will never be able to see you again …"
Acceptance	"I can do this, everyone does …"

Normally the first stage is denial. This is a defense mechanism in which the situation does not seem real. Perhaps the reality is too harsh for the person to accept. The next stage is anger. Sometimes one may have a feeling of unfairness. Bargaining usually follows anger. The person makes promises to himself or herself or to a higher power in the hope of a miracle. Depression may take over at this point, with the realization that nothing is going to change concerning the prognosis. The final phase is acceptance, in which the person concedes his or her own mortality and prepares for eventual death.

Each of these stages can manifest at any time and last for different lengths of time. Therefore it is important that the technician be compassionate to the patient's situation. Most health care workers do not hesitate to help a dying patient; however, the problem is how to identify these patients. Unfortunately, unless the patient decides to share this information, the pharmacy staff does not necessarily know. Some medications indicate an advancing medical condition. These include pain medications such as fentanyl patches or morphine; however, these drugs do not definitively identify a fatal condition. Therefore the pharmacy technician must be objective about each person who enters the pharmacy and realize that he or she does not know what each person is experiencing.

Non–English-Speaking Patients

We live in a culturally diverse society, and technicians often encounter customers who do not speak English as their first language. Technicians who speak multiple languages are in high demand and can play an important role on the pharmacy team. Statistics show that more than 8.6% of the US population speaks English less than "very well." Millions of prescriptions are written for people who have limited English proficiency (LEP) each year. For safety and compliance purposes, it is critical that pharmacy technicians, pharmacists, and LEP patients communicate effectively with each other.

There are many ways pharmacies can help facilitate appropriate communication with the LEP patient. They may employ bilingual staff, provide interpreters, or use software programs that translate the prescription labels and information into various languages. Some pharmacies use pictograms to illustrate a variety of instructions. To view more information on medication pictograms, visit the USP Pictogram Library at *http://www.usp.org/usp-healthcare-professionals/related-topics-resources/usp-pictograms*.

◼ Tech Note!

Consider learning a foreign language, such as Spanish or Chinese, to increase your employment options.

Hearing-Impaired Patients

Approximately 48 million Americans have hearing loss. An estimated one in three cases is caused by excessive noise exposure. One in five American teens has the same degree of hearing loss found in adults 50 to 60 years old. Considering these statistics, there is a high possibility the pharmacy technician will encounter a hearing-impaired patient. Therefore it is important to be aware of any special needs the patient might have as the person approaches the pharmacy counter. If you become aware that the patient's hearing is limited or fully impaired, you must determine a plan of action to best interact with that person. First, ask how he or she prefers to communicate and note the preference on the patient profile in the computer. Some patients may want to use notes, so the technician should write legibly. However, because some hearing-impaired individuals understand only American Sign Language (ASL), it may be difficult for them to read written English. Others may lip-read, so be sure to look at the patient as you speak. Never yell; instead, use a moderately low voice. If the patient is fully hearing impaired, ask whether anyone knows sign language or if a friend or family member can interpret. Remember to direct your communications to the patient and allow him or her to respond to you through the interpreter. It is considered rude in the deaf community not to keep eye contact when speaking.

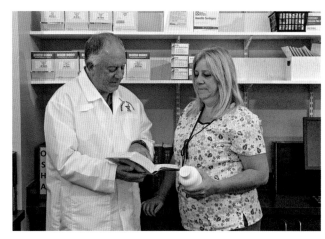

FIG. 4.6 Working together as a team supports providing excellent patient care.

> ### ■ Tech Note!
> Consider enrolling in a local American Sign Language class to enhance your ability to communicate with your hearing-impaired customers.

Remember, if the pharmacy technician treats people equally, regardless of their disposition, the technician is behaving appropriately and professionally. The pharmacy technician can influence the development of a positive atmosphere in the pharmacy setting by maintaining an appropriate attitude. **Attitude** is a mental disposition or feeling a technician adopts toward customers, co-workers, or duties at work.

Allowing customers to express frustration, being a good listener, and doing one's best to help others are important components of acting professionally.

◉ Scenario Checkup 4.2

Jackson is doing a great job answering the phone. His next call is from a hospice nurse, who begins the conversation by giving Jackson a new prescription for Mr. Jones, a terminally ill cancer patient. What is the problem with this situation? How should Jackson handle this call?

Communication With the Health Care Team

Today, the pharmacy technician is an important member of the health care team. In the retail setting, the team may consist of the technician, the pharmacist, the pharmacy manager, counter personnel, and other store employees. In the institutional setting, the team may include technicians, pharmacists and managers, physicians, nurses, and other departmental personnel. In all pharmacy settings, teams work to provide the best patient care possible (Fig. 4.6). The team leadership establishes clear expectations for each member's responsibilities. Trust and communication are key components of a successful team. Here are a few tips to help you become an effective team player:

1. Make sure you clearly understand your job duties and responsibilities.
2. Take time to discuss the pharmacy's goals with the team.
3. Become a positive part of the decision-making process.
4. Stay informed and know the channels of communication.
5. Be loyal and work to build trust.

Eliminating Communication Barriers

Effective communication is challenging in today's workplace. As discussed earlier, there can be many barriers, such as those involving language differences and hearing impairment. The first step in eliminating these barriers is to recognize that they exist. Then, it is the responsibility of each team member to be knowledgeable about the techniques used to overcome these obstacles. We live in the information age and have access to many devices that help us communicate. However, much of this information exchange lacks real meaning. Real communication occurs when both the speaker and the listener are fully engaged. The best defense against any communication barrier is a strong, cooperative team.

> ### ■ Tech Note!
> Technicians must never assume patients understand medical jargon or pharmacy terminology.

Conclusion

When serving patients, technicians should give each person their undivided attention. They should provide all customers with the opportunity to ask questions. Verification of understanding is needed for optimal compliance and patient safety. Technicians should strive to really hear and understand each individual. Effective communication can increase adherence to treatment and decrease adverse effects, which ultimately leads to improved health and safer patient care.

Do You Remember These Key Points?

- The terms and definitions covered in this chapter
- The communication skills a competent pharmacy technician must have to successfully relate to both pharmacy team members and customers
- The communication cycle and how it works
- How to incorporate good listening skills into your daily work routine
- The importance of displaying proper body language and how to interpret the body language of others
- The two parts to verbal communication skills: vocal and verbal
- How to use and improve your vocal and verbal communication skills
- Proper telephone and cell phone etiquette
- The importance of good written communication and its role in preventing medication errors
- How to communicate with special groups of people, such as non–English-speaking individuals, those who are hearing impaired, or terminally ill patients
- How to work as an effective pharmacy team member
- Some common communication barriers technicians face when serving patients

◉ Scenario Follow-Up

As Jackson completes his training, he thanks Catherine for all the important information she has shared. Her tips for communication both with customers and with medical professionals will serve him well throughout his career. He is now considered a pharmacy tech level 1, and the pharmacists and other technicians are pleased with his work. What communication challenges do you think Jackson may face as he continues his job as a pharmacy technician?

Review Questions

Multiple Choice Questions

1. Good communication skills include:
   A. Compassion
   B. Tact
   C. Diplomacy
   D. All of the above
2. Body language should convey an attitude of:
   A. Friendliness and a sense of urgency
   B. Seriousness and professionalism
   C. Helpfulness and concern
   D. Service and dedication

3. This form of communication is judged by others in the first 30 seconds of meeting:
   A. Verbal
   B. Nonverbal
   C. Written
   D. None of the above
4. The primary purpose of having good communication skills is:
   A. To order medications
   B. To relate to pharmacy team members
   C. To relate to customers
   D. All of the above
5. A person's voice can influence how the information is perceived based on:
   A. Inflection
   B. Speed
   C. Volume
   D. All of the above
6. Medication errors have been connected to:
   A. Illegible handwriting
   B. Technician inexperience
   C. Poor phone etiquette
   D. All of the above
7. Which of the following communication tasks is *not* one of the standard technician duties?
   A. Handling angry patients appropriately
   B. Dealing with insurance representatives on the phone
   C. Taking customer refills over the phone
   D. Counseling patients on their medication
8. What is one of the best ways to handle a frustrated customer?
   A. Ask another technician for help
   B. Listen intently
   C. Ask the customer to settle down
   D. All of the above
9. If a technician has tried but is unable to resolve a customer's problem, what step should he or she take next?
   A. Alert the police
   B. Inform the pharmacist
   C. Yell for the technician supervisor
   D. Ask the customer what to do next
10. If any part of a prescription is illegible, technicians should:
    A. Call the prescriber for clarification
    B. Ask another technician for help
    C. See what medication the patient is taking and try to figure it out on their own
    D. None of the above

■ Technician's Corner

Dr. Beth Golden's nurse calls the pharmacy and has the following new prescription for Larry Williams:
- Hydrocodone/acetaminophen tablets #50
- Sig: Take 1 tablet q8h prn severe pain
- 10 refills

The pharmacy technician answers the call. Can the technician take the new prescription over the phone? Determine the laws and regulations in your state regarding this call. What other errors do you find in this order?

Bibliography

Ballington DA. *Pharmacy Practice for Technicians*. 4th ed. St. Paul, MN: EMC/Paradigm; 2009.

George T. Role of the advanced practice nurse in palliative care. *Int J Palliat Nurs*. 2016;22(3):137-140.

Gray Morris D. *Calculate With Confidence*. 6th ed. St. Louis: Elsevier; 2013.

National Association of Boards of Pharmacy. *Survey of Pharmacy Law*. Mount Prospect, Ill: The Association; 2013.

Potter PA, Perry AG. *Fundamentals of Nursing*. 8th ed. St. Louis: Elsevier; 2013.

Proctor DB, Adams AP. *Kinn's the Medical Assistant*. 12th ed. St. Louis: Elsevier; 2013.

Websites Referenced

Communication: An Essential Skill for Pharmacy Technicians. National Healthcare Association. Available at: nhanow.com.

Hearing Health Foundation. Hearing loss and tinnitus statistics. Available at: http://hearinghealthfoundation.org/statistics?gclid5CMbG1dKa1LkCFY9QOgodMksALw.

Hearing Loss Association of America. Hearing loss facts and statistics. Available at: https://www.hearingloss.org/wp-content/uploads/HLAA_HearingLoss_Facts_Statistics.pdf?pdf=FactStats#:~:text=An%20estimated%2050%20million%20Americans,those%20also%20have%20hearing%20loss.

National Health Law Program. Analysis of state pharmacy laws: impact of pharmacy laws on the provision of language services. Available at: https://healthlaw.org/resource/analysis-of-state-pharmacy-laws-impact-of-state-pharmacy-laws-on-the-provision/.

Notable Quotes. John C. Maxwell quotes. Available at: http://www.notable-quotes.com/m/maxwell_john_c.html.

Pew Research Internet Project. Mobile technology fact sheet. Available at: https://www.pewresearch.org/internet/fact-sheet/mobile/.

Rachel Wagner Etiquette and Protocol. Workplace cell phone etiquette—7 smart tips. Available at: http://www.etiquettetrainer.com/cell-phone-etiquette-workplace/.

Rigby A. *Virtual Meeting Etiquette Guide*. October 24, 2023. Available at: https://krisp.ai/blog/virtual-meeting-etiquette/.

The Britannica Dictionary. Available at: https://www.britannica.com/dictionary/perception.

US Pharmacopeial Convention. USP pictograms. Available at: http://www.usp.org/usp-healthcare-professionals/related-topics-resources/usp-pictograms.

CHAPTER 5

Dosage Forms and Routes of Administration

Karen Davis

OBJECTIVES

1. Explain where pharmacy abbreviations originate, list dangerous abbreviations, and explain why these abbreviations are on The Joint Commission's "Do Not Use" list.
2. Recognize the general classifications of medications and the related body systems.
3. Identify various dosage formulations and give examples of each.
4. Identify various routes of administration and give examples of each.
5. Explain the difference between pharmacokinetics and pharmacodynamics.
6. List and explain the absorption, distribution, metabolism, elimination, and bioavailability of drugs in the body. Also, define first-pass metabolism and explain why it is important in drug delivery.
7. Define half-life and describe factors that influence it. Also, define the bioequivalence of drugs and its relationship to the Orange Book.
8. Describe why excipients (additives) are necessary in the production of medications.
9. List three different common drugs and their storage requirements.
10. Discuss the following related to medical terminology: (a) list the segments that make up medical terms and provide examples of each and (b) recognize and interpret common abbreviations as they apply to dosage forms and routes of administration.

TERMS AND DEFINITIONS

Absorption The taking in of nutrients and drugs into the body from food and liquids

Behind the counter (BTC) Nonprescription drugs that are kept behind the pharmacy counter; limited amounts may be sold, or the customer may require the permission of a pharmacist to purchase them

Bioavailability The degree to which a drug or other substance becomes available to the target tissue after administration

Bioequivalence The relationship between two drugs that have the same dosage and dosage form and that have similar bioavailability. Generic versions of a medication must show bioequivalence to the original approved brand product as a requirement of drug approval

Distribution The movement of a medication throughout the blood, organs, and tissues after administration

Elimination The final evacuation of a drug or other substance from the body by normal body processes, such as kidney elimination (urine), biliary excretion (bile to stool), sweat, respiration, or saliva

Enteral A route of administration by way of the intestine, such as orally, rectally, or sublingually

First-pass effect A process in which a portion of the drug dose is metabolized before the drug has a chance to be distributed systemically

Half-life (1) The time required for a chemical to be decreased by half. (2) The time required for half the amount of a substance, such as a drug in a living system, to be eliminated or disintegrated by natural processes. (3) The time required for the concentration of a substance in a body fluid (blood plasma) to decrease by half

Instill To place into; instillation instructions are commonly used for ophthalmic or otic drugs

Legend drugs Drugs that require a prescription; these drugs carry the federal legend: "Federal law prohibits the dispensing of this medication without a prescription"

Metabolism The processes by which the body breaks down or converts medications to active or inactive substances. The primary site of drug metabolism in humans is the liver; however, select drugs are metabolized through other processes

Over the counter (OTC) Medications that can be purchased without a prescription

Parenteral A term used to describe a medication that is usually given by injection into a vein, the skin, or muscle that bypasses the gastrointestinal system

Pharmacokinetics The study of the absorption, metabolism, distribution, and elimination of drugs

Prodrug An inactive substance that is converted to a drug in the body by the action of enzymes or other chemicals

TERMS AND ABBREVIATIONS

DOSAGE FORM	ABBREVIATION/TERM
Buccal tablet or film	Buccal, BUC
Capsule	Cap
Chewable tablet	Chew tab
Diluent	Dil
Elixir	Elix
Enteric-coated tablet	EC tab
Gelatin capsule	Gel cap
Liquid	Liq
Lotion	Lot
Lozenge	Loz
Metered dose inhaler	MDI
Mixture	Mix
Ointment	Ung, oint
Patch, transdermal	Patch, TD
Powder	Pdr
Solution	Sol, soln
Spirit	Sp
Suppository	Supp
Suspension	Susp
Syrup	Syr
Tablet	Tab
Tincture	Tinc
Vaginal cream	Vag cr
Vaginal tablet	Vag tab

MAIN ROUTES OF ADMINISTRATION	ABBREVIATION
Gastrostomy tube	GT
Inhalant	INH (not to be confused with the abbreviation for isoniazid)
Injection	INJ
Intradermal	ID
Intraperitoneal	IP
Intrathecal	IT
Intravenous	IV
Intramuscular	IM
Intravenous piggyback	IVPB
Nasogastric	NG
Nasogastric tube	NGT
Right ear	AD
Left ear	AS
Both ears	AU
Right eye[a]	OD

MAIN ROUTES OF ADMINISTRATION	ABBREVIATION
Left eye[a]	OS
Both eyes[a]	OU
Orally, by mouth	PO
Rectal, per rectum	PR
Small bowel feeding tube	SBFT
Subcutaneous	subcut, SQ,[b] SC[b]
Sublingual	SL
Topical	TOP
Vaginal, per vaginal	PV

[a]The Joint Commission (TJC) recommends that the abbreviations OD, OS, and OU be avoided because of possible medication errors resulting from misinterpretation. TJC suggests that "left ear," "right ear," or "both ears" and "left eye," "right eye," or "both eyes" be written out, for safety purposes.
[b]ISMP recommends avoiding these abbreviations because SC may be mistaken for SL (sublingual) and SQ may be mistaken as "5q" (5 every).
From Institute for Safe Medical Practices. List of error-prone abbreviations. Available at: *https://www.ismp.org/Tools/errorproneabbreviations.pdf*.

◉ Scenario

Mary is a new technician at a local compounding pharmacy. She received an associate in applied science (AAS) degree in pharmacy technology and is eager to put her knowledge into practice. After a few days on the job, she realizes that many of the prescriptions are difficult to decipher because of the physician's handwriting. She hesitates to ask for help. What is the best course of action for Mary?

To become proficient in their jobs, pharmacy technicians must be able to interpret orders correctly. Although it may be true that many physicians' handwriting is referred to as *chicken scratch*, it is the responsibility of the pharmacy technician and the pharmacist to interpret and clarify orders if necessary. Many of the abbreviations used in prescribing medication look very much alike. For instance, mg (milligram) can look much like mcg (microgram) when written quickly. In this chapter, we explore the common abbreviations seen in pharmacy as they apply to dosage forms and routes of administration. In addition to learning the many different types of dosage forms available and the reasons they are necessary, we will discuss the pharmacokinetics related to the manufacturing of dosage forms. We will also present a brief overview of the segments used to compose medical terms and will cover medical and drug abbreviations.

Where Did Pharmacy Abbreviations Originate?

Much of the terminology in pharmacy and medicine comes from the Latin and Greek languages. Because pharmacy began in Europe, most of the abbreviations have their origins in a foreign language. The use of Latin and Greek has continued into the 21st century with little change. Although these abbreviations tend to be confusing at first, they serve an important function. For example, if each pharmacy used its own terminology, it would be virtually impossible for one pharmacy to fill another pharmacy's prescriptions. Therefore the medical community uses terms in Latin and Greek.

These terms serve as a universal language that all medical doctors, nurses, pharmacists, technicians, and other medical personnel can understand. However, the ability to clarify prescribers' orders is still a real dilemma in the United States. The number of errors caused by prescribers' poor handwriting and by inaccurate transcribing of orders by pharmacists and technicians is a great concern (see Chapter 14). Correct interpretation of prescribers' orders by pharmacy staff is obviously extremely important. Interpreting orders can be a time-consuming function of filling prescriptions, and most patients want their medications quickly. This time pressure leaves the pharmacy staff little time to confer or call physicians' offices for every unclear order; however, clarifications must be made if errors are to be avoided. The pharmacy technician must be careful to write the various abbreviations as neatly as possible because other technicians and pharmacists will be reading their writing. Scrolls or stylized or fancy lettering can be easily misinterpreted. The pharmacy technician must learn all of the dosage forms and their abbreviations to decipher prescribers' orders.

"Do Not Use" List

Because of the concern over drug errors that have occurred from the misinterpretation of medication orders, both the Institute for Safe Medication Practices (ISMP) and The Joint Commission (TJC) have provided a "Do Not Use List" that outlines the most commonly misread abbreviations. To reduce the number of mistakes, all practitioners have been informed that these abbreviations should be avoided. In this chapter, these specific abbreviations have been included in the Terms and Abbreviations list at the start of the chapter so that student technicians will recognize them when they encounter them. However, these abbreviations should be avoided and instead spelled out in full. The "Do Not Use List" from TJC is provided in Table 5.1, and the list from the ISMP is provided in Table 5.2, which addresses all the areas that influence drug errors.

TABLE 5.1
The Joint Commission's Official "Do Not Use" List

Do Not Use	Potential Problem	Use Instead
U, u (unit)	Mistaken for "0" (zero), the number "4" (four) or "cc"	Write "unit"
IU (International Unit)	Mistaken for IV (intravenous) or the number "10" (ten)	Write "International Unit"
Q.D., QD, q.d., qd (daily)	Mistaken for each other	Write "daily"
Q.O.D., QOD, q.o.d., qod (every other day)	Period after the Q mistaken for "i" and the "O" mistaken for "i"	Write "every other day"
Trailing zero (X.0 mg)[a] Lack of leading zero (.X mg)	Decimal point is missed	Write X mg Write 0.X mg
MS	Can mean morphine sulfate or magnesium sulfate	Write "morphine sulfate"
MSO$_4$ and MgSO$_4$	Confused for one another	Write "magnesium sulfate"

[a]A trailing zero may be used only where required to demonstrate the level of precision of the value being reported, such as for laboratory results, imaging studies that report the size of lesions, or catheter/tube sizes. It may not be used in medication orders or other medication-related documentation. Applies to all orders and all medication-related documentation that is handwritten (including free-text computer entry) or on preprinted forms.

©The Joint Commission, 2021. *https://www.jointcommission.org/resources/news-and-multimedia/fact-sheets/#first= 10.* Reprinted with permission.

TABLE 5.2
Institute for Safe Medication Practices List of Error-Prone Abbreviations, Symbols, and Dose Designations

Error-Prone Abbreviations, Symbols, and Dose Designations	Intended Meaning	Misinterpretation	Best Practice
Abbreviations for Doses/Measurement Units			
cc	Cubic centimeters	Mistaken as u (units)	Use mL
IU[a]	International unit(s)	Mistaken as IV (intravenous) or the number 10	Use unit(s) (International units can be expressed as units alone)
l ml	Liter Milliliter	Lowercase letter l mistaken as the number 1	Use L (UPPERCASE) for liter Use mL (lowercase m, UPPERCASE L) for milliliter
MM or M M or K	Million Thousand	Mistaken as thousand Mistaken as million M has been used to abbreviate both million and thousand (M is the roman numeral for thousand)	Use million Use thousand
Ng or ng	Nanogram	Mistaken as mg Mistaken as nasogastric	Use nanogram or nanog
U or u[a]	Unit(s)	Mistaken as zero or the number 4, causing a 10-fold overdose or greater (eg, 4U seen as 40 or 4u seen as 44) Mistaken as cc, leading to administering volume instead of units (eg, 4u seen as 4cc)	Use unit(s)
µg	Microgram	Mistaken as mg	Use mcg
Abbreviations for Route of Administration			
AD, AS, AU	Right ear, left ear, each ear	Mistaken as OD, OS, OU (right eye, left eye, each eye)	Use right ear, left ear, or each ear
IN	Intranasal	Mistaken as IM or IV	Use NAS (all UPPERCASE letters) or Intranasal
IT	Intrathecal	Mistaken as intratracheal, intratumor, intratympanic, or inhalation therapy	Use intrathecal

Continued

Institute for Safe Medication Practices List of Error-Prone Abbreviations, Symbols, and Dose Designations—cont'd

Error-Prone Abbreviations, Symbols, and Dose Designations	Intended Meaning	Misinterpretation	Best Practice
OD, OS, OU	Right eye, left eye, each eye	Mistaken as AD, AS, AU (right ear, left ear, each ear)	Use right eye, left eye, or each eye
Per os	By mouth, orally	The os was mistaken as left eye (OS, oculus sinister)	Use PO, by mouth, or orally
SC, SQ, sq, or sub q	Subcutaneous(ly)	SC and sc mistaken as SL or sl (sublingual) SQ mistaken as "5 every" The q in sub q has been mistaken as "every"	Use SUBQ (all UPPERCASE letters, without spaces or periods between letters) or subcutaneous(ly)
Abbreviations for Frequency/Instructions for Use			
HS Hs	Half-strength At bedtime, hours of sleep	Mistaken as bedtime Mistaken as half-strength	Use half-strength Use HS (all UPPERCASE letters) for bedtime
o.d. or OD	Once daily	Mistaken as right eye (OD, oculus dexter), leading to oral liquid medications administered in the eye	Use daily
Q.D., QD, q.d., or qd[a]	Every day	Mistaken as q.i.d., especially if the period after the q or the tail of a handwritten q is misunderstood as the letter i	Use daily
Qhs	Nightly at bedtime	Mistaken as qhr (every hour)	Use nightly or HS for bedtime
Qn	Nightly or at bedtime	Mistaken as qh (every hour)	Use nightly or HS for bedtime
Q.O.D., QOD, q.o.d., or qod[a]	Every other day	Mistaken as qd (daily) or qid (four times daily), especially if the "o" is poorly written	Use every other day
q1d	Daily	Mistaken as qid (four times daily)	Use daily
q6PM, etc.	Every evening at 6 PM	Mistaken as every 6 hours	Use daily at 6 PM or 6 PM daily
SSRI	Sliding scale regular insulin	Mistaken as selective-serotonin reuptake inhibitor	Use sliding scale (insulin)
SSI	Sliding scale insulin	Mistaken as strong solution of iodine (Lugol's)	
TIW or tiw	3 times a week	Mistaken as 3 times a day or twice in a week	Use 3 times weekly
BIW or biw	2 times a week	Mistaken as 2 times a day	Use 2 times weekly
UD	As directed (ut dictum)	Mistaken as unit dose (eg, an order for "dil**TIAZ**em infusion UD" was mistakenly administered as a unit [bolus] dose)	Use as directed
Miscellaneous Abbreviations Associated With Medication Use			
BBA	Baby boy A (twin)	B in BBA mistaken as twin B rather than sex (boy)	When assigning identifiers to newborns, use the mother's last name, the baby's sex (boy or girl), and a distinguishing identifier for all multiples (eg, Smith girl A, Smith girl B)
BGB	Baby girl B (twin)	B at end of BGB mistaken as sex (boy) not twin B	
D/C	Discharge or discontinue	Premature discontinuation of medications when D/C (intended to mean discharge) on a medication list was misinterpreted as discontinued	Use discharge and discontinue or stop
IJ	Injection	Mistaken as IV or intrajugular	Use injection

Error-Prone Abbreviations, Symbols, and Dose Designations	Intended Meaning	Misinterpretation	Best Practice
OJ	Orange juice	Mistaken as OD or OS (right or left eye); drugs meant to be diluted in orange juice may be given in the eye	Use orange juice
Period following abbreviations (eg, mg., mL.)[b]	mg or mL	Unnecessary period mistaken as the number 1, especially if written poorly	Use mg, mL, etc., without a terminal period

Drug Name Abbreviations

To prevent confusion, avoid abbreviating drug names entirely. Exceptions may be made for multi-ingredient drug formulations, including vitamins, when there are electronic drug name field space constraints; however, drug name abbreviations should NEVER be used for any medications on the ISMP List of High-Alert Medications (in Acute Care Settings, Community/Ambulatory Settings, and Long-Term Care Settings). Examples of drug name abbreviations involved in serious medication errors include:

Antiretroviral medications (eg, DOR, TAF, TDF)	DOR: doravirine TAF: tenofovir alafenamide TDF: tenofovir disoproxil fumarate	DOR: Dovato (dolutegravir and lami**VUD**ine) TAF: tenofovir disoproxil fumarate TDF: tenofovir alafenamide	Use complete drug names
APAP	acetaminophen	Not recognized as acetaminophen	Use complete drug name
ARA A	vidarabine	Mistaken as cytarabine ("ARA C")	Use complete drug name
AT II and AT III	AT II: angiotensin II (Giapreza) AT III: antithrombin III (Thrombate III)	AT II (angiotensin II) mistaken as AT III (antithrombin III) AT III (antithrombin III) mistaken as AT II (angiotensin II)	Use complete drug names
AZT	zidovudine (Retrovir)	Mistaken as azithromycin, aza**THIO**prine, or aztreonam	Use complete drug name
CPZ	Compazine (prochlorperazine)	Mistaken as chlorpro**MAZINE**	Use complete drug name
DTO	diluted tincture of opium or deodorized tincture of opium (Paregoric)	Mistaken as tincture of opium	Use complete drug name
HCT	hydrocortisone	Mistaken as hydro**CHLORO**thiazide	Use complete drug name
HCTZ	hydro**CHLORO**thiazide	Mistaken as hydrocortisone (eg, seen as HCT250 mg)	Use complete drug name
$MgSO_4$[a]	magnesium sulfate	Mistaken as morphine sulfate	Use complete drug name
MS, MSO_4[a]	morphine sulfate	Mistaken as magnesium sulfate	Use complete drug name
MTX	methotrexate	Mistaken as mito**XANTRONE**	Use complete drug name
Na at the beginning of a drug name (eg, Na bicarbonate)	sodium bicarbonate	Mistaken as no bicarbonate	Use complete drug name
NoAC	novel/new oral anticoagulant	Mistaken as no anticoagulant	Use complete drug name
OXY	oxytocin	Mistaken as oxy**CODONE**, Oxy**CONTIN**	Use complete drug name
PCA	procainamide	Mistaken as patient-controlled analgesia	Use complete drug name

Continued

Institute for Safe Medication Practices List of Error-Prone Abbreviations, Symbols, and Dose Designations—cont'd

Error-Prone Abbreviations, Symbols, and Dose Designations	Intended Meaning	Misinterpretation	Best Practice
PIT	Pitocin (oxytocin)	Mistaken as Pitressin, a discontinued brand of vasopressin still referred to as PIT	Use complete drug name
PNV	prenatal vitamins	Mistaken as penicillin VK	Use complete drug name
PTU	propylthiouracil	Mistaken as Purinethol (mercaptopurine)	Use complete drug name
T3	Tylenol with codeine No. 3	Mistaken as liothyronine, which is sometimes referred to as T3	Use complete drug name
TAC or tac	triamcinolone or tacrolimus	Mistaken as tetracaine, adrenalin, and cocaine; or as Taxotere, Adriamycin, and cyclophosphamide	Use complete drug names Avoid drug regimen or protocol acronyms that may have a dual meaning or may be confused with other common acronyms, even if defined in an order set
TNK	TNKase	Mistaken as TPA	Use complete drug name
TPA or tPA	tissue plasminogen activator, Activase (alteplase)	Mistaken as TNK (TNKase, tenecteplase), TXA (tranexamic acid), or less often as another tissue plasminogen activator, Retavase (retaplase)	Use complete drug name
TXA	tranexamic acid	Mistaken as TPA (tissue plasminogen activator)	Use complete drug name
ZnSO4	zinc sulfate	Mistaken as morphine sulfate	Use complete drug name
Stemmed/Coined Drug Names			
Nitro drip	nitroglycerin infusion	Mistaken as nitroprusside infusion	Use complete drug name
IV vanc	intravenous vancomycin	Mistaken as Invanz	Use complete drug name
Levo	levofloxacin	Mistaken as Levophed (norepinephrine)	Use complete drug name
Neo	Neo-Synephrine, a well-known but discontinued brand of phenylephrine	Mistaken as neostigmine	Use complete drug name
Coined names for compounded products (eg, magic mouthwash, banana bag, GI cocktail, half and half, pink lady)	Specific ingredients compounded together	Mistaken ingredients	Use complete drug/product names for all ingredients Coined names for compounded products should only be used if the contents are standardized and readily available for reference to prescribers, pharmacists, and nurses
Number embedded in drug name (not part of the official name) (eg, 5-fluorouracil, 6-mercaptopurine)	fluorouracilmercapto-purine	Embedded number mistaken as the dose or number of tablets/capsules to be administered	Use complete drug names, without an embedded number if the number is not part of the official drug name
Dose Designations and Other Information			
1/2 tablet	Half tablet	1 or 2 tablets	Use text (half tablet) or reduced font-size fractions (½ tablet)

TABLE 5.2
Institute for Safe Medication Practices List of Error-Prone Abbreviations, Symbols, and Dose Designations—cont'd

Error-Prone Abbreviations, Symbols, and Dose Designations	Intended Meaning	Misinterpretation	Best Practice
Doses expressed as Roman numerals (eg, V)	5	Mistaken as the designated letter (eg, the letter V) or the wrong numeral (eg, 10 instead of 5)	Use only Arabic numerals (eg, 1, 2, 3) to express doses
Lack of a leading zero before a decimal point (eg, .5 mg)[a]	0.5 mg	Mistaken as 5 mg if the decimal point is not seen	Use a leading zero before a decimal point when the dose is less than one measurement unit
Trailing zero after a decimal point (eg, 1.0 mg)[a]	1 mg	Mistaken as 10 mg if the decimal point is not seen	Do not use trailing zeros for doses expressed in whole numbers
Ratio expression of a strength of a single-entity injectable drug product (eg, **EPINEPH**rine 1:1,000; 1:10,000; 1:100,000)	1:1,000: contains 1 mg/mL 1:10,000: contains 0.1 mg/mL 1:100,000: contains 0.01 mg/mL	Mistaken as the wrong strength	Express the strength in terms of quantity per total volume (eg, **EPINEPH**rine 1 mg per 10 mL) **Exception:** combination local anesthetics (eg, lidocaine 1% and **EPINEPH**rine 1:100,000)
Drug name and dose run together (problematic for drug names that end in the letter l [eg, propranolol 20 mg; **TEG**retol300 mg])	propranolol 20 mg **TEG**retol 300 mg	Mistaken as propranolol 120 mg Mistaken as **TEG**retol 1300 mg	Place adequate space between the drug name, dose, and unit of measure
Numerical dose and unit of measure run together (eg, 10mg, 10Units)	10 mg 10 mL	The m in mg, or U in Units, has been mistaken as one or two zeros when flush against the dose (eg, 10mg, 10Units), risking a 10- to 100-fold overdose	Place adequate space between the dose and unit of measure
Large doses without properly placed commas (eg, 100000 units; 1000000 units)	100,000 units 1,000,000 units	100000 has been mistaken as 10,000 or 1,000,000 1000000 has been mistaken as 100,000	Use commas for dosing units at or above 1,000 or use words such as 100 thousand or 1 million to improve readability **Note:** Use commas to separate digits only in the US; commas are used in place of decimal points in some other countries
Symbols			
ℨ or ♍,[b]	Dram Minim	Symbol for dram mistaken as the number 3 Symbol for minim mistaken as mL	Use the metric system
x1	Administer once	Administer for 1 day	Use explicit words (eg, for 1 dose)
> and <	More than and less than	Mistaken as opposite of intended Mistakenly have used the incorrect symbol < mistaken as the number 4 when handwritten (eg, <10 misread as 40)	Use more than or less than

Continued

TABLE 5.2

Institute for Safe Medication Practices List of Error-Prone Abbreviations, Symbols, and Dose Designations—cont'd

Error-Prone Abbreviations, Symbols, and Dose Designations	Intended Meaning	Misinterpretation	Best Practice
↑ and ↓[b]	Increase and decrease	Mistaken as opposite of intended Mistakenly have used the incorrect symbol ↑ mistaken as the letter T, leading to misinterpretation as the start of a drug name, or mistaken as the numbers 4 or 7	Use increase and decrease
/ (slash mark)[b]	Separates two doses or indicates per	Mistaken as the number 1 (eg, 25 units/10 units misread as 25 units and 110 units)	Use per rather than a slash mark to separate doses
@[b]	At	Mistaken as the number 2	Use at
&[b]	And	Mistaken as the number 2	Use and
+[b]	Plus or and	Mistaken as the number 4	Use plus, and, or in addition to
°	Hour	Mistaken as a zero (eg, q2° seen as q20)	Use hr, h, or hour
φ or ⊘[b]	Zero, null sign	Mistaken as the numbers 4, 6, 8, and 9	Use 0 or zero, or describe intent using whole words
#	Pound(s)	Mistaken as a number sign	Use the metric system (kg or g) rather than pounds Use lb if referring to pounds

[a]These abbreviations are included on The Joint Commission's "minimum list" of dangerous abbreviations, acronyms, and symbols that must be included on an organization's "Do Not Use" list, effective June 2019. Visit http://www.jointcommission.org for more information about this Joint Commission requirement.
[b]Relevant mostly in handwritten medication information.
Other reproduction is prohibited without written permission from ISMP. Report actual and potential medication errors to the ISMP National Medication Errors Reporting Program (ISMP MERP) via the Web at http://www.ismp.org or by calling 1-800-FAIL-SAF(E). Used with permission from the Institute for Safe Medication Practices. © ISMP 2021. Visit http://www.ismp.org; http://www.ismp.org for more medication safety information or to report medication errors or near misses to the ISMP Medication Errors Reporting Program (MERP).

Dosing Instructions

Dosing times are also abbreviated on prescriptions. Although many abbreviations are listed as "Do Not Use," per the recommendations of both TJC and the ISMP, they will be seen in many orders. In addition, many pharmacy computers are programmed to accept these abbreviations.

◉ Scenario Checkup 5.1

Mary continues to enjoy working at the local compounding facility. Her pharmacist gives her a copy of the "Do Not Use" list of abbreviations and asks her to become familiar with it. At first, Mary was skeptical about the value of studying the list. Then, one day as she was compounding a hormone cream, she came across the abbreviation "HS." Did the physician intend for the directions to mean half-strength or at bedtime? At that moment, she realized the significance of the list she had been asked to study. She consulted the pharmacist, who clarified the directions with the physician. What could have been the worst-case scenario in this situation?

Classifications of Medications

Classifications of medications place drugs into groups. Although many medications are used for reasons other than their intended purpose, it is important to know the body system a medication is intended to affect. Each drug can be further broken down into groupings based on pharmacology, intent of use, route of administration, or mechanism of action. Various classifications and attributes of drug therapy are discussed later in this chapter. Table 5.3 presents a generalized list so that students can familiarize themselves with the various classifications of available drugs and the body system with which each classification is associated. Each type of medication may have several dosage forms, giving the consumer or physician a choice in how the drug is administered. For consumers, the choice may be based on which dosage form is easier to take or it may be based on cost. For a physician, the best way to administer medications may be based on how rapidly the medication is needed by the patient.

Classifications of Drug Sales

Three classifications describe drugs' availability to consumers. **Over-the-counter (OTC)** drugs are commonly used and may be purchased without a prescription. **Legend drugs** require a prescription from a prescriber before they can be used and are often denoted as "Rx." **Behind-the-counter (BTC)** drugs do not require a prescription but are

TABLE 5.3
General Classifications of Medications

Body System	Drug Classifications
Cardiovascular	Angiotensin-converting enzyme (ACE) inhibitors, angiotensin II receptor antagonists, antihyperlipidemics, antihypertensives, beta-blockers, calcium channel blockers, diuretics, vasodilators
Circulatory	Anticoagulants, antihemorrhagics, antiplatelets, thrombolytics
Endocrine	Antithyroid agents, corticosteroids, hypoglycemic agents, hypothalamic-pituitary hormones, sex hormones, thyroid hormones
Gastrointestinal	Antacids, antidiarrheals, antiemetics, H_2-antagonists, laxatives, proton pump inhibitors
Immune	Antibiotics, anticancer agents, antifungals, antiparasitics, antivirals, immunomodulators, vaccines
Integumentary	Antipruritics, antipsoriatics, emollients, medicated dressings
Musculoskeletal	Anabolic steroids, antirheumatics, bisphosphonates, corticosteroids, muscle relaxants, nonsteroidal antiinflammatory drugs (NSAIDs)
Nervous	Analgesics, anesthetics, anticonvulsants, antidepressants, antiparkinsonian drugs, antipsychotics, stimulants
Reproductive	Fertility agents, hormonal contraceptives, sex hormones
Respiratory	Bronchodilators, cough medications, decongestants, H_1-antagonists
Other	Antidotes, contrast media, radiopharmaceuticals

kept in the pharmacy; their sales are limited by quantity or may require a pharmacist's approval.

Dosage Forms

Dosage form refers to the means by which a drug is available for use or the vehicle by which the drug is delivered. With individual packaging, the dosage form is given on the package. For example, the form may be a tablet or capsule. However, there are many types of tablets and capsules. Tablets are available in a wide variety of shapes and sizes. For example, they may be scored or unscored (Fig. 5.1) or they may be coated or uncoated (Fig. 5.2). The dosage form of a medication is largely determined by the drug's pharmacokinetic properties. For instance, heparin (an anticoagulant) is available only in parenteral (intravenous [IV] or subcutaneous [subcut]) form because it becomes ineffective when taken orally as a result of its interaction with stomach acids. Manufacturers prepare certain medications with the ability to release the active ingredient over an extended period. This allows the patient to take the medication less often, which increases compliance. Another consideration is the person

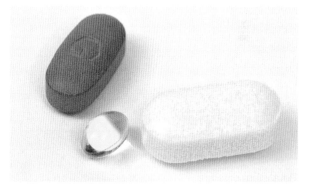

FIG. 5.2 Types of tablets.

taking the drug (eg, age and health status). If a prescription for sulfamethoxazole/trimethoprim (Bactrim) is intended for a child, that dosage form should be available as a liquid, if possible, for ease of administration. The following sections give a brief explanation of the different dosage forms. All of the different forms can be divided into three major categories that comprise subcategories:

1. **Solids:** Tablets, chewable tablets, enteric-coated tablets, extended-release agents, sublingual (SL) tablets, capsules, caplets, lozenges, troches, implant capsules, patches
2. **Liquids:** Syrups, elixirs, sprays, inhalant solutions, emulsions, suspensions, solutions, and enemas
3. **Semisolids:** Creams, lotions, ointments, powders, gelatins, suppositories, inhalant powders

Many of the top-selling drugs are available in several different dosage forms. Different dosage forms give the consumer more options; however, the selection of a dosage form also depends on whether the drug will still be effective in a different form. Twenty-four top-selling generic drugs that are available in at least three different dosage forms are shown in Table 5.4. It is always important to know which dosage form

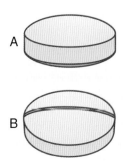

FIG. 5.1 (A) Unscored tablet. (B) Scored tablet.

TABLE 5.4
25 Examples of Drugs With Multiple Dosage Forms

Examples of Drugs Offered in Multiple Dosage Forms	Tablet	Chewable Tablet	Capsule	Caplet	Solution	Gel Caps	Suspension	Syrup	Elixir	Injectable	Topical Patch	Aerosol	Suppositories or Rectal Form	Topical Dosage Forms
Acetaminophen	X	X	X	X	X	X		X	X	X			X	
Acetaminophen/codeine	X						X		X					
Albuterol	X				X			X				X		
Amoxicillin	X	X	X				X							
Carbamazepine	X	X					X							
Clindamycin			X		X					X				X
Diazepam	X				X					X			X	
Digoxin	X								X	X				
Diltiazem	X		X							X				
Diphenhydramine	X		X		X		X	X	X	X				X
Epinephrine					X					X		X		
Erythromycin	X	X	X				X			X				X
Furosemide	X				X					X				
Guaifenesin	X		X		X			X						
Hydrocortisone	X				X					X			X	X
Hydroxyzine	X		X					X		X				
Ibuprofen	X	X	X		X		X			X				
Nitroglycerin	X		X							X	X	X		X
Phenobarbital	X								X	X				
Phenytoin	X		X				X			X				
Potassium chloride	X				X					X				
Prednisone	X				X			X						
Promethazine	X							X		X			X	
Risperidone	X				X					X				

is being requested because each form is dosed in different strengths, depending on the drug's reactive properties and the most suitable form for the consumer. For example, if erythromycin tablets are ordered for a young child, the pharmacist may need to call the physician to request either chewable tablets or an oral suspension.

Tech Note!

Remember that to substitute a different dosage form for the one ordered, the prescriber must give permission. The pharmacist must call the prescriber and explain the reason for the change.

Solids

Solid agents can be contained in various packages, and when administered by the **enteral** route they can be given orally, rectally, or sublingually. When we think of solids, we normally consider medications given by oral or rectal routes rather than parenteral routes. **Parenteral** is a term used to describe a medication that is usually given by injection into a vein, the skin, or a muscle.

Tablets and Caplets

Hundreds of types of tablets are available in a range of sizes, shapes, colors, thickness, and composition. The most common type of tablet contains some type of filler. Fillers are composed of inert substances (no active ingredient) that fill space or cover the tablet (sugar coatings). Sugar coatings improve taste and color or hide unpleasant odors. Certain additives may be used to improve the drug's absorption and/or distribution throughout the body. Some tablets are made to be administered sublingually (under the tongue) or vaginally. Also, some tablets are available in a scored form to allow the dosage to be cut in half if needed. Chewable tablets are convenient for people who have difficulty swallowing tablets and for children who are unable to swallow large tablets. Other tablets are enteric coated to help protect the drug through the acidic environment of the stomach until it reaches the more alkaline intestine. In other cases, the protective covering may delay the release of the drug as it travels through the stomach so that it will not irritate the stomach or become inactive. Orally disintegrating tablets (ODTs) may be dissolved in the mouth without water, easing administration for individuals who have difficulty swallowing medication. Caplet dosage forms are related closely to tablets but are smooth sided and therefore easier to swallow. The word *caplet* refers to the shape of the tablet. Tablets are often identified by shape, color, and imprint codes, which are determined by the manufacturer.

Many medications have extended-release forms and regular forms. The technician must know which form the physician has ordered. Manufacturers have developed controlled-release formulations to enable the patient to take the medication less often. This improves patient compliance. Abbreviations for agents that release medication over different periods of time and in different quantities are as follows:

CD	Controlled diffusion
CR	Continuous/controlled release
CRT	Controlled-release tablet
IR	Immediate release[a]
LA	Long acting[a]
ODT	Orally disintegrating tablet
SA	Sustained action[a]
SR	Sustained/slow release[a]
TD	Time delay
TR	Time release
XL	Extra long[a]
XR	Extended release[a]

[a]Also available in capsule forms.

■ Tech Note!

As a general rule, dosage forms that are specially made to release over time should not be crushed or broken into pieces. This would alter the release process. However, some medications, such as Toprol XL, can be divided if they are scored and approved for such use. Some companies have their own names for extended-release agents. For example, Theo-24 is a theophylline agent that is released over 24 hours, which is why the company named it Theo-24.

Capsules

Capsules are composed of a gelatin container. They can have a hard or soft outer shell. The shells of hard capsules are composed of sugar, gelatin, and water. Their color is determined by the manufacturer and is used primarily for identification, along with the capsule imprint coding. Another type of capsule is the pulvule, which is shaped slightly differently for identification purposes. Spansules are capsules that can be pulled apart to sprinkle the medication onto food for children, making it easier to administer. The medication inside a spansule is specially coated to slow the dissolving rate, allowing the

medicine to be delivered at a particular time (depending on the coating) after the capsule contents are consumed. The medicine inside a spansule should not be crushed or chewed. Soft-gelatin capsules (gel caps) cannot be pulled apart and often hold medications in liquid form. Because of the many capsule sizes available, capsules can be produced to administer medication in many ways. For example, as seen in Fig. 5.3, these capsules can even hold a small capsule or tablet. The reason behind this manufacturing decision is to determine the best absorption and distribution of the medication. Caplets are not capsules; they are simply tablets with a shape similar to that of a capsule that may ease swallowing. More medications are being prepared as caplets to ensure that they are tamper proof. Fig. 5.4 shows more shapes and sizes of capsules.

Capsule sizes Capsules are available in different sizes (Fig. 5.5). They vary in color, transparency, and identifying marks. The larger half of the capsule is known as the *body*, and the shorter half is known as the *cap*. Many companies produce a hard-shelled capsule that cannot be opened, ensuring that it is tamper resistant. Many capsules are designed to be taken orally and swallowed whole. Compounding pharmacies carry empty capsules of varying sizes that can be filled with various amounts of medication; a variety of techniques are used to fill them (see Chapter 11 for more information on compounding).

Some capsules are not intended to be swallowed. For example, Topamax Sprinkles are capsules that hold spheres of anticonvulsant medicine inside the capsule. This specific medication can be sprinkled onto a small amount of soft food immediately before dosing for administration; the sprinkles

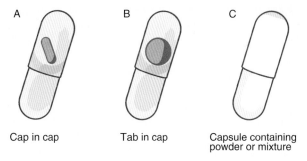

Cap in cap   Tab in cap   Capsule containing powder or mixture

FIG. 5.3 Different types of capsules.

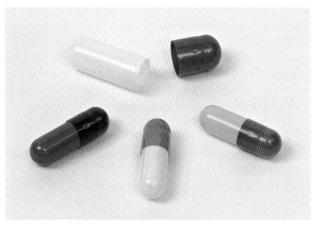

FIG. 5.4 Normal-release and extended-release capsules.

Number	Quantity	Example
000	1.37 mL	
00	0.95 mL	
0	0.68 mL	
1	0.5 mL	
2	0.37 mL	
3	0.3 mL	
4	0.2 mL	
5	0.13 mL	

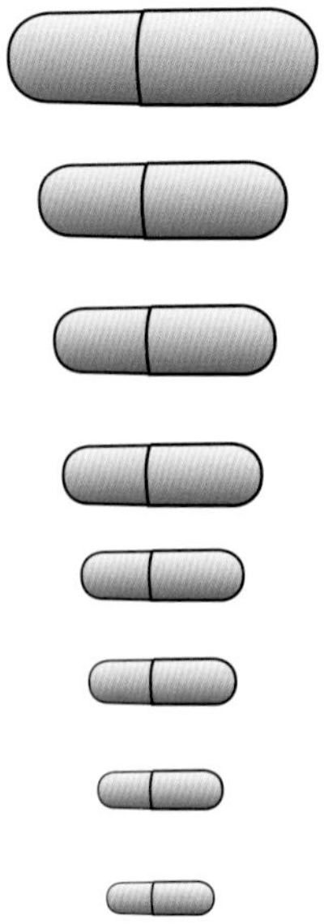

FIG. 5.5 Different sizes of capsules. Eight sizes are available; each holds a specific volume, and each holds a specific amount of medication. The size numbers are 5, 4, 3, 2, 1, 0, 00, 000; 5 is the smallest, and 000 is the largest. (From Clayton B, Stock Y. *Basic Pharmacology for Nurses.* 16th ed. St. Louis: Elsevier; 2013.)

should not be chewed. Pharmacies have capsule dosage forms that hold dry powder medication intended for oral inhalation using inhaler devices; these dosage forms should not be swallowed by the patient.

Examples of caplets and capsules acetaminophen caplets (Tylenol; OTC), hydroxyzine pamoate capsules (Vistaril; Rx)

Lozenges and Troches

Lozenges and troches are other forms of tablets that are not intended to be swallowed; they dissolve in the mouth, which releases the medication more slowly. The medications in lozenges and troches are often aimed at local action in the mouth and/or throat. Many cough drops come in this type of dosage form. Lozenges are similar to hard candy. Troches vary in size. Some are larger than normal-sized tablets and are flat; they usually have a chalky consistency so they can dissolve in the mouth. Clotrimazole troches are normally administered buccally (in the cheek) and left to dissolve, whereas most lozenges are allowed to dissolve in the mouth.

Examples of lozenges and troches benzocaine and menthol lozenge (Cepacol Extra Strength Sore Throat; OTC); clotrimazole troche (Rx), Numoisyn lozenge (Rx)

Biomaterials

Biomaterials are polymers (long chains of hydrocarbons) that combine with or encapsulate a drug; the drug is then released in a predetermined and predictable way. The dosage form of these drugs can be capsules, tablets, or implants. Both pH and solubility can activate the drug and release its contents over a period of from 12 hours (eg, cold medicine) to several

years (eg, Implanon contraceptive implant). These drugs can treat conditions without overdosing or underdosing the patient, and they also promote compliance (patient adherence). These dosage forms help maintain a steady concentration of drug dosing within the accepted therapeutic range or window for the drug. The therapeutic window is essentially a range of concentrations at which a drug is determined to be effective with minimal toxicity to most patients. The top concentration of the range is the maximum concentration for most patients to limit toxicity, and the lowest concentration is the concentration below which the drug is not therapeutically effective for most patients.

Consider two components:
1. Water solubility (eg, ethyl cellulose is water insoluble)
2. pH dependency (eg, sodium alginate is pH dependent, whereas hydroxypropyl methylcellulose is pH independent)

Another consideration with these medications is cost; they are more expensive to manufacture, and that cost is passed along to the consumer.

Implants

Implants are sterile, solid dosage forms that consist of drugs and rate-controlling excipients. They usually are intended for insertion (implantation) into a body cavity or under the skin. Some implants are biosoluble, meaning they degrade in the body over time; others are not and must be removed after a specified time. Many drug-containing implants are actually classified by the US Food and Drug Administration (FDA) as medical devices rather than drugs, such as implantable orthopedic antibiotic beads and various drug-eluting stents for arteries in the heart. Some implants, however, are regulated as prescription drugs. Some popular examples of implants include the Zoladex subcutaneous implant (used for a variety of conditions, including prostate cancer), the Gliadel Wafer (delivers chemotherapy directly to a brain tumor site), and Implanon, a subdermal contraceptive rod (provides birth control that lasts for up to 3 years).

Transdermal Patches

Transdermal patches are solid pieces of material that hold a specific amount of medication to be released into the skin and absorbed into the bloodstream over time. Patches are convenient dosage forms because they are easily applied and eliminate possible upset stomach. Anginal medication, such as transdermal nitroglycerin patches, can be placed on the chest once daily. Some motion sickness patches (eg, Transderm Scop) can be applied and left in place for up to 3 days. Fentanyl, a chronic pain medication, is a transdermal patch with a 3-day delivery time (Fig. 5.6). Nicotine patches help with smoking cessation, and most are available OTC. Many estrogen-containing transdermal patches are suited for hormone replacement therapy or prevention of osteoporosis; most are changed once or twice weekly.

Examples of topical patches nitroglycerin patches (Nitro-Dur; Rx), scopolamine transdermal patches (Transderm Scop; Rx), fentanyl patch

▽ Tech Alert!

Never carelessly discard a medication patch in the trash. The medication present on an unprotected, discarded patch may penetrate the skin of a young child or pet. The best approach is to wrap and discard the patch in such a way that a child or pet would not be able to grasp it. One recommendation is to fold the patch onto itself to cover the adhesive area, then place the patch in a pouch or baggie and discard it out of reach of children or pets.

Liquids

Liquids are composed of various mixtures. Traditional names for these dosage forms relate to the types of liquid with which the medication is mixed. Depending on the type of taste, speed of action, or route of administration intended, a physician can choose the best agent for the job. Liquids can be administered by many routes, which makes them a popular choice for drug delivery. For example, enemas are liquid-filled bottles with a dispensing top that can be placed into the rectum to administer the solution into the lower intestine. Other sterile liquids are used in eye and ear products, which are used to treat a variety of conditions. Solutions also can be used topically to treat skin conditions. The following sections discuss the various types of liquids available (Fig. 5.7).

Syrups

Syrups are sugar-based solutions into which medication has been dissolved. The sugar improves the taste of the drug. Syrups tend to be thicker (more viscous) than water (Fig. 5.8).

Examples of syrups dextromethorphan syrup (Delsym; OTC), hydrocodone and chlorpheniramine syrup (Tussionex PennKinetic; Rx)

Elixirs

Elixirs are clear, sweetened solutions that contain dissolved medication in a base of water and alcohol (hydroalcoholic base). Drugs that are formulated as elixirs usually require alcohol as a solvent for the drug to be placed into solution. Sweeteners are a necessary component of elixirs to improve the taste of the alcoholic mixtures. Unlike syrups, elixirs have the same consistency as water (Fig. 5.9).

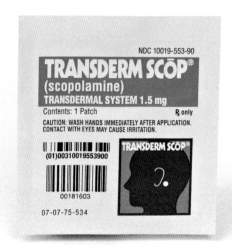

FIG. 5.6 Example of a transdermal patch.

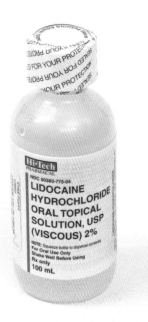

FIG. 5.7 Solution is a universal term for liquid medication. Solutions vary greatly in texture, viscosity, etc. *EG,* Enema; *IV,* intravenous.

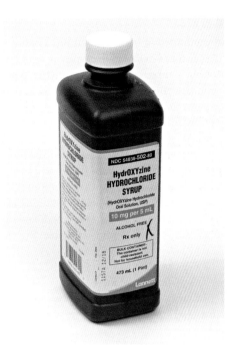

FIG. 5.8 Example of a syrup.

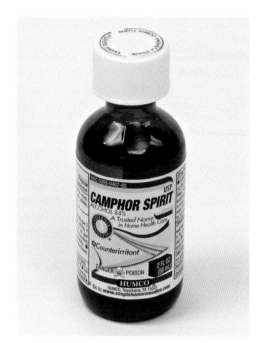

FIG. 5.10 Example of a spirit.

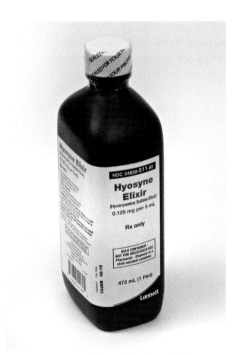

FIG. 5.9 Example of an elixir.

Examples of elixirs brompheniramine/phenylephrine elixir (Children's Dimetapp Cold & Allergy; OTC), theophylline elixir (Elixophyllin; Rx)

Spirits

Spirits are aromatic solutions of drugs designed to evaporate quickly (Fig. 5.10).

Examples of spirits peppermint spirit, camphor, and aromatic spirits of ammonia

Sprays

Sprays are composed of various bases, such as alcohol or water, in a pump-type dispenser. Sprays are available for use in products such as nasal decongestants and topical sunscreens. A nitroglycerin translingual spray also is available for use under the tongue for relief of anginal pain (Fig. 5.11).

Examples of sprays oxymetazoline nasal spray (Afrin; OTC), nitroglycerin SL spray (Nitrolingual Pump-spray; Rx)

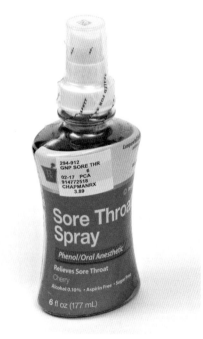

FIG. 5.11 Example of a spray.

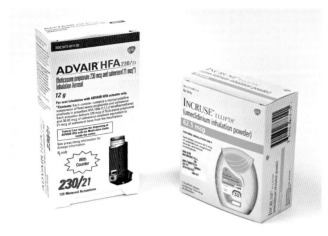

FIG. 5.12 Examples of inhalers.

Inhalants and Aerosols

In certain patients, medications must be delivered directly to the source of inflammation, such as the bronchial tree. Because these areas are so small, the medication particles must be extremely fine to reach them effectively. Inhaler agents are available in a variety of forms, but all must be able to be easily inhaled into the lungs. Common devices of this type, available OTC, are vaporizers that distribute medications when agents are added to a container on the device (Fig. 5.12). In the hospital, respiratory therapists use nebulizers to give breathing treatments to patients; patients also can use nebulizers at home if they or their caregivers are trained in the use of these devices. Proper daily cleaning and care of the nebulizer equipment helps prevent infection (Procedure 5.1). Inhaled anesthetics are solutions inhaled by a patient undergoing surgery; they are administered during surgery by an anesthesiologist.

Many of the prescribed inhalants contain drugs that treat asthma and allergies. Some devices are called *metered dose inhalers (MDIs)* and dispense a specific amount of drug with each puff or inhalation (Fig. 5.13A); the other common type of medication inhaler is a dry powder inhaler. Some aerosols are used to deliver medication into the nasal passages, whereas others are inhaled orally into the respiratory tract. For orally inhaled agents, although the size of the particles is extremely small, unless the patient uses this device correctly, much of the drug is swallowed rather than inhaled into the lungs, where it is needed. Many physicians encourage the use of an Aero-Chamber or other spacer (see Fig. 5.13B) along with traditional MDIs. These allow the patient to take a breath of medication without worrying about poor timing and coordination, which could result in loss of medication. The chamber holds the medication until each puff can be inhaled. Dry powder inhalers can be easier to administer because patients prepare the medication before inhalation, allowing them to focus on the proper breathing and administration technique.

Examples of aerosol and metered dose inhalers albuterol (Proventil HFA; Rx), ipratropium bromide and albuterol sulfate MDI (Combivent Respimat; Rx), Afrezza

---

Procedure 5.1

Cleaning Your Nebulizer Equipment

Goal

To learn the steps for properly cleaning a nebulizer and its tubing to prevent infection.

Equipment and Supplies

- Nebulizer kit (tubing and nebulizer chamber)

Procedural Steps

1. After each treatment, rinse the nebulizer cup with warm water.
   PURPOSE: To wash away any debris or dirt left in the cup.
2. Empty all water from the nebulizer cup and let it air dry.
   PURPOSE: To ensure that no moisture is left in the cup, which could allow bacteria to grow.
3. At the end of the day, wash the nebulizer cup, mask, or mouthpiece in warm, soapy water; rinse; and allow to air dry.
   PURPOSE: To make sure every part is cleaned thoroughly to avoid any debris or moisture that may be left behind after treatments. All parts should air dry to prevent bacteria growth.

4. Every third day, disinfect the equipment using a vinegar and water solution (½ cup white vinegar mixed with 1½ cups water).
   PURPOSE: White vinegar is a mild disinfectant and is used to kill germs and remove odors.
5. Soak for 20 minutes and rinse well under a steady stream of water.
   PURPOSE: Allowing the parts to soak in the vinegar mixture for 20 minutes will ensure that the acid has time to kill any germs and remove any odors. Rinsing well will remove any trace of the cleaning mixture and prevent any cross-contamination.
6. Remove excess water and allow to air dry on a paper towel.
   PURPOSE: To make sure no moisture is left that might grow bacteria.
7. Make sure all equipment is completely dry before storing it in a plastic resealable bag.
   PURPOSE: To avoid any trapped moisture that would be a breeding ground for bacteria.

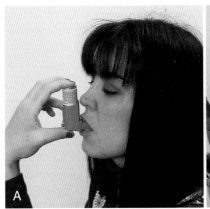
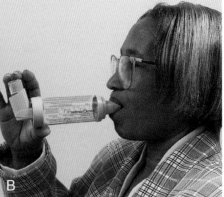

FIG. 5.13 (A) Inhaler. (B) Inhaler attached to an AeroChamber (also known as a *spacer*). (From Potter PA, Perry AG. *Fundamentals of Nursing*, 8th ed. St. Louis: Elsevier; 2013.)

Emulsions

An emulsion is a mixture of two or more immiscible liquids; in an emulsion, one liquid is dispersed throughout the other. Emulsions are fairly unstable; an emulsifier (a substance that stabilizes an emulsion) is often added to improve stability and dispersion. For example, an emulsifier may be used to bind oil and water into a mixture. Many different types of emulsifiers are used, depending on the medication the manufacturer is preparing. A classic example of an emulsion from your kitchen is simple vinaigrette; vinaigrettes quickly separate unless shaken continually. In the pharmacy, calamine lotion is a classic topical emulsion purchased OTC. Propofol injections and IV lipid infusions are prescription medications that are emulsions stabilized with ingredients such as soybean oil and egg lecithin.

Examples of emulsions propofol (Diprivan; Rx), cyclosporine ophthalmic emulsion (Restasis; Rx)

emulsion agents can be given, such as lipids (also known as *fat*), which are used for nutritional parenteral feedings. Various types of emulsion preparations can be administered topically, orally, and even parenterally.

Suspensions

Suspensions are liquid dosage forms in which very small solid particles are suspended in the base solution (Fig. 5.14). Certain active ingredients are unstable when dissolved in a solution but stable in a suspension form. Suspensions such as syrups and other oral solutions can be used orally by children and older individuals because the patient can take the medication more easily. Oral suspensions should have a "Shake Well" auxiliary label that is easily visible on the front of the bottle and in the directions; if the product is prepared (reconstituted) in the pharmacy, proper adherence to the directions for mixing and placement of the date of expiration ("use by"

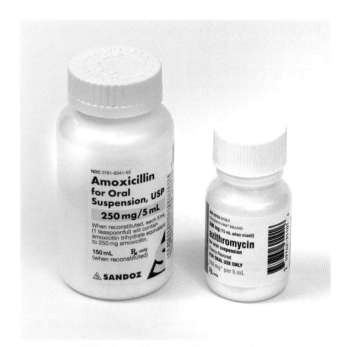

FIG. 5.14 Example of a suspension.

date) on the label or auxiliary label are very important. Suspension dosage forms are also formulated to be used topically, in the eye or ear, rectally, and even parenterally.

Examples of suspensions prednisolone ophthalmic suspension (Pred Forte; Rx), amoxicillin/clavulanate suspension (Augmentin; Rx), ibuprofen suspension (Children's Motrin; OTC)

■ Tech Note!

It is always important to shake oral suspensions well before using. However, care must be taken with injectable suspensions because some drugs, including many biological medicines, are inactivated by vigorous shaking. Always follow the manufacturer's directions for handling. For example, some types of insulin suspensions should be rolled, not shaken, to prevent destruction of the proteins that would result from shaking.

◉ Scenario Checkup 5.2

Mary begins her day at the compounding pharmacy happy to be putting her education into practice. One of the prescriptions she is to fill is amoxicillin for a baby with otitis media. She knows the drug will need to be reconstituted before it is dispensed. This was a call-in prescription, and the baby's parent will be in around noon to pick it up. What is the proper procedure Mary should follow in this situation? What could happen if Mary prepares the amoxicillin before the parent arrives?

Enemas

Enemas may be administered for one of two reasons: retention or evacuation. Retention enemas are used to deliver medication to the body in a manner that bypasses the stomach. Conditions such as ulcerative colitis (inflammation of the intestines) can be treated with antiinflammatory agents in this manner. A rectal diazepam gel (Diastat) is available for certain patients for the immediate treatment of seizures. The most common use of enemas, however, is to evacuate the bowel for a variety of reasons, such as preprocedural care (eg, to prepare for surgeries or examinations involving the intestine) or for women about to give birth. Evacuation enemas can be administered from prefilled squeeze bottles. Some enemas available OTC are used strictly for the relief of constipation. However, because of the dramatic effects of enemas, physicians usually do not recommend them as the first line of treatment for constipation. Enemas are manufactured in a water base, which is faster acting than an oil base. The typical amount of time for an evacuation enema to be effective is less than 10 minutes.

Examples of enemas mesalamine enema (Rowasa; Rx), sodium phosphate enema (Fleet Enema Extra; OTC)

Semisolids

Semisolid agents are different in their composition from liquids or solids. Although they contain solids and liquids, they normally are intended for topical application. Examples include creams, lotions, ointments, gels, pastes, and suppositories.

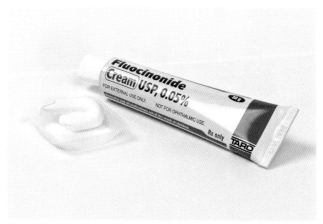

FIG. 5.15 Example of a cream.

Creams

Creams usually have medications in a base that is part oil and part water and is intended for topical or local use. When an emulsifier is added, the water and oil remain combined. Creams are massaged easily into the skin and do not leave a heavy, oily residue. Creams can be formulated to be used vaginally or rectally, taking into account the sensitive tissues to which they will be applied (Fig. 5.15).

Examples of creams hydrocortisone cream 1% (Cortizone-10; OTC), betamethasone cream 0.05% (Diprolene; Rx)

Lotions

Lotions are thinner than creams because their base contains more water. They penetrate well into the skin and do not leave an oily residue after application.

Examples of lotions hydrocortisone 1% lotion (Dermarest Eczema Medicated Lotion; OTC), hydrocortisone lotion 2.5% (Rx)

Ointments

Ointments contain medication in a glycol or oil base, such as petrolatum. Ointments can effectively cover the skin's surface while repelling moisture. Ointments can be used rectally or topically and can be formulated and sterilized for use in the eye as an ophthalmic agent.

Examples of ointments bacitracin/neomycin/polymyxin ointment (Neosporin Original Ointment; OTC), tacrolimus ointment (Protopic; Rx)

Gels

Gels contain medication in a viscous (thick) liquid that easily penetrates the skin and does not leave a residue. Many sunscreens are available in this dosage form. Medications for various skin conditions also are available in gels.

Examples of gels naftifine gel (Naftin; Rx), benzocaine (Orajel Medicated Toothache Pain Relief Gel; OTC)

Pastes

Pastes contain a lesser amount of liquid base than do solids. They are used for topical application and can absorb secretions, unlike other topical agents.

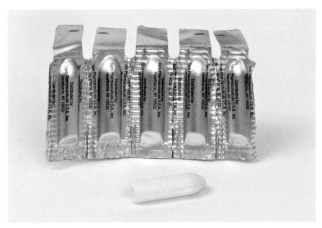
FIG. 5.16 Example of suppositories.

Example of pastes zinc oxide paste 40% (Desitin Maximum Strength; OTC)

Suppositories

Suppositories can be used for rectal, vaginal, or urethral conditions. They can be used for a localized effect (at the site of administration) or a systemic effect (throughout the body). They have several advantages over other dosage forms (Fig. 5.16). Rectal suppositories bypass the stomach, which is important if the patient is experiencing nausea and vomiting. They can relieve these symptoms without the patient having to receive an injection, which is much more invasive. They also are good for relief of constipation. Rectal antiinflammatory suppositories can be used to help treat inflammatory bowel conditions. Vaginal suppositories are used mostly to treat localized conditions of the vaginal area tissues, including yeast infections and atrophy related to menopause.

Examples of suppositories promethazine suppositories (Rx), miconazole vaginal suppositories (Monistat 3; OTC), bisacodyl suppositories (Dulcolax; OTC)

Powders

Powders do not fit neatly into the category of semisolids. Powders are solids, yet they are packaged in some forms that allow them to be sprayed, similar to liquid dosage forms, or inhaled (see Inhalants). Therefore topical powders have been included in the semisolids section. One of the main uses of topical powders is to reduce the wetness in an area. Most antifungal foot agents are available in powdered forms to keep the area as dry as possible, reducing the ability of the fungus to thrive. Powders also can be spread over a wide area if needed.

Examples of powders miconazole powder (Desenex spray; OTC), nystatin powder

Routes of Administration

Although many other types of dosage forms can be made by manufacturers or compounding pharmacies, the types covered in this chapter are those most commonly seen in the pharmacy. Because medications in the pharmacy are stocked according to their different dosage forms, it is important for student technicians to be familiar with all dosage forms so that they can quickly locate a medication. Table 5.5 lists

■ TABLE 5.5
Common Abbreviations Used With Dosage Forms

Abbreviation	Route of Administration	Specific Site of Action	Dosage Forms
BUC	Buccal	In the cheek	Lozenge/troche
IA	Intraarterial	In the artery	Solution
INH	Inhalation	Mouth	Aerosol, solution
IM	Intramuscular	In the muscle	Solution/suspension
IT	Intrathecal	In the space surrounding the spinal cord	Solution
IV	Intravenous	In the vein	Solution/suspension
NAS	Intranasal	Nose	Inhalant, solution, spray
PO	Oral	Absorbed into bloodstream	Capsule, elixir, powder, solution suspension, syrup, tablet, tincture, troche
PR	Per rectum	Rectum	Enema, ointment, solution, suppository
PV	Per vagina	Vagina	Foam, gel, ointment, solution, sponge, suppository
SL	Sublingual	Under the tongue	Sprays, tablet
Subcut	Subcutaneous	Under the surface of the skin	Solution/suspension
TOP	Epicutaneous or percutaneous	On the skin surface	Cream, disk, lotion, ointment, paste, patch, powder, solution, spray
	Transdermal	On the skin surface for delivery through the skin	
Urethral	Urethral	Urethra	Solution, suppository

abbreviations for the most common dosage forms and their routes of administration. The advantages and disadvantages of each type of route of administration determine the physician's final decision on the type of agent the patient should receive. The following sections describe each route of administration and give the advantages and disadvantages of each.

By Mouth (Oral)

A positive aspect of taking tablets or capsules or any agent by mouth (PO) is the convenience of the drug for the patient. Most oral medications can be kept readily available throughout the day in a handy bottle. Tablets and capsules do not need to be measured, which increases their ease of use, and most oral forms are much less expensive than other alternatives. Some oral medications are systemic, which means they are absorbed and dispersed throughout the body, whereas others are not absorbed and act locally in the gastrointestinal tract once swallowed. Oral administration is also one of the safer ways to give medication because if too much is given, there may be time to react before the drug begins to work. The disadvantage of these drugs is that they do not work as quickly as parenteral medications; they take 30 minutes to 1 hour to become active. This can be important, for instance, if the medication is intended for pain relief. Also, some drugs cannot be taken orally because they are not as effective. This complication is due to the acidic pH of the stomach, which breaks down some substances before absorption and makes certain medications of little use orally.

Sublingual and Buccal Agents

Although not many medications are available at this time in the form of sublingual (SL) or buccal (BUC) agents, the few that are commonly used are effective. Nitroglycerin is the most commonly used sublingual tablet (placed under the tongue; Fig. 5.17A) and is used to treat anginal attacks. Angina is a common heart ailment that affects millions of people. Its symptoms include shortness of breath and pain in and around the chest cavity. Nitroglycerin SL tablets bypass the long passage through the gastrointestinal system and are absorbed readily into the bloodstream. This accelerates the drug's action to a few minutes, compared with the longer time required for oral agents. Buccal agents are another type of uncommon dosage form. Buccal tablets are

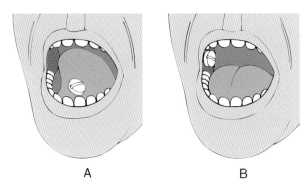

FIG. 5.17 (A) Sublingual tablet placement. (B) Buccal tablet placement. (From Clayton B, Stock Y. *Basic Pharmacology for Nurses*. 16th ed. St. Louis: Elsevier; 2013.)

placed between the gums and cheek (see Fig. 5.17B), where the medication penetrates the mouth lining and then enters the bloodstream.

Rapidly Disintegrating Oral Tablets

Some drugs are available in a newer dosage form that quickly disintegrates when taken orally and may be administered with or without water. This dosage form allows ease of administration for people who do not take larger sized tablets easily and for those with conditions such as nausea and vomiting, in which taking a tablet may induce vomiting. Examples include ondansetron (Zofran ODT) for nausea/vomiting, clonazepam orally for seizures, donepezil (Aricept ODT) for dementia, and rizatriptan (Maxalt-MLT) for migraines.

Rectal Agents

Rectal (PR) agents are used for many different reasons; for example, if a person is vomiting and cannot take oral medications, either suppositories or rectal suspensions can be used to treat the patient's condition. Various preparations are available, depending on the result desired. To reduce inflammation, ointments or creams can be used in addition to suppositories; these types of drugs work locally rather than systemically. However, to treat nausea and vomiting or motion sickness, a systemic-acting suppository can be used. Other agents include rectal solutions that also are used locally for various reasons, usually to clear the intestines of fecal material. The downside is that most people do not feel comfortable using the rectal dosage forms. In addition, depending on the drug and the retention time by the patient, the actual amount of drug absorbed may not be as predictable compared with medications taken orally.

Topical Agents

Many different preparations of topical (TOP) treatments are available. The effects of topical preparations range from systemic to localized (eg, for rashes). The skin is the largest organ of the body because of its large surface area. The skin has many portals through which drugs can pass into the body. Openings include sweat glands, hair follicles, and other small openings in the pores of the skin. Many topical agents fight skin infections, reduce inflammation, and protect the skin from the ultraviolet rays of the sun. Topical agents work at the site of action, which makes them effective for localized use.

In addition, manufacturers have created topical treatments that work systemically, such as medications for angina, blood pressure, hormone replacement, motion sickness, and smoking cessation. These are prepared in a variety of dosage forms, from ointments to patches or small disks that can be applied to the skin. The medication is absorbed through the pores into the bloodstream, where it begins to work.

An advantage of topical agents is the ease of application for the patient. Many topical medications act rapidly at the site of application to relieve itching or inflammation. Patches can be worn all day, which increases patient compliance because the patient does not have to remember to take the medication at various times during the day. In fact, some patches, such as those for motion sickness, can be applied and left in place for days.

The negative aspect of topical drugs is that they may cause skin irritation or may not be adequately absorbed transdermally; therefore many agents cannot be given by this route of administration. Because patches are generally more expensive to produce than other dosage forms, these medications tend to be more costly than their counterpart oral dosage forms.

Parenteral: Intravenous, Intravenous Piggyback, Intramuscular, and Subcutaneous Agents

The word *parenteral* is Greek in origin and means "side of intestine" or "outside the intestine." A wide range of parenteral dosages and administration sites are available. The most common parenteral medications are given intravenously (IV), into the veins; intramuscularly (IM), into the muscles; or subcutaneously (subcut), under the skin. Needles with a very small gauge are used, and the length depends on the site of injection. Parenteral administration has clear benefits, such as the speed of action and completeness of dosing. Parenteral medications such as insulin have allowed millions of people with diabetes to inject themselves daily, allowing them to lead normal and productive lives. In addition, many parenteral drugs work faster than those given by the oral route. This is important for emergency situations, for patients who are unconscious or combative, and for patients who are unable to swallow. In addition, smaller doses may be needed because of the high bioavailability of the agents injected. The disadvantage of parenteral drugs as a group is the increased risk for infection because the techniques for administration are invasive. Any drug injection must be given using as sterile a technique as possible to avoid introducing any microbes into the body. Also, injection is much more expensive than other routes of administration because of the required preparation and administration by trained personnel. Another disadvantage is that, because injectable drugs work quickly, once the drug has been injected, there is little or no time to alter its availability if an unintended dose is given or if an untoward reaction occurs.

Eye, Ear, Nose (Ophthalmic, Otic, Nasal)

A wide variety of agents are used to treat conditions affecting the eyes, nose, and ears. Pharmacy technicians must remember an important fact when preparing and filling prescriptions for agents that treat the ear or eye: physicians often use eye solutions to treat ear conditions; however, because the eye is sterile, ear solutions cannot be used to treat eye conditions. Therefore all ophthalmic drugs (eye preparations) are sterile. Otic drugs (ear preparations) are not necessarily always sterile because many otic agents treat the ear canal and do not typically penetrate a sterile environment. The pharmacy technician may prepare ophthalmic drugs in a laminar flow hood using aseptic technique (see Chapter 12). Technicians must remember that all ophthalmic drugs must be kept sterile.

Different dosage forms are used for the eye, ear, and nose, including ointments, solutions, and suspensions. Most treatments for the ear are for fighting an infection or removing earwax buildup. Most nasal sprays are used to treat symptoms of colds and allergies, whereas eye treatments typically are used for infections, inflammation, and conditions such as glaucoma (increased pressure in the eye). These dosage forms are effective at a specific site rather than involving the whole body. They can be administered with ease because of the small package size of the drug. Instructions for eye and ear preparations should use the word **instill** rather than "take" or "put." The main disadvantage of these drugs is that solutions used for the eye, if not kept sterile, can introduce bacteria into the area being treated. Also, ophthalmic drugs do not last as long as other treatments because of blinking of the eye and tearing, which wash the medication away from the site. Therefore dosing times may be frequent. In addition, most ophthalmic ointments make it difficult to see clearly.

◉ Scenario Checkup 5.3

Mary has been extremely busy in the pharmacy today. She only has 1 hour left on her shift, and she is feeling exhausted. She learned that studies show that mistakes can occur when technicians are overtired. She receives a prescription for Garamycin drops. Why should Mary read the script extremely carefully? What could occur if Mary interprets the order incorrectly?

Inhalants

Many people have lung diseases and use inhalants (INHs) to treat their conditions. As mentioned previously, there are two types of inhalers: those that use a propellant to push the drug to the lungs and those that use dry powder to release the medication as the patient takes a deep, fast breath. The dry powder inhaler may be a dry powder tube inhaler, a powder disk inhaler, or a single-dose dry powder disk inhaler. The choice of inhaler depends on its convenience for the patient and the medication needed. Some agents open the passageways to the lungs (eg, bronchodilators), some reduce inflammation (eg, corticosteroids), and there is even an inhaled insulin.

A positive aspect of inhalants is that most are available in handheld units and are convenient for carrying. The onset of action for short-acting bronchodilators, for example, is quick, which can make a dramatic difference in a person's ability to breathe comfortably. The disadvantage is that if the inhaler is not used properly, little if any of the drug is able to reach the lungs. Breathing in as the inhaler is activated is important, and it may be necessary to shake some inhalers before drug administration. Dry powder inhalants are small and convenient to carry, do not require coordination of breathing at the exact time of medication release, and are not shaken before use, although some models do require cocking the device. Respiratory solutions that are packaged in unit dose ampules or vials are used to deliver a specific amount of drug per treatment with the use of a nebulizer.

Injectables

Injectable medications are normally used to obtain a rapid response. The onset of action of many injectable drugs takes only a few minutes, as opposed to the possible 45 minutes or longer required for oral medications to take effect. People with diabetes may use long-acting insulins along with short-acting insulins. Although people with diabetes are the most

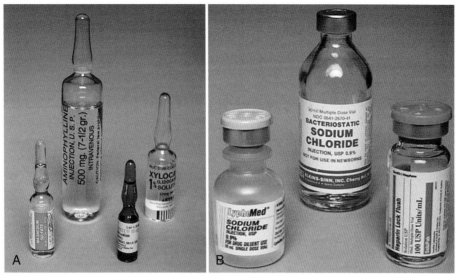

FIG. 5.18 (A) Medication in ampules. (B) Medication in vials.

common users of injectable drugs outside the hospital setting, other types of injectables used in the home are anticoagulants (eg, subcutaneous heparins) and certain injectables for patients with multiple sclerosis.

A variety of long-acting parenteral drugs is available that can be used in place of daily dosing. For example, medroxyprogesterone acetate (Depo-Provera Cl, Depo-subQ Provera 104), which can be used for birth control, must be injected every 3 months. Other parenteral long-acting medications include haloperidol decanoate, which is used monthly for the treatment of schizophrenia, and leuprolide acetate injection suspension (eg, Lupron Depot), which is injected either once monthly or once every 3 months for various hormonal disorders. The technician should note that long-acting depot injectable products are never to be given intravenously.

In the hospital, many oral medications are available in injectable form, and some are *only* available in injectable form. These medications typically are supplied in ampules or vials. Ampules are made of glass (Fig. 5.18A) and can range in volume from 0.5 to 50 mL. (Ampules are opened using the techniques outlined in Chapter 12.) Vials can be made of plastic or glass (see Fig. 5.18B) and range in size from 1 to 100 mL.

A unique type of vial is the ADD-Vantage container, which keeps the medication separate from the diluent until it is time to reconstitute. This saves waste when an expensive drug is used that has a short shelf life after preparation (Fig. 5.19 gives instructions on the use of this type of vial). Other medications that are available in IV form are premade IV bags and those prepared by the technician. Fig. 5.20 presents examples of a large-volume IV and an IV piggyback.

Technicians must pay close attention to the storage requirements for injectable drugs. Some are stored at room temperature, whereas others require refrigeration. For example, phytonadione (vitamin K) must be kept in a light-protected ampule and should be stored at room temperature. Other injectables (eg, ciprofloxacin) must be stored in light-protected bags after being reconstituted into an IV bag. Glass containers are packaged securely to protect them from breakage.

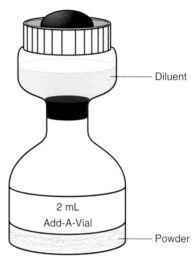

FIG. 5.19 This type of vial is called Add-A-Vial or Mix-O-Vial. The advantage of this type of medication dosage form is its longer shelf life. To use this type of vial: 1. Remove the sterile cap. 2. The powder is below, and the sterile diluent is in the top of the vial. The vial is divided by a rubber stopper in the middle. 3. Push the plunger down, forcing the stopper to fall into the bottom of the vial. This allows the diluent to mix with the powder. Shake well. Once dissolved, the medication is ready to be used.

Miscellaneous Routes

Other common routes of administration include vaginal or urethral dosage forms. These forms are suppositories, creams, ointments, foams, gels, and various inserts, such as rings. These types of delivery systems are used for the treatment of infections and inflammation and, in the case of vaginal foams or rings, for local or systemic birth control, respectively. Although there are clear advantages to the use of these agents, such as bypassing a systemic effect for some medications and affecting the specific site only, they are not necessarily applied easily and can be uncomfortable.

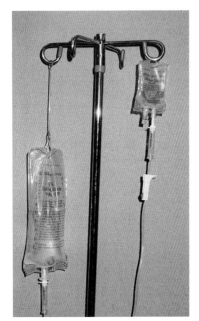

FIG. 5.20 *Left,* A large-volume intravenous bag. *Right,* An intravenous piggyback.

Other Considerations: Form and Function

Dosage forms are created based on the results from many clinical trials that investigate the **pharmacokinetics** of the medication or the function of the drug in experiments.

Pharmacokinetics and Pharmacodynamics

Pharmacokinetics is an all-inclusive word that represents many different components concerning the actions of the body on a drug, as opposed to *pharmacodynamics* (to be discussed later), which describes the effects the drug has on the body. For example, from the time a person takes a tablet, various considerations are examined, such as the levels of the drug in the blood and tissues, the absorption or movement of the drug into the bloodstream, and the overall distribution of the drug throughout the body, in addition to the metabolism and elimination of the drug. This includes the reaction of the drug with other drugs to determine changes that may occur in the course of the drug's time in the body. As these components are tested and refined, the eventual result is a dosage form that is tailor-made to work at its optimal level, while always keeping patient adherence in mind. Patient adherence is the level at which patients will or will not take their scheduled drugs. If a manufacturer can make a drug that can be taken once daily rather than several times a day, the odds increase that the patient will take the medication as directed.

The following sections describe the overall pharmacokinetics or life of the drug in the body. Absorption, distribution, metabolism, and elimination (ADME) are discussed, as well as half-life, bioavailability, and bioequivalence. All information about the pharmacokinetics of a drug and its relation to the proper dosing and use of the drug is listed in several reference books (see Chapter 7) and official drug package inserts.

Absorption

Medications are made specifically to pass through natural body barriers such as the skin, intestines, blood-brain barrier (surrounding the brain), and other membranous tissues. How well the drug passes through these barriers is one factor that determines its ultimate **absorption**, distribution, and effectiveness. Some considerations include whether the barrier is a lipid (fatty) base. Membranes surrounding organs such as the intestine have a variety of proteins and other structures implanted in a membranous protective structure that act as carriers for drug transport or as receptor sites. Important chemicals and drugs are able to pass a lock-and-key mechanism by latching on to receptive sites that allow the chemical or drug to pass into the organ to reach the final site of action intended for the drug (Fig. 5.21).

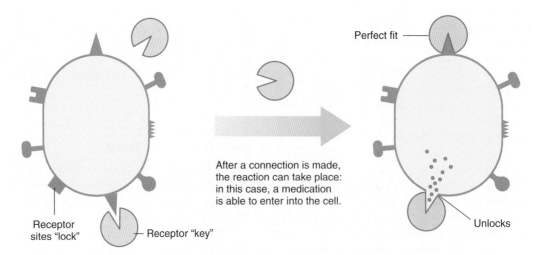

FIG. 5.21 The "lock-and-key" type mechanism that allows absorption to take place in a cell. These common reactions occur naturally throughout the body. Only after the correct receptor makes a connection with the matching receptor site does the cell allow a reaction to take place. Medications often mimic this natural mechanism.

Distribution

After systemic absorption, the medication is distributed throughout the body from the bloodstream into the tissues and, ultimately, into organs of the body. **Distribution** is the location of a medication throughout the blood, organs, and tissues after administration and absorption. For some medications, the distribution of the drug in the blood is measured at certain times throughout the day to keep track of medication concentrations and to ensure therapeutic effectiveness. Clearance (the volume of plasma from which the drug is removed per unit of time) also may be determined from the changes in blood concentrations within the dosing interval. Not all systems are affected equally by the drugs administered; some areas do not allow drugs to infiltrate as rapidly as do other areas. The distribution of a drug therefore is not necessarily equal throughout the body. For example, the blood-brain barrier is a built-in system that functions to keep harmful chemicals away from the brain. Certain medications have to be made that can cross this barrier to help treat diseases. Likewise, many medications that may penetrate the blood-brain barrier can cause unwanted side effects such as confusion. These are just a few of the hurdles drug companies must contend with when creating new medications. Also, most drugs are either weak acids or weak bases, which influences many of their pharmacokinetic characteristics, including their distribution to various body fluids and tissues (Box 5.1).

BOX 5.1 Ionization

Weak acid in weak base is less ionized = Transported more rapidly into lipid membranes
Weak base in weak acid is less ionized = Transported more rapidly into lipid membranes

---

Protein binding is another important factor related to drug distribution. Most drugs bind to blood proteins to some degree. Warfarin (a "blood thinner," or anticoagulant) and phenytoin (an anticonvulsant) are examples of drugs for which alterations in protein binding can become clinically important to the amount of drug available for distribution and therapeutic effect. If a patient is treated with warfarin along with phenytoin, the drugs compete for protein-binding sites and free (unbound) warfarin may increase to an unsafe level.

Metabolism

Drug **metabolism** is the biochemical modification or degradation of drugs in the body. As the drug is distributed throughout the body, some of it reenters the bloodstream and ultimately is transferred to the liver, where most drug metabolism takes place. Metabolism changes the chemical structure of the original drug. A **prodrug** is a drug that is taken in an inactive form and becomes active through the natural metabolic processes. This actually increases the bioavailability of the drug. If a particular drug is poorly absorbed by the body, a prodrug formulation can increase the amount of drug brought into the circulatory system. This is achieved by reducing the number of polar/ionized particles. Prodrugs can carry the medication to the specific site before becoming active, which can reduce the side effects (Fig. 5.22). Table 5.6 presents examples of prodrugs and their metabolites.

Some drugs pass initially through the bloodstream from the gastrointestinal tract to the liver before traveling to other organs of the body, where the strength of the active ingredient is reduced by rapid metabolism. This alters the amount of available drug at the site where it is needed.

Many orally administered drugs travel to the liver, and a proportion of the dose is metabolized before the drug has a chance to be distributed; this is called the **first-pass effect,**

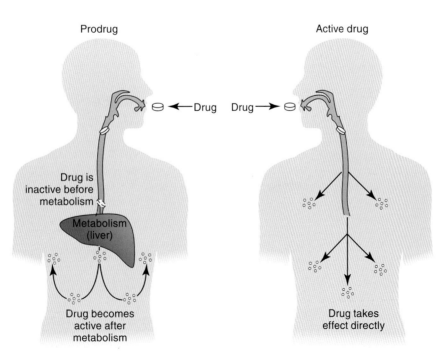

Prodrug

Active drug

Drug is inactive before metabolism

Metabolism (liver)

Drug becomes active after metabolism

Drug takes effect directly

FIG. 5.22 The difference between a prodrug and an active drug.

TABLE 5.6
Examples of Prodrugs and Their Active Metabolites

Prodrug	Active Drug
Prontosil	Sulfanilamide
Levodopa	Dopamine
Talampicillin	Ampicillin
Cyclophosphamide	Phosphoramide mustard
Diazepam	Oxazepam
Azathioprine	Mercaptopurine
Cortisone	Hydrocortisone
Dipivefrin	Adrenaline
Prednisone	Prednisolone
Enalapril	Enalaprilat

Available at: *http://epharmacology.hubpages.com/hub/Pharmacological-Effects-Prodrugs-Definition-Examples-and-Sources-of-Drug-Information.*

which lowers the drug's final bioavailability. Drugs that have a first-pass effect are given in higher doses than their injectable counterparts. Certain oral medications do not have this effect and have good bioavailability from oral or injectable routes. IV agents bypass the first-pass phenomenon because they enter the bloodstream directly. Other drugs do not undergo any change at all and are excreted from the body in the same form in which they were introduced. Different influences can alter metabolism, such as age, sex, genetics, diet, and other chemicals ingested.

Most of the final metabolism of a drug takes place in the liver. This is the final processing center of the body; it extracts toxins and unwanted chemicals and forwards them to the sites of the excretion process (eg, the kidneys). The liver works hard, but the amount it can process in a given time is limited. Individuals with any type of liver damage must be monitored closely when taking various medications to ensure that toxic levels are not present in the liver.

⊙ Scenario Checkup 5.4

As part of Mary's job in the pharmacy, she often helps out with the cashier duties. Mary is waiting on Ms. Black, who is picking up her monthly medications. Ms. Black is an older woman who is taking multiple medications for various conditions. Mary notices that today Ms. Black has some over-the-counter cough and cold products she wants to purchase in addition to her regular prescriptions. When Mary offers pharmacist counseling to Ms. Black, she refuses. What should Mary do next?

Elimination

Elimination is the last phase of a drug's life in the body. Although elimination usually is associated with urination, it is important to know that there are many ways a drug can be excreted from the body. In addition to elimination by the kidneys, drugs also may be expelled in the feces or by exhalation, by the sweat glands, and even in breast milk in women who are lactating. Urination and bowel movements are by far the most common methods of elimination. Remember that drugs that are not eliminated properly may accumulate in the body, which can lead to toxicity. Less common routes of excretion, such as through breast milk, must be considered when a physician prescribes a drug. However, not all drugs are tested by the manufacturer for excretion into breast milk; therefore the physician must rely on his or her judgment on the use of these agents.

Bioavailability

Bioavailability is the proportion of the drug that is delivered to its destination and is available to the site of action for which it was intended. Different drugs clear in different ways and at different times. This is an important consideration when prescribing drugs and determining drug dosing intervals. Drugs that are intended for certain organs or tissues in the body must pass many different obstacles, such as the destructive actions of stomach acids. By definition, an IV injection has a bioavailability of 100% because the drug does not have to be absorbed; however, bioavailability varies for other routes of administration, such as IM, subcut, topical, and oral (PO).

Half-Life

Half-life refers to the time it takes the body to break down and excrete half of the drug. To be more precise, it is the time taken for the plasma concentration of the drug to decrease by 50%. Of course, just monitoring the drug's plasma level is not the only factor that should be considered when determining half-life (eg, muscle, fat, and tissue should be taken into account). After approximately four half-lives, elimination is 94% complete. For example, if a person takes a medication that has a half-life of 10 hours, this means that in 10 hours, half of the drug will be eliminated, and in another 10 hours, another half of the remaining drug will be eliminated. This is an important factor in the creation of all drugs because this information tells the manufacturer how long it takes the body to rid itself of the drug; it also helps determine proper intervals for dosing. If a person takes too much medication or takes doses too close together, the drug can accumulate, which can be dangerous to the patient.

Bioequivalence

Bioequivalence is the comparison of drugs from different manufacturers or from the same manufacturer but different batches (lots). This is an important aspect of a drug because patients assume that every tablet they take is exactly the same as the one before and that all are the exact strength as listed on the label. Generic drug manufacturers strive to achieve equivalence with brand name manufacturers so that they can compete with the original manufacturer. A reference source that can be used to determine whether the generic drug is rated as bioequivalent to the brand name drug is the *Approved Drug Products With Therapeutic Equivalence Evaluations* (the Orange Book).

The Use of Excipients

All medications are prepared with additives (excipients) for many different reasons (Table 5.7). These additives include

TABLE 5.7
Description of Additives

Type of Additive	Example of Chemical	Reason
Antifungal	Benzoic acid	Prevents fungal growth
Base	Petrolatum	A common component to which medication is added for ointments and creams
Buffer	Sodium acetate	Adjusts pH
Coloring	Yellow dye no. 5	Improves visual appearance
Filler	Starch, powdered cellulose	Increases size of dosage form
Flavoring	Cherry	Improves taste
Preservative	Parabens	Increases shelf life
Sweetener	Sucrose	Improves taste
Weak salt acid/base	Hydrochloric acid and sodium hydroxide (base)	Helps drug dissolve more easily once it arrives in the gastrointestinal system

coloring for better appearance of the product and flavorings to disguise taste and/or smell. Many times fillers are used to increase the size of the medication because the amount of drug may be so small that the medication otherwise would be difficult, if not impossible, to handle. Many different types of preservatives are available; each prevents certain microbes from affecting the drug. These preservatives prolong the shelf life after the patient obtains and opens the drug product. Other types of additives include those that either increase the dispersal rate of the drug once it reaches the intestines or decrease the rate of distribution of the medication. As mentioned previously, many components involved in the preparation of dosage forms are added to improve the product for the patient convenience. Patients are more likely to take medication once or twice daily than multiple times per day.

Some patients may be allergic to an ingredient, such as dyes, or may have conditions in which certain ingredients should be avoided. For example, patients with diabetes may be instructed to purchase drug products that are sugar free or alcohol free. Patients with phenylketonuria may need to avoid products containing aspartame as a sweetener. Certain products may be available in the form required, whereas others may not. For patients who need alternative ingredients, a compounding pharmacy may be able to prepare the same drug containing ingredients that are tolerated by the patient.

Manufactured Products

After learning how many different routes of administration there are and the dosage forms used, you may think that is all there is. However, the ever-changing world of drug manufacturing has made available many different choices and has turned a simple compressed powder, known as a *tablet*, into an intricate, complicated, and highly structured format. A tablet is not just a tablet, nor a capsule merely a capsule. There are many different types of dosage forms, depending on the desired effect of the drug in question (Table 5.8). All manufactured types of dosage forms must be approved by the FDA (see Chapter 2). Approval of a drug product includes constant

testing of the product from batch to batch to ensure continuity of the medication. (Injectable dosage forms are discussed further in Chapter 12.) Pharmacies that provide compounded products must comply with the standards of the United States Pharmacopoeia–National Formulary (USP-NF) monographs.

Packaging and Storage Requirements

Medications are packaged according to manufacturers' specifications to ensure the effectiveness and shelf life of the drug. It is important for technicians to learn the various storage requirements of medications. Medications that have specific storage requirements are clearly marked on the container or box in which they are packaged. Certain medications arrive in dry ice and must be unpacked and stored immediately at the temperature indicated. When the outside of a box is labeled "refrigerate or keep frozen," the contents should never be left at room temperature because this can cause the medication to become unusable. Table 5.9 presents some examples of storage requirements for various drugs, along with special considerations. All medications have a package insert that describes the storage and stability of the drug. Technicians should become familiar with this type of information. In addition to manufacturer storage requirements, repackaging medications have their own guidelines, which have been instituted by the FDA and can be found in Chapter 11.

Medical Terminology

Another aspect of working with patients is the ability to understand medical terminology. Just as many medication names are derived from the Greek and Latin languages, so are all medical terms. In this section we will cover the basics of medical terminology. The segments of medical terms, along with terms associated with each body system, are described. Medical terms consist of segments, or word parts, that, when combined, describe all conditions and anatomy known. Table 5.10 presents a sample of abbreviations used in the medical field.

TABLE 5.8
Description of Dosage Forms

Dosage Form	Types	Benefits
Buccal		Dissolves in the cheek and the gum
Capsule	Gelatin cover	Allows for pharmacy-compounded agents; easy to swallow
	Hard gelatin/dry fill	Filled with powder Filled with a tablet inside Filled with pellets Filled with another capsule
	Pulvule	Manufacturer prepared (bullet shaped)
	Soft gelatin/wet fill	Filled with a liquid Filled with a paste
	Spansule	Capsule holds small pellets or beads
Chewable tablet		Chewed
Coated tablet	Caplet	Hard, capsule-shaped tablet
	Colored	Appearance
	Gel	Smaller than a capsule, easier to swallow
	Enteric coated	Delayed release; easier to swallow
	Oral dissolving	Dissolves in mouth on contact
	Sugar added and colored	Protects drug; covers taste
Injectable vial	ADD-Vantage vial	Rubber stopper is depressed, releasing diluents into powder product
	Multiple-dose vial	May be used more than once
	Single-dose vial	Must be discarded after one use
Oral tablet	Compressed	Hard dissolves slower; soft dissolves faster
	Extended release	Releases medication slowly
	Film coated	Protects against stomach acid
	Layered	Slow release
Sublingual	Soft compressed	Dissolves under the tongue

TABLE 5.9
Examples of Storage Requirements

Medication	Location	Considerations
Insulins (Humulin, Novologs)	Refrigerator	Opened 28–30 days; unopened—per package
Latanoprost (Xalatan)	Refrigerator	Stored in refrigerator (2°–8°C) until opened; may be kept up to 6 weeks at room temperature after opening
Mannitol	Room temperature	Mannitol crystallizes at room temperature; do not use crystallized drug; drug must be warmed before using if crystals are present
Metronidazole IV	Room temperature	Stored at 15°–30°C and protected from light
Penicillin IV	Drug shelf or refrigerator	Must be stored in refrigerator after reconstitution
Promethazine Suppository	Drug shelf or refrigerator	Intended to melt at body temperature
Vaccines such as Hib, HepA, HepB, human papillomavirus, DTaP, DT, Td, Tdap, influenza, MMR, meningococcal, pneumococcal, rotavirus	Refrigerator	Kept in refrigerator (2°–8°C)
Vaccines such as MMR, MMRV, varicella-zoster	Freezer	Kept in freezer (<15°C)

DT, Diphtheria and tetanus; *DTaP,* diphtheria, tetanus, and pertussis; *Hep,* hepatitis; *Hib, Haemophilus influenzae* type B; *IV,* intravenous; *MMR,* mumps, measles, and rubella; *MMRV,* mumps, measles, rubella, and varicella; *Td,* tetanus and diphtheria; *Tdap,* tetanus, diphtheria, and pertussis.

TABLE 5.10
Additional Abbreviations

Abbreviation	Meaning	Abbreviation	Meaning
ADHD	Attention-deficit/hyperactivity disorder	HTN	Hypertension
ADR	Adverse drug reaction	ICU	Intensive care unit
AIDS	Acquired immunodeficiency syndrome	IDDM	Insulin-dependent diabetes mellitus
BBB	Blood-brain barrier	KVO	Keep vein open
BUN	Blood urea nitrogen	LBP	Low blood pressure
CABG	Coronary artery bypass graft	LLL	Left lower lobe
CAD	Coronary artery disease	MI	Myocardial infarction
CBC	Complete blood count	MRI	Magnetic resonance imaging
CCU	Coronary care unit	N & V	Nausea and vomiting
CHD	Coronary heart disease	NICU	Neonatal intensive care unit
CHF	Congestive heart failure	NIDDM	Non–insulin-dependent diabetes mellitus
COPD	Chronic obstructive pulmonary disease	NPO	Nothing by mouth
CVD	Cardiovascular disease	OBGYN	Obstetrics and gynecology
DNR	Do not resuscitate	OR	Operating room
DOA	Dead on arrival	PPN	Peripheral parenteral nutrition
DOB	Date of birth	PT	Prothrombin time
DVT	Deep vein thrombosis	RLS	Restless legs syndrome
DX	Diagnosis	SARS	Severe acute respiratory syndrome
EEG	Electroencephalogram	SBO	Small bowel obstruction
EENT	Eye, ear, nose, and throat	SOB	Shortness of breath
ECG	Electrocardiogram	TKO	To keep open
ER	Emergency room	TPN	Total parenteral nutrition
FX	Fracture	TX	Treatment
GERD	Gastroesophageal reflux disease	UNG	Ointment
HBP	High blood pressure	UTI	Urinary tract infection
HIV	Human immunodeficiency virus	WBC	White blood cell count
HPV	Human papillomavirus		

BOX 5.2 Overview of Word Parts of Medical Terminology

Example of how a word is formed:
1. Prefix: placed before each combining form
   Example: peri- (around)
2. Suffix: placed after the combining form
   Example: -itis (inflammation)
3. The root word of the term
   Example: cardia (heart)
4. The combining form
   Example: cardi/o
   Read the suffix first, then go back to the beginning and proceed left to right. Put them together: pericarditis (ie, inflammation around the heart).

Rules
1. Terms can be one to four combinations.
2. Read the suffix first, then go back to the beginning and proceed left to right. Multiple terms can define the same word part.
3. If the combining form has two vowels (eg, i, o) and the suffix begins with a vowel, drop the "o."

It is important to know the basics of how medical terminology applies to various conditions. Terms and drugs fit together like hand in glove. There are four segments, or word parts, as follows:
1. The prefix
2. The suffix
3. The root word
4. The combining form

To combine these word segments, only a few rules must be followed (Box 5.2). A list of common prefixes, suffixes, and root words with their combining forms is shown in Table 5.11.

TABLE 5.11
Common Body System Word Segments

Prefixes

a-	away from, without
brady-	slow
dys-	painful or disordered
hyper-	above, elevated
hypo-	below, low
peri-	around, surrounding
poly-	many
post-	after, behind
pre-	before, in front
sub-	under, less than, below
tachy-	fast

Suffixes

-al	pertaining to
-algia	painful condition
-ectomy	surgical excision
-gram	picture or record
-itis	inflammation
-logist	one who studies
-logy	study of
-megaly	enlargement
-necr/o	tissue death
-plasty	repair through surgery
-pnea	breathing
-rrhage	excessive flow
-rrhea	flow or discharge
-rrhexis	rupture
-scler/o	hardening
-scopy	use an instrument to examine
-sten/o	narrowing
-stomy	opening

Colors

cyan/o	blue
leuk/o	white
melan/o	black
rub/o	red

Cardiovascular System

angi/o, vas/o	blood vessel
arteri/o	artery
capill/o	capillaries
cardi/o	heart
hem/o	blood
phleb/o	vein

Digestive and Hepatic Systems

cholecyst/o	gallbladder
col/o, colon/o	large intestine
enter/o	relating to the intestine
gastr/o	stomach
hepat/o	liver
pancreat/o	pancreas
proct/o, rect/o	anus or rectum
stomat/o	opening

Eyes

ir/o, irid/o	iris
ophthalm/o	eyes
opt/i	eyes
phac/o, phak/o	lens

Ears

acous/o, ot/o	ears or hearing
labyrinth/o	inner ear
myring/o	middle ear
pinn/i	external ear, auricle
tympan/o	membrane of middle ear, eardrum

Endocrine System

adren/o	adrenal glands
gonad/o	gonads (male, female)
parathyroid/o	parathyroid gland
pineal/o	pineal gland
pituit/o	pituitary glands
thym/o	thymus
thyr/o, thyroid/o	thyroid gland

Integumentary/Skin System

cutane/o	skin
dermat/o, derm/o	skin
hidr/o	sweat glands
onych/o	nails
pil/i, pil/o	hair
seb/o	sebaceous glands

Nervous System

encephal/o	brain
mening/o	membranes covering spinal cord and brain
myel/o	spinal cord
neur/o	nerves

TABLE 5.11
Common Body System Word Segments—cont'd

Reproductive System		Musculoskeletal System	
hyster/o	uterus	arthr/o	joints
oophor/o	ovaries	burs/o	bursa
orch/o, test/i	testicles	chondr/o	cartilage
pen/i, phall/i	penis	ligament/o	ligaments
placent/o	placenta	my/o	muscle
salping/o	fallopian tubes	myel/o	bone marrow
Respiratory System		oste/o	bones
alveol/o	alveoli	**Urinary System**	
bronchi/o	bronchi	cyst/o	bladder
laryng/o	larynx	nephr/o	kidneys
nas/o	nose	pyel/o	pelvis or kidney
pharyng/o	pharynx	ur/o, urin/o	urine
rhin/o	nose	ureter/o	ureters
sinus/o	sinus	urethr/o	urethra
trache/o	trachea		

Although this chapter mentioned many competencies in which a technician must be proficient, you will do most of your learning on the job. However, it is important always to keep learning because this both promotes self-development and enables you to advance in your profession. New dosage forms are always being invented for convenience and to achieve the best results. Technicians can stay current on the new trends through additional reading, continuing education, and on-the-job training.

◉ Technician Profile

Emory is a pharmacy purchasing agent for a large area hospital. She is a certified pharmacy technician (CPhT) and has worked in the pharmacy department for more than 15 years. The pharmacy buyer's job is a critical component of a well-run facility and requires an individual who is knowledgeable and dedicated to making sure the patients' needs are met. Most of Emory's duties are performed in an office setting. She procures supplies, materials, and pharmaceuticals for the various pharmacies throughout the hospital. She works with vendors to obtain the highest quality products at the optimum price. Emory is responsible for ensuring dependable, expedient delivery of the merchandise. She has a clear understanding of current market fluctuations and drug shortages. She finds her job demanding but very satisfying.

Do You Remember These Key Points?

- The abbreviations on the "Do Not Use" list and why they are dangerous
- The general classifications of medications and their associated body systems
- The various dosage forms and routes of administration

- The difference between pharmacokinetics and pharmacodynamics
- How drugs are absorbed, distributed, metabolized, and eliminated from the body
- The bioavailability of drugs in the body
- First-pass metabolism and why it is important in drug delivery
- Half-life and the factors that influence it
- The bioequivalence of drugs and its relationship to the Orange Book
- Types of excipients used in manufacturing dosage forms and the reasons for their use
- Packaging and storage requirements of medications
- Segments of medical terms
- Abbreviations for the routes of administration
- Common medical terms and abbreviations

◉ Scenario Follow-Up

As Mary begins to feel more confident in her role as a technician, she finds herself looking forward to the challenges of each new day. Instead of feeling overwhelmed by the sheer number of the different types of drugs and all the various dosage forms she must learn, she understands that with time, she will add to her knowledge base and become a better technician with each passing day.

Review Questions

Multiple Choice Questions

1. Why are sublingual tablets better for relieving angina attacks than traditional tablets?
   - **A.** They will not cause drowsiness.
   - **B.** They bypass the stomach, entering the bloodstream for quicker relief.

    C. They are administered less frequently than traditional tablets.

    D. They are easier to swallow.

2. Why do manufacturers make dosage forms that are effective over a longer time?
   - **A.** To cut down on the cost of making the drug
   - **B.** To save time preparing each dose
   - **C.** To enable the patient to take the medication less often
   - **D.** To meet US Food and Drug Administration standards

3. Parenteral medications are used because:
   - **A.** They work quickly.
   - **B.** They bypass the acidic secretions of the stomach.
   - **C.** The patient is unable to take medication by mouth.
   - **D.** All of the above

4. Which of the following is *not* an example of a semisolid dosage form?
   - **A.** Cream
   - **B.** Gel
   - **C.** Paste
   - **D.** Lozenge

5. Which liquid dosage form has a hydroalcoholic base?
   - **A.** Elixir
   - **B.** Syrup
   - **C.** Enema
   - **D.** Emulsion

6. The organ that performs most of the metabolism of a drug is the:
   - **A.** Kidney
   - **B.** Small intestine
   - **C.** Stomach
   - **D.** Liver

7. If a drug has a half-life of 20 hours, this would mean that:
   - **A.** Half of the drug is eliminated from the body in the first 20 hours, followed by the second half in 20 more hours.
   - **B.** The drug only lasts half as long as needed.
   - **C.** The drug loses half its strength in half of 20 hours.
   - **D.** The drug loses half its strength in 20 hours, followed by half of the remaining strength in the following 20 hours, and so forth.

8. Excipients are used in preparing medications to:
   - **A.** Improve appearance
   - **B.** Disguise taste and/or smell
   - **C.** Increase the size of the medication
   - **D.** All of the above

9. The time taken for the plasma concentration of a drug to decrease by 50% is known as:
   - **A.** Bioavailability
   - **B.** Distribution
   - **C.** Ionization
   - **D.** Half-life

10. Which of the following oral dosage forms should have a "Shake Well" auxiliary label on the bottle?
    - **A.** Suspension
    - **B.** Solution
    - **C.** Syrup
    - **D.** All of the above

☐ Technician's Corner

A 30-year-old woman was brought into the emergency room experiencing shortness of breath and a rash. She told the nurse she had seafood for dinner. The physician ordered a 0.5-mg dose of epinephrine. Shortly after the intravenous infusion, the patient reported chest pain with tingling in her fingers. She was given the *correct* medication but via the *incorrect* route. What should have been the route?

Bibliography

Ansel HC, Allen LV, Popovich NG. *Ansel's Pharmaceutical Dosage forms and Drug Delivery Systems*. 10th ed. Baltimore: Lippincott Williams & Wilkins; 2013.

Brown M, Mulholland J. *Drug Calculations*. 8th ed. St. Louis: Elsevier; 2007.

Drug Facts and Comparisons. 68th ed. St. Louis: Wolters Kluwer Health; 2013.

Gray Morris D. *Calculate with Confidence*. 6th ed. St. Louis: Elsevier; 2013.

Potter PA, Perry AG. *Fundamentals of Nursing*. 8th ed. St. Louis: Elsevier; 2013.

Websites Referenced

Approved drug products with therapeutic equivalence evaluations (Orange Book information). Available at: http://www.fda.gov/cder/ob.

Difference Between.Net. Difference between CFC and HFA inhalers. Available at: http://www.differencebetween.net/science/health/disease-health/difference-between-cfc-and-hfa-inhalers/.

Do Not Use List Fact Sheet | The Joint Commission

Epharmacology. Hub pages. Pharmacological effects, prodrugs (definition, examples) and sources of drug information. Available at: http://epharmacology.hubpages.com/hub/Pharmacological-Effects-Prodrugs-Definition-Examples-and-Sources-of-Drug-Information.

Immunization Action Coalition. (Technical reviewed by CDC 2007). Vaccine handling tips. Available at: http://www.vaccineinformation.org.

Institute for Safe Medication Practices. ISMP's list of error prone abbreviations, symbols, and dose designations. Available at: http://www.ismp.org/tools/errorproneabbreviations.pdf.

Medscape website. Monograph: insulins general statement. Available at: http://www.medscape.com/druginfo/monoinfobyid?cid=med&drugid=5218&drugname=Humulin+R+Inj&monotype=genstatement&monoid=382933&mononame=Insulins%20General%20Statement&print=1.

Miller TC, Gerth J. Dose of confusion. ProPublica. Available at: https://www.propublica.org/article/how-much-acetaminophen-a-day-is-safe-canada-may-decide-its-less.

Newly Developed Prodrugs and Prodrugs in Development; an Insight of the Recent Years. Available at: https://pubmed.ncbi.nlm.nih.gov/32079289/.

WebMD. Asthma Health Center. Nebulizers: home and portable. Available at: http://www.webmd.com/asthma/guide/home-nebulizer-therapy?page=2.

Wisniewski L, Holquist C. *The Absence of a Trade Name Does Not Equal a Generic Drug*. Available at: http://www.drugtopics.com.

CHAPTER 6

Conversions and Calculations

Karen Davis

OBJECTIVES

1. Describe the history of pharmacy calculations.
2. Convert Arabic numbers to Roman numerals.
3. Convert traditional time into international/military time.
4. Convert Fahrenheit temperatures to Celsius temperatures.
5. Use the following to determine medication dosages: (a) multiplication and division, (b) fractions, (c) decimals, (d) percentages, (e) ratio and proportion, (f) dimensional analysis.
6. Demonstrate the ability to convert among the various systems of measurement used in the practice of pharmacy: (a) metric system, (b) household measurement, (c) apothecary system, (d) avoirdupois system.
7. Apply the formulas for calculating doses by body weight and body surface area and for pediatric dosages (Young's Rule and Clark's Rule).
8. Perform calculations involving units and milliequivalents.
9. Calculate infusion rates and drip rates.
10. Understand and apply the calculations involved in dilution.
11. Understand and apply the calculations involved in alligations.

TERMS AND DEFINITIONS

Alligation alternate A mathematical method of solving problems that involves the mixing of two solutions or two solids with different percentage weights to achieve a desired third strength

Apothecary system A system of measurement once used in the practice of pharmacy to measure both volume and weight; this system has been mostly replaced by the metric system

Avoirdupois system A system of measurement previously used in pharmacy for the determination of weight in ounces and pounds; this system has been mostly replaced by the metric system

Conversion factor A fraction with the numerical value of 1, which is used to convert one unit to another without changing the value of the number

Diluent/solvent An inert product, either liquid or solid, that is added to a preparation to reduce the strength of the original product

Dilution The process of adding a diluent or solvent to a compound, resulting in a product of increased volume or weight and lower concentration

Dimensional analysis (DA) A method used to solve complicated pharmaceutical calculations that would require numerous sets of ratio and proportion problems; the main benefit of using DA is the ability to keep track of units during the process

Drip rate (DR) or drop rate The number of drops (gtt) administered over a specific time by an intravenous infusion (eg, gtt/min)

Drop factor The size of drops coming through the tubing; the size is measured in drops per milliliter (gtt/mL) and is found on the tubing package

Household system A system of measurement commonly used in the United States; it measures volumes using household utensils

Infusion rate or flow rate The amount of intravenous (IV) solution administered over a specific period (eg, mL/min, mL/hr, gtt/min); volume/time

International System of Units (SI) A system of measurement based on seven base units with prefixes that change units by multiples of 10; the prefixes for the modern metric system are taken from the French Système International d'Unités and were adopted to provide a single worldwide system of weights and measures

International time A 24-hour method of keeping time; hours are not distinguished as am or pm but rather are counted continuously throughout the day

Markup The amount added to a wholesale price (usually a percentage) to make a profit

Metric system The approved system of measurement for pharmacy in the United States based on multiples of 10; the basic units of measurement are the gram (g) for weight, the liter (L) for volume, and the meter (m) for length

Milliequivalent (mEq) A type of unit used in the United States to express the concentration of electrolytes such as sodium, potassium, magnesium, and calcium

Retail price The wholesale price plus markup

Units A unit of measurement assigned to medications called *biologicals* that have been tested for potency in biological systems; units are specific to each medication; therefore units of one medication cannot be compared with units of a different medication

Volume The amount of liquid enclosed within a container

Wholesale cost The purchase price of a product (in this case, medicine) that is then marked up for resale

◉ Scenario

Victoria is an experienced intravenous (IV) compounding technician. She has worked in her current position at a local hospital pharmacy for 8 years. She is responsible for making IV medications during her shift. Victoria performs many critical calculations on a regular basis. Today she is compounding an antibiotic small-volume parenteral preparation for a patient infected with Staphylococcus aureus. *Why is it important that Victoria's calculations are 100% accurate?*

The ability to manipulate conversions and make calculations is a requirement of pharmacy technicians. Unfortunately, in many cases when math is mentioned to new pharmacy technicians, it can trigger instant stress by reminding students of previous bad experiences. However, pharmaceutical calculations are performed on a daily basis and applied to the medications prepared in class and at work. The repetitiveness of these conversions and calculations reinforces the student technician's knowledge and confidence. It is important to learn and feel comfortable with the basic conversions.

Tech Note!

Although a pharmacist needs to check all transcriptions and calculations, it is important that the technician have a good understanding of these mathematical operations to avoid medication errors.

This chapter describes the types of calculations used throughout history, explains Roman numerals and military time, and presents common math problems involving multiplication, division, fractions, decimals, percentages, and ratios. Other areas of focus include the following:

- Alligation
- Apothecary system
- Avoirdupois system
- Dilution
- Dimensional analysis (DA)
- Dosing using mg/kg and body surface area (BSA) in m^2
- Household system
- Infusion rates, drip rates (DRs), and drop factors
- Metric system

Special calculations for infants, children, and senior citizens also are discussed; these patients deserve special consideration because of the metabolic differences that exist before adolescence and in old age.

Medication dosing is discussed for the following medications and therapies:

- Chemotherapy
- Heparin
- Insulin
- Parenteral nutrition

Make sure you understand each section before moving on to the next.

History of Pharmacy Calculations

Four different measurement systems have been used throughout the history of pharmacy. Most of the systems involve approximate measurements, so the conversion from one system to another is not precise. The pharmacy technician must have a basic understanding of all systems; however, in the

United States, the United States Pharmacopeia (USP) recognizes the **metric system** as the official system of measurement for pharmacy. The metric system (discussed later in the chapter) is based on multiples of 10 and is the most precise of the systems. Technicians in the United States mostly encounter prescriptions expressed in either metric or household systems.

A good way to become familiar with common pharmacy measurements is to start with what you know and build on that knowledge. For example, most people are familiar with the household measurement of a teaspoon. When writing prescriptions, many prescribers prefer to use 5 milliliters (mL) in the metric system rather than 1 teaspoonful (tsp). These two measurements, one in the household system and the other in the metric system, are considered to be equivalent. The pharmacy technician must translate the physician's orders into terms an average person can understand. Always reread what will be printed on the prescription label to consider whether it will make sense to the layperson; never assume that a person understands the meaning of a measurement. This precaution reduces the chance of any misinterpretation of the instructions.

Roman Numerals

Although Arabic numerals (ie, 1, 2, 3, and so on) are commonly used in the United States, physicians do not always use this system when ordering medications. Instead, they may use Roman numerals to indicate the quantity of tablets or capsules, the number of fluid ounces, or the number of refills. Roman numerals may be either uppercase or lowercase letters.

When using Roman numerals, begin with I, II, III (1, 2, 3); then write IV (1 less than 5) to equal 4. Repeat the process at 9 by writing IX (1 less than 10) to equal 9. To write 40, write XL (10 less than 50). However, to write 49, use XLIX (not IL; see rule 9 in the following section). The fraction ½ is written as lower case $\overline{ss}$ (ss with a line over both letters). Table 6.1 presents a comparison of Roman numerals and Arabic numbers.

Rules for Determining Roman Numerals

1. Numbers are represented by combinations of the letters I, V, X, L, C, D, and M, which represent 1, 5, 10, 50, 100, 500, and 1000, respectively.
2. When a numeral is repeated, its value is repeated.
   Examples: II = 2   XXX = 30
3. A numeral may not be repeated more than three times.
   Example: XL = 40, not XXXX
4. V, L, and D are never repeated.
   Example: LL is incorrect for 100 (100 is C)
5. When a smaller numeral is placed after a larger numeral, it is added to the larger numeral.
   Example: CX = 100 + 10 = 110   LXVIII = 50 + 10 + 5 + 3 = 68
6. When a smaller numeral is placed before a larger numeral, it is subtracted from the larger numeral.
   Example: XC = 100 − 10 = 90   XCIX = (100 − 10) + (10 − 1) = 90 + 9 = 99
7. V, L, and D are *never* subtracted. LC is incorrect. (L already is 50)

■ TABLE 6.1
Arabic and Roman Numerals

Arabic Numeral	Roman Numeral
1	I
2	II
3	III
4	IV
5	V
6	VI
7	VII
8	VIII
9	IX
10	X
11	XI
12	XII
13	XIII
14	XIV
15	XV
16	XVI
17	XVII
18	XVIII
19	XIX
20	XX
21	XXI
22	XXII
23	XXIII
24	XXIV
25	XXV
26	XXVI
27	XXVII
28	XXVIII
29	XXIX
30	XXX
40	XL
50	L
60	LX
70	LXX
80	LXXX
90	XC
100	C
500	D
600	DC
700	DCC
800	DCCC
900	CM
1000	M

8. Never subtract more than one numeral!
   Example: 8 = VIII, not IIX
9. When subtracting:
   a. Only subtract powers of 10: I, X, and C (not V or L)
   b. Only use a numeral before the next two higher value numerals:
      • Use I before V and X, X before L and C, and C before D and M
      • *Example:* 40 = XL, but 49 does not equal IL because I and L are too far apart (49 = XLIX)

Example 6.1 Working With Roman Numerals

When working with Roman numerals, remember that if a larger number is placed in front of a smaller one, you must add the two to determine the value.

$$XV = X(10) + V(5) = 15$$

However, if a smaller number is placed before a larger number, you must subtract.

$$IX = X(10) - I(1) = 9$$

Exercise 6.1 Quick Check

Change the following to Arabic numbers.
1. XIV = _____
2. XC = _____
3. XL = _____
4. VIII = _____
5. IV = _____
6. LX = _____
7. IX = _____
8. XX = _____
9. XXIV = _____
10. LXXV = _____
11. XXXIX = _____
12. CXX = _____

International Time (Military Time)

In a hospital or institutional setting, **international time,** also known as military time, is used exclusively. Orders are written 24 hours a day, and a system is needed to ensure that all medical-related caretakers understand exactly when an order was written and when the medication or treatment is to take place. The system is based on 100. Starting at 0000 (midnight) and continuing with 0100 (1:00 am), the clock runs through to 2300 (11:00 pm) and restarts again at 0000 (midnight) (Fig. 6.1). This system is easy for most people to use through 1200 (noon), but then it can become confusing. As the clock hands begin to make their second trip around the face of the clock in the pm hours, the numbers continue. For example, 1300 is 1:00 pm, and 1400 is 2:00 pm. Minutes are added to the hours in the last two places through 59. For instance, 1:32 pm is 1332, and 12:01 am is 0001. When the pharmacy receives orders, the receiver must check the date and time against previous orders to ensure that the most recent order is in effect. Using this system, there is never any

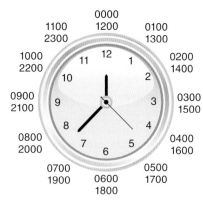

FIG. 6.1 Clock showing regular and military time.

BOX 6.1 Time Conversions

Midnight (12:00 am) = 0000 hr
1:00 am = 0100 hr
2:00 am = 0200 hr
3:00 am = 0300 hr
4:00 am = 0400 hr
5:00 am = 0500 hr
6:00 am = 0600 hr
7:00 am = 0700 hr
8:00 am = 0800 hr
9:00 am = 0900 hr
10:00 am = 1000 hr
11:00 am = 1100 hr
12:00 pm = 1200 hr
1:00 pm = 1300 hr
2:00 pm = 1400 hr
3:00 pm = 1500 hr
4:00 pm = 1600 hr
5:00 pm = 1700 hr
6:00 pm = 1800 hr
7:00 pm = 1900 hr
8:00 pm = 2000 hr
9:00 pm = 2100 hr
10:00 pm = 2200 hr
11:00 pm = 2300 hr

question as to when an order was written or which order supersedes another (Box 6.1).

Exercise 6.2 Quick Check

Convert each time to either international or standard time.
1. 12:00 am = _____
2. 4:30 pm = _____
3. 7:00 am = _____
4. 1:30 am = _____
5. 11:11 am = _____
6. 9:15 pm = _____
7. 2:30 pm = _____
8. 2000 hr = _____
9. 1417 hr = _____
10. 2101 hr = _____
11. 2359 hr = _____
12. 1025 hr = _____

Temperature Conversion Between Fahrenheit and Celsius

The Fahrenheit temperature scale is most commonly used in the United States. Freezing is 32°F, and boiling is 212°F. The Celsius scale is used in countries that regularly use the metric system (discussed later in the chapter). The metric system is based on multiples of 10, and the Celsius temperature scale goes from 0°C as the freezing point to 100°C as the boiling point. It is sometimes necessary to convert between these two scales. Formulas for converting can be written with fractions or decimals as follows.

Fahrenheit to Celsius

$$\text{Fraction equation: } °C = (F - 32) \cdot \frac{5}{9}$$

$$\text{Decimal equation: } °C = \frac{(F-32)}{1.8}$$

◉ Example 6.2

Convert 98.6°F to Celsius:

$$°C = (98.6 - 32)\frac{5}{9} = 37°C \text{ or } °C = \frac{(98.6-32)}{1.8} = 37°C$$

Celsius to Fahrenheit

$$\text{Fraction equation: } °F = \left(\frac{9}{5} \cdot C\right) + 32$$

$$\text{Decimal equation: } °F = (1.8 \cdot C) + 32$$

◉ Example 6.3

Convert 100°C to Fahrenheit:

$$°F = \frac{9 \cdot 100}{5} + 32 = 212°F \text{ or}$$

$$°F = (1.8 \cdot 100) + 32 = 212°F$$

◉ Exercise 6.3 Quick Check

Convert to Fahrenheit or Celsius.
1. 80°C = _____ °F
2. 72°F = _____ °C
3. 65°C = _____ °F
4. 32°F = _____ °C

Basic Math Skills

It is important for pharmacy technician students to review and be comfortable with basic skills such as adding, subtracting, multiplying, and dividing whole numbers, fractions, and decimals before adding new skills. Multiplication is used repeatedly in pharmacy calculations (Table 6.2). Sometimes it is necessary to increase or reduce a prescription. Multiplication by a number greater than 1 is used to increase a formula. Division, which is the same as multiplying by a proper fraction, is used to determine a part or portion of a prescription.

Review your multiplication and division skills. It is *essential* that you memorize multiplication at least through 12 before continuing. Use flash cards if necessary.

Fractions, Percentages, Ratios, and Proportions

Fractions

A fraction consists of a numerator and a denominator: the numerator is the top number in a fraction, and the denominator is the bottom number. The numerator of a fraction shows the number of equivalent parts in the whole, and the denominator shows how many are being considered as the whole.

If an object is divided into four parts, one part can be expressed as ¼, or one part (1) of the whole (4).

If we have a 1000-mg tablet:

½ tablet = 500 mg

¼ tablet = 250 mg

▪ **TABLE 6.2**
Multiplication Chart

	1	2	3	4	5	6	7	8	9	10	11	12
2	2	4	6	8	10	12	14	16	18	20	22	24
3	3	6	9	12	15	18	21	24	27	30	33	36
4	4	8	12	16	20	24	28	32	36	40	44	48
5	5	10	15	20	25	30	35	40	45	50	55	60
6	6	12	18	24	30	36	42	48	54	60	66	72
7	7	14	21	28	35	42	49	56	63	70	77	84
8	8	16	24	32	40	48	56	64	72	80	88	96
9	9	18	27	36	45	54	63	72	81	90	99	108
10	10	20	30	40	50	60	70	80	90	100	110	120
11	11	22	33	44	55	66	77	88	99	110	121	132
12	12	24	36	48	60	72	84	96	108	120	132	144

Types of Fractions

Proper: The numerator is smaller than the denominator, and the *value* is always less than 1.

Example: $^1/_2$

Improper: The numerator is greater than or equal to the denominator, and the *value* is always greater than or equal to 1.

Example: $^5/_2$

Mixed: A whole number and a proper fraction combined.

Example: $5^1/_2$

Converting Fractions to Decimals When converting fractions to decimals, divide the numerator by the denominator.

1. Converting a proper fraction to a decimal: $^1/_2$ equals 1 divided by 2, which equals 0.5
2. Converting an improper fraction to a decimal: $^5/_2$ equals 5 divided by 2, which equals 2.5
3. Converting a mixed fraction to a decimal: $3^1/_2$ equals 3 plus (1 divided by 2 = 0.5), which equals 3.5
   - You can also change $3^1/_2$ to an improper fraction first.
   - Multiply the denominator by the whole number: 2 times 3 equals 6.
   - Add the product to the numerator: 6 plus 1 equals 7.
   - Place new numerator over original denominator: $^7/_2$.
   - $^7/_2$ is 7 divided by 2, which equals 3.5.

⊙ Exercise 6.4 Quick Check

Convert the following fractions to decimals.

1. $^1/_2$ = _____
2. $4^5/_8$ = _____
3. $^3/_4$ = _____
4. $2^1/_2$ = _____
5. $^{55}/_{22}$ = _____
6. $1^1/_8$ = _____
7. $^3/_2$ = _____
8. $^2/_{12}$ = _____
9. $^5/_{20}$ = _____
10. $^9/_5$ = _____

Percentages

The term *percent*, and its corresponding sign, %, means "per 100." Percentages represent a portion of a whole. The number 100 is used to represent the whole; therefore 100% equals the whole.

Converting Decimals and Fractions to Percentages To convert a decimal to a percentage, multiply it by 100, which results in the decimal point moving two spaces to the right; then add a percent sign (%).

$$0.75 = 0.75 \times 100 = 75$$
$$75\%$$

To convert a fraction to a percentage, divide the numerator by the denominator and multiply by 100, which results in the decimal point moving two spaces to the right; then add a percent sign (%).

$$\frac{1}{2} \text{ is 1 divided by 2, which equals } 0.5$$
$$0.5 \times 100 = 50$$
$$50\%$$

In this chapter, round numbers to the hundredths place, which is two places past the decimal point.

Rounding a number.

1. Determine to what whole number or decimal place the number is to be rounded.
2. Look at the number to the right of the value being rounded.
3. If that number is 5 or greater, round up; if less than 5, round down.

Examples.

- Round to whole number—use number in tenths place: 3.**4** = 3
- Round to tenths—use number in hundredths place: 3.4**5** = 3.**5**
- Round to hundredths—use number in thousandths place: 3.45**7** = 3.4**6**
- $^1/_3$ is 1 divided by 3, which is 0.333333333 … (3 repeats indefinitely)
- Round to 0.33 (hundredths place); then: $0.33 \times 100 = 33\%$

Converting Percentages to Decimals To convert a percentage to a decimal, drop the percent sign and divide by 100. This results in the decimal point moving two spaces to the left.

$$60\% = 60 \text{ divided by } 100 = 0.60$$

Converting Percentages to Fractions To convert a percentage to a fraction, drop the percent sign, place the number over 100, and reduce.

$$60\% = \frac{60}{100} = \frac{6}{10} = \frac{3}{5}$$
$$1\% = \frac{1}{100}$$
$$0.5\% = \frac{0.5}{100}$$

This is not an appropriate form, so you must multiply the top and bottom by 10

$$\frac{0.5}{100} \cdot \frac{10}{10} = \frac{5}{1000} = \frac{1}{200}$$

This *does not change the value of the number* because $^{10}/_{10} = 1$; however, it removes the decimal from the numerator.

Converting Decimals to Fractions To convert a decimal to a fraction, place the decimal over 1. Then, as in the previous example, you must multiply the top and bottom of the fraction by a multiple of 10 to remove the decimal point because decimals cannot be part of a fraction.

$$0.02 = \frac{0.02}{1} \cdot \frac{100}{100} = \frac{2}{100} = \frac{1}{50}$$

◎ Practice Quiz 6.1

1. From 0800 to 1500 hours is _____ hours.
2. A dose given at 0600, 1400, and 2200 hours is _____ hours apart.

3. A dose given at 0005, 1430, and 2045 hours would be given at _____, _____, and _____ on a 12-hour clock.
4. Write 4:20 pm, 7:15 pm, and 12:00 am in international time: _____, _____, _____.

Convert international time to 12-hour clock time and vice versa; convert Roman numerals to Arabic numbers and vice versa.

5. 0630 hr = _____
6. 0230 hr = _____
7. 0005 hr = _____
8. 7:00 pm = _____
9. 5:40 pm = _____
10. 9:20 pm = _____
11. XLV = _____
12. CIX = _____
13. IX = _____
14. XXII = _____
15. XCV = _____
16. 24 = _____
17. 59 = _____
18. 2011 = _____
19. 150 = _____
20. 55 = _____

Convert the following temperatures.
21. 40°C = _____ °F
22. Insulin is stored in the pharmacy at 36° to 46°F. What is the range in Celsius?

Convert the following percentages to decimals.
23. 50% = _____
24. 12% = _____
25. 175% = _____
26. 2.5% = _____

Convert the following fractions to percentages.
27. $\frac{1}{8}$ = _____ %
28. $\frac{5}{2}$ = _____ %
29. $\frac{3}{4}$ = _____ %
30. $\frac{4}{10}$ = _____ %

Ratios

A ratio expresses a relationship between two quantities or measurements. The following expression is written as a ratio: 1:2, which is read "one is to two." A ratio also can be written as a fraction, in which the first number is the numerator and the second number is the denominator. This ratio can be written either as $\frac{1}{2}$ or as 1:2. When technicians compound products, they may be required to solve problems using ratios, which can be considered parts or fractions.

Converting Ratios to Percentages To convert ratios to percentages, first express the ratio as a fraction, then convert it to a decimal, and finally multiply the decimal by 100 and add the percent sign.

$$3:4 = \frac{3}{4} = 3 \text{ divided by } 4 = 0.75$$
$$0.75 \times 100 = 75$$
$$75\%$$

If two ratios have the same value, they are considered equivalent.

Proportions

A proportion is an equivalent relationship between two ratios.

$$\frac{1}{2} = \frac{2}{4}$$ A proportion may be written as 1:2::2:4.

This is read "one is to two as two is to four." Most single-step pharmaceutical calculations can be accomplished by using proportions. However, many technicians prefer to use DA (discussed later) to make it easier to keep track of units, especially when performing multiple-step calculations.

Solving Proportion Problems Proportion problems can be solved in two ways. The first method involves cross-multiplying and dividing; the second method is described as "means and extremes." Both methods yield the same answer if set up correctly.

$$\frac{3}{7} = \frac{x}{21}$$ Cross-multiply: $7x = 3 \cdot 21$
$$7x = 63$$

Divide both sides by 7 to get the answer: $x = 9$
3:7:x:21 means and extremes: 7 times x equals 3 times 21 (same solution as earlier)

You may reduce a fraction if possible before solving a proportion.

$$\frac{5}{10} = \frac{x}{40}$$ may be reduced to $\frac{1}{2} = \frac{x}{40}$

to simplify the calculations

The ratio and proportion method also can be used to convert ratios to percentages as follows:

Change the ratio 3:4 to a percentage $\frac{3}{4} = \frac{x}{100}$

$x = 75$; 75 of 100 equals 75%

⊙ Exercise 6.5 Quick Check

Solve the following proportions.
1. $\frac{2}{10} = \frac{4}{x}$ _____
2. $\frac{4}{10} = \frac{x}{100}$ _____
3. $\frac{55}{82} = \frac{35}{x}$ _____
4. $\frac{250}{500} = \frac{750}{x}$ _____
5. $\frac{1}{25} = \frac{40}{x}$ _____

■ Tech Note!
Remember: You must place the proper units, such as mL, L, mg, or g, next to the number amount. This cannot be stressed enough because you may be working with various systems of measurement. Including the units on all numbers helps reduce mistakes.

Working With Word Problems

Many pharmacy technicians have difficulty interpreting word problems. One way you can lessen the confusion of a word problem is by identifying what is known and what is being asked. One of the first things to remember is to dismiss unnecessary information.

In the following ratio and proportion (R&P) examples, identify what strength you have in stock and what strength you need (what the physician is ordering). Next, set up the equation and double-check the calculations. It is important to remember to place the correct units in the correct position. For example, if one side of the equation has milligrams divided by milliliters, the opposite side of the equation must be expressed as milligrams divided by milliliters.

Example 6.4 Single-Step Ratio and Proportion Problem

You receive an order for Ativan 4 mg. You have 2-mg tablets in stock. How many 2-mg tablets will you need to fill this order?

Note that most pharmacists will expect you to be able to answer this type of question quickly, without performing written calculations. This example is being used to demonstrate ratio and proportion calculations.

$$\frac{2 \text{ mg}}{1 \text{ tab}} = \frac{4 \text{ mg}}{x} \quad 2x = 4 \quad x = 2 \text{ tabs}$$

Dimensional Analysis

Dimensional analysis (DA) is a method used to solve more complicated pharmaceutical calculations that would require numerous sets of ratio and proportion problems. The main benefit of using DA is the ability to keep track of units during the process to ensure that the answer has the correct unit and nothing has been overlooked. The steps for DA are as follows:

1. Identify the unit needed in the answer.
2. Write down that unit and an equals sign.
3. Begin the DA equation so that the units you want in the *final* answer are in the numerator of the first fraction of the equation; *do not cancel this unit.*
4. Continue with the next fraction in the equation, placed so that the units of its numerator are the same as the units of the denominator of the first fraction, so they will cancel. Continue until all necessary information has been placed in the problem.
5. Cancel your units and multiply the numbers.

Example 6.5 Dimensional Analysis

You receive an order for amoxicillin 250 mg caps qid × 7 days (4 times a day for 7 days).

How many capsules will be needed?

Once again, most pharmacists want their technicians to perform this type of calculation in their head without having to write out a long equation; however, for practice with the concept of DA, the reasoning is as follows:

$$\text{Capsules} = \frac{1 \text{ cap}}{\text{Dose}} \cdot \frac{4 \text{ doses}}{\text{Day}} \cdot \frac{7 \text{ days}}{1} = 28 \text{ caps}$$

The unit needed in the answer was placed as the numerator of the first fraction and never canceled. Dose canceled dose and day canceled day, leaving the correct unit as capsules.

In this example, the strength of the capsule does not affect the answer and is not used in the calculation.

Example 6.6 Dimensional Analysis

Order: Decadron 3 mg twice a day for 30 days. *How many tablets* are needed to fill this order?

In stock: 1.5-mg tablets

Solve for the total amount of tablets needed for the month.

Set up your equation:

$$\text{Tablets} = \frac{1 \text{ tab}}{1.5 \text{ mg}} \cdot \frac{3 \text{ mg}}{1 \text{ dose}} \cdot \frac{2 \text{ doses}}{\text{day}} \cdot \frac{30 \text{ days}}{1} = 120 \text{ tabs}$$

The unit needed in the answer was placed as the numerator of the first fraction and never canceled; mg canceled mg, dose canceled dose, and day canceled day, leaving the correct unit as tablets.

Tech Note!

Always pay attention to the dosage form. You cannot take one and a half capsules, but you can take one and one half tablets *in some circumstances.* A scored tablet is marked so that it can be split into equal parts. Remember that not all tablets can be split, such as sustained-release or enteric-coated tablets.

Exercise 6.6 Quick Check

Use ratio/proportion, DA, or calculate in your head as appropriate.

1. *Order:* metoprolol tartrate 100-mg tablet twice a day for 30 days.
   In stock: 50-mg tablets. How many tablets will it take to fill this 30-day supply?
2. *Order:* Augmentin 250 mg 4 times a day for 7 days.
   In stock: 250-mg capsules. How many capsules are needed to fill this prescription?
   Determine 1 dose
3. *In stock:* 250-mg tabs. Dosage 125 mg. Give _____ tabs
4. *In stock:* 10-mg capsules. Dosage 30 mg. Give _____ caps
5. *In stock:* 4-mg tablets. Dosage 8 mg. Give _____ tabs

Measurement Systems

For a measurement to make sense, it must have a number and a unit. Different measurement systems use different units. For example, the **household system** uses teaspoons and tablespoons for small volumes, whereas the metric system uses milliliters for this size measurement. All answers must have a unit or they are incorrect. Ordering two per day makes no sense because it could mean two tablets, capsules, teaspoons, milligrams, grams, milliliters, and so on.

Metric System

The USP recognizes the **International System of Units (SI),** or metric system, as the official system of measurement

TABLE 6.3
Metric Prefixes

Prefix	Meaning
nano-	One-billionth of the basic unit
micro-	One-millionth of the basic unit
milli-	One-thousandth of the basic unit
centi-	One-hundredth of the basic unit
deci-	One-tenth of the basic unit
deca-	10 times the basic unit
hecto-	100 times the basic unit
kilo-	1000 times the basic unit

for pharmacy in the United States. The metric system can be used to measure weight, **volume,** and distance. The basic unit of measurement for weight is the gram (g), for volume is the liter (L), and for length is the meter (m). A pharmacy technician will use the prefixes micro-, milli-, and kilo-, along with the base unit (Table 6.3).

In the metric system, each unit of measurement is a multiple of 10. To convert from a larger unit of measurement to a smaller unit of measurement, multiply by a multiple of 10. To convert from a smaller unit of measurement to a larger unit of measurement, divide by a multiple of 10. A technician must know the difference between the various units used in the metric system. If a prescription for 1 mcg of medication was filled with 1 mg, the patient would receive a 1000-fold overdose; there is a 1000-unit difference between these two measurements. This means that 1000 micrograms (mcg) equals 1 mg. It is extremely important for the technician to know how the units relate to one another.

Metric Measurements

1. The most commonly used metric measurements of weight in pharmacy include, from largest to smallest, the kilogram (kg), the gram (g), the milligram (mg), and the microgram (mcg). There is a 1000-fold difference between kg and g, g and mg, and mg and mcg, as seen in the following:
   Metric Measurements of Mass Used in Pharmacy

   $$\text{kg} \underset{\text{1 kg = 1000 g}}{\rule{2.5cm}{0.4pt}} \text{g} \underset{\text{1 g = 1000 mg}}{\rule{2.5cm}{0.4pt}} \text{mg} \underset{\text{1 mg = 1000 mcg}}{\rule{2.5cm}{0.4pt}} \text{mcg}$$

   - There is a 1000-unit difference (three decimal places) between kg and g, g and mg, and mg and mcg.
   - There is a 1,000,000-unit difference (six decimal places) between kg and mg and between g and mcg.
   - There is a 1,000,000,000-unit difference (nine decimal places) between kg and mcg.
2. When measuring volumes, a pharmacy technician uses milliliters (mL) and liters (L).*

   $$1 \text{ L} = 1000 \text{ mL}^*$$

*Some prescribers still use cubic centimeter (cc) for volume (1 cc = 1 mL); however, this unit is on the official "Do Not Use" List because it is easily confused with 00 when written by hand.

3. Meters squared (m^2) are used in drug calculations that are based on BSA, which is calculated by a physician or pharmacist using a BSA calculation chart or a computer program.

▼ **Tech Alert!**

One of the most common errors made in pharmacy is the improper use of the decimal point. Physicians who write medication orders without using a leading zero (eg, .5 g) risk the order being mistaken for 5 g. A leading zero clarifies that the value is less than 1 and helps reduce pharmacy errors (write 0.5 g). The same is true of trailing zeros. An order for 50.0 mg could easily be mistaken for 500 mg. Do not add the decimal point and trailing zero (write 50 mg).

Always seek clarification of an order when it seems that the dose is extremely high or low. When the pharmacy technician performs calculations, he or she must use leading zeros if the number is less than 1. Certain medications given in wrong strengths can harm or even kill the patient (see the following examples). For more information on drug errors, see Chapter 14.

Wrong way: .1 mg could be mistaken for 1 mg.
Right way: 0.1 mg is very clear because of the leading zero.
Wrong way: 25.0 mg could be mistaken for 250 mg.
Right way: 25 mg is very clear because of the lack of decimals and trailing zeros.

Converting Between Units With Dimensional Analysis

Some technicians find it easier to convert between units using DA. DA makes use of a **conversion factor,** a fraction equal to 1, which is used to change the *unit* of a measurement but **not** the *value.*

The following conversion factors are commonly used in the metric system:

$$\frac{1000 \text{ mcg}}{1 \text{ mg}} \quad \frac{1000 \text{ mg}}{1 \text{ g}} \quad \frac{1000 \text{ g}}{1 \text{ kg}} \quad \frac{1000 \text{ mL}}{1 \text{ L}}$$

Regardless of which value is in the numerator and which value is in the denominator, all of these equal 1 numerically, so multiplying by a conversion factor is like multiplying by 1.

Because 1000 mcg = 1 mg,

$$\text{both } \frac{1000 \text{ mcg}}{1 \text{ mg}} \text{ and } \frac{1 \text{ mg}}{1000 \text{ mcg}} \text{ equal 1}$$

5 g equals how many mg?

$$\text{mg} = \frac{1000 \text{ mg}}{1 \text{ mg}} \cdot \frac{5 \text{ g}}{1} = 5000 \text{ mg}$$

Notice that the decimal moved three places to the *right* because there is a 1000-fold difference between *g* and *mg* and *g is larger than mg*

250 mcg equals how many mg?

$$\text{mg} = \frac{1 \text{ mg}}{1000 \text{ mcg}} \cdot \frac{250 \text{ mcg}}{1} = 0.25 \text{ mg}$$

Notice that the decimal moved three places to the *left* because there is a 1000-fold difference between *mcg* and *mg* and *mcg is smaller than mg.*

4.2 g equals how many mcg?

$$\text{mcg} = \frac{1000 \text{ mcg}}{1 \text{ mg}} \cdot \frac{1000 \text{ mg}}{1 \text{ g}} \cdot \frac{4.2 \text{ g}}{1} = 4,200,000 \text{ mcg}$$

Notice that the decimal moved six places to the right because there is a 1,000,000-fold difference between *mcg* and *g* and *g is larger than mcg.*

2500 mL equals how many L?

$$\text{L} = \frac{1 \text{ L}}{1000 \text{ mL}} \cdot \frac{2500 \text{ mL}}{1} = 2.5 \text{ L}$$

The decimal moved three places to the left because *L is larger than mL.*

Metric Rule of Thumb

When converting in the metric system:
- **L**arger unit to **S**maller unit go **R**ight with decimal point (**LSR**)
  Example: Changing kg to g
  6.25 kg = 6250 g
  Moved the decimal three places to the *right* because of the 1000-fold difference between kg and g
  Like multiplying by a multiple of 10, in this case 1000
- **S**maller to **L**arger go **L**eft with decimal point (**SLL**)
  Example: Changing mg to g
  120 mg = 0.120 g
  Moved the decimal three places to the *left* because of the 1000-fold difference between mg and g
  Like dividing by a multiple of 10, in this case 1000
  Remember to place a zero before the decimal point if no other number is there!

Conversions from one metric unit to another become almost automatic once you have practiced them enough. Make sure you know how the units relate to one another.

◉ Exercise 6.7 Quick Check

Solve the following problems using the appropriate conversions.

1. You receive a physician's order for 0.88 mcg of drug A. What is the equivalent in milligrams?
2. You receive a physician's order for 5 g of drug B. What is the equivalent in kilograms?
3. You receive an order for 250 mg of drug C. What is the equivalent in micrograms?
4. You receive a physician's order for 250 mg of drug D. What is the equivalent in grams?
5. You receive a physician's order to prepare 0.5 kg of drug E. What is the equivalent in grams?

Household Measurements

The metric system also can be converted into household liquid measurements. The main dry weight measurements in this system are the pound (lb) and the ounce (oz)—1 lb = 16 oz.

◼ TABLE 6.4
Household Measurements of Volume

	Abbreviation	Equivalent
1 drop	gtt	
1 teaspoon	tsp	60 drops (varies according to dropper size)
1 tablespoon	Tbsp	3 teaspoons
1 ounce	oz	2 Tbsp
1 cup	c	8 oz
1 pint	pt	2 c
1 quart	qt	2 pt
1 gallon	gal	4 qt

◼ TABLE 6.5
Household to Metric Volume Conversions

Household Volume	Metric Volume
1 tsp	5 mL
1 Tbsp	15 mL
1 fl oz	30 mL
1 pt	480 mL
1 gal	3840 mL

Common household measurements of volume are listed in Table 6.4.

The main conversions between household and metric measurements are listed in Table 6.5. Memorize these five conversions. With this information and your knowledge of the household system, you should be able to calculate any volume needed in pharmacy.

The following questions will become easy to answer once you have worked with the measurement systems awhile. They can be performed with ratio and proportion or DA. It is best to use DA if you are performing multistep conversions to keep track of units.

◼ Tech Note!

Remember that you cross-multiply *only* when there is an equal sign between two ratios indicating that they are equivalent. *Never* cross-multiply with DA.

◉ Example 6.7

How many milliliters are in 2 Tbsp? Use 1 Tbsp = 15 mL

$$\text{R \& P:} \frac{15 \text{ mL}}{1 \text{ Tbsp}} = \frac{x}{2 \text{ Tbsp}}$$

Cross-multiply and divide to get 30 mL

$$DA::mL = \frac{15\ mL}{1\ Tbsp} \cdot \frac{2\ Tbsp}{1} = 30\ mL$$

(Tbsp units cancel, leaving mL as the answer)

Example 6.8

How many mL are in 4 oz?

$$R\&P:: \frac{30\ mL}{1\ oz} = \frac{x}{4\ oz}$$

Cross-multiply and divide to get 120 mL

$$DA::mL = \frac{30\ mL}{1\ oz} \cdot \frac{4\ oz}{1} = 120\ mL$$

(oz units cancel, leaving mL as the answers)

Tech Note!

Compare household kitchen measuring devices to metric measurements in milliliters.

Exercise 6.8 Quick Check

1. 3 teaspoons = _____ tablespoons = _____ mL
2. 1 ounce = _____ tablespoons = _____ mL
3. 1 cup = _____ ounces = _____ mL
4. 1 pint = _____ tablespoons = _____ mL
5. 1 quart = _____ pints = _____ mL
6. 1 gallon = _____ teaspoons = _____ mL
7. 40 ounces = _____ tablespoons = _____ mL
8. 32 ounces = _____ cups = _____ mL

Apothecary System

The **apothecary system** of measurement, which originated in Europe, is the traditional system of measurement used by physicians and apothecaries. Although it is now largely of historical significance only, components of this system may still be found on some prescriptions.

The apothecary units used in pharmacy include grain (gr), dram (ʒ), ounce (ℨ), and pound (lb) for dry weight and minim (♏), fluid dram (fʒ), and fluid ounce (fℨ) for volume. When using the apothecary system, place the unit of measurement before the amount and use lowercase Roman numerals for the number; for example, 1 grain is written gr i. Historically, the most common way to write ½ grain is gr s̄s̄. Now that s̄s̄ is identified as a potentially dangerous abbreviation on the list published by the Institute for Safe Medication Practices (ISMP), you should write gr ½. However, prescribers may still use s̄s̄. Never combine Roman numerals and fractions; therefore 3¼ grains would be written gr 3¼ not gr iii ¼.

The following conversion for dry weight is common:

Weight::gr i = 60 mg, 64.8 mg, or 65 mg

(see the following Tech Note!)

Tech Note!

The weight of a grain in the apothecary system varies among 60 mg, 64.8 mg, and 65 mg. Why? When the grain was used in ancient times to determine weight, real grains of wheat were used, and the weight depended on that year's harvest. If the crop was good, it took fewer grains because each piece weighed more. If the crops were bad that year, it took more grains to equal the same weight. Be aware that some medication labels will state that there are 60 mg/gr, whereas others might have 64.8 mg/gr or 65 mg/gr. For example, 60 mg/gr is used with codeine and nitroglycerin (NTG) tablets, whereas 65 mg/g is used with aspirin (ASA), acetaminophen (APAP), and iron tablets.

The following conversions for volume are used occasionally:

Volume::8 fluid drams = 1 fluid ounce = 30 mL = 2 Tbsp

1 fluid dram = 3.7 mL This is often considered to be 5 mL or 1 tsp, which is an approximation

Fig. 6.2 presents examples of volume conversions among household, metric, and apothecary systems in medication cups. The cups show 8 drams equal to 1 fl oz, 30 mL, and 2 Tbsp.

Example 6.9

How many grains are in 325 mg of aspirin (ASA)? Use 65 mg = gr i

$$gr = \frac{gr\ i}{65\ mg} \cdot \frac{325\ mg}{1} = gr\ v$$

Example 6.10

How many milligrams are in gr $^1/_{150}$ of nitroglycerin sublingual (NTG SL) tablets? Use 60 mg = gr i

$$mg = \frac{60\ mg}{gr\ i} \cdot \frac{gr\ 1/150}{1}$$

$$60\ mg \cdot \frac{1}{150} = \frac{60\ mg}{150} = 0.4\ mg$$

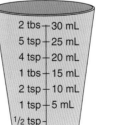
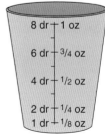

One-ounce medicine cups (30 mL)

FIG. 6.2 Oral cups show equivalent volumes between household and metric and household and apothecary units. (From Gray Morris D. *Calculate with Confidence.* 4th ed. St Louis: Elsevier; 2008.)

Exercise 6.9 Quick Check

Solve the following conversions (refer to Tech Note for conversion factors).
1. NTG gr $^1/_{100}$ = _____ mg
2. NTG gr $^1/_{200}$ = _____ mg
3. codeine gr $^1/_2$ = _____ mg
4. aspirin gr x = _____ mg
5. iron 325 mg = gr _____
6. acetaminophen 130 mg = gr _____
7. 1 oz = _____ fluid drams
8. 1 Tbsp = _____ fluid drams

Avoirdupois System

The **avoirdupois system** is another type of measurement that originated in England. The avoirdupois system is the common system of commerce. It is through this system that items are purchased and sold by the ounce and pound. The avoirdupois system is similar to the apothecary system because it also uses grains, ounces, and pounds for weights. Table 6.6 shows the common avoirdupois weights and volumes.

Avoirdupois Measurements

1. Dry weights use grains (gr), ounces (oz), and pounds (lb).
2. Liquid volumes use fluid ounces (fl oz), pints (pt), and gallons (gal).

Exercise 6.10 Quick Check

Volume
1. 1 fl dram = _____ mL or approximately _____ mL
2. 8 oz = _____ cup(s) or _____ mL
3. 1 gal = _____ mL
4. 5 mL = _____ tsp
5. 30 mL = _____ tsp or _____ Tbsp

   Weight
6. 1 lb = _____ g
7. 1 kg = _____ g or _____ mg
8. acetaminophen gr x = _____ mg
9. 1000 mcg = _____ mg
10. 1 g = _____ mg

TABLE 6.6
Standard Weights and Volumes: Avoirdupois/Metric

Avoirdupois Weight	Metric Equivalent
Dry Weights	
1 lb	454 g
1 oz	30 g
1 gr	64.8 mg
Liquids	
1 fl oz	30 mL
1 pt	473 mL
1 gal	3785 mL

Conversions: 60 minims (℥) = 1 fluidrachm or fluid dram (f℥), 8 fluidrachms (480 minims) = 1 fluid ounce (f℥); 16 fl oz = 1 pint (pt); 2 pt (32 fl oz) = 1 quart (qt); 4 qt (8 pt) = 1 gallon (gal).

Practice Quiz 6.2

1. 5 mL = _____ tsp
2. 15 mL = _____ Tbsp
3. 30 mL = _____ tsp
4. 1 dram = _____ mL or approximately _____ mL
5. 1 L = _____ mL
6. 454 g = _____ lb
7. 4.4 lb = _____ kg
8. 3000 mcg = _____ mg
9. 450 g = _____ mg
10. 25 kg = _____ mg
11. 1.5 L = _____ mL
12. 3 lb = _____ kg
13. 25 lb = _____ oz
14. 2.25 mcg = _____ mg
15. 240 mL = _____ oz
16. 2 pints = _____ quarts
17. 1 gallon = _____ pints
18. 500 mL = _____ L
19. NTG gr $^1/_{100}$ = ____ mg
20. NTG gr $^1/_{150}$ = ____ mg
21. ASA 325 mg = gr _____
22. 9000 mg = _____ g
23. 0900 hr = _____ o'clock (am or pm)
24. 2110 hr = _____ o'clock (am or pm)
25. 1320 hr = _____ o'clock (am or pm)
26. 2350 hr = _____ o'clock (am or pm)
27. 2:30 pm = _____ (international time)
28. 11:00 am = _____ (international time)
29. 9:25 pm = _____ (international time)
30. 4:10 am = _____ (international time)
31. 6 pm = _____ (international time)
32. ix = _____ (Arabic number)
33. viii = _____ (Arabic number)
34. LX = _____ (Arabic number)
35. IV = _____ (Arabic number)
36. XC = _____ (Arabic number)
37. XXX = _____ (Arabic number)

Important Differences Among Systems

You should know how metric system units compare to other units of measure, such as ounces and grains. Most of the time they convert easily, but sometimes there are variances, making conversions between measurement systems approximate in these instances. Because the metric system is the approved system of measurement used in pharmacy, it is the measurement system you should use when preparing a compounded drug. However, you will see differences among manufacturers' products and their weights. For example, some manufacturers consider 473 mL to equal 1 pint, whereas others consider 480 mL to equal 1 pint. The rule is to follow the metric system because it is the approved system of measurement for pharmacy in the United States.

For the following examples, the orders are written in standard abbreviations that indicate how often (frequency) a medication is to be given (Box 6.2).

Calculations With Liquid Medication

Single-step problems with liquid medications can be solved with ratio and proportion.

Order: docusate sodium 20 mg bid
In stock: docusate sodium 4 mg/mL

1. How many milliliters are needed per dose? (Think 4 is to 1 as 20 is to *x*.)

$$\frac{4 \text{ mg}}{\text{mL}} = \frac{20 \text{ mg}}{x} \quad x = 5 \text{ mL}$$

2. How many milliliters are needed per day? 5 mL twice a day equals 10 mL.
   Multiple-step problems can be solved with DA to keep track of the units.

3. How many doses can be taken from the 8-oz bottle?

$$\text{Doses} = \frac{1 \text{ dose}}{5 \text{ mL}} \cdot \frac{30 \text{ mL}}{1 \text{ oz}} \cdot \frac{8 \text{ oz}}{1} = 48 \text{ doses}$$

⬤ Example 6.11 Single-Step Proportion Problem

Prepare 240 mg of gentamicin intravenous piggyback (IVPB) using the pharmacy stock concentration of 40 mg/mL (each mL of stock solution contains 40 mg of gentamicin).

How many mL are needed for one dose?

In this case you need to determine how many *milliliters* of the stock solution are needed to fill the 240-mg order. Write your stock strength or given concentration on the left and the needed amount on the right. Make sure that milligrams are in the numerator and milliliters are in the denominator on both sides. Then cross-multiply and divide; this will give you the necessary milliliters to withdraw from the vial.

$$\frac{40 \text{ mg}}{1 \text{ mL}} = \frac{240 \text{ mg}}{x \text{ mL}} \quad 40x = 240$$

Divide both sides by $40x = 6 \text{ mL}$

⬤ Example 6.12 Single-Step Proportion Problem

Order: clindamycin 450 mg IVPB q12h
In stock: clindamycin 150 mg/mL
How many mL are needed for one dose?

You are solving for *x* because you do not know how much clindamycin to draw up into a syringe. To solve for *x*, you *cross-multiply and divide:*

$$\frac{150 \text{ mg}}{1 \text{ mL}} = \frac{450 \text{ mg}}{x} \quad 150x = 450x = 3 \text{ mL}$$

⬤ Example 6.13 Multiple-Step Dimensional Analysis Problem

Order: theophylline 45 mg PO
In stock: theophylline 80 mg/Tbsp
How many mL are needed for one dose?

$$\text{mL} = \frac{15 \text{ mL}}{1 \text{ Tbsp}} \cdot \frac{1 \text{ Tbsp}}{80 \text{ mg}} \cdot \frac{45 \text{ mg}}{1} = 8.4 \text{ mL}$$

⬤ Example 6.14 Dimensional Analysis

Order: erythromycin suspension 125 mg tid × 10 days. *How many mL are needed to fill this order?*
In stock: 200 mg/5 mL. Interpret order: 125 mg to be taken 3 times per day for 10 days.
Set up your equation:

$$\text{mL} = \frac{5 \text{ mL}}{200 \text{ mg}} \cdot \frac{125 \text{ mg}}{1 \text{ dose}} \cdot \frac{3 \text{ doses}}{1 \text{ day}} \cdot \frac{10 \text{ days}}{1} = 93.75 \text{ mL}$$

The unit needed in the answer (mL) was placed as the numerator of the first fraction and never canceled (mg canceled mg, dose canceled dose, and day canceled day, leaving the correct unit as mL). On a practical note, this would probably be rounded up to 100 mL.

⬤ Exercise 6.11 Quick Check

1. *Order:* 25 mg. *In stock:* 10 mg/mL. Give _____ mL
2. *Order:* 25 mg. *In stock:* 40 mg/mL. Give _____ mL
3. *Order:* 0.6 g. *In stock:* 1.5 g/mL. Give _____ mL
4. *Order:* 500 mg. *In stock:* 25 mg/mL. Give _____ mL
5. *Order:* 250 mg. *In stock:* 500 mg/5 mL. Give _____ tsp

When preparing IV and other parenteral medications, you may need to calculate the correct dose based on weight, in kilograms or pounds, or BSA, in square meters; this is especially true of infants, children, and senior citizens. Chemotherapy medications are often based on the BSA of the patient. Always check your calculations at least three times before asking a pharmacist to check them. The following sections present examples of the most common methods of performing these calculations.

Calculating the Proper Dose Using Body Weight

All official compendia, drug references, and drug manufacturers provide proper dosing regimens. When these are based on kilograms and the patient's weight is provided in pounds, it is necessary to convert pounds into kilograms. It is important to remember that there are 2.2 lb per kilogram.

$$1 \text{ kg} = 2.2 \text{ lb}$$

What is the weight in kg of a 176-lb person?

$$\text{kg} = \frac{1 \text{ kg}}{2.2 \text{ lb}} \cdot \frac{176 \text{ lb}}{1} = 80 \text{ kg}$$

Example 6.15

Dose ordered: 2.5 mg/kg/dose (q8h). Patient weighs 250 lb. How many milligrams per dose?

$$\text{mg/dose} = \frac{2.5 \text{ mg}}{\text{kg/dose}} \cdot \frac{1 \text{ kg}}{2.2 \text{ lb}} \cdot \frac{250 \text{ lb}}{1} = 284 \text{ mg/dose}$$

Observe how the units cancel, leaving the correct unit as mg/dose.

If the answer had been required in g, one more conversion would be necessary, as follows:

$$\text{g/dose} = \frac{1 \text{ g}}{1000 \text{ mg}} \cdot \frac{2.5 \text{ mg}}{\text{kg/dose}} \cdot \frac{1 \text{ kg}}{2.2 \text{ lb}} \cdot \frac{250 \text{ lb}}{1}$$
$$= 0.28 \text{ g/dose}$$

If the question reads: How many g/day, one more conversion would be necessary:

$$\text{g/day} = \frac{1 \text{ g}}{1000 \text{ mg}} \cdot \frac{2.5 \text{ mg}}{\text{kg/dose}} \cdot \frac{1 \text{ kg}}{2.2 \text{ lb}} \cdot \frac{250 \text{ lb}}{1} \cdot \frac{3 \text{ doses}}{\text{day}}$$
$$= 0.85 \text{ g/day}$$

When working the following exercises, take care to read exactly what the question is asking.

Exercise 6.12 Quick Check

1. *Dose ordered:* 125 mg/kg/dose (q24h). Patient weighs 175 lb. How many g per dose?
2. *Dose ordered:* 55 mg/kg/day (q8h). Patient weighs 48 lb. How many mg per dose?
3. *Dose ordered:* 220 mg/kg/dose (q12h). Patient weighs 141 lb. How many g per day?
4. *Dose ordered:* 1.12 mg/kg/day (q6h). Patient weighs 98 lb. How many mg per dose?

Tech Note!

This is how to remember kilogram conversion: Your weight is more than cut in half when measured in kilograms (2.2 lb = 1 kg). If you weighed 200 lb, you would weigh 91 kg.

Calculating Body Surface Area

The BSA method of calculating a patient's dose results in the most accurate dose because it is based on both the *height* and the *weight* of the patient. BSA calculations are extremely important when determining chemotherapeutic and pediatric doses. A *nomogram* is a table used to determine a patient's BSA in meters squared (m^2). Most hospitals use computer-based programs to determine BSA.

Solve BSA calculations in the same way you would a dosing problem based on weight.

Patient: length 20 inches; weight 5 lb; BSA 0.18 m^2; dose 75 mg/m^2

How many mg are required per dose?

$$\text{mg} = \frac{75 \text{ mg}}{m^2} \cdot \frac{0.18 \text{ m}^2}{1} = 13.5 \text{ mg}$$

Exercise 6.13 Quick Check

1. Patient: length 60 inches; weight 85 kg; BSA 1.8 m^2; dose 200 mg/m^2
   How many mg are required per dose?
2. Patient: length 65 inches; weight 150 lb; BSA 1.8 m^2; dose 2.5 g/m^2
   How many g are required per dose?

Tech Note!

Remember to read the dosage instructions carefully to determine whether the medication is dosed in *kg* or *m^2* per dose *or* per day.

Oral and Injectable Syringes

When filling oral liquid prescription orders for pediatric patients and those who cannot take solid dosage forms, you may need to provide an oral syringe with the prescription (Fig. 6.3). A needle cannot be attached to an oral syringe, which reduces the possibility of administration errors. In the case of injectable medications, several possible syringe sizes can be selected to withdraw the correct volume of solution. A needle is attached to this type of syringe.

Pediatric and Geriatric Dosing

Liquid medications are used frequently for children and elderly patients. It is important that the parent understand how much medicine to give a child. Using pharmacy-supplied measuring devices, usually marked in household and metric measurements, increases the accuracy of dosing. Very small amounts may be measured with droppers. The pharmacist, not the technician, should show the parent of a patient how to measure the correct amount. Senior citizens also must be careful to take the correct amount of medication. For oral liquids, dosing devices with large, boldface calibrations may help the geriatric patient see the correct amount. Many of these types of dosing devices are sold over the counter.

Calculating Pediatric Dosages

Pediatrics refers to the practice of medicine in children from childbirth through adolescence. This range of ages is subdivided into various groups:

- *Neonates:* birth to 1 month
- *Infant:* 1 month to 1 year
- *Early childhood:* 1 year through 5 years
- *Late childhood:* 6 years through 12 years
- *Adolescence:* 13 years through 17 years
  Pediatric dosages can be calculated using DA.

Example 6.16

The pharmacy receives an order for a baby girl weighing 7 lb. *Order:* 20 mg/kg/dose.

This means that for every kilogram the child weighs, she should receive 20 mg of medication.

$$\frac{\text{mg}}{\text{dose}} = \frac{20 \text{ mg}}{\text{kg}} \cdot \frac{1 \text{ kg}}{2.2 \text{ lb}} \cdot \frac{7 \text{ lb}}{1} = 63.6 \text{ mg/dose}$$

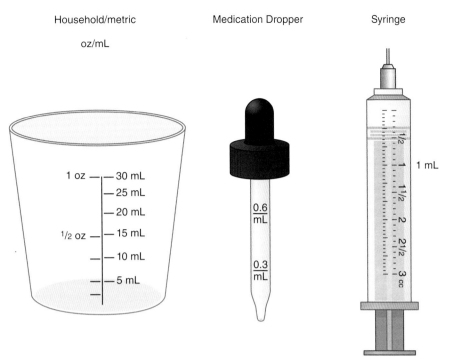

Household/metric
oz/mL

Medication Dropper

Syringe

1 oz — 30 mL
— 25 mL
— 20 mL
1/2 oz — 15 mL
— 10 mL
— 5 mL

0.6 mL

0.3 mL

1/2
1
1 1/2
2
2 1/2
3 cc

1 mL

FIG. 6.3 Common devices used for measuring liquid medications.

Other Methods of Calculating Pediatric Doses

Two other methods can be used to calculate pediatric doses. Clark's Rule uses the child's weight in pounds divided by 150 lb (the average weight of an adult) as the basis for calculating the dose from the adult-recommended dose. Young's Rule uses the child's age in years divided by the child's age in years plus 12 as the basis for calculating the child's dose from the adult-recommended dose. Both of these methods are approximations.

Clark's Rule:

$$\text{Child's dose} = \frac{\text{Weight of child in lb}}{150 \cdot \text{Adult dose}}$$

Young's Rule:

$$\text{Child's dose} = \frac{\text{Child's age in years}}{(\text{Child's age in years} + 12) \cdot \text{Adult dose}}$$

Clark's Rule is preferred over Young's Rule because it is more accurate to use weight than age.

Geriatric Patients

Geriatric medicine encompasses the management of illness or disability in the elderly. A major consideration in the dosing of elderly patients is reduced kidney function, which may result in reduced drug elimination or increased drug accumulation, leading to toxic drug levels and adverse effects. Renal clearance is extremely important when using specific drugs in elderly patients.

High Alert Medications

The ISMP has identified certain medications that require additional checks because of a heightened risk to patients if an error occurs. Two of the medications are heparin and insulin, and there should be special safeguards in place to avoid errors. For a complete listing of medications considered "High Alert," see *https://www.ismp.org/tools/highalertmedicationLists.asp.*

Calculations Involving Units and Milliequivalents

Certain parenteral medications, such as insulin, heparin, and penicillin, are measured in units per milliliter. **Units** are assigned to medications called *biologicals,* which have been tested for potency in biological systems. To prevent errors, health care workers should write out the word *units* rather than abbreviate it as "u." Units are specific to each particular medication because the medication has been tested and shown to produce a specific effect relating to that number of units. Therefore units of heparin have no relationship to units of insulin.

Heparin is an anticoagulant that is available in many different strengths. Be *very* careful when reading heparin orders and labels because it is considered a high-risk medication. It is available in 1000 units/mL, 2000 units/mL, 2500 units/mL, 5000 units/mL, 10,000 units/mL, and 20,000 units/mL. Heparin is also available in 1 unit/mL, 10 units/mL, and 100 units/mL strengths, which are considered heparin lock flushes used to keep a vein open (prevent clotting) so that the IV line remains open for the next dose.

Insulin, a parenteral hypoglycemic medication for lowering the blood glucose level, is also dosed in units. The most common strength used in the United States is U-100, which is 100 units/mL. Regular insulin is the only insulin that can be given intravenously. Other types of insulin, in addition to regular insulin, are given subcutaneously.

Some insulin comes in a U-500 strength, which is used only for patients with extreme insulin resistance.

■ Tech Note!

Insulins and heparin are both considered high-risk medications, and special considerations for storage and administration are usually in place.
   Calculations with units follow the same rules as other calculations.

◉ Example 6.17

Order: heparin sodium 4000 units subcutaneously (subcut)
In stock: heparin sodium 1000 units/mL and heparin sodium 10,000 units/mL

How much of *each* stock volume would be needed for the same dose?

$$\frac{1000 \text{ units}}{1 \text{ mL}} = \frac{4000 \text{ units}}{x} \quad x = 4 \text{ mL}$$

This is too much volume to inject subcut! (see below)

$$\frac{10,000 \text{ units}}{1 \text{ mL}} = \frac{4000 \text{ units}}{x} \quad x = 0.4 \text{ mL}$$

More appropriate amount for a subcut injection

Choose the 10,000 unit/mL stock solution in this case to keep the dose *volume* smaller.

◉ Example 6.18

Order: regular insulin 35 units subcut qam
In stock: regular insulin 100 units/mL
What volume is needed for this dose?

$$\frac{100 \text{ units}}{1 \text{ mL}} = \frac{35 \text{ units}}{x} \quad \text{Cross-multiply and divide.}$$
$$x = 0.35 \text{ mL}$$

Milliequivalents (mEq) are a type of unit used in the United States to express the concentration of electrolytes such as sodium, potassium, magnesium, and calcium. With liquid medications, these strengths are expressed as milliequivalents per milliliter. With solid medications, the strength can be mEq/tablet or mEq/capsule.

Calculations with milliequivalents also follow the same rules as other calculations.

◉ Example 6.19

Order: Add 30 mEq of KCl to 1 L normal saline (NS)
   In stock: KCl 2 mEq/mL. How many mL should be added to the NS IV?

$$\frac{2 \text{ mEq}}{1 \text{ mL}} = \frac{30 \text{ mEq}}{x} \quad \text{Cross-multiply and divide.}$$
$$x = 15 \text{ mL}$$

◉ Exercise 6.14 Quick Check

1. *Order:* 25 units. *In stock:* 100 units/10 mL. Give _____ mL
2. *Order:* 20,000 units. *In stock:* 25,000 units/2 mL. Give _____ mL
3. *Order:* 40 mEq. *In stock:* 20-mEq tablets. Give _____ tablets
4. *Order:* add 45 mEq of KCl to an IV. *In stock:* KCl 2 mEq/mL. Add _____ mL
5. *Order:* 46 units regular insulin. *In stock:* regular insulin 100 units/mL. Draw up _____ mL

◉ Scenario Checkup 6.1

Victoria is nearing the end of a long shift at the hospital. She receives a stat order for 7000 units of heparin subcutaneous to be sent up to the cardiac floor. The supply on hand is heparin 10,000 units per 1 mL. How much will Victoria draw up in the syringe to send to the floor? How quickly must Victoria deliver this medication to the nurse?

Subcutaneous Injections

Subcutaneous (subcut) injections are administered in the subcutaneous or fat layer of the skin. Most subcut doses are less than 1 mL.

Intramuscular Injections

For intramuscular (IM) injections, the needle passes through the cutaneous and subcutaneous layers of the skin, and the injection is delivered into the muscle. Small-volume IM injections are less than 3 mL, and large-volume IM injections are 3 to 5 mL. Larger muscles can handle the larger amounts, but 5 mL is the volume limit on IM injections. Therefore if you calculate an IM dose and your answer is greater than 5 mL, there is probably an error either in the prescribed amount or in your calculations.

Intravenous Medications

Hospital pharmacy technicians prepare and deliver a 24-hour supply of IV solutions to nursing stations daily. Large-volume parenterals (LVPs) contain more than 250 mL of solution, and small-volume parenterals (SVPs) contain 100 mL or less. Most IVPBs are SVPs that are given over 30 to 60 minutes. LVPs for continuous IV administration are "hung" at the patient's bedside and are allowed to drip slowly into a vein either by gravity or through a pump. They must be given at a slow rate because veins can handle only a small volume over a given time. Both LVPs and SVPs must be infused at a constant rate. In either case, the physician determines the infusion, or flow, rate in terms of milliliters per minute, drops per minute, or amount of drug (milligrams, units, or milliequivalents) per hour. The pharmacy technician must be able to calculate the volume needed to last a certain amount of time to calculate how much longer a currently hanging IV solution will last (Fig. 6.4). Depending on the order received, the technician must be able to convert the numbers to determine this information. This ultimately determines the amount of IV solution to be prepared for a 24-hour period.

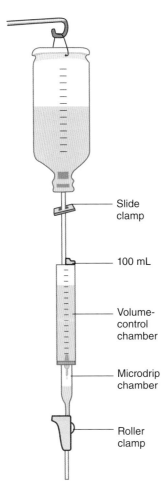

Slide
clamp

100 mL

Volume-
control
chamber

Microdrip
chamber

Roller
clamp

FIG. 6.4 Large-volume intravenous drip with smaller piggy-back attached to tubing on pump.

Intravenous Infusion Rates/Flow Rates

A *rate* is defined as something per unit of time. An **infusion rate** or **flow rate** refers to the amount of IV fluid entering the body over a specific amount of time.

A 1000-mL IV may be ordered to run over 8 hours. The infusion rate would be 1000 mL/8 hr, which reduces to 125 mL/hr.

A 1000-mL IV may be ordered to run at 50 mL/hr.

$$\frac{50 \text{ mL}}{1 \text{ hr}} = \frac{1000 \text{ mL}}{x}\, x = 20 \text{ hr}$$

The infusion would last for 20 hours.

These calculations involve determining the following:
1. The right amount of medication to be given over time
2. The amount of medication needed to last a certain time
3. The amount of time left until an IV is empty
   Basic necessary conversion factors are as follows:

$$1 \text{ hr} = 60 \text{ min}$$
$$24 \text{ hr} = 1 \text{ day}$$

⬤ Example 6.20

Order: Heparin 100 units per 500 mL to run at 10 mL per hour.

How many units will be delivered per hour?

$$\frac{\text{units}}{\text{hr}} = \frac{100 \text{ units}}{500 \text{ mL}} \cdot \frac{10 \text{ mL}}{\text{hr}} = 2 \text{ units/hr}$$

⬤ Exercise 6.15 Quick Check

When using DA, start by identifying the unit needed in the answer.
1. *Order:* 2-L TPN to run at 150 mL/hr. How many hours will this solution last?
2. *Order:* 500-mL solution to run over 24 hours. How many mL per hour?
3. *Order:* 1 L of NS to run at 100 mL/hr. How many hours will this solution last?

A **drip rate (DR),** sometimes called a **drop rate,** represents the number of drops (gtt) administered over a specific time by intravenous infusion. It is a specific type of infusion or flow rate usually measured in gtt/min.

Calculations are affected by the size of the tubing used to deliver the medication. A **drop factor** (gtt/mL) is found on the tubing package. Various drop factors are available: 10, 15, and 20 gtt/mL are called *macrodrip,* and 60 gtt/mL is considered a *microdrip.*

> ### ▪ Tech Note!
>
> Remember, the unit abbreviation for drops is *gtt.* Sizes of drops differ between droppers, and there are various conversion factors with drops that seem contradictory. When calculating a day's supply for insurance company purposes, pharmacists typically use 20 gtt/mL. The household system considers there to be about 60 gtt/tsp, which would convert to 12 gtt/mL.
>
> Also, drops can be intended for drip rates. The number of drops per milliliter in these cases depends on the tubing size of the administration kit.

⬤ Example 6.21 Calculating Infusion Rates and Drip Rates

You receive an order for a 2-L bag to be given over 24 hours. The tubing delivers 15 gtt/mL. What are the drops per minute? To find this out, prepare the problem.

Steps involved in determining drops per minute:
1. Identify the drop factor: 15 gtt/mL
2. How many milliliters will be delivered per hour?

$$2000 \text{ mL}/24 \text{ hr} = 83.33 \text{ mL/hr}$$

3. How many milliliters per minute?

$$\frac{83.33 \text{ mL}}{1 \text{ hr}} \cdot \frac{1 \text{ hr}}{60 \text{ min}} = 1.38 \text{ mL/min}$$

4. What is the drip rate? You can use DA to go directly from the original question to this final answer because that is how this question will usually be phrased.

$$\frac{\text{gtt}}{\text{min}} = \frac{15 \text{ gtt}}{\text{mL}} \cdot \frac{1000 \text{ mL}}{1 \text{ L}} \cdot \frac{2 \text{ L}}{24 \text{ hr}} \cdot \frac{1 \text{ hr}}{60 \text{ min}} = 20.8 \text{ gtt/min}$$
$$(\text{rounds to 21 gtt/min})$$

Note: When performing DA calculations with two units in the answer, as previously with gtt/min, start your solution with the information that contains the numerator of the answer and continue to add information that will cancel the unwanted units. The previous example was begun with gtt/mL because the final answer is needed in gtt/min. Then, each consecutive value canceled unwanted units: mL canceled mL, L canceled L, and hr canceled hr, until you were left with gtt/min.

When expressing gtt/min, the number is always rounded *up* to the nearest whole drop. Whether the answer is 20.1 gtt/min or 20.9 gtt/min, it would be rounded up to 21 gtt/min.

Example 6.22

A 3-L total parenteral nutrition (TPN) bag is being administered to a patient over 24 hours. The tubing size delivers 15 gtt/mL. How many drops per minute will be delivered?

$$\frac{gtt}{min} = \frac{15\ gtt}{mL} \cdot \frac{1000\ mL}{1\ L} \cdot \frac{3\ L}{24\ hr} \cdot \frac{1\ hr}{60\ min}$$
$$= 31.25\ gtt/min = 32\ gtt/min$$

▪ Tech Note!

Technicians and pharmacists do not determine the size of the tubing. This is predetermined by the physician's orders to the nurse.

⊙ Exercise 6.16 Quick Check

1. Aminophylline 500 mg in 1000 mL over 24 hours. The drop factor is 20 gtt/mL.
   a. How many mL would be delivered per hour?
   b. What is the flow rate in drops/min?
2. Heparin 20,000 units in 1 L over 24 hours. The drop factor is 50 gtt/mL.
   a. How many mL would be delivered per hour?
   b. What is the flow rate in drops/min?
3. How many drops per minute would a patient receive at 40 mL/hr using a 20-gtt/mL set?
4. *Order:* 1500 mL of solution over 12 hours. The tubing size is 20 gtt/mL.
   How many drops per minute will be delivered?
5. *Order:* 2.5 L of solution to run over 20 hours. The tubing size is 15 gtt/mL.
   How many drops per minute will be delivered?

▪ Tech Note!

A large-volume bag can hang for a maximum of 24 hours before it must be changed to prevent microbial growth, according to the USP.

Percentage and Ratio Strengths

In the practice of pharmacy, percentage (%) can be expressed in three ways: weight/weight (g/100 g), weight/volume (g/100 mL), and volume/volume (mL/100 mL). Weight/weight % is the number of grams of solute dissolved in 100 g of final product. Weight/volume % is the number of grams of solute dissolved in 100 mL of solution. Volume/volume % is the number of milliliters of solute dissolved in 100 mL of solution.

⊙ Example 6.23 Using Ratio and Percentage

How many g of dextrose are in 250 mL of 10% dextrose solution?

$$\frac{10\ g}{100\ mL} = \frac{x}{250\ mL} \quad 100x = 2500x = 25\ g$$

⊙ Example 6.24

What is the percentage strength of an ointment containing 0.5 g of active ingredient in 50 g?

$$x = 1\ g$$
$$1g/100\ g = 1\%$$
$$\frac{0.5\ g}{50\ g} = \frac{x}{100\ g}$$

▪ Tech Note!

Remember that percent *always* means $x/_{100}$.

A second method of expressing the strength of a substance is by using ratios. Ratio strength is often used to designate the concentration of weak solutions or liquid preparations.

For example, a 1:200 ratio strength is interpreted as the following:
1. Solid in solid (weight to weight, or w/w): 1 g of solute in 200 g of solid preparation
2. Solid in liquid (weight to volume, or w/v): 1 g of solid in 200 mL of solution
3. Liquid in liquid (volume to volume, or v/v): 1 mL of solute in 200 mL of solution

A liquid with a concentration of 1:1000 means there is 1 part active ingredient to 1000 parts total. This could mean 1 gram (g) of drug dissolved in 1000 mL of solution, 1 milliliter (mL) of drug in 1000 mL of solution, or 1 g of drug in 1000 g of product. If you have 25 g of drug dissolved in 100 mL of solution, this can be written as the ratio 25:100, which can be reduced to 1:4.

⊙ Example 6.25 Using Dimensional Analysis

How many mg of medication are in 20 mL of a 1:250 solution?

$$mg = \frac{1000\ mg}{1\ g} \cdot \frac{1\ g}{250\ mL} \cdot \frac{20\ mL}{1} = 80\ mg$$

▪ Tech Note!

Remember that ratio strength is always expressed in the form of 1:*x*.

Converting between percentage and ratio strength is easiest with ratio and proportion as follows.

What is the percentage strength of a 1:1000 solution?

$$\frac{1\ g}{1000\ mL} = \frac{x\ g}{100\ mL} 1000x = 100$$

Divide both sides by 1000 and $x = 0.1$

The answer is 0.1 g over 100 mL, or 0.1%.

The same method can be applied to conversions from percentage strength to ratio strength.

What is the ratio strength of a 5% solution?

$$\frac{5\ g}{100\ mL} = \frac{1\ g}{x\ mL} 5x = 100$$

Divide both sides by 5, so $x = 20$

1 g in 20 mL is a 1:20 ratio strength.

Another method of expressing strength is using fractions such as mg/mL, mEq/mL, and units/mL.

To convert percentage strength to mg/mL with DA, place the unit you want for the answer to the left of the equals sign and line up your known values so that the other units cancel.

Convert 5% (w/v) to mg/mL: 5% means 5 out of 100 and in this case 5 g out of 100 mL.

$$\frac{mg}{mL} = \frac{1000\ mg}{g} \cdot \frac{5\ g}{100\ mL} = \frac{5000\ mL}{100\ mL} = \frac{50\ mg}{mL}$$

To convert ratio strength to mg/mL using DA, place the unit you want for the answer to the left of the equals sign and line up your known values so that the other units cancel.

Convert 1:20,000 (w/v) to mg/mL: 1:20,000 means 1 out of 20,000, and in this case 1 g out of 20,000 mL.

$$\frac{mg}{mL} = \frac{1000\ mg}{1\ g} \cdot \frac{1\ g}{20,000\ mL} = \frac{1000\ mg}{20,000\ mL} = \frac{1\ mg}{20\ mL}$$

1 mg/20 mL reduces to 0.05 mg/mL by dividing the top and bottom of the fraction by 20.

◉ Exercise 6.17 Quick Check

Calculate the strength in the following problems.
1. How many grams of amino acid are in 500 mL of 8.5% solution?
2. 170 g of medication is dissolved in 1 L of water; what is the percentage strength of the solution formed?
3. How many grams of dextrose are in 250 mL of a 5% solution?
4. What is the ratio strength of a 20% solution?
5. How many milligrams of drug are in 20 mL of a 1% solution?

Dilution

The pharmacy often receives a prescription for a liquid or solid medication that is not available commercially in the strength prescribed by the physician. Often the commercial strength is greater than the prescribed strength. In this situation, the pharmacist or pharmacy technician must dilute the commercially available product to a lower strength. In this process, called **dilution,** a pharmaceutical preparation is diluted through the addition of a **diluent** or **solvent** to reach the desired strength. The diluent is an inert substance that does not have a concentration; in other words, it has a concentration of 0%. The diluent adds either volume or mass to the preparation. Sterile water is a common diluent for solutions, and petrolatum is a common diluent for solids.

Liquid dilutions involve adding a diluent (eg, sterile water) with 0% active ingredient to a higher concentration stock solution. During the dilution process, begin with a stock volume (SV) of a particular percentage concentration (SP). Add a diluent to the stock solution to achieve the desired volume (DV) and desired percentage strength (DP). The strengths must always be expressed as percentages, and the volumes must be in the same unit. Usually the volume is requested in mL, but occasionally a physician may request L or oz. The process can be expressed mathematically as:

$$SV \cdot SP = DV \cdot DP$$

Three of the four variables are needed to perform this calculation. The amount of diluent needed can be calculated by using the following equation:

$$\text{Amount of diluent needed} = DV - SV$$

The process is the same when diluting weights. Adding a product such as petrolatum to a stock solid dilutes the preparation to a lower strength because petrolatum has 0% active ingredient. Just change the formulas to read:

$$SW \cdot SP = DW \cdot DP$$

$$\text{Amount of diluent} = DW - SW$$

The technician must remember several important things when using these equations:
1. Convert ratio strengths to percentage strengths before calculating.
2. The stock strength will always be greater than the final strength in a dilution problem.
3. The desired weight or volume will be greater than the initial weight or volume.

◉ Example 6.26

How many milliliters of water must be added to 150 mL of a 25% (w/v) stock solution of sodium chloride to prepare a 0.9% (w/v) sodium chloride solution?

Identify the variables: SV = 150 mL, SP = 25%, DV = ?, DP = 0.9%

Place them in the equation and solve for the desired volume:

$$SV \cdot SP = DV \cdot DP$$

$$150\ mL \cdot 25\% = DV \cdot 0.9\%$$

$$3750 = DV \cdot 0.9\% \text{ Divide both sides by 0.9}$$

$$4167\ mL = DV$$

$$\text{Amount of water needed} = DV - SV$$
$$= 4167\ mL - 150\ mL$$
$$= 4017\ mL$$

Example 6.27

How many milliliters of a 1:50 (w/v) boric acid solution can be prepared from 500 mL of a 10% (w/v) boric acid solution?

First change the ratio strength to a percentage: 1 g/50 mL = x g/100 mL, x = 2 g, so the strength is 2%

Next, identify the variables: SV = 500 mL, SP = 10%, DV = ?, DP = 2%

Place them in the equation and solve for the desired volume:

$$SV \cdot SP = DV \cdot DP$$

$$500 \text{ mL} \cdot 10\% = DV \cdot 2\% \quad DV = 2500 \text{ mL}$$

■ Tech Note!

Remember that the units used for volume must be the same on both sides of the equation.

Exercise 6.18 Quick Check

Solve the following dilution problems.

1. If 200 mL of a 20% (w/v) solution is diluted to 1 L, what will be the percentage strength (w/v)?
2. A pharmacist has weighed 3 g of coal tar (100% strength) and given it to the technician to compound a 1% ointment. What will be the final weight of the correctly compounded prescription?
3. An order calls for 120 mL of a 10% magnesium sulfate solution, and you have a 25% magnesium sulfate solution. How many milliliters of the 25% solution will you use?
4. You are to prepare 50 mL of a 1:100 rifampin suspension from a stock 1:20 rifampin suspension. How many milliliters of the 1:20 suspension will you need?
5. The pharmacist receives a prescription for 100 mL of a 30% hydrochloric acid solution. The pharmacy carries a 90% hydrochloric acid solution. How many milliliters of the concentrated solution are needed to fill the prescription?
6. A stock bottle of Lugol's solution contains 4 oz from the original pint bottle. The technician is able to make four 8-oz bottles of a more dilute 4% solution. What was the original percentage strength of Lugol's solution?

Total Parenteral Nutrition

TPN is covered thoroughly in Chapter 12. The calculations involve determining amounts of dextrose, amino acids, and lipids, in addition to electrolytes, insulin, and other additives.

Example 6.28

Prepare TPN with 400 mL of 10% Travasol, 500 mL of 70% dextrose, and 100 mL of sterile water. What will be the final strengths of the Travasol and dextrose?

This is actually two dilution questions, so use:

$$SV \cdot SP = DV \cdot DP$$

DV for both Travasol and dextrose will be

$$400 \text{ mL} + 500 \text{ mL} + 100 \text{ mL} = 1000 \text{ mL}$$

Travasol:: $400 \text{ mL} \cdot 10\% = 1000 \text{ mL} \cdot DP \quad DP = 4\%$

Dextrose:: $500 \text{ mL} \cdot 70\% = 1000 \text{ mL} \cdot DP \quad DP = 35\%$

Electrolytes to be added to TPNs are mostly supplied in mEq/mL strengths.

Example 6.29

Add 40 mEq of KCl to the TPN. Stock: KCl 2 mEq/mL.

$$\frac{2 \text{ mEq}}{1 \text{ mL}} = \frac{40 \text{ mEq}}{x} \quad 2x = 40 \text{ mL} \quad x = 20 \text{ mL}$$

Add 20 mL to the TPN.

◉ Scenario Checkup 6.2

Victoria is about halfway through her shift when she receives an order for a total parenteral nutrition (TPN). Her company does not have an automated TPN machine, so she will have to make it by hand, which will take longer. The medication is for a baby in the neonatal unit and has several ingredients. Victoria should calculate the ingredients carefully, recheck them, and then have a pharmacist check them. She needs to be extremely careful when preparing a TPN for a neonate!

Alligation Alternate

Alligation alternate is a method used to calculate the number of parts of two different strengths of medication needed to prepare a third strength that is not in stock. For example, if a physician orders 20% potassium chloride (KCl) and you have only 10% and 50% KCl in stock, you can calculate the amount of each solution needed to attain a 20% solution. You can achieve this only when the strength desired is *between* the two strengths being mixed. This means that you cannot make a 20% solution from a 5% solution and a 10% solution. However, you can make a 20% solution from a 5% and a 70% solution. The alligation process is the same when dealing with weight or volume. If a 0% diluent is used, such as water for volume or petrolatum for weight, you can use the alligation method or the equation from the dilution section.

Example 6.30

In stock are a 70% solution and a 20% solution. How much of each are needed to create 1 L of a 40% solution?

This is as simple as tic-tac-toe following these basic rules:
1. Draw a tic-tac-toe board.
2. Place your desired strength in the middle square.
3. Put your higher strength solution in the top left square.
4. Put your lower strength solution in the bottom left square. If you are using water, you will place a zero in this square because water has a concentration of zero.
5. Determine the difference between the number in the top left and middle square and place this new number in the bottom right square. Do the same with the bottom left number and middle square and place this result in the top right square. Always use positive numbers as your answers. Both of these numbers are assigned the unit "parts."
6. Create a fraction by adding the two new numbers (top and bottom right squares) together for a common denominator. Place the top right number over the denominator and do the same for the bottom right number.

$$\frac{20}{20 + 30} \quad \frac{30}{20 + 30}$$

7. Divide each fraction, and then multiply by the total volume you need.
8. Check your answer by adding the two parts. They should equal the total volume.

Answer: 400 mL of 70% solution and 600 mL of 20% solution will create a 1-L solution of 40%.

Tech Note!

Do not read your answer diagonally. Read your answer horizontally!

Exercise 6.19 Quick Check

Solve the following alligation problems.
1. *Order:* 500 mL of 20% KCl. *In stock:* 5% and 70% KCl. How many mL of each solution are needed?
2. *Order:* 8 oz of 2.5% solution. *In stock:* 10% solution and water. How many mL of each solution are needed? *Hint:* Change 8 oz to mL first.

Practice Quiz 6.3

1. 2.5 oz = _____ mL
2. 125 lb = _____ kg
3. 2000 mg = _____ g
4. 0900 hr = _____ o'clock (am or pm)
5. 1 dram = _____ mL
6. 1.5 L = _____ mL
7. 11:00 am = _____ (international time)
8. 15 mL = _____ Tbsp
9. 2 pt = _____ qt
10. gr ii = _____ mg (use gr i = 65 mg)
11. 2:30 pm = _____ (international time)
12. 22,500 mcg = _____ g
13. 25,000 units/2 mL = _____ units/mL
14. 30 lb = _____ kg
15. 2350 = _____ o'clock (am or pm)
16. 240 mL = _____ oz
17. 25 kg = _____ g
18. 10 lb = _____ oz
19. 1.5 g/10 mL = _____ mg/mL
20. 3000 mcg = _____ mg
21. 42 kg = _____ lb
22. 4.4 lb = _____ kg
23. 450 g = _____ mg
24. 908 g = _____ kg
25. 1:1000 = _____ g/_____ mL
26. 6 pm = _____ (international time)
27. 15 mL = _____ tsp
28. 8 Tbsp = _____ mL
29. 50 g/100 mL = _____ mg/mL
30. 2.25 mcg = _____ mg
31. XXX = _____ (Arabic number)
32. 0.02 g = _____ mg
33. *Order:* 90 mg gentamicin. *In stock:* 40 mg/mL. How many milliliters are needed to fill a one-time dose?
34. How many mL of Prozac 20 mg/5 mL are needed to fill a prescription for 10 mg once daily for 30 days?

35. *Order:* 9 mg/kg/dose of amoxicillin. *In stock:* 250 mg/5 mL. If the child weighs 90 lb, how many milliliters are needed per dose?
36. *Order:* digoxin 0.25 mg daily. *In stock:* 125 mcg tabs. How many tablets are needed per dose?
37. *Order:* 1 L of $D_{10}W$ with 20% KCl to run at 100 mL/hr. How many hours will this bag last?
38. *Order:* aminophylline drip 500 mL to run over 24 hours with a drop factor of 25 gtt/mL. How many gtt/min will run?
39. *Order:* make 1 L of a 30% solution. *In stock:* 10% and 40% KCl. How much of each is needed to prepare 1 L?
40. *Order:* 15 mg/kg/day to be given to an infant in three divided doses. If the child weighs 25 lb, how much will each dose be?
41. A pharmacy receives an order for 280 mL of a 5% salicylic acid solution. How much salicylic acid powder is needed to make the solution?
42. The pharmacist weighed 15 g of coal tar and gave it to the technician with instructions to compound a 1% ointment. What will be the final weight of the correctly compounded prescription?
43. The pharmacy has 300 mL of a 50% solution; 200 mL is added to this solution to decrease the concentration. How many grams of active ingredient are in 4 oz of this diluted solution?
44. If 5 g is dissolved in 100 mL of solution, what is the percentage of the solution?
45. If 100 mL of 5% solution is diluted to 500 mL, what is the percentage strength?

Business Calculations

Percentages are used in the pharmacy to identify the strength or concentration of a medication; to perform dilution problems; and to calculate the markup, discounts, net profits, and gross profits in retail pharmacy. Both the Pharmacy Technician Certification Board (PTCB) examination and the Examination for the Certification of Pharmacy Technicians (ExCPT) contain math problems using percentages.

Percentages of Quantities

The easiest method to use for finding percentages of quantities is ratio and proportion because percentage is an amount per 100. Each of the following three questions asks something different, but all can be answered by setting up a ratio and proportion.

What is 50% of 15?

Method 1: Set up a ratio and proportion, cross-multiply, and divide

$$\frac{50}{100} = \frac{x}{15}$$ Reads 50 is to 100 as x is to 15
50 times 15 divided by 100 = 7.5

Method 2: When calculating "what is x percent of" problems, it is also easy to change the percentage to a decimal and then multiply. 50% equals 50 divided by 100 = 0.5

$$0.5 \times 15 = 7.5$$

15 is 60% of what number?

Set up a ratio and proportion, cross-multiply, and divide

$$\frac{60}{100} = \frac{15}{x}$$ Reads 60 is to 100 as 15 is to what?
15 times 100 divided by 60 = 25

You can reduce first:

$$\frac{6}{10} = \frac{15}{x}$$ 15 times 10 divided by 6 = 25

5 is what percent of 20?

Set up a ratio and proportion, cross-multiply, and divide:

$$\frac{x}{100} = \frac{5}{20}$$ Reads x is to 100 as 5 is to 20
5 times 100 divided by 20 = 25

Or reduce first:

$$\frac{x}{100} = \frac{1}{4}$$ 1 times 100 divided by 4 = 25

Most problems in retail pharmacy can be solved with Method 2.

Example 6.31

An invoice from the supplier states that the pharmacy can receive a 1.5% discount if the invoice is paid within 10 days, but the entire amount is due within 30 days. How is the discount determined? The amount due is $500.

Using Method 2, change 1.5% into a decimal by dividing by 100; 1.5 divided by 100 = 0.015, then multiply 500 by 0.015

$$500 \times 0.015 = 7.50;$$ therefore the discount
will be $7.50

The total due within 10 days is $500 − $7.50 = $492.50

Example 6.32

Jane, the inventory technician, was calculating the totals for the day after the pharmacy closed. She calculated $3409.23 as the total income for the day. The pharmacy has an outstanding bill of $8345 with a drug vendor. The vendor requires a minimum payment of 5% of the outstanding bill each month. How much is owed this month?

Change 5% into a decimal by dividing by 100; 5 divided by 100 = 0.05

$$\$8345 \times 0.05 = \$417.25$$

If the pharmacy makes this payment from today's total income, what dollar amount will be left outstanding?

$$\$8345 - \$417.25 = \$7927.75$$

What will be the pharmacy's required payment next month?

$$\$7927.75 \times 0.05 = \$396.39$$

The $3409.23 in income can be ignored because it has nothing to do with the amount due.

Example 6.33

The inventory technician is responsible for figuring out how much the pharmacy can save on invoices if they are paid quickly. The total amount of an invoice is $3500, and the pharmacy is to receive a 2.5% discount.

$$\$3500 \times 0.025 = \$87.50$$

The discount would be $87.50. It does not sound like a big discount but remember that this is only one invoice. A pharmacy could save thousands of dollars a year just by paying the invoices quickly.

Another use of percentages is to calculate the **markup** necessary so the pharmacy can make a profit. Remember, the pharmacy has to make a profit so that it can pay you, pay for rent and utilities, and provide the owner with a profit. The pharmacy purchases medications at **wholesale cost** (ie, the purchase price) and marks them up to the **retail price** (selling price) to make a profit.

Example 6.34

The pharmacy must increase the cost of cold medicines by 56% to make a profit. Determine the markup and then calculate the total retail cost of the product.

Tylenol cough and cold liquid:
$5.50 (wholesale price) × 0.56 = $3.08(markup)
Total retail cost of this medication::
$5.50 + $3.08 = $8.58

Pseudoephedrine tablets::
$2.95 (wholesale price) × 0.56 = $1.65(markup)

Total retail cost of this medication::
$2.95 + $1.65 = $4.60

Similarly, percentages are used to calculate discounts that pharmacies use as incentives to sell products. Once a product has been marked up, a discount may be advertised on the retail price.

Example 6.35

The pharmacy is having a 25% off sale on the medications in Example 6.34. What are the new retail prices?

Tylenol cough and cold liquid::
$8.58 × 0.25 = $2.15 (savings to the customer)

Discounted retail price: $8.58 − $2.15 = $6.43

As you can see, the pharmacy still makes a profit because the wholesale cost was $5.50.

Pseudoephedrine tablets::
$4.60 × 0.25 = $1.15 (savings to the customer)

Discounted retail price: $4.60 − $1.15 = $3.45

Once again, the pharmacy still makes a profit because the wholesale cost was $2.95.

Exercise 6.20 Quick Check

Calculate the dollar amount by using the following percentages.

1. $200 = _____ (25%) _____ (50%) _____ (75%)
2. $956 = _____ (15%) _____ (55%) _____ (85%)
3. $2050 = _____ (20%) _____ (40%) _____ (60%)
4. $10,449 = _____ (2.5%) _____ (5.5%) _____ (7.5%)
5. A discount of 6.2% of a $2100 bill will be given if the bill is paid before the 15th of the month. What is the savings to the pharmacy if the bill is paid early?
6. These products are on sale for 20% off the regular price. Calculate the total amount of savings to the customer:
   Milk of magnesia 4 oz ($3.25)
   Pepcid AC 10-mg tablets ($10.95)
   Motrin suspension 120 mL ($6.50)
   Vitamin C 250-mg tablets #100 ($2.95)

Practice Quiz 6.4

1. The pharmacy's drug wholesaler will give a discount of 2% if the bill is paid within 1 week; calculate the final bill if the amount due is $6544.
2. Your pharmacy is having a big sale on all first aid supplies; take 20% off the following purchase and total the bill.
   Tylenol cold and cough, $8.95
   Bayer aspirin, $1.95
   Pepcid antacid, $18
   Vicks Formula 44, $2.95
   Imodium chewable tablets, $8.50
3. Your pharmacy received an order of 144 bottles; 25% of the bottles were damaged. How many damaged bottles are being returned?
4. All new prescriptions are being given a 15% discount. What is the dollar amount lost by the pharmacy if all the new prescriptions for the day added up to $2339?
5. Your pharmacy has Neosporin ointment on sale at 15% off the price of $2.95 per tube. How much will the customer save?

Scenario Checkup 6.3

Victoria is cross-trained for many positions in the hospital pharmacy. She often fills in wherever she is needed. On this particular day, the pharmacy buyer is out sick. Victoria is helping out by answering the phones and checking in orders. One of the prime vendors must be paid today in order for the hospital to receive a discount. Victoria looks up the information on the computer and finds the following terms: 3%, net in 30. The balance owed is $3200. What will the hospital pay if the bill is taken care of today? What will be owed if Victoria waits until the buyer returns to work?

Do You Remember These Key Points?

- How to convert between Roman numerals and Arabic numbers
- How to convert between the 24-hour clock and the 12-hour clock
- How to convert among fractions, ratios, decimals, and percentages
- The importance of using ratios and proportions in pharmacy calculations
- The importance of using dimensional analysis for tracking units in multistep calculations
- How to convert between units of measurement for weight and volume in the metric system
- The basic measurements of the primary system used in pharmacy—the metric system—in addition to household, avoirdupois, and apothecary units
- The formulas for calculating doses by body weight, body surface area (BSA), Young's Rule, and Clark's Rule
- How to calculate pediatric and geriatric dosages
- Drip rates of intravenous solutions can be expressed either as mL/hr or as gtt/min
- How to determine the duration of an intravenous solution
- Dilution is the process by which an inert substance is added to a preparation so that the final product has a lower concentration than the original product
- Alligation alternate is a method to compound a substance when given two strengths to prepare a third strength in between the two
- All measurements must have units, and it is important to label them correctly while performing calculations and on medication labels to avoid possible errors
- Double-checking calculations is important before preparing medications

Scenario Follow-Up

As Victoria continues to excel at the hospital pharmacy, she has learned that it is imperative to check and double-check her calculations. She understands that she can be held accountable for any medication errors she makes. She is diligent in making sure all her work is thoroughly checked by a pharmacist before it reaches the patient.

Review Questions

Convert the following units to percentages.

1. $\frac{1}{5}$ = _____
2. 0.25 = _____
3. $\frac{10}{25}$ = _____
4. 2.275 = _____

Convert the following fraction of grains into milligrams.

5. NTG gr $\frac{1}{300}$ = _____ mg

Write the Arabic numbers in Roman numerals and the Roman numerals in Arabic numbers:

6. 20 = _____
7. 50 = _____
8. 59 = _____
9. CXL = _____
10. XC = _____
11. XXXIV = _____

Convert the following temperatures:

12. 37°C = _____ °F
13. 86°F = _____ °C

Convert the following metric units into the units indicated:

14. 5 cc = _____ tsp

15. 1 mcg = _____ mg

16. 15 cc = _____ tsp

17. 1000 mg = _____ g

18. 30 mL = _____ tsp

19. 900 mL = _____ oz

20. 1000 mL = _____ L

21. 0.25 L = _____ mL

22. 2 kg = _____ lb

23. 0.25 mg = _____ mcg

24. *Order:* cimetidine 300 mg tab qid × 30 days. *In stock:* cimetidine 150 mg tablets.

How many tablets will you need to fill this order?

25. *Order:* tobramycin IV 60 mg in D₅W 50 mL. *In stock:* tobramycin 40 mg/mL in 2-mL vials.

How many milliliters are needed to fill the order?

26. *Order:* vancomycin IV 750 mg bid in D₅W 250 mL. *In stock:* vancomycin 1 g per 20-mL vial.

How much will you take from the 1-g vial?

27. *Order:* 10% dextrose solution 1 L. *In stock:* 5% and 50% dextrose bags.

How much of each solution will it take to make a 1-L bag of 10% dextrose?

28. *Order:* 0.5 L of a 30% amino acid solution. *In stock:* 70% amino acids and sterile water.

How much of each solution is required to prepare a 30% solution?

29. Convert the following ratios into grams per milliliter and also to percentage strengths:

A. 1:10

B. 2:100

C. 1:1000

30. *Order:* dispense ibuprofen liquid 40 mg/kg per day; give qid. *In stock:* ibuprofen liquid 100 mg/5 mL.

How much will this patient receive *per dose* if the patient's weight is 10 lb?

How much liquid is needed to fill a 7-day supply?

31. Heparin 500 mL is to be given over 20 hours. The tubing size delivers 10 gtt/mL.

How many drops per minute are being delivered to the patient?

32. What is the percent strength of a 1:25 (w/v) solution?

33. You add 40 g of salicylic acid to white petrolatum to make a total of 800 g.

What is the percentage strength of the product?

34. What is the initial strength of a solution that is made by adding 200 mL of purified water to make 600 mL of a 25% solution?

35. If you dilute 60 mL of a 30% solution to 480 mL, what is the percentage strength of the new solution?

36. How many milliliters of pure alcohol (w/v) are required to make 480 mL of a solution containing 30% alcohol?

37. You need to mix magic mouthwash that has a ratio of 1:1:1. Using diphenhydramine, Maalox, and lidocaine, how much of each do you need to make 8 oz? Give your answer in milliliters.

☐ Technician's Corner

An order comes to the pharmacy with the following directions:
- D₅W 250 mL with heparin 10,000 units IV at 500 units/hr
- Calculate the flow rate in mL/hr

Bibliography

Brown M, Mulholland JM. *Drug Calculations: Process and Problems for Clinical Practice.* 8th ed. St. Louis: Mosby; 2008.

Gray Morris D. *Calculate with Confidence.* 5th ed. St. Louis: Elsevier; 2010.

Mizner JJ. *Mosby's Review for the Pharmacy Technician Certification Examination.* 3rd ed. St. Louis: Mosby; 2014.

CHAPTER 7

Drug Information References

Karen Davis

1. Demonstrate the appropriate way to research drugs and other information from reference books, journals, and electronic resources.
2. Describe the information contained in the following references: *American Drug Index; American Hospital Formulary Service Drug Information; Approved Drug Products With Therapeutic Equivalence Evaluations* (otherwise known as the *Orange Book*); *Clinical Pharmacology* and other Gold Standard/ Elsevier products; *Drug Facts and Comparisons; Drug Topics Red Book; Geriatric Dosage Handbook; Goodman & Gilman's The Pharmacological Basis of Therapeutics; Handbook of Nonprescription Drugs; Ident-A-Drug; Martindale's The Complete Drug Reference; Micromedex Healthcare series; Pediatric and Neonatal Dosage Handbook; Physicians' Desk Reference (PDR); Remington's Pharmaceutical Sciences: The Science and Practice of Pharmacy; Trissel's Handbook on Injectable Drugs; United States Pharmacist's Pharmacopeia; United States Pharmacopoeia–National Formulary (USP-NF).*
3. Explain the importance of carrying a pocket-sized reference book.
4. List types of electronic reference materials.
5. Demonstrate the appropriate way to research drugs and other information on the Internet.
6. Explain the importance of journals and news magazines as they pertain to pharmacy and continuing education.
7. Describe different considerations when choosing a reference.

Brand name Trademark of a drug or device held by the originating manufacturing company

Chemical structure The makeup of a chemical, including the elements, the shape, the bonding types, the molecular configurations, charges, and so on; the nature of the chemical's structure has much to do with the chemical's stability, reactivity, and physical and chemical properties

Drug classification Categorization based on various characteristics, including the chemical structure of a drug, the action of a drug, and/or the therapeutic or anatomical use of a drug

Drug Facts and Comparisons Reference book found in pharmacies that contains detailed information on more than 22,000 prescription and 6000 over-the-counter medications; drugs are divided into therapeutic groups for easy comparison

Formulary A list of approved drugs to be stocked by the pharmacy; also a list of drugs covered by an insurance company

Generic name Name assigned to a medication or nonproprietary name of a drug

Monograph Comprehensive information on a medication's actions within that class of drugs; also lists generic and trade names, ingredients, dosages, side effects, adverse effects, how the patient should take the medication, and foods or other drugs (eg, over-the-counter medications, herbals) to avoid while taking the medication

Nonformulary A list of drugs that are not included in the list of preferred medications that a committee of pharmacists and physicians deems to be the safest, most effective, and most economical; they are drugs not included in the drug list approved for reimbursement by the health care plans

Package insert The official prescribing information for a prescription drug; the medication information sheet provided by the manufacturer that includes side effects, dosage forms, indications, and other important information

Trade name The proprietary or brand name given to a drug by the company that developed it; the trade name may be related to the function or main use of the drug

⊙ Scenario

Robert is an experienced technician at a busy retail pharmacy. He has been certified with the Pharmacy Technician Certification Board (PTCB) for 6 years. One of his responsibilities is to update the Drug Facts and Comparisons *loose-leaf binder with the new drug inserts each month. Robert finds this task tedious and time-consuming and often wishes his pharmacist would use an online drug database. Do you think Robert should suggest this change to his supervisors? What would be the best way to approach this subject with the pharmacist? What are the pros and cons of using electronic drug databases in the pharmacy?*

Drug information reference books are some of the most important tools used in pharmacy (Fig. 7.1). Physicians, nurses, and other health care professionals call the pharmacy daily to ask questions about various medications. Pharmacists rely on credible, accurate, and up-to-date reference resources to help give the correct information to others. Although a few of the books in pharmacy are highly technical, most give basic information on drugs. Knowing which book to choose for referencing and how to access the information is an important skill for pharmacists and technicians. This chapter covers the references that are more commonly used in a pharmacy. In addition, other types of referencing materials that can be of help specifically to the technician are listed.

Researching a Drug

Before you begin to look for information, take these key points into consideration. First, what exactly is the purpose of your search? What is the question that needs to be answered? Do you need to know the generic drug name only, the drug's interactions and classification, or perhaps the drug's appearance?

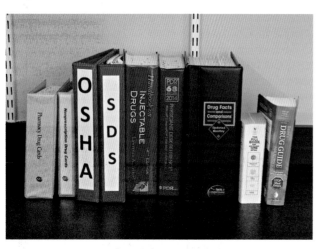

FIG. 7.1 Drug information references.

▽ Tech Alert!

It is important for technicians to be proficient in accessing accurate drug references and materials; however, technicians should not provide patients with information about side effects, dosing, or compatibility. This is out of the technician's scope of practice.

Let's begin with the process of developing, manufacturing, and naming drugs to learn the importance of each one of these components.

■ Tech Note!

Technically, all generic drug names are spelled in lowercase letters, whereas trade or **brand names** are capitalized. *For example:* atenolol (generic) and Tenormin (brand).

When a new drug is in the experimentation phase, the creators or the company give the drug a generic or investigational drug name based on its chemical attributes; the name also prepares the drug for recognition during future marketing after approval. Later, when the drug has been approved by the US Food and Drug Administration (FDA), a **monograph,** or official label, is created to include important findings such as side effects that were reported during clinical trials.

The **drug classification** is important because it places the drug into proper categories based on its **chemical structure,** mechanism of action, anatomical function, and/or therapeutic use. Many times, drugs in the same class have the same mechanism of action. This information can assist the prescriber and pharmacist in determining the expected therapeutic effect and possible adverse reactions.

The indications list the main conditions for which the chemical is used. A contraindications list is also an important part of a drug monograph. This list identifies types of individuals who should not be given the medication. Reasons may range from certain serious drug-drug interactions to conditions that conflict with the action of the drug. After all the studies have been done and the data have been analyzed, contraindications still may be discovered in postmarket use; these are updated in the drug's monograph. It is always helpful to ensure that you are reading the most recent information on a drug. The last date of update is listed directly on the official product labeling.

The founding company assigns the chemical name, **generic name,** and **trade name,** which are found in the product's official label. The chemical name is a scientific name given to a chemical in accordance with the nomenclature system developed by the International Union of Pure and Applied Chemistry, Chemical Abstracts Service, or another authoritative agency. Many times generic names are closely related to the chemical name of the drug but not always. The trade name (proprietary or brand name) is determined by the company that developed the drug and is therefore the exclusive property of that company. Some trade names may be related to the function or main use of the drug (Box 7.1). Examples of generic names are presented in Box 7.2.

The US Adopted Names Council has established a list of word stems (prefixes, root words, and suffixes) that identify a drug's classification. These word parts reflect a specific drug classification (see Box 7.2). Knowing these word parts makes it easier to learn what a specific drug does.

Tech Note!

Generic drug names do not typically begin with J or W because those letters do not exist in the languages of many countries other than the United States that use generic drugs. Trade names can reflect the drug's primary characteristics or use but cannot imply a cure of a specific part of the body.

References Used in Pharmacy

In addition to being familiar with the official label of a product, technicians should be adept at using basic pharmacy drug references. A better understanding of medications and diseases allows for safer patient care; however, consult with the pharmacist before sharing any information with a patient. Most references have a section on how to use the text or online "help" sections to aid the reader in the use of computerized resources. It is helpful for the technician to be familiar with performing a reference search before it is required. Knowing how to use the reference properly allows the technician to find the correct information in a timely manner.

Although many different types of reference materials are available, this chapter describes only the most common types seen in a pharmacy setting.

Many reference materials are available to technicians and pharmacists in a variety of formats, and it should be noted that online interfaces, such as *Micromedex* and *Lexicomp*, are increasingly more prevalent in the pharmacy setting. The following examples of commonly used reference materials are normally available in more than one form. All of the books can be found at online booksellers, such as amazon.com. At the end of each description is a list of available product formats.

Drug Facts and Comparisons

Drug Facts and Comparisons is one of the resources available in both print and online, most frequently used by pharmacists. This reference book was first published in 1946 and was created for quick and accurate reference and drug comparison. Because of its vital information and ease of use, it is a very popular pharmacy reference. *Drug Facts and Comparisons* has five sections.

At the front of each classification section is extensive information on various aspects of that class of drugs. Included under each drug listing are indications for use. In addition, a chart lists all of the dosage strengths, dosage forms, sizes, and manufacturers. Most pharmacies carry the unbound book to allow for monthly updates. *Drug Facts and Comparisons* answers many basic questions for the pharmacist. It is available in hardback, loose-leaf hardback, pocket size, or as an electronic subscription (Facts and Comparison eAnswers). An example of how to locate an over-the-counter (OTC) drug such as Prilosec would start with locating the drug name in the index under either the generic or the trade name. Once you find the page, the information will contain the usual dosage, strengths, and forms it is available in and patient information. When dispensing in a pharmacy, other useful information, such as the type of auxiliary label that is needed and drug interactions, is also provided.

Physicians' Desk Reference

The *Physicians' Desk Reference (PDR)* is a popular reference found in most physicians' offices and pharmacies. The *PDR* has been in publication for more than 50 years. It has six sections. The pages are color coded and contain information regarding manufacturer, product specifics, and diagnostic information.

Each drug referenced in the *PDR* has a complete description, including its chemical structure and study results. This book is a compilation of **package inserts** (official labels) provided by manufacturers who have paid a fee for inclusion in the reference; not all package inserts are available. Package inserts can be difficult to read. Although most pharmacies have a *PDR*, physicians are the primary users, and, again, the *PDR* lists only FDA-approved drugs that the manufacturers choose to send for inclusion. This book is not as important in a pharmacy setting as it is in a physician's office. The *PDR* does contain useful drug manufacturer contact information, such as addresses and phone numbers. However, manufacturer information now is available in many other online drug information subscription programs. The *PDR* is available in

hardback and electronic formats. Online subscription is free to prescribers.

Drug Topics Red Book

One of the longest published reference guides is the *Drug Topics Red Book*. This book is updated monthly and is a good source of information pertaining to average and wholesale drug costs and prices. The *New Red Book* has 10 sections. Information contained within each describes useful information for pharmacy personnel from drug information such as whether they can be crushed or whether they are sugar free. This reference also provides information that technicians use in dispensing such as reimbursement; disease information; color photos and look-alike, sound-alike drugs; and even an herbal reference. Community pharmacies, rather than hospital pharmacies, are more likely to use this book.

Red Book contains valuable information, in the form of quick referencing charts, that technicians can use, such as drugs that should not be crushed, drugs that are sugar free and alcohol free, and drugs excreted in breast milk. In addition, *Red Book* includes convenient tables showing pharmacy calculations and dosing instructions translated into Spanish. Although *Red Book* has an extraordinary amount of information, it is not an easy book to reference without knowing the abbreviations for the drug sections. An added feature of *Red Book* is a listing of all nontraditional doctor of pharmacy (PharmD) programs, along with requirements and current enrollment numbers. This is information that few, if any, other books contain. This book is available in softcover and electronic formats.

Approved Drug Products With Therapeutic Equivalence Evaluations: The Orange Book

The *Orange Book* is a comprehensive list of approved drug products with therapeutic equivalence evaluations that is provided by the FDA. This is the book to use for determining whether a generic drug is the same as a brand drug. Other information includes discontinued drug products, orphan product designations, and approval lists. Information searches can be accessed by several different means: active ingredient, patent number, proprietary name, applicant holder, or application number. The *Orange Book* publication is updated annually. Frequent updates are made to the online version, and it can be accessed free of charge.

The Purple Book: A Compendium of Biological and Biosimilar Products

The *Purple Book* is a comprehensive list of approved biological products with biosimilar and interchangeable products, similar to the FDA's *Orange Book*.

American Hospital Formulary Service Drug Information

Used mainly by hospitals, the *American Hospital Formulary Service Drug Information (AHFS DI)* provides drug monographs that list drug information, including the following:

- Acute toxicity
- Adverse reactions

- Drug interactions
- Laboratory and test references
- Mechanism of action
- Pharmacokinetics
- Pharmacology
- Preparations, chemistry, and stability
- Specific dosage and administration information
- Spectrum and resistance for antibiotics
- Uses and off-label uses

This information is derived from experts in the fields of medicine, pharmacy, and management, through an independent editorial review process. This book is available in hardback, electronic, and a mobile application version.

United States Pharmacopoeia–National Formulary

The *United States Pharmacopoeia–National Formulary* (USP-NF) provides access to official standards of the FDA. It is a guide for the specifications—tests, procedures, and acceptance criteria—required for pharmaceutical manufacturing and quality control. This book aids compliance with standards and lists new product development and approvals. It is available in hardback, electronic form, or online with a subscription.

United States Pharmacists' Pharmacopeia

United States Pharmacists' Pharmacopeia is a comprehensive compilation of information on compounding products and ingredients and their safety, in addition to products used to treat specific medical conditions. Also included are the most recent sterile preparation guidelines for USP, the most common **nonformulary** agents, veterinary compounding, dietary supplements, and laws pertaining to compounding. This book is available in hardback or online with a subscription.

Clinical Pharmacology and Other Gold Standard/Elsevier Products

Clinical Pharmacology is an electronic drug compendium commonly encountered in retail and health system pharmacies. Similar to *Drug Facts and Comparisons*, the reference is very popular because of its ease of use and quick access to needed information. The information can be provided to the pharmacy or health system by online, intranet, electronic, or mobile applications. The reference can be used by physicians, pharmacists, nurses, and other allied health professionals. Similar to the American Society of Health-System Pharmacists (ASHP) and *Micromedex DRUGDEX*, *Clinical Pharmacology* is a compendium officially recognized by the Centers for Medicare & Medicaid Services (CMS) because of its extensive amount of drug information, including off-label drug uses supported by clinical evidence. Data are continuously updated, making this reference a very timely resource for current drug information. *Gold Standard Drug Database* by Elsevier also has a complement of other products that can be bundled to the subscription to enhance the base compendia product. The following are examples of the various types of information available:

- Alchemy
- Comprehensive drug details, including pharmacology, pharmacokinetics, contraindications, boxed warnings,

precautions, pregnancy category, breastfeeding, indications and dosage for all populations, off-label uses, and adverse events
- Consumer medication information: MedCounselor sheets
- Drug interactions (available in professional and consumer-friendly reports)
- Drug product comparison reports
- FDA-approved drugs and "how supplied" data for generic, trade name, prescription (Rx), and nonprescription (non-Rx) products; drug product images are included
- Herbals and dietary supplements, including multivitamin and nutritional product listings
- Identification of drug products: Drug IDentifier (includes imprint codes, colors, shapes, scoring, and images)
- Integrated drug product data, including clinical decision support and pricing modules:
  - International listing of drugs: Global Drug Name Index
  - Intravenous (IV) compatibility report
  - Material safety data sheets: ToxED
  - Toxicology and poisoning management: ToxED

Fig. 7.2 presents a screen shot of a *Clinical Pharmacology* drug monograph.

Ident-A-Drug

Ident-A-Drug lists tablet and capsule identifications. Most tablets and capsules have a code or number stamped on them by the manufacturer for identification purposes. *Ident-A-Drug* includes more than 38,000 listings. The drugs are not listed by pictures but by identifiable codes, colors, and shapes and also by whether the tablet is available scored. After these characteristics have been identified, the book provides the name of the manufacturer, generic and brand names, strength, and use of the drug. *Micromedex's* IDENTIDEX and *Clinical Pharmacology's* Drug IDentifier are also useful resources that are currently available in many pharmacies (both hospital and retail). *Micromedex* is an online interface that has pictures to aid in identifying drugs quickly and accurately. This type of referencing is very helpful when patients do not know the name of the drug they are taking but have a capsule or tablet of the drug to use as a reference. Emergency departments often have patients who have overdosed on an unknown drug. If one tablet or capsule is brought in with the patient, the pharmacy probably can identify the drug using the *Ident-A-Drug* book, *Micromedex's* IDENTIDEX, or *Clinical Pharmacology's* Drug IDentifier (Fig. 7.3). Although some books such as *Drug Facts and Comparisons* have some pictures of tablets and capsules, these are not extensive and are not the first choice to use in identifying a drug. *Ident-A-Drug* is available as a softcover book, mobile application, and online with a subscription. With today's artificial intelligence capabilities, the ability to take a picture of the tablet using auto capture can also be used. Smart Pill ID is offered through drugs.com for android and iOS devices.

◉ Scenario Checkup 7.1

Robert had a very productive meeting with his supervisors about using more computerized drug references. He is excited to hear that his

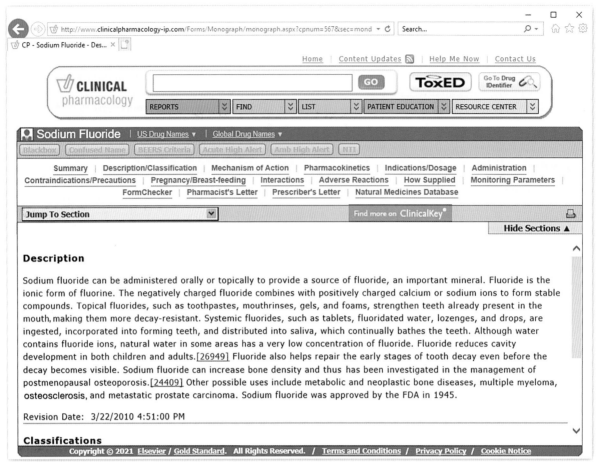

FIG. 7.2 Screenshot from *Clinical Pharmacology* showing a drug monograph.

pharmacy will now be using the Clinical Pharmacology *electronic database from Elsevier. Today Robert is busy filling prescriptions when the phone rings. The call is from a middle school counselor. She has just found a handful of pills in one of the student's backpacks. She describes the pills to Robert, noting the color, shape, and numbers on each tablet. Using a resource discussed above, what could Robert do to help identify the drug and assist the counselor?*

Micromedex Healthcare Series

Micromedex Healthcare Evidence and Clinical Xpert provides an online and mobile application that can be used by physicians, pharmacists, and nurses in a health care facility. The information is provided through several different software programs that can be purchased. The following list includes examples of the various types of information available with the specific software programs:

- Comprehensive drug details: DRUGDEX
- Dosing information and parenteral nutrition solutions for infants: NeoFax
- Drug information for more educated patients: Detailed Drug Information for the Consumer
- Drug interactions: DRUG-REAX
- Drug pricing: ReadyPrice
- FDA-approved drugs: PDR
- Formulary management for hospitals: Formulary Advisor
- Herbals, supplements, and alternative therapies: AltMedDex

- Identification of capsules and tablets: IDENTIDEX
- International drugs: Index Nominum
- Management of medication reconciliation throughout the hospital workflow: Clinical Xpert Medication Reconciliation
- Monographs for pharmacy and therapeutics (P&T) evaluations: P&T QUIK
- Pharmacokinetics calculators: KINETIDEX
- Proper drug usage and precautions: DrugNotes
- Safety data sheets: Pharmaceutical SDS
- Verification of IV compatibility: IV INDEX

Trissel's Handbook on Injectable Drugs

Mostly used in the hospital setting, the *Handbook on Injectable Drugs** by Lawrence Trissel is a well-known reference used for information on parenteral agents. The monographs discuss products, administration, stability, and compatibility with infusion solutions and other drugs. Although technicians cannot relay information from this book to physicians or nurses, they can find the information and have it ready for the pharmacist. In this way, they can facilitate a rapid response from the pharmacy to the necessary medical personnel. This book is available in hardback, electronic, mobile application, and online formats and is updated yearly.

---

*Many online drug compendia, including *Clinical Pharmacology* and *Micromedex*, have incorporated the online Trissel databases into their product offerings.

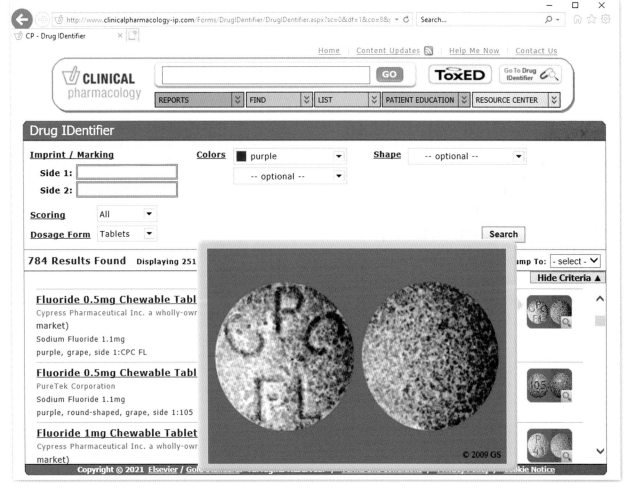

FIG. 7.3 Screenshot from *Clinical Pharmacology* showing a pill using the Drug IDentifier.

American Drug Index

The *American Drug Index* contains listings for more than 24,000 drugs, both Rx and OTC. Information includes the following:

- Active ingredients
- Dosage forms
- Drugs that should not be crushed or chewed
- Look-alike or sound-alike drugs
- Manufacturers' names
- Normal laboratory values and more
- Packaging and uses
- Pronunciation of drug names
- Storage requirements for USP drugs
- Strengths
- Trademark glossary
  The book is available in hardback or electronic format.

Goodman & Gilman's The Pharmacological Basis of Therapeutics

The following is a list of some of the information provided in *Goodman & Gilman's The Pharmacological Basis of Therapeutics:*

- Drug metabolism pharmacogenomics
- Drug transport/drug transporters
- Pharmacokinetics and pharmacodynamics
- Principles of therapeutics in all areas of the body system
  This book is available in hardback format or as an online subscription.

Handbook of Nonprescription Drugs

The *Handbook of Nonprescription Drugs*, a reference published by the American Pharmacists Association (APhA), provides self-care options for the following:

- Complementary and alternative medicine
- Complementary and alternative therapies
- FDA-approved dosing information and evidence-based research on efficacy and safety considerations of nonprescription, herbal, and homeopathic medications
- Medical foods
- Nondrug and preventive measures for self-treatable disorders
- Nonprescription medications
- Nutritional supplements
  This book is available in hardback format or as an e-book (textbook is downloaded onto a computer).

Martindale: The Complete Drug Reference

Martindale: The Complete Drug Reference provides information on drugs in clinical use worldwide, in addition to the following:

- Contrast media and diagnostic agents
- Disinfectants
- Drugs of abuse and recreational drugs
- Herbal and complementary medicines
- Medicinal gases
- Pesticides
- Pharmaceutical excipients
- Radiopharmaceuticals
- Selected investigational and veterinary drugs
- Toxic substances
- Vaccines
- Vitamins and nutritional agents

The book is available in hardback or electronic format.

Remington's Pharmaceutical Sciences: The Science and Practice of Pharmacy

Remington's Pharmaceutical Sciences: The Science and Practice of Pharmacy covers the entire scope of pharmacy, from the history of pharmacy and ethics to the specifics of industrial pharmacy and pharmacy practice. The following specific areas are included:

- Disease state management
- Immunology
- Manifestations and pathophysiology of diseases
- Professional communication
- Specialization in pharmacy practice
- Various aspects of patient care

The book is available in hardback format.

Pediatric and Neonatal Dosage Handbook

The *Pediatric and Neonatal Dosage Handbook*, published by Lexi-Comp, provides information on suggested current dosages for pediatric patients. The 20th edition features 983 drug monographs. It is alphabetically organized and cross-referenced by US and Canadian brand names. An appendix is provided that contains comparative charts, tables, and other supportive information. A Therapeutic Category and Key Word index also are included. The book is available in hardback format.

Geriatric Dosage Handbook

The *Geriatric Dosage Handbook*, published by Lexi-Comp, provides information on suggested current dosages for geriatric patients. The brand and generic drug names are alphabetically organized and cross-referenced by page number to the generic drug monograph. Geriatric-sensitive information is provided, along with the latest Beers Criteria (updated 2013). Beers outlines drugs to avoid or to use with caution in older adults. It is available in hardback format.

In addition to these well-known books, many specialty reference books are available, such as those covering information on drugs in pregnancy and breastfeeding, psychotropic medications, and antibiotics. Many pharmacies have a wide range of these types of reference books available (Table 7.1).

Pocket-Sized Reference Books

Technicians traditionally have not carried pocket versions of drug books. However, as roles expand at work, the pharmacy technician needs to have his or her own reference books. Some manufacturers produce small pocket versions of trade/generic name drug books, but the drugs listed often are limited to their drug line only. It is becoming more important for technicians to carry a good pocket guide not only of trade and generic names but also of drug classifications, indications, and side effects. Before purchasing a pocket guide, technicians should examine a variety of different guides to determine the one that is most pertinent to their jobs. One of the best books to keep is one in which a drug can be looked up by trade or brand name without having to check the index. The cost of these pocket handbooks generally ranges from $5 to $10. The disadvantage is that they are softbound and must be updated yearly to incorporate new drugs or discontinued ones. The advantage is that most of the drugs remain the same over time.

There are also apps for many of the references such as Micromedex or drugs.com that can be downloaded for iPhone and Android devices.

◉ Scenario Checkup 7.2

Robert is a dedicated technician who likes to keep up on the most recent new drugs. His friend Haley suggests he invest in an updated pocket drug guide. Robert tells Haley he would prefer to download one of the new drug apps for his iPhone, but he is not sure whether he would be allowed to use it. Employees are not supposed to have their phones out during work. How can Robert solve this dilemma?

Electronic Referencing

Electronic devices, such as smartphones and tablets, are becoming more popular and economical. An assortment of drug databases and other reference materials can be downloaded onto a handheld device for easy access. Several companies offer short-term trial periods for these reference materials before requiring the user to purchase a subscription. Others offer a limited amount of information for free. One example is Epocrates *(http://www.Epocrates.com)* which offers a basic free drug information package that can be downloaded onto a smartphone or other handheld device. The following information is included:

- Classification
- Dosing
- Indications
- Interactions
- Manufacturer's contact information
- Medication and study updates
- Pill identification
- Provider directory
- Resource center
- Trade and generic name reference

The smartphone with the most drug database options is the iPhone/iPad, followed by the Android platform.

TABLE 7.1
Pharmacy Reference Books

Reference Book	Publisher	Available in	Updated
Drug Facts and Comparisons	Wolters Kluwer Health	Hardbound book Loose-leaf book Electronic Mobile application	Yearly Monthly Current updates Current updates
Physicians' Desk Reference	Thomson Healthcare	Hardbound book Mobile application	Yearly Current updates
Drug Topics Red Book	Medical Economics	Softbound book	Yearly and monthly
Orange Book	FDA	Electronic	Current updates
USP-NF	USP	Three-volume hardbound Online CD	Monthly Current updates Monthly
Ident-A-Drug	Therapeutic Research Faculty	Softbound book Online Mobile application	Monthly Current updates Current updates
Goodman & Gilman's The Pharmacological Basis of Therapeutics	McGraw-Hill	Hardbound Electronic Mobile application	Every 5 years Current updates cut/paste With electronic subscription
Remington's Pharmaceutical Sciences: The Science and Practice of Pharmacy	Lippincott Williams & Wilkins	Hardbound and online	Every 5 years
United States Pharmacopoeia–National Formulary (USP-NF)	USP	Hardbound and online	Yearly
Drug Information	ASHP	Softbound	Yearly
American Hospital Formulary		Electronic	Current updates
Trissel's Handbook on Injectable Drugs	ASHP	Hardbound and online	Yearly
Pediatric Dosage Handbook	Lexi-Comp/Wolters Kluwer Health APhA	Hardbound Softbound Online	Yearly Yearly
Geriatric Dosage Handbook	Lexi-Comp/Wolters Kluwer Health APhA	Hardbound Softbound	Yearly Yearly
Purple Book	FDA	Online searchable reference	Current updates

APhA, American Pharmacists Association; ASHP, American Society of Health-System Pharmacists; FDA, US Food and Drug Administration; USP, US Pharmacopeial Convention.

The following are several free drug reference apps:

Drugs.com (https://:www.drugs.com): provides easy drug lookup information, an identifier, and drug interaction check.

- Fingertip Formulary (http://www.fingertipformulary.com/): Provides drug formulary information listed by state. A free version is available for most platforms, and extra drug monograph information is available for licensed providers.
- IBM Micromedex Drug Information: An extensive drug database with detailed information, including pharmacokinetics, toxicology, and clinical teaching pearls. It is available for iOS, Android, and Windows devices.
- Medscape Mobile: A combination drug reference and database that includes a drug-drug interaction checker. It is available for download on both iOS and Android platforms.
- mobilePDR (https://www.pdr.net/resources/mobilePDR/): This is an electronic version of the paper book that is published annually. It has a pill search function that includes pictures, and access to thousands of drug summaries continually updated by PDR within a week of manufacturers' updates. This app is free to all US health care professionals (registration required) and is available on both iOS and Android devices.

The Internet

Referencing should not be limited to books alone. The Internet has a lot of information; however, it is up to the reader to determine whether the information is reliable and accurate. Finding websites at universities and through publishing companies is a good way to look for information. Accessing personal websites may give you a person's perspective but may not provide medically sound information. A list of reputable websites for news concerning medications is provided at the end of this chapter.

Pharmacy organizations have websites on the Internet, and many have weekly news boards that reference important information concerning pharmacy. Because pharmacy is constantly evolving, much of the information cannot be included in journals. The news links are listed on the website. Many databases have up-to-date information and links (Table 7.2). These are valuable tools for keeping members updated with accurate information. In addition, these association sites have links to other pharmacy sites that may be of interest. Pharmacy associations also may offer Internet links where the user can have questions answered by other members.

Many websites provide continuing education (CE) in the form of online examinations and live CE courses. With the online CE courses, the student sometimes can download and study the information before taking the examination online; other online courses require live participation. After the course has been completed, the certificate is mailed, e-mailed, or provided online to the student. CE certificates should be filed for reference when obtaining recertification. Often these CE courses are offered free of charge, and although a certain number of CE units are required for recertification, there is no limit to the number of CE courses a person may take. Upon completion of the CE examination, you receive notification of your score, and a certificate can be printed and filed in your records as a recertification reference. Starting in 2015, CE courses began to be coded for technicians specifically. For more information on CE sources, see Chapter 3.

▣ TABLE 7.2
Websites and Databases Helpful for Pharmacy Technicians

Website	Name of Organization or Site	Type of Information
http://www.cdc.gov	Centers for Disease Control and Prevention	Current health issues
http://www.cms.gov	Centers for Medicare & Medicaid Services	Reimbursement information
https://dailymed.nlm.nih.gov/dailymed/	Online database	Includes package inserts for more than 5000 drugs available in the United States
https://www.drugs.com	ASHP, Cerner Multum, and Watson Micromedex	Comprehensive drug guide with over 24,000 listings and medical information
http://drugtopics.modernmedicine.com/	Online information	Up-to-date medical news and pharmacy issues
http://www.FDA.gov	US Food and Drug Administration (FDA)	Drug, food, and cosmetics safety information
http://www.fda.gov/drugs/default.htm	FDA drug evaluation and research development	Links to *Orange Book, Purple Book, MedWatch, NDC Directory,* and new drug approvals
http://www.Health.nih.gov	National Institutes of Health	Health issues and studies
http://www.MayoClinic.org	Mayo Clinic	Information on conditions and diseases, lifestyle health issues
http://www.medicare.gov/part-d/coverage/part-d-coverage.html	US Department of Health and Human Services	Information on Medicare Part D, formulary index
http://www.medscape.com	Online database	Information on diseases; links to medical journals and continuing education (CE) courses
http://www.nlm.nih.gov/medlineplus	National Library of Medicine database	Health and drug information, medical dictionary and encyclopedia
http://www.PDRhealth.com	*Physicians' Desk Reference* online	Interactions database for both legend and over-the-counter (OTC) drugs and also herbs and supplements; information on conditions and diseases
http://www.Rxlist.com	Online database	Both prescription and OTC drug information
http://www.webmd.com	Online database	Up-to-date health topics, conditions, and diseases and drug information

Journals and News Magazines

Nearly every pharmacy subscribes to journals and news magazines that pertain to pharmacy. They may be paper journals or electronic versions. These can be informative to the pharmacy technician. When a technician becomes nationally certified, he or she must complete CE units and may at some point use these journals to complete some if not all the necessary units. Journals offer CE at a reasonable cost; in addition, they allow the technician to stay current on the most recent drugs being developed. Journals and newsletters may be published monthly, bimonthly, quarterly, or even weekly. They contain articles on new drugs, technicians, the future of pharmacy, and various legislative changes that may be taking place. The information they can provide about the field of pharmacy can be beneficial. Many different journals, newsletters, and magazines are available. Other journals that technicians may not see in the pharmacy setting are those written by pharmacy technician associations. These journals are geared specifically to technician issues. Table 7.3 provides a sample of the types of journals and pharmacy magazines available.

⊙ Scenario Checkup 7.3

As a certified pharmacy technician, Robert must complete 20 hours of continuing education (CE) every 2 years. He has read that the National Pharmacy Technician Association (NPTA) provides free CE for its members. He also found that with the yearly membership, he would receive the Technician Today *magazine. Robert is considering asking his company to pay for his NPTA membership. Do you think this is a good idea? Why or why not?*

Additional Types of Information

In addition to large desktop books, pocket handbooks, journals, and the Internet, other sources of information can keep you current and on the cutting edge as a pharmacy technician. For examples of additional references geared to technicians and health care workers, see Table 7.4. Another way to obtain new drug information is to join an association. Membership can be rewarding and can serve as a good source of information and a way to network. Many associations offer webinars, both live and recorded, for members. CE credits can be earned while learning new material. The associations listed in Box 7.3 currently provide CE and information for technicians.

All of these organizations offer a great way to stay current on new drugs, devices, and current and future pharmacy issues. In addition, they usually offer a way to order pharmacy technician certification review books and other reference books, sometimes at a reduced membership rate. These reference books can be found on their websites or at their bookstores (this information may be found at their seminars). The information and support they can provide is limited only by how much they are used. In addition, many pharmacist associations, such as the ASHP and APhA and their chapters, have specific divisions for pharmacy technicians, providing technicians with additional sources for learning new information. You must inquire about your local pharmacy associations to determine what they offer. Some technician divisions are active in supplying CE courses to technicians and host various functions for networking and unifying pharmacy technicians from different types of pharmacies. For more information on all associations, refer to Chapter 3.

▣ TABLE 7.3
Pharmacy Publications

Publication	Published	Continuing Education Included	Website	Association
AAPT	6 times yearly	Yes	*https://www.pharmacytechnician.com/*	Yes
Computer Talk	6 times yearly	No	*http://www.computertalk.com*	No
Hospital Pharmacy	Monthly	Yes	*http://www.hospitalpharmacyjournal.com*	No
Drug Topics	Monthly	Yes	*http://drugtopics.modernmedicine.com*	No
Today's Technician	6 times yearly	Yes	*http://www.pharmacytechnician.org*	Yes
Pharmacy Times	Monthly	Yes	*http://www.pharmacytimes.com*	No
Pharmacy Today (JAPhA)	Monthly	Yes	*http://www.pharmacytoday.org*	No
The Script	Monthly	No	*http://www.pharmacy.ca.gov*	No
U.S. Pharmacist	Monthly	Yes	*http://www.uspharmacist.com*	No
AJHP	Twice monthly	Yes	*http://www.ajhp.org*	Yes
Journal of Pharmacy Technology	6 times yearly	Yes	*http://pmt.sagepub.com*	No

AAPT, American Association of Pharmacy Technicians; *AJHP,* American Journal of Health-System Pharmacy; *JAPhA,* Journal of the American Pharmacists Association.

Additional Reference Books for Pharmacy Technicians[a]

Name	Useful Information
Gray Morris D. *Calculate With Confidence*. 8th ed. St. Louis: Elsevier; 2022 ISBN 978-0-323-75157-5	Math calculations for all types of dosage forms
Potter PA, Perry AG. *Fundamentals of Nursing*. 11th ed. St. Louis: Elsevier; 2021 ISBN 978-0-323-81035-7	How nurses approach patients In-depth information on disease states
Mosby's Dictionary of Medicine, Nursing and Health Professions. 11th ed. St. Louis: Elsevier; 2022 ISBN 978-0-323-63914-9	Anatomical diagrams along with definitions
Gerdin J. *Health Careers Today*. 7th ed. St. Louis: Elsevier; 2023 ISBN 978-0-323-73355-7	Good description of more than 45 vocations in the medical field Gives technician a better understanding of health fields
Perry AG, Potter PA, Ostendorf W. *Nursing Interventions & Clinical Skills*. 7th ed. St. Louis: Elsevier; 2020 ISBN 978-0-323-54701-7	In-depth information on disease states

[a]Technicians may find these references helpful for understanding various aspects of health care.

BOX 7.3 Pharmacy Associations That Provide Continuing Education and Information

American Association of Pharmacy Technicians (AAPT): *http://www.pharmacytechnician.com*
American Pharmacists Association (APhA): *http://www.pharmacist.com*
American Society of Health-System Pharmacists (ASHP): *http://www.ashp.org*
National Pharmacy Technician Association (NPTA): *http://www.pharmacytechnician.org*
Society for the Education of Pharmacy Technicians (SEPhT): *http://www.thesepht.org*

For additional associations, look in the *Red Book* under Associations or search the Web under Pharmacy Associations.

Seminars and CE dinners, provided by pharmacy associations, are sometimes sponsored by drug companies and are another good source of information on drug topics, new drugs, and fulfilling CE requirements. You do not need to be a member of an association to attend, but the cost usually is lower for members. Although seminars normally are held once or twice yearly, depending on the association that is presenting the seminar, CE dinners may be hosted monthly by the local chapter of an association. At seminars, many of the technician classes include math, aseptic technique, the future of pharmacy technicians, law updates, and more. Monthly CE dinners or events usually have a limited amount of space available; depending on the drug company sponsoring the event, there may be a speaker and a meal for a low cost or (more rarely) no cost. These costs usually are predetermined by the chapter of the association. All of these seminar classes and CE dinners can be applied to CE credit for pharmacy technicians.

■ Tech Note!

Before you join an association, check out its website for information on the level of involvement of the association with its technician members. Many associations do not have a technician division or offer continuing education (CE) classes specifically for technicians. Most, but not all, have yearly seminars and a bimonthly journal containing CE and other useful information pertaining specifically to technicians. Becoming familiar with the various patient conditions and understanding the terminology are essential for becoming a competent pharmacy technician. Table 7.4 lists books that represent various aspects of health care. All health care workers should constantly pursue the acquisition of new information.

○ Technician Profile

Ann is a freelance writer for a national pharmacy technician magazine. She is a career hospital technician and has more than 20 years of pharmacy experience. Ann is able to share her knowledge by writing on various topics near and dear to her heart. Many of the duties Ann performed in the hospital pharmacy align well with her freelance job description. Both require attention to detail, love of the technician field, and a willingness to serve. Ann is expected to maintain a high degree of accuracy and to meet all productivity deadlines efficiently. Ann maintains active memberships in her local, state, and national technician associations. These connections allow her to stay current on the issues affecting her peers. She finds being a freelance writer gives her a sense of purpose and accomplishment, and she enjoys the challenge.

Considerations When Choosing a Reference

At times, technicians may need to use a reference for obtaining information on a drug or for billing purposes. Knowing the proper book to reference is important, not only for finding the correct information but also for saving time and avoiding frustration.

The references listed previously are large reference books that are provided for the staff in the pharmacy. Some online subscription contracts in the pharmacy may have codes that allow you individual access to use the reference at home; check with your employer. If you choose to buy your own reference books or online subscriptions for home use or pocket versions for use at work, you should consider some basics. If your main use of the reference will be to determine generic and trade names, indications, and side effects, a reference such as *Drug Facts and Comparisons* or drugs.com are good choices. As pharmacies update their reference books, you might be able to obtain a free copy of some print references. Some pharmacies that subscribe to electronic resources also receive complimentary access for their employees' use at home; check with your employer. In addition, check bookstores on the Internet for the previous year's edition of a desired resource. Older editions can be sold at a reduced price and may contain most of the information you require. However, you should consider the need to have updated information because drug information changes very quickly. You might check other book companies for similar information. Many reference books contain the same type of information as *Drug Facts and Comparisons*. Another consideration may be the size of the reference book. For instance, although *Drug Facts and Comparisons* is a complete and up-to-date book, it is large and will not fit in your pocket for easy access; however, a pocket version is available. Other publishers also offer pocket versions of their references, including mobile versions for various devices.

Tech Note!

If a technician needs to find a drug price and manufacturer for a drug such as Tenormin and its generic version, a book such as the *PDR* is not helpful because the drugs are listed by manufacturer and the reference does not give prices. *Drug Facts and Comparisons* references drugs by trade or generic name but also does not list prices. *Red Book* is an excellent source to find drug prices using the trade name. It provides prices for the trade name and generic equivalents.

Avoid books that reference drug names in only one way (eg, only by trade or generic names) because their use can become time-consuming. Most drugs have many names, depending on the drug company that manufactures them. If you are going to keep the book at home or in your office, you might be looking for a larger book. If your space is limited, you may be more interested in a handbook. Remember that smaller books contain less information or have print that is more difficult to read. If you are going to purchase a reference book at a bookstore, take a wide variety of drug names with you to reference in the store. If the book has all the drugs you are looking for and is easy to read, you will use the book more often. Table 7.4 presents additional reference books that are informative for the pharmacy technician. These range from information on various topics in the medical field to resources that can help you practice pharmacy calculations.

Do You Remember These Key Points?

- The appropriate way to research drugs
- The appropriate way to reference drugs
- The major sources of information a technician most often uses in pharmacy
- The key attributes of each of the reference books explained in this chapter
- The importance of carrying a pocket-sized reference book
- Types of electronic reference materials
- The importance of journals and news magazines as they pertain to pharmacy and continuing education
- Different considerations when choosing a reference
- The benefits of joining a pharmacy association

Scenario Follow-Up

Robert was thrilled when his company paid for his NPTA membership. He has already learned a great deal from reading the technician journal. He knows that to be the best technician possible, he must have access to the most current and accurate drug information available. He now uses the online PDR, the Clinical Pharmacology *electronic database, and the* Epocrates *website on a regular basis.*

Review Questions

Multiple Choice Questions

1. Which book provides package inserts from manufacturers?
   A. *Drug Facts and Comparisons*
   B. *Goodman & Gilman's The Pharmacological Basis of Therapeutics*
   C. *Red Book*
   D. *Physicians' Desk Reference*

2. Which book or books is/are the best source for locating manufacturers' addresses?
   A. *Red Book*
   B. *Physicians' Desk Reference*
   C. *Goodman & Gilman's The Pharmacological Basis of Therapeutics*
   D. *Drug Facts and Comparisons*
   E. A, B, and D

3. If you need to find the average wholesale price (AWP) of a drug, the best source to look in is:
   A. *American Drug Index*
   B. *Drug Facts and Comparisons*
   C. *Red Book*
   D. A journal

4. The book that is available both hardbound and loose-leaf to allow for monthly updates is:
   A. *Drug Facts and Comparisons*
   B. *Red Book*
   C. *Goodman & Gilman's The Pharmacological Basis of Therapeutics*
   D. None of the above

5. The most widely used reference book in pharmacy is:
   A. *Goodman & Gilman's The Pharmacological Basis of Therapeutics*
   B. The dictionary
   C. *Remington's Pharmaceutical Sciences: The Science and Practice of Pharmacy*
   D. *Drug Facts and Comparisons*

6. If you need to identify a specific tablet or capsule only by the markings, color, and shape, you would look in:
   A. *Drug Facts and Comparisons* loose-leaf version
   B. *Ident-A-Drug*
   C. *American Drug Index*
   D. *Red Book*

7. All of the following are updated at least yearly *except*:
   A. *Drug Facts and Comparisons*
   B. *Red Book*
   C. *Goodman & Gilman's The Pharmacological Basis of Therapeutics*
   D. *Physicians' Desk Reference*
   E. All of the above books are updated yearly.

8. All of the following information can be found in *Drug Facts and Comparisons* (F&C) *except*:
   A. Schedule of a narcotic
   B. Storage and stability
   C. Patient information
   D. All of the above information can be found in F&C.

9. Information about pharmacy technician associations can be found:
   A. Online
   B. In journals
   C. In the *Red Book*
   D. A and C

10. All of the following can be found in free downloaded materials from Epocrates *except*:
    A. Contraindications
    B. Herbals
    C. Pill identification
    D. B and C

■ Technician's Corner

A patient arrives at the pharmacy holding a single capsule in her hand and explains that she has lost her Rx bottle. She needs to have the medication refilled. The capsule is white and has the markings "Watson 369" on one side and "5 mg" on the opposite side. What is this drug, and what is its intended use?

Bibliography

Adult Drug Information Handbook. 31st ed. St. Louis: Wolters Kluwer Health; 2023.

Billups NS. *American Drug Index*. Philadelphia: Lippincott Williams & Wilkins; 2016.

Brunton L, Dandan H, Knollman B. *Goodman & Gilman's the Pharmaceutical Basis of Therapeutics*. 13th ed. New York: McGraw-Hill Professional; 2018.

Drug Topics Red Book. 32nd ed. Montvale, NJ: Thomson; 2021.

Gennaro A. *Remington's Pharmaceutical Sciences: The Science and Practice of Pharmacy*. 22nd ed. Philadelphia: Lippincott Williams & Wilkins; 2022.

Jellin J, ed. *Ident-A-Drug Reference: For Tablet and Capsule Identification*. Stockton, CA: Therapeutic Research Faculty; 2023.

Krinsky D. *Handbook of Nonprescription Drugs: An Interactive Approach to Self-Care*. 20th ed. Washington, DC: American Pharmacists Association; 2020.

Physicians' Desk Reference Inc. *Red Book: Pharmacy's Fundamental Reference*. Montvale, NJ: Thomson Reuters; 2023.

Trissel L. *Handbook on Injectable Drugs*. 2023 ed. Elk Grove Village, IL: American Society of Health-System Pharmacists; 2023.

United States Pharmacopeia: USP 43: *the National Formulary: NF 43*. Rockville, MD: US Pharmacopeial Convention; 2022.

Websites Referenced

Drug names. Available at: http://www.webmd.com/drugs/.

Drugs@FDA database. Available at: http://www.fda.gov/Drugs/InformationOnDrugs/ucm135821.htm.

Gold standard clinical pharmacology. Available at: http://www.clinicalpharmacology.com/.

Micromedex information. Available at: http://www.micromedex.com/products/hcs/.

Orange Book: Approved Drug Products With Therapeutic Equivalence Evaluations. 33rd ed. Available at: http://www.fda.gov/cder/ob.

United States Pharmacopeia, usp.org. Official standards for compounding.

CHAPTER 8

Community Pharmacy Practice

Karen Davis

1. List and describe the different types of community pharmacies.
2. Explain the pharmacy technician's role in the medication use process.
3. Define *prescription* and list the advantages of e-prescribing.
4. List the information needed to have a prescription filled at a pharmacy, and define various pharmacy abbreviations.
5. Explain the pharmacy technician's role in prescription processing.
6. Describe the pharmacy technician's role in prescription preparation, including (a) accurately count or measure finished dosage forms as specified by the prescription/medication order, (b) identify all situations in which the patient requires the attention of a pharmacist, (c) identify situations in the screening of refills and renewals in which the technician should notify the pharmacist of potential inappropriateness.
7. Describe other pharmacy technician duties, such as refilling prescriptions and transferring a prescription.
8. Describe the layout of the pharmacy and list the important areas.
9. Discuss effective verbal and written communication skills, including listening skills.
10. Examine strategies for communicating with patients who are non-English speakers or who have other special needs, such as vision or hearing problems, a low reading level, or difficulty understanding instructions. Demonstrate a respectful attitude with diverse groups of people.
11. Identify state laws and regulations regarding the technician's role in immunizations. Explain the purpose of monitoring a patient's medication therapy and discuss home health care and long-term care services.

Adjudication The process by which a prescription is submitted electronically to a third-party payer for the pharmacy to be reimbursed for the medication dispensed

Aphasia A communication disorder that results from damage or injury to the language parts of the brain; it is more common in older adults, particularly those who have had a stroke

Auxiliary label A label that provides supplementary information about proper and safe administration, use, or storage of a medication

Bank identification number (BIN) A six-digit number on a prescription drug card that is used for routing and identification to process a prescription claim

Behind-the-counter (BTC) medications Medications kept behind the pharmacy counter that require a pharmacist's intervention before dispensing to a patient; BTC medications are not considered prescription medications

Chain pharmacy A corporate-owned group of pharmacies that share a brand name and central management and usually have standardized business methods and practices

Dispense as Written (DAW) codes A numerical set of codes, created by the National Council for Prescription Drug Programs (NCPDP), that is used when filling prescriptions; they can affect reimbursement amounts from insurance companies

Drug Enforcement Administration (DEA) number An alphanumeric number consisting of two letters and seven numbers that is assigned to prescribers authorized by the US Drug Enforcement Administration to prescribe controlled substances

Drug utilization evaluation (DUE) (Formerly known as drug utilization review) An authorized, structured, ongoing review of health care provider prescribing, pharmacist dispensing, and patient use of medication

Dysarthria A speech deficiency that interferes with the normal control of the speech mechanism

e-Prescribing The computer-to-computer transfer of prescription data among pharmacies, prescribers, and payers

Federal Legend A statement required on the labeling of all prescription medications: "Federal law prohibits dispensing without a prescription"

Franchise A form of business organization in which a firm that already has a successful product or service (the franchisor) enters into a continuing contractual relationship with other businesses (franchisees) operating under the franchisor's trade name and usually with the franchisor's guidance, in exchange for a fee

Help Desk A toll-free hotline to an insurance company, available 24 hours a day, 7 days a week, so that pharmacists can call in specific questions about insurance claims and coverage and pharmacy-specific inquiries

Inscription The name, dosage form, strength, and quantity of the medication prescribed

National Drug Code (NDC) number A unique 10- or 11-digit number, composed of three segments, that is assigned to a medication. The first four/five digits identify the drug manufacturer, the next four identify specifics about the product, and the last two identify the drug packaging

National Provider Identifier (NPI) A unique 10-digit identification number for covered health care providers that is issued by the Centers for Medicare & Medicaid Services

Nonproprietary (generic) name A short name coined for a drug or chemical that is not subject to proprietary (trademark) rights and is recommended or recognized by an official body

Over-the-counter (OTC) medication A medication that does not require a physician's order or prescription for the patient to purchase

Prescription An order for medication issued by a physician, dentist, or other properly licensed practitioner, such as a physician assistant or nurse practitioner

Proprietary (brand or trade) name A brand name or trademark under which a drug product is marketed

Refills Permission by a prescriber to replenish a prescription

Repackage To reduce the amount of medication taken from a bulk bottle

Signatura (*signa* or *sig*) The directions on a prescription that explain how the patient is to take the prescribed medication; a Latin expression meaning to "write on label"

Sole proprietorship An unincorporated business owned by one person

Subscription The part of the prescription that provides specific instructions to the pharmacist on how to compound the prescription

Superscription The heading of a prescription, represented by the Latin symbol Rx, meaning "take thou" or "you take"; the symbol has come to represent prescription or pharmacy

Therapeutic alliance A trust relationship between a health care professional and a patient, incorporating patient perceptions of the acceptability of interventions and mutually agreed upon goals for treatment

⊙ Scenario

Andrew is a new pharmacy technician working at a local community pharmacy. During his orientation, he is introduced to the several other pharmacy technicians who are performing various pharmacy activities. He observes one technician accepting new prescriptions from a patient, another pharmacy technician entering information into the pharmacy's computer information system, and one technician checking in a pharmacy order from a drug wholesaler. Andrew is completely overwhelmed by the operations. He asks the pharmacist, "Where do I begin?"

A community pharmacy, also known as a *retail or ambulatory care pharmacy*, is a vital component of our health care delivery system. There are many types of community pharmacies, including independent, franchise, and chain pharmacies (eg, CVS and Walgreens).

The independent pharmacy originally was known as the "corner drugstore" in a community. Often these pharmacies were classified as a **sole proprietorship.** A sole proprietor is someone who owns an unincorporated business by himself or herself, according to the Internal Revenue Service. The owner of an independent pharmacy was normally the pharmacist in charge of the pharmacy. The services provided in an independent pharmacy varied based on the pharmacist, the location of the pharmacy, and the patient population. Many independent pharmacies are compounding pharmacies. Independent pharmacies may also sell or rent durable medical equipment. In addition, they now may provide immunizations to the public.

A **franchise** is an authorization, granted to a person or group of people, that allows them to operate under a franchisor's well-established trade name and usually under the franchisor's guidance. A franchise pharmacy is a business organization in which a pharmacy with a successful product or service (the franchisor) enters into a continuing contractual relationship with other pharmacies (franchisees) in exchange for a fee. Examples of franchise pharmacies include Medicine Shoppe, Good Neighbor Pharmacy, and Care Pharmacy.

A **chain pharmacy** is a corporate-owned group of pharmacies that share a brand and central management and usually have standardized business methods and practices. A chain must have at least two locations and have a central headquarters that is overseen by a board of directors. CVS and Walgreens are the two largest pharmacy chains in the United States. According to the National Association of Chain Drugstores (NACDS), in 2019, chain pharmacies filled over 3 billion prescriptions, which is more than 73% of the total number of prescriptions filled. Chain pharmacies may be classified as mass merchandisers (eg, Target), discounters (eg, Walmart), and membership stores (eg, Costco and BJ's Wholesale Club). Many grocery stores have a pharmacy department (eg, Safeway).

The pharmacy technician plays an instrumental role in our prescription processing system. Pharmacy technicians assist licensed pharmacists, prepare prescription medications, provide customer service, and perform administrative duties in a community pharmacy. They are generally responsible for receiving prescription requests, inputting prescriptions into the pharmacy information system, counting tablets, labeling bottles, maintaining patient profiles, preparing insurance claim forms, and performing administrative functions, such as answering phones, stocking shelves, and operating cash registers. The success of a community pharmacy depends heavily on the knowledge and training of its pharmacy technicians. This chapter focuses on the role of and responsibilities delegated to a pharmacy technician in a community pharmacy.

◎ Scenario Checkup 8.1

Andrew is manning the prescription drop-off counter at the pharmacy. A patient presents his prescription to Andrew. Andrew collects information from the patient, including the patient's address, contact telephone number, birth date, and prescription drug card coverage. He reads the name of the medication on the prescription, which states that the prescriber wrote for Bayer Aspirin 81 mg. Andrew is bewildered because he has purchased Bayer Aspirin 81 mg in the past for his mother, and he wonders if Bayer Aspirin 81 mg is now a prescription medication. What would you tell him?

Role of the Pharmacy Technician

The primary role of the pharmacy technician in a community pharmacy is the same as that in an institutional pharmacy or any other pharmacy setting: *to assist the pharmacist*. A community pharmacy technician may be assigned a specific duty or many different responsibilities in the pharmacy (Fig. 8.1). The following are some of the more common duties:
- Provide customer service
- Take the information needed to fill a prescription from customers or health professionals
  - Visually scan new prescriptions to ensure they contain all of the required information

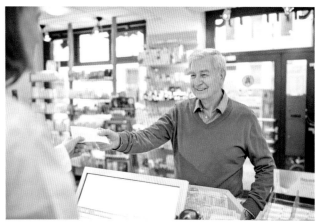

FIG. 8.1 Pharmacy technicians have a variety of roles in the community pharmacy, including talking with customers, processing and reviewing prescriptions, counting medications, labeling containers, restocking supplies, and other administrative duties. (Copyright © Alverez/Getty Images.)

- Answer the telephone
- Obtain refill information from the patient
- Input various types of data into a pharmacy information system
  - Add a prescriber to a database
  - Add a new patient to a database
  - Update a patient's profile or prescriber's information
  - Add insurance plans to a database
  - Add a drug to the database
  - Enter a new prescription
  - Obtain a refill authorization
  - Process a new prescription for prior drug approval
  - Refill, transfer (with a pharmacist's assistance), file, or reverse a prescription
  - Run various productivity reports
- Compound prescriptions
  - Perform necessary calculations before compounding a prescription
  - Weigh or measure amounts of medication for prescriptions
  - Clean equipment after compounding
- Package and label prescriptions
  - Count the prescribed quantity of medication
  - Select the appropriate container
  - Apply both the prescription and the auxiliary label to the container in a professional manner
  - Print the appropriate literature for each prescription to give to the patient
  - Return the medication to the shelf
- Price medications
- Organize inventory and alert pharmacists to any shortages of medications or supplies
  - Reorder medications and pharmacy supplies
  - Check the ordered medication against the packing slip
  - Place ordered medication in its appropriate place on the shelf
  - Check pharmacy stock for medication that may have short dating

- Accept payment for prescriptions and process insurance claims
- Arrange for customers to speak with the pharmacist if customers have questions about medications or health matters
- Perform pharmacy housekeeping tasks

These duties vary, depending on the size of the community pharmacy and the experience of the pharmacy technician.

Prescription

A **prescription** is an order for medication issued by a physician, dentist, or other properly licensed practitioner, such as a physician assistant or nurse practitioner. In some states, other practitioners have been licensed with a limited scope of practice. A prescription designates a specific medication and dosage to be administered to a particular patient at a specific time. Often the prescribed medication is referred to as a prescription.

There are two broad legal classifications of medications: those that can be obtained only by a prescription, or legend medications, and those that can be obtained without a prescription, or an **over-the-counter** (OTC) **medication.** A prescription medication is also known as a legend medication because it bears the **Federal Legend,** which states: "Federal law prohibits dispensing without a prescription." OTC medications are deemed safe for an individual to take without being under a physician's supervision. As a result of the Combat Methamphetamine Epidemic Act of 2005, a subclassification of OTC medications has been established; these drugs are known as **behind-the-counter** (BTC) **medications.** BTC medications are OTC medications that contain ephedrine, an ingredient used to make methamphetamine, which is a schedule I controlled substance. Individuals who want to purchase products containing ephedrine must buy them at the pharmacy counter under the supervision of a pharmacist and provide proper identification. The purchaser must be at least 16 years of age. An individual may purchase up to 3.6 g of products containing ephedrine (eg, pseudoephedrine) in 1 day or no more than 9 g within a 30-day period.

A prescription written by a physician may be given to the patient to take to the patient's pharmacy or mailed to a mail-order pharmacy. A physician may designate an employee of the practice to telephone a prescription into the pharmacy; in this case, the pharmacist must create a written form of the telephoned order. A physician's office may fax a patient's prescription to the pharmacy. In some states it is legal for a patient to fax his or her prescription to the pharmacy; however, the patient must provide the pharmacy with the original prescription before receiving the medication.

A prescription also may be sent to the pharmacy electronically; this is known as e-prescribing. **e-Prescribing** is the computer-to-computer transfer of prescription data between pharmacies, prescribers, and payers. It is not the use of an email message or a facsimile transaction. e-Prescribing functions include messages about new prescriptions, prescription changes, refill requests, prescription fill status notification, prescription cancellation, and medication history. e-Prescribing involves a wide range of participants in the health care system: individual practitioners, clinics, hospitals, provider associations, pharmacies, software vendors, trade and professional associations, laboratories and ancillary services, state and federal governments, standards development organizations, terminology and code set organizations, health plans, payers, and processors.

e-Prescribing has many advantages, such as the following:
- Enabling prescribers to receive on-screen prompts for drug-specific dosing information
- Expediting refills
- Facilitating data exchange between the physician and the pharmacist and ultimately their patients
- Linking information from a patient's medical file to a patient's prescription file
- Notifying the prescriber if a drug product is covered by the patient's insurance plan when the order is generated rather than when it is presented at the pharmacy
- Reducing or eliminating errors associated with illegible handwriting

Prescription Information

In most situations it is the pharmacy technician who has the initial contact with the patient when the person drops off a new prescription or requests a refill of a prescription. The first thing a pharmacy technician does when receiving a new prescription is determine whether the patient has had prescriptions filled at that pharmacy previously. If the patient has filled prescriptions previously at that pharmacy, the pharmacy technician verifies the accuracy of the information in the patient's profile. If the patient has never had a prescription filled at that pharmacy, the pharmacy technician collects the necessary information, which includes the following:
- Patient's full name
- Patient's home address (street, city, state, and ZIP code)
- Patient's telephone numbers (home, work, and mobile)
- Patient's birth date
- All allergies (drug and food)
- Patient's current physical condition
- Prescription drug card information (group number, member number, and relationship to the cardholder)
- Whether the patient wants to receive generic medications
- A list of any OTC and BTC medications the patient takes
- A list of any herbal supplements the patient takes

This information is used to develop a patient profile for the individual.

A patient profile is a list of the patient's prescriptions and all related information, including the original date of fill, refill dates, and the prescribing practitioner. The Omnibus Budget Reconciliation Act of 1990 (OBRA '90) requires that every ambulatory pharmacy maintain patient profiles. A patient profile is a tool that can help eliminate medication errors. The patient profile is extremely valuable when drug utilization evaluation (DUE) is performed. During this evaluation, an accurate patient profile can reduce potential drug-food interactions, drug-disease interactions, drug–environmental chemical interactions, and drug-laboratory interactions. In addition, the patient profile can identify multiple pharmacological effects caused by medications being prescribed, distinguish multiple physicians that a patient may be using, detect patient nonadherence to the drug regimen, and disclose possible drug abuse by the patient.

Originally prescriptions were written using Latin abbreviations, and measurements were expressed using the apothecary and avoirdupois systems. Some Latin abbreviations are still used in the practice of pharmacy today (Table 8.1). The metric system (Table 8.2) is the official system of measurement for weights and volumes in the United States; however, some older physicians continue to use the apothecary and avoirdupois systems in writing prescriptions (see Chapter 6).

TABLE 8.1
Pharmacy Abbreviations

Abbreviation	Meaning	Abbreviation	Meaning
aa	of each	gt(t)	drop (drops)
ac	before meals	HA	headache
AD	to, up to	HBP	high blood pressure
ad^a	right ear	HR	heart rate
ad lib	at pleasure, freely	hs	at bedtime
AM	morning	HTN	hypertension
Amp	ampule	ID	intradermal
Aq	water	Inj	injection
as^a	left ear	IV	intravenous
au^a	each ear	IM	intramuscular
bid	twice a day	IU^a	international units
BM	bowel movement	JRA	juvenile rheumatoid arthritis
BP	blood pressure	KCl	potassium chloride
BPH	benign prostatic hypertrophy	Kg	kilogram
BS	blood sugar	L	liter
BSA	body surface area	mcg	microgram
c̄	with	mEq	milliequivalent
Ca	calcium	mg	milligram
CAD	coronary artery disease	mg/kg	milligram per kilogram
Cap	capsule	mg/m^2	milligram per square meter
CHF	congestive heart failure	mL	milliliter
COPD	chronic obstructive pulmonary disease	mOsm	milliosmole
Dil	dilute	N&V	nausea and vomiting
Disp	dispense	noct	at night
Div	divide	non rep	do not repeat
DJD	degenerative joint disease	NS	normal saline
DM	diabetes mellitus	OA	osteoarthritis
Dtd	give of such doses	OCD	obsessive compulsive disorder
DW	distilled water	od^a	right eye
Dx	diagnosis	os^a	left eye
Elix	elixir	ou^a	each eye
Ft	make	pc	after meals
g (gm)	gram	PM	afternoon
GERD	gastroesophageal reflux disease	PO	by mouth
GI	gastrointestinal	Pr	by rectum
GU	genitourinary	PRN	as needed
gr	grain	pulv	powder

Continued

TABLE 8.1
Pharmacy Abbreviations—cont'd

Abbreviation	Meaning	Abbreviation	Meaning
PVCs	premature ventricular contractions	Sx	symptom
PVD	peripheral vascular disease	Syr	syrup
q[a]	every	Tab	tablet
qd[a]	every day	TB	tuberculosis
Qh	each hour	Tbsp	tablespoon
qid	4 times a day	TED	thromboembolic disease
qod[a]	every other day	TIA	transient ischemic attack
Qs	a sufficient quantity	tid	3 times a day
qs ad	a sufficient quantity to prepare	Tiw	3 times a week
RA	rheumatoid arthritis	Top	topical
$\bar{s}$	without	tsp	teaspoon
subcut, SC,[a] SQ,[a] SubQ[a]	subcutaneous	U[a]	unit
		UA	uric acid; urinalysis
Sig	write on label	UC	ulcerative colitis
SL	sublingual	Ud	as directed
SLE	systemic lupus erythematosus	ung	ointment
SOB	short of breath	URI	upper respiratory infection
Sol	solution	ut dict	as directed
$\bar{ss}$	one-half	UTI	urinary tract infection
stat	immediately	WA	while awake
supp	suppository	Wk	week
susp	suspension		

[a]Included in The Joint Commission (TJC) "do not use" list of abbreviations; however, physicians still use them in writing prescriptions.

TABLE 8.2
Metric-Household Conversions

Metric (volume)	Household Equivalent
5 mL	1 teaspoon (tsp)
15 mL	1 tablespoon (Tbsp)
30 mL	1 fluid ounce (fl oz)
240 mL	1 cup
480 mL	1 pint (pt)
960 mL	1 quart (qt)
3840 mL	1 gallon (gal)

Prescriber Information

A valid prescription must contain specific information (Figs. 8.2 and 8.3). Every prescription is required to have prescriber information, patient information, a superscription, an inscription, a subscription, and a signa. A prescriber's information includes the prescriber's name, office address, and telephone number. If the prescribed medication is a controlled substance, the physician's **Drug Enforcement Administration (DEA) number** must be included. Some states may require the physician's **National Provider Identifier (NPI) number** and/or medical license to be included on the prescription.

Patient Information

The patient's information includes his or her full name, home address, and birth date. The patient's birth date is used as an identifier to ensure that the correct patient is receiving the correct medication. At times an illegible prescription will be presented to the pharmacy. The individual who accepts the prescription is responsible for verifying that the information is correct. If the patient's name is not spelled correctly, the patient may question whether he or she is receiving the correct prescription.

Date

The date the prescription was written by the prescriber must appear on the prescription. If there has been a time lapse between the date the prescription was written and when it was received by the pharmacy, the pharmacist may question the intent of the physician and whether the patient's needs are being met. Some medications, such as controlled substances, must be filled or refilled within 6 months of the date the prescription was written. It is the responsibility of the pharmacy

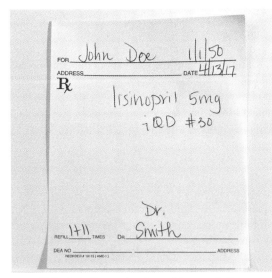

FIG. 8.2 Example of a valid prescription.

technician to be aware of any state regulations regarding the amount of time that may lapse from the date the prescription was written to the date it is presented for filling.

For noncontrolled prescriptions, there are no federal guidelines so the life of the prescription can vary from state to state. Thirty-six states give it a year from the date written, NOT the date filled. There are eight states that do not have a defined expiration date.

Tech Note!

If a person waits a month before filling a new prescription, the life of the prescription still begins from the original date written.

Superscription

The **superscription** (Rx symbol) is a contraction of the Latin verb *recipe*, meaning "take this drug." It is used as the heading on a prescription and usually precedes the inscription. Presently, the Rx symbol represents prescription and the pharmacy.

Inscription

The **inscription** contains the medication name, dosage form, strength, and quantity. Today most medications are already prepared by the pharmaceutical manufacturers. However, the pharmacy may receive a prescription for a nonsterile or sterile compound for which the names and quantities of each ingredient are listed. In this situation the medication or ingredient is listed by its nonproprietary, or generic, name. The quantities should be listed using the metric system; however, some older prescribers may use the apothecary system.

Subscription

The prescription's **subscription** consists of directions to the pharmacist or pharmacy technician on how to compound a

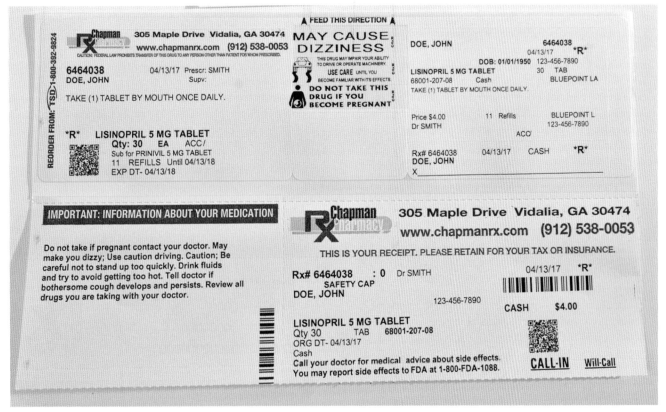

FIG. 8.3 Example of valid prescription label.

prescription. Many of the medications dispensed today do not require compounding and therefore do not contain a subscription.

◉ Scenario Checkup 8.2

A new patient arrives at the pharmacy with a prescription from a local health care provider. The pharmacist asks Andrew to set up a new patient profile in the pharmacy's computer system. What information does Andrew need from the patient to set up a new profile?

Signatura (Signa or Sig)

Signatura (**signa or sig**) is a Latin expression meaning to "write on label." The *signa* is the instruction to the patient on how to take the prescribed medication. These directions are written using English or Latin abbreviations or a combination of the two. They are transcribed by either the pharmacist or the pharmacy technician when this information is entered into the pharmacy's computer system. The *signa* tells the patient how much, when, and how long to take the medication.

Prescription Processing

Intake

A pharmacy may receive a new prescription by a variety of methods. The patient may bring the prescription to the pharmacy, a designated employee from a physician's office may telephone a new prescription into the pharmacy, the physician's office or patient may fax the prescription, or the prescription may be submitted electronically (e-prescribing) from the physician's office. e-Prescribing is not the same as a faxed prescription. Pharmacy technicians must be familiar with their state's pharmacy regulations for receiving new prescriptions.

Often the pharmacy technician is the first individual to come in contact with a new prescription brought in by the patient. The pharmacy technician should accept the prescription in a professional manner and review it to ensure that the patient's name, address, and any other required information are on the prescription. If the patient has never had a prescription filled at that pharmacy, the pharmacy technician must collect detailed information from the patient, including medications the patient is currently taking (prescription, nonprescription, vitamins, and herbal supplements), medical conditions, and allergies. Many pharmacies have a form for the patient to complete that requests this information so that a patient profile can be created.

Data Input

Computer systems are standard in pharmacies today because they can provide the following:
- Improved efficiency
- Information to the pharmacist at a moment's notice
- Online prescription claim approval
- Reduction in prescription errors
- Speed in processing prescriptions

Patient Information

The pharmacy technician is responsible for inputting the patient's information into the pharmacy's computer information system. Although pharmacy information systems may vary, the system prompts the user for the necessary information. If the information is not entered, the system will not permit the user to continue with the process. Patient information includes the following:
- Full name
- Home address (number, street, city, state, and ZIP code)
- Telephone numbers (home, mobile, and work)
- Birth date
- Sex
- Allergies
- Generic preference
- Request for non–child-resistant container

A thorough and accurate patient profile can help eliminate possible adverse drug events.

Prescription Drug Benefits

Today many individuals receive prescription drug coverage through medical insurance. Many companies offer prescription drug coverage as an employee benefit. The prescription drug benefit defines the drug coverage that is provided to the member. An individual who is covered under a prescription drug benefit receives a prescription drug card (Fig. 8.4).

The National Council for Prescription Drug Programs (NCPDP) provides a guide for the information found on a card. This card contains the necessary information for the pharmacist or pharmacy technician to process the prescription. Information contained on a prescription drug card includes the following:
- Complete electronic transaction routing information (RxPCN). This is a specific identifier used to transmit the claim to third parties.
- A group number, which identifies the coverage for a group of individuals under one contract; normally the group consists of a company's employees.
- A subscriber number, which identifies the individual who pays the premiums.
- A person code, which identifies the specific individual covered. Some plans use "01" to identify the card holder, "02" for the card holder's spouse, and "03" for the first child dependent. Person codes may vary according to the plan.

Prescription Savings Card

RxBIN: 000000

RxPCN: 0000

Group #:   00000000

ID #:   00000000000

This is NOT insurance - Discount only

FIG. 8.4 Prescription drug card.

- A **bank identification number (BIN),** which is a field in the telecommunication standard that is used for the routing and identification of pharmacy claims. The NCPDP assigns a six-digit BIN to process a prescription claim.
- A Help Desk telephone number, which is a 24-hour service that enables a pharmacy to obtain assistance in processing a prescription claim.

Unfortunately, there is no uniform standard for the information or its format on a prescription drug card.

Prescriber Information

The pharmacy technician must verify that the prescriber's information is accurate in the computer system. The prescriber's information includes his or her name, office address (street number, street, city, state, and ZIP code), office telephone number (including area code), and DEA number for controlled substances only. Depending on state regulations, the NPI number and state medical license number also may be required.

Medication

The pharmacy technician must enter the name of the medication, its strength and quantity, and the number of refills indicated on the prescription. All quantities ordered are to be expressed in metric quantities. For example, 4 fluid ounces would be entered as 120 mL, and 1 pound would be 454 g.

Calculating the Day's Supply

After the quantity has been entered, the pharmacy technician must calculate the day's supply of medication being dispensed to the patient. The day's supply can be calculated using the following formula:

Day's supply = Total quantity dispensed ÷

Total quantity taken per day

When calculating the day's supply for either ophthalmic or otic drops, the technician should use the conversion of 20 drops per milliliter and calculate according to the following formula:

Day's supply = (20 gtts/mL × Number of mL) ÷

Number of drops instilled per day

For inhalation products, use the following formula:

Day's supply = Number of inhalations per container ÷

Number of inhalations breathed

each day

In all situations, the day's supply is always rounded to the nearest whole number.

Directions for Use

The directions for use by the patient must be entered into the pharmacy's computer system. Often the prescriber writes the directions using pharmacy abbreviations, and the pharmacy technician must transcribe the directions. Each computer system has developed specific shortcuts that allow the user to use abbreviations that are translated into English when entering the prescription's signa. By becoming familiar with these shortcuts, the user can save time by not having to enter each word. Several hints for inputting the directions for use include the following:
- Begin with a verb
- Do not use abbreviations
- Identify the dosage form
- Indicate the route of administration
- Use terminology in everyday language so that the patient understands it

If a prescriber writes "as directed" for the directions, the technician should promptly inform the pharmacist of this, and the pharmacist will call the prescriber for explicit directions.

Prescription Refills

The pharmacy technician must enter the approved number of **refills** from the prescriber into the computer system. The prescriber must provide a specific number of refills for the prescription. Some prescribers may indicate "prn" refills on a prescription. In this situation, the technician must be aware of the state's regulations regarding "prn" refills. The pharmacy technician enters zero refills if a prescriber does not enter any refills on the prescription.

Generic Substitution

If the prescriber authorized a generic drug to be dispensed, the technician will dispense the generic version of the medication. Some states require the prescriber to write "Dispense as Written" or "Brand Name Medically Necessary" in their own handwriting on the prescription; other states may allow the prescriber to check a box on the prescription. The pharmacy technician must be familiar with the state's pharmacy regulations regarding generic substitution.

Dispense as Written Codes

Dispense as Written (DAW) codes are a numeric set of codes, created by the NCPDP, that are used when entering prescriptions into the computer (Box 8.1). If a pharmacist or pharmacy technician fails to submit a prescription claim using the correct DAW code, the pharmacy may not be reimbursed properly for the medication that was dispensed. In addition, a pharmacy may be audited by a third-party provider to verify that the DAW code used was correct. If a third-party audit reveals that a pharmacy is improperly using DAW codes, the pharmacy may be held responsible for refunding claims that were submitted incorrectly.

Prescription Adjudication

Prescription **adjudication** is the process by which a prescription is submitted electronically to a third-party payer so that the pharmacy can find out whether it will receive reimbursement for the medication. The pharmacy is notified of the status of the claim within a few seconds of submission. Most of the time, the pharmacy will be reimbursed for the medication; however, in some situations the prescription claim is rejected. This can occur for a variety of reasons, such as the medication is not covered, the refill was requested too

BOX 8.1 Dispense as Written Codes

0	No product selection indicated
1	Substitution not allowed by provider
2	Substitution allowed—patient requested product dispensed
3	Substitution allowed—pharmacist selected product dispensed
4	Substitution allowed—generic drug not in stock
5	Substitution allowed—brand drug dispensed as generic
6	Override
7	Substitution not allowed—brand drug mandated by law
8	Substitution allowed—generic drug not available in marketplace
9	Other

TABLE 8.3
Prescription Claim Rejection Codes

Rejection Code	Meaning
5	Missing or invalid pharmacy number
6	Missing or invalid group number
7	Missing or invalid cardholder ID number
8	Missing or invalid person code
9	Missing or invalid birth date
11	Missing relationship code
19	Missing days' supply
22	Missing or invalid Dispense as Written (DAW)/product selection code
25	Missing or invalid prescriber ID
26	Missing or invalid unit of measure
54	Nonmatched National Drug Code (NDC) number
60	Drug not covered for patient
75	Prior authorization required
79	Refill too soon

soon, or the patient is an invalid card holder. If the prescription claim is rejected, the pharmacy is notified of the reason with a one- or two-digit rejection code (Table 8.3).

The prescription claim must be corrected before it is resubmitted. The correct information can be obtained from the patient or the patient's representative or by contacting the Help Desk associated with the third-party provider. A **Help Desk** has a 24/7 toll-free hotline for pharmacists to address specific questions relating to claim rejections, payment status, prior authorization procedures, explanation of DUE messages, and pharmacy-specific inquiries.

Drug Utilization Evaluation

The pharmacist is responsible for reducing medication errors and drug-related illnesses. As a result of OBRA '90, the pharmacist is responsible for obtaining information from Medicaid patients or their caregivers, with the goal of identifying and resolving potential medication-related issues. Patient profiles are created and contain the following information, which the pharmacist uses in reviewing a patient's medication therapy:

- Adverse drug reactions
- Allergies
- Comprehensive list of medications being taken
- Disease states
- Patient demographic information
- Pharmacist's comments regarding a patient's drug therapy

A prospective drug use review is conducted during a **drug utilization evaluation** (**DUE**) (formerly known as drug utilization review [DUR]). This review examines all the patient's medication records before dispensing is conducted. During this review, the following factors are evaluated:

- Clinical abuse or misuse
- Drug allergy problems
- Drug overutilization
- Drug underutilization
- Drug-disease contraindications
- Drug-drug interactions
- Incorrect dosages
- Incorrect duration of drug treatment
- Therapeutic duplication

Pharmacy technicians may be involved with prescription data entry and adjudication, and they should notify the pharmacist immediately of any issues regarding medication. The pharmacist will make a clinical decision based on the information available as to whether the prescription should be processed. It is not within the scope of the pharmacy technician's responsibilities to make judgment decisions regarding medication use.

Scanning the Prescription

Many pharmacies scan the original prescription; therefore a digital copy of the prescription is available when a prescription is refilled. Also, if the original prescription is misfiled, a digital copy is available for the pharmacist to review. Scanning of prescriptions is a quality assurance tool that can help reduce medication errors.

Prescription Labeling

Every prescription filled should have a visually appealing and professional label (see Figs. 8.2 and 8.3). It is extremely important that the pharmacist or pharmacy technician affix the label neatly to the prescription container. This professional appearance conveys to the patient that care was taken in filling the prescription.

A legal prescription label is required to have several pieces of information:
- Name, address, and telephone number of the dispensing pharmacy
- A prescription number (which is used to identify a particular prescription order and to refill the prescription)
- Prescriber's name
- Patient's name

- Date the prescription was dispensed
- Name, strength, and quantity of the medication dispensed
- Directions for use (should be in a format that the patient can easily understand)
- "Federal Legend" usually preprinted on purchased labels

Some states may require the name or initials of the individual who dispensed the medication. Often the number of refills may appear on the prescription label. Some pharmacies may list the drug manufacturer's lot number on the label; this makes it easier to identify a medication that has been recalled from the drug manufacturer. In some communities with a large Hispanic population, the prescription label may appear in Spanish.

Auxiliary Labels

Auxiliary labels are normally printed with the pharmacy label (Table 8.4). An **auxiliary label** provides the patient with additional information about taking the medication. Auxiliary labels may indicate when it is best to take a medication (eg, before a meal) or a potential side effect ("may cause drowsiness" or "avoid sunlight"), or they may remind the patient to discard the medication after a given time (as with a reconstitutable antibiotic). Auxiliary labels should be affixed to the prescription container so that no important information, such as the **National Drug Code (NDC) number**, lot number, or expiration date, is covered (Fig. 8.5).

Patient Product Information

The federal government has required that patient product information (PPI) be provided to the patient when specific medications are dispensed. The purpose of the PPI sheet is to ensure that the patient is provided with information on the proper use of the medication. Examples of medications requiring an accompanying PPI include oral contraceptives,

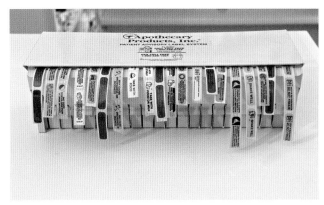

FIG. 8.5 Auxiliary labels include additional information on how and when to take medications.

estrogens, and nonsteroidal antiinflammatory drugs (NSAIDs). Information contained on a PPI includes the following:

- **Proprietary (brand or trade) name** and **nonproprietary (generic) name** of the product
- Clinical pharmacology
- Indications and use
- Contraindications
- Warnings
- Precautions
- Adverse reactions
- Drug abuse
- Overdosage
- Dosage and administration
- How supplied

Almost all pharmacies provide supplemental printed instructions to the patient.

⊙ Scenario Checkup 8.3

Andrew is responsible for inputting the prescription into the pharmacy's computer system and billing the patient's pharmacy benefits manager. During the adjudication process, he receives the following message: #60—Drug Not Covered for Patient. Andrew knows the medication is a prescription drug. What should he do?

Prescription Preparation

After reading and checking the prescription order, the pharmacy technician should decide on the exact procedure to be followed in dispensing or compounding the product. Many of the medications are already prepared for the pharmacy by the drug manufacturers. Pharmacy technicians should take the prescription label with them when they go to the shelf to gather the medication. They should compare the NDC number on the prescription label with the NDC number on the manufacturer's drug label (Fig. 8.6). The technician should pull the medication from the shelf and return it to the dispensing area of the pharmacy. The pharmacy technician must take great care in selecting the prescribed dosage form and strength and the number of dosage units dispensed.

The prescription label should be checked with the original prescription and the manufacturer's label. The prescription

TABLE 8.4
Commonly Used Auxiliary Labels for Side Effects

Classification	Commonly Used Auxiliary Label
Contraceptives	Take as directed
Nonsteroidal antiinflammatory drugs (NSAIDs)	May cause dizziness/drowsiness Take with food
Narcotics	Do not drink alcohol, and/or drinking may increase the effects of the drug
Macrolide antibiotics	Take on an empty stomach Take with plenty of water
All antibiotics	Take until gone
Sulfa antibiotics	May cause sensitivity to light Take on an empty stomach Take with plenty of water
Warfarin	Do not take aspirin unless prescribed

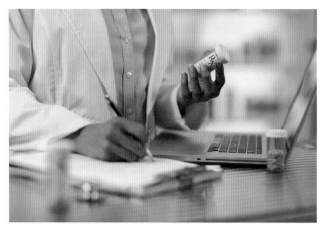

FIG. 8.6 Technicians should always verify any prescription information with the label on the manufacturer's container. (Copyright © Steve Cole Images/Getty Images.)

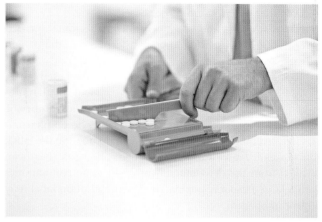

FIG. 8.8 Counting trays may be used to more easily count and pour tablets into medication vials. (Copyright © People Images/Getty Images.)

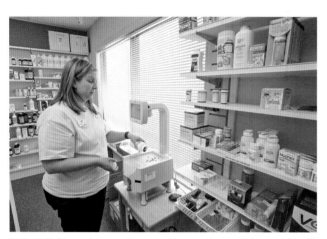

FIG. 8.7 Narcotic counting machine performs automated verification with laser. Pharmacist double counts what the ACD counted and checks the prescription against the label prepared.

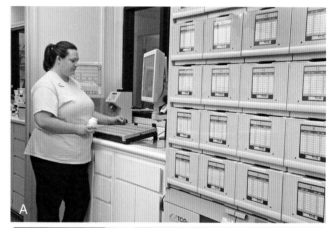

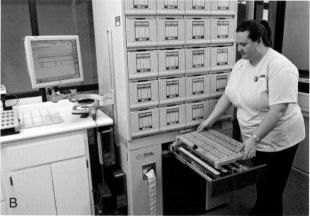

FIG. 8.9 (A) The technician fills a tray with a patient's medications, which packages them in strip packaging form. (B) The technician places the tray in the machine once filled with correct medications.

should be checked a second time with the prescription and the drug manufacturer's bottle. A final check should be performed before the prescription is bagged for pickup. Any medication that appears to have deteriorated or has passed the manufacturer's date should never be dispensed.

Many pharmacies use automated filling machines that include verification by laser technology (Fig. 8.7). The pharmacist reviews a finished product by scanning the bottle and checking NDC, bar code, and drug chosen against a prescription. In some instances the pharmacy may not have the medication on hand to fill the prescription. The pharmacy technician should promptly tell the pharmacist. The patient should be informed of the situation, and the pharmacy should offer to order the medication for the patient or to locate it at another pharmacy.

Many pharmacies use a tray with a spatula to count solid dosage forms (Fig. 8.8). It is best to count the dosages in multiples of five. To prevent contamination of tablets and capsules, the counting tray should be wiped clean after each use because powder from tablets may remain on the tray. Some pharmacies may use automatic counting machines during dispensing. High-volume community pharmacies may use

automatic dispensing equipment (eg, a Baker Cell) to dispense medications (Fig. 8.9).

Although extemporaneous compounding is still performed in community pharmacies, the percentage of compounded prescriptions is relatively small. However, the pharmacy technician must perform the necessary calculations and have them checked before compounding the medication. The pharmacy technician may need to weigh substances or measure liquids before compounding and use the appropriate techniques when adding the ingredients. Extemporaneous compounding is discussed in Chapter 11.

Scanning the Manufacturer's Bottle

Many pharmacies use equipment to scan the bar code on the drug manufacturer's bottle and compare it to the NDC number of the medication selected. If the scanned bar code does not coincide with the medication's NDC number, the pharmacist is notified. This process is used as a quality assurance measure to help eliminate medication errors.

> **Tech Note!**
>
> The Drug Supply Chain Security Act requires the FDA to create and implement a national tracking system to be used by manufacturers and bar coding technology to introduce and track medications entered into the FDA system.

Packaging the Prescription

When dispensing a prescription, the pharmacy technician may select a container according to size, color, and composition; the selection is based on the type and quantity of the medication being dispensed. A variety of medication containers is used in the community pharmacy, including the following:

- Applicator bottles: Used for topical medications
- Dropper bottles: Used for dispensing ophthalmic, otic, nasal, or oral liquid medications
- Ointment jars and collapsible tubes: Used to dispense ointments, creams, and gels
- Prescription bottles: Used for dispensing liquids
- Round vials: Used primarily for solid dosages (eg, tablets, capsules, and caplets)

Many of these containers are amber in color and are made of either glass or plastic. The amber color protects the medication from breaking down because of exposure to sunlight. It is extremely important that the pharmacy technician package the medication in a container that ensures the drug's strength, quality, and purity. Plastic containers have several advantages over glass ones: they are lighter in weight, are more resistant to breakage, and are more adaptable in design.

The Poison Prevention Packaging Act (PPPA) requires the pharmacist to dispense a prescription in a container that has safety closures unless the prescribing physician or patient requests otherwise. This request for a non–child-resistant container may be for a single prescription or for all of a patient's prescriptions. It is the responsibility of the pharmacy staff to obtain a signed waiver from the patient making this request, and this information should be entered into the pharmacy's information system. The PPPA does make exceptions for specific medications not to be dispensed in child-resistant containers. These medications include nitroglycerin (because the patient must have immediate access to the medication in an emergency), oral contraceptives, and various oral and nasal inhalers (because of their unique design and construction). The prescription label should be affixed to the medication container and should convey a professional appearance.

Checking the Prescription

The pharmacist is responsible for checking the final prescription before it is dispensed to the patient to eliminate the possibility of a medication error. The prescription should be checked to verify that the actual medication and strength is being dispensed according to the prescriber's original prescription. The pharmacist should verify the patient's name, the prescription's directions for use, the prescription number, the date, and prescriber's name.

Filing Prescriptions

The pharmacy's information system maintains an electronic record of all filled and refilled prescriptions. The pharmacy is required by law to maintain the actual "hard copy" of the prescription. The Controlled Substance Act provides the following two options for filing filled prescriptions.
1. Option 1 (three separate files)
   - A file for schedule II controlled substances dispensed
   - A file for schedules III, IV, and V controlled substances dispensed
   - A file for all noncontrolled drugs dispensed
2. Option 2 (two separate files):
   - A file for all schedule II controlled substances dispensed
   - A file for all other drugs dispensed (noncontrolled and those in schedules III, IV, and V). If this method is used, a prescription for a schedule III, IV, or V drug must be made readily retrievable by use of a red "C" stamp not less than 1 inch high in the lower right-hand corner of the prescription. If a pharmacy has an electronic record-keeping system for prescriptions that permits identification by prescription number and retrieval of original documents by prescriber's name, patient's name, drug dispensed, and date filled, the requirement to mark the hard copy with a red "C" is waived.

Electronic Prescription Records

- If a prescription is created, signed, transmitted, and received electronically, all records related to that prescription must be retained electronically.
- Electronic records must be maintained electronically for 2 years from the date of their creation or receipt.

> **Tech Note!**
>
> *Remember:* The Patient Protection and Affordable Care Act (ACA) requires insurance companies to cover all applicants with certain standards, and electronic health record (EHR) and the process of medication management therapy are components of that requirement. As a technician, it is critical that your patient has a complete medication record, including over-the-counter or herbal medications.

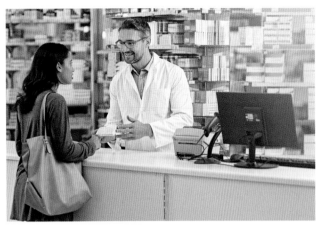

FIG. 8.10 Patient consultations are performed by the pharmacist at the agreement or request of the patient. (Copyright © Grady Reese/Getty Images.)

Patient Counseling

OBRA '90 requires that an offer to counsel be made to every Medicaid patient who receives a new prescription. Many states have since adopted this to apply to *all* new prescriptions and refills. Often it is the responsibility of the pharmacy technician to ask a patient whether he or she has any questions for the pharmacist. If a patient has questions about his or her medication, the pharmacy technician should promptly inform the pharmacist. The pharmacist is responsible for identifying and resolving any problems involved with medication use. Only the pharmacist is legally permitted to counsel a patient (Fig. 8.10).

Prescription Payment

Often it is the responsibility of the pharmacy technician to collect a patient's payment for the amount due for the prescription. The pharmacy determines the available payment methods. The patient often has the option of paying for the prescription with cash, a check, or a credit card. The person collecting payment for the medication must know how to use the cash register and credit card machine and how to return correct change to the patient if required.

◎ Scenario Checkup 8.4

The pharmacy receives a prescription for amoxicillin 250 mg/5 mL 150 mL. The pharmacist asks Andrew to go to the shelf to obtain a bottle. While visually scanning the prescription for completeness, Andrew notes that the prescription calls for 150 mL. Where would he find the amoxicillin in the pharmacy?

Other Pharmacy Technician Duties

Prescription Refilling

Instructions for refilling a prescription are provided by the prescriber on the original prescription or by verbal communication to the pharmacist. A patient may call the pharmacy or walk in to the pharmacy to request a prescription refill.

The pharmacy technician must obtain the following information from the patient:
• Patient's name
• Patient's contact telephone number
• Prescription number
• Medication name and strength
• Physician's name
• Whether the patient will wait or return for the prescription
   Many pharmacies use telephone refill trees, which allow the patient to call in 24 hours a day to refill prescriptions. The patient must enter the prescription number and is prompted to verify specific information about the prescription.

Requesting Prescription Refill Authorization

Many states permit a pharmacy technician to contact the prescriber's office for authorization of a refill. Depending on the system used by the pharmacy, the pharmacy technician may submit a refill request electronically, transmit a facsimile of the prescription, or use the telephone to call the prescriber's office. It is important for the technician to be familiar with the schedule category of a medication before requesting a refill authorization. Pharmacies are not permitted to refill schedule II medications; these require a new, handwritten prescription. In addition, specific medications such as isotretinoin, clozapine, and thalidomide have special processes that must be followed.

Transferring a Prescription

Both federal and state laws govern the transfer of a prescription from one pharmacy to another pharmacy. A pharmacy technician may pull the original prescription from its file or pull it up on the computer system, but the pharmacist is responsible for ensuring that the information transferred is correct. Once the prescription has been transferred from one pharmacy to another pharmacy, the original prescription becomes void. The transferring pharmacist must record the following information from the receiving pharmacist:
• Date of the transfer
• Name, address, and telephone number of the receiving pharmacy
• Name of the pharmacist at the receiving pharmacy
• Number of refills transferred
• National Association of Boards of Pharmacy (NABP) number for the receiving pharmacy
• DEA number of the receiving pharmacy (controlled substances only)
   This information must appear on the back of the original prescription or in the computer system. The receiving pharmacist must record the following information from the transferring pharmacist:
• Date of the transfer
• Name, address, and telephone number of the pharmacy where the prescription was originally filled
• Name of the pharmacist at the original pharmacy
• Number of refills received
• Original date of the written prescription
• NABP number for the originating pharmacy

- DEA number of the originating pharmacy (controlled substances only)

Many states allow a prescription to be transferred only one time.

⊙ Scenario Checkup 8.5

A patient calls the pharmacy and informs Andrew that she would like to transfer her prescription for hydrochlorothiazide 50 mg, which was originally filled at Ambitious Anthony's Pharmacy, to Andrew's pharmacy. Is it possible for Andrew to transfer the prescription for hydrochlorothiazide 50 mg to his pharmacy? If so, what information would Andrew need to obtain from the patient?

Pharmacy Layout

The state board of pharmacy (BOP) regulates the practice of pharmacy for that state. Their regulations determine the physical standards for all pharmacies. The standards include the minimum amount of space for the prescription department of the pharmacy. The pharmacy must be well lit and ventilated, and the proper storage temperature must be maintained to meet the specifications of the *US Pharmacopoeia: National Formulary* (USP-NF) for drug storage. The prescription counter should be used only for compounding, dispensing of drugs, and necessary record keeping. The prescription department must have a sink with hot and cold running water. The pharmacy must have adequate refrigeration equipment with a monitoring thermometer for the storage of drugs requiring cold storage temperature if the pharmacy stocks such medications. The pharmacy department must be maintained in a clean, sanitary manner and in good condition. The pharmacy also must have adequate trash receptacles.

The state board requires that each pharmacy maintain a current dispensing information reference source that is consistent with the practice of the pharmacy. Regardless of the state, every pharmacy is required to have a current copy of the Controlled Substances Act, a current copy of the USP-NF, and any other reference mandated by the state's BOP. A pharmacy is required to have a prescription balance that is sensitive to 15 mg and weights or an electronic scale if the pharmacy engages in activities that require weighing of ingredients. The pharmacy must maintain equipment and supplies that are consistent with the pharmacy's practice.

A community pharmacy is required to have a security system that detects attempts to break into the pharmacy. The purpose of the security system is to protect the pharmacy department when it is closed. The security system must meet current alarm industry standards and may be a sound, microwave, photoelectric, ultrasonic, or any other generally accepted device. The alarm system must have an auxiliary source of power and must be capable of sending an alarm signal to the monitoring company if the main line of communication is not working.

The prescription department of the pharmacy is required to have enclosures that protect the prescription drugs area from unauthorized entry and theft, regardless of whether a pharmacist is on duty. Only authorized personnel, such as pharmacists, pharmacy interns, or pharmacy technicians, are permitted in the pharmacy.

Prescription Intake Window

The prescription intake window is where a patient drops off the prescription to be filled. It is at this location that a pharmacy technician collects the necessary patient information that will be used in developing the patient profile.

Pharmacy Bench

The pharmacy bench is the work area of the pharmacy (Fig. 8.11). Numerous tasks are performed at the bench, including the following:

- Entering patient and prescriber information and prescriptions into the pharmacy's computer information system
- Adjudicating prescription claims
- Scanning prescriptions into the pharmacy's information system
- Pouring and counting medication
- Scanning the manufacturer's drug container for quality assurance purposes
- Packaging and labeling the prescription
- The pharmacist checking the final product against the original prescription order
- Bagging the patient's prescription

A state BOP may require the pharmacy bench to be a specific length. The pharmacy technician must maintain a clean and clutter-free work area to reduce the possibility of errors. After the pharmacist has checked the pharmacy technician's work and final product, the remaining medication should be returned to its proper location on the shelf.

Pharmacy Stock Area

A community pharmacy stocks many different dosage forms, and the medications are often arranged alphabetically for the various dosage forms. Some pharmacies may arrange the medications on the shelf alphabetically by brand name, whereas other pharmacies may arrange them alphabetically by their generic name (Fig. 8.12). Many pharmacies have a designated area for oral dosage forms (tablets and capsules), oral liquids, reconstituted liquids (antibiotics), oral contraceptives, inhalation products, topical agents, ophthalmic and otic

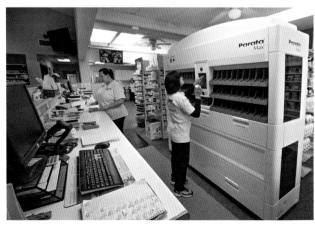

FIG. 8.11 Technicians filling prescriptions.

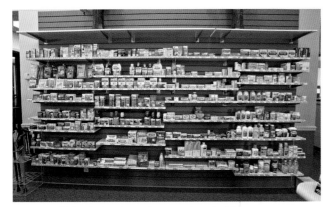

FIG. 8.12 Over-the-counter shelving area.

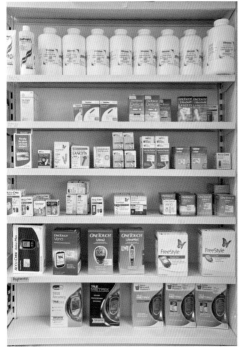

FIG. 8.13 Stock shelving and filling area.

products, vaginal and rectal products, and refrigerated products. Some community pharmacies have an area designated for "fast movers," which are the more commonly dispensed medications for that pharmacy (Fig. 8.13).

A retail pharmacy has a locked safe to ensure that schedule II medications are kept secure at all times. This safe may have a combination lock or a key lock, or it may be opened through biometrics if approved by the state BOP. Other controlled substances should be dispersed throughout the pharmacy.

If a retail pharmacy stocks drugs that require a cold storage temperature, the pharmacy must have adequate facilities, including a monitoring thermometer, for storage of these drugs in the prescription department. If a pharmacy has controlled substances that must be refrigerated, a separate refrigerator is required for the controlled substances. Pharmacists and pharmacy technicians should *never* place their lunch or a beverage in a refrigerator designated for medications.

Every pharmacy must check its inventory to ensure that all medications are in date. Often the pharmacy's standard operating procedure states when this must be performed. If the pharmacy staff identifies medication that has expired, the medication must be removed from the shelf and placed in a designated area in the pharmacy where expired and recalled medications are kept. These medications cannot be dispensed or sold and must be separated from the other stock used for dispensing. These medications should be maintained in this designated area until they are properly discarded.

Nonsterile Compounding Area

The nonsterile compounding area should be away from other workflow to minimize distractions to the compounder and contamination of the product. The area should be kept clean and free of clutter at all times. It should have a controlled temperature and proper ventilation. All equipment and supplies used in nonsterile compounding should be easily accessible to the compounder. All equipment should be examined for cleanliness before use and washed immediately after use to prevent any cross-contamination between ingredients and the final product. Isopropyl 70% alcohol is often used to clean the compounding area. It is recommended that a log be maintained to show when equipment was cleaned.

A sink with hot and cold running water and proper drainage is required by all state BOPs. Cleaning products, such as sponges and brushes of various sizes, should be kept next to the sink. Disposable paper towels should be kept adjacent to the sink. Trash receptacles should be kept a distance away from the compounding procedures. All trash should be disposed of safely and properly, including personal protective equipment (PPE) and hazardous waste (Fig. 8.14).

Some of the equipment used in nonsterile compounding includes the following:
- Balances
- Beakers
- Brushes
- Graduated cylinders
- Evaporating dishes
- Funnels
- Graduates
- Metric weights

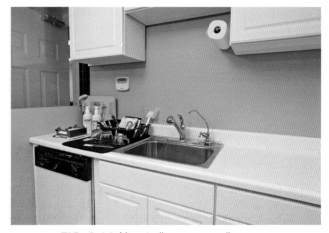

FIG. 8.14 Nonsterile compounding area.

- Mortar and pestles
- Pipettes
- Sharps containers
- Spatulas
- Spray bottles
- Stirring rods
- Weighing papers or boats

The pharmacy technician should have a firm understanding of *United States Pharmacopeia* <795> (USP <795>), the equipment used in nonsterile compounding, and the appropriate techniques.

Sterile Compounding Area

Some retail pharmacies may have a sterile compounding area if the pharmacy administers vaccines or provides intravenous medications to its patients. This area must comply with the *United States Pharmacopeia* <797> (USP <797>). USP <797> has established specific guidelines for maintaining sterility in compounding and for addressing medication errors. The American Society of Health-System Pharmacists (ASHP) and the National Coordinating Committee on Large Volume Parenterals (NCCLVP) also have released guidelines describing the conditions and practices needed to process compounded sterile preparations so as to prevent harm or even death as a result of cross-contamination.

Pharmacy Order Check-in Area

Many pharmacies have a designated area where warehouse and wholesaler deliveries are received and checked in by the pharmacy technician. The pharmacy technician checks the medication received against the accompanying packaging slip to ensure that everything ordered was received. The pharmacy technician places the medications in their proper places on the pharmacy shelves or in the refrigerator.

Reconstitution Area

All community pharmacies have an area where medication is reconstituted. Reconstitution is the process in which a dehydrated product is returned to a liquid state. The most common type of medication that is reconstituted in a retail pharmacy is oral liquid antibiotics (see Chapter 11). Distilled water is used to reconstitute oral liquid antibiotics. Medications that require reconstitution are not reconstituted until the patient arrives to pick up the prescription because reconstituted medications are good only for a predetermined number of days, as outlined by the drug manufacturer on the bottle. Many reconstituted antibiotics must be refrigerated after mixing with distilled water. Auxiliary labels are affixed to the bottle reminding the patient to shake the bottle before using it and to refrigerate the medication if necessary.

Repackaging Area

Some community pharmacies may **repackage** medications if they provide pharmacy services to long-term care (LTC) facilities. These pharmacies may have unit dose packaging equipment to prepare unit dose medications for these facilities. The pharmacy must maintain accurate records for repackaged medications; these records are found in the repackaging log. Table 8.5 presents information contained in a repacking log.

A beyond-use date (BUD) is assigned by the pharmacy to replace the drug manufacturer's expiration date. The USP has changed its beyond-use dating method for nonsterile solid and liquid dosage forms that are packaged in single-unit and unit dose containers; the BUD is 1 year or less, unless stability data or the manufacturer's labeling indicates otherwise. BUDs are nearer than expiration dates to account for the fact that the manufacturer's original container has been opened in the repackaging process, thereby exposing the pharmaceutical article to ambient atmospheric conditions. This exposure,

■ TABLE 8.5
Repackaging Log Information

	Description
Date	Date the drug is repackaged, which includes date, month, and year
Drug	Drug name, usually by generic and then brand name, if indicated on the repackaging log sheet
Dosage form	Examples include tablet, capsule, spansule, troche, suspension, elixir, solution
Drug manufacturer	Drug manufacturer (usually abbreviated)
Drug manufacturer's lot number	Control number located on the side of the label or on the bottom of the bottle
Drug manufacturer's expiration date	Located with the lot number; remember that if the date indicates only the month and year, the medication is good through the end of the month
Assigned pharmacy lot number	Each item repackaged in pharmacy is given a number consecutive to the previous batch prepared
Pharmacy beyond-use date (BUD)	New date assigned to repackaged medications according to *United States Pharmacopeia* <795> guidelines
Pharmacy technician	Must initial logbook entry
Pharmacist	Must check off each item repackaged

and the fact that containers into which dosage forms are repackaged may not have the integrity of the original package, necessitates a shortening of the expiration period from that originally set by the manufacturer.

Pharmacy Records

All community pharmacies must maintain the original prescription on file for the minimum time required by the state BOP, including the daily prescription record with the signatures of the filling pharmacists. The pharmacy must maintain all controlled substance invoices for a minimum of 2 years, according to federal regulations. These records include completed DEA Form 222, DEA Form 41, DEA Form 106, biennial inventories, and change of the pharmacist in charge.

Patient Bins

Once a prescription has received its final check from the pharmacist, it is placed in a bin awaiting pickup by the patient (Fig. 8.15). These prescriptions may be placed in a secured area outside the prescription department, not accessible by the patient, where access to the prescriptions is restricted to individuals designated by the pharmacist. The patient bins are normally arranged in alphabetical order. It is very important that a patient's prescription be placed in the appropriate bin. State pharmacy regulations determine whether a pharmacy technician may provide a patient with his or her medication when the pharmacist is not present.

Prescription Pick-Up Window

Some retail pharmacies have a separate pick-up window for prescriptions. Other pharmacies may have the patient pick up the prescription at the drop-off window. Regardless of the arrangement, there is at least one cash register at this point. Often the pharmacy technician rings up the patient's prescriptions and collects payment. The patient acknowledges receipt of the prescription by signing an electronic device for insurance purposes. When the patient comes to pick up the prescription, the pharmacy technician asks whether he or she has any questions for the pharmacist. If the patient has questions about the medication, the pharmacy technician notifies the pharmacist.

Consultation Area

As the result of changes made through OBRA '90, a pharmacy must have an area designated for patient consultation (Fig. 8.16). Depending on the state BOP's regulations on counseling, the offer to counsel may be made in any manner the pharmacist thinks appropriate, in his or her professional judgment, and may include any one or a combination of the following:
- Face-to-face communication with the pharmacist
- A sign posted so that it can be seen by patients
- A notation affixed to or written on the bag in which the prescription is to be delivered
- A notation on the prescription container
- By telephone

If the offer to counsel is accepted by the patient, the pharmacist counsels the person, presenting the prescription to the extent the pharmacist feels appropriate in his or her professional judgment. Information provided during counseling may include the following:
- The name and description of the medication
- The dosage form, dosage, route of administration, and duration of drug therapy
- Special directions and precautions for preparation, administration, and use by the patient
- Common adverse or severe side effects or interactions and therapeutic contraindications that may be encountered, including their avoidance and the action required if they occur
- Techniques for self-monitoring drug therapy
- Proper storage
- Prescription refill information
- Action to be taken in the event of a missed dose

Some pharmacies may have a separate area where the pharmacist can counsel the patient. The consultation area should allow the pharmacist and patient to speak in privacy, away from other patients. Each state BOP establishes its own criteria.

Drive-Through Window

Within the past two decades, many retail pharmacies have established a drive-through window, where patients can drop

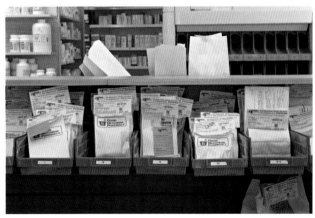

FIG. 8.15 The patient bins should be in alphabetical order, clearly labeled, and easily accessible to the pharmacy staff.

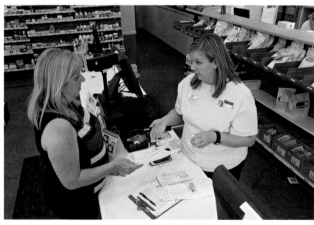

FIG. 8.16 Patient consultation area.

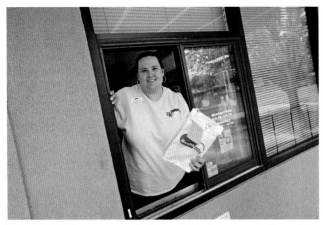
FIG. 8.17 Pharmacy technician delivering prescription at the pharmacy drive-through window.

off a new prescription, request a refill, or pick up a prescription without leaving their vehicle (Fig. 8.17). The drive-through window is an added customer convenience that saves patients time because they do not have to park their vehicles and walk into the pharmacy. If the pharmacy has a drive-through window, the individual responsible for that area is responsible for collecting all the necessary patient information when a new prescription is presented and payment when it is purchased.

◎ Scenario Checkup 8.6

Andrew is working at the pharmacy bench, and he notices one of his co-workers has left random papers and candy wrappers in her work area. Andrew knows it is important to keep the bench clean and organized. How should he handle this situation? What can he do to help his co-worker and the pharmacy maintain the necessary standards of cleanliness?

Communication

Pharmacy technicians have very strong technical skills that are essential in the practice of retail pharmacy. These skills include a strong knowledge base of diseases and their treatment with medication or through behavior modification, solid use of math in performing the necessary pharmacy calculations for compounding, the ability to transcribe a prescriber's order for medications, sound computer skills, and excellent techniques for both sterile and nonsterile compounding. One asset that is just as important as those just mentioned is interpersonal communication skills.

Interpersonal communication skills are necessary in the process by which messages are generated and transmitted by one individual and subsequently received and translated by another individual. Communication consists of five important components: sender, message, receiver, feedback, and barriers. The sender transmits a message to another person. The message is the component that is transmitted from one person to the other person. A message may be a thought, an idea, an emotion, information, or other factors that can be transmitted either verbally or nonverbally. Nonverbal communication

includes facial expressions (eg, smiling, frowning, or grinning) and hand motions. The receiver receives the message from the sender. Feedback is the process by which the receiver communicates back to the sender his or her understanding of the message. Barriers affect the accuracy of the communication.

Nonverbal communication consists of a complex mix of behaviors and psychological and environmental interactions through which a person consciously and unconsciously relates to another individual. A study by Pyothos reported that 55% to 95% of all communication can be attributed to nonverbal communication. Nonverbal communications are distinctive because they mirror an individual's innermost thoughts and feelings. In addition, they are difficult to fake during interpersonal communication.

There are numerous barriers in nonverbal communication, including the following:
- Body position in relation to the patient (eg, closed or open stance, folded arms, or slouching)
- Facial expressions (eg, wandering eyes)
- Lack of eye contact
- Tone of voice (eg, being sarcastic or using a threatening tone)

Although these may be interpreted as barriers in our culture, they may not be a barrier in another culture. Therefore an understanding of cultural behaviors can be helpful to pharmacy technicians if they have a diverse patient base.

All communication between health professionals and patients has two principal purposes:
1. To establish an ongoing rapport between the provider and patient
2. To provide the exchange of information necessary to assess a patient's health condition, apply the treatment of a medical problem, and evaluate the effects on a patient's quality of life

Interacting With the Pharmacist

The pharmacist is responsible for communicating with the technician in a clear and concise manner. Using the proper terminology ensures that the pharmacist and pharmacy technician share common definitions associated with the circumstance. Individuals assign meanings to their words based on their background, values, and experiences. In this situation, the pharmacy technician is responsible for listening intently to the pharmacist. The pharmacist should check with the technician to ensure that he or she understood the communication. It is the pharmacy technician's responsibility to request any clarification of the message. Neither the pharmacist nor the pharmacy technician should ever make assumptions because false assumptions may adversely affect the patient's outcome. Sometimes there is a disconnection between the pharmacist and the pharmacy technician because although the words mean one thing, the nonverbal communication demonstrates something else. Feedback is essential in communications between the pharmacist and the technician. Conversely, when the pharmacy technician is initiating the communication, the pharmacist is responsible for listening and providing feedback to the technician.

Pharmacists play an integral role in making certain their patients obtain the desired outcomes with their medication therapy. The role of the pharmacist has evolved from medication-centered to patient-centered care. To establish a patient-centered care environment, it is essential that the pharmacist develop a trusting relationship with the patient. This allows the pharmacist and patient to be actively involved in the treatment and leads to the desired outcome.

The National Academy of Medicine (formerly the Institute of Medicine [IOM]) defines patient-centered care as "providing care that is respectful of and responsive to individual patient preferences, needs, and values, and ensuring that patient values guide all clinical decisions." To provide patient-centered care, the pharmacist must be able to:

- Build a **therapeutic alliance** with patients to meet mutually understood goals of therapy
- Develop a self-awareness of personal effects on patients
- Foster an unrestricted relationship with the patient
- Identify the patient's experience as unique
- Understand the patient's illness experience

The efforts of the pharmacy technician aid pharmacists in performing their clinical pharmacy activities.

Interacting With the Patient

Often pharmacy communication is delayed because of challenges from distinctive obstacles posed by particular groups of patients. Many communication barriers exist within each of these groups of individuals. As a pharmacy technician, it is vital that if you sense an individual has a specific problem, you check your perception of that individual. If you are dealing with elderly patients, what is your initial perception of them? Are they forgetful? Do you consider them to have visual or auditory issues? Based on your perceptions, you make assumptions about this group of patients.

Tech Note!

The pharmacist role is now more clinical than ever, and the technician is an integral part during communication or the initial encounter with a patient. Any concerns or observations should be shared with the pharmacist, so that they can provide better overall counseling.

Elderly Patients

The elderly population is increasing and living longer as a result of advances in the treatment of diseases and disorders with medication and behavioral modification. The elderly experience more chronic conditions than do younger individuals and therefore take a greater number of medications. As individuals age, they may experience a loss in their communication skills (Fig. 8.18).

Also, as individuals age, they tend to process information at a slower rate than younger individuals. The rate of speech and the amount of information an elderly patient receives at one time must meet the individual's ability to understand this information. Also, the elderly person's short-term memory, recall, and attention span may be reduced. Elderly patients may perceive things differently from individuals in other age groups and may have specific expectations.

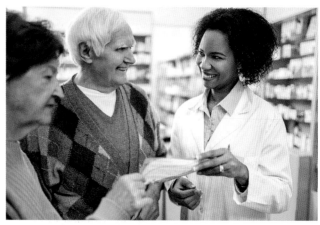

FIG. 8.18 A technician should be aware of communication issues that may affect elderly patients. (Copyright © 2014 SkyNesher Getty Images.)

Elderly patients may experience physical changes in their bodies that affect their communication skills. The elderly patient who has experienced a decrease in vision may have difficulty reading the font size of written materials. Therefore it may be necessary to explain to the individual how to take or store the medications.

An elderly patient may develop hearing impairments. Hearing impairments may occur when something blocks the conduction of sound into the ear's sensory nerve centers, when damage occurs in the sensory center of the inner ear, or when the nerve centers of the brain are affected. A loss of hearing may be due to birth defects, injuries, or chronic exposure to loud noises. The amount of hearing loss varies among individuals. Some individuals may actually hear words and sounds yet not be able to comprehend the meaning of the words.

Some patients with hearing difficulties depend on speech reading; they watch a person's lips, facial expressions, and gestures to improve their communication skills. As a pharmacy technician, you should position yourself 3 to 6 feet from the hearing-impaired individual. You should never speak directly into the patient's ear because the sound may become distorted. If the patient is experiencing difficulty understanding what you are telling him or her, you should not repeat the sentence, but rather rephrase it in shorter and simpler sentences.

As a pharmacy technician, you may encounter patients with speech impairment. Speech impairments may be caused by a variety of factors, including birth defects, injuries, or other illnesses. **Dysarthria** is a speech impairment involving interference with the normal control of the speech mechanism because of damage to specific facial muscles. Dysarthria can be caused by Parkinson's disease, multiple sclerosis, strokes, and accidents. Often patients with a speech impairment may communicate through the use of notes or sign language. A pharmacy technician should always have a pad of paper at the prescription intake or pick-up station for patients who want to communicate by writing.

Another speech issue that may occur after a patient has experienced a stroke or other adverse event is known as aphasia. **Aphasia** is a complex condition in which an individual has a reduced ability to understand what others are saying and express himself or herself. Depending on the severity of the problem, an individual may have no speech or may have difficulty with names or words. Other individuals may experience difficulty putting words in the proper sequence in a sentence. These patients may encounter problems in understanding oral directions, reading, writing, and the use of numbers. Patients with aphasia may have normal hearing; therefore speaking loudly to them will not improve the situation. When dealing with a patient who has aphasia, it is best to speak with the patient's caregiver.

Patients With Mental Health Problems

According to a finding in 2012 by the National Institute of Mental Health (NIMH), 43.7 million (18.6%) adults have some form of mental illness. Unfortunately, many pharmacists and pharmacy technicians experience difficulty communicating with patients with mental disorders because they do not know what to say to them. There are many stereotypes about patients with mental health problems that some members of the pharmacy team may believe.

Some patients with mental health disorders may be hesitant to speak with members of the pharmacy staff for a variety of reasons. These reasons may include a poor self-image and hesitancy to interact with other people. These patients may think that they have a condition that may make some individuals feel uncomfortable. Some patients may not feel comfortable interacting with health care professionals.

The pharmacy staff may also have difficulty relating to these individuals. They may feel uncertain about how much information they should provide to the patient. In addition, the pharmacy staff may not know what the prescriber has told the patient about his or her condition.

When speaking with patients with mental health issues, it is best to use open-ended questions. Patients with mental illness should not be treated any differently from any other patient who has a condition such as hypertension, chronic obstructive pulmonary disease, diabetes, or thyroid disease. Every patient should be treated with the same dignity and respect.

Terminally Ill Patients

Many individuals find it difficult to interact with terminally ill patients. They may feel uncomfortable discussing the topic of death and experience difficulty finding the correct words to use. Most terminally ill patients need a supportive relationship with family, friends, and health care providers, including both pharmacists and pharmacy technicians. Often the pharmacy team may be the only health care providers in the community that a patient may encounter frequently.

In 1969, Elisabeth Kübler-Ross wrote *On Death and Dying*, which identified five stages of grief: denial, anger, bargaining, depression, and acceptance. By understanding these five stages, a health care professional is better able to understand what a patient is experiencing. In addition to the patient, the person's family also may be experiencing the five stages of grief. Terminally ill patients may be hesitant to discuss various issues, but they may become more receptive as time passes.

Communicating with terminally ill patients and their families is extremely important. You should never avoid talking to them unless you sense they do not want to discuss the illness. Furthermore, not talking to them isolates the individual and may endorse the idea that talking about death is uncomfortable.

Patients With Health Literacy Issues

According to the American Medical Association (AMA), health literacy is defined as the ability to read, understand, and act on health care information. According to the National Patient Safety Foundation (NPSF):
- According to the Center for Health Care Strategies, a disproportionate number of minorities and immigrants are estimated to have literacy problems:
  - Fifty percent of Hispanics
  - Forty percent of African Americans
  - Thirty-three percent of Asians
  - More than 66% of US adults age 60 or older have either inadequate or marginal literacy skills.
- Annual health care costs for individuals with low literacy skills are four times higher than for those with higher literacy skills.
- Limited health literacy increases the disparity in health care access among exceptionally vulnerable populations (eg, racial and ethnic minorities and the elderly).
- Literacy skills are a stronger predictor of an individual's health status than age, income, employment status, education level, or racial/ethnic group.
- Ninety million people in the United States may be at risk because of the difficulty some patients experience in understanding and acting on health information.
- One of five American adults reads at the 5th grade level or below, and the average American reads at the 8th to 9th grade level, yet most health care materials are written above the 10th grade level.
- Patients with low literacy skills were observed to have a 50% increased risk for hospitalization compared with patients who had adequate literacy skills.
- Problems with patient compliance and medical errors may be based on poor understanding of health care information. Only about 50% of all patients take medications as directed.

Patients with low health literacy are often uncomfortable and fail to inform their pharmacist or pharmacy technician of this situation. Without this knowledge, the pharmacy team is unable to properly assess a patient's understanding of the information they provide. To help these patients, the USP has developed pictographs that illustrate common medication instructions and precautions (see Fig. 14.1 and Chapter 14 for more information on pictographs).

Caregivers

Communication issues develop when information is provided to the caregivers of patients with chronic conditions, parents who take care of children with acute illnesses, family members, or friends. A caregiver must understand a patient's condition and treatment and how to effectively communicate the special instructions to the patient. It is extremely important for the caregiver to understand the importance of refilling the patient's medication. Often it is best to give the caregiver written information so that it can be given to the patient at home.

Patients visit the pharmacy because they need to obtain a medication to treat a current condition or to prevent a condition from occurring. As a pharmacy technician, it is extremely important that you demonstrate empathy toward the patient. By demonstrating to the patient that you understand his or her feelings, you will be able to develop a caring, trusting relationship with the patient. Demonstrating empathy allows patients to understand their own feelings about their conditions and makes it easier for them to solve their own problems. Empathy enables patients to place their trust in the pharmacy team because they have confidence the team will work in their best interest.

A survey conducted in 1997 by the National Harris Survey revealed that many patients do not seek medical attention because of the sensitivity of their condition. A pharmacy technician should be aware that a patient may have difficulty discussing topics such as breast or prostate cancer, contraception, depression, hemorrhoids, incontinence, menopause, and sexual dysfunction. Discreetly approach these sensitive issues, taking the patient's feelings into account to avoid making the person uncomfortable. It is also important to be aware that patients may not adhere to their drug regimens if the situation or the side effects of the medication are difficult for them to discuss.

The pharmacy technician should apply the following techniques when addressing any patient:
- Avoid using professional jargon
- Avoid using words with more than one meaning
- Develop a sense of trustworthiness with the patient by demonstrating friendliness, a sense of ethics, sociability, and fairness
- Recognize that there are differences in cross-cultural styles of speaking
- Use simple ideas and words when obtaining information from the patient

Customer Service

Customer service is defined as the provision of service to customers before, during, and after a purchase. Customer service in health care is different from that in other industries because the customers are recipients of medical services that are critical to their health. The pharmacy provides OTC, BTC, and prescription medications to its customers and patients. In addition, the pharmacist provides information to patients to maximize the therapeutic effects of the medications they are prescribed.

The "five rights" of medication administration used by nurses also apply to pharmacy practice. They are:
- *Right patient:* The patient's identity must be verified against the prescription order to ensure that the correct patient is receiving the medication.
- *Right medication:* It must be verified that the medication written on the prescription order is the same as the medication being prepared for the patient.

- *Right time:* The pharmacist must ensure that the medication is to be taken by the patient at the correct time it was ordered by the physician.
- *Right dose:* The medication dose being prepared must be confirmed against the written medication order before it is dispensed.
- *Right route of administration:* The pharmacist must verify the correct route for delivering the ordered medication to the patient by reading the order and preparing the medication appropriately.

In recent years, the medical profession has added some additional rights of administration to include:
   Right to refuse: Give the patient the autonomy to decide whether or not to take the medication.
   Right history and assessment: Include allergies, drug interactions, or previous history before medication administration.

In 2011, J.D. Power and Associates conducted a National Pharmacy Study of all patients who filled a prescription at a pharmacy over a 2-month period. The study ranked the customer satisfaction of more than 12,300 customers, using a 1000-point scale for their ranking. Customers were asked about their experiences and perceptions as a pharmacy patient, including their satisfaction with the store environment, prescription drop-off and pick-up process, costs, and interactions with pharmacists and other staff. Rick Millard, J.D. Power senior director of the health care practice, said, "Customers are expecting more from their brick-and-mortar pharmacy; not just in terms of wait time, but also in terms of contact with the pharmacist and pharmacy staff."

As a pharmacy technician, you will encounter many unique individuals. Some of these individuals may not fully understand the prescription filling process, the legal requirements of filling a prescription, or their prescription coverage. Box 8.2 presents some complaints that you might hear from your customers.

Given the shrinking margin in prescription profits because of managed care agreements, it is easy to see the importance of customer service in retail pharmacy. Developing excellent customer service skills is important in any job and even more important as a pharmacy technician. Customers who come to your pharmacy will remember if you were rude, uninformative, helpful, or courteous. Your attitude can have a direct effect on whether a pharmacy customer comes back, and it can also alter your image as a technician. Here are some helpful tips you can use on the job.
- *Appearance:* Individuals who shop and pick up their prescriptions at your pharmacy appreciate a well-groomed pharmacy technician. The way you look has an impact on how others see you.
- *Attitude:* Courtesy and knowledge are important. Be sure to keep up with the pharmacy field and know your subject.
- *Efficiency:* It is imperative to complete your work efficiently and correctly the first time. Mistakes in pharmacy can cause serious illness or even death.
- *Helping out:* Going the extra mile and assisting other co-workers when they are overwhelmed will make you a star worker. Co-workers will also return the favor when you need it.

BOX 8.2 **Common Pharmacy Customer Service Complaints**

- I called in my prescription refill 2 days ago; why isn't it ready?
- My doctor said they would call the prescription in right away!
- My doctor told me that I would be on this medication the rest of my life; what do you mean that there are no refills left on the prescription?
- The prescription was for 90 days, and you gave me only a 30-day supply; what do you mean my prescription card will pay only for a 30-day supply?
- The wait time to fill a prescription is too long.
- What do you mean my prescription card will not pay for this medication?
- What do you mean my prescription coverage will not pay for my medication? I am going on a trip and need to have my prescription refilled before I leave.
- What do you mean, that if I want the brand name drug, I will have to pay more for it?
- Why did my doctor prescribe this medication if it is on back order?
- Why didn't someone call me to tell me that my doctor wants to see me?

BOX 8.3 **Customer Service Statistics**

- The main reason for customer turnover is poor customer service, not price.
- One negative experience requires 12 positive experiences to change customer opinion.
- Ninety-six percent of dissatisfied customers do not complain.
- Ninety-one percent of dissatisfied customers leave and do not come back.
- Seventy percent of customer opinion is based on how customers feel they were treated.
- One unhappy customer tells between 9 and 15 people about a bad experience.
- Thirteen percent of unhappy customers will tell more than 20 people.
- One happy customer will only tell between 4 and 6 people about the good experience.
- Fifty-five percent of customers would pay more if it meant improved service.

Data from Digby J. 50 Facts about customer experience. *Return on Behavior Magazine.* October 25, 2010. Retrieved from http://returnonbehavior.com/2010/10/50-facts-about-customer-experience-for-2011/.

Box 8.3 shows key customer service statistics that you should keep in mind when serving pharmacy customers.

⊙ Scenario Checkup 8.7

Andrew is responsible for the prescription drop-off window when a Hispanic customer enters the pharmacy to drop off his prescription. Andrew scans the prescription and notices that there is no address on it. Andrew attempts to ask the patient his address and quickly realizes the patient does not speak English. Andrew checks the pharmacy's computer system to see whether the patient has ever filled a prescription at Andrew's pharmacy before and finds that the patient has not. How should Andrew handle the situation?

Other Pharmacy Services

Immunizations

Many community pharmacies provide immunizations to their patients. These include immunizations for influenza, pneumococcal infection, hepatitis A and B, herpes zoster, and varicella. Pharmacists can administer vaccines in most states, but with the release of the COVID-19 vaccine, many state boards have changed to allow trained technicians to immunize. Pharmacy technicians can also facilitate the programs, including billing, scheduling, and reporting and documentation requirements, to reduce some of the barriers to providing personal counseling services by the pharmacist. Technicians can also take an active role in pharmacy-based immunization programs by obtaining cardiopulmonary resuscitation training and certification and completing the required immunization training per each state's guidelines.

Did You Know?

There are several state and national organizations offering immunization training or certificates to include the Pharmacy Technician Certification Board (PTCB).

Medication Therapy Management

Another requirement of the ACA is medication therapy management (MTM). This is medical care provided by pharmacists whose aim is to optimize drug therapy and improve therapeutic outcomes for patients. MTM covers a broad range of professional activities, including but not limited to performing a patient assessment and/or a comprehensive medication review, formulating a medication treatment plan, monitoring the efficacy and safety of medication therapy, enhancing medication adherence through patient empowerment and education, and documenting and communicating MTM services to prescribers to maintain comprehensive patient care. Overall wellness and disease prevention is now an integral part of the pharmacist's role, and the technician role often includes gathering information from the patient to complete a medication and disease history that provides counseling documentation.

As the pharmacy profession embraces extensive patient counseling in the form of MTM, many aspects of the practice of pharmacy must evolve to ensure the success of the MTM program. Time constraints limit the ability of pharmacists to handle administrative tasks and represent a major barrier to the implementation of MTM programs. Technicians can do some of the work to reduce this barrier. With proper training, technicians can assist pharmacists in the tasks that do not require the professional judgment of a pharmacist, freeing pharmacists to focus on clinical activities and making an MTM program more sustainable. For example, technicians can help in areas such as scheduling and patient reminders through phone calls. Medication histories and health histories also can be documented by technicians, as can chart construction, filing, and the documentation of release forms and health histories. Additional steps can be taken to further increase efficiency in the MTM process, including the creation of a flow map and cross-training of all pharmacy staff.

Synchronization of Medications

Patient adherence programs such as packaging medications for times of administration is very common today. Even companies such as Amazon offer PILL PACK (*https://www.pillpack.com/*).

Offer monthly delivery of medications that are presorted and ready at the time of each required dose. This allows the patient to adhere to specific dosing without removal of bulk medications from prescription bottles.

Patients taking routine or maintenance medications should take advantage of medication synchronization, which allows for more accurate dosing and medication compliance (see Fig. 8.9). Medications are packaged in individual packets per the dose they are to be taken. For example, if the dose is 2 tablets in the am, there will be 2 tablets in a single packet marked, "Take in am." Technicians play a critical role in patient safety and compliance and assist the pharmacist by observing a patient's medication adherence. Maybe there are medications on the patient's profile that are not being regularly refilled due to cost or side effects the patient has experienced. Using the strip packaging with clear instructions per each dose rather than a bulk bottle with loose pills makes it easier for the patient to take the medication correctly.

Technician Profile

Roberto has been certified as a pharmacy technician by the PTCB since 1997. He is the lead pharmacy technician at an independent pharmacy in Falls Church, Virginia. Roberto is fluent in Spanish, which is helpful when he is dealing with the pharmacy's Hispanic customers. Recently the pharmacist has begun providing medication therapy management services to his patients. Roberto understands that he may not counsel patients, but he is able to assist the pharmacist in performing medication therapy management for their patients.

Durable and Nondurable Supplies and Equipment

Often patients will need to purchase equipment or supplies to use at home. They may have been hospitalized and now need further care that can be done at home with or without additional caregivers. Community pharmacies often have a part of their business that supplies these products known as durable and nondurable equipment and supplies (Fig. 8.19). An example of durable equipment would be a hospital bed or wheelchair. A nondurable product may be Jobst stockings or diabetic or ostomy supplies. Today's community pharmacy provides even more of these products or services for their patients for a variety of reasons, as follows:

- The number of elderly patients has increased, resulting in a growing need for these products and services.
- Patients prefer to be treated and to convalesce in their homes.
- Services at home are less expensive than staying in a hospital or assisted living facility.
- The patient is able to maintain his or her independence.
- Technology has evolved such that traditional treatments now can be performed in the patient's home.
- Managed care supports the discharge of patients from a hospital to the home.

Most community pharmacies have provided crutches, canes, and walkers for their patients. Within the past several decades, some pharmacies have expanded their inventory of home health care products. These products include the following:

- Antiembolism stockings (eg, thromboembolism-deterrent hose [TED stockings])
- Durable medical equipment (eg, wheelchairs, hospital beds, and commodes)

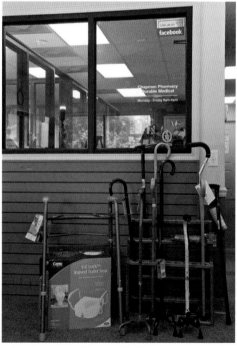

FIG. 8.19 A nondurable supply display at local pharmacy.

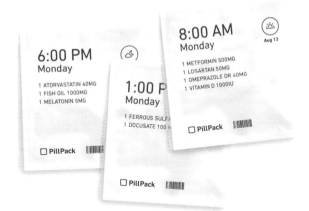

6:00 PM
Monday

1 ATORVASTATIN 40MG
1 FISH OIL 1000MG
1 MELATONIN 5MG

□ PillPack

1:00 P
Monday

1 FERROUS SULF
1 DOCUSATE 100

□ PillPack

8:00 AM
Monday
Aug 13

1 METFORMIN 500MG
1 LOSARTAN 50MG
1 OMEPRAZOLE DR 40MG
1 VITAMIN D 1000IU

□ PillPack

- First aid supplies
- Home diagnostic products (eg, glucometers and diabetic supplies)
- Medical instruments (eg, stethoscopes and blood pressure kits)
- Nutritional therapy (eg, Ensure, Sustacal)
- Orthopedic supplies (eg, braces)
- Ostomy and incontinence products
- Oxygen therapy (eg, oxygen tanks)
- Prescription medications not for self-administration (eg, respiratory drugs)
- Prosthetic devices
- Wound care and decubitus ulcer (bed sore) products

Pharmacy technicians who work in community pharmacies that provide home health care products are able to provide excellent customer service if they have received the proper training in the use of these products.

Tech Note!

This service is part of the overall wellness and disease management of the patient, which is now a significant part of changing pharmaceutical practice.

Long-Term Care Services

Some community pharmacies have contracts with long-term care facilities to provide medications for their residents. Long-term care facilities include subacute care facilities, correctional facilities, assisted living facilities, and board and care homes. As in a traditional community pharmacy, technicians assist the pharmacist in providing long-term care services. Packaging for long-term care services is different from the traditional bottles of 30-day supplies of medication. The packaging is in blister cards or strip packaging to make it easier for dispensing and changes to orders. Long-term care facilities use 30-day cards with individual pockets for medications so that each dose is separated and given individually. The unopened blisters or pockets remain untouched and therefore can be returned for order changes if necessary. In addition, the patient takes a "pocket contents" and gets the correct dose instead of counting from a bottle of loose medication (Fig. 8.20).

Often a pharmacy will dedicate a part of their business to packaging for contract long-term care facilities.

Another type of packaging is commonly referred to as "strip packaging," and this is performed by a robot or machine. The technician keeps the canisters stocked and manually operates the tray for certain medications. Each "pouch" contains a time of day medication such as breakfast, lunch, or dinner. The pouch lists the medications inside and they are perforated but remain in a roll. The roll is placed in a box and the patient tears off the pouch when it is time to take that time's medications. These packages are delivered to the patient's home monthly.

For example, a patient is prescribed a multivitamin, Lasix 40 mg, and Synthroid at breakfast time. These medications will be in one single pouch and can be taken together.

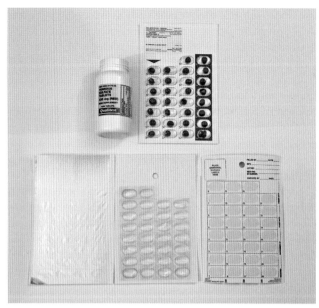

FIG. 8.20 Cold-seal and heat seal packaging can be done for community and hospital pharmacy long-term care packaging.

Pharmacy technicians perform many of the dispensing tasks associated with packaging for long-term care medications that were previously done by pharmacists. Some of the responsibilities assigned to pharmacy technicians include the following:

- Billing prescription, OTC, and nondrug services
- Entering computer data on prescription drug and nondrug orders
- Maintaining a drug library
- Maintaining computerized information to include patient profiles and drug information requests
- Maintaining delivery records
- Maintaining repackaging equipment
- Ordering, receiving, and stocking medications and supplies
- Packaging and labeling prescriptions
- Performing general pharmacy housekeeping
- Processing returned medications for reuse
- Providing the necessary forms to the long-term care facility
- Repackaging and labeling medications
- Transporting medications to the facility

As the population continues to age, the need for pharmacy services for long-term care facilities will continue to expand, creating additional employment opportunities for pharmacy technicians in community and retail pharmacy.

Wellness and Disease Prevention

Many of today's community pharmacy settings have incorporated wellness and disease-prevention roles for technicians. The pharmacist is now an integral part of the patient's overall well-being and disease management for diseases such as diabetes or heart conditions, and these are included in the prescription dispensing process. Technician duties also include point-of-care testing (POCT), which offers patients assistance with real-time testing such as A1c, glucose monitoring, pregnancy, drug screening, and immunizations. Many pharmacies have clinics in the stores staffed with a team of health care personnel to allow patients to obtain routine treatment and care. Technicians in many states can now administer immunizations with the proper training.

Current patient medication histories allow the pharmacy team to have accurate electronic records. Information such as disease states, immunizations, current conditions, providers, and medication are recorded and maintained, often by a technician.

For example, a patient is a smoker and has been instructed by the physician to stop. The patient may have questions about patches or other forms that best suit them. A patient with diabetes may need to purchase a meter and has no idea about which one or how to test. The technician could help choose a meter and align the strips and lancets that go with the product chosen.

Other OTC medication options is another area that patients may need assistance with in the community setting. Technicians must understand that OTC medications, and even herbals or vitamins, can have interactions with other medications being prescribed, and helping to maintain an electronic record of these is essential to a complete profile.

Do You Remember These Key Points?

- The different types of community pharmacies
- The pharmacy technician's role in the medication use process
- State laws and regulations related to receiving and screening prescription orders
- Assessing prescription orders for completeness and authenticity when receiving orders via paper or electronic systems
- Efficiently obtaining information to complete a prescription order
- Special procedures pharmacy technicians are responsible for in preparing, storing, and distributing controlled substances
- The pharmacy technician's role in preparing medications for distribution
- The process of creating a new patient profile or entering data into an existing patient profile
- Accurately counting or measuring finished dosage forms as specified by the prescription/medication order
- The protocol to assemble appropriate patient information materials
- Collecting needed information from the patient profile
- Identifying situations in which the patient requires the attention of the pharmacist
- Applying effective verbal and written communication skills, including listening skills
- Effective strategies for communicating with patients who are non–English speakers or who have other special needs, such as vision or hearing problems, a low reading level, or difficulty understanding instructions

- Using a respectful attitude with diverse patient groups
- Recognizing effective interpersonal and teamwork skills in working with health care teams
- The pharmacy technician's role in assisting in the administration of immunizations in a community pharmacy
- The purpose of monitoring a patient's medication therapy

Review Questions

Multiple Choice Questions

1. Which term refers to the name of the prescription?
   A. Inscription
   B. Subscription
   C. Superscription
   D. Signa

2. What Dispense as Written (DAW) code is assigned to a prescription for "No product selection indicated"?
   A. DAW 0
   B. DAW 1
   C. DAW 2
   D. DAW 3

3. Which of the following may be identified during a prospective drug review?
   A. Drug-disease contraindication
   B. Drug duplication
   C. Therapeutic duplication
   D. All of the above

4. Which of the following is *not* one of the patient's rights?
   A. Right patient
   B. Right drug
   C. Right price
   D. Right dosage form

5. Which of the following may a pharmacy technician not do regarding immunizations?
   A. Administer the immunization
   B. Bill the patient for the immunization
   C. Collect patient information
   D. Draw the correct amount of vaccine into the syringe

6. What does this signa mean: 1 tsp PO qid ac & hs?
   A. Take 1 teaspoonful by mouth four times a day after meals and at bedtime.
   B. Take 1 teaspoonful by mouth four times a day before meals and at bedtime.
   C. Take 1 tablespoonful by mouth four times a day before meals and at bedtime.
   D. Take 1 tablespoonful by mouth three times a day before meals and at bedtime.

7. Which of the following may a pharmacy technician *not* do in a retail pharmacy?
   A. Accept a new prescription over the telephone from the physician's office
   B. Accept a new prescription from the patient at the intake window
   C. Order medications from a wholesaler
   D. Check medications received from a wholesaler

8. Which of the following should a pharmacy technician *not* demonstrate to a pharmacy patient?
   A. Empathy
   B. Sarcasm
   C. Sensitivity
   D. Understanding

9. Which information may a pharmacist provide to a patient during counseling?
   A. Proper storage
   B. Prescription refill information
   C. Action to be taken in the event of a missed dose
   D. All of the above

10. What is adjudication?
   A. The process by which a prescription is submitted electronically to a third-party payer so that the pharmacy can be reimbursed for the medication dispensed
   B. A number assigned to a medication that indicates the drug manufacturer, drug entity, and drug packaging
   C. A number required to dispense a controlled substance
   D. A number assigned to a health care provider that allows them to be reimbursed by Medicaid or Medicare

☐ Technician's Corner

One day while you are inputting prescriptions into the pharmacy's computer system, you receive a prescription for ciprofloxacin 500 mg for a Marty Smith who lives at 11608 Happiness Lane in Washington, DC. The pharmacy technician who accepted this prescription failed to obtain the patient's birth date or telephone number. When you search the patient database, you find that you have three Marty Smiths who live at 11608 Happiness Lane in Washington, DC. One of them is 13 years of age, one of them is 45 years old, and the other one is 72 years old.

- How would you handle this situation?
- Is this medication appropriate for all three patients?
- Which of the three patients should not receive ciprofloxacin and why?
- What type of additional training should be provided to the pharmacy technician who accepted the prescription?

Bibliography

Baker DW, Parker RM, Williams MV, et al. Health literacy and the risk of hospital admission. *J Gen Intern Med*. 1998;13:791.

Center for Health Care Strategies. *Health Literacy and Understanding Medical Information Fact Sheet*. Available at: https://www.chcs.org/media/Health_Literacy_Role_of_Culture.pdf.

DAA Enterprises, Inc. *Pharmacy Management Software for Pharmacy Technicians*. 3rd ed. St. Louis: DAA Enterprises; 2018.

Davis K. *Sterile Processing for Pharmacy Technicians*. 2nd ed. St. Louis: Elsevier; 2022.

Doak CC, Doak LG, Friedell GH, Meade CD. Improving comprehension for cancer patients with low literacy skills: strategies for clinicians. *CA Cancer J Clin*. 1998;48:151-162.

Institute of Medicine (US) Committee on Quality of Health Care in America. *Crossing the Quality Chasm: A New Health System for the 21st Century*. Washington, DC: National Academies Press; 2001.

Kirsch I, Jungeblut LJ, Kolstad A. *A First Look at the Results of the National Adult Literacy Survey*. National Center for Education Statistics; 1993. Available at: https://nces.ed.gov/pubs93/93275.pdf.

Maizes V, Rakel D, Niemiec C. *Integrative Medicine and Patient-Centered Care. Commissioned for the IOM Summit on Integrative Medicine and the Health of the Public*. February 2009. Available at: http://www.nacds.org/pdfs/comm/sfc-statement-on-fy2014-budgetapril2013.pdf.

National Association of Chain Drug Stores. *Statement of the National Association of Chain Drug Stores for U.S. Senate Committee on Finance. Hearing on the President's Budget for Fiscal Year 2014*. Available at: http://www.nacds.org/pdfs/comm/sfc-statement-on-fy2014-budget-april2013.pdf.

National Council for Prescription Drug Programs. *NCPDP Health Care Identification Card Fact Sheet Pharmacy and/or Combination ID Card*. Available at: https://www.ncpdp.org/NCPDP/media/pdf/NCPDPpharmacyIdCardFactSheet.pdf.

Okeke CC, Bailey L, Medwick T. Revised USP standards for product dating, packaging, and temperature monitoring. *Am J Health Syst Pharm*. 2000;57(15):1441-1445.

Pharmacy Times. *6 Surprising Pharmacy Laws*. Available at: https://www.pharmacytimes.com/contributor/timothy-o-shea/2015/07/6-surprising-pharmacy-laws.

Pyothos F. *New Perspectives in Nonverbal Communication*. New York: Pergamon Press; 1983.

University of the Sciences in Philadelphia. *Remington: The Science and Practice of Pharmacy*. 21st ed. Philadelphia: Lippincott, Williams & Wilkins; 2005.

Weiss BD, ed. *20 Common Problems in Primary Care*. New York: McGraw Hill; 1999.

Weiss BD. *Health Literacy: A Manual for Clinicians*. Chicago: American Medical Association/American Medical Association Foundation; 2003:7.

Websites Referenced

An Overview of Aphasia. Available at: http://www.webmd.com/brain/aphasia-causes-symptoms-types-treatments.

Dysarthia. Available at: http://www.nlm.nih.gov/medlineplus/ency/article/007470.htm.

Stats At-a-Glance. Available at: http://www.npsf.org/wp-content/uploads/2011/12/AskMe3.

Statistics. Available at: https://www.nimh.nih.gov/about/organization/dar/hiv-prevention-and-care-continuum-co-morbidities-and-translational-research-branch.

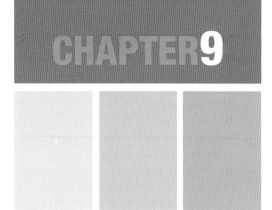

CHAPTER 9

Institutional Pharmacy Practice

Karen Davis

1. Define the most common tasks performed by hospital pharmacy technicians.
2. Identify different types of hospital pharmacy settings.
3. Discuss different hospital pharmacy standards and procedures and identify the difference between formulary and nonformulary medication lists.
4. Explain the importance of a good relationship between the pharmacy and the nursing staff.
5. Identify different regulatory agencies that govern the operations of hospitals, including pharmacies in the hospital.
6. Discuss the following related to hospital orders: (a) list various ways orders are processed by the pharmacy; (b) identify the difference among stat, ASAP, and standing orders; and (c) describe how point-of-entry (POE), computerized physician order entry (CPOE), bar code point-of-entry (BPOE), and computerized adverse drug event monitoring (CADM) systems are used in medication ordering.
7. Identify the responsibilities of an institutional pharmacy technician.
8. Describe the technician's role in the investigational new drug (IND) process.
9. Describe the advantages of using automated dispensing systems (ADSs).
10. Discuss the following related to controlled substances: (a) explain the importance of counting, dispensing, and tracking controlled substances and (b) explain what periodic automatic replenishment (PAR) levels are and who is responsible for maintaining them.
11. Identify the difference between hazardous and nonhazardous intravenous preparations and explain the importance of aseptic technique for the technician preparing compounded sterile preparations (CSPs).
12. Discuss the following related to maintaining stock and supplying specialty areas: (a) identify the duties involved in ordering and maintaining the stock levels of the pharmacy; (b) recognize the differences in floor stock, depending on the area of the hospital; and (c) identify specialty areas of the hospital for which the pharmacy stocks or orders medication.
13. Describe the importance of ongoing technician education and identify professional organizations that institutional technicians can join.

ASAP order As soon as possible but not an emergency

Aseptic technique Procedures used in the sterile compounding of hazardous and nonhazardous materials to minimize the introduction of microbes or unwanted debris that could contaminate the preparation

Automated dispensing system (ADS) Computerized cabinets and integrated systems that control inventory on nursing floors, in emergency departments, and in surgical suites and other patient care areas

Computerized physician order entry (CPOE) Computerized order entry

Crash carts Moveable carts containing trays of medications, administration sets, oxygen, and other materials used in life-threatening situations such as cardiac arrest; also known as *code carts*

Electronic medication administration record (E-MAR) A computer program that automatically documents the administration of medication into certified electronic health record (EHR) systems; the report serves as a legal record of medications administered to a patient at a facility by a health care professional

Floor stock Drugs not labeled for a specific patient and maintained at a nursing station or other department of the institution (excluding the pharmacy) for the purpose of administration to a patient of the facility

Formulary A list of drugs approved for use in hospitals by the pharmacy and therapeutics committee of the institution that have become the standard stock carried by the pharmacy and other departments

Institutional pharmacy A pharmacy in facilities in which patients receive care on site (eg, hospitals, extended-living homes, long-term care, and hospice facilities); institutional pharmacies are also found in government-supported hospitals run by the Department of Veterans Affairs, Indian Health Service, and Bureau of Prisons

Investigational drug A drug that has not been approved by the US Food and Drug Administration (FDA) for marketing but is in clinical trials; also, an FDA-approved drug seeking a new indication for use

Medication order A prescription written for administration in a hospital or institution

NKA No known allergies

NKDA No known drug allergy

Nonformulary medications Drugs that are not approved for use within an institution unless specific exceptions are filed and accepted by institutional protocols

Parenteral medication Medication that bypasses the digestive system but is intended for systemic action; the term *parenteral* most commonly describes medications given by injection such as intravenously or intramuscularly

Periodic automatic replenishment (PAR) A set level of certain medications kept on hospital floors

prn From the Latin term *pro re nata*, meaning "as needed"

Protocol A set of standards and guidelines by which a facility operates

Pyxis An automated dispensing system often used in hospitals

Satellite pharmacy A specialty pharmacy located away from the central pharmacy, such as an operating room (OR), emergency department (ED), or a neonatal pharmacy; satellite pharmacies typically are staffed by a pharmacist and a pharmacy technician

Standing order Written procedure for drug or treatment that is to be used in a specific situation

Stat order A medication order that must be filled immediately, as quickly as is safely possible to prepare the dose, usually within 10 to 15 minutes

SureMed An automated dispensing system often used in hospitals

The Joint Commission An independent, nonprofit organization that accredits hospitals and other health care facilities in the United States; the facility must be accredited to receive Medicare and Medicaid payment

Unit dose (UD) Individualized packaged doses used in institutional practice settings

United States Pharmacopeia (USP) A compendium of drug information, published annually, comprising enforceable guidelines for the safe preparation of sterile products

◉ Scenario

Marcus is employed as a certified pharmacy technician II in a 500-bed hospital. Some of his duties include picking and preparing medications, restocking supplies, delivering supplies and medications to various floors, and refilling the Pyxis machines. During the morning staff meeting the pharmacy manager explains that The Joint Commission will be visiting the pharmacy the next week. What is The Joint Commission, and what will the visit entail?

Probably one of the most challenging settings in which a pharmacy technician can work is a hospital pharmacy, also known as an **institutional pharmacy.** The dynamics of this environment can be exhilarating and exhausting, depending on the circumstances. Because there are fewer hospital pharmacies than community pharmacies, there are fewer job openings for pharmacy technicians in hospitals. However, as a result of the current changes in the pharmacist's role in hospitals, the number of highly skilled technicians needed has increased. Pharmacists once prepared all intravenous (IV) antibiotics, chemotherapy drugs, and large-volume parenteral medications, in addition to other inpatient tasks. Because of the increase in patient volume and the need for pharmacy interventions and evaluations as they pertain to patient profiles, today's pharmacists do not have time to perform many of the important tasks they did in the past. Technicians have assumed control of these tasks, which include preparing IV medications, loading patient medication drawers or **Pyxis** machines, and entering patient data into the pharmacy computer systems. This chapter outlines the daily tasks of a pharmacy technician, lists the various areas or departments of a hospital that require medication supply from the pharmacy, and describes The Joint Commission (TJC) standards relevant to pharmacy and medication use. As the health care industry changes and improves, so will the vital roles required of pharmacy technicians as they strive to provide improved health care services.

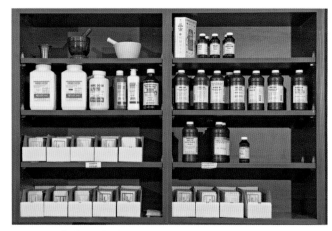

Bulk and unit dose medications in a hospital/community.

Types of Hospitals

Depending on the function of the hospital (facility), patient populations vary. The size of a hospital may be thought of in terms of the number of beds available for patient use. Many small cities or towns may have small facilities, with a capacity of 50 beds or fewer. Larger urban areas have facilities that can range from 50 to more than 250 beds. There are nonprofit and for-profit hospitals. A nonprofit hospital is a facility that does not pay either state or local property taxes or federal income taxes because it is considered a charity. Nonprofit organizations must meet certain criteria established by state and federal guidelines. A for-profit or investor-owned hospital is a facility owned by private investors or owned publicly by shareholders. For-profit hospitals issue shares of stock to raise funds for the expansion of hospital activities.

Other factors that differentiate hospitals from one another are their capabilities for diagnosis, surgery, and outpatient services. For instance, many hospitals do not have the funds to house computed tomography (CT) scanners. CT scanners use a computer that takes data from several radiographic images of structures inside the body. The multiple views create a cross-sectional image of the bones and soft tissue on the computer screen. If a facility does not have a CT scanner, patients who need such scans must be sent to another hospital to have procedures or diagnostic examinations performed.

Another important difference between hospitals is the organization of their pharmacies. Many older hospitals may have one central inpatient pharmacy that is responsible for supplying the entire hospital and all clinics. Larger hospitals and those with specialized areas may have a central pharmacy and smaller **satellite pharmacies** throughout the facility. For instance, a large teaching facility may have specialized areas of treatment, such as pediatrics, burn units, intensive care units (ICUs), investigational drugs, surgery (OR), and cancer units. Because of the large volume and specialty of the medications needed for these areas, these units may have small pharmacies that stock specific medications in both bulk and unit dose (UD) packaging (Fig. 9.1). This practice can accelerate the distribution of commonly used medications and allow the pharmacists to work directly with physicians,

nurses, and patients on an individualized basis to address specific medical problems.

Hospitals are funded by various entities. Health insurance companies and Medicare pay for services in many institutions; others are funded by donations (eg, Shriners Hospitals for Children treat children whose families cannot afford treatment in mainstream hospitals). Other institutions are managed completely by the government (eg, Veterans Affairs hospitals). Table 9.1 lists hospital facilities and types of pharmacy arrangements.

Hospital Pharmacy Settings

As mentioned, in addition to the typical inpatient pharmacy, hospitals may have other types of pharmacies that are more specialized. For instance, more hospitals are incorporating satellite pharmacies to expedite order preparation and delivery. Specialty medications can be stocked in these pharmacies, as is the case for units such as oncology, pediatrics, and intensive care. Certain hospitals interconnect inpatient and discharge pharmacies; this is an area where a technician may work with both inpatients and outpatients concurrently (Fig. 9.2).

Satellite Pharmacies

Satellites are small specialty pharmacies that supply a clinic, such as the emergency department (ED), or an entire floor of a hospital. Larger hospitals, such as teaching institutions, use satellite pharmacies because obtaining the medication from one centralized pharmacy can be too time-consuming. The number of satellites varies depending on the size of the facility, but most are small and minimally staffed. The satellites fill most of the daily medications for patients on their floors. They may be equipped with a laminar air flow workbench (LAFW) or IV hood for the preparation of parenteral products; they also are used to replace any missing medications in the automated systems or in the patients' cassette drawers. Most of the **floor stock** used by the satellites is supplied by the hospital's large central pharmacy. The pharmacist's role is to monitor regulatory compliance and oversee all medications dispensed from the particular satellite to ensure optimal

TABLE 9.1
Examples of Various Sizes and Types of Hospitals

Type	Bed Capacity	Usually One Pharmacy	Central Pharmacy and Satellites	Pharmacies Independent From One Another	Type of Care Given
Small	25–50	X			Limited, minor surgeries; critical care is temporary
Medium	50–100	X			Most surgeries, a coronary care unit, and an intensive care unit
Large	100	X	X	X	Treats most conditions; physical therapy, intensive care unit, coronary care unit; may have specialty areas such as a burn or pediatric unit
Teaching	100	X	X	X	Covers all conditions and has specialty areas for teaching purposes; trains physicians and other health care providers
Institutional	10–100	X		X	Care ranges from treating severe emergencies to continuing treatment but also may include triage to a larger facility that specializes in a particular area; found in institutions such as prisons and mental health facilities
Convalescent or long-term care	100	X			Depending on type of convalescent home, level of care may vary; some patients are sent to a hospital for surgery and recovery and then are sent back to their main residence or home

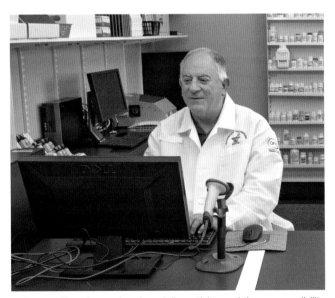

FIG. 9.2 Entering orders is a daily activity and the responsibility of the pharmacy technician.

patient care. A pharmacist working in a satellite facility must have a thorough knowledge of all medications used in that specialty setting. Technicians who work in the satellites are responsible for filling all medication orders and delivering them to the nurses' stations. Other duties include answering

phones, keeping satellites stocked, filling stat orders, preparing IV medications, replacing missing doses, and replenishing pharmacy stock.

Discharge Pharmacies

Many hospitals have a discharge and/or outpatient pharmacy that fills prescriptions in the same manner as a community pharmacy except that it is located in the institution. Physicians' orders are written on special discharge order forms that are sent to the pharmacy with other orders by fax machine, pneumatic tube, or delivery by staff. Other hospitals have designated pharmacies where patients can pick up their discharge medications. The discharge orders may be sent by the hospital computer to the outpatient pharmacy for filling. Once a discharge order has been sent, the pharmacy fills the order by the same process used in any community pharmacy. This includes determining the patient's address, phone number, and insurance coverage.

Pharmacy technicians normally process the prescription just as they would an outpatient pharmacy prescription. After the patient information has been entered into the computer system, the order is filled. All required auxiliary labels are attached before a final check by the pharmacist. Once these orders are complete, the medication can be sent back to the floor for the nurse to give to the patient; alternatively, if the drug is a controlled substance or a new medication for the patient, the nurse can transport the patient directly to the pharmacy to receive the medication and consult the pharmacist if necessary. If the orders are sent to an outpatient pharmacy, they are filled in the same manner but then placed in a holding bag for pickup. These are kept in alphabetical order according to the patient's last name. Depending on the protocol of the hospital and the location of the pharmacy, filled prescriptions may remain in the pharmacy for 3 or more days before they are returned to stock. A large hospital may have an adjacent pharmacy that functions both as a discharge pharmacy and as a community pharmacy.

Hospital Pharmacy Standards and Procedures

Policies and Standard Operating Procedures

All pharmacies have a policies and procedures (P&Ps) manual (also known as *standard operating procedures* [SOPs]). This manual contains the policies and the rules of the facility and the procedures that explain how, when, and/or why the policies are to be executed—in other words, the **protocol** of the facility. These rules apply to all pharmacy employees. Adherence to these P&Ps keeps patients safe and the P&Ps comprise the department's quality assurance and quality control plans. For example, information contained in the P&P manual concerns daily work routines and responsibilities, benefits, protocols for emergency situations, mandatory training, and other important and useful information. Technicians should be familiar with the P&P manual for their facility.

> **Tech Note!**
>
> All pharmacy employees are responsible for knowing the P&Ps and the SOPs of the pharmacy where they are employed. During your externship, be sure to familiarize yourself with the specific rules and regulations of the pharmacy by reading the P&P manual.

Hospital Protocol

Protocol also defines the guidelines within the hospital, such as the **formulary** medications (those that are approved for use) and **nonformulary medications** (those not approved). Formularies are developed by a group of physicians and pharmacists from a variety of medical specialties who do not work for the entity requiring the formulary. These group members review new and current medications to evaluate selections based on the cost, effectiveness, and safety of the drugs and patient demographics. If the recommended criteria are not met, the drug is considered nonformulary and is not included on the approved list.

These rules must be enforced and updated constantly. The Pharmacy and Therapeutics Committee—composed of pharmacists, physicians, nurses, other health care workers, and administrators—meets on a routine basis to discuss appropriate changes to the protocol. The purpose of the committee is to choose the best medicine for patients at the best cost. A drug education coordinator is a pharmacist who helps educate the health care providers about the changes in protocol concerning drug coverage and helps the hospital pharmacy implement these changes. Not all hospitals have the extra help needed to perform these duties; sometimes the tasks of the drug education coordinator may be part of the job description of staff pharmacists or the pharmacy manager.

> **Tech Note!**
>
> The abbreviation **NKA** means "no known allergies"; the abbreviation **NKDA** indicates "no known drug allergies." Both of these abbreviations are used in the pharmacy and by hospital personnel. Allergy information and any other previous history of a serious adverse drug event must be entered into the computer system before any medications can be released to the nursing floors; this information includes any specific allergies to foods, dyes, preservatives, or inactive ingredients because these allergies may also pertain to medications. Proper recording of this information in the patient's computer profile helps ensure that the patient does not experience any preventable allergic or untoward reactions. All pharmacy staff members are responsible for making sure the patient information is maintained and updated on a regular basis.

Pharmacy and Nursing Staff Relationship

The pharmacy staff probably works more with nurses than with anyone else in the hospital (Fig. 9.3). Nurses are the pharmacy's primary customers and should be given the highest level of support. They depend on the pharmacy for all their medications; they generally are responsible for more than 80% of the total calls or electronic contacts with the inpatient pharmacy. The subjects of these inquiries include the status of their patients' medications and requests for information about drug interactions, dosing ranges, and pharmacy calculations. By far the most common question asked of the pharmacy is, "Where are the medications I ordered?" Any pharmacy technician can answer this question by simply accessing the computer system to see whether the medication was sent or by checking the orders that have not yet been entered. The technician can also check the **automated dispensing system (ADS)** to see whether the stock is empty; this can be done from the main pharmacy ADS machine. All other questions should be referred to the pharmacist.

As a result of the newer technology, many facilities receive fewer phone calls and more computerized communications about missing medications. The technician can look into the ADS machine to see whether the stock is empty and fill the missing medication. The technician then can notify the nurse (by computer) that the order is being processed.

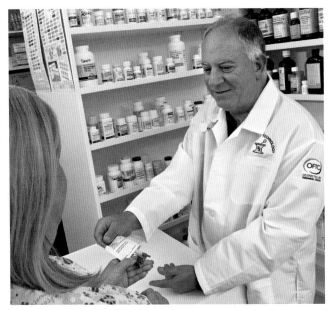

FIG. 9.3 Interaction between nurses and pharmacy staff occurs often.

Today's approach to health care is a value-based system that is determined by outcomes rather than the amount of services provided. The health care team works together to increase the patient's overall wellness through education, medication adherence, preventive testing, and changes in lifestyle. This starts with the pharmacy and nursing working together to maintain electronic records, current patient history, and discharge planning, Using ADS technology and interfacing with electronic health records (EHRs) allows each provider in the health care system to track and view a current patient history in real time.

Remember, collaboration between nurses and pharmacy teams is important to ensure that medication errors are prevented. Teamwork opens channels of communication and improves patient care.

> **■ Tech Note!**
>
> Clearly identify yourself as a technician when answering the phone. Immediately let callers know whether you can help them. This information prevents the caller from having to repeat a possibly lengthy question.

Regulatory Agencies

All hospitals must meet federal and state guidelines if they are to be reimbursed for patients who have Medicare or Medicaid insurance coverage. Various agencies, such as the US Department of Health and Human Services (DHHS), ensure that hospitals meet all standards of safe operation. Each state's board of pharmacy may inspect pharmacies to guarantee that all personnel are working within legal guidelines. The board has the authority to fine, and even close, any pharmacy that is noncompliant with current laws.

The following are some of the agencies that govern or offer voluntary accreditations for the operations of hospitals.

- **The Joint Commission**. This independent, nonprofit organization offers special certifications and accreditations to organizations willing to go through a process and pay a fee for certifications or accreditation to show quality and patient safety. TJC surveyors visit accredited health care organizations a minimum of once every 39 months (2 years for laboratories) to evaluate standards compliance. This visit is called a *survey*, and all accreditation surveys are unannounced. TJC can require compliance with applicable local rules and regulations, so it can indirectly enforce **United States Pharmacopeia (USP)** guidelines in states that have adopted USP in their pharmacy rules and regulations.
- *Centers for Medicare & Medicaid Services (CMS)*. This agency was formerly known as the Health Care Financing Administration (HCFA). It regulates and administers Medicare, Medicaid, the Children's Health Insurance Program (CHIP), the Health Insurance Portability and Accountability Act (HIPAA) standards, and several other health-related programs. The CMS inspects facilities and must give approval for hospitals to provide care and receive reimbursement for patients covered by Medicaid and Medicare.
- *Department of Health and Human Services (DHHS)*. This department is the primary agency that protects the health of the American people and provides essential human services. It includes more than 300 agencies, covering areas such as infection and disease, preventive care, and disaster preparedness.
- *Department of Public Health (DPH)*. Each state's DPH inspects hospitals and hospital pharmacies to ensure that they are in compliance with DPH regulations.
- *State Board of Pharmacy (BOP)*. Each state's BOP develops, implements, and enforces pharmacy practice standards in that state for the purpose of protecting the public. State BOPs regulate the pharmacists and pharmacy technicians that work in each hospital facility.

◉ Scenario Checkup 9.1

Marcus and the entire pharmacy staff are continually preparing for a possible TJC visit. The hospital's goal is to meet or exceed the standards outlined by TJC and to provide the highest level of patient care possible. Marcus is assigned to verify the refrigerator temperature logs. What does this duty involve and why is it important?*

Hospital Orders

Flow of Orders

When a physician visits a patient in the hospital, he or she may write a medication order for the patient. A **medication order** is a prescription written for administration in a hospital or institutional setting. Fig. 9.4 shows a visual representation

*For information about TJC's standards for medication management, see the commission's website at *https://www.jointcommission.org/resources/news-and-multimedia/blogs/ambulatory-buzz/2017/08/new-medication-management-standards-effective-jan-1-2018/.*

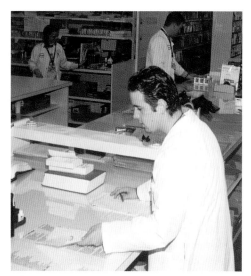

FIG. 9.4 The flow of orders. As orders arrive, they are entered into the computer. If an order is unclear or if there is a question, the pharmacist contacts the physician.

UNIVERSITY HOSPITAL AND MEDICAL CENTER

PHYSICIAN ORDER SHEET   Patient name: *Jonathan Simmons*
                         Medical Record Number: *88454959 - 2*
                         Physician: *Dr. Cynthia Gardella*

Medication or Patient Treatment

Date	Time	• Press firmly using a ball point pen • White copy remains in patient record. Fax copy to pharmacy • Do not enter antibiotics or TPN orders on this sheet
6/23/2014 1020		V.O. Dr. Gardella → C. Kipton, RN Percocet 5mg tabs ?? po Q4 hrs for pain C. Kipton, RN 1020

FIG. 9.5 Example of a physician's order. Note the medical record number in place of a prescription number. Also, the patient's room number and allergies should be listed (not shown). (Modified from Perry AG, Potter PA, Elkin MK. *Nursing Interventions and Clinical Skills*. 5th ed. St. Louis: Elsevier; 2012.)

of the flow of orders. The order is written on a physician's order sheet and is placed in the patient's chart (Fig. 9.5). The chart is a record that contains all the medical orders written by medical staff, along with nursing assessments and notes, medication administration records, laboratory results, and other vital information about the patient's admission. The chart remains in the patient care area where the patient is admitted. The unit clerk or nurse periodically checks all records for new orders that must be sent to various areas of the hospital. These include dietary restrictions to be sent to the dietary department, laboratory test requests to be sent to the laboratory, and orders for medications to be sent to the pharmacy. Pharmacists review each patient's profile and the history, progress, and laboratory values for each to monitor

the effectiveness of the prescribed medications. The physician, nurse, or unit clerk must include all the necessary information on the patient's admitting record and subsequent medication orders to ensure that the orders are filled correctly. This includes the patient's full name, date of birth, medical record number, room number, diagnosis, weight, and, of course, drug allergies.

Some hospital pharmacies are not open 24 hours a day or on weekends or holidays, whereas others are open all day, 365 days of the year. For those that are not staffed by pharmacy personnel at all times, contingent policies and regulations allow specific nursing personnel to have limited inpatient pharmacy access to obtain needed medications. In other facilities, an "on-call" pharmacist may provide the necessary services in times of less than full operation. Still other facilities may have off-site pharmacies that provide courier services to deliver needed orders.

Various methods are used to send orders to the pharmacy. **Computerized physician order entry (CPOE)** is a new technology by which the medication order is sent electronically to the pharmacy. (More detailed information on CPOE systems can be found in Chapter 14.) Another method is a pneumatic tube system that allows a person to send orders and other small items by an air-propelled tube. In this system, cylindrical canisters can carry IV bags and other medications to the hospital floor (Fig. 9.6). A disadvantage of this system is that the carrier can get jammed or the item can accidentally be sent to the incorrect department. In addition, fragile items (eg, those encased in glass), controlled substances, expensive medications, and protein-derived medications require special packaging to be sent safely by the pneumatic tube system because they can break during the rough ride. Some pharmacies may receive orders by a fax machine. Although the fax machine is an effective way to send orders to the pharmacy quickly, it is being replaced by computerized order entry.

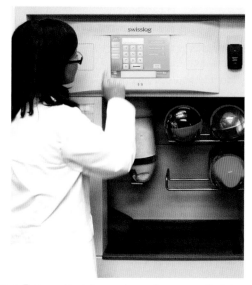

FIG. 9.6 Pneumatic tube system. A pneumatic tube system is used to transport orders to the pharmacy and medications to hospital floors. (Courtesy Swisslog Healthcare Solutions, Buchs/Aarau, Switzerland.)

Another method of transmitting physicians' orders is to have a staff member deliver the order to the pharmacy. This normally is done when a system (eg, the pneumatic tube system) breaks down or if the facility is extremely small.

Once the orders have been received in the pharmacy, they must be processed in the same way a regular prescription is processed. However, instead of using the name, address, and phone number for identification, the pharmacy uses the patient's medical record number. Even though this method is the primary way patients are identified, all information, including name and room number, should always be verified against the order. In this way, errors are reduced, especially when two patients with the same last name are on the same floor. In such a situation, the pharmacy uses name-alert stickers, which are placed on the patient's drawer and medication. Many computer systems also have name-alert functions to help distinguish between patients with similar identifying characteristics.

Most computer systems allow pharmacy technicians to enter the patient's medical record number and drug orders. In many hospitals, the pharmacist enters the order because if the information is entered by the technician, it must be checked by the pharmacist to ensure accuracy before a label is released. Many pharmacists think that the work is doubled if the technician enters an order and then the pharmacist must reread and approve the order. After an order is signed off, a printer produces a label that has the patient's name, medical record number, and room number along with the medication information. The name of the drug, strength, dosage form, route of administration, dose, quantity, and dosing interval are included on the printed label. Because the labels are produced continually, the technician usually pulls them off the printer and fills the order from the UD pick station. A variety of medication and dosage forms is always kept in stock for starter doses and for medications not stocked in the ADS.

To make sure the technician retrieves the correct medication, a bar coding system must be used. The technician uses a handheld device to scan the medication's National Drug Code (NDC) to verify that the correct item has been selected. If it is correct, the label will print and the medication can be given to the pharmacist for final verification. (For additional information on bar coding technology and regulations, see Chapter 14.) Patient drug labels should be placed so that medications can be checked visibly against the label by the pharmacist before they are placed in a pneumatic tube or taken to the patient's floor.

Stat, ASAP, and Standing Orders

Medication orders that must be filled within minutes are referred to as **stat orders.** When the pharmacy receives a stat order, it should take precedence over all other orders. Normally, a stat order can be filled in less than 10 minutes, depending on the preparation time required for the medication. Some stat orders can be filled quickly using stock off the shelf, whereas others may require special preparation, such as the mixing of a parenteral preparation. In such cases, the medication is made as quickly as possible using proper aseptic technique. Stat orders can mean the difference between life and death; they must be taken seriously. If possible, a stat order should be hand-delivered to ensure that it arrives at the correct destination safely and quickly.

An **ASAP order** is not normally as urgent as a stat order. However, these orders should be put in front of the new orders to ensure fast processing by the pharmacist. If the order has any discrepancies, it is the pharmacist's responsibility to contact either the nurse or the physician caring for the patient. Once the orders have been cleared, they are entered, verified, and sent.

Standing orders are written procedures for drugs or treatment that are to be used in a specific situation. For example, if a procedure is to be performed, a preprinted order with the list of medications to be administered is on file for the physician to use. This saves the physician from having to write the same order each time he or she performs the procedure. These also may be used in surgery cases to allow for medications to be removed from the automated medication dispensing systems while the patient is in the OR. Standing orders can include orders for **prn** (as needed) drugs that can be given in case the patient needs additional medication. A standing order may include a variety of prn medications with dosage forms, routes of administration, and dosing times that require only the physician's checkmark and signature.

Point-of-Entry Systems

Published reports from many error-prevention studies are responsible for a complete revamping of order entry. According to the 2006 Institute of Medicine report "Preventing Medication Errors," it was estimated that 1.5 million preventable medication errors occur annually in the United States alone. One major change that can counteract errors is the implementation of electronic systems that can quickly and clearly transfer patient information to and from the pharmacy. Point-of-entry (POE) systems provide electronic access to medical information and drug information data and allow physicians, nurses, and pharmacists to communicate directly with one another, limiting errors of transcription. Systems used include CPOE, IV smart pumps for infusible medications, computerized adverse drug event monitoring (CADM), and bar code point-of-entry (BPOE) medication systems. These systems are a technologic step above the previous systems, called *computers on wheels (COWs)*, which are computers on stands located at the patient's bedside. These new COW systems are used mainly in specialty units such as ICUs, where it is important that the nurse remain near the patient. However, their usefulness is limited because they do not have bar code reading abilities and are much larger than handheld devices.

Computerized Physician Order Entry

Although CPOE technology is still new and is not used in every hospital, it is becoming more popular because it eliminates the need to decipher physicians' handwriting, and the order is sent safely to the pharmacy for processing by computer entry. The Health Information Technology for Economic and Clinical Health (HITECH) Act, enacted as part of the American Recovery and Reinvestment Act of 2009, was signed into law in February 2009. It promotes the adoption and meaningful use of health information technology. After the HITECH Act Enforcement Interim Final Rule began, penalties of up to $1.5 million could be assessed for noncompliance.

With the use of CPOE, the number of errors is reduced because medication orders can be clearly identified, and the computer systems check new medications against current medications for interactions or contraindications. If an interaction is possible, the computer shows an alert icon on the screen, and the order cannot proceed until the problem is resolved. The systems may also check for proper dosage selection based on patient parameters and diagnoses. Physicians can enter all laboratory results, dietary requirements, medications, and special notes in the computer, which makes the information of all patients accessible to them at one time. Medication orders are sent directly to the pharmacy, thus eliminating the possibility of a lost order.

Bar Code Point of Entry

Nurses are now electronically connected to the pharmacy through the use of bar codes. The nurse can ensure accuracy of medication dosages at the patient's bedside before any medications are given. Each UD medication is bar coded (Fig. 9.7) and can be scanned with a handheld device. Information is linked to pharmacy and to **electronic medication administration record** (**E-MAR**) systems. The nurse is alerted to any special notes or warnings as each dose is verified for the patient. If there is any discrepancy between the current orders and the medications sent for the patient, it is detected by the scanner and the nurse is alerted to the specific problem. For example, a medication is sent to the floor

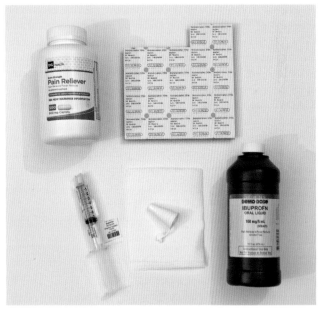

FIG. 9.7 When medications are repackaged, the pharmacy technician places each dose in a separate package and records bulk bottle information on the packaging. Medication is provided with a specific bar code and beyond-use date.

for administration, the nurse scans the tablet's bar code, and the BPOE system informs the nurse that the order has been discontinued. An error has been averted.

Orders are sent to the nurse in "real time" on the nurse's handheld device, along with any notes. Once the order has been sent to the nurse, it must be verified before administration. If there is a discrepancy, the nurse can send a note to the pharmacy for clarification. This constant communication between nurses and the pharmacy staff ultimately benefits patient care. The E-MAR is useful for documenting the patient's vital signs and other chart notes, which can be entered from the bedside directly onto the E-MAR. For example, the patient's blood pressure, respiration rate, and pain levels can be entered. The nurse's ability to verify dosages at the patient's bedside helps ensure that the Five Rights of medication safety (Right person, Right dose, Right time, Right drug, Right route) are followed, reduces the time required for charting, and creates less paperwork, so the nurse can spend more time attending to the patient.

> ### ▮ Tech Note!
>
> Every medication should be bar code scanned as part of the CPOE tracking system, and technicians have the ability to create codes if the product does not have one from the manufacturer.

Computerized Monitoring for Adverse Drug Events

CADM systems detect and monitor adverse drug events. Although pharmacy has used this type of system for years, it is now being integrated into the CPOE and EHR systems. This allows for a more comprehensive health care practice.

The overall change with the use of these new systems is not without problems. Pharmacies must make sure all medications are bar coded for identification, and the information in the computer must accurately reflect how the dosage form is to be given. The usual workflow of personnel is often affected and must adjust to accommodate the new technologies. The training of pharmacists, physicians, and nurses to use these electronic systems is a significant task and must be analyzed continually for accuracy and interactions between systems already in place. Most people find major changes in their daily routine very difficult to accept; therefore it is important to implement a system that is not too difficult to use. More hospitals are implementing these systems as new versions are developed for ease of use and accuracy.

Systems such as DoseEdge (Baxter Healthcare, Deerfield, IL) are designed specifically for the technician to prepare IV medications by using scans and bar coding of each ingredient before the final product is completed. For example, the technician is to make an IV of dextrose 100 mL with gentamicin 80 mg. Each component is scanned during the process, and the final syringe of gentamicin drawn up is verified by a pharmacist before entry into the dextrose 100-mL bag.

Institutional Pharmacy Technicians

Pharmacy technicians must have many skills in today's pharmacy; because the roles of pharmacists are continually expanding, so must the roles of the pharmacy technician. Because pharmacists now have more interaction with the proper dosing of medications and implementation of formularies, the pharmacy technician completes many of the daily tasks that were previously delegated to the pharmacist. The institutional pharmacy has many different functions that depend mostly on the size of the hospital and number of pharmacies in operation. Many hospitals have 24-hour pharmacies. Technicians need to be flexible to work all shifts, including holidays. They also need to be multifunctional because there are usually half as many technicians and pharmacists employed during night and weekend shifts in most hospital pharmacies. However, the patient load may remain the same or even increase during these times. Therefore it is essential that the technician be able to perform all the functions necessary for all shifts.

Table 9.2 outlines a variety of institutional pharmacy technician jobs and their descriptions. Because institutional pharmacies need to be staffed around the clock, it is important to have employees who can function in all areas. Technicians who are cross-trained in a variety of institutional settings become more valuable employees.

Specialty Tasks

In addition to the previously outlined tasks that technicians commonly perform, there are other duties that require the

TABLE 9.2
Job Descriptions for Institutional Pharmacy Technicians

Technician Responsibilities	Description
Chemotherapy	Prepares cytotoxic agents and other medications that may accompany these agents
Controlled substances	Gathers all controlled substance inventory sheets from all areas of the hospital; technician also may fill and deliver all controlled substances; pharmacist is required to verify pharmacy inventory daily
Discharge pharmacy	Fills prescription orders as patients are discharged from the hospital; medications are sent to the floor for patients, or patients may come to the pharmacy window to pick up medications
Filling requisitions	Fills all requisitions sent to pharmacy; stocks inventory; orders pharmacy stock; controls opioids inventory and audits opioids if required; transports medications throughout hospital facility
Inventory	Orders all medications and supplies for the pharmacy; also may order specialty items for other areas of the hospital; handles all returns and recalled items that must be sent back to the manufacturer; responsible for handling all invoices and for putting all stock in appropriate bins; rotates stock, performs nursing floor inspections, and inspects other pharmacy supply areas for outdated drugs and inventory levels; restocks these areas if necessary; this may include the operating room, postoperative area, preoperative area, and other sterile areas
IV room	Prepares all parenteral IV preparations, including large-volume drips and parenteral nutrition; prepares drugs that are under investigational trial and logs these special medications in appropriate manner as required by law
Medication reconciliation	Reviews and documents patient's arrival medication (for pharmacist review), ensuring appropriate dose, route, frequency, and duration of therapy; may review records for drug-drug interactions, duplication, and drug-allergy interactions; assists with arrival medication order entry; participates in hospital committees relevant to practice area
Miscellaneous duties	Able to work in all areas of the pharmacy as needed; answers phones, trains new technicians and pharmacist interns; works on a team with other technicians, clerks, and pharmacists
Patient medication	Fills medication drawers on a pharmacy cart that will deliver filled medications to all hospital patients; also may deliver carts to all patient areas and restock any floor stock medications; if hospital uses an automated medication dispensing system instead, technician must fill this unit on all floors; fills prescriptions for patients who will be discharged on an as-needed basis
Preparation of medication	Fills unit dosing bulk medications; compounds drugs for ointments, creams, and solutions
Satellite pharmacy	May be responsible for all tasks related to a small, isolated pharmacy, such as answering phones, ordering and putting away stock, preparing parenteral medications, transcribing and pulling all medication orders, and making deliveries to nursing stations

skills of a technician. These duties include assisting with clinical duties such as medication reconciliation assistance and anticoagulant therapy tasks.

Some hospitals have already implemented reconciliation as a way to prevent adverse drug events (ADEs). This is done at admission, transfer, and discharge intervals. Technicians can assist by performing an interview or recording the medications on specific forms before the pharmacist's review.

> **■ Tech Note!**
>
> There are opportunities for advanced positions in many facilities for medication reconciliation technicians.

Some hospitals that have nuclear medication pharmacies are using technicians to prepare these medications. These agents may be used in diagnostic procedures. Some hospitals employ investigational drug technicians. An **investigational drug** is an agent not yet approved by the US Food and Drug Administration (FDA). After a drug has finished prehuman testing, and if the results are positive, the next phase involves testing with human volunteers. The drug company must apply for permission through the FDA. The application is referred to as an Investigational New Drug (IND) application. The FDA must approve the use (through clinical trials) of an investigational drug to ensure that the patient would not be exposed to high risks. If the drug is approved, patients can apply to participate in a clinical trial. Under certain circumstances the clinical trial may be performed in the hospital.

People want to participate in a clinical trial for many reasons. Common reasons include that they have exhausted all other currently approved treatments and they think the investigational drug will be more effective than what they are currently using. Others may want to participate in the study to simply promote the future development of medicine.

Hospitals frequently treat patients with investigational drugs. Depending on the hospital, this practice may be more or less common. TJC regulations must be met, and strict protocols regulate the ordering, storing, inventory, and final disposal of the drug or drugs. All investigational drugs are delivered to the central pharmacy, where they are signed in by the pharmacist and stored separately from other drugs. Each drug has a logbook that must contain the following information:

- Drug name
- Drug strength
- Unit size
- Protocol title and numbers
- Principal investigator
- Manufacturer's lot number
- Identification
- Date dispensed
- Units and/or doses dispensed
- Stock balance
- Pharmacist's initials

The investigational drug technician assists in preparing, maintaining, monitoring, and auditing investigational drug study agents and related pharmacy documentation.

Once the study is complete, the remaining drugs are returned to the sponsor along with the log records. Copies of the records are kept by the pharmacy under "closed studies."

> **■ Tech Note!**
>
> Institutional technicians can join the American Society of Health-System Pharmacists (ASHP). This national organization has more than 40,000 members, including pharmacists, pharmacy technicians, and pharmacy students who serve patients in hospitals, health systems, and ambulatory clinics. For more information on membership, visit the society's website at *http://www.ashp.org*.

◉ Scenario Checkup 9.2

Today Marcus is busy supervising the Pyxis refills. Marcus works in a state that allows certified technicians to check the work of fellow technicians. He begins to check the cassette drawers of his co-worker, Janet. Janet is normally a very hard-working and responsible technician. Today she seems distracted. Marcus finds several errors in the drawers Janet has completed. How should he handle this situation? Do you think technicians should be allowed to check other technicians' work? Explain your answer.

Patient Cassette Drawers and/or Pyxis Machines

A long-standing daily task of pharmacy technicians is loading the patient cassette drawer from a pick station. These stations in the pharmacy can be quite extensive, depending on the hospital's needs. All UD medications are arranged in order by generic name and are located in sections that separate solid oral dosage forms, liquids, suppositories, and other miscellaneous types of medication containers. Even though pick stations can hold many medications, some patients may require medications that must be taken from the normal stock area, such as injectable dosage forms.

After a new order is received, a starter dose is sent to the floor. The medications that will be needed for the next day are loaded in the patient cassette drawer. The technician reads the daily medication record printed each morning and fills the necessary medications into the cassettes. Normally, routine medications are placed in these drawers in the front, and as-needed (prn) doses are put in the back, separated by a divider. Routine medications are taken on a schedule every day, whereas prn medications are taken only if needed. For example, most acetaminophen (Tylenol) is ordered as needed for headache or fever.

The patient cassette drawers are held in large pushcarts so they can be delivered to the various floors each day. All medications are delivered to the patient floors using two carts that are rotated daily. Before the patients' drawers are loaded with the next 24-hour supply, all previous medications are emptied from the drawer. This is done to reduce the possibility of errors. Many hospitals use a combination of patient cassette drawers and an ADS (discussed in the next section). Commonly used medications are stocked in the automated machines, whereas specialty or uncommon medication dosages are loaded in the cassettes.

One type of automated system used by large hospital pharmacies is the robot dispensing machine. It uses mechanical arms to scan bar codes on each UD medication to identify the correct dose. (Dose information is fed into the machine by computer input from the pharmacist or technician.) The machine fills each patient's medication cassette with 99% accuracy as the cassette moves along a conveyer belt. Once the order has been filled, the cassette is delivered by the technician, who returns the previous day's cassette for the next day's filling.

Although some hospitals still use the patient cassette system only, most facilities use an ADS and robotics. These systems accelerate delivery of medication to the patient and help ensure accuracy. Automated floor dispensing systems used in hospital settings include Pyxis and **SureMed.** Both Pyxis and SureMed are machines on the nursing floor that are preloaded with a variety of commonly used medications. The pharmacist need only enter the order and verify it; the nurse then can retrieve the medication on the patient's floor by using a thermal fingerprint for access. These dispensing systems require continual filling and updating, which are among the duties of properly trained technicians.

Automated Dispensing Systems

An example of an ADS is the Pyxis MedStation 4000 system (Fig. 9.8). This automated system uses a biometric user identification security system. This means the user's fingerprint is scanned and verified before the system grants the user access. Many automated systems similar to the Pyxis MedStation system rely on passwords or identification swipe cards to control access. This approach puts security at risk because the card could be given to or stolen by unauthorized personnel. The advantage of the Pyxis MedStation 4000 system is that it helps ensure the security of the system and ultimate control over access to medications. Once the fingerprint scanner verifies the user, the user can access the drawers in the station for filling or dispensing purposes according to the privileges the user is assigned.

After obtaining access to the station, the nurse selects the patient for whom he or she wants to obtain medication by touching the name of the patient and the name of the medication on the display screen. The appropriate drawer with the medication then opens. When the drawer is closed, the amount of medication removed is recorded for inventory tracking purposes. The pharmacy can generate reports that identify who accessed the station, when the station was accessed, which medication was removed, and how much of each medication was supposedly removed. This information is valuable in solving discrepancies and managing inventory.

Other products offered by the Pyxis Products division of Cardinal Health (Dublin, Ohio) include the Pyxis CII Safe system and the Pyxis Oral Solid Packager. The Pyxis CII Safe system is a controlled substance management system that creates detailed tracking and reporting for each transaction to improve inventory management. This system is separate from the Pyxis MedStation 4000 system, but the inventory

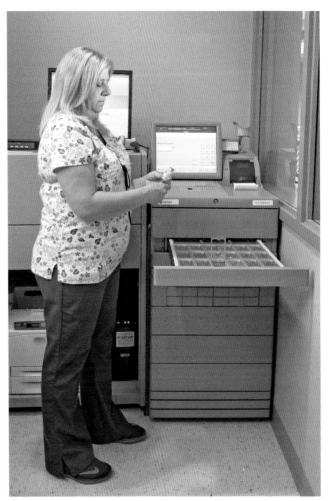

Example of a medication in unit dose form, individually packaged for dispensing.

management functions between the two systems can be integrated. The Pyxis Oral Solid Packager is an automated packager and bar code labeling system.

Most hospitals have incorporated automated dispensing machines to hold all types of stock. These containers are available in many different sizes, from countertop models to 6-foot-tall cabinets that hold tubing, large-volume IV lines, and dressings. The three main advantages of this type of cabinet are as follows:

- *Inventory control:* Inventory sheets can be generated in the pharmacy. Also, the patient can be charged exactly as each item is dispensed from the ADS machine.
- *Reduced wait time:* Nurses can directly access the patient's drugs from the ADS. No starter dose needs to be sent to the floor from the pharmacy.
- *Accuracy:* Nurses who access the ADS machines are allowed to take only the specific medication or medications ordered for their patients. In this way, an incorrect medication is less likely to be dispensed.

Several companies supply ADS machines, but all the machines operate on the same principle. The central unit is located in the pharmacy, where stock levels can be generated for any department at any time. Depending on the size and activity of the hospital, stock levels may have to be replenished once daily or several times a day. PAR levels are predetermined for each drug. When the count is lower than the PAR level, the technician can pull the amount needed to restore the original count. All orders must be checked against the pull list before delivery by either a qualified technician or a pharmacist. All opioids are kept in drawers that are physically separated from other medication, although all medications are open for removal when the main drawer opens. Box 9.1 lists various manufacturers of ADS machines and their websites.

Larger facilities may receive daily stock from an electronically produced inventory sheet that is sent to the distributor, such as Cardinal Health. For example, Cardinal Health pulls every UD ADS medication, identifies the intended location on each bag, and sends the bags to the hospital each day at a specific time. The pharmacist checks the order, and the technician merely needs to fill the ADS machines. This saves time for the technician because only a fraction of each drawer needs to be filled.

Unit Dose Medications

Another important daily task technicians perform is the preparation of **unit dose (UD)** medications that are not available from the manufacturer or stocked by the pharmacy. Although many premade UD containers are available from manufacturers, not all drugs are available in UD form. In other cases, the hospital may prefer to make its own UD packaging because it can be less expensive and the hospital can make specific amounts to reduce waste (see Fig. 9.8).

Technicians are responsible for determining which medications need to be made based on the use of stock by patients, documenting all necessary information per protocol, and preparing the doses. The final check is done by the pharmacist. Bulk bottles of medication are pulled from stock shelves and made into UD oral syringes and other dosage forms. Many different types of methods and machines can aid in the preparation of UD medications (see Chapter 11). Only medications used on a regular basis are made into UDs. For uncommon medication orders or unusual dosage strengths, the technician must prepare individual dosages as patient needs arise.

Unit Dose Liquids

In the past, bulk liquid items were sent to the floor for several days' use. For example, if a physician ordered Mylanta 15 mL five times daily, the pharmacy would send an 8-oz bottle that would stay on the patient's floor until empty. This minimized the need to place several UD cups in a small cassette drawer. As a result of new standards implemented to reduce drug errors (see Chapter 14), TJC now requires hospitals to make all medications specific to the patient's dose. This means that every liquid dose must be prepared in a UD package and labeled before it is sent to the patient's room. A hospital may have a separate room dedicated to the preparation of all oral liquid medications and may use oral syringes to prepare each dose. Other pharmacies may make all their own UD cups from their bulk stock; this would be done by a technician following repackaging guidelines outlined in Chapter 11.

Controlled Substances

The task of counting, dispensing, and tracking controlled substances is a critical job that requires perfection. Many hospitals use pharmacy technicians to restock and fill opioids for the entire hospital. In each hospital unit that stocks controlled substances, two nurses must conduct an actual count before the beginning of each shift. Therefore all controlled substances are counted two or three times daily, depending on the length of a nursing shift. One nurse counts the controlled substances while the other nurse confirms the count on the controlled substance sheet or on the ADS record. If the opioids are documented on paper, the count is transferred to a new inventory sheet each morning and the last day's sheet is sent to the pharmacy for filing. PAR levels are written at the top of the controlled substance sheets, identifying the amounts of medications that should be kept on the floor at all times. Often the technician is responsible for retrieving these sheets daily from all units and beginning assessment of how many controlled substances of various sizes and strengths must be provided to keep the unit at its PAR level. If ADS machines are used, a PAR list is generated daily that records the current count of opioids. Opioids that are not being used may be returned to the pharmacy at the time of delivery.

In the pharmacy, controlled substances are normally kept in a locked room or vault, which may be under surveillance. All written records must be in pen. A registered pharmacist must verify all inventories.

Each hospital has its own system for delivering controlled substances, but one of the most important aspects is to keep the controlled substances nonidentifiable. For example, hospitals without ADS units might place controlled substances in brown paper bags that are stapled shut; most people would never suspect that controlled substances were being delivered in this type of package. Even so, the pharmacy technician should never let these controlled substances out of sight when delivering them throughout the hospital. Other hospitals may have lockboxes for opioids delivery.

After the technician has confirmed the pharmacy's controlled substances count for the day, he or she must sign out each drug onto a dispensing sheet that is used to deliver the controlled substances. A pharmacist must check all opioids before they leave the pharmacy. A pharmacist must also verify all final counts. Monthly or bimonthly inventories are taken, depending on state regulations.

All controlled substances are signed into the nursing department by adding them to the department's controlled substances sheet. A technician and nurse must observe the addition or return of stock. State laws vary as to which nursing staff (RNs or LPNs) can sign in controlled substances. All controlled substances then must be countersigned onto or off of the pharmacy inventory sheet by both the technician and the nurse. The nurse and pharmacy technician should perform an actual count of the current levels of controlled substances to verify all existing controlled substances before adding additional ones into stock. In addition to delivering controlled substances, the technician may be asked by the nurse to return certain substances to the pharmacy. The same validation system is used to enter onto the pharmacy inventory sheet any drugs that are to be returned to the pharmacy.

An ADS machine verifies the count as the technician enters the narcotic to be added. An electronic record is maintained that includes the time the drawer was accessed, the name of the person accessing the drawer, the count before opening the drawer, the amount added or deleted, and the final count. In many hospitals, an RN is still required to countersign on the delivery sheet to verify that it is the correct drug and the correct beginning and ending inventory, in addition to the correct ADS station. All additions and deletions are documented by the ADS machine, which shows who opened the cabinet, when the cabinet was opened, and in which drawer the additions or deletions were made. The technician must count first, then add or remove items, and then recount afterward. Only one type of narcotic dosage form is allowed per drawer container. The stock is put into the ADS, and a receipt is printed. This verification receipt is taken to the pharmacy and kept in the narcotic count area.

When returned to the pharmacy, all controlled substances must be signed back into the pharmacy stock, along with the receipt from the ADS if one has been used. This normally is done by a technician and verified and countersigned by a pharmacist. One of the most important parts of this job is to verify that all numbers are correct. The pharmacist must never sign in controlled substances without first visually counting the existing and returned stock.

Opioids are normally filed in stock under their generic names and by their schedule. All controlled substances are confined in the same area. Binders may be used to keep

inventory of each drug. As stock is removed, the amount is taken off the inventory sheet, and the remainder must be counted and correct. Certain scheduled drugs are also stored in a refrigerator, and in the pharmacy a small refrigerator is often kept in the locked room or vault for this purpose. Nursing units have a lockbox in their medication refrigerator for scheduled drugs.

◉ Scenario Checkup 9.3

Marcus continues preparing for TJC's visit. His pharmacist has asked him to look over the controlled substance logs to check for any errors or irregularities. He also must do a count of the current controlled substance inventory along with the supervising pharmacist. During the review, Marcus finds that one particular technician had an unusually high number of accesses to the controlled substance drawer. What could this mean? What precautions should Marcus take during this review?

Intravenous Preparations

At certain intervals throughout the day, IV labels representing all current orders are printed from the computer system. All changes in IV medication information are kept updated by the technician and the pharmacist who work in the IV room. Only specially trained and properly garbed pharmacy personnel are allowed into the clean room.

Normally, the technician labels all premade IV antibiotics and other IV medications and the pharmacist answers the phones and enters new and changed orders. Pharmacists are also responsible for contacting the nurse or physician if a problem arises with an order. For example, if an order is sent to the pharmacy for ampicillin/sulbactam (Unasyn) and the patient is allergic to penicillin, the pharmacist contacts the physician and asks the physician to replace this antibiotic with one that will not cause an allergic reaction.

Orders in an inpatient pharmacy are affected by the time of day. For example, in the early morning several preoperative (preop) medications may be ordered, and later in the morning postoperative (postop) medications may be ordered for surgical patients. Also, more diagnostic examinations are performed in the morning or afternoon hours than in the evening. Medications that are required for these diagnostic tests usually must be sent by the pharmacy.

The pharmacy technician is responsible for stocking the IV room with all the supplies needed for the day. The technician also must make sure the work area stays clean. Usually the same technician prepares all IV medications, and at the end of the shift, he or she delivers them to the nursing floors. When the IV medications are delivered to the nursing stations, the unused IV medications are returned to the pharmacy. If they have not expired, they are placed in the refrigerator or back into stock for future use; otherwise, they are logged and discarded properly according to pharmacy policy. Because each IV preparation must be registered and justified, most pharmacies keep a binder or book in which information about all wasted IV preparations is written. Technicians must remember that it is important to complete all tasks before the end of the shift and to replace all stock items as best they can for the next shift.

Aseptic Technique

Aseptic technique is a set of guidelines and procedures used to prevent the contamination of an object by microorganisms. Use of this technique is important in the preparation of all IV medications, IV nutrition solutions, chemotherapy products, and compounded ophthalmic medications. All personnel preparing sterile preparations must be tested periodically on the proper guidelines of aseptic technique; this usually is done by management at the yearly evaluation. Samples normally are taken from a newly prepared parenteral medication and are sent to the laboratory for testing, or media fill kits may be used to test on site. This testing is performed to ensure that microbial contamination is not present in medications that must be sterile. Aseptic technique is discussed in detail in Chapter 12.

Nonhazardous Intravenous Preparation

An IV technician is responsible for preparing various **parenteral medications.** Parenteral medications bypass the digestive system and are intended for quick systemic action. Parenteral medications are given by injection using the intramuscular or IV route. This includes piggyback antibiotics, large-volume IV solutions (eg, sodium chloride, dextrose, amino acid infusions), and other parenteral medication orders. Some hospital pharmacies are responsible only for the large volumes of IV medications that must be prepared with special additives; the nurses on the floor maintain a floor stock of premade, large-volume bags that can be supplied by central supply or by the pharmacy. Typical antibiotics and other IV admixtures can be prepared in a horizontal laminar flow hood after the proper personnel cleansing procedures and garbing order have been followed (Procedure 9.1).

IV preparation areas are required to have a clean room outside the compounding area that meets federal standards. These clean rooms buffer the IV admixture room and allow preparation of IV labels and stock to be maintained in a clean yet separate area. They also must meet USP standards. Only the necessary supplies should be carried into the buffer room, and the room must be cleaned with specific cleaning solutions and devices.

Many hospitals cannot convert their compounding areas to USP standards; therefore they have begun to contract out the bulk of their IV preparations to USP-certified compounding pharmacies. The policies vary from hospital to hospital.

Horizontal laminar air flow hoods are cabinets that direct filtered air horizontally toward the opening of the cabinet,

Procedure 9.1

Personnel Cleansing and Garbing Order for Sterile Compounding

Goal

To learn the steps required to cleanse and garb up to properly prepare compounded nonhazardous sterile preparations (CSPs).

Equipment and Supplies

- Antiseptic hand cleanser
- Face mask or eye shield
- Head and facial hair cover
- Nonshedding gown
- Shoe cover
- Sterile powder-free gloves
- Surgical scrub

Procedural Steps

1. Remove all personal outer garments.
   PURPOSE: Outer garments such as jackets or coats may have shedding fibers or hairs that could contaminate the compounding area.
2. Remove all cosmetics and jewelry (no artificial nails are allowed).
   PURPOSE: Cosmetics can flake off and jewelry and artificial nails can have dirt and other debris on and under the surface. These contaminants can be carried into the compounding area if not removed.
3. Put on personal protective equipment (PPE) in the following order:
   a. Shoe covers
   b. Head and facial hair covers
   c. Face masks/eye shields

   PURPOSE: Shoe covers help prevent any germs that may be on your shoes from entering the compounding area. Head and facial hair covers are used to keep any hairs from falling into the compounding area. Face masks and eye shields are used to protect the technician from exposure to medications that may splash or may accidentally spill during the compounding process.
4. Perform aseptic hand cleansing procedures with a surgical scrub.
   PURPOSE: Proper hand washing with a surgical scrub helps lessen the bacteria found on the hands before beginning the compounding process.
5. Put on a nonshedding gown.
   PURPOSE: A nonshedding gown serves to prevent any contaminants that may be on the technician's clothes from getting into the compounding area. Most gowns are resistant to penetration by moisture, which helps protect the technician if a spill occurs.
6. Put on the sterile powder-free gloves.
   PURPOSE: Gloves protect the compounding area from the skin that is constantly shedding from our hands. They also protect the technician from exposure to medications that may be used in the compounding process. Double gloving is recommended when hazardous drugs or chemicals are being compounded.

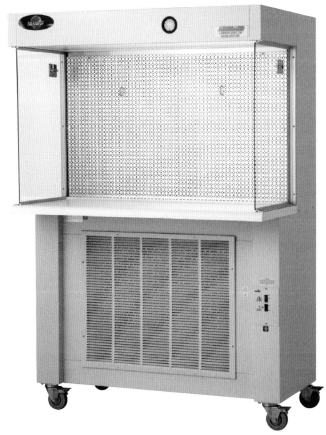

FIG. 9.9 Horizontal laminar flow hood clean bench (Airegard 301). (Courtesy NuAire, Plymouth, Minn.)

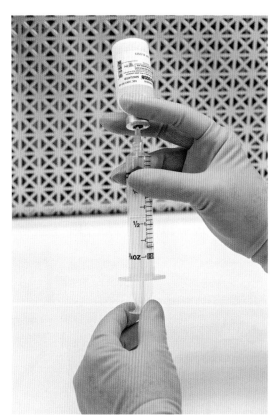

FIG. 9.10 The technician must ensure that his or her hands are not blocking the required air flow.

which provides a sterile environment for preparing parenteral medications (Fig. 9.9). There are other types of hoods, such as partially covered vertical hoods and biological safety cabinets (BSCs). Each type meets specific environmental requirements. (For more information on flow hoods and their uses, see Chapter 12.)

A horizontal flow hood or LAFW is used for preparing non-hazardous IV medications. A high-efficiency particulate air (HEPA) filter is located at the back of the hood. When the technician is working inside the horizontal flow hood, the orientation of the hands must not block the flow of first air. First air is the air issuing directly from the HEPA filter. This means that hands cannot be moved between the vial, needle, or IV bag and the first air (Fig. 9.10). Blocking the flow of first air can allow contamination of the preparation. Technicians must practice and master proper aseptic technique. Nonhazardous IV preparations can also be made by robotic systems.

The hospital technician may be responsible for preparing chemotherapeutic medications. The same aseptic techniques are used in preventing contamination when preparing any parenteral medication. However, a few differences between the IV and chemotherapy environments should be noted. All chemotherapy compounds are prepared within a vertical flow hood BSC, glove box, or a compounding aseptic containment isolator (CACI).

USP regulations state that compounding should take place in an International Standards Organization (ISO) class 8 or better clean room. There are different levels of clean rooms. The ISO ranks clean rooms as ISO class 1 (the cleanest) through ISO class 9. The lower the ISO rating, the cleaner the environment. Contamination is measured by particle count. HEPA filters capture the contaminated particles. An ISO class 8 environment means that the filter captures 3,520,000 parts per cubic meter that measure greater than 0.5 mcg.

There also must be an anteroom for gowning and degowning and movement of personnel into and out of the clean room. Additionally, a hood known as the primary engineering control providing an ISO class 5 or better environment must be used to perform compounding activities.

Building and operating a clean room can be expensive and may not be in the budget for smaller hospitals. Fortunately, glove box isolators (or barrier isolators) can now be added to comply with USP requirements.

There are different classes of glove boxes, but they are all based on the same principle, that all medication preparation is performed in a closed, sterile environment (Fig. 9.11). Glove boxes have been found to reduce the possibility of contamination, which is a major concern in error prevention. All materials are placed in a side cabinet attached to the main cabinet and then transferred into the main cabinet for preparation. The hood must be cleaned both before and after each use with special cleaning cloths and 70% isopropyl alcohol. Guidelines for proper use and cleaning are provided by the manufacturer.

Glove boxes can be used for higher risk IV admixtures per USP regulations. Air is filtered through a HEPA filter and

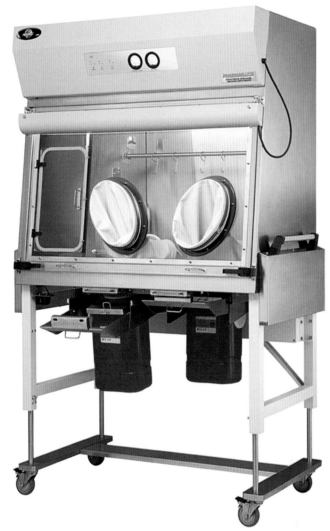

FIG. 9.11 Glove box for IV admixture (Pharmagard 797). (Courtesy NuAire, Plymouth, Minn.)

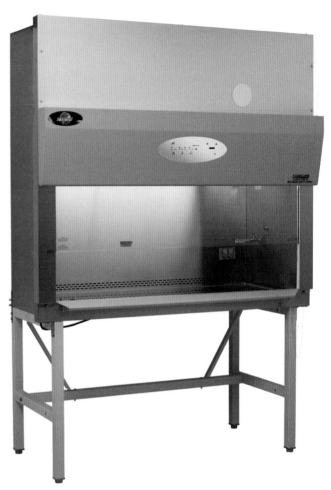

FIG. 9.12 Biological safety cabinet with vertical flow hood (Labgard 437). (Courtesy NuAire, Plymouth, Minn.)

then through a final HEPA filter before it is exhausted to the outside of the facility (not into the work area). The technician never directly contacts the medication while manipulating it in the hood. This is a closed system, unlike the partially shielded vertical flow hood or horizontal flow hood. In a glove box the air flow is also vertical; therefore hands must not move over the top of any vial, needle, or IV bag. If the hands do move into these areas, aseptic technique has been broken. Regardless of which hood is used, it is most important that aseptic technique is always practiced (see Chapter 12).

Hazardous IV preparations follow the USP 800 guidelines and in some facilities can be made by robotic systems such as CYTOCARE. The BSC (see Fig. 9.6) is the proper hood to use in a room with negative air pressure. Personnel who handle hazardous drugs must follow specific guidelines, including proper garbing attire, disposal of used supplies, delivery, and techniques.

BSCs are partially open front vertical air flow hoods used to prepare chemotherapeutic agents (Fig. 9.12). The air is pulled down toward the tabletop filter from the ceiling of the hood, which contains the first HEPA filter. The chemotherapy hood does not allow the air to leave the container compartment; instead, the air is recycled through a second HEPA filter that removes any particulate matter before the air is recirculated into the work environment. The flow of air vertically helps protect the person preparing the agents from unwanted exposure. To maintain sufficient air flow, hands should not move over or above the items in the vertical flow hood. Technicians must follow the standard personnel cleansing and garbing regulations, with a few extra precautions. For safety, a special impervious chemotherapy gown must be worn, along with eye protection and double gloves (latex or nonlatex) or special chemical safety gloves (nitrile or neoprene rubber and polyurethane). The first pair is worn under the wrist cuff of the gown and the second pair is pulled over the wrist cuff of the gown.

▽ **Tech Alert!**

Safe practices recommend that gloves used to prepare chemotherapeutic agents should not be worn longer than 30 minutes. Hands must always be washed before and after removal of gloves.

◎ Scenario Checkup 9.4

Today Marcus is working in the IV compounding area. He receives an order for intravenous immunoglobulin (IVIG) for Ms. Wallace, who comes in once a month to the outpatient care unit. Marcus knows that this is a very expensive medication, and he has never compounded it before. How should he approach this challenge? What makes this IV preparation different from most compounded sterile preparations (CSPs)?

Labeling

The proper placement of labels is important to ensure visibility of the parenteral solution and contents (Fig. 9.13). All labels must be placed squarely onto the medication and should be clear and easy to read.

The technician must initial all medications, even if the label is placed on a premade bag. Before IV piggybacks and drips are delivered to the appropriate floors, the pharmacist must check each medication and countersign with his or her initials. Labels usually contain the same type of information regardless of the facility. In addition to labeling parenteral medications, the technician must be aware of additional information, such as medications that need to be placed in light-protected bags and those requiring refrigeration. The technician must know the storage requirements and the stability of the medications he or she prepares.

▽ Tech Alert!

Gloves must be surface cleaned before you wipe down the final preparation, place the label on the preparation, and move the preparation to the pass-through area for removal from the sterile parenteral preparation room. The inner pair of gloves (for preparing chemotherapeutic agents) is used to affix labels and place the agent in a sealable containment bag for transport; this must be done within the BSC. You must put on a new pair of gloves before handling the completed preparation to avoid any exposure to the agent by yourself or others.

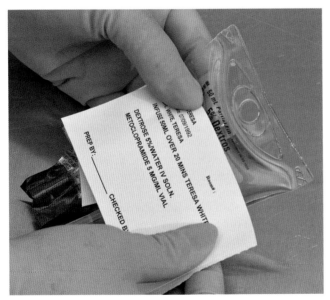

FIG. 9.13 Proper placement of any type of labeling should never cover the actual drug information.

All drugs must be labeled before they leave the pharmacy. The required parts of a label include the patient's name, patient's medical record number and room number, name of the drug, strength of the medication, name of the solution with which the medication was mixed, and the rate of infusion. The pharmacy technician must check this information several times before he or she applies the label to the medication. Additional information on a label includes the time the dose should be given, the date, and the expiration date. Expiration dates are important because many IV preparations are returned to stock if not expired.

Several references can provide stability information:
- *Trissel's Stability of Compounded Formulations*
- *Trissel's Handbook of Injectable Drugs*
- *USP Dispensing Information*
- *Journal of Pharmaceutical Sciences*
- *American Journal of Health-System Pharmacy*
- *Remington: The Science and Practice of Pharmacy*

Beyond-use dating is described in the USP as consisting of two components: chemical stability and microbial sterility. Storing a compounded sterile preparation for an extended period before use creates the potential for microbial growth and pyrogen formation. Therefore the risk level is based on the duration of storage.

When IV preparations are delivered to the floor, the technician checks the remaining supplies for unused medications. If the preparation was not used, it is picked up by the pharmacy at the time of the daily delivery and returned to stock for later use. IV preparations that have expired are logged into a log book. The solution is emptied (normally into the sink) and the Viaflex bag is disposed of in the garbage. Viaflex bags are made of flexible polyvinyl chloride (PVC). If the drug removed from the bag is a potential environmental hazard or biohazard, it must be disposed of according to certain regulations. These regulations vary by state and local requirements and also by rules established by federal agencies, including the FDA, Environmental Protection Agency (EPA), Department of Transportation (DOT), and Occupational Safety and Health Administration (OSHA). The technician should always be familiar with the disposal regulations of the facility before emptying any medications into sewage systems.

Maintaining Stock and Supplying Specialty Areas

In several areas of a hospital the pharmacy must maintain a PAR level of medications. Technicians must recognize each of the abbreviations representing the units and clinics that require medication from the pharmacy (Box 9.2). The supplies kept on hand in these units are referred to as *floor stock*. The technician must be fully aware of the types of medications used in each of these areas because each unit, ward, or clinic has its own special stock. Because of the special needs of each area, many pharmacies have special forms that are preprinted with complete descriptions of commonly used drugs. This helps reduce the incidence of stock being sent to the wrong areas in the hospital. The pharmacy normally receives the supply ordering forms from the specialty areas daily. Although they are not a high-priority task, these orders

BOX 9.2 Examples of Primary Units and Areas That Require Medication From the Pharmacy

CCU	Coronary care unit
Clinics	Patients may visit a clinic to be seen by a physician, physician's assistant, or nurse practitioner
ED or ER	Emergency department; area of hospital where patients can receive emergency care; physicians and nurses are on staff 24 hours a day
ICU	Intensive care unit
L&D	Labor and delivery; unit where a woman goes through labor and delivers a baby
MED-SURG	Medical unit for patients who have undergone surgery or who may be under observation
NICU	Neonatal intensive care unit; can also stand for neurologic intensive care unit
NSY, NUR	Nursery; unit where babies are taken for care and observation by nurses
OB/GYN	Obstetrics/gynecology; unit that takes care of expectant mothers or those who have just given birth
ONCOLOGY	Unit that takes care of patients with cancer
OR	Operating room
ORTHO	Orthopedics unit; takes care of patients who may need treatment or surgery on bones or joints
PACU	Postanesthesia care unit
PED	Pediatrics; unit for children younger than age 14 years
POSTOP	Unit where patient is kept after an operation or procedure
PREOP	Unit where patient is kept before an operation or procedure
UROLOGY	Unit that takes care of patients who may need treatment, surgery, or procedures on the urinary system

should be filled before the end of the day. In addition, the technician may need to deliver the medications and check various areas of the hospital for any outdated medications. This task should be done monthly, preferably before the end of the month. Outdated medications normally can be returned to the pharmacy if they will expire within 3 months. Expired medications may be returned to the manufacturer for credit (most manufacturers accept returned expired medications in batches of 100), or they may be taken by an independent company and destroyed in a proper manner. This depends on the contract between the hospital and the manufacturer. Some hospitals contract with an outside company that specializes in drug inventory to visit the pharmacy periodically and document all expired medications before they are destroyed.

Each department (eg, preoperative, postoperative, operating room, wards, and clinics) is stocked with specific medications, depending on the type of services it provides. Because of the many different areas throughout a hospital, the pharmacy must stock a wide variety of medications in different dosage forms. Therefore the pharmacy technician must have a good understanding of which medications are appropriate for each department. Departments such as the ED, OR, and ICU stock many drugs in injectable form and a wide variety of oral and injectable controlled substances. The pediatrics department uses many of the same medications used in the other departments except in smaller doses and medications in special pediatric dosage forms. The labor and delivery department stocks injectables and other drugs used for women in labor, contractions, and cesarean births. The tasks of collecting and filling all floor stock medications are part of the daily routine of a technician. As always, it is necessary that all orders be verified and initialed by a pharmacist before they can be delivered to the correct departments unless the tech-check-tech process has been approved under hospital protocol.

▽ Tech Alert!

In refilling a crash cart, *never* assume that the unused drugs left inside the tray are correct. A prime example is the common error of failing to differentiate between pediatric and adult strengths of lidocaine. As another example, epinephrine is always stocked on a crash cart. Both adult and pediatric strengths are packaged in prefilled syringes, and they have a similar appearance. *Note: the dose of pediatric-strength epinephrine (1:1000 [1 mg/mL]) is an order of magnitude different from adult-strength epinephrine (1:10,000 [0.1 mg/mL]). Placing adult-dose epinephrine into a pediatric tray is a common error. If that should occur, it could cause a death rather than save a life.* Always remove all medications and start anew. Following the prepared list, check all the strengths of the medications and their expiration dates.

Emergency Carts

Another important pharmacy task is the refilling of emergency carts, or **crash carts.** These are trays used by all areas of the hospital. They contain injectable medications used for a code situation (eg, cardiopulmonary distress) (Fig. 9.14). Each hospital has a set of codes (Box 9.3). It is the responsibility of each employee to know the hospital's code names. The naming of the code varies from hospital to hospital. Table 9.3 lists examples of the types of injectable drugs commonly used on crash carts. The pharmacy stocks extra trays in case of a stat call for another tray. The three types of trays are adult, pediatric, and neonatal. Each type of tray contains a different strength of drug. When a tray has been used, the pharmacy technician takes a new tray, retrieves the used tray, and refills the missing contents. Also at this time the technician checks expiration dates on all medications. These dates are listed on a preprinted form. All crash cart medications

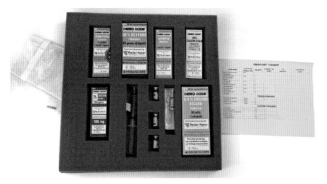

FIG. 9.14 Emergency medication tray (crash cart tray).

▣ TABLE 9.3
Commonly Used Crash Cart Medications and Their Classification

Medication	Classification/Indications	Common Dosage Forms Stored on Cart
Adenosine	Antiarrhythmic	Vial
Amiodarone	Antiarrhythmic	Ampule, vial
Atropine sulfate	Anticholinergic	PFS
Calcium chloride	Electrolyte	PFS
Dextrose	Carbohydrate	IV solution bags[a]
Dextrose 50%	Carbohydrate	PFS
Digoxin	Cardiac glycoside	Ampule
Dobutamine	Vasopressor	Vial
Dopamine	Vasopressor	Vial, IV bag[a]
Enalapril	ACE inhibitor	Vial
Epinephrine	Vasopressor	PFS
Furosemide	Loop diuretic	Vial
Glucagon	Glucose-elevating agent	Vial
Heparin	Anticoagulant	IV bag,[a] vial
Lidocaine	Antiarrhythmic	PFS, IV bag[a]
Magnesium sulfate	Electrolyte	Vial
Mannitol	Osmotic diuretic	Vial, IV bag[a]
Metoprolol	Beta-blocker	Ampule
Naloxone	Narcotic antagonist	Ampule
Nitroglycerin	Antianginal	Vial
Nitroprusside	Antihypertensive	Vial
Norepinephrine	Vasopressor	Ampule
Procainamide	Antiarrhythmic	Vial
Propranolol	Beta-blocker	Vial
Sodium bicarbonate	Alkalinizing agent	PFS
Sodium chloride	Electrolyte	Vial, IV solution bags[a]
Vasopressin	Vasopressor	Vial
Verapamil	Calcium channel blocker	Vial

[a]IV bags may be kept in a drawer different from the medication tray.
ACE, Angiotensin-converting enzyme; *IV,* intravenous; *PFS,* prefilled syringe.

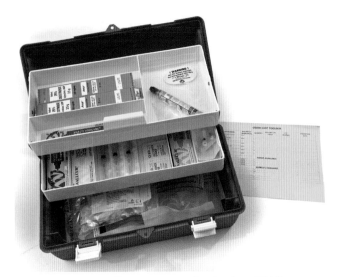

FIG. 9.15 Emergency medication box (EMS).

BOX 9.4 Special Departments Stocked by the Pharmacy

Anesthesia	Physicians or nurse anesthesiologists administer medications used before and throughout surgery
Injection clinic	Nurses administer adult and pediatric immunizations and may also perform allergy skin tests
Radiology or imaging department	Technicians and physicians may administer dyes for imaging and may need to use a medication cart (known as a *crash cart*) for adverse reactions or incidents
Respiratory	Therapists administer breathing treatments to hospitalized or clinic patients

should always be placed in the tray in the same order. The familiar order enhances the ability of nurses and physicians to quickly grab a needed medication. If all crash carts were in a different order, the nurse would have to search for the life-saving medication. As always, it is necessary that all orders be verified and initialed by a pharmacist before they can be delivered to the correct departments. All crash carts are wrapped in a perforated plastic bag or assigned a lock, which is broken at the time of use. Each lock is imprinted with a number controlled by the pharmacy, and the location of every crash cart is documented.

In addition to filling crash carts or trays for hospital use, the department may be responsible for the emergency boxes used by EMS once a call has been completed. The box is brought to the pharmacy for replenishment (Fig. 9.15).

Supplying Nonclinical Areas

Nonclinical areas of a hospital can include areas that a patient never sees or areas that are used as temporary patient care areas. Some examples of these special areas of the hospital, along with the types of medications the pharmacy may be responsible for ordering and stocking, are presented in Box 9.4.

◉ Scenario Checkup 9.5

Today Marcus and Janet are preparing to update all the crash carts. TJC will be checking for accuracy and any outdated medications. While filling the crash cart, Marcus notices that Janet has the correct medication but she is putting it into the tray in a different order than usual. When he discusses this with Janet, she becomes defensive and insists that her order is correct. What should Marcus do next? What are the dangers associated with this situation?

Central Supply

Another area that stocks supplies for the hospital is central supply. Usually boxes of large-volume IV preparations and mixtures are kept here, in addition to dressings, tubing, and

instruments used by various departments. The pharmacy orders stock normally on a daily basis from central supply. The type of stock ordered includes sterile water and various strengths of solutions, such as premade potassium chloride (KCl) bags or lactated Ringer's solution. These are supplied in case-size boxes that can weigh almost 15 lb each. They are ordered early in the morning and are delivered within a few hours. It is the responsibility of the stock person to ensure that all stock was delivered. The parenteral technician normally obtains his or her order from the stock delivered and restocks the pharmacy's IV room. At the end of the day, the stock for the next day must be ordered by contacting the order clerk. Drugs are not stocked in central supply; they must be ordered directly from the manufacturer or distributor.

The Future of the US Health Care System

Since early 2020 the COVID-19 pandemic has changed the health care system significantly. The focus on improving the individual's overall health is even more critical. Chronic conditions such as heart disease, diabetes, obesity, and respiratory illnesses have proven to show the importance of a preexisting disease affecting recovery. Technicians can play an important role in assisting pharmacists with identifying risk factors, providing immunizations, and documenting medication histories. Telehealth and virtual physician care allows patients to receive medical care closer to home. Programs such as "hospital at home" utilize trained technicians as part of the team.

Value-based care allows for teams and innovative approaches to include increasing numbers of trained technicians in the workforce. The ASHP Pharmacy Practice Model Initiative (*http://www.ashpmedia.org/ppmi/*) recognizes pharmacy technicians as a cornerstone of the future of pharmacy practice. This initiative recommends increased educational requirements for technicians to prepare them for expanded roles and increased responsibilities. The benefits of technician education are numerous. Technicians play an integral role in the institutional pharmacy practice. With continuing education, they become more engaged in their work, which leads to better accountability and greater job satisfaction. The technician who has experience in many different settings and a broad knowledge of pharmacy practices will be in high demand.

● Technician Profile

Dana is a pharmacy technician manager and recruiter for a large teaching hospital. She is certified with the Pharmacy Technician Certification Board (PTCB) and has 10 years of experience as a technician. She holds a bachelor's degree in health care administration and an associate's degree in pharmacy technology. Her job is to provide operations management and support to specialized areas. In this position, she worked to develop a career ladder for technicians that allowed for increased pay for advanced education and training. Dana supervises the new-hire orientation process and is responsible for overseeing the technician schedules for 10 different pharmacies in the hospital complex. She works side by side with many dedicated pharmacists who support and encourage advanced roles for technicians. Dana believes that broadening the responsibilities of pharmacy technicians is a critical component to improving patient care and safety.

Do You Remember These Key Points?

- The different types of hospital pharmacies and what differentiates them from one another and how that affects the overall services they may provide
- What an SOP and a P&P include
- The difference between formulary and nonformulary medication lists
- The importance of a good relationship between the pharmacy and the nursing staff
- Which agencies monitor hospitals, including pharmacies in the hospital
- The various ways orders are processed by the pharmacy
- The difference among stat, ASAP, and standing orders
- How POE, CPOE, BPOE, and CADM systems are used to reduce drug errors
- The various duties of an institutional pharmacy technician, including the areas described in this chapter
- The technician's role in the IND process
- How ADS machines function in the hospital setting and how they are stocked
- The steps in and frequency of filling automated medication dispensing systems
- The importance of counting, dispensing, and tracking controlled substances
- What PAR levels are and who is responsible for maintaining them
- How often medications are supplied to nursing units using a cart-filling method
- The difference between hazardous and nonhazardous preparation of parenteral drugs
- The importance of aseptic technique for the technician preparing CSPs

- Duties involved in ordering and maintaining the stock levels of the pharmacy
- Hospital areas that the pharmacy stocks
- Specialty areas of the hospital for which the pharmacy stocks or orders medication
- Why technician education is important and the name of a professional organization that institutional technicians can join

● Scenario Follow-Up

TJC's visit is over, and Marcus is proud to report that the pharmacy received only one finding. The commission found an outdated flu vaccine in the back of the pharmacy refrigerator. Several technicians and pharmacists had checked for out-of-date medications, but somehow one was missed. Everyone understood the danger of possibly administering an outdated vaccine and is determined to be more diligent in the future to prevent the same mistake. Overall, the visit was a success, and the pharmacy staff was proud of their efforts to ensure high-quality patient care.

Review Questions

Multiple Choice Questions

1. P&P manuals contain information pertaining to all of the following *except:*
   A. Employees' weekly schedule
   B. Emergency situations
   C. Training
   D. Daily work routines
2. TJC does *not* inspect or accredit:
   A. Long-term care pharmacies
   B. Hospital pharmacies
   C. Retail pharmacists
   D. All of the above are inspected and accredited by TJC
3. Hospital orders contain which information?
   A. Drug interactions
   B. Dietary restrictions
   C. Medication orders
   D. All of the above
4. What is the meaning of the acronym CPOE?
   A. Computerized pharmacy operating element
   B. Counseling program offering education
   C. Counseling pharmacy operations elective
   D. Computerized physician order entry
5. Hospital technicians must be available to:
   A. Work various shifts
   B. Work weekends
   C. Fill different jobs per operational needs
   D. All of the above
6. Technicians have all of the following responsibilities *except:*
   A. Printing labels for IV medications before filling the container
   B. Preparing antibiotics
   C. Discontinuing intravenous medications per physician's orders
   D. Contacting the physician for order clarification

7. Which statement about investigational drugs is false?
   A. An IND application must be filed with the FDA before the clinical study.
   B. All investigational drugs must be disposed of on site at the hospital where the study has taken place.
   C. A log book containing all required information on the investigational drug must be maintained by the pharmacy.
   D. A clinical trial with investigational drugs is the last phase before a drug is approved by the FDA.

8. Stat orders should be filled within:
   A. 10 minutes
   B. 20 minutes
   C. 25 minutes
   D. 30 minutes

9. Which of the following provides guidelines and regulations for the compounding of sterile preparations?
   A. HHS
   B. USP
   C. ADS
   D. DPH

10. Which is *not* an ADS?
    A. Pyxis
    B. Glove box
    C. SureMed
    D. SmartCart

◼ Technician's Corner

You receive an order for Ms. Jeni Gilbert. Only her name and her room number are written on the order. The order is for ceftriaxone 1 g q4h.

● Is this an appropriate dosing regimen for this medication?
● What information must you have before you can process this order?
● What actions should you take concerning the dosing regimen for this medication?

Bibliography

Ansel H, Allen L, Popovich N. *Pharmaceutical Dosage Forms and Drug Delivery Systems*. 9th ed. Baltimore: Lippincott Williams & Wilkins; 2011.

Elkin M, Perry A, Potter P. *Nursing Interventions and Clinical Skills*. 5th ed. St. Louis: Elsevier; 2011.

Harrison M. *5 Ways to Improve the U.S. Health Care System*. 2021. Available at: advisory.com.

United States Pharmacopeia. *Pharmaceutical Compounding: Sterile Preparations*. Rockville, MD: United States Pharmacopeial Convention; 2013. Revision Bulletin.

Websites Referenced

American Society of Health-System Pharmacists. *Compounding Sterile Preparations*. Available at: ashp.org.

American Society of Health-System Pharmacists. *Medication Reconciliation and Pharmacy Technicians*. Available at: https://www.ashp.org/pharmacy-technician/about-pharmacy-technicians/advanced-pharmacy-technician-roles/medication-reconciliation-technician.

eHow. *What Is the Meaning of Non-formulary Drugs*. Available at: http://www.ehow.com/about_6749588_meaning-non_formulary-drugs_.html?ref=Track2&utm_source=ask.

Healthcare IT News. *Is CPOE Getting Better—or Just Bigger?* Available at: http://www.healthcareitnews.com/news/cpoe-getting-better-%E2%80%93-or-just-bigger.

Lionheart Publishing. *Patient Safety and Quality Healthcare. Healthcare-Associated Infection Reports*. Available at: https://www.thefreelibrary.com/%22Patient+Safety+%26+Quality+Healthcare%22+from+Lionheart.-a0127012742.

Society of Nuclear Medicine and Molecular Imaging. *Frequently Asked Questions About USP*. Available at: http://www.snmmi.org/.

UNC Eshelman School of Pharmacy. *Prescriptions & Medication Orders | Pharmlabs*. Available at: unc.edu.

University of Kentucky Hospital Chandler Medical Center. *Department of Pharmacy Policy*. Available at: https://ukhealthcare.uky.edu/hospitals-clinics/albert-b-chandler-hospital.

Wyoming State Board of Pharmacy. *Wyoming Pharmacy Act, Rules and Regulations. Institutional Pharmacy Practice Regulations*. Available at: http://pharmacyboard.state.wy.us/laws/Chapter_12_Pharmacy_Act.pdf.

CHAPTER 10

Additional Pharmacy Practice Settings and Advanced Roles for Technicians

Karen Davis

OBJECTIVES

1. List and describe the roles, requirements, and responsibilities of an inventory and purchasing agent.
2. List and describe the roles, responsibilities, and requirements of a medication reconciliation pharmacy technician, prior approval or investigational drug coordinator, and managed care pharmacy technician.
3. List and describe the roles, responsibilities, and requirements of a pharmacy technician educator or trainer.
4. List and describe the roles, responsibilities, and requirements of a pharmaceutical sales representative.
5. List and describe the roles, responsibilities, and requirements of a nuclear pharmacy technician.
6. List and describe the roles, responsibilities, and requirements of a telepharmacy/remote pharmacy technician.
7. List and describe the roles, responsibilities, and requirements of a pharmacy informatics pharmacy technician.
8. List and describe the roles, responsibilities, and requirements of a lead pharmacy technician.
9. Evaluate how advanced education and responsibilities of the pharmacy technician play a part in patient safety and discuss future opportunities for the pharmacy technician. Describe the changing roles of future pharmacy technicians and the initiatives for education and advanced or specialized training.

TERMS AND DEFINITIONS

Interdisciplinary team Consists of a health care team from different disciplines, including pharmacy technicians, and is designed to provide care for the patient's total needs

Managed care An organized health care delivery system designed to improve both the quality and accessibility of health care, including pharmaceutical care, while containing costs

Medication reconciliation The process of preparing a complete and accurate listing of patient's medications and all related medical information such as allergies

Pharmacy benefit management (PBM) The development and management of broad and cost-efficient prescription drug benefits for a large group of patient populations

Pharmacy informatics Practice that includes the use of information technology designed to ensure optimal medication use

Telepharmacy The provision of pharmaceutical care to patients at a distance through the use of telecommunications and information technologies

213

Scenario

John is a certified pharmacy technician at a local hospital. Recently the department added a new technician role, medication management technician. John is very interested in this position and wants to apply for it. He has the required 2 years of experience in the pharmacy and a good understanding of brand and generic medication names. What other attributes would make him successful in this position?

As the field of pharmacy evolves, so do the responsibilities of and opportunities for the pharmacy technician. The expected employment growth rate for pharmacy technician careers between 2021 and 2031 is 5%. There are several reasons for this increase in the need for technicians with advanced qualifications, such as medication safety regulations, the increasing development of new medications, and the rapid growth of the elderly population, who have polypharmacy (the simultaneous use of multiple drugs to treat a single ailment or condition) concerns.

The role of the pharmacy technician was once considered a clerk-type position—stocking shelves and running the register. However, the technician's role has grown into a position with important responsibilities and most states require the pharmacy technician to be licensed or registered with the state board of pharmacy. In some cases, national certification is required to obtain a position as a pharmacy technician. More than 66% of pharmacy technicians work in the traditional settings, such as community pharmacies and hospitals. However, with the increase in qualified, experienced, and well-trained technicians, many other opportunities at an advanced level have become available to pharmacy technicians. Previous chapters have discussed the job responsibilities and requirements for an entry-level position. This chapter discusses advanced-level opportunities and the requirements for obtaining these positions.

Advanced or Specialized Pharmacy Technician Opportunities

Employers hiring pharmacy technicians in an advanced-level pharmacy setting often look for individuals who have had previous formal training and often certification. Technicians applying for the types of positions discussed in the following sections should keep in mind that the more entry-level experience they have, the more competitive their resume will be.

In 2010 the American Society of Health-System Pharmacists (ASHP) began promoting the Practice Advancement Initiative (PAI) through the Pharmacy Practice Model Initiative. The future of health care includes an interdisciplinary approach to ensure the wellness and overall optimum health of patients. Some of the PAI technician-related initiatives include the following:

- Pharmacy technicians are urged to seek nontraditional roles and advanced certifications.
- Pharmacy technicians should perform traditional preparation and distribution activities to allow pharmacists the time for more direct patient interaction.

Leadership and advanced training or certification provides the certified technician with additional knowledge and skills to play a larger significant part of an **interdisciplinary team**, who, along with assisting the pharmacists, works closely with other health care team members to ensure the best overall care of a patient. The technician workforce of tomorrow will begin with education and certification for entry-level positions, followed by advanced specialty positions for technicians.

> ### ■ Tech Note!
>
> As one of the fastest growing jobs in the United States, over 420,000 pharmacy technician positions existed in 2018. By 2023, over 447,300 jobs were held by pharmacy technicians in the United States. (*https://www.bls.gov/OOH/healthcare/pharmacy-technicians.htm#tab-3*).

Inventory and Purchasing Agent

With the increasing number of medications being prescribed, pharmacies need at least one employee to do the purchasing for the department. Most commonly found in an institutional setting, pharmacy purchasing agents also can work in retail, nuclear, or mail-order settings (Fig. 10.1). Also known as the *pharmacy procurement specialist* or *pharmacy buyer,* the pharmacy purchasing agent has several responsibilities, including the following:

- Placing daily orders to keep the department stocked so that patients' needs can be met
- Meeting with pharmaceutical sales representatives to discuss new and alternative medications
- Negotiating prices and contracts
- Planning ahead for the demand for certain products
- Establishing cost-effective practices
- Working closely with pharmacy management to take advantage of cost-saving opportunities

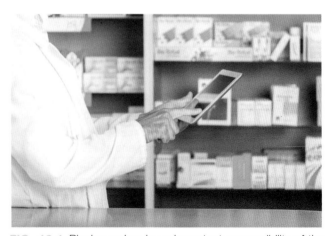

FIG. 10.1 Placing orders is an important responsibility of the pharmacy purchasing agent. (iStock/Getty Images Plus.)

- Ensuring bar codes are available and integration with electronic health records (EHRs) and automated dispensing systems inventory are current
- Working with outside entities such as disaster planning agencies; emergency medical services; and fire, safety, and public health departments to maintain specific inventories
- Maintaining required documentation for returns, wastes, recalls, and regulatory agencies

This position includes automation and a working knowledge of integration with other systems. Patient dispensing is usually done through automation, and identification methods include bar coding and National Drug Code numbers. The constant verification of drug names and identifying markers is essential to quality, safety, and accuracy. The EHR is shared with multiple team members internally and externally, and the information recorded must be accurate.

Records for dispensed medications, charges and credits, and regulatory information are part of the daily responsibilities of this advanced position. By 2023, the requirement for establishing an electronic tracking system, known as the Drug Supply Chain Security Act (DSCSA), will require the establishment of an interoperable system to track certain prescriptions per the US Food and Drug Administration. This is to improve the detection of harmful or dangerous products and then the deletion from the pharmacy supply chain. Along with maintaining the records for this, the technician must record and maintain controlled substance information, recalls, investigational medications, and reverse distributor records.

In most facilities, the requirements for the position of pharmacy purchasing agent usually include up to 2 years of experience as a pharmacy technician and related on-the-job training. Additional requirements may include one or more pharmacy technician certifications. In addition, an associate's or bachelor's degree, although not required, is often preferred. A person interested in this type of position should have general clerical and computer knowledge and excellent communication skills.

Medication Reconciliation Technician

Medication reconciliation is defined as "the process of preparing documentation with brand, generic, and drug use information to ensure accuracy of the patient current regimen." Other pertinent information, such as allergies and conditions or diseases, is also included to provide a complete patient profile. Typically this is done through an interview process with a medication reconciliation technician.

The pharmacy medication reconciliation technician is an essential factor in patient safety. The goal of this position is to prevent medication errors. Adverse drug events (ADEs) are preventable, and according to the FDA, there are more than 400,000 drug-related injuries that happen in the hospital setting because of medication errors.

Performing **medication reconciliation** (med recon) can prevent drug omissions, duplications, errors in dosing, drug-drug interactions, and ADEs (Fig. 10.2). In one study,

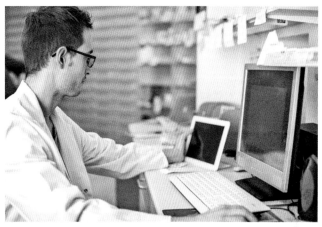

FIG. 10.2 A medication reconciliation technician must be sure to compare information for all of the patient's prescriptions to ensure that everything is correct and there are no conflicts or interactions. (iStock/Getty Images Plus.)

there was an overall 67% reduction on medication errors in hospital settings. The process of medication reconciliation has shown to reduce medication errors (eg, prescribing, dispensing, and administering) and is currently a task trained pharmacy technicians play a significant role in.

The step-by-step medication reconciliation process is as follows:
1. Developing a list of current medications.
2. Developing a list of medications to be ordered/prescribed.
3. Comparing the information on the two lists.
4. Making clinical decisions.
5. Communicating the new list to appropriate individuals.

The technician's responsibilities begin with interviewing patients about their at-home medications, including prescription and over-the-counter medications, vitamins, and herbal supplements. This can be done in the emergency department before admission to the floor, during a preoperative registration for a procedure, or on discharge. The list should include the drug name, dosage, frequency of administration, and any notes included with the medication. The technician may have to call different sources to get all the information required to complete each patient's list. Calls are frequently made to pharmacies, prescriber's offices, long-term care facilities (eg, assisted living facilities and nursing homes), and other health care settings. Once a patient's list is complete, the technician is responsible for entering the information into the computer system, being careful to avoid any errors, so that it is available to the health care provider. This information helps the provider make informed decisions about the patient's medication regimen.

Although additional education is not required for the position of medication reconciliation technician, the pharmacy technician is always at an advantage if he or she is certified. Medication reconciliation technicians must be familiar with medications and possible side effects and/or drug-drug interactions or food-drug interactions. As a result, the technician must have significant experience in the pharmacy field. Medication reconciliation technicians also must have good communication skills and a strong sense of professionalism because they communicate with the patient in person.

Once the listing is complete, the technician's role does not stop. As part of the interdisciplinary team, the next step may include filling the prescriptions and delivery at bedside before a discharge. It can also include collaboration with nursing and pharmacy for reviews or future improvement of plans of care or transfers to other facilities. In addition, criteria-based screening is often used to alert the pharmacist of an intervention need, which requires critical thinking and advanced knowledge of pharmacology and disease profiles.

Prior Approval or Investigational Drug Coordinator

This position may be a separate job or part of the medication reconciliation technician position, because certain medications require special documentation before dispensing. The technician must maintain inventory, keep records, and, under the direct supervision of a pharmacist, work directly with manufacturers, physicians, nurses, and patients on a daily basis.

Patients who participate in a study or clinical trial have to be located and require extensive interviewing and medical history documentation. Medications needing prior approval (PA) can require prior regimens of other trials of less expensive medications. This may be due to third-party requirements, manufacturer recommendations, or the inability of the patient to afford the medication. In all of these cases, a working knowledge of pharmacology, a basic knowledge of data entry, and good writing and communication skills are needed. In addition, dispensing of investigational drugs, prior-approved drugs, or indigent medications requires separate inventory control and documentation and often advanced or specific ordering and return protocols.

Managed Care Pharmacy Technician

The definition of **managed care** is "an organized health care delivery system designed to improve both the quality and the accessibility of health care, including pharmaceutical care, while containing costs." Congress passed the Health Maintenance Organization Act in 1973, creating health maintenance organizations (HMOs). When HMOs started up, the cost of prescription medications accounted for only about 5% of health care costs. However, because of improved health care and the discovery of more effective treatments for medical conditions and diseases, the number of elderly patients has increased. Most elderly patients take multiple medications, increasing the need for the management of prescription drug use. As a result, **pharmacy benefit management** (PBM) companies were created (eg, ClearScript). The purpose of PBMs is to develop and manage broad and cost-efficient prescription drug benefits for a large group of patient populations.

The responsibilities of a pharmacist in a PBM setting include building formularies, creating drug benefit plans, and negotiating contracts with community pharmacies. The role of the pharmacy technician in this setting varies even more

broadly. Managed care pharmacy technicians work mainly in an office, and their responsibilities include the following:
- Providing benefit information to the patient or client
- Determining the proper use of benefits
- Receiving and entering clinical data
- Processing claims for members according to their benefits
- Troubleshooting rejected claims
- Entering and preparing mail-order prescriptions

Although no additional formal education is required for the position of managed care pharmacy technician, companies usually require experience in the pharmacy field and prefer call center experience. The training required for this position is most commonly company-based training.

◉ Scenario Checkup 10.1

John was given the new position of medication reconciliation technician in his department. He really enjoys his new role and wants to stay current with all the new medications coming out. What is the best way for him to stay current with new drugs on the market?

Pharmacy Technician Educator or Trainer

Another specialty area for a pharmacy technician is education or training. An experienced pharmacy technician can take on a role as an educator at an accredited school or lead training for new pharmacy employees (Fig. 10.3).

As a pharmacy technician trainer, a technician must have adequate experience in the practice area he or she is teaching. A trainer's responsibility is to provide on-the-job training for new employees or for technicians in new roles. The training usually continues until the trainer and the new employee both feel confident that the new employee can perform the task with minimal supervision. In some instances, the trainee may have to take a test to prove that he or she understands some tasks and can competently complete the work.

The pharmacy technician educator is most commonly found working for an accredited college or university, either on campus or online. Some community pharmacies (eg, Walgreens and CVS) offer a training course that is certified

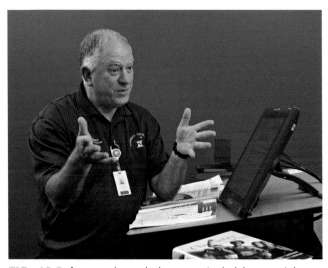

FIG. 10.3 An experienced pharmacy technician can take on the role of a trainer for new employees.

by ASHP and the Accreditation Council for Pharmacy Education (ACPE) and differs from on-the-job training. The responsibilities of a pharmacy technician educator include teaching pharmacy technician students the knowledge and skills they need to pass an ASHP/ACPE-approved national certification examination and become certified pharmacy technicians. Subjects taught by pharmacy technician educators include the following:

- Personal/interpersonal knowledge and skills
- Foundational professional knowledge and skills
- Processing and handling of medications and medication orders
- Sterile and nonsterile compounding
- Procurement, billing, reimbursement, and inventory management
- Patient and medication safety
- Technology and informatics
- Regulatory issues
- Quality assurance

Most schools with campuses provide a hands-on laboratory where students learn and demonstrate compounding techniques, intravenous (IV) solution admixture, prescription processing, and the correct way to handle products in the pharmacy setting. All pharmacy technician programs are moving toward becoming ASHP/ACPE approved, which requires the programs to teach the required goals and objectives of an accredited program found on the ASHP website *(http://www.ashp.org)*.

Technicians interested in a rewarding career as a pharmacy technician educator must have national certification, meet their state's regulations for practice, have at least an associate's degree, and have a minimum of 5 years of experience in the pharmacy setting. Most employers look for candidates with retail and hospital pharmacy experience, and individuals with a bachelor's degree tend to be more competitive.

Pharmaceutical Sales Representative

Although a pharmaceutical sales representative career is a more nontraditional setting for a pharmacy technician, it has its advantages. The pay for a pharmaceutical sales representative is significantly higher than that for a pharmacy technician in a traditional setting. A good knowledge base of pharmacology, good communication, and organizational skills are key to this role. Most pharmaceutical companies offer their employees a company car and a great benefits package.

The responsibilities of pharmaceutical sales representatives include traveling to the clients' sites and promoting their assigned medications (Fig. 10.4). The representative should have on hand important information on the medication he or she is trying to sell, including up-to-date reports on clinical studies and side effects, in addition to a pharmacological knowledge of the drug. The ultimate goal of a sales representative is to do everything possible to sell specific products, often by persuading the buyer that the products are the best on the market.

The requirements for a pharmaceutical sales representative include an associate's or a bachelor's degree in fields such as biology, chemistry, marketing, business, or a related field.

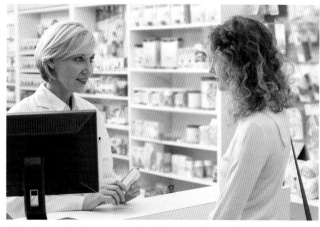

FIG. 10.4 A pharmacy technician may have the opportunity to become a pharmaceutical sales representative or may be in communication with various sales representatives as part of a job in a community pharmacy. (iStock/Getty Images Plus.)

The candidate also must have excellent communication skills. Other qualifications for a candidate in the pharmacy sales industry include self-motivation and self-confidence. Experience in business relations is preferred. This area of pharmacy does not require national certification; however, a candidate who is knowledgeable about the policies and procedures of pharmacy is at an advantage.

Nuclear Pharmacy Technician

As defined by the Department of Pharmacy Practice at Purdue University, *nuclear pharmacy* is a "a specialty area of pharmacy practice dedicated to compounding and dispensing of radioactive materials for use in nuclear medicine procedures." Nuclear pharmacy developed after the specialty of nuclear medicine was recognized by the American Medical Association (AMA). With the increase in the use of nuclear products, it became evident that individuals were needed to prepare these products. Larger hospitals were able to accommodate this activity. However, many smaller hospitals did not have the staff or capability to handle the radioactive materials, resulting in the concept of centralized, freestanding nuclear pharmacies.

When an order or prescription is written and presented for a particular radioactive product, it is entered by the pharmacist, just as it would be in a traditional setting. The pharmacy technician, taking specific safety precautions, prepares the product as ordered. The final product is checked by the pharmacist and dispensed or shipped to its destination using proper procedures to reduce the risk for exposure.

Radiopharmaceuticals are a special class of drugs used in the nuclear pharmacy. The Mayo Clinic defines radiopharmaceuticals as "agents used to diagnose certain medical problems or to treat certain diseases [that] may be given by mouth, by injection, or placed into the eye or into the bladder." Examples of these types of medications are fluorodeoxyglucose, diethylenetriamine pentaacetic acid, and pertechnetate, to name a few. The technician must be aware of special risks such as exposure to radioactive material when preparing and handling these materials, and specialized training is required for everyone handling these products, including the pharmacist and pharmacy technician. The University of Arkansas for Medical Sciences, the University of New Mexico, Purdue University, and The Ohio State University are the only schools that offer an approved training program for nuclear pharmacy technicians.

Because of the strict guidelines required to perform the duties of a nuclear technician, many nuclear pharmacies send new employees to attend these programs to complete their training. Some very important competencies required of the nuclear pharmacy technician include the following:

- A thorough knowledge of the terms, abbreviations, and symbols often used in the prescription of radiopharmaceuticals
- The ability to differentiate between therapeutic and diagnostic use of radiopharmaceuticals
- A knowledge of procedures related to the reconstitution, packaging, labeling, aseptic compounding, and validation of parenteral admixture techniques
- The ability to perform the calculations required to compound the preparation
- A knowledge of the record-keeping procedures for the compounding and dispensing of radiopharmaceuticals, including those involving quality control and testing

Because of the risks associated with the nuclear pharmacy setting, the pay in this area of pharmacy is most often higher than in a traditional pharmacy setting. Furthermore, because of the specialized nature of this practice, opportunities in the nuclear pharmacy setting are very limited.

◉ Technician Profile

Justin is a nuclear pharmacy technician for a large company. He graduated from a program accredited by the ASHP/ACPE and obtained his certification from the Pharmacy Technician Certification Board (PTCB) during the program. He had 5 years of experience before obtaining this position, and after he was hired, he went to the University of Arkansas for additional training in nuclear practice. Justin's job includes working with radiopharmaceutical drugs and preparing sterile preparations every day for delivery. He takes orders over the phone and uses his knowledge of pharmacology and aseptic technique to prepare products for techniques such as magnetic resonance imaging and other diagnostic procedures. Justin is a very detail-oriented technician who finds his job challenging and rewarding.

◎ Scenario Checkup 10.2

John recently had a patient encounter with an individual who was taking more than 15 medications. As a result of his reading and knowledge of some recently released medications, John notices that one of the medications the patient has been taking for a long time is very similar to a new medication she recently started. He is concerned about the duplication. What should he do to help the patient?

Remote/Telepharmacy Technician

Since the early 2000s, the National Association of Boards of Pharmacy (NABP) has included **telepharmacy** in its Model

Pharmacy Act defining pharmacy practices. The Model Pharmacy Act, updated every August, provides the boards of pharmacy with model language that may be used when developing state laws or board rules. The NABP defines telepharmacy as "the provision of pharmaceutical care through the use of telecommunications and information technologies to patients at a distance."

Telepharmacy has expanded nationwide since its start in rural areas of North Dakota. This system has had positive results serving communities that have been without pharmacies for years. Within the past decade, a total of 16 states have written rules and regulations that allow this practice. Other states are considering moving forward with rules and regulations to begin the telepharmacy practice, and no state laws prohibit the practice of telepharmacy.

As the practice of telepharmacy grows, it is no longer restricted to rural areas. Veterans Affairs health care organizations across the country are using the technology of telepharmacy in their community-based clinics.

A telepharmacy consists of a centralized pharmacy, where the pharmacist is located, and a community pharmacy, where the technician is located. The centralized pharmacy is connected to the community pharmacy by audio and/or visual technology, allowing the pharmacist to communicate with the pharmacy technician while remaining in the community pharmacy (Fig. 10.5). The technology also allows the pharmacist to communicate with the patient and to check and verify the prescriptions being dispensed.

The job responsibilities of a pharmacy technician in a telepharmacy setting are much like those of the technician in a community or hospital pharmacy. However, because the pharmacist is not physically on site with the technician, a candidate for this position must have experience, self-motivation, and self-confidence. In some states, a "tech-check-tech" procedure is an approved practice when the pharmacist is not available; one technician can check another technician's work. No extra formal education is required for a telepharmacy technician position, although a candidate who is certified is preferable.

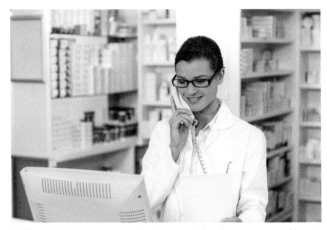

FIG. 10.5 Telepharmacy helps provide pharmacy services to communities through the use of technology to link pharmacists in a central location with technicians at local pharmacies. (iStock/Getty Images Plus.)

Pharmacy Informatics

Pharmacy informatics is a specialty practice of pharmacy that focuses on the use of information technology and drug information to optimize medication use. With the requirements set forth by the government to help reduce medication errors through the use of technology, informatics has become an increasingly important field.

The main responsibility of a pharmacy informatics technician is to provide support for pharmacy information in clinical systems. The technician assists in building new systems to be used by the pharmacy staff and also must be available to help troubleshoot if anything needs to be fixed. In this setting, the technician should build in relevant pharmacy information (eg, pharmaceutical, formulary, financial, and operational information) into informatics materials.

No additional education is required for the position of pharmacy informatics technician; however, most employers look for candidates with a bachelor's degree, preferably in computer science, and a knowledge of pharmacology. A minimum of 2 years' experience in a community or hospital pharmacy is required for a prospective candidate in pharmacy informatics.

Lead Pharmacy Technician

This position requires national certification, proven leadership skills, and experience as a working certified technician. Sometimes an advanced degree also may be required. The position includes daily responsibilities such as the following:

- Interviewing, identifying, and assessing baseline skills levels for technicians
- Scheduling training and task assignments for the technicians in a department or even multiple sites
- Performing audits for compliance such as United States Pharmacopeia (USP), patient safety, and quality to ensure optimum workflow
- Serving as additional team member when department is short of employees or as workload requires

In some states, technicians can check another technician's work in certain dispensing situations known as *tech-check-tech*. In North Carolina, for instance, a lead technician could check another registered technician's filling of floor stock or unit dose medications in a hospital setting.

In addition to good leadership and communication skills, a basic understanding of all technician roles in traditional and nontraditional settings is needed. Multitasking and organizational skills are also key to managing other technicians and managing projects.

Medication Adherence or Compliance Technician

There are more than 4 billion prescriptions being dispensed in the United States yearly that are never filled or taken as prescribed. Nonadherence costs the industry and can be linked to more than 125,000 deaths each year. Technicians are often the first and last contact point at a pharmacy, and this interaction can greatly influence how the patient will take their medication.

Advanced trained technicians can recognize roadblocks such as financial hardship, language barriers, or other issues that may lead to nonadherence.

Some of the qualities needed for this position include the following:

- Ability to problem solve
- Good verbal and written skills
- Knowledge of pharmacology
- Ability to research and analyze data

These positions may be found at inpatient facilities, community pharmacy, or even at home. Companies employ technicians to educate and inform patients on the services they offer and communicate any concerns to the pharmacist if needed. This may include completing a medication history or updating an electronic profile.

Certified technicians should complete additional continuing education or specialty certifications in the areas of medication reconciliation and stay current on new drugs and pharmacy regulations.

Other similar positions for advanced technicians are discussed in case studies found on the ASHP website at *https://www.ashp.org/Pharmacy-Technician/About-Pharmacy-Technicians/Advanced-Pharmacy-Technician-Roles?loginreturnUrl=SSOCheckOnly*.

Future Opportunities for the Pharmacy Technician

Advances in technology are making new medical treatments ever more available, a growing population of elderly requires more medications, and the health care industry in general is rapidly expanding. As a result of all of these factors, pharmacy technician employment is expected to continue to grow. As new treatments are discovered and new technology is created, the role of the pharmacy technician also will evolve. Education and experience are common requirements for the current and future practice settings of pharmacy, but professionalism is the most important characteristic of a candidate seeking any health care position.

Since 2020, PTCB has required graduation from an ASHP/ACPE (see Chapter 3) accredited technician training program or from a PTCB-approved program to sit for the Pharmacy Technician Certification Exam (PTCE). This comes after much debate and discussion among the pharmacy profession and education community.

The current eligibility requirements are for taking the PTCE are as follows:

Pathway 1: a recognized PTCB-approved program (or completion within 60 days)
Pathway 2: equivalent work experience (minimum of 500 hours)

Beginning in January 2023 there is no longer an age requirement for testing. If the candidate is under 18, they must have a minor's consent who must give a verbal consent and possess a valid ID.

Future models from ASHP advocates a minimum of an associate's degree from an accredited source. Education and ongoing competence for technicians will ensure the continuing knowledge and quality of care for patients. The advancement of roles, specific training, assessment of accuracy for a position, and specialty certifications also began to be offered by PTCB. Additional certificates continue to be added. Currently, PTCB offers specialty certifications to certified pharmacy technicians (CPhTs) as the following: Immunization Administration, Controlled Substances Diversion Prevention Program, Hazardous Drug Management, Billing and Reimbursement, Compounded Sterile Preparation (CSPT), Technician Product Verification (TPV), Medication History, Nonsterile Compounding, Point-of-Care Testing, and Supply Chain and Inventory. A CPhT in good standing who completes PTCB requirements will have the ability to earn a new designation called *CPhT-Adv.*

There are also several continuing education courses offered by other organizations that cover medication therapy management, veterinary medications, diabetes management, and both sterile and nonsterile compounding, with more on the horizon. The future is bright, and beginning with entry-level knowledge, technicians can advance in careers and become very successful.

Tech Note!

According to the *Occupational Outlook Handbook,* the pharmacy technician salary in 2022 was $36,740 and the projected change in employment or average growth rate is 5% between 2021 to 2031.

Do You Remember These Key Points?

- The roles and responsibilities of a pharmacy purchasing agent
- The requirements for becoming a pharmacy inventory and purchasing agent
- The roles and responsibilities of a medication reconciliation pharmacy technician
- The requirements for becoming a medication reconciliation pharmacy technician
- The roles and responsibilities of a managed care pharmacy technician
- The requirements for becoming a managed care pharmacy technician
- The roles and responsibilities of a pharmacy technician educator
- The requirements for becoming a pharmacy technician educator
- The roles and responsibilities of a pharmaceutical sales representative
- The requirements for becoming a pharmaceutical sales representative
- The roles and responsibilities of a nuclear pharmacy technician
- The requirements for becoming a nuclear pharmacy technician
- The roles and responsibilities of a telepharmacy/remote pharmacy technician

- The requirements for becoming a telepharmacy/remote pharmacy technician
- The roles and responsibilities of a pharmacy informatics pharmacy technician
- The requirements for becoming a pharmacy informatics pharmacy technician
- How each additional role of the pharmacy technician plays a part in patient safety

Scenario Follow-Up

John has been working as a medication reconciliation technician now for 1 year and doing a great job. He has learned so much and has helped many patients with their medications and compliance. Staying current with the medications has really made a difference, and the future is bright.

Review Questions

Multiple Choice Questions

1. Which pharmacy setting does *not* have a pharmacist on site?
   A. Pharmacy informatics
   B. Telepharmacy
   C. Nuclear pharmacy
   D. Managed care pharmacy

2. Employment of pharmacy technicians is expected to grow by _____ from 2021 to 2031.
   A. 5%
   B. 10%
   C. 15%
   D. 8%

3. Providing benefit information to the patient is a responsibility of which pharmacy technician practice?
   A. Pharmaceutical sales representative
   B. Managed care pharmacy technician
   C. Pharmacy technician educator
   D. Telepharmacy pharmacy technician

4. Which professional works closely with the pharmacy management in implementing cost-saving opportunities?
   A. Pharmaceutical sales representative
   B. Managed care pharmacy technician
   C. Pharmacy purchasing agent
   D. Nuclear pharmacy technician

5. When health maintenance organizations were created in 1973, the cost of prescription medications was about _____ of health care costs.
   A. 2%
   B. 32%
   C. 10%
   D. 5%

6. A specialty area of pharmacy practice dedicated to compounding and dispensing of radioactive materials is:
   A. Pharmacy informatics
   B. Nuclear pharmacy
   C. Managed care pharmacy
   D. None of the above

7. Telepharmacy began in rural areas of:
   A. South Dakota
   B. North Dakota
   C. Maine
   D. Montana
8. Which pharmacy technician position requires the technician to interview patients about their medications?
   A. Pharmaceutical sales representative
   B. Telepharmacy technician
   C. Medication reconciliation technician
   D. Pharmacy informatics technician
9. A pharmacy technician may be employed by the information technology department of a health care organization in which type of pharmacy practice?
   A. Telepharmacy
   B. Pharmacy informatics
   C. Pharmacy purchasing agent
   D. Pharmacy technician educator
10. The pharmacy field highly prefers a candidate to have experience in business and business relations for the position of:
    A. Pharmacy purchasing agent
    B. Pharmacy informatics
    C. Pharmaceutical sales representatives
    D. Pharmacy technician trainer

◼ Technician's Corner

Pamela is a pharmacy technician in a telepharmacy setting. There has been a power outage in the area. Mr. Jones, a patient, has a very important question for the pharmacist about his medication. Pamela cannot get through to the pharmacist, and Mr. Jones is anxious. What can Pamela do to make sure Mr. Jones's question is answered?

Bibliography

Frederick J. *Technicians Join the Fight to Boost Rx Adherence*. Available at: https://drugstorenews.com/pharmacy/technicians-join-fight-boost-rx-adherence.

Levitz MD. Med recon: The role of the pharmacy Technician. Pharmacy Times. Available at: https://www.pharmacytimes.com/view/medication-reconciliation-the-role-of-the-pharmacy-technician.

Mekonnen AB, McLachlan AJ, Brien JA. Effectiveness of pharmacist-led medication reconciliation programmes on clinical outcomes at hospital transitions: a systematic review and meta-analysis. *BMJ Open*. 2016;6(2):e010003. doi: 10.1136/bmjopen-2015-010003.

North Dakota State University. *Telepharmacy*. Available at: http://www.ndsu.edu/telepharmacy/.

Purdue University. *Nuclear Pharmacy Program: What is Nuclear Pharmacy?* Available at: http://nuclear.pharmacy.purdue.edu/what.php.

Pharmacy Technicians: Occupational Outlook Handbook: U.S. Bureau of Labor Statistics. Available at: https://bls.gov.

UNM Health Sciences Center. *Schools That Offer Nuclear Pharmacy Technician Programs*. Available at: http://www.ehow.com/list_7230135_schools-nuclear-pharmacy-tech-programs.html.

Websites Referenced

Available at: https://www.bpsweb.org/bps-specialties/nuclear-pharmacy/.

Available at: http://www.himss.org/library/pharmacy-informatics.

Available at: http://www.pharmacypurchasing.com/.

Available at: http://www.ptcb.org.

Available at: http://www.thesepht.org.

Jacobson A. *Medication Error Statistics* 2024. January 24, 2024. Available at: SingleCare.

NABP | National Association of Boards of Pharmacy | NABP Login. Available at: http://www.nabp.net.

Pharmacy Technicians. Available at: https://www.ashp.org/.

CHAPTER 11

Bulk Repackaging and Nonsterile Compounding

Karen Davis

1. Explain the need for packaging products in the appropriate type and size of container.
2. List the steps in the bulk repackaging of medications.
3. List five reasons pharmacies often repackage bulk medications into unit dose packages.
4. Describe the proper handling of medications during bulk repackaging.
5. Demonstrate how to complete a repacking logbook with the necessary information.
6. Explain the importance of the accurate labeling of pharmaceuticals.
7. Explain the calculations used to determine the beyond-use date when repackaging and discuss long-term care packaging, including blister card packaging.
8. Define nonsterile compounding, discuss its history, and list the common reasons that patients need compounded medications.
9. Explain the important considerations in the storage and stability of compounded products and list the types of dosage forms that can be compounded under USP-NF <795>.
10. Describe the equipment used in compounding drugs and differentiate among the types of scales used to weigh compounds.
11. Discuss additional supplies used in compounding and list the competencies a pharmacy technician must possess to reduce the possibility of errors when compounding.
12. Demonstrate compounding procedures related to weighing techniques, measuring liquids, preparing solutions, reconstituting premade suspensions, tablet additives, calibrating molds, compounding for molded tablets, and nasal preparations.
13. Discuss packaging for compounded products.
14. Keep accurate records for compounded medications.
15. Describe the importance of safety, professionalism, and quality control related to compounding.
16. Describe the types of dosage forms compounded for animal use.

API Active pharmaceutical ingredient

Beyond-use date (BUD) Date after which a compounded preparation should not be used, which is determined from the date the compound was prepared

Bubble pack (blister card) A preformed card with 28-, 30-, and 31-day depressions that can hold medications; the medication is sealed into the pack with a foil card backboard; this type of packaging usually is used for long-term care medications

Bulk repackaging The process by which the pharmacy transfers a medication manually or by means of an automated system from a manufacturer's original container to another type of container

Calibration Determining graduations (measurements) on a device such as a scale

Compounded nonsterile preparation (CNSP) Preparation created by combining, admixing, diluting, or reconstituting any way other than how the manufacturer lists in the package insert information

Compounding The act of mixing, reconstituting, and packaging a drug

Compounding record (CR) The form that documents a nonsterile compounding process

Containment ventilated enclosure (CVE) Often referred to as a "powder hood," this is where weighing, measuring, or any other manipulations with active pharmaceutical ingredient must occur

Cream A hydrophilic base

Elixir A base solution that is a mixture of alcohol and water

Emulsion A mixture of two or more liquids that do not usually blend using a stabilizing agent; the process of making an emulsion is called emulsification

Excipient An inert substance added to a drug to form a suitable consistency for dosing

FDA Acronym for the US Food and Drug Administration

Good manufacturing practices (GMPs) Federal guidelines that must be followed by all entities that prepare and package medication or medical devices

Hydrophilic Having a strong affinity for water; any substance that easily mixes in water

Hydrophobic Lacking an affinity for water; any substance that does not mix or dissolve in water

Master formulation record (MFR) A detailed record of procedures used to describe how a CNSP is to be prepared

Mortars and pestles Bowls and tools with a rounded knob used to grind substances into fine powder or to mix liquids

Nonsterile compounding The compounding of two or more medications in a nonsterile environment (no clean room or hood is required)

Ointment A hydrophobic product, such as petroleum jelly

Oleaginous base An ingredient used in compounding that does not dissolve in water

Periodic automatic replacement (PAR) levels Minimum set amounts of stock that must be kept on hand

Punch method Manual filling of capsules with powdered medication that has been premixed

Reconstitution The mixing of a liquid and a powder to form a suspension or solution

Solute The ingredient that is dissolved into a solution

Solution A water base in which one or more ingredients are dissolved completely

Solvent The greater part of a solution that dissolves a solute

Suspension A solution in which the powder does not dissolve into the base; the solution must be shaken before use

Syrup A sugar-based liquid

Triturate To grind or crush powder, such as a tablet, into fine particles

Troches Flat, disklike tablets that dissolve between the gum and cheek

Unit dose A single dose of a drug

Unit dose packs or strip packs Strip of heat-sealed packets, each packet holding one tablet or capsule; used in the bulk repackaging process

USP <795> General chapter in the defining practices and guidelines for nonsterile compounding

Scenario

Judy recently began her career as a technician at a long-term care pharmacy. She graduated from a technician training program accredited by the American Society of Health-System Pharmacists (ASHP). She is cross-trained in many different areas, including order entry, repackaging, extemporaneous compounding, and intravenous (IV) admixture. During her training, she compounded many different dosage forms, such as troches, ointments, creams, and suspensions, in an actual laboratory setting. What are the advantages of this type of hands-on training?

There are several different pharmacy settings, and each stocks specific types of medications and dosage forms that best suit its functions. This chapter discusses methods of providing single or unit doses for patients in institutional settings such as hospitals, nursing homes, or long-term care facilities.

Repackaging medications into single doses, known as **bulk repackaging,** and preparing patient-specific medication doses or formulas, known as **nonsterile compounding,** are two common tasks performed in modern pharmacies. **Compounding** may be done in a specialty or compounding pharmacy or in a community or retail pharmacy that provides this service. These pharmacies are equipped to prepare a wide assortment of solutions, ointments, creams, suppositories, and other drug delivery systems. Compounding pharmacies also prepare medications in various dosage forms and strengths for animals. Although the types of products compounded may differ, many of the same rules apply for medications compounded for both humans and animals. This chapter covers the skills, formulas, equipment, procedures, and documentation necessary for repackaging and compounding nonsterile products.

Bulk Repackaging

Institutional pharmacies often purchase medication in bulk quantities. These are large-count bottles, containing up to 1000 doses each, that are sold at a much lower cost because of their size. For example, a bottle of 100-count aspirin, 81-mg tablets can be packaged into 100 individual containers. The department employs technicians to repackage these medications into single doses, or what is commonly referred to as *unit dose medication*, to save a substantial amount of money and to create an inventory of medications for the automated dispensing machines. These unit doses are dispensed to specific patients one dose at a time when they are needed per the physician's order. Even liquids can be divided into single 15- to 30-mL dose cups to allow the nurse to dispense just the correct amount for a single dose. This process is called bulk repackaging, and it can be done manually or by means of an automated system, transferring medications from a manufacturer's original container to another type of container before the need arises to dispense a prescriber's order. Prepackaged medications may be in unit dose, single dose, bubble or blister pack, or a container used in a traditional dispensing system.

One dose is referred to as a unit dose. Hospitals use unit dose containers ordered from the manufacturer or make their own when necessary. Examples include **unit dose packs** or **strip packs** and liquid cups that contain one medication for one dose. Nursing and home health care facilities may use a **blister card** or **bubble pack** (ie, punch cards) (see Fig. 8.20), which may contain one to several tablets or capsules for dosing several days of medication.

Only one drug product at a time should be prepackaged in a specific work area. All federal and state laws and regulations must be followed. Label requirements include the proprietary and nonproprietary names, dosage form, strength, strength of an individual dose, total contents delivered, beyond-use date (BUD), and lot number. Proper procedures must be followed in the repackaging of medications; these require accuracy, technique, and documentation.

The following are five possible reasons a pharmacy may repackage bulk medication:

1. Certain medications are not available unit dosed.
2. The cost of repackaging bulk medication may be less than purchasing it unit dosed.
3. Repackaging may allow the pharmacy to provide a patient with a new medication more quickly, rather than having to order the drug and wait for it to be delivered.
4. Labeling each individual dose reduces the chance of errors.
5. If unit dose medication is not used, it can be returned to stock and used for another patient at a later time.

■ TABLE 11.1
Examples of Good Manufacturing Practice Guidelines for Repackaging

Item	Guidelines
Drugs and labels	All medications must be checked by a registered pharmacist
Equipment	In good condition and clean
Beyond-use date	One year from the date repackaged or the expiration date on the manufacturer's container, whichever is earlier (unless stated otherwise in the manufacturer's literature)
Package	Appropriate for the drug
Preparation	Not more than one item prepared at a time
Records	All items repackaged are logged for reference

Although packaging guidelines are not exactly the same between pharmacies and manufacturers, both entities must use good manufacturing practices. **Good manufacturing practices (GMPs)** are guidelines established by the US Food and Drug Administration (**FDA**) to guarantee safe and effective products for consumers. Examples of GMP guidelines that the technician and pharmacist should follow when preparing unit dose medications are listed in Table 11.1. GMP guidelines that should be followed when repackaging include the type of packaging used. Some medications degrade on exposure to sunlight. Other regulatory agencies, such as US Pharmacopeia (USP) <795> and the Occupational Safety and Health Administration (OSHA), must be considered as well when preparing medications from bulk or compounding medications for a specific patient. Specific labeling, techniques, equipment cleaning and maintenance, assigning BUDs, and record-keeping are required.

Unit dose medications must be repackaged in amber-colored containers. Examples of the types of containers used in repackaging are listed in Table 11.2. Each type of container holds specific amounts and types of medications (Fig. 11.1). When a medication is not available from the manufacturer in single doses, liquids normally are placed in glass or plastic bottles, syringes, or plastic or foil cups. Tablets and capsules are usually placed in individual plastic "cups" or strip packs (Fig. 11.2A).

■ Tech Note!

It is common practice to use only amber-colored containers to avoid possible degradation of medication, although clear unit dose packs are available.

Bulk Repackaging Equipment

Types of unit dosing equipment vary, depending on the number of drugs to be repackaged. Large pharmacies that supply many patient medications may use automated packaging

◼ TABLE 11.2
Unit Dose Containers

Type of Container	Medication Types	Volume/Size
Amber blister packs	Tablets, capsules	1 unit dose
Amber glass	Liquids	5, 10, 25, 30 mL
Applicators	Suppositories, creams, ointments	1 application
Foil cups	Liquids, suspensions	5, 10, 30 mL
Heat-sealed strip packs	Tablets, capsules, troches	1 unit dose
Oral syringes	Liquids	1, 3, 5, 10 mL
Plastic cups	Liquids, suspensions	5, 10, 15, 30 mL
Plastic suppository shells	Suppositories	1- to 5-g sizes in different colors
Syringes	Parenterals, oral liquids, transdermal gels	0.5, 1, 3, 5, 10, 15, 20, 30, 60 mL
Various sizes of bubble packs	Tablets, capsules, troches	1–3 medications

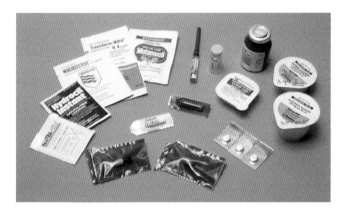

FIG. 11.1 Sample of unit dose containers.

machines. These machines not only fill the unit dose containers but also may generate bar coded labels for the drugs and apply them to the containers as they pass through the machine (see Fig. 11.2B). Other types of equipment are much less high tech. A technician can manually place each tablet or capsule into the individual blister pack and then apply the label. Although this type of repackaging is considered non-sterile, the technician should carefully use appropriate aseptic techniques to keep the process of preparing medications as clean as possible.

Bulk Repackaging Techniques

Sterile technique is not required for repackaging. However, technicians must observe the following rules for garments, techniques, and equipment to ensure that the environment is as clean as possible:

- Wear a lab coat.
- Pull the hair back.
- Wash the hands.
- Wear a face mask when appropriate.
- Wear gloves if the tablets or capsules will be touched.
- Use a pill counting tray and spatula if the tablets will be dispensed from the tray.

All equipment should be kept clean and in good condition at all times. The process of repackaging should take place in a designated area of the pharmacy, away from high-traffic

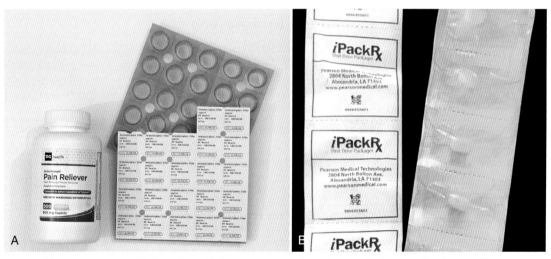

FIG. 11.2 (A and B) Samples of blister pack containers for a unit dose medication. (B, From Pearson Medical Technologies, LLC, Alexandria, LA.)

areas. This reduces air flow over the medication, which may cause contamination. If the technician is using manual methods to load medications into blister packs, it is important that he or she wear gloves after washing the hands. If a pill tray is used to guide tablets or capsules into their containers, the tray should be washed with alcohol after each use. If tablets or capsules are to be unit dosed, it is important to have enough packages and labels ready for use. In addition to having these supplies, keeping medications separate from one another is important. Only one item at a time should be prepared because leaving multiple drugs on a countertop leads to errors. Keeping the area clean and well organized not only helps avoid contamination of drugs but also reduces the chance of errors.

Tech Note!

To reduce cross-contamination of patients' prescriptions, pill counting trays should be cleaned after each use. If residue is left behind on the pill counter and the next patient is allergic to the previously counted medication, that patient may have an allergic reaction. When chemotherapy medication is counted, a tray marked specifically for counting chemotherapeutic drugs should be used to avoid cross-contamination. All trays are cleaned with alcohol prep pads.

Documentation

Keeping track of the products you are repackaging is a major step that must not be overlooked. Just as manufacturers must document all drugs they have packaged, so must the pharmacy.

If a manufacturer recalls a drug that has been repackaged, it is essential to have an accurate count of how many unit doses were made with the recalled product and to be able to identify them by the lot number on each. Therefore documentation for repackaged drugs must include the information shown in Table 11.3. Table 11.4 provides examples of how the drug manufacturers' names normally are abbreviated. It is important to enter as much information as possible on the unit dose log record, which is usually a separate binder used for record-keeping. Fig. 11.3 shows an example of a unit dose log record.

Scenario Checkup 11.1

Today Judy is assigned to work in the repackaging station. As she gets ready to begin her shift, she notices that her co-worker is filling blister packs by hand without wearing gloves. Judy knows that even though repackaging is considered nonsterile, gloves should be worn to limit contamination possibilities. Should Judy discuss this with her co-worker? What is the best way to handle this situation?

Labeling and Checking Bulk Repackaged Medications

Common dosage forms of drugs that normally are repackaged in a pharmacy include oral medications such as tablets, capsules, and liquids. Tablets may be cut in half and repackaged per facility protocol.

Many different types of computer labeling programs are used to generate unit dose labels in the pharmacy. The pharmacy technician is responsible for determining which drugs are needed to replenish the pharmacy stock according to **periodic automatic replacement (PAR)** levels and then preparing the necessary

■ TABLE 11.3
Example of Unit Dose Record Log Sheet Information[a]

Item	Description
Date	Date the drug is repackaged, which includes day, month, and year
Drug	Drug name, usually by generic and then brand name if indicated on log sheet
Dosage form	Tablet, capsule, spansule, troche, suspension, elixir, solution
Manufacturer	Manufacturer of drug, usually abbreviated
Manufacturer's lot number	Control number located on side of label or on bottom of bottle
Manufacturer's expiration date	Located with lot number; remember that if the date indicates only the month and year, the drug is good through the end of the month
Pharmacy lot number	Each item repackaged in the pharmacy is given a number consecutive to the previous batch prepared
Pharmacy beyond-use date	One year from the date packaged or the expiration date on the manufacturer's container, whichever is earlier
Technician	Must initial MFR and CR records
Pharmacist	Each item repackaged must be checked off by a pharmacist

[a]Much less information is required on the label of the unit dose item than in the logbook, but it is just as important. The components necessary on a typical unit dose label include the name of the drug, generic name, trade name (the trade name is commonly given for easy identification of the proper medication), strength, dosage form, lot number, and beyond-use date.
CR, Compounding record; *MFR*, master formula record.

TABLE 11.4
Examples of Manufacturer Abbreviation Codes

Manufacturer	Code	Manufacturer	Code
3M Pharmaceuticals	3MP	Johnson & Johnson	JJ
Abbott Laboratories	ABB	Lederle	LED
A.H. Robins	ROB	Marion Merrell Dow	MMD
AstraZeneca	AZN	Mead Johnson Nutritionals	M/J
Barr Laboratories	BRR	Merck & Co	MSD
Bausch & Lomb	B-L	Novartis Pharmaceuticals	NVR
Bayer Pharmaceuticals Corp	BYR	Novo Nordisk	NNP
Boehringer Ingelheim	B-I	NovoPharm	NOV
Burroughs Wellcome	BW	Parke-Davis	P-D
Ciba Pharmaceuticals	CIB	Pfizer Pharmaceuticals	FD
Colgate Oral Pharmaceuticals	COP	Pharmacia & Upjohn	UPJ
Dey LP	DEY	Procter & Gamble	PG
DuPont Pharmaceuticals	DUP	Purdue Pharma	PUR
Econo-Med Pharmaceuticals	ECO	Roche Laboratories	ORC
Eli Lilly and Company	LY	Roxane Laboratories	ROX
Endo Pharmaceuticals	END	Rugby Laboratories	RUG
Eon Laboratories	EON	Sandoz	SAN
Fujisawa Pharmaceutical	FUJ	SmithKline Beecham Pharmaceuticals	SKF
G & W Laboratories	G&W	Taro Pharmaceuticals	TRO
Geigy Pharmaceuticals	GEI	Teva Pharmaceuticals	TEV
Geneva Pharmaceuticals	GG	Upsher-Smith Laboratories	UPS
Glaxo Wellcome	GLX	Wyeth-Ayerst	WY
Hoechst Marion Roussel	HMR	Zenith Goldline Pharmaceuticals	Z/G
ICN Pharmaceuticals	ICN		

	Date	Drug (generic)	Strength	Dosage form	Amount	MFG	MFG lot#	MFG exp date	Pharmacy expiration date	Pharmacy lot #	Tech	RPH
1	2/11/2018	aspirin	81 mg	tab	100	Bayer	JGH405	7/15/2020	6/16/19	A1001	LP	TG
2	2/12/2018	perphenazine	2 mg	tab	100	Schering	XYZ124	12/1/2020	7/16/19	A1002	TK	DS
3												
4												
5												
6												
7												
8												
9												

FIG. 11.3 Example of a unit dose log record.

medications. Technicians must calculate the correct BUD, document the essential information, generate the labels, fill the medication, and apply the label neatly on the container. Finally, the pharmacist checks the completed work to ensure that the label, drug, and logging of the medication are correct.

In specific situations, a technician who has received specialized training may check another technician's work; this is referred to as tech-check-tech. Certain states allow pharmacy technicians to check the work of other technicians. This is limited to checking repackaged unit doses, floor stock, and patient medication drawers. Even if your state has approved the use of the tech-check-tech process, each pharmacy can choose whether to adopt the process and provide the necessary training (see Chapter 3).

Storage and Stability

Medications in a solid form (eg, tablets) usually have a longer shelf life than liquid forms because it is easier for a liquid product to degrade or for its components to separate. The FDA is responsible for providing guidelines for all manufacturers that package medications. Expiration dates are determined on the basis of tests conducted by manufacturers and the FDA; however, these rules do not apply to medications repackaged in a hospital setting for individual patient use. *Once the medication is removed from its original packaging, the expiration date changes.* The BUDs assigned to repackaged products are established according to the guidelines in USP, "Pharmaceutical Compounding—Nonsterile Preparations" (USP <795>). Items repackaged for use in a hospital or for a specific patient's use cannot be mass produced. Only drug manufacturing companies following FDA guidelines may mass produce medications.

Expiration Dates and Beyond-Use Dating

There is an important distinction between expiration dates and BUDs. Expiration dates are assigned by the manufacturer. When reading a manufacturer's expiration date, such as 9/21, it means that the drug is effective through the last day of the month, in this case September 2021. BUDs are calculated by the pharmacy when repackaging or compounding medications. Assigning BUDs is an important process. Once a bulk bottle is opened and the medication is repackaged, the manufacturer's expiration date may no longer be valid.

Determining Beyond-Use Date

The **beyond-use date** (**BUD**) of a repackaged nonsterile solid or liquid dose is 1 year from the date repackaged or the expiration date on the manufacturer's container, whichever is earlier (unless otherwise stated in the manufacturer's literature). The manufacturer's expiration date is the exact amount of time the drug is usable. Once repackaged, this may be different. This applies to unit dosing and filling prescriptions in a retail pharmacy. Example 11.1 shows this calculation for proper dating.

◉ Example 11.1: Beyond-Use Dating

Acetaminophen 500-mg tablets
Today's date: December 15, 2021
Per the manufacturer, the medication expires in December 2024

Because the manufacturer's expiration date is more than 1 year away, you may give this drug a 1-year BUD of December 15, 2022.

◉ Scenario Checkup 11.2

Judy continues her work at the long-term care pharmacy. She is busy finishing up the repackaging for the day. It is her responsibility to check her partner's work before it goes to the pharmacist for final approval. Judy notices that the BUDs have been calculated incorrectly. What steps should she take to correct this error? What if the mistake had been overlooked entirely?

Long-Term Care Packaging

Often patients need their medications packaged in 28- to 31-day cards for ease of individual administration and accuracy in dosing. The method is often referred to as *blister packing* or *bubble packaging.* The medications prescribed by a physician are put into individual pockets in a card that holds a month's worth of medication. Morning doses and night doses can be placed in different cards, and each dose is put in an individual pocket. This method has many advantages for patients and health care providers. For example, it makes compliance easier for patients in taking their medication correctly, and it allows timely monitoring by health care team members (Fig. 11.4). In addition, the unsteady hands of an elderly patient can get one tablet from the card without spilling the entire contents of a bottle or touching the other tablets in the card. If a dose is changed (and with long-term care patients this is often the case because of their chronic or multiple disease states), the remaining uncontaminated medications in the card can be returned and reused. The card is a visible way to easily identify missed doses and to aid the patient in medication compliance.

Nonsterile Compounding

History

The art of compounding dates back more than 4000 years, beginning with medicinal mixtures using plants, animals, and minerals. Historians have found recipes for various treatments written on scrolls from 1500 BCE, and **mortars and pestles** have been unearthed that were used in the early Egyptian and Roman societies. Early pharmacists compounded each prescription individually. In the United States the first pharmacopoeia was published in 1820 and listed more than 80% of the prescriptions that were made; all were compounded products at that time. As the pharmaceutical business grew, more drugs were manufactured in common dosages by drug companies, which reduced the number of products that needed to be compounded by the pharmacy. It was not until the late 1990s that compounding once again became popular.

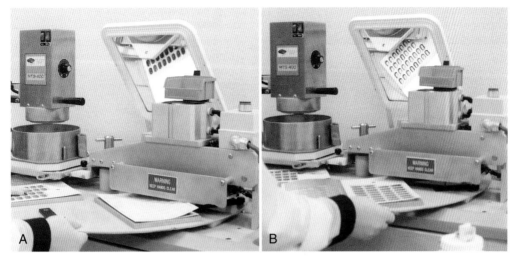

FIG. 11.4 **A technician is responsible for the proper preparation and labeling of all repackaged medications.** (A) The empty 30-day long-term care card is rotated under the hopper, where the medication is placed into the card. The medication card is then rotated to the heating element, where the seal is made to enclose each tablet. (B) The technician uses a mirror to verify that each sheet is filled completely.

Premade dosages are not always appropriate for everyone; each person is different because of other concurrent conditions or physiologic factors that affect the drug prescribed. This is evident in pediatrics, in which dosages must be calculated and provided based on the weight of the child because the metabolic rate of children is quite different from that of adults. Dosages that are much easier for a child to take also are needed. Examples of these dosage forms include ice pops and lozenges that deliver medications. Hospice patients, who may not be able to swallow oral medications or have injections, require a different dosage form that is not available by a manufacturer. A list of reasons for compounding medications is given in Box 11.1. People who would benefit from a combination drug that is not already packaged can have a combination drug made specifically for them. For example, women who are menopausal can have compounded medications made specifically for their hormone supplementation needs.

BOX 11.1 Why Compound Medications?

Medications may need to be compounded by a pharmacy for several reasons, including the following:
- The medication is no longer manufactured by the drug company.
- The patient is allergic to a preservative, dye, or other additive in the normal drug.
- A specialized dosage or strength is needed for a patient with unique needs (eg, an infant or a patient with diabetes).
- Combining several medications will increase patient compliance.
- The patient cannot ingest the normal dosage form.
- The medication requires flavorings and/or additives to make it more palatable for patients, most often children.

Use of Nonsterile Compounding

Nonsterile compounding consists of compounding two or more medications in a nonsterile environment. Aseptic technique (sterile compounding) is discussed in depth in Chapter 12. Most community pharmacies do not have the staff, the wide variety of supplies, or the time to compound various dosage forms and medication strengths. This type of task is performed by specialized compounding pharmacies. However, the average technician will perform some basic types of nonsterile compounding when working in institutional settings or community pharmacies. Compounding standards, common preparations prepared in most pharmacies, and types of items prepared in specialized compounding pharmacies are discussed.

The FDA requires that nonsterile compounded products meet the *United States Pharmacopoeia: National Formulary* (USP-NF) standards, although they do not specifically regulate compounding. Compounding pharmacies must follow each state's board of pharmacy (BOP) regulations in addition to USP-NF standards. Other standards that must be followed involve the quality and stability of ingredients, assigning BUDs, the policies and procedures used during preparation, the equipment required, and the quality control and documentation guidelines that must be followed (per the BOP). Box 11.2 lists the types of dosage forms that can be compounded under the USP-NF.

Determining Beyond-Use Dating for Nonsterile Compounds

Unless there is specific information available in the literature for a particular nonsterile compounded drug preparation, USP <795> provides general guidelines to follow. The **USP <795>** guidelines for determining BUDs for nonsterile compounding are shown in Table 11.5; however, more stringent specific state requirements may dictate the method used. This information should be outlined in each facility's policies

◼ TABLE 11.5

USP <795> Guidelines for Beyond-Use Dating With Nonsterile Compounding

Nonpreserved aqueous dosage forms ($a_w \geq 0.60$) =	**14 days**
Preserved aqueous dosage forms ($a_w \geq 0.60$) =	**35 days**
Oral liquids (nonaqueous) ($a_w < 0.60$) =	**90 days**
Other nonaqueous dosage forms ($a_w < 0.60$) =	**180 days**

From US Pharmacopeial Convention, General Chapter <795>, Pharmaceutical Compounding - Nonsterile preparations. Revised (published November 1, 2023). Available at: https://online.uspnf.com/uspnf/document/1_GUID-98DCB48D-DC23-4A63-AD2E-01CA8979FB7E_6_en-US?source=TOC

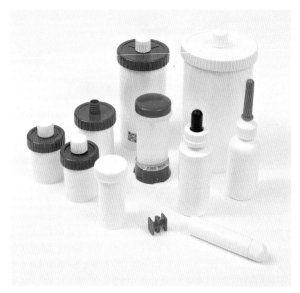

FIG. 11.5 Nonsterile compounding containers.

and procedures manual. According to USP <795>, a nonsterile compound has three main parts: the active ingredient, medication, or active pharmaceutical ingredient (**API**); the inactive ingredient; and the diluent or vehicle. When the shelf life or BUD of a compound is determined, the dosage forms are taken into consideration.

Compounding Area

Certain criteria established by USP <795> must be met in setting up a compounding area. Although the compounding area and its supplies can be located in a pharmacy, the compounding area must be kept separate from areas not directly related to compounding. The compounding surfaces should be nonporous, smooth, and in good condition, and good lighting should be provided. Overhanging shelves or ledges should not be located over the workspace because dust can accumulate in these spaces. There should be a source of hot and cold water with an accessible sink located close to the compounding site for hand washing and cleaning. Purified water should be used to rinse equipment and utensils. When in use, all surfaces should be cleaned on a routine basis, between compounding procedures and at the beginning and the end of the day, to avoid cross-contamination. The temperature and humidity should be monitored to avoid decomposition of chemicals.

Equipment

Types of compounding equipment include personal protective equipment (PPE), measuring and weighing devices, an assortment of containers, and labels (Fig. 11.5). The minimum required equipment list is provided by each state BOP (see your state's requirements), although pharmacies may want to stock additional types of equipment for preparing products (Table 11.6). This determination normally is made on the basis of the amounts and types of nonsterile products the pharmacy provides. The maintenance, **calibration,** and cleaning of each piece of equipment is required according to the manufacturer's specifications, and documentation, in the form of logs, is required by USP <795> (Fig. 11.6). Various types of compounding equipment required for specific uses are discussed in the following sections.

Containment Ventilated Enclosure

Preparation, weighing, measuring, or any other manipulations of APIs must occur in the containment ventilated enclosure (CVE). In the "powder hood," the air is controlled and allows for exhaust to be directed away from the compounder to prevent inhalation of powders. The CVE must be certified annually. Cleaning should be done at the beginning of each shift, if a spill or known contamination has occurred. Scales and other equipment may remain inside the hood at all times and be cleaned and calibrated therein (Fig. 11.7).

TABLE 11.6

Examples of Compounding Equipment

Equipment	Use/Description
Autoclave	For sterilization
Balance	Class A balance, torsion digital balance
Beakers	1, 5, 10, 20, 50, 100, 500, 1000 mL
Blender	Electric
Capsule molds	For making multiple capsules
Containers	Spray bottles, ointment tubes, plastic jars, vials, bottles, stick containers, ophthalmic containers
Crimpers	For sealing tubes and glass bottles
Disposable weighing devices	Papers (glycerin), boats (plastic)
Droppers	Sterile and nonsterile
Filters	0.5 and 0.2 μm
Foil wraps	For wrapping suppositories
Funnels	For transferring liquids
Glass stirring rods	For stirring/mixing liquids
Glass tile	For mixing ingredients
Graduated cylinders	For performing various measurements
Heat gun	For sealing packages
Hot plate	For melting ingredients
Magnetic stir plate	Automatically stirs for long periods
Magnetic stirrers	Used in beaker to stir contents
Metal measuring scoop	For transferring powders to scale
Molds	Capsules, tablets, lozenges, troches, suppositories, ice pops, lollipops
Mortar and pestle	Glass, porcelain
Ointment mill	For increasing the overall surface area of the active substance, thereby maximizing the benefit to the patient; produces very smooth and elegant ointments
Paper sheets, 12 × 12 inches	For levigation and mixing ingredients
Pipettes	For adding minute amounts of liquids: 50 micrograms (mcg) to 1 mL
Refrigerator	For storage
Rubber grippers	For removing glass from hot plates
Sieves	For removing particles
Sink	For washing all equipment
Solvents	For cleaning surface area of compounding room
Spatulas	For moving and mixing ingredients
Thermometers	For ingredients that must be prepared at a certain temperature
Tongs	For removing hot contents
Wash bottle	For rinsing
Weights	Brass weights used on Class A balance

Personal Protective Equipment

PPE is used to ensure the sterility of the product and to protect the technician from spills while working. The following are considered necessary PPE:

- Gloves
- Goggles
- Gown
- Hair cover
- Lab coat
- Mask
- Shoe covers

Measuring Devices

Graduated cylinders (Fig. 11.8) are available in various sizes (from 1 mL to 1 L), types (eg, glass and plastic), and shapes (eg, conical and cylindrical) to measure liquids (Table 11.7).

Title of SOP: Room Cleaning Procedures—Compounding Room	SOP No. 5.008

Original: ☐ Yes ☐ No   Revision: ☐ Yes ☐ No   Revision No.: _____

Responsibility:

The pharmacist-in-charge and the support staff or contract labor are responsible for this procedure.

Purpose:

The purpose of this standard operating procedure is to establish appropriate guidelines and documentation for the maintenance of the compounding room.

Equipment/Supplies Required:

- Cleaning items designated for compounding room cleaning only—mop, bucket, floor soap, proper cleaning attire
- Cleaning Maintenance Log

Procedure:

General

A. Use cleaning items that are designated for compounding room cleaning only. ***WARNING:*** *Do not use cleaning items that are designated for clean room cleaning only. Do not perform cleaning procedures during a compounding process.*

B. Clean areas immediately following any repairs or spills.

Preparation of Cleaning Solutions

A. Prepare cleaning solutions on the day of use. ***WARNING:*** *Do not combine cleaning solutions or use in concentrations other than those outlined in the appropriate SOPs and/or the manufacturer's instructions.*

B. Discard any unused cleaning solutions immediately after the cleaning has been completed.

Cleaning Schedule

A. Document all cleanings on the Cleaning Maintenance Log.

B. Perform the following daily cleaning duties:

   1. Empty all waste receptacles.

   2. Sweep the floors.

   3. Clean the counter tops as needed.

   4. Wash dishes, utensils, and drain items.

C. Perform the following weekly cleaning duties:

   1. Damp mop the floor.

D. Perform the following monthly cleaning duties:

   1. Clean the shelving and items stored on the shelving.

Approved by _____ Date _____

Implemented by _____ Date _____

A

FIG. 11.6 (A) Guidelines for cleaning the compounding room.

Cleaning Maintenance Log								

Room Description: (Check one) ☐ IV room ☐ Compounding laboratory ☐ Anteroom ☐ Ancillary room ☐ IV infusion room

Check activity as completed

Month _____ Year _____

Date	Daily				Weekly	Monthly		Signature
	Waste removal	Sweep floors	Clean counter tops	Wash dishes, utensils	Mop floor	Check out-of-date drugs	Clean and disinfect shelves of bulk drug	
1								
2								
3								
4								
5								
6								
7								
8								
9								
10								
11								
12								
13								
14								
15								
16								
17								
18								
19								
20								
21								
22								
23								
24								
25								
26								
27								
28								
29								
30								
31								

Approved by _____ Date _____

Implemented by _____ Date _____

B

FIG. 11.6, cont'd (B) Log used to record cleaning activities. (Courtesy Karen Davis.)

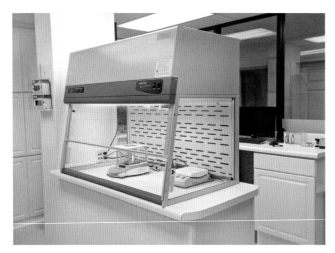

FIG. 11.7 Containment ventilated enclosure (CVE) "powder hood" used for nonsterile compounding.

▣ TABLE 11.7
Types of Graduated Cylinders

Type	Use
Conical	Wider platform is more stable when measuring viscous liquids and makes it easier to mix solutions; however, because sides flare outward, reading meniscus is more difficult, which affects accuracy of measurement
Cylindrical	Used to measure liquids more accurately
Glass	Used for hot liquids or liquids not compatible with plastic devices
Plastic	Used for cold liquids

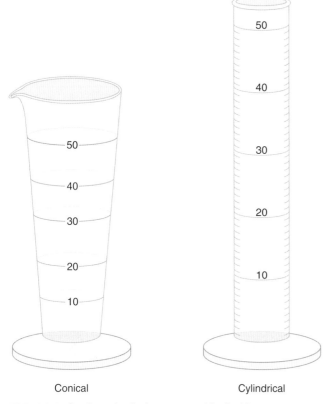

Conical　　　　Cylindrical

FIG. 11.8 Graduated cylinders are used for liquid measurement.

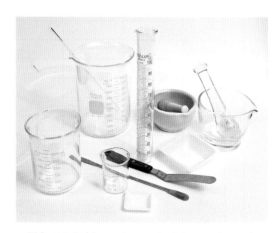

FIG. 11.9 Measuring and mixing equipment.

▣ TABLE 11.8
Types of Compounding Mixing Equipment

Mortars and Pestles

Glass	Used for preparing liquids such as solutions and suspensions and for mixing oily or staining materials
Porcelain	Used for blending powders and pulverizing soft aggregates or crystals

Spatulas

Plastic	Used for mixtures that may react with metal
Metal	Used for mixing ointments or creams and handling dry chemicals
Long (>6 inches)	Used for ointments or creams and powder blends for capsules
Short (≤6 inches)	Used in handling dry chemicals

Other types of measuring instruments can range from syringes (for small volumes) and pipettes (for minute volumes) to large, automated measuring machines. These electronic machines, ointment mills, and capsule-filling machines are used in compounding pharmacies to prepare large amounts of medications. Capsule-filling machines normally fill 100 to 300 capsules at a time.

Mixing Equipment

Various sizes of glass and porcelain mortars and pestles are necessary, depending on the types of ingredients to be prepared (Fig. 11.9). Various spatula types include metal and plastic (Table 11.8). Automated mortars and pestles, used for ointments and creams, have settings for mixing times and speed (Fig. 11.10). These allow the preparer to set up the machine for a time to mix according to

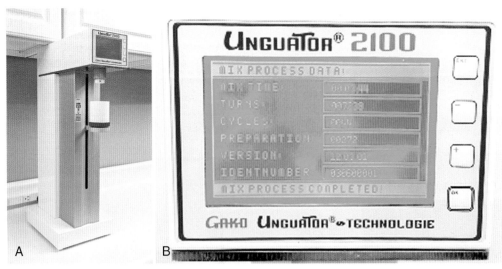

FIG. 11.10 (A) Electronic mortar and pestle (Unguator). (B) Operator can choose various settings for mixing on the screen. (Courtesy Karen Davis.)

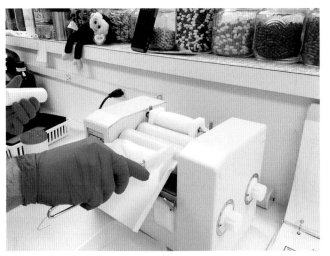

FIG. 11.11 A three-roll ointment mill in operation. (Courtesy Karen Davis.)

a formulation compound or recipe. An automated ointment mill also is available for mixing creams and ointments (Fig. 11.11).

Weighing Equipment

One of the most expensive pieces of compounding equipment is the balance or scale used to weigh powders. Scales differ in their range of weight and style. A Class III balance, also called a Class A balance (Fig. 11.12A), is a torsion balance. This type of scale uses a counterbalance (weights) to determine the weight of the substance being measured and is referred to as a mechanical scale (required by most state BOPs). This type of scale has special weights that are labeled in a range of milligrams and grams (see Fig. 11.12B). The minimum weighable quantity for a Class A balance is 120 mg. Weights used on this type of scale should be stored in a hard-shelled container and should be handled only with the accompanying tweezers.

Another style of balance is the analytical electronic balance (Class II) (see Fig. 11.12C), which provides a digital read-out of the weight. No weights are used with this balance; instead, the calibrations are electronic. Digital balances are more commonly used than two-pan torsion balances. They can weigh heavier substances than the Class III balance, as shown in the following comparisons:

- *Digital balance/Class II:* Capacity 100 g; readable to 0.0001 g (eg, Sartoris GD503)
- *Digital balance/Class II:* Capacity 200 g; readable to 0.01 g (eg, PCE-LSM200)
- *Digital balance/Class II:* Capacity 410 g; readable to 0.01 g (eg, Adventurer Pro) (Fig. 11.13)
- *Class III balance:* Capacity 60 to 120 g; sensitivity of 6 mg or less (eg, DRX-3 Torbal)

Appropriate calibration, care, and cleaning of these sensitive instruments are the responsibility of the person using them and should be performed before, during, and after use.

▼ Tech Alert!

Always place and use a scale outside of direct air flow to obtain the most accurate reading.

Additional Supplies

Mold Forms

Various suppository molds can be used to prepare suppositories. These include the traditional metal molds, in which cavity openings range from 1 to 2.5 g. Different mold sizes (6–100) allow for different numbers of suppositories to be prepared. The molds are held together by nuts and screws while the ingredients solidify. Another option is hard rubber molds, which are similar to the metal molds. Hard rubber molds are held together by screws that are loosened when the suppositories are solid. Flexible rubber molds in strips that can be placed in the refrigerator, if necessary, are also available.

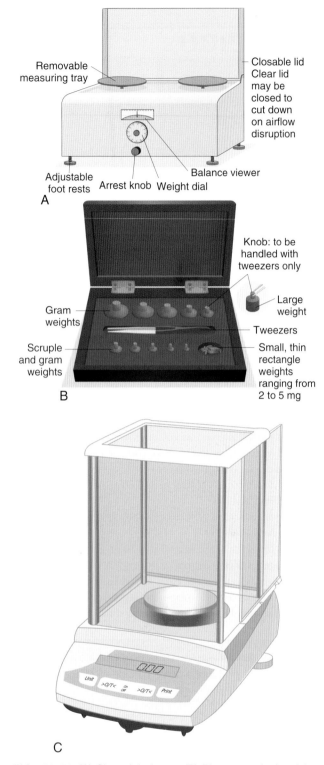

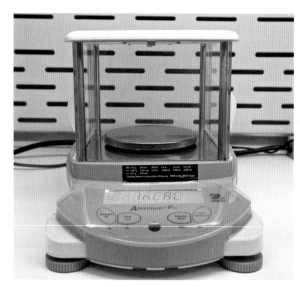

FIG. 11.13 Digital balance/Class II Adventurer Pro.

FIG. 11.12 (A) Class A balance. (B) Pharmaceutical weights. (C) Analytical balance.

When strips of molds are used, the exact number of suppositories can be removed to fill a prescription, and the remainder can be left in the refrigerator for the next order.

Excipients

Excipients are inert (not medicinally active) ingredients that are added to preparations to achieve the required consistency, effectiveness, and functional properties to form a suitable dosage form for administration (Table 11.9). They are used in a variety of dosage forms, such as liquids, suspensions, tablets, and capsules. Chemicals may be used to alter the pH and solubility of the active medication as needed.

Taste

Flavorings are often added to medications to mask the bad taste of the ingredients. The tongue recognizes four basic tastes: sweet, sour, salty, and bitter. Masking the taste becomes more difficult as the distaste increases. Flavorings such as saccharin impart a bitter taste followed by a sweet taste, whereas sucrose gives an immediate sweet taste. Sucrose flavorings are the most commonly used because of this property. Preservatives can alter the properties of flavorings, causing different results in taste. Many of the flavorings have a color additive; for those that do not, dyes can be used, although they are not absolutely necessary. Colors should match the flavor; for example, cherry flavor should be colored red. Each recipe indicates which flavorings and/or colors can be mixed into the compounded product. Examples of the types of agents used as flavorings when compounding antibiotics, antihistamines, barbiturates, decongestants, and electrolytes are shown in Table 11.10. Consideration always must be given to the stability and solubility of the additives. In addition, the patient's record must be checked for any allergies before preparation. Children's medications are often flavored with types of flavors similar to those found in candy and drinks.

Personal Preparation

Before beginning the compounding process, the technician should tie back long hair and put on a lab coat and gloves to reduce contamination of the product. In addition to these personal considerations, a technician who is sick or has any open wounds should not compound any products. For commonly compounded items, pharmacists and technicians use a

TABLE 11.9
Common Additives

Additive	Description
Coatings	Surrounding layer of polymeric material that coats a tablet, capsule, or pellet. This is done to change color; protect active ingredient from moisture, light, pH of stomach; and hide bad taste or odor when taken by mouth. Film coatings can provide functional properties that enable the creation of a sustained- or delayed-release dosage form.
Disintegrants	Added to a tablet or capsule blend to help break up compacted mass when put into a fluid environment; especially important for rapid-release agents.
Emulsifying agents	Maintain dispersion of finely divided liquid droplets in a liquid vehicle; made from two or more immiscible liquids (eg, water and oil) and can be a liquid or semisolid (creams and lotions).
Gums	Naturally occurring plant derivatives that are water soluble. They provide a variety of properties, including gelling, thickening, and film forming.
Lubricants	Additive for a powder blend to prevent compacted powder mass from sticking to equipment during the process of making tablets or capsules.
Plasticizers	Blend of plasticizers in acrylic emulsion coatings. They have a wide variety of functional properties (eg, retarding drug release) and allow for flexibility in coating.
Suspending agents	Insoluble particles that are dispersed in a liquid; they act by increasing the viscosity of the liquid vehicle. This reduces the rate of sedimentation of the particles in a suspension.

TABLE 11.10
Common Flavoring Additives for Taste[a]

Drug Class	Most Suitable Flavorings
Antibiotics	Citrus flavors, cherry, pineapple, orange, berry, banana, strawberry-vanilla, banana-vanilla, lemon custard, fruit cinnamon
Antihistamines	Cherry, cinnamon, grape, lime, peach-orange, raspberry, root beer, wild cherry, apricot
Barbiturates	Lime, orange, banana-vanilla, banana-pineapple, peach-orange, root beer
Decongestants and expectorants	Cherry, lemon, loganberry, gooseberry, orange-peach, apricot, strawberry, pineapple, raspberry, tangerine, custard-mint-strawberry
Electrolytes	Cherry, grape, lemon-lime, raspberry, wild cherry
Geriatrics	Black currant, grenadine-strawberry, lime, root beer, wild strawberry

[a]Additional flavorings include menthol, monosodium glutamate (flavor enhancer), peppermint oil, spearmint oil, and wintergreen.

recipe book or formula cards listing compounds, their weights, and step-by-step instructions. The pharmacy technician should be competent in several skills to reduce the possibility of errors when compounding (Box 11.3).

Weighing Techniques

When using a Class A balance, begin by gathering the necessary ingredients and supplies, such as glycerin paper or weighing boats and weights. The balance has adjustable legs for leveling it on the compounding surface, if necessary. Each balance also has an arrest knob that is used to lock the scale in place, which reduces the possibility of damage to the balance. The proper setup of a balance involves six steps (Procedure 11.1), and each step is critical to obtaining the proper weight of a substance. Inside the container that holds the weights is a pair of tweezers for grasping the brass or metal weights. Use of these tweezers prevents hand oils from being transferred to the surface of the metal. Oils can corrode the metal, altering the exact weight.

Pharmacy balances are very sensitive. Regardless of the substance you are weighing, it is important to keep air flow around the balance to a minimum. Even the motion of a person walking by can set the balance into a rocking motion, making calibration difficult. Pharmacy balances have a glass lid that can be used to impede air currents while compounds are weighed. As the balance levels, it is important to add less and less substance to it. One way of doing this is to use a spatula and pick up a small amount of substance, then lightly tap the side of the spatula

To reduce the likelihood of errors and to maximize the quality of the compounded preparation, the pharmacy technician should follow several steps, including the following:

1. Identify the equipment needed to prepare the medication.
2. Wear the proper gear.
3. Wash hands appropriately.
4. Clean the compounding area and necessary equipment with antibacterial solvent.
5. Assemble all necessary materials before beginning the compounding process.
6. Perform all necessary calculations to determine the amounts of ingredients necessary.
7. Determine the intended use, safety, and legal limitations of the prescription to be compounded.
8. Compound only one preparation at a time.
9. Compound the preparation according to the prescription or formula (recipe).
10. Assess the weight variation; consistency of mixture; and color, odor, clarity, and pH of preparation.
11. Determine the beyond-use dating for the product prepared.
12. Complete the log sheet and add a notation to describe the appearance of the formulation.
13. Label the prescription container, making sure to include all required information.
14. Immediately clean and store all equipment used.
15. Thoroughly clean surface areas.

Before compounding, ensure that you know your state's laws for compounding. If you have any questions on how to prepare a product, ask the pharmacist before you begin the compounding process, not in the middle of it.

Procedure 11.1

Instructions for Using a Class A Balance

Goal

To learn the steps involved in using a Class A balance.

Equipment and Supplies

- Class A balance
- Lightweight papers
- Log to record weight
- Material to be weighed
- Weighing boats
- Weights

Procedural Steps

1. Turn the arrest knob to arrest the balance. Make sure the balance is steady on the counter.
2. Level the balance from front to back using the adjustable legs.
   PURPOSE: The balance must be level to ensure accuracy.
3. Turn the calibrated dial to zero to set the internal weights.
   PURPOSE: The weights must start at zero to ensure accuracy.
4. Level the balance from left to right using the adjustable legs.
   PURPOSE: The balance must be level to ensure accuracy.
5. Add lightweight papers or weighing boats to both sides of the balance.
   PURPOSE: Papers or weighing boats protect the weighing plates and hold the substance being weighed.
6. "Zero out" the balance.
   PURPOSE: This prevents the paper from being included in the weight of the drug.
7. Place weights on the right side of the balance and set the balance to reflect the proper weight.
   PURPOSE: The balance should indicate the correct amount of the weights; if it does not, make the necessary adjustments before weighing the material.
8. Place the substance to be measured on the left side of the balance and view the pointer. Add and/or remove material until the pointer is in the center.
   PURPOSE: The pointer is in the center if the right side and the left side of the balance contain exactly the same weight.

For more details and to watch a video of this procedure, visit the following website: *http://pharmlabs.unc.edu/labs/measurements/balance_operate.htm.*

(from behind the substance) to flick on a few granules at a time. This technique is easier with powders than with other substances. Compounding is time-consuming. It is important to always strive for accuracy. Thus you must take your time.

Tech Note!

Always place the weights on the right side of the balance using a weighing boat or paper. This is done to ensure continuity of measurement.

Measuring Liquids

Measuring liquids requires a few simple steps to ensure the proper volume. Because water molecules cling to the sides of a container (called *capillary action*), the amount of liquid appears to be more than the actual amount. When reading the calibrations of a beaker or graduated cylinder, you must have the liquid at eye level. You must read the graduated cylinder at the bottom of the liquid line, also known as the *meniscus* (Fig. 11.14).

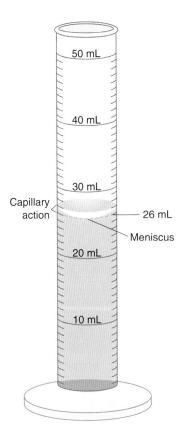

FIG. 11.14 **The meniscus is the level at which liquids are measured and recorded.** For accuracy, always have the container at eye level when determining the volume.

When choosing a container in which to measure your liquids, remember that it is best to choose the size closest to the volume required because the calibrations are more accurate than in larger containers. For maximum accuracy in measuring liquids, use the 20% rule: measure no less than 20% of the capacity of any graduate. For example, a 100-mL graduated cylinder should be used to measure no less than 20 mL (20% of 100) of liquid. Likewise, a 250-mL cylinder should be used to measure no less than 50 mL (20% of 250). In the case of small or extremely small amounts, a syringe or micropipette is used. It would not be accurate to measure 1 mL of liquid in a 10-mL graduated cylinder because 20% of 10 mL is 2 mL. This amount is much more accurately measured with a 3-mL syringe.

Depending on the type of product being prepared, different techniques are required. Each type of compounded product requires specific steps that must be carefully followed, including appropriate labeling. Pharmacy technicians often prepare compounded products and should be familiar with the behavior of each type of additive and of the final product.

Preparing Solutions

When preparing solutions, you must understand the major parts of the liquid: the **solvent** is the vehicle used to dissolve something, the **solute** is the ingredient or agent dissolved in the solvent, and the **solution** is the result, the final mixture of the solute and solvent. Most solutions are compounded by adding the solute to the solvent in portions for proper mixing

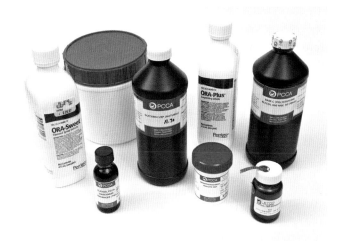

FIG. 11.15 Basic suspensions, syrup, and powders used in nonsterile compounding.

or by adding two solutions together. Two of the most important techniques of mixing solutions are to measure carefully and mix thoroughly. Solutions are prepared in all types of pharmacy settings. Always check the final solution for any precipitation or discoloration.

Solubility

A drug's solubility dictates the type of dosage form that must be prepared. For example, if the drug is water soluble, a **syrup** or solution can be prepared; however, if it is insoluble, an **elixir,** a **suspension,** or possibly an **emulsion** can be made (Fig. 11.15). The pH also affects the solubility of a drug; in such cases buffers may be used to maintain the correct solubility characteristics. Buffers are solutions that resist pH changes when either acids or bases are added to the solution. Factors that affect solubility characteristics are listed in Box 11.4.

▊ Tech Note!

When orders indicate a solution to be a specific strength with instruction to "qs" to a final volume, this means that the solution is to yield a final volume and final strength exactly as ordered by the physician. The "qs" (quantity sufficient) means to add a sufficient quantity of liquid to reach that final required volume.

BOX 11.4 Solubility Characteristics

1. Small particles dissolve faster than large particles.
2. Stirring increases the dissolution rate.
3. The more soluble the drug, the faster it dissolves.
4. Viscous liquids decrease dissolution rates.
5. Increased temperature normally increases the dissolution rate.
6. Mixing an electrolyte with a nonelectrolyte drug can either increase or decrease the dissolution rate.

Reconstituting Premade Suspensions

The only type of compounding that may be done away from the compounding area is the **reconstitution** of premade oral suspensions. Reconstituting involves mixing a diluent (liquid) into a powder to form a solution or suspension. These products are simple to prepare and do not need to be logged or labeled in the same manner as compounded products.

When prepackaged drugs are reconstituted (eg, an amoxicillin suspension), the label is already attached to the product. All the technician must do is read the side panel and follow the directions indicating the proper amount of sterile water (SW) to be mixed with the powder. The BUD that must be applied to the product after reconstitution is marked clearly on the side of the medication, which is active as soon as the suspension is mixed. Therefore, after mixing the drug, the technician should write the BUD on the front of the label. In addition, the patient information and any necessary auxiliary labels must be attached (Table 11.11).

Suspensions are different from solutions because they mix a **hydrophobic** (not water soluble) ingredient into a **hydrophilic** (water soluble) solution. When you reconstitute a suspension, if the manufacturer suggests 110 mL of distilled water to be mixed with the powder in the bottle, you should at first add only part of the water, as the manufacturer directs. This allows the powder to mix with the water in enough free space in the bottle; this lower volume in the bottle makes it easier to mix in the remaining amount. The powdered ingredient is suspended in SW after mixing. Therefore all suspensions must be shaken well before each use to mix the powder evenly, allowing delivery of the proper amount of medication. Many antibiotics, but not all, must be refrigerated after mixing.

Solids: Tablets, Capsules, and Lozenges

Tablets, capsules, and lozenges can be compounded by pharmacy technicians. These preparations have the advantage of providing a custom-made medication for each patient's specific needs. Molds are used to make these oral dosage forms. A product can be made accurately using careful measuring, weighing, and mixing procedures.

Technicians must have great skill and experience to prepare these dosage forms.

Pharmacies can provide individualized strengths and dosage forms to meet the needs of the patient. Molded tablets can be prepared using a tablet **triturate** mold. Compressed tablets are made using a pellet press or single-punch tablet-making machine. Tablets by far are the most common dosage form used because of their ease of administration; they can be taken orally, sublingually, or as a buccal dose, or they can be prepared similar to troches and wafers.

Molded Tablets

Molded tablets disintegrate quickly when they are exposed to moisture. Because molded tablets are small, they are limited to substances that require a smaller dose. Ingredients used in the preparation of molded tablets include a base, additives (Box 11.5), and the active drug.

Tablet molds Tablet molds are made of metal and consist of a top plate (ie, cavity plate) with holes and a bottom plate (ie, peg plate) with pegs. Capacities for tablet molds can range from 60 to 100 mg.

Steps necessary for preparation of molded tablets Because molds have a fixed volume, they must be calibrated (Procedure 11.2). This is because each base used in preparing a molded tablet has a different density, which changes the capacity of each hole in the mold plate. Procedure 11.3 presents the process used to compound molded tablets.

Compressed Tablets and Lozenges

To prepare tablets or lozenges, a single-punch tablet press can be used to make one dose at a time, or a metal punch press can be used to make multiple doses. These presses are available in a variety of sizes to make various strengths of tablets or lozenges. Types of lozenges include hard or soft, and tablets can be chewable, effervescent, or disintegrating. The metal punch press is composed of two parts: the bottom

■ TABLE 11.11
Common Auxiliary Labels Placed on Medication Containers

Dosage Form	Auxiliary Label
Ointments, creams, lotions	For topical use For external use only
Ophthalmic preparations	For the eye
Otic preparations	For the ear
Patches	Apply to skin
Suppositories	For rectal use For vaginal use
Suspensions	Shake well

BOX 11.5 Tablet Additives

Diluent bases: These can be combined to increase the firmness of the tablet.
- Dextrose
- Lactose
- Mannitol
- Sucrose

For drugs that react chemically with sugars, the following can be added:
- Bentonite
- Calcium carbonate
- Calcium phosphate
- Kaolin

Liquids can be added to moisten and mold powder:
- Mixture of alcohol and water in different percentages (50%–80% alcohol): Alcohol accelerates drying, and water causes sugar to dissolve and bind the tablet. If the ingredients dissolve in water quickly, adding water can be omitted.

■ Procedure 11.2

Calibrating the Mold

Goal

To be able to calibrate the mold before making molded tablets.

Equipment and Supplies

- Calculator
- Mold
- Pencil/pen

Procedural Steps

1. Make tablets that contain only a powder base first. Weigh the entire batch and then average the weight per tablet.
   PURPOSE: It is important to know what each tablet will weigh once it is molded to confirm that it has been properly made.
2. Determine the average weight of only the active drug; fill a few cavities in the mold and average the weight per tablet.
   PURPOSE: Knowing the average weight of the active drug can help determine the proper weight of the molded tablet.
3. The quantity of the total prescription is divided by the average weight of each tablet's active ingredient.

PURPOSE: This gives the percentage of the cavity volume required by the active drug, which affects the amount of other material used in the molded tablet.

4. Subtract the percentage in step 3 from 100%; this equals the volume (%) available for the base.
   PURPOSE: Knowing the volume is necessary to determine the correct amount of base to include in the molded tablet.
5. Use percentages of both the active drug in the cavity and the base in the cavity to calculate the amount of base and drug to weigh. (For example, if the mold holds 10 cavities, each holding 100 mg, then 1000 mg of mixture is needed to fill the entire mold.) From this calculation, calculate the base and drug to weigh. (For example, multiply 1000 by the two different percentages from steps 3 and 4.)
   PURPOSE: This calculation provides the amount of active drug and the amount of base needed for the entire batch. Once those amounts have been determined, the mixture can be prepared and placed in the mold (see Procedure 11.3).
6. Prepare 5% to 10% excess mixture.
   PURPOSE: Creating excess mixture allows for powder loss and any variance in the capacity of the molds.

For more details and to watch a video of this procedure, visit the following website: *http://pharmlabs.unc.edu/labs/tablets/molded.htm.*

has a small cavity in one end of the tube; the top has a rod that pushes through the cavity. The rod does not extend totally through the cavity; instead, it leaves a small gap. The punch fits into the press. As the handle is depressed and then released, the rod moves in and out of the bottom piece.

Making a tablet The following steps are used to make a compressed tablet:

1. Place the powder in the bottom piece.
2. Depress the handle and then release. The powders are compressed and will occupy the gap left in the press.
3. Let the tablets harden; then remove them from the punch press.

Compounding capsules Various sizes of capsules are kept in stock for the compounding of encapsulated drugs. Advantages of capsules include masking of ingredients' taste and ease of swallowing compared with tablets. After the proper proportions have been prepared, the powder is then blocked. With a steel spatula, the powder is gathered and compressed onto a flat surface, making it easier to fill the capsule using the **punch method.** The body (ie, the longer and thinner part of the capsule) is punched, attached to the cap (ie, the shorter and wider part of the capsule), and then weighed to make sure each capsule is filled with the same amount of drug. The error rate is calculated by recording each capsule's weight and determining the average weight. According to quality control measures from USP <795>, capsules, powders, lozenges, and tablets must not weigh less than 90% or more than 110% of the calculated weight for each unit.

In larger pharmacies, automated capsule-filling machines can quickly and accurately fill various capsule sizes, saving the pharmacy staff hours of compounding and allowing them to fill other orders or prepare more difficult mixtures. The punch method is used when smaller quantities of capsules are prepared. Capsules are composed of vegetable-based or gelatinous materials. Great care must be taken to load the capsule accurately (Fig. 11.16). Table 11.12 shows the sizes of capsules and the quantity of medication each one holds.

Other solids include minitabs (mostly used for pediatric patients), troches, and lozenges. **Troches** are larger than tablets and are intended to dissolve slowly in the mouth. Troches often are placed in the cheek (buccal) for administration.

Troches Troches, often called lozenges, are made by molding or compression and have several advantages (Fig. 11.17). They are normally made with flavors to enhance their taste. They also can be used as buccal tablets that are absorbed through the buccal lining of the mouth when the appropriate ingredients are used. Children have a much easier time taking gummy-type lozenges than other dosage forms because they look like candy. Lozenges either dissolve or disintegrate slowly in the mouth.

The following traditional ingredients are used to make lozenges:

- Benzocaine
- Cetylpyridinium chloride
- Phenol

Compounding Procedure for Molded Tablets

Goal

To be able to accurately compound pharmaceutically elegant tablets with a mold.

Equipment and Supplies

- 80- to 100-mesh sieve
- Alcohol
- Hard rubber spatula
- Ointment tile or glass plate
- Powder mixture
- Tablet mold
- Water

Procedural Steps

1. Prepare the powder mixture using proper techniques for that specific recipe; then sift the mixture through the 80- to 100-mesh sieve.
   PURPOSE: The sieve is used to reduce the particle size. A good powder formulation has a uniform particle size distribution. If the particle size distribution is not uniform, the powder can segregate according to the different particle sizes, which may result in inaccurate dosing or inconsistent performance.
2. Moisten the mix (alcohol/water) until it adheres to the pestle.
   PURPOSE: To make sure the mixture sets up properly.
3. Place the cavity plate on either an ointment tile or a glass plate.

PURPOSE: To make sure the cavity plate is on an even surface before filling.

4. Take the molded form and press the mixture into the cavity plate using a hard rubber spatula. The choice of material for the spatula depends on any reaction with the ingredients.
   PURPOSE: To evenly distribute the tablet material throughout the cavity plate.
5. Apply sufficient pressure to each cavity to make sure all cavities are entirely filled.
   PURPOSE: To ensure uniformity of all the tablets.
6. Inspect the cavity plate to ensure that all cavities are filled to capacity (there should be very little mixture left unused).
   PURPOSE: To visually check for consistency and accuracy.
7. Align the cavity plate onto the peg plate and then slowly press down evenly on the peg plate.
   PURPOSE: To use the mold to form tablets.
8. The cavity plate will fall, having pushed out the tablets onto the pegs.
   PURPOSE: To use the tablet mold to form individual, uniform tablets.
9. Leave the tablets on the pegs until dried. This typically takes 1 to 2 hours.
   PURPOSE: To allow the tablets to dry so they can be easily removed.
10. Invert the plate and press the tablets off.

To watch a video of this procedure, visit the following website: *http://pharmlabs.unc.edu/labs/tablets/videos.htm.*

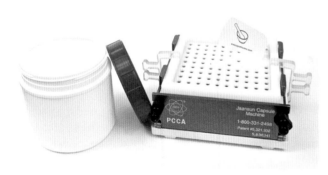

FIG. 11.16 Automated 100-count capsule machine.

- Sodium phenolate
- May also contain anesthetics, antimicrobials, antitussives, antiemetics, and decongestants

Molding mixtures are used to prepare different types of lozenges and may contain the following ingredients:

- Gelatin to form a chewable lozenge
- Polyethylene glycol (PEG) to form a soft lozenge
- Sugars to form a hard lozenge

Hard lozenges Hard lozenges can be made into the traditional round shape or manufactured to look like a lollipop or sucker. A combination of sugars is mixed with other

■ **TABLE 11.12**
Capsule Sizes

Number	Contains Approximate Amount (mg)	Example
000	1000	
00	750	
0	500	
1	400	
2	300	
3	200	
4	150	
5	100	

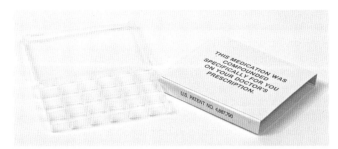

FIG. 11.17 Packaging for troches or lozenges.

ingredients and the medication, and the mixture is poured into a mold and allowed to cool before removal. When the various ingredients are heated together, great care must be taken in monitoring the temperature, moisture content, and pH of the final product.

Considerations in preparing hard lozenges include the following.
- Drugs that may degrade in high heat cannot be made into hard lozenges.
- The dosage form needs a low moisture content, between 0.5% and 1.5%.
- Certain syrups cannot be stirred until a specific temperature is reached.
- Between 55% and 65% sucrose and between 35% and 45% corn syrup must be used to avoid a grainy consistency.
- The use of acidic flavorings lowers the pH; calcium carbonate, sodium bicarbonate, or magnesium hydroxide must be used to raise the pH to 5 or 6.

◉ Example 11.2: Hard Lozenge Formula
- Corn syrup: 46 g
- Drug: 2 g
- Mint extract: 2 mL
- Powdered sugar: 70 g
- Water: 48 mL

Use food coloring to confirm adequate mixing in the laboratory.

Soft lozenges Soft lozenges can be made relatively quickly and then colored and flavored. They can be chewed or dissolved in the mouth. Ingredients include PEG 1000 or 1450, chocolate, or a sugar/acacia base. Lozenges can be hand rolled and cut into pieces or poured while warm into a plastic troche mold. After the mold cools, a spatula is used to level the excess solution; using a hair blow-dryer gives a smooth appearance.

Softeners are mixed and heated to 50°C; mixtures may include the following ingredients:
- 9 parts NutraSweet and 1 part saccharin
- Acacia gel: Used to add texture and smoothness
- Flavoring
- Food extracts
- Silica gel: Used as a suspending agent to keep materials from settling to the bottom of the mold

- Sweeteners
- Syrup flavor concentrates
- Volatile oils

◉ Example 11.3: Soft Lozenge Formula
- Aspartame: 20 packets
- Drug: 1 g
- Mint extract: 1 mL
- PEG: 10 g
- Color: qs

Chewable lozenges Gummy-type lozenges are made primarily for children. The formulations consist of glycerinated gelatin and water. Fruit flavoring is used to sweeten the ingredients and disguise the taste of glycerin, which is very acidic. After the ingredients have been combined, they are heated at a low heat until a fluid forms; the fluid is then poured into preshaped gummy molds and cooled.

◉ Example 11.4: Chewable Lozenge Formula
- Drug: 0.5 g
- Flavoring oil: 3 to 4 gtt
- Gelatin: 18 g
- Glycerin: 70 mL
- Methylparaben: 0.4 g
- Water: 12 mL
- Color: qs

Semisolids

Ointments (Box 11.6), pastes, and creams each have different consistencies, depending on the amount of solids used. Pastes have more solids than ointments and creams. A **cream** is a semisolid emulsion that is similar to an **ointment,** but it is opaque (cloudy) instead of translucent. All three final forms have smooth consistencies.

Semisolids are prepared in all types of pharmacy settings. It is important to mix all ingredients in the right order, following the recipe exactly for uniformity.

Medication Sticks

Medication sticks provide another way of administering medication. Agents such as antibiotics, local anesthetics, sunscreens, antivirals, and oncologic drugs can be manufactured as medication sticks and applied directly to the site on the body that needs treatment. They also can be applied to certain epidermal sites for a systemic effect (ie, affecting the whole body).

Various waxes are used to make either hard or soft sticks; specific blends and temperatures are used to achieve the desired consistency. Additional ingredients, such as resins, polymers, oils, and gels, determine the texture and appearance (ie, clear or opaque) of the finished product.

When combining two or more ingredients that have different ranges of melting points, melt the ingredients sequentially from highest to lowest melting point. Reducing the temperature on the hot plate prevents overheating.

BOX 11.6   **Classifications of Ointment Bases**

Absorption Bases

Properties: Absorb water; highly compatible with medications; increased stability to heat; greasy; most not washable. Examples include:
- Hydrophilic (water-loving) petrolatum bases (USP)
- Petrolatum-based ointment (Aquaphor)

Emulsion Bases

Properties: Insoluble in water; not washable unless mixed with water-in-oil (w/o) base; subject to water loss; washable and nongreasy when in an oil-in-water (o/w) base; more prone to mold growth unless a preservative is added. Examples include:
- Cold cream for w/o and Dermabase for o/w
- Hydrophilic ointment
- Lanolin
- USP (o/w)
- Vanishing creams (o/w)

Oleaginous Bases

Properties: Insoluble in water; good compatibility with a variety of medications; difficult to remove from clothing and skin; difficult to determine the amount of medication released on application. The following are types of oleaginous bases:
- Able to withstand a wider range of temperatures before melting

- All bases are greasy
- Consistency can be altered by adding mineral oil or white wax
- Jelene (Plastibase)
- Jelly-like consistency
- Melting point between 38°C and 60°C
- Mixture of hydrocarbons in both liquid and wax types
- Petrolatum (Vaseline)
- Polymers of silicon and oxygen
- Protect skin from moisture
- Releases medication faster than petrolatum base
- Silicones
- Stable bases that mix well with most substances
- Will not absorb much water unless mixed with cholesterol

Water-Soluble Bases

Properties: Both absorb and dissolve in water; nongreasy and therefore washable; not susceptible to mold or microbial growth; color of the base can change in the presence of certain drugs unless cetyl alcohol is added. Example:
- Polyethylene glycols (also called carbowaxes): Consistency depends on molecular weight, which is noted by a number; the increasing number relates to the solidity of the agent. Carbowax 300 is a liquid at room temperature, whereas 1540 is a solid.

Filling Ointment Jars

An appropriately sized container should be selected for an ointment preparation. Containers range in size from ¼ oz to 1 lb. Using a small spatula, pack the ointment carefully into the bottom and sides of the container and then fill the center (see Fig. 11.9). The jar can be tapped to release any trapped bubbles. As the final step, top off the jar, smoothing the ointment level at the top. For melted ointments, pour the ointment into the jar while still warm, let the ointment solidify, and then smooth off the top using a heated metal spatula.

Filling Ointment Tubes

Ointment tubes are available in different sizes. First roll the ointment (on glassine paper) into a cylinder slightly smaller than the circumference and length of the appropriately sized tube (see Fig. 11.9). Before placing the roll into the back of the tube, take off the cap to release the displaced air when the ointment is inserted. Place both the ointment and the rolling paper into the tube; then cover the end of the tube with a spatula and carefully pull out the paper, leaving the ointment inside the tube. Fold the end of the tube over twice, use crimpers to seal the end of the tube, and label the product.

Soft Sticks

Soft sticks can be clear or opaque; they spread the medication evenly when applied, soften at body temperature, and do not leave a residue on the skin after application (see Fig. 11.9). Ingredients used in soft sticks include the following:

- Cocoa butter
- Gels
- Oils
- PEG
- Petrolatum
- Polymers
- Waxes

Example 11.5: Soft Opaque Stick Formulation

- Active drug: qs
- Aquabase T: 20 g
- Butyl stearate: 5 mg
- Carnauba wax: 1 g
- Castor oil (tasteless): 2 mL
- Cetyl alcohol: 8 g
- Cocoa butter: 6 g
- Perfume: 0.9 mL
- Petrolatum: 13.5 g
- Preservative: 0.1 g
- White beeswax: 30 g

Example 11.6: Soft Clear Stick Formulation

The example given here is an analgesic stick; methyl salicylate is the active ingredient for topical pain relief.
- Menthol: 15%
- Methyl salicylate: 35%

- Propylene glycol: 25%
- Sodium stearate: 13%
- Water: 12%

Hard Sticks

Hard sticks contain crystalline powders that are held together either by heat or by a binding agent. This type of stick must be moistened before it becomes active, and it leaves a white residue when applied (see Fig. 11.9).

⊙ Example 11.7: Hard Stick Formulation

The example given here is a styptic stick, which stops bleeding from minor cuts, such as razor cuts.
- Aluminum sulfate: 27 g
- Ammonium chloride: 7 g
- Copper sulfate: 26 g
- Ferric sulfate: 40 g

The following are additional types of ingredients that can be used in sticks:
- Castor oil
- Corn oil
- Cottonseed oil
- Lubricants
- Oleic oil
- p-Aminobenzoic acid (PABA)
- Paraffin
- Peanut oil
- PEG 300 or 400
- Skin care additives
- Soybean oil
- Sun protection agents
- Vitamin A
- Vitamin E
- Zinc oxide

Sizes and styles of applicators differ, depending on their intended use. Lip balms are prepared in small, cylinder-shaped plastic applicators. To fill the applicators without leaving an indentation in the top (caused by the cooling process), follow these steps:

1. Turn the base of the applicator two full turns to raise the bale (the bottom platform).
2. Slightly overfill the tube with the base. Do this when the mixture has cooled as much as possible to avoid shrinkage.
3. Top the base by pressing a warm spatula on the top of the base to cover any hole that may have appeared during the cooling process.
4. Turn the base of the applicator downward and place the cap on top.

Suppositories

Several sizes and shapes of suppositories are used to administer medications to vaginal, rectal, and urethral areas; suppositories are made with either solutions or ointments. Suppositories can be prepared in three ways: hand rolling, compression, and fusion molding. The various bases used in suppositories serve two purposes: they provide a medium that can carry the medication to the site of absorption, and they allow the medication to be released over different lengths of time. Common bases used are listed in the following sections.

Oleaginous bases An **oleaginous base,** such as cocoa butter or a synthetic triglyceride, can be used because it remains solid at room and body temperatures and melts at a warm temperature. However, care must be taken when heating suppositories made with cocoa butter. If a suppository is heated above 35°C (95°F), its properties change, and it will not keep a solid form when the temperature rises to 30°C (77°F). Synthetic triglycerides are more stable, although they are more expensive. Stepan (Northfield, Illinois), the manufacturer of Wecobee, makes several bases from coconut oil with a melting point temperature range of 33.9°C to 40.5°C, depending on which formula is used. Other triglyceride products by different manufacturers include Dehydag, Hydro-Kote, Suppocire, and Witepsol. Because of the temperature range at which suppositories melt, they should be stored in a cool place or in the refrigerator.

Water-soluble bases PEG polymers or glycerinated gelatins can be used in the manufacturing of suppositories. These types of ingredients dissolve in body fluids and are not as dependent on temperature; therefore they can be stored at room temperature. PEG polymers are a popular choice because of their properties: they are nonirritating, they can be used to make suppositories either by molding or by compression, and they have a wide melting point range. Different weights of PEG bases are normally mixed together or with another base to form different levels of solidity and dissolving lengths. The combinations include the following:
- PEG 300 (60%) and PEG 8000 (40%)
- PEG 1000 (75%) and PEG 3350 (25%)
- PEG 1450 (2.3 g) and silica gel (25 mg)
- PEG 1450 (30%) and PEG 8000 (70%)

Glycerinated gelatins Glycerinated gelatins are often used for vaginal suppositories and have a wide range of additives such as zinc oxide and boric acid. Their properties include an ability to disperse slowly in mucous secretions; they are translucent and gelatinous solids. They must be kept in a cool, dry place because they decompose in humid environments. If they are to be kept for an extended period, preservatives are added, such as methylparaben, propylparaben, or a combination of the two. They should be dipped in water before administration to activate the gelatin.

Preparing suppositories

Using molds. If suppository molds are used, they must be kept at room temperature because the rapid cooling of refrigeration can cause the suppositories to break. The formulation should be poured into each mold cavity in a steady and consistent manner to prevent a layered appearance. Also, pouring the ingredients just before they reach their congealing point allows for a solid suppository. Pouring the mixture too soon (after heating) can produce a hole in the top of the suppository as a result of contraction. Hard molds, such as metal or rubber, require a lubricant, which aids in removal of the suppositories. For this purpose, a light coat of vegetable oil spray can be applied to the mold before the mixture is poured.

When filling molds, pour to the top of each one; filling slightly over the mold is also permissible because the excess can be removed with a heated metal spatula. A black light (to improve visualization) is used to fill suppository shells (unit dose) to ensure that the ingredients are filled to the proper line. These shells may be filled either by pouring or by using a syringe, which limits spillage and allows better control over the volume filled. It is important to be very careful when removing suppositories; the two halves should not be pried apart; instead, they should be pushed away from one another by placing the top of the screws on the table and pushing down on the mold (Fig. 11.18).

Hand-rolling method. Another way of preparing only a few suppositories is to roll them by hand. For this method cocoa butter is used as a base because it does not have to be melted. Triturate the grated cocoa butter, along with the active ingredient, in a mortar. Form a ball-like shape using the palm of your hands; then roll the suppository into a cylinder using a large spatula or a small flat board on a pill tile. The cylinder is cut into suppository segments, which are then rolled on one end to form a conical shape.

Packaging suppositories. If plastic shells are not used, each suppository must be wrapped separately, using foil wrappers that are available in different sizes and colors.

⊙ Scenario Checkup 11.3

Judy is looking forward to her day because she has been assigned to the compounding station. She loves to prepare medications by following the formula! It is always a challenge to make the most pharmaceutically elegant (the special use of a finishing technique to give the final product a professional look) product possible. Her first task is to measure a liquid in a graduated cylinder. What should Julie remember about measuring liquid in a cylinder? What process should she follow to determine the proper amount of liquid?

Nasal Preparations: Ointments, Suspensions, Gels, and Solutions

Nasal preparations can be compounded as jellies, gels, ointments, solutions, or suspensions. They can be used for topical application (eg, ointments, gels, jellies), as sprays, as inhalers, or as drops. Excipients used include buffers, preservatives, tonicity-adjusting agents, gelling agents, and antioxidants, all of which must be nonirritating. These are the same types of agents that are used in ophthalmic formulations. They are quickly absorbed into the bloodstream for rapid onset of activity.

Common preservatives used in nasal products include the following:
• Benzalkonium chloride
• Benzethonium chloride
• *p*-Hydroxybenzoates
• Phenylmercuric acetate
• Phenylmercuric nitrate
• Thimerosal

The preparation method for each type of dosage form begins with accurate measuring and weighing of each ingredient.

Preparing Solutions

1. Dissolve ingredients into three-fourths of the total amount of SW for the injection to be used; mix well.
2. qs with SW to the total volume required.
3. Determine the pH, clarity, and other quality control factors from a sample of the solution.
4. Filter through a sterile 0.2-μm filter into a sterile nasal container.
5. Package and label.

Preparing Suspensions

1. Repeat steps 1 through 3 under Preparing Solutions.
2. Package in an appropriate container for autoclaving.
3. Autoclave, cool, and then label (this step is optional, depending on the recipe).
4. Choose a random sample to check for quality of product (eg, sterility, pH).
5. Package and label; shake well before using.

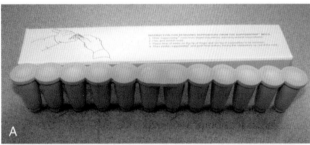
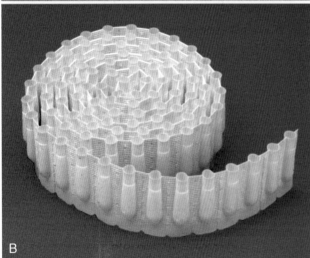

FIG. 11.18 Suppository molds can be used in addition to the hand-rolled method. (A) Suppository molds prepared in the pharmacy. (B) Suppository packaging. (B, Courtesy Total Pharmacy Supply, Inc., Arlington, TX.)

Preparing Ointments

1. Repeat step 1 under Preparing Solutions.
2. Sterilize each ingredient using an appropriate method.
3. Mix each of the ingredients with the sterile vehicle.
4. Perform quality control on a sample of the mixture.
5. Package and label; for topical use only.

Preparing Gels

1. Repeat step 1 under Preparing Solutions.
2. Filter through a 0.2-μm filter into a sterile container.
3. Add the (sterilized) gelling agent and mix well.
4. Add SW for injection to volume/weight and mix well.
5. Perform quality assurance (QA) on sample.
6. Package and label; for topical use only.

> ▼ **Tech Alert!**
>
> Ophthalmic, inhalant, otic, and nasal preparations carry a high risk for cross-contamination if used by more than one patient. Patients should be advised never to share these agents because they are considered sterile.

Packaging

The types of containers used for compounded products must be appropriate. The container must protect the contents and have a child-resistant cap (if applicable), the appropriate label, and any auxiliary labels required. Once mixed to the proper concentration, all products are filled into the appropriately sized container. This should be done neatly to avoid waste. Containers vary in size and in manufactured materials, depending on the circumstances in which the drug is used (Table 11.13). Containers used to package compounded products include glass and plastic bottles, syringes, dropper bottles, and jars of various sizes. Containers in a variety of sizes are used to hold medications and suppository molds for rectal preparations.

Syringes sometimes are used to prepare oral, vaginal, or parenteral compounds. Once the drug has been loaded into the barrel of the syringe, a cap is placed over the top to keep the contents inside. For items that should not be injected, an oral syringe or other syringe to which a needle cannot be attached should be used; using an oral/nonparenteral syringe reduces dosage administration errors.

Certain containers do not have childproof caps or lids; therefore the patient must be instructed by the pharmacist to keep these types of containers out of the reach of children. The following are some examples of these types of containers:

- Cream or ointment jars
- Dropper bottles
- Ointment tubes
- Syringes

> ■ **Tech Note!**
>
> Read all instructions before beginning to compound materials. Make sure that all the ingredients are available to avoid a delay in product preparation. Also, it is important to reorder stock after ingredients have been depleted so that the ingredients are available for the next prescription.

Stability

Several factors affect the stability of a drug. The amount of light and air, the temperature, and even the pH alter the longevity of a drug. Legally, the date given to a pharmacy-prepared product cannot be longer than that for any of the ingredients in the product. The pharmacist or the pharmacy technician must find the appropriate BUD in the manufacturer's literature if it is not already provided. In addition to this reference, many compounding books contain calculations that determine appropriate BUDs. Prepared recipes contain all necessary information. The BUD of a preparation is set from the time of compounding, not from the time when the medication is dispensed. If no literature is available to determine the BUD, USP <795> provides guidelines that can be used to set the appropriate date (see Table 11.5).

Documentation

As in the case of repackaging, documentation of compounded medications is important. Keeping accurate records ensures the integrity of the product dispensed and meets FDA guidelines for quality assurance. According to USP <795>, there should be documentation to describe the process for creating the compound. The **master formulation record (MFR)** is a detailed record of procedures to describe how the **compounded nonsterile preparation (CNSP)** is prepared. It includes a list of ingredients, the preparation methods, safety requirements, BUD information, description of the final product, storage, and references for the preparer. This documentation ensures that the procedures are consistent and can be reproduced (Fig. 11.19). In addition to the MFR, pharmacies are required to have a **compounding record (CR),** or log

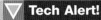
TABLE 11.13
Containers and Sealants and Associated Dosage Forms

Container/Sealant	Dosage Forms
Amber blister packs[a]	Tablets, capsules
Amber bottles	Tablets, capsules, liquids
Foil paper	Suppositories
Heat-sealed strips[a]	Tablets, capsules
Metal tubes	Ointments and semisolids
Polystyrene	Solids in bottles and jars

[a]For institutional use only.

Progesterone 100 mg SR Capsules Size #0 (LoxOral™)

SUGGESTED FORMULA FOR
Progesterone 100 mg SR Capsules Size #0 (LoxOral™)
Version: 1.0
100 Capsules

PROGESTERONE USP, PCCA SPECIAL MICRONIZED	10 g
METHOCEL® E4M PREMIUM CR [HYPROMELLOSE USP]	14 g
BASE, PCCA LOXORAL™	14.857 g

SUGGESTED COMPOUNDING PROCEDURE

Note: It is recommended that you follow USP <795> recommendations for potency testing which states "... each preparation shall contain not less than 90.0% and not more than 110.0% of the theoretically calculated and labeled quantity of active ingredient...". In order to provide some guidance in this area, please contact Eagle Analytical Services regarding the use of Skip Lot testing.

Note: This is a theoretical formula and has not been tested in the PCCA lab.

Note: This formula was calculated using the following capsule packing statistics:

Progesterone USP, PCCA Special Micronized:
Lot #C151637, 327 milligrams in a size #0 capsule
Methocel ® E4M Premium CR (Hypromellose USP):
Lot #C104616. 350 milligrams in a size #0 capsule
Base, PCCA LoxOral™:
Lot #PILOT, 505 milligrams in a size #0 capsule

Pack stats will vary from lot to lot so it is recommended that you perform your own packing statistics before proceeding with this formulation. Please contact PCCA's Pharmacy Consulting Department for further assistance.

1. Using the Principles of Geometric Dilution, mix Progesterone, Methacel E4M and PCCA LoxOral Base together with trituration in a mortar and pestle.
2. Capsule formulations should have powders where the particle size is the same throughout. Once powders are thoroughly mixed, sieve through an 80 mesh sieve (PCCA #35-3125) to ensure even particle size. Do not force large particles through the sieve as this destroys the integrity of the sieve. Instead, any particles remaining in the sieve should be triturated in a mortar and pestle to reduce particle size, and ALL powders should be sieved again.
3. Encapsulate in size #0 capsules.

Progesterone 100 mg SR Capsules Size #0 (LoxOral™) (10802)

Page 1/2

FIG. 11.19 Master formulation record.

Principles of Geometric Dilution:

This procedure should be followed when mixing an ingredient of a larger quantity (L) with a second ingredient of a smaller quantity (S). L is to be mixed into S in small proportions.

First, add a portion of L which has the same volume of that of S followed by thorough mixing. You will get a mixture (M1).

Then, add another portion of L which has the same volume of that of M1 followed by thorough mixing. Do the mixing based on the above principle until L is mixed into S completely.

Under no circumstance should the entire quantity of L be added at once to S in the expectation that uniform dispersion of the latter will be more expeditiously achieved on brief trituration of the mixture.

WARNING!
SAFETY WHEN COMPOUNDING:

Precautions should be taken when compounding hormone and other steroids, as they can be absorbed through skin, mucous membranes and lungs. Wear appropriate lab apparel, eye protection and respirator. Use an appropriate filter system to reduce the amount of airborne chemical particles in your lab. Monitor to ensure there is no direct exposure to the compounder. Consider using Flow Sciences Vented Balance Safety Enclosures - PCCA #35-3310 or PCCA #35-3311. Pregnant women and compounders with hormone related cancer should not compound hormone therapy.

See PCCA #35-3020, Pharmacy Safety Kit in catalog, and review "Safety in the Compounding Pharmacy" Video PCCA #35-3025, CD-ROM PCCA #35-3120. (These two are available at no charge or they may be viewed on the PCCA Members Only Website.) Call PCCA Pharmacy Consulting Department with questions.

Note: No claims are made as to the safety or efficacy of this preparation. This formulation is provided solely at the unsolicited request of the pharmacist.

Note: Beyond Use Dates of preparations are conservative estimates by the formulator using reference books, peer reviewed literature, intended duration of therapy, formulation from commercially available products, organoleptic stability observations and current USP guidelines. Compounders may have stability tests performed by a reputable laboratory if they wish to extend the Beyond Use Date.

Note: Beyond Use Date after compounding is estimated to be 180 days.

10802
Revised: Fri Oct 18, 2013

Progesterone 100 mg SR Capsules Size #0 (LoOral™) (10802)

Page 2/2

FIG. 11.19, cont'd

sheet, that is a record of finished compounds and includes all ingredients in the mix, the BUD assigned, the preparer, and assigned lot numbers (Box 11.7). Also required are Safety Data Sheets (SDSs) for all chemicals and drug substances, either in hard copy or as electronically accessible forms. However, if commercial products are used in preparing the medication, the package insert may be used.

Once the label has been affixed to the container, all necessary auxiliary labels are chosen. Many auxiliary labels not only instruct the patient in the intended use of the product but also indicate the appropriate storage requirements. In addition, some labels allow for BUDs to be added.

◉ Scenario Checkup 11.4

Judy is in the middle of her shift in the compounding area. She is documenting her completed prescription in the compounding record (CR). She notices that the technician who worked the previous shift forgot to list the lot numbers on her last two medications. Why are the lot numbers so important? What should Judy do next?

Safety

All chemicals should be safely stored inside cabinets or behind shelf brackets to avoid spillage. Several additives can be harmful if they are inhaled or come in contact with the eyes or skin. Every pharmacy has an SDS binder with information about all chemical products and how to handle spillage or contact. It is important to know where the SDS binder is kept in the pharmacy department.

Cleaning up excess ingredients appropriately is important; the method of cleaning up and disposing of agents or any equipment used depends on the type of agents used. Hazardous chemicals must be discarded properly according to pharmacy protocol. Nonhazardous chemicals normally can be discarded in a regular trash container. Any glass or needles must be placed in a sharps container.

Compounding Professionalism

Pharmaceutical elegance is the special use of a finishing technique to give the final product a professional look. Great care must be taken when topping off jars of creams and ointments. By holding the spatula very straight across the top of the ingredients and slowly turning the container, the top achieves a smooth appearance. Then slowly lift the spatula, as you are turning, to leave a small curl in the center of the cream or ointment.

Regulatory and Quality Control

The repackaging and compounding of pharmaceutical products are subject to regulatory control. The manner in which the medication is packaged affects both the product inside the package and the user's compliance with the physician's orders for taking the medication. Many medications can degrade with ultraviolet (UV) light exposure; therefore they must be placed in amber-colored containers to protect the medication. Storage is another consideration for a prepared product in a specific type of container. All labeling requirements must be followed, or the prescription is considered misbranded. Under the Food and Drug Administration Modernization Act of 1997, the following restrictions were placed on pharmacies:

- Compounded drugs may be made in limited quantities.
- Compounded products must be made from approved ingredients that meet manufacturing and safety standards.
- The drug product must not be identified by the FDA as a product that presents demonstrable difficulties for compounding in terms of safety or effectiveness.

Veterinary Medications

The FDA regulates animal medications under the *Food, Drug, and Cosmetic Act*. In 2020, the *Compounding Animal Drugs from Bulk Drugs Substances #256* was enacted to provide additional guidance for those compounds made from bulk substances. This applies to drugs compounded when an FDA-approved drug cannot be used as the source of active ingredient.

If the compound is made of FDA-approved medications, the FD&C Act provides guidance just as human compounds are regulated.

Many owners must medicate their animals. Administering oral medications to a pet can be difficult. Many delivery systems have been developed to avoid forcing a tablet down the throat of an animal. For example, dog treats can be made that have the medication mixed into the treat; other forms of dosing include liquids and transdermal routes of administration. Sticks can be prepared to administer antibiotics to the inside of the ear; liquids poured onto a pet's food reduce the stress on both the animal and the owner. Labeling requirements for compounded veterinary products are listed in Box 11.8.

Compounding pharmacies provide many more choices for patients to administer their medications in the appropriate strength and dosage form to their pets (Table 11.14).

Technician Profile

Shevala is a certified compounding technician at an independently owned pharmacy. She has worked in this position for 7 years. Her responsibilities include using a computerized compounding system, weighing and recording chemicals, combining chemicals into appropriate dosage forms per formula instructions, and properly using and calibrating all laboratory equipment, including scales, electronic meters, and IV pumps. Shevala is also responsible for following all safety and USP <795> guidelines, recording daily refrigerator and freezer temperatures, and ordering medication and supplies as needed. She has the strong math skills and basic knowledge of compounding laws and regulations that are essential to this position. She enjoys her job and the opportunity to help individualize medications to optimize the patient's health.

Personnel Training

Pharmacy programs must include supportive personnel (technicians) with adequate training to perform the necessary functions of compounding. To enable technicians to build and maintain a high skill level, training programs should be offered periodically. Instructions on compounding should include the following:

- Calculations
- Compounding equipment
- Dosage forms
- Interpretation of symbols
- Literature
- Safety
- Techniques

These programs may include watching instructional videos or observation and dialog between instructor and personnel. The instruction should also include either a written test or a quality control test of finished preparations. The highest level of competency in compounding procedures is ensured if pharmacies provide initial training followed by recurrent training in methods, regulations, and techniques of compounding. In this way, the pharmacy can provide the customer with the highest product quality.

BOX 11.8 Labeling Requirements for Animal Prescriptions

1. Name and address of veterinarian
2. Active ingredient or ingredients
3. Date dispensed and beyond-use date
4. Name of pet
5. Directions for use specified by practitioner and the class/species or identification of the animal
6. Dosage
7. Frequency
8. Route of administration
9. Duration of therapy
10. Any warnings and information on side effects must be given by the veterinarian and/or the pharmacist to ensure safety
11. Name and address of the dispenser (pharmacy/pharmacist)
12. Prescription number
13. Date filled
14. Caution: Federal law restricts this drug to use by or on the order of a licensed veterinarian

---

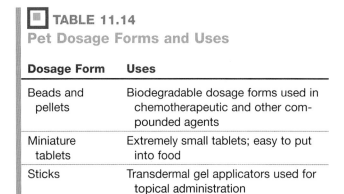

TABLE 11.14
Pet Dosage Forms and Uses

Dosage Form	Uses
Beads and pellets	Biodegradable dosage forms used in chemotherapeutic and other compounded agents
Miniature tablets	Extremely small tablets; easy to put into food
Sticks	Transdermal gel applicators used for topical administration
Treats	Chewable flavored tablets (beef, chicken, turkey) for oral doses

Compounding Calculations

Many formulas are already documented in a compounding recipe book; however, in some situations the final product may have to be prepared in a strength or volume different from that listed in the recipe, or products of different strengths may need to be used to prepare a final percentage solution. In such cases the pharmacist or technician must perform calculations to attain the correct weights and/or volumes for the final product. The following sections discuss calculation procedures for reducing or increasing formulas, determining partial dosage units, changing stock solutions, mixing products of different strengths, performing solubility expressions, and converting units to weights.

Example 11.8: Increasing a Formulation's Quantity

Recipe is for 100 mL of 2% ibuprofen gel.

By definition a 2% gel means 2 g per 100 mL of gel, so set up a ratio and proportion to determine how much ibuprofen powder is required to prepare 240 mL of gel.

$$\frac{2 \text{ g}}{100 \text{ mL}} = \frac{x}{240 \text{ mL}}$$

$$(x)(100 \text{ mL}) = (2 \text{ g})(240 \text{ mL})$$

$$x = (2 \text{ g})(240 \text{ mL})/(100 \text{ mL})$$

$$x = 4.8 \text{ g of ibuprofen powder needed}$$

Example 11.9: Reducing (Decreasing) a Formulation's Quantity

Recipe is for 100 mL of 2% ibuprofen gel.

How much ibuprofen powder is required to prepare 40 mL of gel?

$$(x)(100 \text{ mL}) = (2 \text{ g})(40 \text{ mL})$$

$$x = (2 \text{ g})(40 \text{ mL})/(100 \text{ mL})$$

$$x = 0.8 \text{ g of ibuprofen powder needed}$$

Example 11.10: Reducing a Formulation's Quantity

Recipe is for 100 mL of 5 mg/mL of drug D.

Ingredients:

- Drug D: 50-mg tablets #10
- SW for injection: 4 mL
- Artificial banana flavoring: 3 mL
- Simple syrup (with suspending agent) mixture: qs to 100 mL

Reduce this recipe to 35 mL of drug D, 5 mg/mL suspension.

The new volume ordered (35 mL) divided by the amount in the recipe in the original (100 mL) gives the final percentage to alter the formula. Reduce the entire formula to 35% of the original by multiplying each ingredient by 0.35.

$$\frac{35}{100} = 0.35$$

Drug D: 10 tablets $\times$ 0.35 = 3.5 tablets

Sterile water: 4 mL $\times$ 0.35 = 1.4 mL

Banana flavoring: 3 mL $\times$ 0.35 = 1.05 mL

Sterile water for injection: qs to 35 mL

Example 11.11: Determining Partial Dosage Units

Recipe: Mixture M, the original formula, calls for 125 mg of active ingredient M.

- Active ingredient M: 125 mg (need 5 capsules at 25 mg each)
- Ora-Plus: 60 mL
- Ora-Sweet: qs 120 mL

Using 25-mg capsules, determine the amount needed to make only 120 mg:

$$\frac{25 \text{ mg}}{1 \text{ cap}} = \frac{120 \text{ mg}}{x}$$

$$(x)(25 \text{ mg}) = (1 \text{ cap})(120 \text{ mg})$$

$$x = (1 \text{ cap})(120 \text{ mg})/(25 \text{ mg})$$

$$x = 4.8 \text{ caps}$$

Then:

1. Empty 5 capsules onto a weighing boat or paper and weigh.
2. Determine how many grams you need to remove.

If the weight of 5 capsules of active ingredient and filler is 1600 mg:

$$\frac{1600 \text{ mg}}{5 \text{ caps}} = \frac{x}{4.8 \text{ caps}}$$

$$(x)(5 \text{ caps}) = (1600 \text{ mg})(4.8 \text{ caps})$$

$$x = (1600 \text{ mg})(4.8 \text{ caps})/(5 \text{ caps})$$

$$x = 1536 \text{ mg needed}$$

3. Remove 64 mg from the balance to retain the necessary 1536 mg.

Example 11.12: Changing Stock Solutions

Order: Prepare three 15-mL bottles of medicated solution with 0.01% ingredient A.

In stock: 17% ingredient A solution

How much of the 17% ingredient A solution is needed?

Note: 0.01% final strength needed = 0.01 g/100 mL; ingredient A 17% = 17 g/100 mL.

$$15 \text{ mL} \times 3 = 45 \text{ mL}$$

$$\frac{0.01 \text{ g}}{100 \text{ ml}} = \frac{x}{45 \text{ ml}}$$

$$100 \text{ mL} \times x = 0.01 \text{ g} \times 45 \text{ mL}$$

$$x = 0.0045 \text{ g of ingredient A needed}$$

$$\frac{17 \text{ g}}{100 \text{ mL}} = \frac{0.0045 \text{ g}}{x}$$

$$17\text{g} \times x = 0.0045 \text{ g} \times 100 \text{ mL}$$

$$x = 0.026 \text{ mL of } 17\% \text{ solution needed}$$

Use 0.026 mL of 17% solution and qs with appropriate liquid to 45 mL.

An easier way to approach this question is to use the equation from Chapter 6 for diluting stock solutions: SV:SP = DV:DP.

$$\text{Identify the variables: SV} = ?$$
$$\text{SP} = 17\% \quad \text{DV} = 45 \text{ mL} \quad \text{DP} = 0.01\%$$

$$\text{SV} \cdot 17\% = 45 \text{ mL} \cdot 0.01\% \text{ SV} = 0.026 \text{ mL}$$

Example 11.13: Mixing Products of Different Strengths

Order: 120 g of 0.1% ointment B

In stock: 1 oz of 0.1% ointment B base

   0.5 oz of 0.15% ointment B base

   2.5 oz of 0.005% ointment B base

If these three ingredients are mixed together, how much of ointment powder drug B must be added to prepare the prescription to attain 120 g of 0.1% ointment B?

Note: This cannot be done using the SV:SP = DV:DP equation or the alligation alternative method because three strengths are being combined.

Use dimensional analysis to determine how many milligrams of ingredient B are in each amount. Remember from Chapter 6 to begin with the conversion that has the unit of your desired answer (milligrams) in the numerator and add information to cancel unwanted units with each subsequent fraction.

$$\frac{1000 \text{ mg}}{1 \text{ g}} \times \frac{0.1 \text{ g}}{100 \text{ mL}} \times \frac{30 \text{ mL}}{1 \text{ oz}} \times \frac{1 \text{ oz}}{1} = 30 \text{ mg}$$

$$\frac{1000 \text{ mg}}{1 \text{ g}} \times \frac{0.15 \text{ g}}{100 \text{ mL}} \times \frac{30 \text{ mL}}{1 \text{ oz}} \times \frac{0.5 \text{ oz}}{1} = 22.5 \text{ mg}$$

$$\frac{1000 \text{ mg}}{1 \text{ g}} \times \frac{0.005 \text{ g}}{100 \text{ mL}} \times \frac{30 \text{ mL}}{1 \text{ oz}} \times \frac{2.5 \text{ oz}}{1} = 3.75 \text{ mg}$$

Total amount = 56.25 mg

(120 mg − 56.25 mg = 63.75 mg additional ingredient B powder needed)

⊘ Example 11.14: Performing Solubility Expressions

Order: Prepare 150 mL of a 1:15 strength solution of drug X. How much of drug X is required to fill this order?

This is a single-step problem that is easy to solve with ratio and proportion.

$$\frac{1 \text{ g}}{15 \text{ ml}} = \frac{x}{150 \text{ ml}} \quad x = 10 \text{ g}$$

⊘ Example 11.15: Converting Units to Weights

Order: 150,000 units of drug N per gram of ointment; quantity: 60 g to be dispensed

How much of drug N should be weighed (based on 4400 [USP] units/mg)?

This is a multistep problem, so use dimensional analysis to keep track of units.

$$\frac{1 \text{ g}}{1000 \text{ mg}} \times \frac{1 \text{ mg}}{4400 \text{ units}} \times \frac{150,000 \text{ units}}{1 \text{ g}} \times \frac{60 \text{ g}}{1} = 2.045 \text{ g}$$

Do You Remember These Key Points?

- The need for packaging products in the appropriate type and size container
- The proper steps to follow in the repackaging of bulk medication
- Five reasons pharmacies often repackage bulk medications into unit dose packages
- The proper handling of medications during bulk repackaging
- The documentation necessary for repackaged and compounded products
- Information required on labels
- Common auxiliary labels used on compounded products
- How expiration and beyond-use dates are determined when repackaging
- Common reasons for using unit dose medications
- The various types of containers used in repackaged and compounded products
- Definition of nonsterile compounding
- Common reasons patients need compounded medications
- The various types of equipment used in compounded medications
- The various types of scales used in compounding
- How to complete a compounding sheet with necessary information
- The proper steps to follow when compounding a product

- Types of additives that are used to improve the taste and appearance of oral solutions
- The sizes of capsules used in compounding
- How ointments, suppositories, nasal sprays, and other dosage forms are prepared
- Good manufacturing practices used when preparing compounded products
- Regulations pertaining to compounding pharmacies on limits of quantities
- The use of compounded products for animals

Review Questions

Multiple Choice Questions

1. According to the USP <795> guidelines, the BUD for solid dose form is:
   A. 14 days
   B. 90 days
   C. 35 days
   D. 180 days

2. To grind or crush powders into fine particles using a mortar and pestle best describes:
   A. Trituration
   B. Levigation
   C. Mixing
   D. Stirring

3. Determine the beyond-use date of a liquid drug to be repackaged into unit doses that has a manufacturer's expiration date of 10/01/20. If today's date is 10/01/18, the BUD is:
   A. 10/01/19
   B. 10/14/18
   C. 11/01/18
   D. 4/01/18

4. The type of balance(s) that can weigh 10 g of powder accurately is (are):
   A. Class A
   B. Class B
   C. Both A and B
   D. None of the above

5. A meniscus is best described as:
   A. A beaker filled with a small amount of water
   B. Water molecules attaching to the sides of a container
   C. A container used to measure very small amounts of liquid
   D. The lowest level of liquid, which is the point that should be used to assign a measurement

6. The arrest knob on a balance is used to:
   A. Measure the weight of a compound
   B. Balance the feet of the balance
   C. Adjust the balance's weights
   D. Lock the balance

7. Emulsion bases are:
   A. Absorbent
   B. Insoluble in water
   C. Greasy
   D. Not susceptible to mold growth

8. Which type of medication can be compounded for animal use?
   A. Tiny tablets
   B. Transdermal sticks
   C. Transdermal patches
   D. All of the above
9. According to FDA regulatory guidelines, compounding pharmacies are *not* allowed to:
   A. Advertise their compounding products
   B. Prepare large quantities of compounded product
   C. Prepare transdermal medications
   D. None of the above
10. Beyond-use dating differs from expiration dates because:
    A. Beyond-use dating is used only when compounding, and expiration dates are used for repackaging
    B. Beyond-use dating is used when repackaging or compounding products, whereas only manufacturers use expiration dates
    C. Expiration dates are used only for medications, whereas beyond-use dating applies to all additives
    D. None of the above

◼ Technician's Corner

You receive an order for 50 g of 2.5% hydrocortisone cream. You have hydrocortisone powder and Dermabase in stock.
- How many grams of hydrocortisone powder are needed?
- How much Dermabase do you need to qs to 50 g?
- What documentation is required for these items?
- What information would you place on the label (include auxiliary labels needed)?

Bibliography

Allen L. *The Art, Science, and Technology of Pharmaceutical Compounding*. Washington, DC: American Pharmaceutical Association; 2002.

American Society for Health System Pharmacists. Technical assistance bulletin on compounding nonsterile products in pharmacies. American Society of Hospital Pharmacists. *Am J Hosp Pharm*. 1994;51(11):1441-1448.

Ansel H, Allen L, Popovich N. *Pharmaceutical Dosage forms and Drug Delivery Systems*. 8th ed. Baltimore: Lippincott Williams & Wilkins; 2004.

Leon S, Mutnick AH, Swanson LN, Souney PF. *Comprehensive Pharmacy Review*. 7th ed. Baltimore: Lippincott Williams & Wilkins; 2009.

USP Bulletin. Compounding pharmacies at the forefront of personalized medicine. 2007;96:6. https://www.usp.org/sites/default/files/usp/document/public-policy/What%E2%80%99s%20Next%20for%20Compounded%20Medicines%20%281%29.pdf

Websites Referenced

Allen Jr L. Compounding oral liquids. *Secundum Artem*. 5(1). Available at: http://www.paddocklabs.com/forms/secundum/volume_3_1.pdf.

American Society of Consultant Pharmacists. Guidelines for prepackaging of medications. Available at: http://www.ascp.com/resources/policy/upload/Gui98-Prepackaging%20meds.pdf.

Compounding nasal preparations. *Secundum Artem*. 7(1). Available at: http://www.paddocklabs.com/images/PadSec7-1.pdf.

Compounding rectal dosage forms. II. *Secundem Artem*. 14(1). Available at: http://www.paddocklabs.com/forms/secundum/Volume 14.4.pdf.

Excipients category list. Available at: http://www.pformulate.com/labclass/categories.htm.

Limited FDA survey of compounding drug products. Available at: http://www.fda.gov/Drugs/GuidanceComplianceRegulatoryInformation/PharmacyCompounding/ucm155725.htm.

Pharmaceutics and Compounding Laboratory. Pharmaceutical solutions. III. Ophthalmic solutions. Available at: http://pharmlabs.unc.edu/labs/ophthalmics/objectives.htm.

Accuracy in Measurement | Pharmlabs (unc.edu).

USP & Compounding. Compounding pharmacy resources. Available at: https://www.fda.gov/animal-veterinary/unapproved-animal-drugs/animal-drug-compounding

Wedgewood Pharmacy. Veterinary dosage forms. 2009. Available at: https://www.wedgewoodpharmacy.com/medications/.

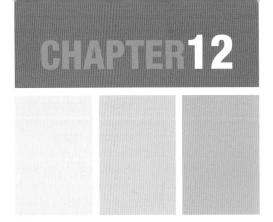

Aseptic Technique and Sterile Compounding

Karen Davis

OBJECTIVES

1. Explain why certain medications must be sterile.
2. Define common terms used in sterile compounding.
3. Describe Standard Precautions necessary when preparing compounded sterile preparations.
4. Discuss the following as they relate to supplies and equipment used to prepare compounded sterile preparations: (a) describe standard supplies and equipment used to prepare compounded sterile preparations, (b) explain the anatomy of a syringe and needle, (c) list the sizes of syringes and needles used in the pharmacy setting, (d) explain when and why filters are used in sterile compounding, and (e) list the types of stock used within a clean room.
5. Describe various medication delivery systems.
6. Discuss the following as they relate to the *United States Pharmacopeia* (USP) <797>: (a) explain the history of USP <797>, (b) list the main components of USP <797> regulations, and (c) list the categories of drug preparation determined by USP <797>.
7. Discuss the following as they relate to hood cleaning and maintenance: (a) explain the differences between the various types of hoods, (b) describe how often hoods must be inspected, and (c) describe how to properly clean various types of hoods and prepare them for use.
8. Describe proper aseptic technique.
9. Demonstrate the steps in drawing up medication from an ampule and from a vial.
10. Discuss the following as they relate to aseptic technique: (a) describe different types of intravenous parenteral medications, (b) discuss hyperalimentation, (c) list types of parenteral additives, (d) discuss compatibility considerations for parenteral medications, (e) list components of a label for an intravenous medication, and (f) describe how to properly dispose of needles, vials, and cytotoxic supplies.
11. List two key components of USP <800> regulations and the proper steps that need to be taken for a pharmacy technician to be competent in compounding hazardous preparations.

TERMS AND DEFINITIONS

Anteroom The room adjacent to the "clean room" used for donning all personal protective equipment (PPE) and wiping down all supplies that will be used in the compounding area

Aseptic technique The procedures used to eliminate the possibility of a drug becoming contaminated with microbes or particles

Beyond-use date (BUD) Defined by USP <797> as the date or time after which a compounded sterile preparation (CSP) shall not be administered, stored, or transported; it is determined from the date the preparation is compounded

Biological safety cabinet (BSC) A vertical flow hood that should be used for making hazardous sterile preparations in the clean room

255

Clean room In pharmacy, a contained and controlled environment in the pharmacy that has a low level of environmental pollutants (eg, dust, airborne microbes, aerosol particles, and chemical vapors); the clean room is used for preparing sterile medication products

Compounded sterile preparations (CSPs) Preparations prepared in a sterile environment using nonsterile ingredients or devices that must be sterilized before administration

Compounding aseptic containment isolator (CACI) ISO Class 5 compounding area used to prepare hazardous drugs

Critical site Any surface or area exposed to first air, which is exposed or at risk for touch, or direct air (ie, vial tops, open ampules, needle hubs, or injection ports)

First air Air exiting the high-efficiency particulate air (HEPA) filter in a unidirectional air stream

Gauges The sizes of needle openings

Hazardous drug Any drug that has been proven to have dangerous effects during animal or human testing; it may cause cancer or may harm certain organs or pregnant women

Hazardous waste Any waste that meets the Resource Conservation and Recovery Act (RCRA) criteria of ignitability, corrosiveness, reactivity, or toxicity

Health care–associated infection (HAI) An infection that patients acquire during the course of receiving treatments for other conditions in an institutional setting

Horizontal laminar flow hood An environment for the preparation of compounded sterile preparations in which air originating from the back of the hood moves forward across the hood and into the room

Hyperalimentation Parenteral nutrition for individuals who are unable to eat solids or liquids

Infection control Policies and procedures put in place to minimize the risk for spreading infections in hospitals or other health care facilities

Laminar air flow workbench (LAFW) An environment for the preparation of sterile products

Parenteral medications Medications that bypass the digestive system but are intended for systemic action; the term parenteral most commonly describes medications given by injection, such as intravenously or intramuscularly

Peripheral parenteral Injection of a medication into the veins on the periphery of the body instead of into a central vein or artery

Peripheral parenteral nutrition (PPN) Intravenous nutrition administered through veins on the periphery of the body rather than through a central vein or artery

Precipitate To separate from solution or suspension; a solid that emerges from a liquid solution

Primary engineering control (PEC) A device or zone that provides a Class 5 environment for sterile compounding (ie, hoods)

Reconstituted A substance that has had a diluent (eg, saline or sterile water) added to a powder

Standard operating procedures (SOPs) Written guidelines and criteria that list specific steps for various competencies

Standard Precautions (Universal Precautions) A set of standards that reduce the possibility of contamination and the risk for transmission of infectious disease; these standards are used throughout a health care facility, including to prepare medications

Sterile preparation A preparation that contains no living microorganisms

Total parenteral nutrition (TPN) Large-volume intravenous nutrition administered through a central vein (eg, subclavian vein), which allows for a higher concentration of solutions

United States Pharmacopeia <797> (USP <797>) Chapter 797, "Pharmaceutical Compounding—Sterile Preparations," of the USP National Formulary. It contains a set of enforceable sterile compounding standards; describes the guidelines, procedures, and compliance requirements for compounding sterile preparations; and sets the standards that apply to all settings in which sterile preparations are compounded

United States Pharmacopeia <800> (USP <800>) Chapter 800, a new general chapter created to identify the requirements for receipt, storage, mixing, preparing, compounding, dispensing, and administration of hazardous drugs to protect the patient, health care personnel, and the environment (*https://www.usp.org/compounding/general-chapter-hazardous-drugs-handling-healthcare*)

Vertical laminar flow hood An environment for the preparation of chemotherapeutic and other hazardous agents in which air originating from the roof of the hood moves downward (over the agent) and is captured in a vent on the floor of the hood

Scenario

Ken is a total parenteral nutrition (TPN) technician specialist at a prominent hospital pharmacy. He received his training on the job and has more than 20 years of experience. Ken is nationally certified with the Pharmacy Technician Certification Board (PTCB) and is an active member of the American Society of Health-System Pharmacists (ASHP). He works rotating shifts, in which he is scheduled one weekend per month in addition to his normal work week. Ken has seen many changes in the hospital pharmacy over the years. He remembers when the TPN medications were made by hand, which was very time-consuming and labor-intensive. He enjoys his job and thinks that his department plays an important role in providing high-quality patient care. Why is it important that all parenteral medications be prepared by well-trained pharmacy technicians?

Proper preparation of **parenteral medications** is one of the most crucial responsibilities of the hospital pharmacy technician because these medications enter the bloodstream directly, usually through injection. Preparation of all parenteral medications in a manner that reduces the chance of contamination is important. This is possible only through the proper manipulation of materials used within the appropriate hood. Various sizes and types of hoods are available; all are capable of excluding bacteria and other unwanted particulates if the technician uses proper aseptic technique. **Aseptic technique** involves procedures used to eliminate the possibility of a drug becoming contaminated with microbes or other unwanted particles.

The pharmacy technician may prepare **compounded sterile preparations** (**CSPs**) in pharmacy settings such as home health services and long-term care facilities. This chapter predominantly focuses on the technician working in a hospital pharmacy. The regulations of **United States Pharmacopeia <797> (USP <797>)**, "Pharmaceutical Compounding— Sterile Preparations," are explored, as are policies established by other organizations to monitor compliance in the **sterile preparation** of compounded products.

Wider varieties of parenteral medications are used in the hospital than in any other setting. In the hospital, the pharmacy technician may be responsible for many daily tasks related to compounding sterile preparations. Each skill has its own set of guidelines, which are outlined in the three risk levels of USP <797> (discussed later).

This chapter explores several types of parenteral medications, including the terminology and equipment commonly associated with medications and the various methods used in their preparation. The student technician must understand many important aspects of sterile preparation of medications before filling an order, including the type of drug to be prepared, equipment used, sterilization steps per USP <797>, expiration dates, storage, and proper disposal of equipment. These are the technician's responsibilities in producing a compounded sterile preparation; in addition, technicians must be competent in using drug abbreviations and performing calculations that may be required to prepare medications. These are all important skills of a pharmacy technician.

Terminology Used in Pharmacy

Solutions, medications, and supplies may be required when preparing sterile products. The terms used to identify these items often are abbreviated in prescribers' orders and on supply lists. Pharmacy technicians need to understand these terms and abbreviations to interpret orders and fill stock levels in the intravenous (IV) room. Table 12.1 lists some of the most common terms and abbreviations used for IV supplies.

Standard Precautions for a Health Care Worker

When working in a hospital setting all employees must comply with the policies of **Standard Precautions (Universal Precautions)**. To prevent the dissemination of highly contagious diseases, hospitals usually require an employee to receive both tuberculosis testing and an immunization against influenza annually. Standard Precautions are practices followed to prevent the transmission of infection and contamination; they are based on the principle that all blood, body fluids, secretions, excretions (except sweat), nonintact skin, and mucous membranes may contain infectious agents. Based on the anticipated exposure to potentially infectious substances, each area in the hospital has specific **infection control** guidelines (which can be found in the facility's policies and procedures manual); employees are expected to meet these requirements, including hand washing, orderliness, and cleanliness. The pharmacy does not supply blood or blood products. However, pharmacy personnel must participate in training sessions on blood-borne pathogens so that they not only understand various aspects of contamination but also are aware of ways to prevent exposure and transmission of infections. For example, training includes the interpretation of room signs that indicate patient isolation (eg, droplet or contact isolation) and the precautions and procedures that should be followed if access to these rooms is necessary.

Other hospital-wide standards include the following:
- Employees are not to use patient restrooms; they should use only employee restrooms.
- Medication refrigerators and freezers may hold only medications; they should not be used to store food or drink.
- Eating is prohibited in any drug preparation or patient care areas.

The following are examples of procedures specific to the pharmacy:
- All injectable drugs and other compounded sterile preparations must be made in a "clean room" under laminar flow hoods.
- All flow hoods are recertified every 6 months by an independent contractor or anytime the hood is moved.
- Routine maintenance of hoods includes cleaning all work surfaces and prefilters.
- Records of all inspections are to be kept on file in the pharmacy department.

Abbreviations and Descriptions of Pharmacy Stock

Types of Containers Used for Preparing Parenteral Medications

Amp	Ampule; 1- to 50-mL glass container
Flexible bag	Plastic container (empty or filled with various fluids ranging from 50 to 3000 mL)
MDV	Multidose vial; holds multiple doses of medication
SDV	Single-dose vial; holds one dose of medication
Vial	0.5- to 100-mL glass or plastic container with a stopper

Common Types of Solutions Used/Ordered for Parenteral Agents

D_5NS	5% dextrose in normal saline
$D_{5\frac{1}{2}}NS$	5% dextrose and 0.45% normal saline contained in the same bag of solution
D_5W	5% dextrose in water
$D_{10}NS$	10% dextrose in normal saline
$D_{10}W$	10% dextrose in water
Diluent	Agent used to dilute medications; can be sterile water, normal saline (NS), or others
LR	Lactated Ringer's solution; isotonic solution containing sodium, potassium, calcium, acetate, and chloride
0.45 NaCl	One-half normal saline; has a concentration of 0.45% sodium chloride
NS	Normal saline; has a concentration of 0.9% sodium chloride
¼NS	One-fourth normal saline (concentration of 0.225% sodium chloride)
SWFI	Sterile water for injection; usually used to reconstitute other medications

Routes of Administration for Parenteral Agents

ID	Intradermal injection up to 1 mL into the upper layers of the skin
IM	Intramuscular; into the muscle
IT	Intrathecal; into a sheath (hollow tube), such as the lumbar sheath located at the base of the spine
IV	Intravenous; into the vein
IV push	Into the vein directly from a syringe
Subcut	Subcutaneous; under the skin

Miscellaneous Terms Used With Parenteral Medications

Drip or infusion	An IV bag medication that is infused over a specified amount of time but is not given IV push
NPO	Nothing by mouth
On call	Physician wants dose to be ready when he or she decides to give the medication; most anesthesiologists order on-call preoperative medications
Postop	Medication to be given after surgery (eg, pain control or antiemetic)
Preop	Medication to be given before surgery (eg, sedative or antiemetic)
prn	Medication to be given as needed
qs	Quantity sufficient; adding enough diluent or medication to attain the correct amount needed

⊙ Scenario Checkup 12.1

Ken begins his shift by donning the proper personal protective equipment (PPE) and preparing to clean the hood. He cleans all work surfaces with sterile 70% isopropyl alcohol and checks the prefilters. He notices that the hood certification expires in 30 days. What should Ken do before the end of the month? Why must hoods be inspected every 6 months?

Supplies

Before discussing the actual techniques required to prepare injections, IV drips, chemotherapeutic drugs, and other compounded sterile preparations, the types of supplies and equipment necessary for these processes should be explained. Different types of equipment are available for IV preparation, depending on the amount or volumes to be prepared. For instance, many different types of automated pumps automatically fill IV bags and other sterile containers. These pumps range in complexity and cost. For example, if large multiadditive automated machines are rented by the pharmacy, only the tubing required for that specific pump needs to be purchased. Small pumps, such as Baxa's Repeater pump, are used to administer smaller reconstituted volumes into single-dose vials (SDVs) or larger volumes into multidose

TABLE 12.2
Commonly Used Intravenous Room Supplies

Supplies	Common Description
70% isopropyl alcohol	Antiseptic for cleaning the hood
Ampule breaker	Plastic device on which one end is smaller for small ampules, the other end is used for larger ampules; helps prevent crushing of the glass or cutting oneself when opening ampules
Filter needles	Needle that includes a filter; it prevents glass from entering the final solution when drawing from an ampule
Filter straws	Used for withdrawing medication from ampules
Filters	Used for specific medications to trap particles 0.22–5.0 μm from entering intravenous fluids
Forceps	Instruments that lock; used to obstruct tubing while transferring medications
Male/female adapter	Universal size; fits a syringe on each end for mixing two contents
Minispike	Large-bore spike that is pushed into vial with a syringe attachment at the other end
Sterile 70% alcohol pads	Alcohol on pads for convenience
Syringe caps	A sterile cap used to prevent contamination of syringes during transportation out of pharmacy
Syringe needles	Most common bore sizes used in pharmacy are 16–20 gauge
Syringes	Instrument that holds 0.5–60 mL for administration of medications
Transfer needles	A needle on both ends used to transfer a vial to a bottle
Tubing for pumps	Tubing is specific to manufacturer's machine
Tubing transfer sets	Blood transfer sets; used to transfer the contents of large containers into empty containers

vials (MDVs). In addition, a wide variety of supplies used in the **clean room** must be kept in stock for daily use (Table 12.2). For this reason, the technician must inventory these supplies and reorder stock daily, anticipating the stock needed for the next day.

Syringes

Syringes used in the pharmacy are available in eight basic sizes: 0.5, 1, 3, 5, 10, 20, 30, and 60 mL. As the size of the syringe increases, the accuracy decreases (Fig. 12.1). For parenteral products, the exact amount of drug ordered must be obtained. Syringe tips are available in two types. A tension-type syringe has a 1-mL volume. In this case the needle is attached by friction only (Fig. 12.2A). This type of syringe can be used for withdrawing insulin and other medications that require volumes of 1 mL or less. However, tension-type tips cannot be used when preparing doses of chemotherapeutic

drugs because of the risk for the needle detaching from the syringe and causing a spill or a possible needle stick to the technician. On all other sizes of syringes, the needle is held in place by a locking mechanism, commonly referred to as a Luer-Lok (see Fig. 12.2B). This ensures a safe seal for withdrawal of the medication.

Most syringes are made of plastic and must be discarded after one use. Glass syringes rarely are used in the pharmacy, although they can be used when a patient is allergic to plastics. Glass syringes, unlike plastic syringes, can be sterilized and reused.

Another type of syringe is a Tubex or Carpuject (Fig. 12.3). These cartridge systems can hold a variety of medications and are available in volumes from 0.5 mL up to 3 mL. The bottom of the cartridge is screwed into the system's syringe holder. The syringe cartridge holders for these systems are reusable and normally are dispensed to the nursing units by the pharmacy

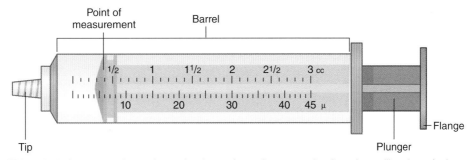

FIG. 12.1 Anatomy of a syringe. As the syringe decreases in size, the calibrations (volume markers) become larger, allowing a more accurate dosage.

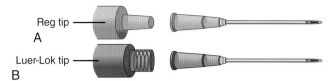

FIG. 12.2 Two types of syringes. (A) Regular tip syringe. The regular tip is held in place by pressure, as seen in the 1-mL syringe. (B) The Luer-Lok syringe has spirals to secure the needle, as seen on a larger 3-mL syringe. (From Potter PA, Perry AG. *Fundamentals of Nursing*. 8th ed. St. Louis: Mosby; 2013.)

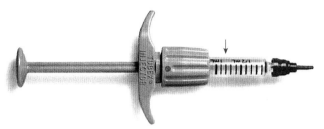

FIG. 12.3 Tubex holders are intended to be reused. They hold the disposable Tubex or Carpuject cartridges. Each cartridge is prelabeled with the medication name, strength, volume, and concentration. The pharmacy stocks holders and cartridges.

on request. The Tubex or Carpuject cartridge is discarded after use; if desired, the holders may be autoclaved for sterility.

Needles

Needles are made of aluminum or stainless steel and are available in many different **gauges** (sizes) and lengths. Higher gauge needles (eg, 20–25 gauge) are used by nurses to administer injections. The nurse determines which gauge and needle length to use according to the injection site. In the pharmacy, needles are used to draw solutions into a syringe, not to administer medications to patients. A limited number of needle gauges are available in the pharmacy, and the lower gauge needles make drawing medications easier. The most common needle sizes used for preparing IV medications are 19, 18, and 16 gauge, which are used to draw solutions from vials or other containers (Fig. 12.4). These needles are normally 1 to 1.5 inches long. The gauge (size) number of a needle is inversely proportional to the bore (opening) size of the needle. This means that as the bore size increases, the gauge decreases. For example, a 25-gauge needle has a much smaller opening than a 19-gauge needle. The *bore size* refers to the circumference of the needle opening; as this increases, so does the probability of coring or cutting out a piece of rubber from the vial's rubber stopper. When a vial is cored, a chunk of rubber is dislodged and may fall into the vial. To avoid coring, the bevel edge should face upward. If coring does occur, a filter needle must be used to prevent the piece of cored rubber from entering the parenteral solution. No part of a needle below the hub should be touched (Fig. 12.5). The point and shaft must remain sterile.

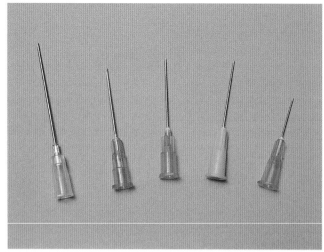

FIG. 12.4 *Left to right,* Needle sizes 19, 20, 21, 23, and 25 gauge. Technicians may use a 19-gauge needle for small volumes, such as 1 mL or less. Larger gauges (not shown) include 18 and 16 gauge for larger volumes. (From Potter PA, Perry AG. *Fundamentals of Nursing*. 8th ed. St. Louis: Mosby; 2013.)

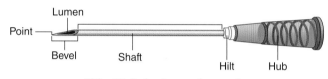

FIG. 12.5 Anatomy of a needle.

> ### ■ Tech Note!
>
> You should not wipe needles with sterile 70% alcohol. If you touch the needle with alcohol or something unintended (eg, the outside of a vial), the needle must be discarded and replaced with a new one.

Filters

Different types and sizes of filters can be used when preparing parenteral medications. Filters are located within the hub of the needle, depending on the type used. Typical filter sizes are 10, 5, 1, and 0.45 micrometer (μm); the smallest filter is 0.22 μm, which removes all unwanted particles from the solution. If use of a filter needle is necessary, the technician must follow the manufacturer's guidelines regarding filter needles suggested for the specific medication. Some medications should never be filtered because filtering would remove active drug from the solution. Filter needles are for single direction use only and cannot be used to both withdraw and inject a solution.

Another type of filter is the filter straw. This strawlike needle can withdraw a larger amount of solution quickly, sifting it through a filter in the hub of the needle. The filter straw often is used to remove any fine particles of glass from an ampule. The filter straw must be replaced with a normal needle before the medication is pushed into the final container. Fig. 12.6

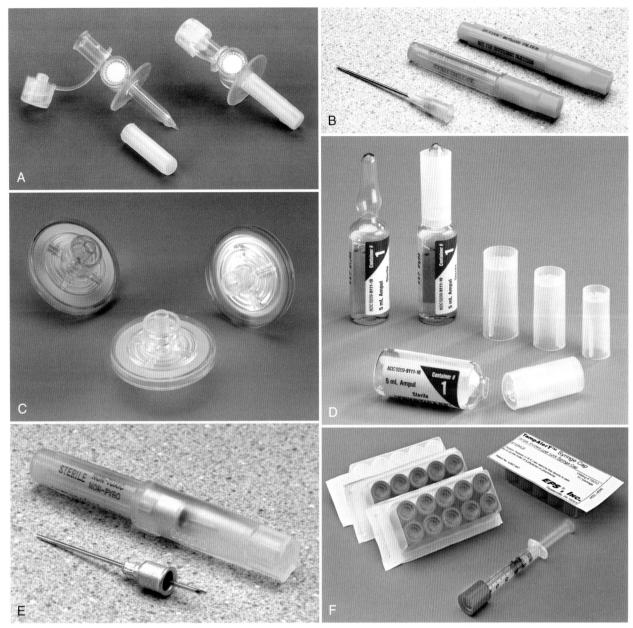

FIG. 12.6 (A) Minispikes used in multidose vials. (B) Filter needles. (C) Filter sizes. (D) Ampules and ampule breakers. (E) Transfer needle. (F) Syringe and caps. (Courtesy Medi-Dose/EPS.)

shows the other types of filters and other materials used in the IV room.

Stock Levels

All the items stored in the IV room of the pharmacy must be kept in stock above their minimum levels at all times. Current USP <797> standards (revised in 2019) require that a minimum number of supply items be kept in the clean room. Only items that will be used immediately for direct compounding should be in the clean room. Supply items must be wiped down with an appropriate cleaning solution before they are brought into the clean room.

Before and after each shift, the IV technician is responsible for reordering and restocking the clean room for the next shift. Some IV supplies may be ordered from the central supply area

of the hospital and arrive by the next shift. However, most supplies are ordered directly from the pharmacy wholesaler, and delivery can take 2 days to 1 week. Therefore, to ensure that required pharmacy stock is always on hand, the technician must be knowledgeable about delivery options.

Many IV antibiotics are available in premade bulk packs; for example, 12 or 24 packs are frozen in boxes. Although these are convenient, they are more expensive than those prepared by technicians. Most of the time, technicians prepare the IVs needed throughout the week. Certain IV medications can be frozen in either IV solutions or syringes, but each bag must be marked with the date of reconstitution, the **beyond-use date (BUD),** the concentration/strength, and the preparer's initials. The expiration dates for frozen, refrigerated, or room-temperature products are determined by using the manufacturer's information, the known stability data, and other pharmaceutical specialty publications and research. Large, temperature-controlled refrigerators may be used to store thawed IV medications. Antibiotics and other medications in MDVs can be stored in the refrigerator after opening, sometimes for days, and used as determined by USP guidelines for MDVs. All of these items should be visually checked each day for stock levels and out-of-date medications.

Routes of Administration

Because prepared solutions differ in their volumes and/or concentrations, understanding the routes of administration (ROAs) is important. For example, if a dose of ceftriaxone 1 g is to be given intramuscularly (IM), it is normally divided into two syringes for the nurse to inject into each side of the hip area. Injections can be given on several areas of the body. The route of administration of each type of medication must be stated on the label (this is discussed later in the chapter).

Medication Delivery Systems

Many different types of containers are used to deliver medications. Advanced technology includes "smart" pumps, which contain databases of drug information, concentrations, and dosing units and limits. There are also special containers developed to be stable and easy to use. In addition, because many medications are not premade for final use by the manufacturer and must be prepared in the pharmacy, it is important to determine whether the medication must be discarded (ie, wasted) if not administered to the patient in a timely manner. For example, once a medication has been **reconstituted,** it must be used within a certain time or it expires, resulting in lost revenue for the pharmacy. Sometimes the drug may not be given to the patient for whom it was prepared; the physician may have decided to use a medication of a different dose, type, volume, and solution. This type of waste only adds to the high costs of health care. Systems can be used to eliminate waste, such as the ADD-Vantage system. Although these systems are expensive, they can be beneficial by reducing waste and ultimately adding cost efficiency. These systems and others are discussed later.

Piggyback Containers

Flexible bags and bottles are the two main types of piggyback containers. Most IV bags are made of polyvinyl chloride (PVC), which consists of several flexible layers of plastics. Other types of IV bags are made with non-PVC materials such as ethylene vinyl acetate (EVA). The EVA bags are not as flexible as PVC bags. Piggyback IVs are intended to be placed on top of a primary IV using tubing connection sets (Fig. 12.7). Containers can be purchased prefilled with solutions or may be empty and filled with a custom-made IV solution. The sizes and types of piggyback containers and solutions range from 50 to 250 mL. Examples of specialized containers used for medication dispensing include large- and small-volume drips, syringe pumps, and miscellaneous dispensing systems. Many controlled substances also are

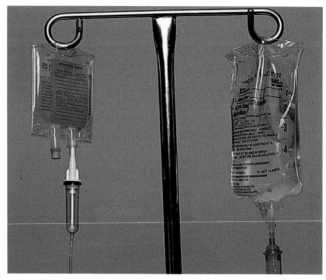

FIG. 12.7 This gravity pump system intravenous piggyback setup shows a 100-mL Viaflex container *(left)* piggybacked to a large-volume 1-L IV line *(right)*. (From Potter PA, Perry AG. *Fundamentals of Nursing*. 8th ed. St. Louis: Mosby; 2013.)

prepared in such systems and are dispensed to the nursing floor after they have been documented according to established procedures for controlled substances.

Large-Volume and Small-Volume Drips

Large-volume drips include Viaflex bags in 500-mL and 1-, 2-, and 3-L volumes. Volumes greater than 1 L are often reserved for use with parenteral nutritional formulas. Bottles are also available in various sizes ranging from 500 mL to 1 L. These can deliver a variety of fluids, including parenteral nutrition. Parenteral nutrition is a combination of essential nutrients that is administered through a drip system for several hours or up to 24 hours. (Parenteral nutrition solutions are discussed later in the chapter.) Small-volume piggyback containers and solutions are available in 50-, 100-, 150-, and 250-mL volumes. Small-volume drips can be piggybacked onto large-volume drips. All Viaflex bags have a 10% overfill of solution. To attain an accurate final concentration of drug, some mixtures require that a volume of base solution equal to the volume of medication being added, plus the solution overfill, be removed during the mixing process. This type of procedure usually occurs with critical care medication drips, in which small changes in drug concentration may greatly influence the dosage given to the patient and the subsequent patient response.

> ### ■ Tech Note!
>
> All dosage forms of controlled substances that are delivered to nursing floors must be signed out of the pharmacy stock and into the floor stock of the receiving station. Documents registering controlled substances should be kept up to date, and all controlled substances should be counted at the end of every shift to account for all opioid use or waste.

Continuous Analgesic Delivery Systems

Patients who require analgesics after major surgery and individuals who are in hospice normally have their medications prepared in the pharmacy. In the hospital setting, nursing stations stock various strengths of controlled substances intended to relieve extreme pain. Depending on the physician's order, the nurse can prepare IM or IV push doses from the controlled substances cabinet.

When a patient is in severe pain, physicians often order analgesic medications such as morphine or fentanyl (both schedule II [C-II] drugs) on a schedule (eg, every 6 or 8 hours). When this strength of analgesic is given in larger doses to patients who have no history of opioid use, the initial effects of the medication may be extreme, causing side effects such as nausea, vomiting, and in some cases difficulty breathing. Toward the end of the 6 or 8 hours, some patients are once again experiencing pain and waiting for the next dose to be administered. To provide a more constant degree of comfort and to limit unwanted side effects, some patients may be given either an implantable port or a catheter system attached to a portable electronic pump system that administers a steady flow of analgesics to control the patient's pain more effectively. These pumps are used to dispense controlled substances at a specific rate of infusion. Two types of portable electronic pumps can be used to deliver controlled substances: a syringe system or a cassette system. Technicians may prepare either syringes or cassettes that are placed into a pump that automatically delivers the medication over a predetermined time. These pumps can be programmed for short or long durations to deliver medication, not to exceed a 24-hour period. These devices are especially effective for patients who require constant pain control and those discharged home with this type of medication. Another type of dispensing system that uses syringes relies on gravity for delivering the solution. The syringes are placed in a freestanding IV pump system on wheels; these are used only in the hospital.

Patient-Controlled Analgesia Syringe System

Patient-controlled analgesia (PCA) is a method of administration that allows the patient to control the rate at which the drug is delivered for the relief of pain. The PCA pump holds a syringe of pain medication that is attached to the IV line and is regulated by a computerized device that automatically dispenses the medication. The pump may be programmed to deliver a small, constant dose of pain medicine, and the patient has the option of receiving additional doses (bolus) if necessary. This is done by depressing a button attached to a line on the machine. The boluses are preset for amount and frequency; even if the patient presses the button many times, he or she receives only the predetermined amount of drug. For example, if the dose is set at 1 mg/mL with dosing intervals every 6 minutes and a 1-hour lockout dose of 10 mg, regardless of how many times the patient presses the button within 6 minutes, he or she receives only 1 dose. The 1-hour lockout limits medication administration to a total dose of 10 mg in 1 hour. This safeguards the patient from overdosing. The PCA syringe device is normally used in a hospital setting

for acute postoperative pain control. Children ages 7 years and older can typically use this pump device independently once they are familiar with it. Young or debilitated patients need assistance from a nurse or caregiver to receive their dosing. Many manufacturers provide prefilled PCA syringes that may be used directly from the packaging in these pumps. Alternatively, pharmacy technicians (using aseptic technique in a **horizontal laminar flow hood**) can prepare the syringes for PCA pumps. Each syringe must be labeled, capped, and checked by the pharmacist before delivery. When the pharmacy technician is ready to have a prepared medication inspected by the pharmacist, he or she should include the finished product, along with the syringe, the opioid analgesic container, and the diluent used in its preparation.

Patient-Controlled Analgesia Syringe Systems

The following are some manufacturers of PCA syringe systems:
- Aitecs: *http://www.aitecs.com*
- B Braun: *http://www.bbraunusa.com*
- Smiths Medical (Medfusion): *http://www.smiths-medical.com*

Patient-Controlled Analgesia Cassette System

Cassette pumps are another type of PCA system that can be used at home. The programmed pumps work similarly to the syringe pumps in that they are preset for dosage administration. Additional boluses may be programmed into the pump per the physician's orders and cannot be altered by the patient. A *bolus* is a predetermined amount of drug that can be administered by the patient at one time when pain intensifies. The cassettes are available in various sizes, such as 50- or 100-mL volumes. The pharmacy may prepare the cassettes. A short piece of tubing with a Luer-Lok can be connected to a 60-mL syringe that is used to load the proper amount of solution. After the cassette has been filled, the line (tubing) must be primed. To prime a line, the tubing is allowed to fill with solution so that there is no air in the tubing; the tubing then is secured with a twist cap. This is usually done by the pharmacy at the time the medication is prepared. Fig. 12.8 shows an example of a PCA device.

Patient-Controlled Analgesia Cassette Systems

The following are examples of manufacturers of PCA cassette systems:
- CADD pumps: *http://www.smiths-medical.com*
- ambIT infusion pumps for home use: *https://ambitpump.com/*

United States Pharmacopeia <797>

History of *United States Pharmacopeia* <797>

The USP is responsible for providing safety guidelines for the preparation of parenteral and other sterile medications. In the 1970s, because of the dramatic increase in nosocomial infections, the National Coordinating Committee on Large Volume Parenterals (NCCLVP) provided guidelines for the preparation of parenteral medications. A nosocomial infection, or **health care–associated infection (HAI),** is an

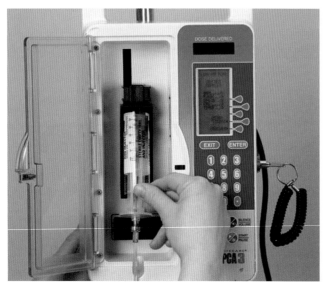

FIG. 12.8 Patient-controlled analgesia device with cartridge. (From Perry AG, Potter PA, Ostendorf WR. *Clinical Nursing Skills and Techniques*. 8th ed. St. Louis: Elsevier; 2014.)

TABLE 12.3
Environmental Cleaning Schedule

Site	Minimum Frequency
Laminar air flow workbench, biological safety cabinet, compounding aseptic isolator, compounding aseptic containment isolator	Start of each shift, start of each batch, at least every 30 min, and after spills or when surface is contaminated
Counters and work surfaces	Daily
Floors	Daily
Walls, ceilings, and storage shelves	Monthly

infection that originates in a hospital. Later, in the 1980s, the efforts of the NCCLVP were replaced by several other organizations as they began to establish standards for pharmacists and technicians in the safe preparation of parenteral medications. These organizations included the ASHP, the National Association of Boards of Pharmacy (NABP), and the United States Pharmacopeial Convention. Through the 1990s these organizations wrote both recommendations and guidelines for safe standards, but they were not monitored or enforced. In the mid-1990s it was determined through health system surveys that very few pharmacies followed these standards explicitly. For example, most pharmacies did not perform quality assurance checks or solution tests on a regular basis for prepared parenteral medications, and many did not provide education and training for personnel on a periodic basis. In addition, various IV medications were reported contaminated with bacteria because of poor aseptic technique. The reports of patient harm from improper preparation of medications by pharmacies continued through the 1990s.

In 2004 the USP <797> regulations were written with the intent that they would constitute an enforceable standard. The USP <797> standards must be met in all practice settings where sterile products are compounded. The USP, ASHP, and The Joint Commission (TJC) outlined a timeline for total compliance, realizing that it would take time for pharmacies to implement all the changes mandated. Pharmacies and other areas that prepare compounded sterile preparations must research, create, and document their **standard operating procedures (SOPs)** for meeting USP <797> regulations.

In June of 2019 the USP <797> released the current version for industry, effective December 2019. A number of changes were made, including clarification regarding the use of alternative technologies when preparing a compounded sterile product (CSP). A comprehensive list of definitions, including the terms used in this chapter, was provided. The risk categories of CSPs were revised, with two instead of three, based on conditions under which they were made and the time period in which they would be used (Table 12.3). More information on the revisions can be found at the USP website *(http://www.usp.org)*. In 2013, as a result of the fungal meningitis tragedy at the New England Compounding Center, a group of executives from the sterile compounding industry formed the Specialty Sterile Pharmaceutical Society (SSPS). It was founded to support more stringent standards of practice regarding quality control and to ensure the safety and welfare of individuals receiving CSPs. (For more information about SSPS standards and activities, visit the website *https://www.steri-pharma.com/*.) In November 2022 USP made revisions to the guidelines which became official in November 2023.

Sections of *United States Pharmacopeia* <797>

USP <797> has the following major sections:

1. Scope: List of sterile compounds, specific practices, risk factors
2. Personnel Qualifications: Proficiencies, training, evaluation
3. Personal Hygiene and Personal Protective Equipment: Hand hygiene, garbing,
4. Building and Facilities: Facility design and environmental controls
5. Environmental Monitoring: Air quality and surface sampling procedures
6. Cleaning and Disinfecting: Surfaces and tools used
7. Equipment and Components Packaging: Ingredients
8. Sterilization and Depyrogenation: Process for sterilizing and filtering of CSPs
9. Standard Operating Procedures and Master Formula Records and Compounding Records: Documentation explained
10. Release Testing: Final product inspection processes
11. Labeling: Required information for CSPs
12. Establishing Beyond-Use Dates and In-Use Times: Methods for establishing BUDs
13. Quality Assurance and Quality Control: Programs and documentation required for compounding pharmacies

TABLE 12.4
Terms and Abbreviations Used in Pharmacy

Terms	Definition
Ante area	An area in which all preparations for intravenous (IV) admixture are gathered, including labels, gowning, and drug materials
Beyond-use date (BUD)	The date or time a drug or material can no longer be used; the drug is ineffective after this date
Biological safety cabinet (BSC)	A cabinet with a high-efficiency particulate air (HEPA) filter for laminar air flow
Buffer area	An area in which hoods are kept and IV preparation takes place
Clean room	A space where microbial containment is kept at a specific level of safety to ensure a certain level of cleanliness
Compounding aseptic isolator (CAI)	An isolator cabinet designed to contain all contaminants; prevents contaminants from escaping IV lines and being transferred to the surrounding area
Critical site	An area exposed to air or touch, such as a vial, a needle, or an ampule
Direct compounding area (DCA)	A critical area within the hood (International Standards Organization [ISO] Class 5) where compounding materials are exposed to filtered air; also known as *first air*
First air	The air from the HEPA filter that passes over materials; this air is contaminant free
Hazardous drugs	Drugs that have been proven to have dangerous effects during animal or human testing; they may cause cancer or harm to certain organs or to pregnant women
Media-fill test	A test performed on compounded products to ensure that no contamination has taken place during preparation phase
Multidose container/vial (MDV)	A vial or container that can be used for more than one admixture; MDVs normally contain preservatives; the maximum dating is 28 days unless specified by the manufacturer
Negative pressure room	A room that has lower pressure than the adjacent rooms; net air flow is into the room
Positive pressure room	A room that has a higher pressure than the adjacent rooms; net air flow is out of the room
Primary engineering control (PEC)	A practice in which an ISO Class 5 system is in place that provides safety for admixtures; this includes laminar flow hood, glove boxes, vertical flow hoods, or compounding aseptic isolators
Single-dose container/vial (SDV)	A vial or container that can be used only once

14. Compounded Sterile Preparations Storage, Handling, Packaging, and Transport: Proper methods for CSP handling
15. Documentation: Requirements per USP for compounding facilities

Table 12.4 presents many of the terms and abbreviations used in USP <797> standards.

Categories of CSPs Levels

Following an update in November 2022, USP <797> has identified three categories that are based on various criteria per USP.

Category 1 CSPs

Category 1 CSPs are those assigned a maximum BUD of 12 hours or less at controlled room temperature or 24 hours or less and must be compounded in an International Organization for Standardization (ISO) Class 5 environment. Technicians must wear gown, gloves, hair covering, and mask during manipulation; these items of clothing are typically referred to as personal protective equipment and must be provided by the facility (Fig. 12.9). The technician must verify all ingredients and instructions and visually inspect the solution after preparation (Fig. 12.10A). Each person's knowledge of aseptic technique and proper manipulations

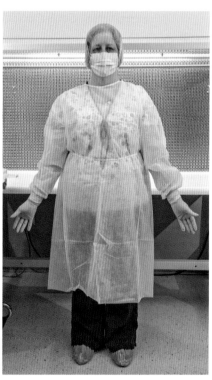

FIG. 12.9 Personal protective equipment shown. Start at feet first.

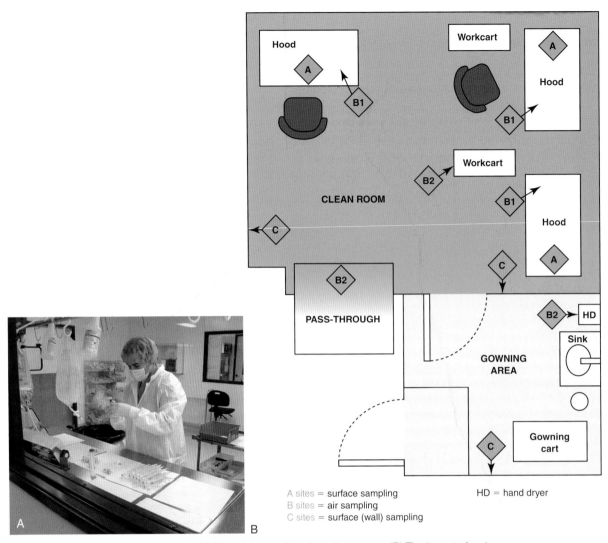

FIG. 12.10 Clean room. (A) Technician working in a clean room. (B) The layout of a clean room. (B, From Davis K. *Sterile Processing for Pharmacy Technicians*. St. Louis: Elsevier; 2014.)

A sites = surface sampling
B sites = air sampling
C sites = surface (wall) sampling

HD = hand dryer

must be monitored and verified quarterly. In addition, a quarterly media-fill test must be done for each person compounding products in the hood. Environmental compliance such as surface sampling and proper testing and certification of environment and equipment also must be performed.

Category 2 CSPs

Category 2 CSPs are those that have been prepared aseptically with all sterile components and untested for sterility. These CSPs have a BUD of 4 days at room temperature, 10 days if refrigerated, and 45 days if frozen. These CSPs also must meet the same aseptic techniques, procedures, and environmental controls as category 1 CSPs.

Category 3 CSPs

These CSPs must be prepared aseptically and have passed all sterility and applicable testing as assigned by USP <797> standards. The BUD is 60 days at room temperature, 120 days refrigerated, and 180 days frozen.

All categories MUST follow aseptic preparation guidelines, training, and testing to minimize potential contamination.

Requirements for Compounding

All personnel who prepare parenteral medications are required to be trained and monitored for compliance with techniques on a periodic basis. This includes ensuring that the drug ingredients, containers, labeling, and equipment are correct. Products must be stored according to manufacturer guidelines or other scientific findings. In addition, pharmacists must determine the risk level of each type of preparation. Although USP <797> outlines risks, the standards do not rate every type of manipulation; the standards outline basic guidelines. The hoods and clean room, in addition to the pharmacy rooms adjacent to these rooms, must be within the guidelines of USP <797>. It is essential that any contamination be kept away from these areas. The guidelines for air standards in IV areas and individual hoods are listed in Table 12.5.

Intravenous Environment

Most pharmacies can easily meet the educational and training aspects of USP <797>; however, this is not true of the new regulations related to the areas where these products are prepared. Each type of environment in the pharmacy is required

TABLE 12.5
United States Pharmacopeia <797> Air Standards Based on 0.5-μm Particle Size

BSC or Room	Description	Number of Particles/m³	Area in Pharmacy	Required Testing for Compliance
ISO Class 8	Class 100,000	3,520,000	Nonhazardous room	Checked every 12 months
ISO Class 7	Class 10,000	352,000	Clean room (ie, buffer room and anteroom)	Checked every 12 months
ISO Class 6	Class 1000	35,200	Anteroom	Checked every 6 months
ISO Class 5	Class 100	3520	IV hood	Checked every 6 months

BSC, Biological safety cabinet; *ISO,* International Standards Organization.

to meet minimum standards pertaining to air flow, microbe and particle size, and quantity. According to studies conducted by USP, using a **laminar air flow workbench (LAFW)** in an open room is no safer than preparing products on a countertop. This has been one of the most significant changes in pharmacy. As a result of the enormous expense required to create these new areas, many hospitals now contract out to specialized pharmacies to prepare their compounded sterile preparations. Facilities that have been able to meet USP standards must also test the air periodically to ensure that guidelines are met. The terms and definitions used to describe types of environments are listed in Box 12.1.

The **anteroom** is adjacent to the buffer room (or clean room) and is sometimes called the gowning/degowning area. The maximum size of air particles allowed in the anteroom is 0.5 μm, and air pressure is monitored. All donning of PPE occurs in the anteroom. The clean room, where the technician actually prepares compounded sterile preparations, must meet more stringent requirements for air particulate size (see Fig. 12.10B).

USP <797> also requires specific types of hoods to be used for compounding specific sterile products (Fig. 12.11). Laminar flow workbenches that have only positive (horizontal) air flow may be used to prepare nonhazardous sterile compounds (CSPs) (see Fig. 9.9), whereas a negative (vertical) air flow environment may be used to prepare hazardous products per USP guidelines (see Fig. 9.12). A **biological safety cabinet (BSC)** is a totally enclosed environment that is available with either positive or negative air flow; these cabinets are known as glove boxes or barrier isolator hoods (see Fig. 9.11). All types of hoods have high-efficiency particulate air (HEPA) filters, although the way in which they expel the air differs. Proper use of these hoods requires additional training. The hoods must be verified and certified every 6 months or whenever moved to ensure their ability to filter contaminants. Both anterooms and clean rooms must be within standards. Assessments must be completed by a certified outside source; any movement of the equipment requires additional inspection.

Pharmacies must use special equipment and chemicals to sterilize the anteroom and clean room; specialty knowledge about the proper way to clean each room is also required. For example, hoods and surface areas must be cleaned and sterilized daily and the walls and floor must be cleaned and sterilized

BOX 12.1 Environment Terminology

Air lock: A space of separation between two different air pressures; may be a pass-through chamber or room; a door must be present to prevent loss of pressure in the room with higher pressure
Air pressure: Can be either positive or negative; positive air pressure environments may be used only for nonhazardous sterile preparation; negative air pressure environments can be used to prepare both nonhazardous and hazardous sterile preparations
Anteroom: Space adjacent to the clean or buffer room
Biological safety cabinet (BSC): A hood that should be used for hazardous sterile preparation in the clean room
Clean or buffer room: Space adjacent to the primary engineering control room where sterile preparation takes place
Compounding aseptic containment isolator (CACI): Another type of Class III CAI glove box that exhausts 100% of the air through a high-efficiency particulate air filter; to be used for preparation of hazardous medications; may also have either negative or positive air pressure
Compounding aseptic isolator (CAI): A Class III glove box that can have either negative or positive air pressure
Laminar air flow workbench (LAFW): A hood that should be used for nonhazardous sterile preparation in the clean room
Primary engineering control (PEC): Space or hood where sterile preparation takes place

weekly. SOPs must be written and studied, and all who work in these areas must take evaluation examinations.

Primary Engineering Controls

Air Flow

Three types of hoods are used depending on the sterile product being prepared: the horizontal flow hood such as an LAFW; the **vertical laminar flow hood,** such as a BSC or **compounding aseptic containment isolator (CACI);** and the isolator hood, also referred to as a glove box (see Fig. 9.11).

LAFWs (ie, hoods) are used for many types of parenteral or sterile product preparations. Horizontal hoods provide positive air pressure, moving the filtered air outward toward the preparer.

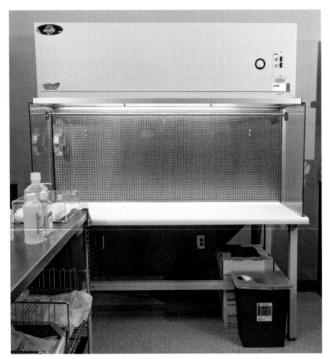

FIG. 12.11 Specific area kept clean. Certain requirements per *United States Pharmacopeia* <797>.

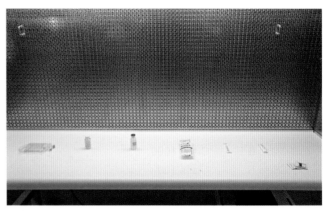

FIG. 12.12 Items in hood must be 6 inches apart and 6 inches from the side and front of the hood per *United States Pharmacopeia* <797>.

For chemotherapeutic agents, a type of vertical flow hood, known as a BSC or CACI, is used because of the direction of the air flow and the specifications of the hood. A vertical flow hood provides negative air pressure, circulating the air through an additional HEPA filter and then through a vent away from the preparer.

Another version of a vertical flow hood can be used to mix nonchemotherapeutic agents if needed, such as nonsterile compounds; however, *hazardous drugs such as chemotherapeutic agents should never be mixed in a LAFW or any type of horizontal flow hood* (see Fig. 11.7).

Isolator hoods, also known as glove boxes, are closed systems (see Fig. 9.11) that use a HEPA filter and a sophisticated venting system. These provide the greatest amount of safety to the preparer because of the containment ability. With all systems, strict aseptic technique and care must be used because spillage can still occur on the surface of the IV bag or container and can cause contamination or unwanted exposure on removal from the hood.

In a horizontal flow hood, or LAFW, the outside air flow starts in the back of the hood, passes through a special filter, and circulates out toward the opening across the deck or direct compounding area (DCA). This special filter is a HEPA filter that traps all particles larger than 0.2 μm. The sides of the hood and items within the hood create a disruption of air flow. For this reason, the technician must work at least 6 inches from the sides and front of the hood (Fig. 12.12). In addition, movement within the hood should be kept to a minimum to reduce disruption of air flow.

The concept is similar for a vertical flow hood, although air cannot be released back into the room. For this reason, vertical hoods have a Plexiglas shield that separates the technician from the inside work surface. In a vertical flow hood, such as a BSC or CACI for compounding a **hazardous drug**, the air enters the HEPA filter vertically and flows down, passing into the HEPA filter and then onto the workspace area. A grid at the front of the tabletop draws in the air and filters it once again through a HEPA filter before it is released into the workspace area or is vented to the outside, depending on the type of venting system used.

Regardless of a vertical or horizontal hood air flow, the technician must not block the flow of air while working. This air is considered **first air,** and it must remain free of obstruction to ensure the critical areas are free of microbes.

Tech Note!

Remember to alter your hand placement and technique based on the air flow of the **primary engineering control (PEC)** being used. Try identifying the best spot on the deck to perform your manipulations in each of the hoods you regularly use.

It is best practice to leave primary engineering controls (PECs) turned on at all times, but if this cannot be accomplished, an LAFW must be turned on at least 30 minutes before use, every 30 minutes while in continuous use, when there are spills, or when there is suspected contamination. In addition, daily cleaning is required and is best performed at the end of the day. The cleaning must be performed by trained compounding personnel, not environmental departments or outside sources.

As mentioned, there is also a PEC known as a glove box or barrier isolator. It is becoming the most popular type of hood for sterile preparation. It reduces the risk for contamination caused by accidental mishandling of drugs during compounding and reduces the number of environmental microbial contaminants, thus increasing the sterility of the prepared product. This ultimately protects patients from possibly harmful medications. If it is a BSC, it also protects the person preparing a hazardous or chemotherapeutic agent because these medications can be harmful if they are inhaled or come in contact with the skin.

The air is redirected through a HEPA filter, and an additional air flow system helps decontaminate the medication preparation. Daily monitoring of the pressure gauge, flow indicators, or alarms should be documented.

A BSC must be turned on at least 10 minutes before use. After the technician washes his or her hands and cleans the hood properly, all the necessary materials and medications can be placed inside a sterile holding chamber. Using the attached gloves, the technician takes the materials from the sterile chamber and transfers them into the main hood. All products and supplies should be placed at least 4 inches inside the sash. At this point, the technician may prepare the medication. Any high-risk medication can be prepared in this type of hood. Inspections should be performed every 6 months. In an effort to comply with USP <797> guidelines, more pharmacies are using these types of hoods.

Cleaning and Maintaining Primary Engineering Controls

All hoods in the pharmacy must be thoroughly cleaned using the appropriate solvent and cleaning methods (see Table 12.3 for the cleaning schedule). Procedure 12.1 lists systematic instructions for cleaning a laminar air flow workbench, and Procedure 12.2 lists the instructions for cleaning a vertical flow hood. Cleaning of BSCs differs from the cleaning of horizontal and vertical flow hoods, as described in Procedure 12.3.

Procedure 12.1

Cleaning a Horizontal Laminar Air Flow Hood

Goal
To learn to properly clean a horizontal laminar air flow workbench (hood)

Equipment and Supplies
- Horizontal laminar air flow hood
- Lint-free wipes or gauze
- Sterile 70% alcohol
- Sterile water

Remember
- Procedures for cleaning and disinfecting the hood should be developed, implemented, and practiced by trained compounding personnel. These procedures must follow *United States Pharmacopeia* <797> guidelines and should be written in the facility's standard operating procedures.
- Cleaning and disinfecting are to be completed before any compounding is performed.
- The hood should be turned on and running at least 30 min before cleaning.
- Follow proper hand washing procedure and technique.
- Put on appropriate apparel, following proper garbing technique.

Procedural Steps
1. Remove any items from within the hood.
   PURPOSE: The hood should be completely empty so that all surfaces can be cleaned. Unnecessary items clutter the workspace and may contaminate the area.
2. Clean all surfaces inside the hood with a lint-free wipe and sterile water.
   PURPOSE: To make certain all surfaces are clean and free from any loose material or residue.
3. Inspect all surfaces for any crystallized solutions. Clean these with sterile water before continuing.
   PURPOSE: To make certain nothing is left on the surface that may contaminate the compounded sterile preparations (CSPs).

4. Moisten a 4- × 4-inch gauze or other lint-free cloth with sterile 70% alcohol.

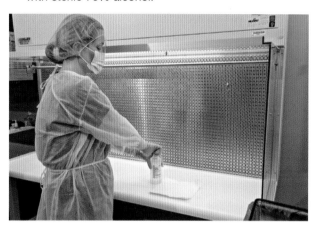

PURPOSE: To prepare to disinfect the surfaces in the hood. If used properly, sterile 70% alcohol reduces the probability of contamination.
Remember to use a new wipe moistened with sterile 70% alcohol on each section of the hood cleaned.[a]

5. Wipe the top of the hood first. Clean in a side-to-side motion from left to right, working from back to front.

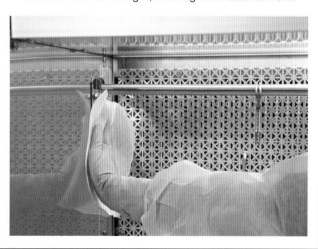

Continued

Cleaning a Horizontal Laminar Air Flow Hood—cont'd

PURPOSE: To ensure uniformity of the cleaning procedure from shift to shift and person to person. This also follows the method of cleaning from top to bottom to ensure nothing falls from a higher surface to contaminate a lower surface.

6. Wipe the horizontal intravenous (IV) pole and any hooks or brackets using a smooth motion from left to right.

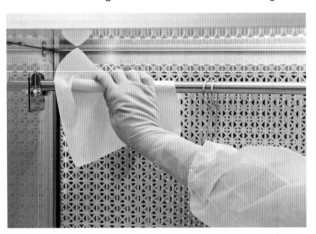

PURPOSE: To ensure that the IV pole is disinfected and ready to use if any items need to be attached during the compounding process.

7. Wipe from top to bottom on each side of the hood. Always work from the back to the front.

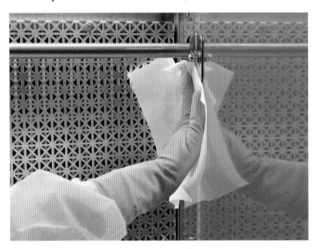

PURPOSE: To disinfect the sides of the hood to prepare for the compounding process.

8. Wipe the rear wall of the hood using a side-to-side motion from left to right, beginning at the top and working down to the bottom.

PURPOSE: To disinfect the rear wall of the hood to prepare for the compounding process. Remember, the high-efficiency particulate air (HEPA) filter is delicate and easily damaged. Never put too much pressure on the filter cover when cleaning. This could drive one of the aluminum separators into the filter, causing damage that can be detected only through testing.

9. Finally, wipe the flat work surface area using a side-to-side motion from left to right, working from back to front.

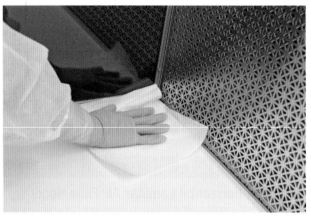

PURPOSE: To disinfect the work surface area of the hood to prepare for the compounding process.

10. Pull the used cloths out of the hood. NEVER reenter or wipe an area with the used cloths.

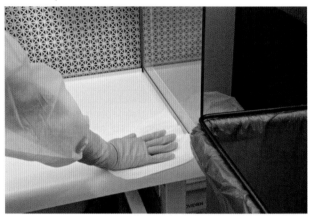

11. Allow the sterile 70% alcohol to remain on surfaces to be disinfected for at least 30 seconds before such surfaces are used to prepare CSPs.

PURPOSE: To kill organisms that may contaminate the CSPs. If the alcohol is not allowed to dry completely, it may itself act as a vehicle for the transfer of contaminants.

[a]Never attempt to clean the high-efficiency particulate air (HEPA) filter or spray any solutions toward the HEPA filter. Also, discard alcohol bottles when empty and be sure to disinfect the spray head if transferring it to a new bottle to avoid contamination.

Cleaning a Vertical Air Flow Hood

Goal
To learn to properly clean a vertical laminar air flow hood.

Equipment and Supplies
- Lint-free wipes or gauze
- Sterile 70% alcohol
- Sterile water
- Vertical air flow hood

Remember
- Procedures for cleaning and disinfecting the hood should be developed, implemented, and practiced by trained compounding personnel. These procedures must follow *United States Pharmacopeia* <797> guidelines and should be written in the facility's standard operating procedures.
- Cleaning and disinfecting are to be completed before any compounding is performed.
- The hood should be turned on and running at least 30 min before cleaning.
- Follow proper hand washing procedure and technique.
- Put on appropriate apparel, following proper garbing technique.

Procedural Steps
1. Remove any items from within the hood.
   PURPOSE: The hood should be completely empty so that all surfaces can be cleaned. Unnecessary items clutter the workspace and may contaminate the area.
2. Clean all surfaces inside the hood with a lint-free wipe and sterile water.
   PURPOSE: To make certain all surfaces are clean and free from any loose material or residue.
3. Inspect all surfaces for any crystallized solutions. Clean these with sterile water before continuing.
   PURPOSE: To make certain nothing is left on the surface that may contaminate the compounded sterile preparations (CSPs).

4. Moisten a 4- × 4-inch gauze or other lint-free cloth with sterile 70% alcohol.
   PURPOSE: To prepare to disinfect the surfaces in the hood. If used properly, sterile 70% alcohol reduces the probability of contamination.
   Remember to use a new wipe moistened with sterile 70% alcohol on each section of the hood cleaned.[a]
5. Wipe the horizontal intravenous (IV) pole and any hooks or brackets using a smooth motion from one side to the other.
   PURPOSE: To ensure that the IV pole is disinfected and ready to use if any items need to be attached during the compounding process.
6. Wipe from top to bottom on each side of the hood. Work side to side with overlapping strokes.
   PURPOSE: To disinfect the sides of the hood to prepare for the compounding process.
7. Wipe the rear wall of the hood and inside the front shield using a side-to-side motion from left to right, beginning at the top and working down to the bottom.
   PURPOSE: To disinfect the rear wall and front shield of the hood to prepare for the compounding process.
8. Finally, wipe the flat work surface area using a side-to-side motion from left to right, working from back to front. Start with the "ceiling," then generally from top to bottom and back to front. Follow this by the back, IV poles and hangers, and then items on deck and the deck. Always use overlapping strokes.
   PURPOSE: To disinfect the work surface area of the hood to prepare for the compounding process.
9. Allow the sterile 70% alcohol to remain on surfaces to be disinfected for at least 30 seconds *and dry completely* before such surfaces are used to prepare CSPs.
   PURPOSE: To kill organisms that may contaminate the CSPs. If the alcohol is not allowed to dry completely, it may itself act as a vehicle for the transfer of contaminants.

[a]Never attempt to clean the high-efficiency particulate air (HEPA) filter or spray any solutions toward the HEPA filter. Also, discard alcohol bottles when empty and be sure to disinfect the spray head if transferring it to a new bottle to avoid contamination. Treat cleaning supplies as hazardous waste for disposal purposes.

Tech Note!

When applying 70% isopropyl alcohol to gloves, always allow to dry completely, and spraying should be avoided inside a hazardous drug PEC because of the action possibly spreading any residue that remains.

Aseptic Technique

When CSPs are prepared, aseptic techniques must be used. Normally nurses do not have the advantage of using a laminar flow hood; however, they sometimes must prepare products for immediate use and they still must use strict aseptic technique. Aseptic technique is directly associated with Universal Precautions (also known as Standard Precautions). Universal Precautions are guidelines followed by all health care workers when exposure to body fluids or blood products is likely. These precautions involve washing hands and putting on gloves and gowns (ie, PPE) when in the presence of any body fluids. Similarly, aseptic technique is used when both hazardous and nonhazardous products are prepared. Products that have been tested and shown to cause adverse or toxic effects in humans are classified as hazardous. Examples of these types of medications include chemotherapeutic agents, radioactive compounds, and various hazardous chemicals, such as phenol and glacial acetic acid.

Cleaning a Biological Safety Cabinet

Goal

To learn to properly clean a biological safety cabinet.

Equipment and Supplies

- Biological safety cabinet
- Lint-free wipes or gauze
- Sterile 70% alcohol
- Sterile water

Remember

- Procedures for cleaning and disinfecting the biological safety cabinet should be developed, implemented, and practiced by trained compounding personnel. These procedures must follow *United States Pharmacopeia* <797> guidelines and should be written in the facility's standard operating procedures.
- Cleaning and disinfecting are to be completed before any compounding is performed.
- Biological safety cabinets are intended to operate 24 hr/d. They must be cleaned every 30 min while continuous compounding is taking place.
- Follow proper hand washing procedure and technique.
- Put on appropriate apparel, following proper garbing technique.

Procedural Steps

1. Remove any items from within the biological safety cabinet.
   PURPOSE: The biological safety cabinet should be completely empty so that all surfaces can be cleaned. Unnecessary items clutter the workspace and may contaminate the area.
2. Clean all surfaces inside the biological safety cabinet with a lint-free wipe and sterile water.
   PURPOSE: To make certain all surfaces are clean and free from any loose material or residue.
3. Inspect all surfaces for any crystallized solutions. Clean these with sterile water before continuing.
   PURPOSE: To make certain nothing is left on the surface that may contaminate the compounded sterile preparations (CSPs).

4. Moisten a 4- × 4-inch gauze or other lint-free cloth with sterile 70% alcohol.
   PURPOSE: To prepare to disinfect the surfaces in the biological safety cabinet. If used properly, sterile 70% alcohol reduces the probability of contamination.
   Remember to use a new wipe moistened with sterile 70% alcohol on each section of the biological safety cabinet cleaned.[a]
5. Wipe the horizontal intravenous (IV) pole and any hooks or brackets using a smooth motion from left to right.
   PURPOSE: To ensure that the IV pole is disinfected and ready to use if any items need to be attached during the compounding process.
6. Wipe from top to bottom on each side of the biological safety cabinet. Work side to side with overlapping strokes.
   PURPOSE: To disinfect the sides of the biological safety cabinet to prepare for the compounding process.
7. Wipe the rear wall of the biological safety cabinet and inside the front shield using a side-to-side motion from left to right, beginning at the top and working down to the bottom.
   PURPOSE: To disinfect the rear wall and front shield of the biological safety cabinet to prepare for the compounding process.
8. Finally, wipe the flat work surface area using a side-to-side motion from left to right, working from back to front.
   PURPOSE: To disinfect the work surface area of the biological safety cabinet to prepare for the compounding process.
9. Allow the sterile 70% alcohol to remain on surfaces to be disinfected for at least 30 seconds before such surfaces are used to prepare CSPs.
   PURPOSE: To kill organisms that may contaminate the CSPs. If the alcohol is not allowed to dry completely, it may itself act as a vehicle for the transfer of contaminants.

[a]Never attempt to clean the high-efficiency particulate air (HEPA) filter or spray any solutions toward the HEPA filter. Also, discard alcohol bottles when empty and be sure to disinfect the spray head if transferring it to a new bottle to avoid contamination. Treat cleaning supplies as hazardous waste for disposal purposes.

These precautions are used to prevent contamination by a product or to a product.

For pharmacy technicians, the importance of using aseptic technique cannot be stressed enough. Do not touch your face or glasses with sterile gloves, because touch contamination is the most common way to introduce microbes to a CSP. A medication that contains any microbes or unwanted debris can cause a dangerous infection, or even death, when administered to a patient. The steps used in aseptic technique begin with hand hygiene (Procedure 12.4), followed by proper donning of gloves and gown, cleaning of the flow hood, and, finally, preparation of the parenteral medication. Procedure 12.5 lists the preparation required for aseptic technique; except for putting on the surgical face mask immediately before entering the hood, all of these steps should be completed outside the clean room. On leaving the IV area, the technician must remove the hair cover, gloves, and face mask. Another consideration is the preparation of the rooms and equipment used in preparing CSPs. Accuracy in performing calculations and measuring medications is paramount; all calculations and measurements should be double-checked and must be verified by a pharmacist (Figs. 12.13 and 12.14).

Proper Hand Hygiene

Goal

To learn to follow proper hand washing procedures to prevent the spread of infection.

Equipment and Supplies

- Facility-approved hand cleanser
- Nail brush or scrub sponge
- Nonshedding disposable towels or an electronic hand dryer
- Warm water
- Waterless alcohol-based hand rub

Remember

- Personal electronic devices, such as cell phones or iPods and any associated attachments, must be removed before hand washing and should not be used in the sterile compounding area.

Procedural Steps

1. Remove all visible jewelry and cosmetics before beginning the hand washing process.
   PURPOSE: To minimize the risk for bacterial contamination by minimizing the number of particles introduced into the sterile compounding area.
2. Wash the hands, nails, wrists, and forearms up to the elbows for at least 30 seconds with a brush and/or sponge, warm water, and a facility-approved cleansing agent.
   PURPOSE: To make certain all surfaces are clean and free from any residue. The cleansing agent should remain in contact with the skin for at least 20 seconds to complete the bactericidal activity.
3. Rinse thoroughly with the hands and forearms in an upright position, beginning with the fingertips down to the elbows.
   PURPOSE: To make certain contaminants flow away from the hands and all cleansing residue is removed.

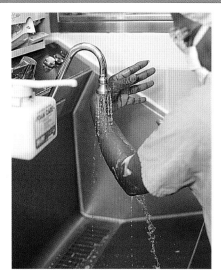

4. Dry the hands and arms with a nonshedding or lint-free cloth or with an electronic hand dryer.
   PURPOSE: To ensure that no contaminants are transferred from the towel to the clean hands.
   Remember to leave the water running while you dry your hands and arms and do not touch any part of the sink or dryer surfaces.[a]
5. After the hands and arms are completely dry, throw away damp towels and use a new towel to turn off the running water.
   PURPOSE: To ensure that clean hands and arms are not contaminated by touching any unclean surfaces.
6. Sanitize the hands by applying a waterless, alcohol-based hand rub and allow it to dry completely before putting on sterile gloves.
   PURPOSE: To prohibit regrowth of bacteria after hand washing.

[a]Touch is the most common source of contamination. Hands and gloves remain sterile only until they touch something.

Hand Placement

Regardless of the type of hood used, the placement of the hands is one of the most important aspects to consider when preparing sterile medications. The technician should practice some simple yet important techniques that reduce the possibility of contamination and errors when preparing CSPs to avoid compromising first air. Fig. 12.15 outlines the necessary steps for withdrawing a liquid from a vial while working in the hood. When working in a horizontal hood, you must not block the air flow or contaminate a **critical site** or area at any time; to prevent this, grasp the vial or ampule by the front; avoid placing the hands or fingers right behind the top of the container. When holding up the vial or ampule, keep the fingers from blocking air flow. This technique takes time to perfect and should be practiced constantly until it becomes second nature. When working in a vertical flow hood, avoid placing the hands and fingers over the container because this would break air flow. It is also important not to overload the hood with drugs and supplies, which can lead to a break in aseptic technique and increases the likelihood of drug errors. When using a BSC, you must follow strict protocol in handling and transferring solutions.

 Tech Alert!

Never recap the used needles; instead, discard each syringe in a sharps container, along with the uncapped needle, after use. Syringes cannot be reused when changing from one drug to another. This reduces the chance of drug-to-drug contamination.

Personnel Cleansing and Garbing Order

Goal

To learn the steps required to cleanse and garb up to properly prepare compounded sterile preparations

Equipment and Supplies

- Antiseptic hand cleanser
- Face mask or eye shield
- Head and facial hair cover
- Nonshedding gown
- Shoe covers
- Sterile powder-free gloves
- Surgical scrub

Procedural Steps

1. Remove all personal outer garments.
   PURPOSE: Outer garments such as jackets or coats may have shedding fibers or hairs that could contaminate the compounding area.
2. Remove all cosmetics and jewelry (no artificial nails are allowed).
   PURPOSE: Cosmetics can flake off and jewelry and artificial nails can have dirt and other debris on and under the surface. These contaminants can be carried into the compounding area if not removed.
3. Put on personal protective equipment in the following order:
   a. Shoe covers
   b. Head and facial hair covers
   c. Face masks/eye shields

PURPOSE: Shoe covers help prevent any germs that may be on your shoes from entering the compounding area. Head and facial hair covers are used to keep any hairs from falling into the compounding area. Face masks and eye shields are used to protect the technician from exposure to medications that may splash or may accidentally spill during the compounding process.

4. Perform aseptic hand cleansing procedures with a surgical scrub.
   PURPOSE: Proper hand washing with a surgical scrub helps lessen the bacteria found on the hands before beginning the compounding process.
5. Put on a nonshedding gown.
   PURPOSE: Donning a nonshedding gown serves to prevent any contaminants that may be on the technician's clothes from getting into the compounding area. Most gowns are resistant to penetration by moisture, which helps protect the technician if a spill occurs.
6. Put on the sterile, powder-free gloves.
   PURPOSE: Gloves protect the compounding area from skin that is constantly shedding from our hands. They also protect the technician from exposure to medications that may be used in the compounding process. Double gloving is recommended when compounding hazardous drugs or chemicals.

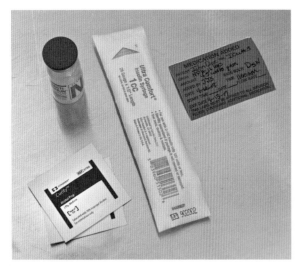

FIG. 12.13 The technician prepares supplies and medications (staging) and the pharmacist approves.

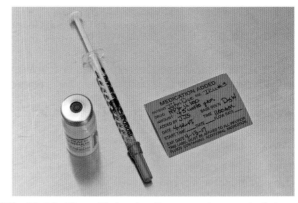

FIG. 12.14 After withdrawing the correct amount of drug for the syringe, the final product with the drug used is staged for the pharmacist to verify.

Use of Ampules to Prepare Medications

IV push or IM medications can be prepared by the nurse at the nursing station or at the patient's bedside; however, the pharmacy does prepare some IV push and IM medications.

These agents are placed in a syringe and sealed with a syringe cap until it is time to administer the medication (see Fig. 12.14).

The technician must follow the steps outlined in the following sections and shown in Fig. 12.16 when preparing these syringes from ampules; the procedures differ from those followed when using a vial. Once the medication is withdrawn, replace the filter needle or straw used with a regular needle and inject the drug into the IV solution; however, if the drug

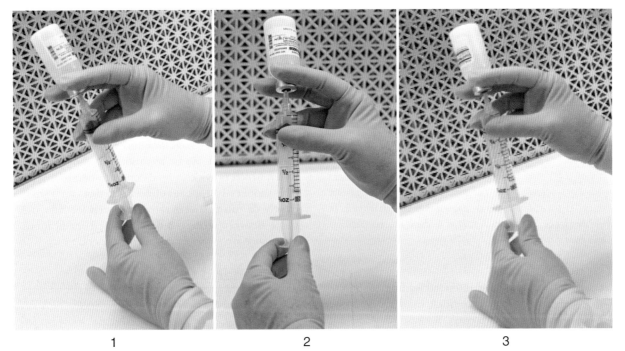

FIG. 12.15 The process for drawing medication from a vial. (1) After using sterile 70% alcohol, wipe the top of the vial and place the needle bevel side up and push it into the rubber stopper of the vial. (2) Preload the syringe with the necessary amount of air to replace solution. (3) Invert the vial and syringe 180 degrees. Push in the air from the syringe and pull out the solution.

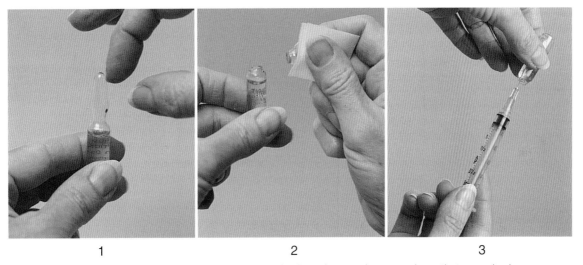

FIG. 12.16 Proper manipulation of an ampule. Ampules are glass containers that range in size from 1 to 50 mL. For larger ampules, an ampule breaker is suggested. For smaller ampules, follow these steps: (1) Tap the top of the ampule to empty the top of the container. (2) Using a sterile 70% alcohol swab, wipe the neck of the ampule and snap it open (away from you). (3) Tilt the ampule at an angle (the solution will not spill) and withdraw the required amount of drug using a filter needle. (From Potter PA, Perry AG. *Fundamentals of Nursing*. 8th ed. St. Louis: Mosby; 2013.)

is to be transported in the syringe, remove the needle and cap the end of the syringe. Label the container and place it in the proper location for the pharmacist's inspection.

Technique

When solution is pulled from an ampule, there is no positive or negative pressure because this is an open system; that is, the container is open and able to allow air to enter it, replacing the missing volume of solution. However, it is important to remember to use a filter needle when transferring drug from an ampule because small pieces of the ampule may detach and fall into the solution when the ampule is broken. A filter needle may be used only for one draw (push or pull); either it can be replaced by a regular needle before the drug is pushed into a piggyback or a regular needle can be used to withdraw the solution and then a filter needle can be used to push the filtered solution into the piggyback. Otherwise, the glass trapped in the filter needle is pushed into the final solution.

⊙ Scenario Checkup 12.2

After cleaning the hood and the Automix compounder, Ken gathers his orders and supplies to begin his TPN compounding. It is extremely important that all TPN medications be prepared in a manner that reduces the possibility of contamination. The first order calls for magnesium chloride as one of the additives; this is supplied in a 10-mL ampule. In addition to the syringe, what will Ken need to draw up this additive? Why is this extra step critical?

Vials

The two types of vials are those intended for immediate use (single-dose vials [SDVs]) and those that can be used more than once (multidose vials [MDVs]). Because they are not discarded after one use, MDVs contain preservatives. Volumes for SDVs and MDVs range from 1 mL up to 100 mL, and vials may contain either solution for withdrawal or powder for reconstitution. When an MDV solution is used, the date the vial was opened must be written on the label, along with the initials of the person who opened the vial.

■ Tech Note!

Never use an unmarked reconstituted vial because the amount of diluent is unknown. Instead, discard unmarked reconstituted vials. Frozen parenteral products must be thawed slowly, using either a cool bath or a thawing platform. They should never be placed in hot water or in a microwave oven. Once such medications have been thawed, they must be marked with the new expiration date per literature or the manufacturer's guidelines.

Reconstituting a medication is the addition of a diluent such as sterile water to convert the medication into solution form. If an antibiotic MDV portion has been used, the following information must be indicated on the vial: the date the vial was opened, the date the vial expires, the diluent used (if applicable), the concentration (eg, milligrams per milliliters), and the technician's initials. Bulk vials can be reconstituted in varying concentrations per the manufacturer's instructions to provide multiple IV bags for future use. For example, a cefazolin 10-g bulk vial can be reconstituted with 45 mL of sterile water, which provides a final concentration of 1 g per 5 mL. This supplies 10 1-g bags of cefazolin that can be used immediately or can be refrigerated or frozen for later use. BUDs differ between frozen and refrigerated medications. Many antibiotics are available in bulk containers.

⊙ Scenario Checkup 12.3

Ken is preparing to inject the next additive into the TPN mixture. He notices that the additive is from a multidose vial, which has been opened. The date the vial was opened is missing. What should Ken do in this situation? What could be the result if he uses the vial without proper documentation?

Specialized types of vials, such as the ADD-Vantage system (Fig. 12.17), can be placed on a small piggyback solution with an adapter; these are not mixed with the solution until immediately before administration. The pharmacy technician is responsible for proper attachment of the vial to the proper solution, but the nurse is responsible for breaking the adapter seal between the vial and the piggyback and mixing the powdered drug with the solution. Because the medication does not mix with the solution until the seal is broken, the IV can be returned to the pharmacy if it is not used. This greatly reduces the amount of wasted medication.

A controlled-release infusion system (CRIS) is another type of delivery system in which the vial is reconstituted (mixed) but is not added to the piggyback. At the time of administration,

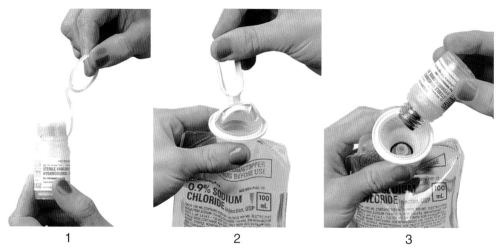

1   2   3

FIG. 12.17 ADD-Vantage system. To prepare an intravenous (IV) medication, follow these three steps: (1) Remove the top of the vial. (2) Pull up the flange, removing the seal on the IV bag. (3) Screw the vial into the port. Do not break the seal between the vial and the bag.

the vial is attached to a special port on the side of the tubing set that allows the medication to enter the piggyback, from which it then is delivered through the IV tubing.

Parenteral Antibiotics and Solutions

Manufacturers have suggested guidelines for dosing regimens and volumes of solutions that most physicians follow (Table 12.6). Pharmacies have a chart that instructs the person preparing the medication as to the type and amount of diluent needed, the normal dosing times, and expiration dates. Antibiotics also differ in how they should be prepared and how long it takes the powder to dissolve in the diluent. Once the drug has been reconstituted, the solution should be checked for color and clarity.

Technique

When a diluent is added to a powder, an equal amount of air must be removed from the vial or positive pressure is created, which causes pressure resistance in the syringe. For example, if you are adding 10 mL of diluent to a powder, push on the syringe until you feel a very slight resistance and then stop and withdraw an equal amount of air from the vial to relieve the positive pressure. Repeat this until all the diluent has been added. To work with negative pressure, first withdraw air from the vial until you feel resistance and then allow the vial to pull diluent out of the syringe. Never let go of a syringe. This type of technique works well because there is less chance of a spill.

Hyperalimentation

Hyperalimentation, or parenteral feeding, is a term for large volumes of parenteral nutrition solutions normally prepared for individuals who cannot orally consume nutrition (ie, they cannot eat). Some reasons for this inability to eat include the following:
- Recent stomach or intestinal surgery
- Unconsciousness (coma)
- Various conditions that may adversely affect the gastrointestinal system

■ TABLE 12.6
Examples of Suggested Dosing Times, Solutions, and Appropriate Volumes for Antibiotics

Generic Name	Trade Name	Common Dosing Regimens (hour)	Common Solutions	Common Volumes
Ampicillin	Omnipen[a]	q6–q8	NS	Less than 1.5 g (50 mL), more than 1.5 g (100 mL)
Cefazolin	Ancef[a], Kefzol[a]	q6–q8	D_5W or NS	Less than 2 g (50 mL), more than 2 g (100 mL)
Cefotaxime	Claforan[a]	q6–q12	D_5W or NS	Less than 2 g (50 mL), more than 2 g (100 mL)
Ceftazidime	Fortaz	q6–q8	D_5W or NS	Less than 2 g (50 mL), more than 2 g (100 mL)
Ceftriaxone	Rocephin[a]	q8–q24	D_5W or NS	Less than 2 g (50 mL), more than 2 g (100 mL)
Doxycycline	Vibramycin	q12	D_5W or NS	250 mL
Erythromycin	E-Mycin[a]	q6–q24	NS	250 mL[b] (10 mg) or 500 mL (20 mg) lidocaine
Gentamicin	Garamycin[a]	q8–q18[c] based on glycoside levels	D_5W or NS	Less than 100 mg (50 mL), more than 100 mg (100 mL)
Imipenem–cilastatin	Primaxin	q6–q12	NS	Less than 500 mg (100 mL), more than 500 mg (250 mL)

[a]Brand discontinued; now available only as generic.
[b]Erythromycin stings when given intravenously; therefore it is commonly mixed with lidocaine to relieve the pain.
[c]See Chapter 25 for more information on antibiotics.
D_5W, 5% dextrose in water; *NS*, normal saline.

Two main types of hyperalimentation are prepared in the pharmacy: **total parenteral nutrition (TPN)** and **peripheral parenteral nutrition (PPN)**. A **peripheral parenteral** injection is administered into the veins on the periphery of the body (arms, hands, or feet) instead of into a central vein or artery.

In a hospital setting, after the initial TPN has been prepared and hung, daily laboratory tests of electrolyte levels are drawn from the patient to determine necessary changes. For example, if a patient's potassium levels begin to drop, the next TPN is altered to compensate for this decrease. In this way, the patient receives exactly the nutrients needed each day. Home health clinics and some hospitals prepare hyperalimentation solutions that last 1 week. If this is done, the vitamin additive must be added daily to the TPN because this is one limiting factor for the bag's 24-hour expiration. Electrolyte levels are tested weekly instead of daily. Some patients may receive this type of nutrition for many months. Fig. 12.18 shows a TPN preparation connected to an automatic infusion pump system.

Many different protocols are used to prepare parenteral nutrition. The following is a list of typical solutions prepared in a hospital pharmacy. The large-volume components (eg, protein, carbohydrates, and fats) are premixed and ordered in cases from the manufacturer. Added to these solutions are the various electrolytes and other compatible medications requested by the patient's attending physician:

- TPN normally contains 50% dextrose, 10% amino acids, and 20% fat.
- PPN normally contains 25% dextrose, 10% amino acids, and 10% fat.
- TPNs are prepared for neonates, children, and adults.

Because of the regulations established by USP <797>, many pharmacies contract out their TPN/PPN orders to specialized compounding companies. Bags can range in volumes from 50 mL for neonates up to 3 L for adults. It is important to note that neonatal and pediatric additives differ in concentration from adult formulas; therefore great care must be taken when pulling the correct medication for preparation if your facility prepares these products.

◉ Scenario Checkup 12.4

Ken is now compounding a TPN for a baby in the intensive care unit. The physician's TPN order included directions to add zinc in a concentration of 200 mcg/100 mL. The automated compounder requires entry of zinc in a mcg/kg dose. What will happen if the pharmacist enters the zinc dose into the pharmacy computer as mg instead of mcg? What should Ken do if he discovers the error? A scenario similar to this one actually happened. For more information on the story, visit the website http://www.ncbi.nlm.nih.gov/pmc/articles/PMC3171817/.

> **Tech Note!**
>
> Some chemicals can **precipitate** other chemicals, creating solid flakes in the IV solution. Always check your IV bag for clarity after you finish preparing the solution.

Because of their range of concentrations, PPN solutions are administered differently from the higher concentration TPN solutions. TPN is administered intravenously by the subclavian vein and superior vena cava because of the higher concentration of nutrients. Patients must have a catheter surgically inserted for this procedure. PPN is administered via a peripheral vein, either in the back of the hand or in another peripheral area in the upper extremity, and therefore is a less complicated procedure. Most facilities have a standard order to initiate patient hyperalimentation. The volume of hyperalimentation typically ranges from 2 to 3 L. The physician determines the rate of infusion over the course of 24 hours. Regardless of how many milliliters run per hour, the hyperalimentation must be changed at least every 24 hours to ensure the sterility of the solution. If standard rate of infusion is 100 mL/hr, then 2400 mL may be used over the course of a day. Most hyperalimentation preparations are tailor-made for each patient. Fig. 12.19 gives an example of a protocol order.

> **Tech Note!**
>
> The final product must always be checked for color, clarity, and evidence of precipitation.

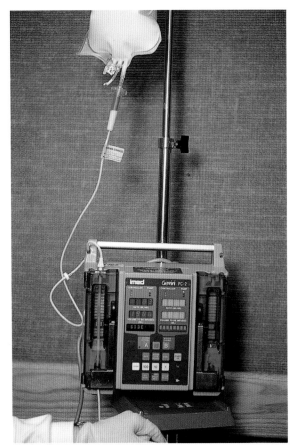

FIG. 12.18 Total parenteral nutrition preparation connected to an infusion set. (From Perry AG, Potter PA, Elkin MK. *Nursing Interventions and Clinical Skills*. 5th ed. St. Louis: Elsevier; 2012.)

HOME HEALTH		DATE	
PATIENT		ADDRESS	

TPN FORMULA:

AMINO ACIDS: ☐ 5.5% ☐ 8.5% ☑ 10%	425 mL
☐ WITH STANDARD ELECTROLYTES	
DEXTROSE: ☐ 10% ☐ 20% ☐ 40% ☐ 50% ☑ 70%	357 mL
(check one)	
LIPIDS: ☐ 10% ☑ 20%	125 mL
FOR ALL-IN-ONE FORMULA	

FINAL VOLUME		
qsad STERILE WATER FOR INJECTION	400mL	1307 mL

Calcium Gluconate	0.465m Eq/mL	5	mEq
Magnesium Sulfate	4m Eq/mL	5	mEq
Potassium Acetate	2m Eq/mL		mEq
Potassium Chloride	2m Eq/mL		mEq
Potassium Phosphate	3m M/mL	22	mM
Sodium Acetate	2m Eq/mL		mEq
Sodium Chloride	4m Eq/mL	35	mEq
Sodium Phosphate	3m M/mL		mM
TRACE ELEMENTS CONCENTRATE	☐ 4 ☐ 5 ☐ 6		mL

Patient Additives:

☐ MVC 9 + 3 10 mL Daily

☐ HUMULIN-R __10__ u Daily

☐ FOLIC ACID _____ mg
_____ times weekly

☐ VITAMIN K _____ mg
_____ times weekly

☐ OTHER: __MVI 12 1.5mL/daily__

☐ OTHER: _____

Directions:

INFUSE: ☑ DAILY

☐ _____ TIMES WEEKLY

OTHER DIRECTIONS:

_____

_____

_____

_____

Rate:	☐ CYCLIC INFUSION:	"	☐ CONTINUOUS INFUSION:	"	☑ STANDARD RATE:
	OVER _____ HOURS	"	AT _____ mL PER HOUR	"	AT __110__ mL PER HOUR
	(TAPER UP AND DOWN)	"		"	FOR __12__ HOURS

LAB ORDERS:

☐ STANDARD LAB ORDERS
SMAC-20, CO2, Mg+2 TWICE WEEKLY
CBC WITH AUTO DIFF WEEKLY
UNTIL STABLE, THEN:
SMAC-20, CO2, Mg+2 WEEKLY
CBC WITH AUTO DIFF MONTHLY

☐ OTHER: _____

_____

_____

VALIDATION:

_____

DOCTOR'S SIGNATURE

Print Name: _____

Office Address: _____

_____

Phone: _____

WHITE: Home Health   CANARY: Physician

FIG. 12.19 Total parenteral nutrition order.

Types of Parenteral Additives

Abbreviation	Meaning	Concentration	Notes
CaGluconate	Calcium gluconate	0.465 mEq/mL	
KAc	Potassium acetate	2 mEq/mL	Used to balance[a]
KCl	Potassium chloride	2 mEq/mL	
KPO_4	Potassium phosphate	Potassium 2 mEq/mL; phosphate 3 mEq/mL	Always determine phosphate concentration first
$MgSO_4$	Magnesium sulfate	1 mg/mL	
NaAcetate	Sodium acetate	2 mEq/mL	Used to balance[a]
NaCl	Sodium chloride	2 mEq/mL	Used to balance[a]
$NaPO_4$	Sodium phosphate	2 mEq/mL	
Miscellaneous Additives			
MTE	Multiple trace elements		Both adult and pediatric dosing
MVI	Multivitamin		Both adult and pediatric dosing
Regular insulin	Insulin		Can be added to TPN and PPN
Se	Selenium		
Zn	Zinc		
Other Nonsupplements Added to TPN or PPN Solutions			
Generic Name	**Trade Name**	**Concentration**	
Famotidine	Pepcid	20 mg/mL	

[a]*To balance* means the pharmacist determines the amount to be added.
PPN, Peripheral parenteral nutrition; *TPN,* total parenteral nutrition.

Electrolytes and Additives

All TPN preparations contain dextrose and amino acids; both ingredients help nourish the body. The metabolism of dextrose (ie, sugar) provides calories and a quick energy source for the body, whereas amino acids are the essential components the body uses to synthesize protein, needed enzymes, and other important molecules. Lipids commonly are added to give the body the fat needed for synthesis of important cell components, such as cell membranes. The rest of the additives are additional electrolytes (Table 12.7). These components can be determined daily if the patient is in a hospital. Other medications such as cimetidine or famotidine (both histamine-2 antagonists), which help patients with stomach problems, also can be added to hyperalimentation. Besides stomach medications, insulin often is added in quantities up to 100 units per bag. Only regular insulin is added to hyperalimentation preparations because it is the only insulin product that may be given intravenously.

Compatibility Considerations of Parenteral Medications

Many different types of medications are prepared in a clean room. Some medications must be protected from light, whereas others must be kept in bottles (as discussed previously). Table 12.8 presents additional considerations in the preparation of parenteral drugs. Special instructions for the preparation of many types of parenteral medications can be found in reference books in IV rooms. The IV technician

must become familiar with the idiosyncrasies of medications to ensure that all solutions he or she makes are effective and safe.

■ Tech Note!

Each type of medication has its own unique properties. For example, ceftazidime produces gas when reconstituted. Therefore, to prevent the solution from shooting out of the vial, the gas must be released first. This can be done by puncturing the vial membrane with a needle to allow venting of the gas. Erythromycin powder is difficult to dissolve into the diluent; therefore it is important to allow additional time when reconstituting erythromycin. Allow the vial to sit in the hood (and shake it occasionally) until the powder turns into a solution.

Components of a Label for Intravenous Medication

The final step in preparing parenteral medications is the application of the label. First, check the label against the medication and the physician's orders to ensure that the right medication is being given to the right patient. Although each pharmacy prepares its own label, all labels require the same minimum information (Fig. 12.20).

All labels produced for parenteral medications must be initialed by the technician who prepares them. A registered

TABLE 12.8
Additional Considerations for the Preparation of Drugs

Medication	Special Instructions
Amiodarone	D_5W
Ciprofloxacin	Protect from light
Insulin	NS or ½NS; must be placed in glass container
Lorazepam	Protect from light; stable longer in glass than in plastic
Nitroglycerin	D_5NS or NS; must be placed in glass container

D_5NS, 5% dextrose in normal saline; D_5W, 5% dextrose in water; NS, normal saline.

```
HOME INFUSION PHARMACY

Patient A                    Date: 03/26/2018
RX#37856

Amino*Acids 10%=425 mL  Dextrose*70%=357 mL
Ster*Water=400 mL  Lipids*20%=125 mL
MVI=10 ml/day  *Additives per liter*
Sod*Chlor=35 mEq  Pot*Phos=15 mM  Calcium=
5 mEq  Magnesium=5 mEq

Qty#     TPN 40-51GM Protein+Lipids
Infuse nightly 8pm to 8am thru IV PICC line via sigma
pump. *****Add 10 units Humulin-R to each bag just
prior to infusion***** **Note: contains TPN soln+lipids:
rate adjusted**  Settings: rate=104 mL/hr
volume=1248 mL

***REFRIGERATE***

Expiration date: 04/01/18
```

FIG. 12.20 Intravenous medication label.

pharmacist is responsible for the final label inspection. If the medication is not used, perhaps because of a discontinued order, it often can be recycled for use with another patient.

After the labels have been applied, the IV preparations are left for the pharmacist to check, along with the vial or container of medication used to make the IV preparation. When this check has been completed, the IV preparations are loaded onto a cart or delivery vehicle that delivers them to their destinations. In a home health setting, a delivery service may be used to transport the medications to the patient's home. In a hospital, this task normally is done by the technician. When the IV preparations are placed in the correct nursing unit, all unused IV preparations are collected and returned to the pharmacy for recycling. As long as the IV preparations are within their expiration dates and are kept at proper temperature, they can be used to fill new orders.

Disposal

Once the technician has finished using the hood area, he or she should clean all unused materials and discard any used products. To clean a horizontal flow hood, wipe down the surface with a sterile 70% isopropyl alcohol swab and then allow the surface to air dry. Dispose of all paper products in a trash bin; dispose of needles, syringes, and vials in a sharps container. Most sharps containers are made of heavy-duty plastic; they have a separate lid that can be locked into place on top of the container and a one-way opening in the lid for the disposal of needles and other sharps. Normally a 7-gallon size is used and is located outside the hood. When cleaning a vertical flow hood, discard needles, syringes, and vials in a small sharps container placed inside the hood area. Wrap all other materials to be discarded into the spill-proof pad and place inside a chemotherapeutic protective bag. This may be discarded in a special hazardous materials bin located outside the hood. All materials used in the BSC, including disposable needles and syringes, must be placed in appropriate sharps disposal containers and discarded as infectious waste. This is located inside the hood area.

For all hoods, the last step is to clean the entire area with the proper sterile 70% alcohol solution as appropriate for the type of cabinet involved. Sharps containers are to be replaced when two-thirds full and must be picked up or delivered to an approved "red bag" or medical waste treatment site.

Tech Note!

Always check the pharmacy protocol for the disposal of sharps containers. This information can be found in the policies and procedures handbook. Never insert your hand into a sharps or hazardous waste container! This could result in a needle stick or exposure to a hazardous chemical.

Chemotherapeutic Agents

In February 2016 a proposed set of guidelines known as **United States Pharmacopeia <800> <USP 800>** was added to deal with hazardous drugs in health care settings. Special considerations apply in the preparation of chemotherapeutic agents, both in preparation and in administration. The following two key changes from USP <797> were addressed:

1. Hazardous drugs must have separate storage and preparation from nonhazardous drugs.
2. USP <800> requires the use of closed-system transfer devices for administration of hazardous drugs. This minimizes exposure to nurses and patients receiving the medications. Because of the risks involved in handling chemotherapy drugs, technicians must be thoroughly trained in chemotherapy admixture technique to reduce the chances of exposure to hazardous medications should be prepared only in a safe environment, such as a vertical flow barrier hood or a BSC. Pharmacy technicians should always follow chemotherapy guidelines and should be trained in proper disposal of hazardous substances. Special chemotherapy gowns and gloves are worn to repel any substances that might spill or drip onto the technician during the compounding process (see Fig. 12.21 for proper setup [staging] and Fig. 12.22 for supplies used). Double gloves are worn for extra protection. Face and eye shields

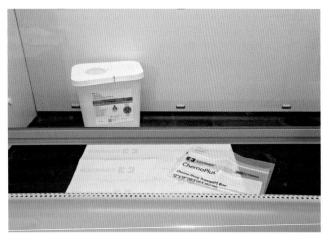

FIG. 12.21 BSC staging (setup) for hazardous preparation. Biological safety cabinet preparation area.

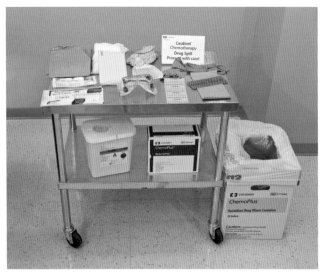

FIG. 12.22 Special chemotherapy supplies and equipment used in the preparation of a hazardous medication.

help the technician avoid contamination of the eyes. Masks are worn to prevent inhalation of any dangerous chemicals. When chemotherapeutic agents are compounded, preparation and cleanup must be done slowly and carefully, and the proper documentation should be completed.

Spills

If a spill occurs in a horizontal flow hood, it may be cleaned using a gauze pad and sterile 70% isopropyl alcohol. The gauze can be discarded in a regular trash bin. Always wear the proper protective equipment for the type of spill to be handled. If a small spill occurs in a vertical flow hood, it should be cleaned with sterile gauze and 70% isopropyl alcohol and discarded inside a marked hazardous bag. If a small spill occurs in a BSC, wipe up the spill with a disinfectant-soaked paper towel and then clean the surface with 70% isopropyl alcohol. The outer pair of gloves must be replaced after cleaning up a spill (see Fig. 12.22). Dispose of the materials in the appropriate container. For specific information on spill size and cleaning techniques, see the policies and procedures binder.

⊙ Scenario Checkup 12.5

Ken is required to complete an aseptic validation certification each year to maintain his position. He must complete a media-fill simulation test that demonstrates his ability to use aseptic procedures to compound sterile pharmacy products. He must meet the verification and sterility testing requirements as detailed in USP <797>. What should be his margin of error? Should he be allowed more than one attempt? What should be the consequence of failing this simulation test?

Education and Training

Both pharmacists and technicians must be able to show competency in compounding. Before compounding is permitted, the pharmacist and technician must complete video and written and practical instruction, followed by observations, a media-fill test, and a written examination. Training and testing must be repeated quarterly for all compounding personnel.

Although individuals who prepare sterile products must receive training on standards of sterile compounding, those instructions differ depending on the number and type of manipulations performed. Normally physicians, nurses, and emergency medical technicians (EMTs) prepare only low-risk products. Pharmacy technicians and pharmacists must be instructed on all standards if they are to prepare all types of compounded sterile preparations.

Several steps must be accomplished to complete the proper training. By viewing instructional videos from the ASHP, technicians can learn safe handling of compounded sterile preparations. In addition, aseptic technique verification services, such as Valiteq Products, provide training packets for various risk levels. Both ASHP and Valiteq have compounding manuals that can be used throughout the training period. Valiteq includes media-fill tests (Box 12.2) and a written examination, in addition to a visual check-off list for observation of the preparer. Once the preparation is complete, the growth medium is incubated according to set requirements and tested at various times for any abnormal growth. No growth is acceptable for a passing score. These validations must be completed and passed before the technician is permitted to prepare compounded sterile preparations. Personnel who fail any of the tests must repeat instruction and reevaluation. According to UPS <797>, the following schedule applies for gloved fingertip, thumb sampling, and media-fill testing of compounding personnel:

- Compounding personnel must complete competency evaluations no fewer than three separate times initially and one time for subsequent evaluations.
- A sample form (Fig. 12.23) lists the standards required of personnel who prepare CSPs. To ensure compliance, an observer must rate each standard while preparations are being compounded.

BOX 12.2   Media-Fill Tests

What Is a Media-Fill Test?

For a media-fill test, a microbial growth medium (eg, trypticase soy broth [TSB]) solution is substituted for the actual drug to simulate the admixture compounding technique. After the TSB is injected into the compounded sterile product, the final container is incubated at 20°C to 25°C for 7 days followed by 7 more days at 30°C to 35°C and then checked for turbidity. A positive test result confirms the presence of microbial contaminants.

How Often Are Media-Fill Tests Performed?

Per *United States Pharmacopeia* <797> regulations, a series of three media-fill tests must be completed at the time of hire. Thereafter, it must be performed at least quarterly.

Under What Conditions Is a Media-Fill Test Performed?

It is suggested that the test be performed in a manner to mimic a real case scenario—for example, at the end of the day when the preparer is tired or at stressful work times during the day.

What Happens if the Test Results Are Positive?

The written policies for the pharmacy include steps that should be taken for positive test results; they include retraining in aseptic techniques with a mentor and then repeating the media-fill test with passing results at a minimum of three times. If the test results are positive after the retest, it is suggested that the clean room and hoods be tested for any contamination. All results should be documented.

COMPOUNDING EVALUATION CHECKLIST
(circle answer)

No jewelry	YES	NO	N/A
Hair tied back	YES	NO	N/A
All calculations done prior	YES	NO	N/A
All products gathered prior	YES	NO	N/A
Washes hands appropriately	YES	NO	N/A
Gowns appropriately	YES	NO	N/A
Cleans hood 70% isopropyl alcohol	YES	NO	N/A
Cleans hood appropriately	YES	NO	N/A
Puts all items into the hood properly	YES	NO	N/A
Uses aseptic manipulation in the hood	YES	NO	N/A
Works within 6" radius of hood	YES	NO	N/A
If left the hood, sterilizes gloves prior to re-entering	YES	NO	N/A
Checked label 3 times	YES	NO	N/A
Uses proper equipment while in the hood	YES	NO	N/A
Uses foil cover on port after adding medication	YES	NO	N/A
Checks final product for color, clarity	YES	NO	N/A
Places label properly on product	YES	NO	N/A
Label is correct	YES	NO	N/A
Calculations are correct	YES	NO	N/A
Expiration date given	YES	NO	N/A
Signature of preparer signed	YES	NO	N/A
Disposes of vial and used packages appropriately	YES	NO	N/A
Cleans hood after use	YES	NO	N/A
Did not spill any contents	YES	NO	N/A
Did not break airflow	YES	NO	N/A
Checked for any particulates in diluted solution	YES	NO	N/A

Name _____   Date_____Time _____

Evaluator _____

Comments:_____

FIG. 12.23 Compounding evaluation checklist.

Do You Remember These Key Points?

- Why certain medications must be sterile
- Common terms used in sterile compounding
- The Standard Precautions necessary when preparing compounded sterile preparations
- The standard supplies and equipment used to prepare compounded sterile preparations
- The anatomy of a syringe and needle
- The sizes of syringes and needles used in the pharmacy setting
- When and why filters are used in sterile compounding
- Types of stock used in a clean room
- The various medication delivery systems
- The history of the USP <797>
- The main components of USP <797> regulations
- The categories of CSPs determined by USP <797>
- The various types of hoods
- How often environmental controls must be inspected
- How to properly clean various types of hoods and prepare them for use
- The proper aseptic technique
- The steps in drawing up medication from an ampule
- The steps in drawing up medication from a vial
- Different types of intravenous parenteral medications
- How to properly dispose of needles, vials, and hazardous supplies

⊙ Scenario Follow-Up

Ken completes his yearly aseptic validation certification and receives his results. He is delighted to see that his compounded parenteral products were 98% particulate free. He knows the only way to ensure product quality is to continually demonstrate proper procedure. His goal is to produce 100% contaminant-free TPN and IV admixtures. Do you think this is an attainable goal? Why or why not?

Review Questions

Multiple Choice Questions

1. The smallest filter that can be used is a:
   A. Filter straw
   B. Filter needle
   C. 5-μm filter
   D. 0.22-μm filter
2. Laminar flow hoods should be cleaned:
   A. With 70% isopropyl alcohol
   B. At least 30 minutes before using
   C. After any spill
   D. All of the above
3. Chemotherapeutic agents should be disposed of:
   A. In a plastic chemotherapy bag
   B. In a sharps container
   C. Only at the end of a shift
   D. By a biohazard team of professionals

4. HEPA stands for _____, which traps particles larger than _____:
   A. Heated environmental parenteral air filter; 2 μm
   B. High-environmental particulate air filter; 0.2 μm
   C. Horizontal-efficiency particulate air filter; 0.2 μm
   D. High-efficiency particulate air filter; 0.2 μm
5. How far should you be working in the hood when compounding?
   A. At least 12 inches
   B. At least 6 inches
   C. Just past the front grill
   D. At least halfway between the front grill and the HEPA filter
6. A room adjacent to the clean room must meet standards classified as:
   A. ISO Class 5
   B. ISO Class 6
   C. ISO Class 8
   D. ISO Class 10
7. First air refers to:
   A. The air from the HEPA filter that passes over the materials
   B. The first air that you breathe in the clean room
   C. The air contained inside a vial
   D. The air contained inside a syringe
8. Category 1 CSPs may have an assigned BUD of ____ hours or less if kept at refrigerated temperatures:
   A. 7
   B. 14
   C. 24
   D. 30
9. Horizontal flow hoods should be inspected every:
   A. Month
   B. 3 months
   C. 6 months
   D. 12 months
10. SOP means:
    A. Safe operating protocol
    B. Safe operations policy
    C. Standard operating policy
    D. Standard operating procedure

■ Technician's Corner

Laura recently moved to a new city and was hired as an IV technician for the local hospital. She has 5 years of IV room experience and is a certified pharmacy technician with the PTCB. During her first week at her new job, she notices that some of her co-workers do not always follow proper aseptic technique. A few wear makeup and jewelry into the compounding area on a regular basis. Laura knows that these behaviors put the patients at risk. How should she handle this dilemma?

Bibliography

Bachenheimer BS. *Manual for Pharmacy Technicians*. 4th ed. Bethesda, MD: American Society of Health-Systems Pharmacists; 2010.

Ballington D. *Pharmacy Practice for Technicians*. 5th ed. St. Paul, MN: EMC/Paradigm; 2014.

Baxa Corporation. *USP <797> Training Requirements: 2011 Course Schedule*. Englewood, CO: The Corporation; 2010.

Holmes CJ, Ausman RK, Kundsin RB, et al. Effect of freezing and microwave thawing on the stability of six antibiotic admixtures in plastic bags. *Am J Hosp Pharm*. 1982;39:104. Available at: http://www.ncbi.nlm.nih.gov/pubmed/6798865.

Perry A, Potter P, Elkin M. *Nursing Interventions and Clinical Skills*. 5th ed. St. Louis: Elsevier; 2012.

Potter P, Perry A. *Fundamentals of Nursing*. 8th ed. St. Louis: Mosby; 2013.

Simmons H. Best practices for aseptic media-fill testing. *Pharm Purch Prod*. Available at: http://www.pppmag.com/documents/V4N8/p2_4_5.pdf.

Websites Referenced

Centers for Disease Control and Prevention. *2014 Biosafety and Operations Management*. Available at: https://www.cdc.gov/labs/BMBL.html.

USP. Available at: go.usp.org/USP_GC_797_FAQs.

USP. Available at: https://go.usp.org/usp-bud-factsheet.pdf.

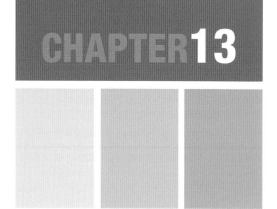

Pharmacy Billing and Inventory Management

Karen Davis

OBJECTIVES

1. Discuss the importance of pharmacy billing and inventory management to the pharmacy practice.
2. Discuss the following related to formulary and drug utilization: (a) explain the function of a drug formulary in insurance plans, (b) describe the role of the pharmacy technician in the drug utilization evaluation, and (c) discuss how a drug formulary or an approved/preferred product list affects pharmacy billing and inventory control.
3. Assess the differences between generic and trade name (proprietary) drugs in pharmacy billing.
4. Discuss the following related to private and group medical insurance plans: (a) list the primary types of private and group medical insurance plans and (b) describe how each type of private and group insurance manages drug coverage.
5. Discuss the following related to government-managed insurance programs: (a) differentiate among Medicare, Medicaid, and Medigap programs; (b) list the four parts of Medicare coverage; (c) differentiate between TRICARE and Civilian Health and Medical Program of the Department of Veterans Affairs (CHAMPVA) benefits; and (d) describe workers' compensation coverage.
6. Explain the purpose of third-party billing, describe the purpose of point-of-sale billing, and describe the role of prior authorization in claims processing. List the information found on a prescription card.
7. Determine the information needed to complete a patient profile for a pharmacy database.
8. Discuss the following related to claims: (a) identify the information needed to complete a universal claim form, (b) list and discuss reasons for claim rejections, and (c) describe the process of resubmitting rejected claims.
9. Discuss the types of plan limitations common in managed care.
10. Explain the various prescription payment methods, including self-pay, discount programs or coupons, private plans, and health savings accounts/flexible spending accounts.
11. Explain the importance of inventory management, define the periodic automatic replenishment level and describe how it affects inventory management, and describe the role of an inventory control technician.
12. Explain the inventory ordering and receiving processes, including special orders, bar coding, automated dispensing systems, manual ordering, and new stock.
13. Describe storage requirements for various types of inventory.
14. Outline the steps for handling recalled, returned, or expired medications.
15. List the types of suppliers of pharmacy stock.
16. Identify any special considerations related to drug ordering and storage.

Adjudication Electronic insurance billing for medication payment

Average wholesale price (AWP) The average price at which a drug is sold; the data are compiled from information provided by manufacturers, distributors, and pharmacies; the AWP is often used in calculations related to medication reimbursement

Civilian Health and Medical Program of the Department of Veterans Affairs (CHAMPVA) A program for veterans with permanent service-related disabilities and their dependents and for the spouses and children of veterans who died of service-connected disability; also known as the Veterans Health Administration (VHA)

Closed formulary Tight restriction of medication use to the medications included on the formulary list; medications that are not listed as preapproved drugs per the health plan provider or pharmacy benefits manager are not reimbursed except under extenuating circumstances and with proper documentation

Copayment The portion of the prescription bill that the patient is responsible for paying

Deductible The amount paid by a policyholder out of pocket before the insurance company pays a claim

Direct manufacturer ordering Pharmacies may join a group purchasing organization and contract directly with the manufacturer to obtain better pricing

Drug utilization evaluation (DUE) or review (DUR) An ongoing review by a pharmacist of the prescribing, dispensing, and use of medications, based on predetermined criteria, to decide whether changes need to be made in a patient's drug therapy

Formulary A list of preapproved medications that are covered under a prescription plan or within an institution

Health Insurance Portability and Accountability Act (HIPAA) Federal guidelines for the protection of a patient's personal health information

Health Maintenance Organization (HMO) An insurance plan that allows coverage for in-network–only physicians and services and uses the primary care physician (or provider) as the "gatekeeper" for the patient's health care; patients often have copays to defray the costs of medical care and prescription drugs

Inventory The amount of product a pharmacy has for sale

Just-in-time ordering A system that orders a product just before it is used

Medicaid A government-managed insurance program that provides health care services to low-income children, the elderly, the blind, and those with disabilities

Medicare A government-managed insurance program composed of several coverage plans for health care services and supplies; it is funded by both federal and state entities, and individuals must meet specific requirements to be eligible; individuals must be 65 years or older, be younger than 65 with long-term disabilities, or have end-stage renal disease

Medicare Modernization Act (MMA) The enactment of prescription drug coverage provided for individuals covered under Medicare

Medigap plan Supplemental insurance provided through private insurance companies to help cover costs not reimbursed by the Medicare plan, such as coinsurance, copays, and deductibles

National Drug Code (NDC) A 10-digit number given to all drugs for identification purposes; in health and drug databases, the NDC is represented as an 11-digit number, in which placeholder zeros are inserted in the proper order in the code for the purpose of standardizing data transmissions

National Provider Identifier (NPI) A number assigned to any health care provider that is used for the purpose of standardizing health data transmissions

Open formulary A formulary list that is essentially unrestricted in the types of drug choices offered or that can be prescribed and reimbursed under the health provider plan or pharmacy benefit plan

Patient profile A document listing necessary patient personal and health information, including comprehensive information on the medications the patient is taking, disease states, and any food or drug allergies the person might have

Periodic automatic replenishment (PAR) The PAR of stock levels to a certain number of allowed units

Pharmacy and therapeutics committee (P&T committee) Medical staff composed of physicians, pharmacists, pharmacy technicians, nurses, and dieticians who provide necessary information and advice to the institution or insurer on whether a drug should be added to a formulary

Point of sale (POS) A system that allows inventory to be tracked as it is used

Preferred provider organization (PPO) An insurance plan in which patients choose a provider from a specified list, resulting in reduced costs for medical services

Prime vendor A large distributor of medications and retail products that contracts with the pharmacy to deliver the bulk of their medications in exchange for lower prices; examples of prime vendors are McKesson, Cardinal Health, and AmerisourceBergen

Prior authorization Insurance-required approval for a restricted, nonformulary, or noncovered medication before a prescription medication can be filled

Safety Data Sheets (SDSs) Information sheets supplied to the pharmacy from the manufacturer of chemical products; the SDS lists the hazards of the product and procedures to follow if a person is exposed to that product

Trade, brand, or proprietary drug name The name a company assigns for marketing and identification purposes to a commercial drug product; most brand names are trademarked and belong to originator products; the named products are often protected for a time by patents

Treatment authorization request (TAR) The process used by Medicare and Medicaid for authorization of assistive technology devices costing more than $100; durable medical equipment (eg, wheelchairs and walkers) also requires a TAR; similar to a preauthorization form

TRICARE (formerly CHAMPUS) A health benefit program for active duty and retired personnel in all seven uniformed services; it also covers dependents of military personnel who were killed while on active duty

Wholesalers Companies that stock a variety of drug manufacturers' medications and normally have a "just-in-time" turnaround for ordered drugs; this means that drugs ordered today arrive the next day

Workers' compensation Government-required and government-enforced medical coverage for workers injured on the job, paid for by the employer; the programs are managed by each state in accordance with the state's workers' compensation laws

◉ Scenario

Brian is a technician at a large retail pharmacy. He is nationally certified with the Pharmacy Technician Certification Board (PTCB) and is registered with his state board. Brian has been working in his current position for 2 years, and he is classified as a level 2 technician. His company requires completion of additional training materials, which will be evaluated by his supervising pharmacist, to advance to the senior level 3 technician. What else could Brian do to enhance his job performance while pursuing the higher level position?

Everyone working in the pharmacy is responsible for maintaining the **inventory** stock. This is an essential part of the daily tasks of pharmacy staff. As stock is depleted, it is important to order replacement inventory. Although many different systems are available for ordering stock, the task of ordering may be delegated to a specific person in the pharmacy. It is then the responsibility of the staff to inform the inventory control person of decreasing stock levels. One method of replenishing the stock is **just-in-time ordering.** This is an inventory strategy in which medications are ordered and received only as they are used.

Along with ordering stock, pharmacy technicians help manage the third-party billing process. Knowledge of proper billing procedures is a skill that normally is learned by experience over time as a technician works in the pharmacy. Because each pharmacy contracts to accept different insurance companies, the technician must become acquainted with the normal billing procedures of that particular pharmacy and its associated insurance companies. Common types of billing practices are covered in this chapter to help you understand the proper information needed to file a claim for reimbursement.

In addition, the chapter introduces the pharmacy technician to basic information about the major types of insurance coverage. A firm knowledge of terminology and guidelines must be in place for proper ordering and billing practices. This chapter begins with a discussion of formularies and the knowledge needed about insurance companies. Also discussed are pharmacy inventory, some major types of devices used to keep track of inventory, and ways to handle special obstacles as they occur.

Formulary and Drug Utilization

A formulary is analogous to a backbone. The **formulary** is a list that describes all the medications covered under a specific insurance plan approved for use in an institution, such as a hospital. It may also offer alternative medications if the first choice is not covered. For medications to become part of a formulary, they must meet certain requirements, such as effectiveness and cost. These are determined by pharmacists, pharmacy technicians, physicians, nurses, and administrators who are members of the **pharmacy and therapeutics committee (P&T committee).** Formularies are not the same at all institutional pharmacies or for all health plans. An institution can have an **open formulary,** which means any drug can be ordered and stocked for patient use; a **closed formulary** places certain restrictions on the drugs ordered.

Often retail pharmacies stock a variety of medications to accommodate both their patients and the many different insurance companies for which they are contracted providers. Each insurance company has its own formulary, with recommendations for therapeutic alternatives when a drug is not covered under a particular plan. A therapeutic alternative is a drug that may differ chemically from the one prescribed but provides the same effect when administered to the patient. Many insurance companies have a variety of prescription plans and formularies that coincide with the many different types of health plans they provide. Specific formulary information can usually be found on insurance company websites. A hospital or home health care pharmacy is more likely to have a closed formulary or a specific list of drugs to be kept on hand and dispensed to the patients and health plans served by the pharmacy.

Drug utilization evaluation (DUE), formerly known as **drug utilization review (DUR),** is an important process in ensuring that the correct drug is prescribed for a condition. Pharmacists must perform this function, but pharmacy technicians play an important role in the DUE process. When technicians are inputting prescriptions, DUE alerts interrupt the process if a drug interaction or duplicate therapy is found. Technicians must *never* override these warnings on the computer! They must notify the pharmacist immediately so he or she can screen the medication order for potential problems such as drug-drug interactions, duplicate therapy, or other possible errors. This is done before the drug is dispensed, which reduces the risk for the patient receiving the wrong treatment.

Many formulary drugs are generic versions of proprietary (brand name) products. These drugs are as effective as the brand name drugs. They meet the same bioequivalence requirements but are less expensive. A health plan or prescription plan committee composed of pharmacists, physicians, and other health care administrators reviews drugs that have been approved by the US Food and Drug Administration (FDA) to ensure that they are cost-effective. In addition, consideration may be given to drug companies that bid or give rebates when their drug is chosen for a formulary. This decrease in price to the pharmacy ultimately saves money for both the insurance company and the patient. Although most insurance companies cover most of the cost of a generic drug, some do allow the patient to choose the brand name drug. However, if the patient selects the brand name drug, he or she is responsible for the amount due based on calculation of the copay as outlined in the third-party agreement. For example, if the normal **copayment** is $5 per prescription and the patient chooses a brand name medication that costs $10 more than the generic equivalent, the patient must pay $15. The dollar amount of a prescription also depends on orders such as Dispense as Written (DAW) drugs that require specialty codes. The three DAW codes that are most often used in the pharmacy setting are 0, 1, and 2.

- DAW 0 indicates that the physician authorizes a therapeutic alternative and the pharmacy can dispense the generic drug to the patient. If a generic is not available, the trade name product must be given; however, the DAW code must still be zero because this indicates that if a generic becomes available at a later date, the physician has given permission to the pharmacy to make the substitution. The pharmacist can find the therapeutic equivalent in the *Orange Book*.
- DAW 1 indicates DAW and is usually used by the physician to indicate that the trade or brand name medication is in some way medically necessary for the successful treatment of the patient. Often patients must have proof that other therapies have been tried but failed. Sometimes, such as in the case of the drug Celebrex, a patient must be age 50 or older. Physicians must write either "Brand Name Medically Necessary" or "Dispense as Written" in their own handwriting.
- DAW 2 indicates that the physician has approved the generic substitution of the medication prescribed; however, the patient has insisted on receiving the brand name medication.

Tech Note!

Technicians must be aware of and understand the proper use of DAW codes for accurate insurance billing.

Other DAW codes are assigned very infrequently and should be used only under the direction of the pharmacist. It is important to pay attention to the DAW codes and to use the correct one.

Insurance companies audit pharmacies; they specifically verify whether DAW 1 claims sent by the pharmacy have prescriptions in which the physician specifically indicates a brand name drug be dispensed. The selection of proper DAW codes is easy to overlook and can cause seemingly simple mistakes. However, if these mistakes are found in an audit, they can cause the reversal and repayment of the inaccurate claims and may result in the insurance company terminating its contract with a pharmacy.

Formularies are constantly changing. If and when new generic drugs are introduced, cost and other factors are reviewed again. Typically, the types of drugs not included on a formulary are new drugs, uncommon drugs, and extremely expensive drugs. However, if a nonformulary drug can be justified as a medically necessary substitution by the physician, it may be approved for reimbursement under the insurance plan.

In some instances, there are medications such as clozapine and isotretinoin that require certain documentation testing or blood levels before dispensing. Refer to Chapter 2 for more information.

Generic Versus Trade Name Drugs

The terms **trade, brand,** and **proprietary** are used interchangeably to refer to the name of a drug product that was first patented and marketed by the owner or manufacturer. Another name for such a product is *innovator product*. After a certain time passes, the patent expires. Eventually other drug companies can apply for the right to produce the same drug product, although not all drugs will be available in generic form. For example, it is usually not advantageous to drug companies to make generic medications that are used by a small percentage of the population. Brand name drugs that are produced by nonproprietary companies as an alternative to the proprietary product are considered "generic." A common example in pharmacy is the many different generic brands of birth control pills. Although the FDA approves generic drugs as equivalent to the trade name drug, the drugs often have different appearances because of different manufacturing procedures. Brand name drugs generally are protected for 17 to 20 years (depending on a drug company's petition to the FDA) before patents expire (Center for Drug Evaluation and Research [CDER]). After generic competition is introduced, prices can drop 50% to 80%. Drug price competition and patent term restoration expedite the availability of less costly generic drugs by permitting the FDA to approve applications to market generic versions without repeating the research needed to prove them safe and effective. At the same time, the brand name companies can apply for up to 5 years of additional patent protection for the new medicines they developed or for a new indication of a medication to compensate for the time lost while their products were undergoing the FDA approval process.

Types of Private and Group Medical Insurance Plans

Many different types of medical insurance plans are available. Understanding the policies and procedures of these plans is challenging, especially because their guidelines change regularly. Therefore this chapter covers the most basic information applied to the major types of insurance. Technicians must be able to differentiate between the different types of insurance, obtain the necessary information from the insurance card, determine whether the patient has prescription (Rx) coverage and who should be billed, and transmit the claim correctly. The types of medical insurance plans and cards currently in use include the following:

- CHAMPVA card
- Drug discount card
- Medicaid card
- Medical insurance ID card
- Medicare Advantage card
- Medicare card
- Medigap card
- Pharmacy benefits card (has "Rx Yes" printed on it)
- Prescription coupon card provided by drug manufacturers to patients: Coupon cards are provided either as an incentive for the patient to try the drug or as an aid to patients who meet certain income requirements
- TRICARE
- Workers' compensation (no card is required)

Health Maintenance Organization

A **health maintenance organization** (**HMO**) has specific features that distinguish it from traditional insurance programs. An HMO is an effective method of controlling health care costs. Aetna, Anthem, United Healthcare, and Kaiser are just a few examples of the many insurance companies that offer HMO coverage. HMOs include the following:

1. *Primary care physician (PCP):* The insurance company requires the patient to choose a primary physician to coordinate all of the patient's medical needs.
2. *Independent physician association (IPA):* The provider offers a discounted rate to the patient through the contract made with the insurance company. In return, the physician accepts a lower payment than normally is charged for the procedure performed. These are contracted providers; examples of contracted providers are certain hospitals, clinics, and medical groups.
3. *Copay:* The insurance company requires the patient to pay a predetermined amount for office visits, emergency department visits, and drugs, regardless of the final cost. The rate varies, depending on the patient's coverage plan. The insurance company is responsible for the remainder of the cost.
4. *Capitation:* Some physicians are independent and see both HMO policyholders and nonmembers in their practice.

In this situation the HMO pays the physician a fixed amount for each member patient regardless of how many times the patient visits the physician. This method of payment is known as capitation.

What if Your Patient Has Health Maintenance Organization Insurance?

If a patient has HMO insurance, the technician must obtain information from the patient such as address, date of birth, insurance number, and full name. The technician also must obtain the patient's prescription insurance card and verify that the pharmacy is a contracted provider for that particular insurance company and group. The pharmacy bills the insurance company first, through online adjudication, and receives an authorization number and copay information for the patient. **Adjudication** is the processing of claims over a computerized system. If the insurance claim is rejected, the pharmacy either must troubleshoot the issues or have the patient pay full price for the medication. It is then the patient's responsibility to contact the insurance company and attempt to obtain reimbursement. The patient is responsible for the entire cost only if the insurance company denies coverage based on eligibility or authorization not received before service. HMOs may require **prior authorization** on certain medications per their formulary guidelines. State regulations regarding the types of forms used to approve such medications may vary. The prescriber must justify the therapeutic basis for the prescribed medication. This prior authorization must be entered into the system before payment is approved. One example is Botox. Botox is used to treat muscular disorders but also can be used cosmetically. If a patient's plan does not cover cosmetic services but the drug is prescribed to treat a muscular disorder, a prior authorization is required. Technicians are crucial personnel in securing the prior authorization for the patient. They may call the physician's office and/or the insurance companies to ensure that the patient's needs are met.

There are opportunities to specialize and work specifically as a prior authorization technician. These technicians are considered experts in prior authorization and provide customer service support to members, customers, and/or providers. They take incoming requests for prior authorizations for both formulary and nonformulary medications. Requests can be received by fax or telephone, from providers' offices, and from pharmacists. The position provides clinical review for authorizations in keeping with legal and contractual requirements, including but not limited to turnaround times and service level agreements (SLAs). The technician must provide the information clearly, accurately, and in a professional manner. Interactions with callers must be documented per contractual and various regulatory and legal requirements.

⊙ Scenario Checkup 13.1

Brian has begun working on the level 3 technician learning materials. He has passed the first three chapters with flying colors, and his pharmacist is impressed with his work. A co-worker is also vying for the tech 3 spot. While contemplating how he can improve his productivity, Brian decides to develop a plan that will reduce time spent dealing with securing prior authorizations. What are some ideas Brian might implement?

Preferred Provider Organization

A **preferred provider organization (PPO)** provides health care for members for a discounted fee. The benefit is that the patient can choose a physician from the insurance plan's list of contracted providers or may choose to consult any specialty physician without PCP referrals. There are no requirements to choose a specific PCP.

Aetna, Anthem, United Healthcare, State Farm Insurance, and others offer PPO plans. Patients choosing a PPO may have a higher copay for their office visits than an HMO copay. Members of a PPO may have to meet a yearly **deductible** (the amount that the patient must pay before the insurance company pays). The insurance then pays a certain percentage of the medical expenses and medication bills if the patient's claims meet the criteria (ie, charges were incurred by a contracted provider and the service provided was within the allowed amount of the PPO). This helps control the cost to the insurance company because the patient pays everything the insurance company does not pay.

What if Your Patient Has Preferred Provider Organization Insurance?

You must determine whether the patient has medication coverage through the PPO plan. In addition, you must establish whether the patient pays the complete cost for the medication and then files for direct reimbursement, has a deductible, or has a copay. This is determined from the information on the patient's health insurance card and through the online billing process. An example of a health insurance card is shown in Fig. 13.1. After the information is transmitted to the insurance provider, an approval code is sent to the pharmacy. If the patient has a copay or deductible, the insurance company should monitor the patient's obligation. If the patient must self-bill the insurance company for reimbursement, the patient needs the receipt to submit to the insurance company.

From the pharmacy perspective, the billing processes for an HMO and a PPO are similar. The difference is that if the patient has a PPO, he or she may have a deductible to meet before the cost share (such as a percentage) or copay becomes activated. Most HMO and PPO insurance plans have separate deductibles for medical and prescription services. Often patients forget they have a deductible to meet, or they do not realize it resets at the beginning of the year. In addition, they may not realize that each family member may be required to meet his or her own deductible before the insurance pays that individual's portion. For example, for a family of four with a $1000 individual deductible, if one family member receives $1000 of medical services, the insurance pays a portion of that family member's medication for the remainder of the year. However, if another family member then needs medication, the second family member's $1000 deductible must be met before the insurance pays a portion of the second family member's medication.

Government-Managed Insurance Programs

Programs such as Medicare and Medicaid are examples of state-managed and federally managed medical insurance plans. Each employee in the United States pays the government a percentage of his or her income toward Medicare. A percentage of each state budget is applied toward Medicaid. Each plan has specific guidelines that must be followed precisely for patients to qualify for reimbursement.

History of Medicare and Medicaid

Both Medicaid and Medicare were implemented in 1965. **Medicaid** provided health care services to low-income children, the elderly, the blind, and people with disabilities. Until 1977, Medicaid was associated with the Social Security Administration. Later, in 1986, coverage was expanded to infants of pregnant women with low incomes and became state regulated. Through the following years, many revisions were made, including increasing the eligibility age of children and covering certain individuals who were disabled or unable to return to work. Medicaid is funded by both federal and state governments, and the benefits vary widely. Each state is responsible for payment to health care providers. Participants must prove that their income and financial resources are at or below national poverty levels. Although each state may vary in its scope of coverage, the state must provide a minimum level of benefits according to federal guidelines. The following benefits are included:

- Home health care
- Hospital inpatient services
- Laboratory services
- Outpatient services
- Physician services
- Radiology services
- Skilled nursing care

In 1966 more than 19 million people enrolled in the newly formed **Medicare** program. Coverage consisted of several parts (Box 13.1). In 1972 Medicare eligibility was extended to include people older than age 65, those younger than 65 with long-term disabilities, and individuals with end-stage renal disease (ESRD).

In 1987 both Medicare and Medicaid required health care providers to include patient privacy provisions if they were to

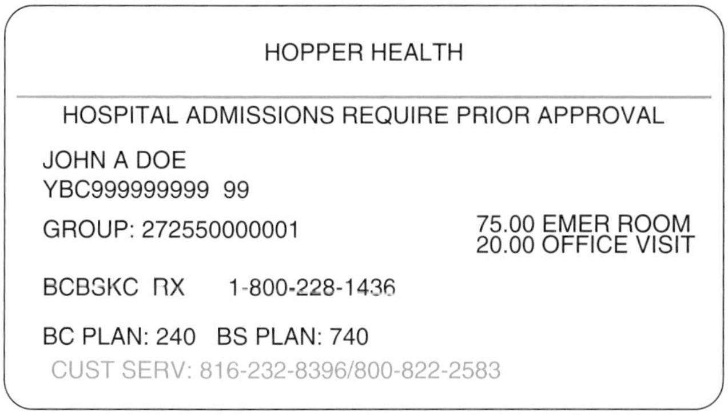

HOPPER HEALTH

HOSPITAL ADMISSIONS REQUIRE PRIOR APPROVAL

JOHN A DOE
YBC999999999 99

GROUP: 272550000001   75.00 EMER ROOM
                                20.00 OFFICE VISIT

BCBSKC ℞   1-800-228-1436

BC PLAN: 240   BS PLAN: 740

CUST SERV: 816-232-8396/800-822-2583

FIG. 13.1 Example of a health insurance card.

Part A: Covers institutional costs if the participant meets the criteria established by federal and state regulations.

Part B: Covers physician and other outpatient services, including diabetes testing, physical therapy, and other preventive costs.

Part C: Also known as Medicare Advantage, this is an optional plan to Parts A and B. It is a private plan that uses Medicare and must be equivalent to coverage provided by Parts A and B. Some Part C plans cover certain prescription drugs. A person should have either Part C or Medigap because the two are not cumulative in coverage.

Part D: Specifically covers prescription drugs. The coverage is provided by individual private insurance plans that are overseen by Medicare. A monthly premium is paid, and the plan chosen by the patient may have an annual deductible. Once the deductible has been paid, the insurance plan pays either all or some of the remaining costs. After the maximum benefit has been reached, there is a gap in the coverage of drug costs and the patient must pay for prescriptions out of pocket.

participate in the government-sponsored programs. Medicare revised its coverage in 1988, implementing prescription drug benefits, along with a cap on patient liability. In 1996 the **Health Insurance Portability and Accountability Act (HIPAA)** (linked to the Employee Retirement Income Security Act of 1974) provided new rules for improving portability (continuity) of coverage and simplified standards for electronic transactions, among other changes.

In 1997 Medicare implemented additional changes, including the following:

- Expanded education; new information helped participants make a more informed choice about their health care
- Expanded preventive benefits
- Four new payment systems for services:
  1. Home health services
  2. Hospital outpatient services and rehabilitation
  3. Inpatient rehabilitation hospital or unit services
  4. Skilled nursing facility services

A significant change was made in 2003 with the **Medicare Modernization Act (MMA)** and the creation of prescription drug discount cards, which allowed competition between health plans, benefiting participants. In 2006 Medicare Part D was enacted; this requires the federal government to provide subsidies to participants whose income is less than 150% of the federal poverty limit. Those with higher incomes would pay a greater share of drug costs as of 2007. Certain individuals may be covered under both Medicaid and Medicare and are known as "dual eligible"; Medicaid supplements Medicare coverage. In 2010 the Patient Protection and Affordable Care Act (ACA) was signed into law and has had a significant impact on Medicare and Medicaid services. According to *WalletHub*, as of September 2020, over 70 million Americans were enrolled in Medicaid (see Chapter 2 for more information on the ACA).

Many savings programs assist low-income participants with out-of-pocket health care costs. Each state has its own programs for assistance and may or may not include services such as home-delivered personal care and other community-based services for the disabled. Table 13.1 presents a timeline that explains various changes in the coverage and events in both Medicare and Medicaid programs.

Tech Note!

In 1997 both Medicaid and Medicare were reorganized and became subsidiaries of the Health Care Financing Administration (HCFA), now called the Centers for Medicare & Medicaid Services (CMS). In 2010 the ACA was signed into law. It will be implemented in phases, and changes related to the practice of pharmacy will begin to occur. Technicians should familiarize themselves with the language of the ACA, particularly changes dealing with medication management and Medicare Part D.

Current Use of Medicare and Medicaid Insurance

Medicare

Medicare is a federally sponsored program for seniors, the disabled, and patients on dialysis. It functions much like an HMO and a PPO. The patient must see a provider who accepts Medicare, but the patient has a yearly deductible and a percentage share of the cost. The share of the cost is similar to a deductible and copay combined. The patient is responsible for paying a deductible up to a certain amount in a hospital setting. Medicare has four parts: Parts A, B, C, and D.

- **Medicare Part A** *(Hospital Insurance):* Part A helps cover inpatient care in hospitals, skilled nursing facilities, and critical care hospitals. It also helps cover hospice and some home health care. Patients who are eligible for Social Security benefits are automatically enrolled in Medicare Part A. Most people do not pay a premium, but those who are 65 or older who do not qualify for Social Security benefits may enroll with the understanding that they will be required to pay a premium to obtain benefits.
- **Medicare Part B** *(Medical Insurance):* Part B helps pay for physicians' services and outpatient care. It helps pay for services that Part A does not cover, such as durable medical equipment (DME) and even physical and occupational therapists when deemed medically necessary. This coverage is optional, and most people pay a monthly premium.

Tech Note!

If a patient has Medicare Part B, the technician should ask the patient for the most current card at each visit. Some states require Part B to be renewed monthly, so it is important to verify that it has not expired. Medicare Part B also includes coverage for DME.

■ TABLE 13.1

Chronological Changes in Medicare and Medicaid Coverage

Year	Description
1965	Medicaid and Medicare were signed into law.
1966	Nineteen million people requested Medicare benefits.
1972	Medicare expanded coverage to include individuals younger than age 65 with low income and those with end-stage renal failure.
1977	Medicaid and Medicare were placed under the control of the Social Security Administration.
1980	Medigap was introduced to fill a gap in Medicare coverage; patients could choose among 12 different Medigap plans.
1986	Medicaid expanded coverage to include infants and pregnant women of low income.
1987	Medicare and Medicaid payment was linked to the Omnibus Budget Reconciliation Act of 1987 (OBRA '87) and specifically addressed poor conditions of nursing homes.
1988	Medicare introduced a prescription drug benefit plan.
1990	OBRA '90 required that all health care personnel participating in Medicare and Medicaid programs protect patient privacy; it also required patient consultation with pharmacists.
1996	The Health Insurance Portability and Accountability Act (HIPAA) implemented patient privacy rules for Medicare payment and provided electronic payment methods.
1997	Medicare made several important changes that expanded coverage and developed five new payment systems.
1997	Both Medicare and Medicaid were placed under the control of the Health Care Financing Administration.
2003	The Medicare Modernization Act (MMA) provided drug discount cards to eligible individuals.
2004	A temporary Medicare-approved drug discount card program began, along with a transitional assistance program to provide a $600 annual credit to low-income Medicare beneficiaries without prescription drug coverage in 2004 and 2005.
2005	Medicare began covering a "Welcome to Medicare" physical, along with other preventive services, such as cardiovascular screening blood tests and diabetes screening tests. Medicare begins education and outreach activities to implement the 2006 prescription drug benefit.
2006	Medicare Part D was enacted, requiring the federal government to provide subsidies to participants whose income was less than 150% of the federal poverty limit.
2010	Medicare spending was reduced; Medicaid enrollment and spending were increased; and new payment and reimbursement guidelines for Medicare and Medicaid services were introduced. These changes were associated with the Health Care and Education Affordability Reconciliation Act (HCERA) of 2010.
2011	Medicare began covering preventive care services such as mammograms and colonoscopies without charging Part B coinsurance or deductibles. Yearly "wellness" visits were also covered.
2011	Effective July 1, 2011, federal payments were prohibited to states for Medicaid services related to certain health care–acquired conditions.
2012	States received 2 more years of funding for the Children's Health Insurance Program (CHIP) to continue coverage for children not eligible for Medicaid.
2013	Effective January 1, 2013, until December 31, 2014, the Patient Protection and Affordable Care Act (ACA) requires an increase in Medicaid payments for primary care physician services. This increase is fully funded by the federal government.
2014	Affordable insurance exchanges were created and implemented. Individuals and small businesses can sign up and buy affordable health benefit plans. The new system will determine eligibility and coordinate enrollment for Medicaid and the CHIP.
2015	Effective October 2015, federal matching funds for CHIP will increase by 23 percentage points, with a cap of 100%, to help states pay for coverage of uninsured children.
2020	Part D donut hole is closed and newly eligible Medicare members are no longer eligible for Medigap C or Plan F. Because of COVID-19, vaccines and testing are covered for Part D members.

- **Medicare Part C** (*Medicare Advantage*): Part C allows participants in Medicare Parts A and B to obtain additional insurance through private HMOs or PPOs. The MMA changed the rules for contracting with these private health insurance companies to provide participants with better benefits and lower costs.
- **Medicare Part D** (*Prescription Drug Plan*): Part D provides people who are eligible for Medicare a voluntary prescription drug plan. This plan covers medications, insulin, vaccines, and certain medical supplies. Most enrollees pay a monthly premium for the discounted prices, and not all medications are covered. Technicians, along with the pharmacist, can assist patients in choosing the best prescription drug plan based on their particular medications. Most Medicare prescription plans have a coverage gap known as the "donut hole." This means that there is a limit to how much a particular plan covers for drugs. In 2014, once you and your plan had spent $2850 on covered medications, which included your deductible, you were in the coverage gap. This amount varies from year to year. For 2014, once you had reached the coverage gap, you had to pay out of pocket 47.5% of the price for brand name drugs and 72% of the price for generic drugs. Starting in 2025, out of pocket prescription drug costs will be capped at $2000.

Medicare services were expanded in 1980 with the creation of the **Medigap plan,** which is also regulated by the federal government. The last significant update to Medigap plans was in June 2010, when Medicare SELECT was introduced in some states. This required participants to use specific hospitals and specific providers for full coverage.

The traditional Medigap plan offers optional insurance policies that can be purchased through privately owned insurance companies. The plans are intended to fill the gap in the Medicare program coverage. However, if you have Medicare Part C, Medigap cannot be used. There are 12 different Medigap policies, labeled A through L. Most of the insurer plans do not differ significantly in their policies. Each person must purchase his or her own policy. Medicare is the primary payer, and the Medigap carrier is secondary. There is also a 6-month open enrollment for Medigap coverage (Box 13.2).

What if Your Patient Has Medicare Insurance?

Any changes in Medicare drug coverage increase the number of consultations by the pharmacist because pharmacists must explain different issues caused by a change in medications. In addition, people may need to have their prescriptions filled at a different pharmacy. This is because of the time it takes to register the patient in the Medicare database. Pharmacies must apply for a **National Provider Identifier** (**NPI**) from the CMS. All providers who bill electronically must use an NPI, which is required by HIPAA. Any pharmacist who provides services such as consultation and does not bill for this time under a pharmacy with an NPI must have his or her own NPI. The NPI number may be assigned either per person or per pharmacy, depending on each state's laws. For example, in Nevada, individual pharmacists must apply for an NPI number to process prescriptions covered by Medicare, whereas in California, this number is assigned for each pharmacy. If a patient is not in the system yet and the physician has ordered a drug that is not covered, the pharmacist may call the physician for a substitute if possible or the patient may pay out of pocket for the medication and try to obtain reimbursement when he or she is in the system.

An important "bottom line" approach to consider is this: the patient will be encouraged to receive generic drugs. Brand name drugs are often covered at a much higher cost if a generic is available, and this cost may be prohibitive enough to force many people into using the generic versions. Typically, brand name drugs are covered at the generic price and the patient is responsible for paying the difference. For a drug such as Zocor (generic name, simvastatin), this difference in cost can be as much as $100. The overall use of generic drugs has increased greatly under Medicare Part D.

In the past, open enrollment for Medicare plans ran from November 15 to December 31. This period was changed in 2011 to ensure that Medicare has enough time to process plan choices so that coverage begins at the beginning of the new year. Currently, the election period begins on October 15 and ends on December 7 each year. This is when a patient can change plans.

Because different items are covered under different parts of the plan, it is important for the technician to obtain not only the Medicare Part D card (Fig. 13.2) for pharmacy billing but also a copy of the Part A and Part B cards in case other items are needed (Box 13.3).

◉ Scenario Checkup 13.2

Brian has completed approximately half of the required lessons for tech 3 status. He is in the middle of a busy work day when he encounters an elderly customer who wants to pick up her prescription. Brian rings up the medication on the register and explains to the patient that her portion of the cost is $50. She explains that she now has Medigap insurance and should not have to pay any money out of pocket. How should Brian handle this situation?

Medicaid

Medicaid is a federal assistance program based on income and other circumstances. Individuals earning below the national poverty level are eligible for health care services. Each state has its own Medicaid program for low-income residents. This also includes uninsured pregnant women and

---

BOX 13.2 Medigap Coverage

A patient has Medicare Part D prescription coverage. This sample plan shows that the patient typically pays for generic medications or brand name drugs, with a yearly maximum payout of $1200. If the patient purchases $1200 in medication in the first 3 months of the year, the patient's insurance will not pay for any medication prescribed during the remainder of the year. At this point, the patient can apply for coverage for this "gap." This coverage can help pay the deductible or copay on Medicare Parts A, B, and D. The patient must determine whether Medigap would be beneficial.

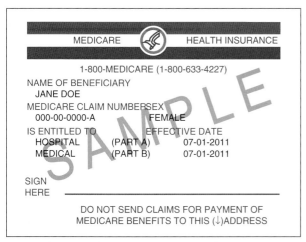

FIG. 13.2 Example of a Medicare Part D card.

MEDICARE HEALTH INSURANCE

1-800-MEDICARE (1-800-633-4227)

NAME OF BENEFICIARY
JANE DOE
MEDICARE CLAIM NUMBER SEX
000-00-0000-A FEMALE
IS ENTITLED TO EFFECTIVE DATE
HOSPITAL (PART A) 07-01-2011
MEDICAL (PART B) 07-01-2011

SIGN
HERE

DO NOT SEND CLAIMS FOR PAYMENT OF
MEDICARE BENEFITS TO THIS (↓)ADDRESS

BOX 13.3 Various Supplies Covered by Medicare

Typical supplies or prescriptions that may be covered under specific parts of Medicare insurance include the following:
- Blood glucose testing strips (Part B)
- Heparin for home dialysis (Part B)
- Hospital stay (Part A)
- Insulin (Part D)
- Lancets (Part B)
- Lasix (generic only, Part D)
- Nebulizer solutions

---

those with certain disabilities. Medicaid is funded by both the state and the federal government. Depending on a state's level of unemployment and poverty, it may receive matching funds from the federal government. Medicaid can be used with Medicare if the person qualifies. In addition, each state may have many different programs that help defer the cost of health care and medication. The following are the three major levels of coverage in the Medicaid system:

1. The patient may not be responsible for any cost.
2. *Share of cost:* The patient's plan requires that the patient pay a deductible (ie, a specific dollar amount must be met before the insurance company pays). For instance, the patient may be responsible for the first $1000, but any remaining amount is paid by Medicaid.
3. *Geographical managed care program:* A geographical managed care plan allows patients to belong to a medical group with which Medicaid has a contractual agreement. This includes HMOs, thus allowing patients to have Medicaid benefits similar to benefits offered by HMOs. The regulations may vary from state to state.

Effective January 1, 2014, Medicaid benefits were expanded to include individuals age 19 to 65 with incomes up to 138% of the federal poverty level. For a single person, that translates into an annual income of $15,856. This change opened up Medicaid for many childless adults who were not previously eligible.

States must provide certain mandatory benefits for Medicaid participants, such as the following:
- Family planning services
- Home health services
- Inpatient hospital services
- Laboratory and x-ray services
- Outpatient hospital services
- Physician services
- Prenatal and nurse midwife services
- Smoking cessation for pregnant women

States can also choose to provide optional benefits for Medicaid participants, such as the following:
- Chiropractic services
- Dentures
- Eyeglasses
- Physical therapy
- Prescription drugs
- Respiratory care

What if Your Patient Has Medicaid Insurance?

You must know whether the patient has Medicaid benefits. If the patient is covered under Medicaid, you need a copy of the patient's insurance card. This card identifies the program under which the patient is covered. Because different states authorize coverage at varying durations, it is important for the technician to verify eligibility each time the patient has a prescription filled. Many states use the Electronic Medicaid Eligibility Verification System (EMEVS), which verifies coverage by electronic transmission or by telephone.

Other Government Medical Insurance Plans: TRICARE and CHAMPVA

TRICARE

TRICARE is a health care program for military personnel and their families. This includes approximately 9.6 million active duty service members, National Guard and Reserve members, and retirees. TRICARE is managed by the Defense Health Agency and covers beneficiaries in the Army, Navy, Marines, Air Force, and Coast Guard. TRICARE eligibility is tracked through a worldwide database known as the Defense Enrollment Eligibility Reporting System (DEERS). Active duty and retired service members are automatically entered into DEERS, but family members must be registered separately. This system helps eliminate fraudulent claims. Fig. 13.3A shows an example of a TRICARE Prime card; Fig. 13.3B shows an example of a uniformed services ID card, which must be presented with the TRICARE card.

CHAMPVA

The **Civilian Health and Medical Program of the Department of Veteran Affairs (CHAMPVA)** (also known as the Veterans Health Administration [VHA]) is a health benefits program in which the VA shares the cost of certain health care services with eligible participants. This includes families of veterans who are totally or permanently disabled as a result of service-related injuries. To be eligible for CHAMPVA, an individual cannot be eligible for TRICARE.

TRICARE Prime Enrollment Card

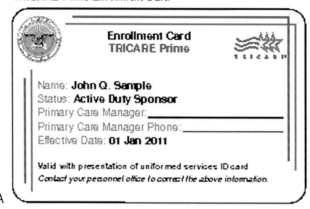

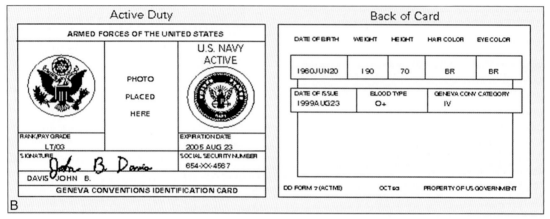

FIG. 13.3 (A) Example of a TRICARE Prime card. All TRICARE cards are valid only when accompanied by a uniformed services ID card (B). (From Fordney M. *Insurance Handbook for the Medical Office*. 13th ed. St. Louis: Elsevier; 2014.)

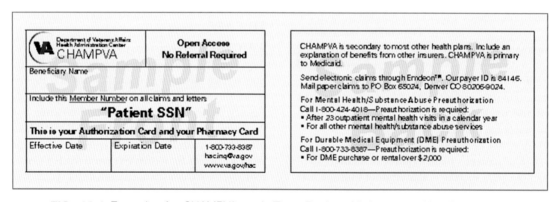

FIG. 13.4 Example of a CHAMPVA card. (From Fordney M. *Insurance Handbook for the Medical Office*. 13th ed. St. Louis: Elsevier; 2014.)

In most cases, CHAMPVA pays comparable to Medicare/TRICARE rates. Drugs and medications are covered under CHAMPVA when the following conditions are met:
- The medication has a valid **National Drug Code** (**NDC**).
- The drug has been approved by the FDA for the condition being treated.
- The drug is medically necessary.
- The drug is prescribed by an authorized prescriber and dispensed lawfully.

Fig. 13.4 shows an example of a CHAMPVA card.

Workers' Compensation

Workers' compensation is a type of insurance paid by employers to entirely cover injuries suffered by employees while on the job. Federal law requires employers with a certain number of employees to offer workers' compensation. Insurance coverage is provided by private insurance carriers.

Anyone who works for a company that pays into workers' compensation may be eligible to use this insurance if he or she has a work-related injury. The patient does not have to pay anything. Instead, claims are filed electronically or on

TABLE 13.2
Minimum Information Required by Insurance Companies

Required by Insurance Company	Reason
Patient's name	To verify insurance coverage
Date medication is filled	To process claim for reimbursement purposes; must be done within a specific period determined by provider
Pharmacy name and address	To pay pharmacy
Medication prescribed	To verify whether drug is on the formulary and is covered
Dosage	To determine cost of medication
Date of birth	To verify medication is dispensed to correct patient
Identification number	To provide authorization of coverage

hard copy to the insurance companies. If the patient arrives at the pharmacy with a workers' compensation claim, it is important to obtain billing information before dispensing medication, if possible. This may involve contacting the patient's employer, obtaining the billing information over the phone from the human resources department, and then calling the workers' compensation insurance company for further information. To avoid any billing errors, it is important to keep detailed notes regarding communication when processing workers' compensation claims. Be sure to include the name of the person who was consulted, the date of the consultation, and detailed notes about your conversation. It is also important to follow HIPAA guidelines. The only people who need to know that the patient is injured or ill are those in the human resources department. They do not need to be given a specific diagnosis from the pharmacy; they just need to provide the billing information.

Third-Party Billing

The term *third-party billing* refers to the portion of payment reimbursed by insurance companies. The three entities that are responsible for payment include the patient, the pharmacy, and the insurance company. It is customary for the pharmacy to bill the insurance company on behalf of the patient. The patient is often responsible for meeting the copayment or deductible at the time the medication is dispensed, and the pharmacy must collect the rest of the drug cost from the insurance based on contracted rates and dispensing fees. A copay is a predetermined amount the patient always pays when a medication is dispensed, whereas a deductible is the amount of out-of-pocket cost the patient must pay before his or her insurance coverage is activated. Copays can be a fixed dollar amount or a fixed percentage. Because there are so many different insurance

companies, each with different billing requirements, it often takes more than 1 year for a technician to become proficient in third-party adjudication, or claim billing.

The information needed by insurance companies to process a claim from the pharmacy or to reimburse the patient is the same as the information required on a pharmacy label, plus date of birth, insurance group number, and identification number. All information must be verified before the medication is dispensed. After the patient's information has been entered into the pharmacy computer system, it is important to keep that information updated both for the pharmacy and for the insurance company (Table 13.2).

Point of Sale Billing

Pharmacies that send claims electronically to an insurance company participate in **point-of-sale (POS)** billing. Electronic billing is performed by a secure data and transactional network to ensure patient confidentiality. The insurance company verifies eligibility, identifies covered drugs, prices a claim, and returns a response to submitting pharmacies within seconds during the prescription processing functions.

Prior Authorization

Often an insurance company pays for a medication only if a prior authorization is first received. Prior authorization is needed for a variety of reasons; for example, the drug of choice may not be included in the formulary or the insurance company may have determined that less costly methods of treatment are available and the patient must use those first. Two types of forms are used: a prior authorization form (or **treatment authorization request [TAR]**) or an eTAR, which is an Internet-based, paperless process for submitting an electronic TAR for payment. Most insurance companies

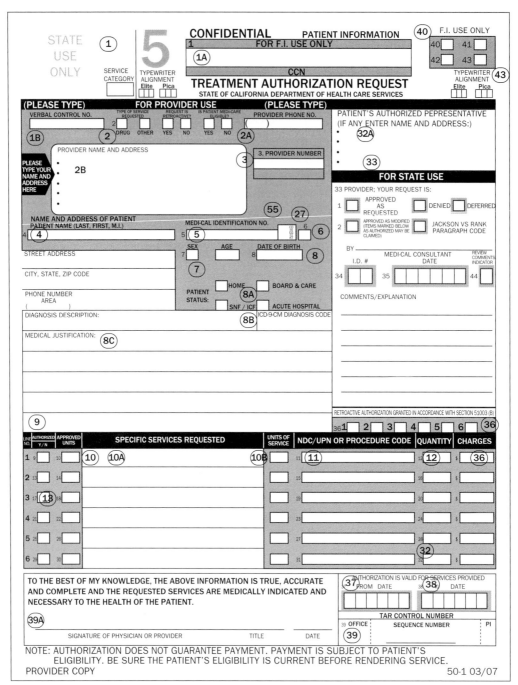

FIG. 13.5 Treatment authorization request form.

require a prior authorization form. The pharmacy typically does not contact the insurance company about prior authorization. If a third-party claim is rejected as "prior authorization required," the pharmacy either contacts the patient's physician or directly notifies the physician's office. The physician's office then contacts the insurance company to request the prior authorization. Policies may vary, depending on the insurance provider and the medication prescribed. For Medicare and Medicaid the TAR form is used, which requires the same information as forms used for standard insurance companies (Fig. 13.5).

The physician often must produce documentation explaining why a specific course of therapy is needed, such as "The patient tried the other therapies, and they were ineffective"; "The patient has allergies to certain medications"; or "The patient must undergo diagnostic tests that require the requested therapy." All of this information must be provided by the physician because the pharmacy does not have access to the patient's records. The insurance company either approves or denies the authorization in 24 to 48 hours. Rarely does the insurance company or the physician alert the pharmacy when authorization has been approved; therefore the pharmacy should attempt to rebill the claim in 48 to 72 hours. If the claim is still denied, the pharmacy may need to contact the physician's office or the insurance company to determine whether the authorization was submitted and

BOX 13.4 **Information Included on a Prescription Card**

Each insurance card contains information about the coverage plan, the patient's name and identification number, and the phone number of the insurance company. The basic information needed to bill a third-party claim is provided on the card. If any additional information is needed, the insurance company or provider should be contacted.

- *Pharmacy Benefit International Identification number (RxBIN):* Used much like an Internet protocol (IP) address to direct the claim to the correct third-party provider. All network pharmacy payers have an RxBIN.
- *Pharmacy Benefit Processor Control Number (PCN):* Some, but not all, network pharmacy payers use this number, labeled RxPCN, for network pharmacy benefit routing, along with the RxBIN. If used, this number is required for specialized health care coverage plans such as those that begin with the letter U, W, X, or Y. For example, dental coverage plans are identified by a PCN identifier with the letter "W." This has been used increasingly in the past few years because of the greater number of plans available to patients.
- *Prescription group number (Rx Grp #):* Directs the claim to the specific insurance benefits for that group. Groups are usually organized by collections of people who work for the same company or have similar benefits packages.

- *Identification number (ID #):* A unique identification number that is specific to each member or member family group. Some insurance companies, such as Kaiser, issue an ID number to each person in the plan. Some issue one to the cardholder and each member of the family has the same ID number.
- *Person code:* Each member of the family has the same ID number; however, an individual code is used to differentiate family members from one another. Often the cardholder, or the primary person on the insurance, is person 00 or 01. The spouse or other insured adult is person 01 or 02. The children covered under the plan are listed in numerical order according to their birth order.
- *Date of birth (DOB):* Must match the date the insurance company has on file for each patient.
- *Sex code:* Must match sex filed by insurance company. The insurance company also rejects claims for drugs if the sex code is incorrect. For instance, if the technician submits a claim stating that Mary Clein is a man and attempts to bill her insurance for Ortho Tri-Cyclen, the claim may be rejected by the insurance company because males typically are not prescribed birth control pills.

---

whether a special override code is needed to bill the claim. Regardless of whether the claim is approved or denied, the patient should be contacted within 3 days so that he or she is not waiting for a medication that has been denied.

Each plan has its own formulary, limitations, and exclusions. In addition to these variances, each pharmacy has certain insurance types that it accepts or rejects. This means that if the pharmacy accepts the copayment as payment in full, the pharmacy bills the insurance company for the cost of the medication. Otherwise, the pharmacy may not accept the insurance based on the limits of payment. Insurance cards have all the information necessary to perform the billing process. An explanation of the information contained on an insurance prescription card is presented in Box 13.4.

Tech Note!

Identify each insurance card as a prescription discount card, prescription coupon card, or insurance card. For each card, identify the payer and the Pharmacy Benefit International Identification Number (RxBIN), the Pharmacy Benefit Processor Control Number (RxPCN), and the group and ID numbers.

◉ Scenario Checkup 13.3

Brian is working with Ms. Jones, a new patient at the pharmacy. He begins by explaining to Ms. Jones that he will need to get some important information from her before he can begin filling her prescription. Brian brings up a new patient profile on the computer. What questions do you think he will ask Ms. Jones?

Patient Profiles

Each pharmacy has its own specific computer system, which details each **patient profile.** Fig. 13.6 shows an example of a pharmacy patient profile database. This profile must be kept updated for proper billing. Basic information that can be viewed on this computer system includes the following:

- Name
- Date of birth
- Address
- Phone number
- Sex
- Allergies (both drug and food)
- Insurance provider's information: provider's phone number and insurance number (per hospital or institution policies)
- Over-the-counter (OTC) medications
- Diagnoses or disease states

If the information contains a mistake, the insurance claim may be rejected.

If the patient does not have insurance, he or she must pay full price for prescriptions. The cost of a prescription can vary greatly. Many pharmacies offer certain generics at a lower cost, $4 for a 30-day supply or $10 for a 90-day supply. The use of generic drugs can reduce the medication cost greatly.

If the patient has insurance, determining the guidelines of the program is of primary importance if the pharmacy is to receive reimbursement. The process by which all claims are processed over a computerized system is referred to as adjudication. The insurance determines the amount of coverage per medication based on various criteria, such as the following:

- **Average wholesale price (AWP):** The AWP can be found in *Drug Topics Red Book,* or this information may be

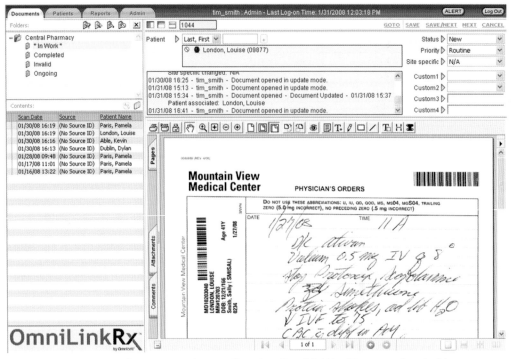

FIG. 13.6 Computer patient profile using OmniLinkRx. (Courtesy Omnicell.)

contained in a portion of the pharmacy database. Use the *Red Book* to determine the price of a medication based on the listed price. The *Red Book* is available electronically, and the online databases supply real-time updates to medication price changes.

• *Copay:* A relatively small fixed fee required by the health insurer to be paid by the patient at the time of each office visit, outpatient service, or filling of a prescription.

Processing Claims

When handling a patient's medication claim, the pharmacy technician may be responsible for using the insurance company claim form to relay the necessary patient information. Because each company requires its forms to be filled out entirely and correctly, the technician must know the specific needs of the company. Universal claim forms (UCFs) (Fig. 13.7) are used in certain circumstances. For instance, because a compounded medication does not have an NDC number, it cannot be submitted in the normal manner, as are manufactured products. However, it can be submitted using a UCF. Sometimes patients arrive at the pharmacy with a claim form that the pharmacy needs to complete for reimbursement. Claims are filed electronically. The general types of information required may include the following:

• Processor: Typically the insurance company
• Member's identification number: Can be either the assigned number specific to that patient or the Social Security number; however, fewer insurance companies are using Social Security numbers because of the potential for identity theft
• Group number (if applicable)
• Plan code (if applicable)
• Insurance carrier

Claim Problems

A prescription may not be covered for the insured patient for many reasons. For example, the NDC may not be covered. The NDC number is organized into three sections: the labeler code, the product code, and the package code (Fig. 13.8). All medications have an NDC number. When a prescription is not covered, it can be frustrating for both the patient and the technician and even for the insurance company representative. Other common reasons that a prescription may not be covered are as follows:

• Coverage has expired.
• Coverage limits have been exceeded.
• Patient is trying to refill a prescription too early.
• The cardholder's information does not match the processor's information.
• The physician who wrote the prescription is not the patient's PCP.
• The prescription is written for an invalid amount of medication; most insurance companies cover only a 30-day supply unless it is mail order, which covers a 90-day supply. Many insurance companies are now requiring patients to use mail order for certain maintenance medications.

Coverage Expiration Policy for Drugs

If the patient has lost his or her coverage, the claim is rejected. Following HIPAA regulations, the pharmacy does not have access to information about the reason for rejection and only a termination date is disclosed. Patients often are unaware of why coverage has been discontinued and may want the pharmacy to investigate. Pharmacy personnel are not permitted to call the patient's insurance carrier about these types of inquiries. Patient confidentiality would be breached, and legal action could result. The only recourse is

NCPDP UNIVERSAL CLAIM FORM (UCF)

TYPE OR PRINT ALL INFORMATION NEATLY AND COMPLETELY IN APPROPRIATE SPACES

I.D. _____ GROUP I.D. _____

NAME _____ PLAN NAME _____

PATIENT NAME _____ OTHER COVERAGE CODE (1) _____ PERSON CODE (2) _____

PATIENT DATE OF BIRTH ___ ___ ___ MM DD CCYY   PATIENT (3) GENDER CODE _____   PATIENT (4) RELATIONSHIP CODE _____

PHARMACY NAME _____

ADDRESS _____   SERVICE PROVIDER I.D. _____ QUAL (5) ___

CITY _____   PHONE NO.( )_____

STATE & ZIP CODE _____   FAX NO. ( )_____

FOR OFFICE USE ONLY

WORKERS COMP. INFORMATION
EMPLOYER NAME _____

ADDRESS _____

I have hereby read the Certification Statement on the reverse side. I hereby certify to and accept the terms thereof. I also certify that I have received 1 or 2 (please circle number) prescription(s) listed below.
PATIENT/ AUTHORIZED REPRESENTATIVE _____

CITY _____   STATE _____ ZIP CODE _____

CARRIER I.D. (6) _____   EMPLOYER PHONE NO. _____

DATE OF INJURY ___ ___ ___ MM DD CCYY   CLAIM (7) REFERENCE I.D. _____

ATTENTION RECIPIENT PLEASE READ CERTIFICATION STATEMENT ON REVERSE SIDE

1

PRESCRIPTION/SERV. REF. #	QUAL (8)	DATE WRITTEN MM DD CCYY	DATE OF SERVICE MM DD CCYY	FILL#	QTY DISPENSED (9)	DAYS SUPPLY

PRODUCT/SERVICE I.D.	QUAL (10)	DAW CODE	PRIOR AUTH # SUBMITTED	PA TYPE (11)	PRESCRIBER I.D.	QUAL (12)

DUR/PPS CODES (13)	BASS COST (14)	PROVIDER I.D.	QUAL (15)	DIAGNOSIS CODE	QUAL (16)

OTHER PAYER DATE MM DD CCYY	OTHER PAYER I.D.	QUAL (17)	OTHER PAYER REJECT CODES	USUAL & CUST. CHARGE

1

INGREDIENT COST SUBMITTED
DISPENSING FEE SUBMITTED
INCENTIVE AMOUNT SUBMITTED
OTHER AMOUNT SUBMITTED
SALES TAX SUBMITTED
GROSS AMOUNT DUE SUBMITTED
PATIENT PAID AMOUNT
OTHER PAYER AMOUNT PAID
NET AMOUNT DUE

2

PRESCRIPTION/SERV. REF. #	QUAL (8)	DATE WRITTEN MM DD CCYY	DATE OF SERVICE MM DD CCYY	FILL#	QTY DISPENSED (9)	DAYS SUPPLY

PRODUCT/SERVICE I.D.	QUAL (10)	DAW CODE	PRIOR AUTH # SUBMITTED	PA TYPE (11)	PRESCRIBER I.D.	QUAL (12)

DUR/PPS CODES (13)	BASS COST (14)	PROVIDER I.D.	QUAL (15)	DIAGNOSIS CODE	QUAL (16)

OTHER PAYER DATE MM DD CCYY	OTHER PAYER I.D.	QUAL (17)	OTHER PAYER REJECT CODES	USUAL & CUST. CHARGE

2

INGREDIENT COST SUBMITTED
DISPENSING FEE SUBMITTED
INCENTIVE AMOUNT SUBMITTED
OTHER AMOUNT SUBMITTED
SALES TAX SUBMITTED
GROSS AMOUNT DUE SUBMITTED
PATIENT PAID AMOUNT
OTHER PAYER AMOUNT PAID
NET AMOUNT DUE

FIG. 13.7 Universal claim form.

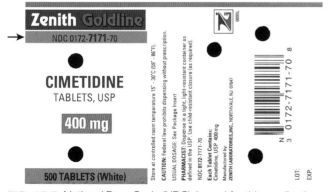

FIG. 13.8 National Drug Code (NDC) (arrow) for this medication.

to explain to the patient that he or she must contact the insurance company to resolve the issue. In the interim, the patient must pay full price for the medications. If there has been an error, reimbursement is made after the insurance company corrects the problem.

Limitation of Plan Exceeded

The phrase *limitation of plan exceeded* refers to a patient who has exhausted his or her pharmacy benefits for the specified time period or quantity limitation on a drug.

If a prescription requests a greater quantity of the drug than is allowed by the insurance plan, the plan limits are exceeded. For example, some government insurance plans limit the number of prescriptions that can be filled per month or per year. If the prescription is written for a specific quantity of medication that exceeds the maximum amount to be filled per day, the prescription is rejected and the patient must contact the insurance company for special permission to obtain the drug. "Limit exceeded" could also mean that the patient has met a yearly or lifetime benefit amount.

Some patients are exempt from these types of limitations because of their illness. These include individuals who have diabetes and those who have been diagnosed with human immunodeficiency virus (HIV) infection or acquired immunodeficiency syndrome (AIDS). People with diabetes mellitus require a continuous refill of lancets and blood-testing strips to monitor their blood glucose levels. In addition, they must refill their insulin syringes monthly. In the case of patients treated for HIV infection or AIDS, the medication is expensive, and these patients usually have to take many medications simultaneously. When a claim is rejected because the maximum limits of the insurance are exceeded, the technician must explain the problem to the patient. The patient is ultimately responsible for contacting the insurance company to dispute the problem.

Tech Note!

Only a pharmacist can contact the physician to request a change in medication.

Handling Nonformulary Drugs or Noncovered National Drug Codes

Formularies tend to be specific. This includes the decision on which drugs are included in the member's plan. These drugs are identified by their NDC, a code assigned to every drug in the United States. If the code submitted is not in the formulary, the claim is rejected by the insurance company. In pharmacy, these types of medications are referred to as *nonformulary drugs*. In this case two options can be explored. First, the pharmacist can contact the physician and request that the prescription be changed to a drug that is covered under the patient's insurance plan. Second, the physician can submit a prior authorization form to the insurance company indicating why the patient must take the nonformulary drug. The type of prior authorization form varies, depending on insurance company guidelines. Physicians normally complete and submit the prior authorization form for approval. This approval process can take up to 2 weeks. Therefore the patient can either purchase the medication for immediate use or wait to have the prescription filled after approval or rejection is given by the insurance company. If the patient pays upfront and the medication is approved, the patient is reimbursed by the insurance company after the pharmacist completes a reimbursement form for the patient. The form is sent to the insurance company to reimburse the patient for the covered drug cost.

Filling a Prescription Too Soon

Patients attempt to have their prescriptions refilled for several reasons when they still have medication remaining. Most of the time it is not a problem to obtain a refill 1 week before the prescription's refill date; however, there are instances in which the patient may request a refill as early as 1 week after having the prescription filled. For example, the patient may be leaving the country for an extended time and wants to ensure that sufficient medication is available until he or she returns. Most insurance plans allow extra refills in circumstances such as vacations or the occurrence of devastating events. For example, when Hurricane Sandy devastated the East Coast of the United States, many insurance companies allowed early refills and replacement fills on prescriptions and even permitted patients to be treated by physicians outside their medical plan.

If the patient's insurance will not pay, the patient is responsible for the cost of the medication. Prescriptions normally are written for a 30-, 60-, or 90-day supply, depending on the condition treated. Mail-order companies usually fill up to a 90-day supply for certain maintenance drugs, such as diabetes or heart medications. Sometimes the amount of medication prescribed is limited because of safety or legal issues regarding the dispensing of a specific medication. Because certain medications are dangerous, they may not be prescribed for more than 30 days. Examples include US Drug Enforcement Administration (DEA) schedule II controlled substances and a specific drug, isotretinoin (an acne medication), which has been linked to teratogenicity if given to pregnant women. Many insurance plans allow additional savings if refills are ordered by mail-order pharmacies that are on their list of participating pharmacies.

Sometimes a physician instructs the patient to increase the dosage, thus forcing the refill process before its allotted time. In this case a new prescription order must be submitted to the insurance company. In some cases the technician must contact the insurance company "Help Desk" to explain the circumstances of the prescription change. However, some insurance companies may require a direct response from the patient's physician before granting approval.

Nonidentification Match

Probably one of the most common problems arises when the cardholder's information does not match the processor's information, thus resulting in a claim rejection. To determine whether this is the case, the technician should always recheck the information submitted to the insurance company. Items to double-check include the following:
- Health plan card number, identification number, and insurance number
- Patient's name, date of birth, and relationship to the insured person

The relationship of the patient to the cardholder is important because he or she may be a new spouse or adopted child, or other significant changes may have occurred. In this case the technician may be able to ask for a new insurance card for the member through the insurance Help Desk.

⊙ Scenario Checkup 13.4

Brian is learning a great deal from the training materials he has been studying. He just completed a lesson on how to effectively resolve rejected insurance claims. Today at work, a new technician asks if Brian can help her with a billing problem. When she sends the prescription to the insurance company for adjudication, it comes back with a "nonidentification match" rejection code. When Brian double-checks the patient's name, date of birth, and relationship to the insured person, he finds that the information entered is correct. Upon further investigation, he learns that the patient is one of a set of identical twins who have the same birth date and same first name but different middle names. What can Brian do to help the new technician get this prescription processed?

Resubmitting Rejected Claims

Sometimes an insurance company mistakenly rejects a valid claim. When this happens, the pharmacy technician can resubmit the claim. Special attention should be paid to the rejection codes provided by the payer in the remittance information. Next, the insurance company determines whether the issue has been resolved and the claim can be processed and paid. It is the responsibility of the pharmacy to keep records of claims that are submitted until they are processed or denied. Follow-up is the key to ensuring that payment is received.

Plan Limitations

Often insurance carriers enact plan limitations to control drug use and reduce drug costs. Some examples include:
- Maximum amounts on medication that can be dispensed at one time.
- Days' supply restrictions: 30 days for retail and 90 days for mail-order supplies.
- Refill limits.
- Requiring prior authorization for certain medications.
- Step therapy: One or more cheaper medications must be demonstrated to be ineffective before more expensive medications may be used.

These limits are sometimes called "cost utilization measures" and are designed to reduce health care costs.

Tech Note!

Fraud involving pharmacy insurance claims is a serious issue and should not be taken lightly. Falsely billing charges for medication that was not dispensed is a crime.

Other Methods of Payment

Self-Pay

Some patients do not have insurance coverage and are solely responsible for their prescription cost. These patients can pay with cash, check, or credit or debit card.

Drug Discount Cards or Drug Coupon Cards

Patients can obtain drug discount cards from a variety of sources. These do not offer insurance benefits but instead allow the patient to obtain medications at the contracted provider rate. For example, if a drug discount card contracts

with a pharmacy to pay the AWP -10% plus a \$2 dispensing fee for a drug that would normally be sold at retail for AWP $+15\%$ plus a \$5 dispensing fee, the patient can obtain the medicine at the less expensive rate through a prescription discount card.

Drug manufacturers provide drug coupon cards to patients either as an incentive for the patient to take the drug or as an aid to patients who meet certain income requirements. Both types of cards are billed as a third-party claim for the pharmacy to receive reimbursement and the patient to receive his or her discount.

Private Plans

With a private plan, the patient obtains a prescription drug card from a pharmacy benefits manager. Usually these plans are very expensive.

Health Savings Account and Flexible Spending Account

Health savings accounts and flexible spending accounts are something like a savings account that can be used to pay medical bills before a deductible has been met, along with copays for prescriptions and office visits. The government has put limits on the amounts that can be put into these accounts per calendar year. There is also a "use it or lose it" component. Some employers contribute to these accounts and some do not. Restrictions are placed on what is covered. Participants must be knowledgeable about the regulations affecting these types of accounts.

Many times pharmacists must explain the various types of benefits to patients. Technicians play an important role in helping patients understand their coverage. They should keep themselves updated on any changes in the system to ensure that the billing process goes smoothly. Technicians must have patience and good communications skills to explain technical issues or terms, such as *coverage, formulary,* and *generic availability,* in language the patient can understand.

Inventory Management

Proper inventory management is the key to an efficiently run pharmacy. Having the needed medications and supplies on hand to serve the patients' needs is a top priority. Minimizing the carrying cost of the pharmacy's inventory investment enhances the pharmacy's ability to earn a profit. Inventory management focuses on ordering stock, proper storage of medication and supplies, repackaging, disposal of used and unused pharmaceutical products, and distribution systems.

Pharmacy Stock

Everyone working in the pharmacy is responsible for maintaining the inventory stock. This is an essential part of the daily tasks of pharmacy staff. As stocks are depleted, it is important to order replacement inventories. Although many different systems are available for ordering stock, the task of ordering can be delegated to a specific person in the pharmacy. It is then the responsibility of staff to inform the inventory control person of decreasing stock levels.

Each pharmacy orders drugs that include formulary drugs and a limited amount of nonformulary or less commonly used drugs. The established level of medication stock kept on hand at any given time is referred to as the **periodic automatic replenishment (PAR)** level. This is the minimum amount of medication that should be maintained in the pharmacy at any given time. Just as insurance billing has become a common task of pharmacy technicians, so has the responsibility of ordering medications. Different systems are available that can keep an updated inventory of medications and alert the technician when new stock must be ordered. This can be done in several ways, such as at the POS, by order cards, or by handheld inventory computers. Because so many different types of systems are currently in use, this section of the chapter explores the main characteristics of various systems and explains when and how stock arrives at the pharmacy. Proper storage of all drugs is also discussed. In addition, this chapter discusses how recalls are addressed and how returns are processed.

Although some pharmacies may contract out the job of processing returns and sending them to the manufacturer, this function is usually assigned to a pharmacy technician who is an employee of the pharmacy. Typically, an inventory technician is in charge of all aspects of ordering, restocking, and returning stock in the pharmacy.

Inventory Control Technician

Most hospitals have a technician who is in charge of maintaining stock levels and completing the special ordering of medications. The technician who orders the stock is responsible for the actual ordering, billing, and restocking of the pharmacy shelves; however, it takes a group effort in the pharmacy to maintain stock levels and avoid having to borrow items from another hospital or special order them at a higher cost.

Many methods of keeping stock at necessary levels are available. Before current electronic stocking methods became available, a hospital pharmacy used ordering cards to reorder stock when it was low. Each person was responsible for pulling the card (normally kept with the medications) and placing it in a designated area where the inventory technician could place the order. When the order arrived, the card was put back into the box along with the new stock. For the electronic stocking method typically used today, a handheld device that reads bar codes is used for electronic ordering. In this case the inventory technician must check visually to see which medications need to be ordered.

A third method of stocking requires each item to be tagged with a manufacturer's sticker as it arrives in the pharmacy. Stickers are provided by the manufacturer and must be affixed to each item before it is placed on the shelf. This sticker lists the stock number of the medication along with the price. When an item needs to be reordered, the sticker is taken off the container and placed on an ordering sheet, also known as a "want book." It is then entered into an electronic device for transmission by phone or by online ordering.

Duties

Every day the pharmacy depletes some of its stock of drugs and supplies. Although pharmacies have different systems of ordering the medications, most orders normally are placed using a computer. Depending on the location of the warehouse or manufacturer, the turnaround time for the shipment may vary. For example, if a supplier is thousands of miles away, that medication must be ordered earlier than a medication from the pharmacy's warehouse (which usually takes less than 24 hours). Knowing the right time to order medications is a skill that pharmacy technicians must acquire; it is crucial to keep the pharmacy completely stocked with necessary medications.

When the shipment arrives, all included medications and supplies must be verified against the inventory list; initialing and writing "received" on each invoice are important. Some medications are backordered; these items are currently not in stock from the manufacturer but will be sent as soon as they are available. If the medication is one that cannot be left out of stock for any length of time, it may be necessary to borrow from another pharmacy. This can be done by calling a pharmacist at a neighboring hospital and asking whether that pharmacy has enough to share. A loan/borrow sheet is filled out, and either a taxi or a hospital courier normally is sent to carry the medication from one location to the other. After the original ordered stock arrives, replacements for the borrowed items are returned to the lending pharmacy.

Placing stock on the shelves is another important duty of the pharmacy technician; it is the point at which the stock is rotated (Fig. 13.9). Placing medications with later expiration dates farthest back on the shelf ensures that the medications with the earliest expiration dates are used first. The inventory technician is also responsible for returning damaged items and expired agents and handling recall items according to the manufacturer's guidelines.

Timing is probably one of the most important aspects of keeping inventory at a constant level. The technician can order appropriately if he or she learns the pharmacy protocol for ordering, compensates for items that take longer to ship, and considers upcoming holidays. Patient load also directly

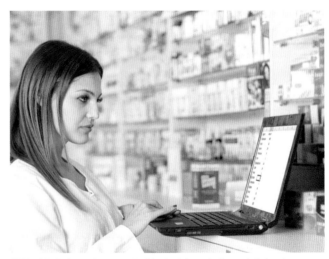

FIG. 13.9 Inventory control technicians help maintain pharmacy stock by ordering drugs, stocking shelves, and managing returns. (iStock/Getty Images Plus.)

relates to the types of medications to be ordered. It is a well-known fact that during the winter months, hospitals have more patients because more people become ill at this time of year. The elderly are especially at risk. In addition, certain hospitals have primary functions such as burn centers, rehabilitation, or specific surgeries, and their specialties influence the overall increase in the use of medications specific to those patients' needs.

Ordering Process

Maintaining a PAR level in the pharmacy is important for several reasons. Many manufacturers do not fill orders on weekends or holidays. Thus, if the pharmacy depletes its stock during this time, it may have to wait until the following delivery day to receive the necessary stock. It is serious if a patient cannot obtain an essential medication because the pharmacy is out of stock. Patients visiting a community pharmacy may be able to go elsewhere to have prescriptions filled, but hospitalized patients rely on the hospital pharmacy to stock medications.

If stock will not arrive until the following Monday or Tuesday, the only recourse is to use an express delivery company contracted by the pharmacy or to borrow the medication from another pharmacy. Express delivery can range from delivery of a medication by courier to air delivery of the medication. In some cases, pharmacies even contact other stores in the area to "borrow" stock for patients. Of course this is done only in case of an emergency, when all other options have been exhausted. Express delivery is also expensive and in many cases unnecessary if the pharmacy staff understand when to reorder a specific drug. Shipping time varies, depending on the type of drug ordered. This is when pharmacy personnel must demonstrate their teamwork. It is improper and inappropriate to assume that medication ordering is another team member's responsibility.

Special Orders

When a pharmacy does not carry a medication (perhaps it is new or uncommon), it may be ordered from a drug wholesaler. It is important to know the length of time needed for the wholesaler to deliver a medication and to follow the order's progress. Special-order prescriptions should be filed in a specific location in the pharmacy. The technician must check for special orders each time stock arrives. This ensures that the patient is not waiting for a medication that was received by the pharmacy a week ago. In addition, if a medication has not been delivered by the expected date, the wholesaler should be contacted to determine whether there is a backorder, ordering problem, or other issue. Notification of any ordering issues as soon as possible means that patients will not have therapy delayed any longer than necessary.

More pharmacies rely on computerized systems that are programmed to order medications. This is by far one of the best ways to maintain appropriate stock levels, although not all pharmacies have this system. Three main systems are discussed in this chapter, although there are many more types. All systems are similar to those discussed in the following sections.

Bar Coding

Most manufacturers identify their products with bar codes that can be scanned. This process accelerates the input of information because one pass of the bar code device identifies the drug, strength, dosage form, quantity, cost, package size, and any other information necessary to fill the medication or device. Pharmacies also can use these bar codes. The medication is scanned at the register, known as the POS, and electronically deleted from the computerized inventory list. When the in-stock quantity drops below the PAR level, it is reordered automatically. Other devices used to scan drugs are handheld components that identify the necessary drug information. The technician needs to enter only the quantity to be ordered. The information from this handheld set then is transferred to the main computer ordering system.

Automated Dispensing Systems

Automated dispensing systems (ADSs) involve technology designed to reduce labor and increase patient safety. ADSs store medications and control electronic dispensing.

ADSs are used in community pharmacies to monitor the inventory as tablets and capsules are dispensed into a drug vial from a bulk bin. As the pills pass a beam of light, they automatically are removed from the inventory. An example of this type of system is a Baker Cell system. Technicians are responsible for filling, cleaning, and troubleshooting these systems when a problem occurs. In the hospital the pharmacy is responsible for stocking the various clinics and nursing units. To avoid a stock shortage, dispensing systems that link the nursing units to the pharmacy computer system allow the stock levels to be viewed at any time. Each time the nurse indicates the type and amount of drug taken from these drug cabinets, it is deducted from the current stock levels in the cabinet, and this information is transferred electronically to the pharmacy unit. Various reports can be generated from this centralized unit, which can provide an overall stock inventory for a specific drug. In addition to the inventory status, such units monitor controlled substance use and inventory. All individuals adding drugs to or taking drugs from the unit are identified, and a log is kept of all users. This also ensures the proper use of controlled substances and detects any discrepancies. Examples of these types of ADSs are hospital units such as Pyxis (see Chapter 9), OmniRx (Fig. 13.10), or Baker Cell systems. Again, technicians are responsible for the maintenance of these systems, including filling, cleaning, and troubleshooting when necessary. Technicians also run various reports needed for filling the medication drawers and other reconciliation procedures.

■ Tech Note!

Automated systems in hospitals are being transitioned from personal codes entered by nurses and pharmacy personnel to biometric identification, making it more difficult to misuse the system.

Manual Ordering

Although manual ordering is being eliminated slowly as the primary ordering technique, it is still important in the

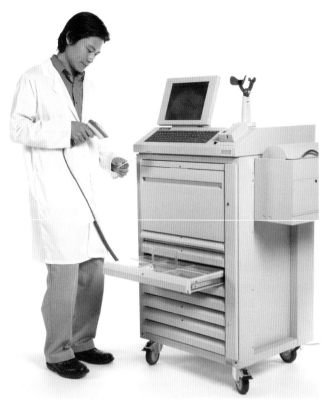

FIG. 13.10 OmniRx. (Courtesy Omnicell.)

- *Special orders:* These are drugs typically used by only a few patients, but they may be important for proper treatment. It is easy to forget to order these drugs because of their infrequent use. Usually they are ordered at the time of use, and some of these drugs may be nonformulary.
- *Time of year:* The drugs that are part of this category vary, depending on the time of year. Many medications that are fast movers during a particular time of year may need their PAR levels raised during that period. For example, albuterol inhalers are normally fast movers in the spring, when allergy symptoms and consequently asthma or respiratory tract symptoms increase. Antiviral medications used to treat influenza are prescribed more often during the flu season, from fall to spring. All pharmacy staff must be aware of the types of medications used during different times of the year and understand how levels fluctuate.

New Stock

Stock normally arrives daily at the pharmacy (excluding weekends and holidays) from different sources (except for central supply in a hospital setting, which functions 7 days a week). For billing purposes, it is important that all stock be checked completely against the packing list when first received. Procedure 13.1 presents a step-by-step approach that should be used when receiving stock.

Proper Storage

As stock arrives, it is important to follow the manufacturer's requirements for storage. Certain medications must be frozen at temperatures between $-20°C$ and $-10°C$, refrigerated at temperatures between $2°C$ and $8°C$, or stored at room temperature ($23°C$). Light or humidity can also affect the stability of the medication; therefore care must be taken to protect stock from

continued monitoring of stock levels. Some pharmacies still visually note that stock is getting low or use ordering cards that stay inside the medication box. These cards list the drug information, including the ordering number and the necessary PAR levels, to aid the technician in ordering the proper amount. Using the card system or simply writing down the right amount of stock to be ordered depends on the PAR levels or special orders.

Just-in-time ordering allows for just enough stock to be ordered to avoid excess inventory sitting on the shelves. For example, when one bottle is used up, just a single bottle is ordered just in time to replace it.

More commonly, orders are processed electronically by the computer or handheld computers that transmit the order. The following list categorizes the drugs stocked by many pharmacies:

- *Formulary:* In a hospital pharmacy, these drugs, normally stocked by the pharmacy, are approved by a P&T committee. In a retail pharmacy a specific formulary indicates which drugs are on the approved list of a patient's insurance company. Because there are many different insurance companies and thus many different formularies, retail pharmacies stock a wide range of products.
- *Fast mover:* These drugs typically are kept in a separate area from the normal stock because of the high volume of use. These must be ordered in larger quantities, keeping the overstock in close proximity, or must be ordered more often.
- *Slow mover:* These drugs are prescribed regularly by a few physicians but are not commonly prescribed. They must be checked before ordering and periodically to ensure that the drugs are not close to expiring.

Receiving Stock in the Pharmacy

Goal

To learn the steps involved in properly receiving and checking in pharmacy stock.

Equipment and Supplies

- Clipboard and pen
- Manufacturer or warehouse invoice
- Medication to be checked in

Procedural Steps

1. Retrieve the manufacturer or warehouse invoice.
   PURPOSE: You must have the appropriate invoice to accurately check in the order.
2. Account for all boxes.
   PURPOSE: To make certain that if the invoice indicates there are five boxes, you verify that there are indeed five boxes.
3. Inspect all boxes for storage requirements.
   PURPOSE: To make certain that if any box is marked "Refrigerate" or "Freeze," you immediately comply with the instructions to avoid product damage.
4. Check all information against the invoice, which includes the drug name, strength, dosage form, and quantity. Also check that the expiration date is not too soon.
   PURPOSE: To confirm that all information on the invoice matches the product you are checking in.
5. Compare the invoice with the order form to ensure that only the items requested were received.
   PURPOSE: To ensure that no drugs are missing or shorted and that you have no extra items you did not order.

6. Sign and date the invoice and forward it for processing per pharmacy protocol.
   PURPOSE: To ensure that the invoice is forwarded and stored appropriately for future reference and accounting purposes.
7. Place the stock in the correct location per pharmacy protocol, placing new stock behind existing stock, with the most current expiration dates in the front.
   PURPOSE: To rotate stock appropriately to avoid accumulation of expired drugs that may be used accidentally.
8. Return inventory cards to the medication box for future use.
   PURPOSE: To prevent medication inventory from becoming depleted because of failure to properly reorder out-of-stock items.

Note!

- Proper inventory control is very important. Marking stock shelves clearly reduces the probability of drug errors. For example, if a drug is accidentally placed in a box intended for a different drug with a similar sounding name, it may be used to fill a prescription for the sound-alike drug and ultimately affect the patient's health and well-being.
- Checking the expiration date is important. Drugs that are used rarely and have short expiration dates may stay on the shelf and expire before use.

---

either light sources or excessive humidity. If these guidelines are not followed, the medication is compromised, rendering it unusable. Just as it is important to return unused stock to its proper location when it is returned from the nursing floors (in hospital pharmacy), it likewise is essential that the pharmacy technician place new stock items in their respective areas of storage as soon as possible. Chemicals such as phenol and other toxic materials are usually kept behind cabinet doors and low to the ground. It is not wise to leave these types of materials exposed to the public because they are toxic. Read the packaging on all medications and follow the manufacturer's requirements for storage. Storing medications in the proper location is the responsibility of everyone working in pharmacy.

Returns

Medication is returned to the warehouse or manufacturer for four main reasons:

1. Drug recalls
   - *Class I:* Recalls for drugs that may pose a serious threat to users' health or even death
   - *Class II:* Recalls for drugs that may cause a temporary health problem and have a low risk for creating a serious problem

- *Class III:* Recalls for drugs that violate FDA regulations concerning container defects or have a strange taste or color
2. Damaged stock
3. Expired stock
4. Medication is about to expire; the pharmacy may return the drug to the wholesaler for credit or full price if the drug has at least a 9-month expiration date later than the date of return.

Depending on the reason, certain documentation must accompany the medication. Pharmacy policies and procedures should list the steps involved for returns. Except for scheduled drugs that fall under the jurisdiction of the DEA (see Chapter 2), most medications can be returned by the technician without a pharmacist's signature.

Drug Recalls

Manufacturers are required by law to recall any product that has been found to violate any of the following guidelines:

- Labeling is incorrect.
- Product was not packaged or produced properly.
- Drug batch was contaminated.

- The FDA has required removal of the drug from the market as a result of safety risks.
- Any other change occurs that causes the drug to fall outside the FDA or manufacturer's guidelines.

Recall notices may arrive at the pharmacy by mail, e-mail, or fax. Notices should identify the necessary information about the drug or device in question and describe the necessary steps to follow the recall procedure. This information includes the drug name and the reason it is being recalled. One of the most important pieces of information provided is the *lot number* of the drug. Lot numbers are assigned by the drug manufacturer to identify a specific batch of medication. This is the key to identifying the recalled medication. Retail pharmacy corporations and hospitals often have detailed procedures and teams of people who ensure the documentation, implementation, and completion of recall procedures, including final notification to the manufacturer and the FDA of the completion of removal of the recalled product. Upon receipt of the recall notification, pharmacy staff should immediately inspect and remove all stock from shelves, refrigerators, and freezers. If a pharmacy finds recalled medication on its shelves, a report is normally generated identifying the patients who may have received the medication within the past 30 days, and the patient is notified. The prescriber should be notified if a patient has received any of a recalled medication.

The pharmacy should place the recalled medication in a designated area or container for return to the manufacturer or disposal in accordance with the recall notice. Technicians are responsible for checking all the drug stock throughout the pharmacy and facility to ensure that the recalled drug is not in stock. If this is the case, the recall form is initialed to indicate that the item is not in stock. If pharmacy stock does include a drug with the recalled lot number, the pharmacist must be notified in case a patient has been issued one of these products. Prescribers also are notified by manufacturers and the FDA in the same manner as the pharmacy. It is the responsibility of the prescriber to notify patients currently using a recalled medication or device if treatment is to be discontinued or altered. The pharmacy can help facilitate the patient's return or disposal of a recalled medication. Although the FDA can issue mandatory drug recalls, most are voluntary recalls issued by the manufacturers. All recalls monitored by the FDA are included in a weekly Enforcement Report and are classified as to the level of hazard involved. These Enforcement Reports are available on the FDA website *(http://www.fda.gov)*. You can sign up to receive the reports by e-mail. Box 13.5 presents an example of a recall notification.

Damaged Stock

If you notice that some drugs were damaged en route to the pharmacy but you were not aware of damage at the time of delivery, it is not too late to return the damaged stock to the manufacturer. It may be necessary to first contact the manufacturer and obtain an authorization before the damaged goods are returned. The patient may also notice damaged stock. Sometimes EpiPen or Imitrex injections have bent needles, broken plungers, or other issues. In these cases the patient returns the medications and the pharmacy replaces the item. The pharmacy must then contact the manufacturer, who sends a replacement to the pharmacy directly and may or may not collect the damaged merchandise.

Expired Stock

Some pharmacies have a policy to pull any medication that expires in 3 months or sooner. This ensures that no drugs on the shelves are close to their expiration date. Depending on the contract between the pharmacy and the manufacturer, it may be acceptable to return items as long as they can be bundled into a minimum package size rather than as partials. For instance, if the stock of cimetidine expires within 3 months, the manufacturer may allow it to be returned for full or partial credit if a box of 100 tablets can be returned at one time. Following manufacturers' guidelines for returns is important. Hazardous chemicals, including cytotoxic agents, must be repackaged carefully to avoid breakage during transport.

Pharmacy personnel can also pull and return slow-moving stock that has 9 to 12 months before expiration; the pharmacy can receive credit from the wholesaler, who in turn may be able to resell the drug to another pharmacy. This applies only to unopened bottles, and regulations vary according to the wholesaler's or manufacturer's specific operating policies.

Many pharmacies have a service that processes returns to drug companies for a percentage of the credits obtained. These companies visit the pharmacy at various times, ranging from once every 3 months to once a year, and complete all the paperwork and documentation for returning expired inventory.

Tech Note!

Patients should be instructed in the proper disposal of unused medications. For many drugs, it is advisable to mix them with either coffee grounds or kitty litter and then place them in the garbage. Used transdermal patches and other novel dosage forms will need special care for disposal to prevent accidental exposures. Certain pharmacies allow patients to return to the pharmacy any expired or unused prescriptions found in their medicine cabinets. Check with your pharmacy supervisor to see whether your pharmacy offers this service. Medications should never be emptied into a toilet or a drain because the drugs can infiltrate the water supply. The DEA initiated a National Prescription Drug Take-Back Day in 2010 and since then has been holding take-back days twice yearly. The program provides a safe, convenient, and responsible means of disposing of prescription drugs while educating the public about the potential for medication abuse. For more information about this program in your state, visit the website *http://www.deadiversion.usdoj.gov/drug_disposal/takeback/*.

Automated Return Companies

Some companies' sole job is to process returns for hospitals, wholesalers, pharmacy chain stores, and independent retailers. They are responsible for all records and recalled items and for disposal of hazardous waste. Pharmacies contract with these companies for regular pickups; it is the pharmacy's

BOX 13.5　Recall Notification

The Harvard Drug Group, LLC Issues Voluntary Nationwide Recall of Dronabinol Capsules, USP, 2.5 mg and Ziprasidone Hydrochloride Capsules, 20 mg Due to Label Mix-up

For Immediate Release
June 13, 2023

Contact
Consumers: 1-888-759-6904
Media: 800-875-0123

Announcement
The Harvard Drug Group, LLC d/b/a Major Pharmaceutical and Rugby Laboratories is initiating a voluntary recall of a single lot of Dronabinol Capsules, USP, 2.5 mg and Ziprasidone Hydrochloride Capsules, 20 mg to the consumer level. The Harvard Drug Group, LLC received a customer complaint from a distributor, that some unit dose cartons labeled as Ziprasidone Hydrochloride Capsules, 20 mg were found to contain blister packages labeled as and containing Dronabinol Capsules, USP, 2.5 mg for Lot T04769. Accordingly, The Harvard Drug Group, LLC is recalling all of Lot T04769, Dronabinol Capsules, USP, 2.5 mg, which may be in outer cartons that read Dronabinol Capsules, USP, 2.5 mg OR Ziprasidone Hydrochloride Capsules, 20 mg.

Risk Statement: There is a reasonable probability that patients who mistakenly take Dronabinol Capsules, USP, 2.5 mg instead of Ziprasidone Hydrochloride, 20 mg capsules, can experience serious adverse events from 1) missing their ziprasidone dose and 2) taking an unexpected dose of Dronabinol. Patients missing doses of Ziprasidone can experience exacerbation of underlying health issues such as bipolar disorder, schizophrenia, agitation, aggression, or delirium. This can result in mental illness instability with possible consequences of self-harm or harm to others which could result in medical or psychiatric hospitalization. Taking an unexpected dose of Dronabinol may cause mental and cognitive effects that result in impairment of mental and/or physical abilities. This can include worsening of symptoms in patients with mental illness disorders and limitation of patients' abilities to safely complete hazardous activities (e.g., driving a motor vehicle, operating machinery). Elderly patients or those taking other medications that affect mental function may be particularly at risk for these reactions. The Harvard Drug Group, LLC has not received any reports of adverse events related to this recall.

Ziprasidone Hydrochloride Capsules, 20 mg, is used for the treatment of schizophrenia, as monotherapy for the acute treatment of bipolar manic or mixed episodes, and as an adjunct to lithium or valproate for the maintenance treatment of bipolar disorder.

Dronabinol Capsules, USP, 2.5 mg, is used as (1) an anorexia associated with weight loss in patients with Acquired Immune Deficiency Syndrome (AIDS) and (2) nausea and vomiting associated with cancer chemotherapy in patients who have failed to respond adequately to conventional antiemetic treatments.

Both Ziprasidone Hydrochloride Capsules, 20 mg and Dronabinol Capsules, USP, 2.5 mg are labeled with lot T04769 EXP. 2024/12 and can be identified on the outer carton labeling as follows:

Product Name	Package Description	Brand Name	Lot Number	NDC	Expiration Date
Dronabinol Capsules, USP, 2.5 mg	100 Unit Doses per Carton (10 × 10 blister packs)	Major	T04769	0904-7144-61	2024/12
Ziprasidone Hydrochloride Capsules, 20 mg	40 Unit Doses per Carton (10 × 4 blister packs)	Major	T04769	0904-6269-08	2024/12

Ziprasidone Hydrochloride Capsules, 20 mg are capsules with a lavender opaque cap and flesh opaque body, imprinted "RDY" on the cap and "356" on the body.

Dronabinol Capsules, USP, 2.5 mg are white capsules imprinted with "M2."

Images of the outer carton labeling of both Ziprasidone Hydrochloride Capsules, 20 mg and Dronabinol Capsules, USP, 2.5 mg and in addition, images of the blister packages of Dronabinol Capsules, USP, 2.5 mg found in cartons labeled as Ziprasidone Hydrochloride Capsules, 20 mg, can be found below.

Products were distributed Nationwide to Wholesalers starting April 5, 2023.

The Harvard Drug Group, LLC is notifying all impacted direct accounts via mail of this voluntary recall and is arranging for return of all recalled products listed above. Wholesalers, Distributors and Retailers that have the affected product which is being recalled should stop distribution of the product and consumers should stop using this affected product, return it to the place of purchase, and contact their physician or healthcare provider.

Consumers with questions regarding this recall can contact Sedgwick, Inc. by phone at 1-888-759-6904 (8:00 am–5:00 pm EST Monday through Friday) or by e-mail address harvarddrug6068@sedgwick.com. Consumers should contact their physician or healthcare provider if they have experienced any problems that may be related to taking or using this drug product.

Adverse reactions or quality problems experienced with the use of this product may be reported to the FDA's MedWatch Adverse Event Reporting program either online, by regular mail, or by fax.

Complete and submit the report
Online: *http://www.fda.gov/medwatch/report.htm*
Regular Mail or Fax: Download form *http://www.fda.gov/MedWatch/getforms.htm* or call 1-800-332-1088 to request a reporting form, then complete and return to the address on the preaddressed form or submit by fax to 1-800-FDA-0178.

This recall is being executed with the knowledge of the U.S. Food and Drug Administration.

See *https://www.fda.gov/Safety/Recalls-market-withdrawala-safety-alerts*

responsibility to choose a licensed, qualified business to perform these services. Some examples of automated return companies are Return Solutions, Guaranteed Returns, and PharmaLink.

Tech Alert!

No medications taken out of the pharmacy by a patient can be returned to stock!

Nonreturnable Drugs and Waste Management

Many items cannot be returned to manufacturers. Some examples of nonreturnable drugs are any drug that is reconstituted or compounded in the pharmacy, partially used bottles of medication, and any drugs that have been repackaged by the pharmacy. These drugs, including most reconstituted agents (eg, amoxicillin suspension), can be discarded in the pharmacy garbage. They should not be allowed to infiltrate the water supply. In most cases, especially in chain pharmacies, the drugs are sent to a central location for destruction or returned to the manufacturer for credit.

There are special storage and disposal considerations from the Environmental Protection Agency (EPA) based on environmental hazards. The EPA has a P listing that includes specific drugs that must be discarded in special containers. Toxic agents such as chemotherapy waste must be discarded in a yellow sharps container. Drugs such as nitroglycerin must be put into a "black" container along with neostigmine, warfarin, and phentermine. Purple is used for live vaccines or hazardous waste, and nonhazardous intravenous agents should be discarded in a standard blue and white sharps container marked for proper disposal.

For environmental concerns regarding medications getting into the water supply or just removal from the residence to avoid accidents, rather than flush the drug, encourage patients to use your store's drug disposal program or a sponsored Drug Take-Back program.

Controlled substances must be counted and cosigned by a pharmacist before they are destroyed. Before any scheduled medications are destroyed, the DEA must be contacted for specific instructions concerning their destruction. A pharmacist always must be present to cosign for the disposal of controlled substances and must return required information about the disposal to the DEA. The DEA issues a receipt for schedule II merchandise destroyed. This receipt must be kept for 2 years from the date of receipt or disposal with the schedule II inventory.

Returns of Patient Medications Not Picked Up

In addition to regular inventory returns, technicians must routinely check patient medications ready for pick up that have not been picked up by or for the patient. They may be not picked up because of unknown changes in medication, hospitalizations, or cost. Those that were charged to insurance must be reversed to the third party by electronic submission to credit the patient and remove the prescription from the insurance. Once the completed prescriptions are removed, names and other pertinent information are blacked out and

labels are placed in a HIPAA trash container. Medications that have never left the pharmacy may then be returned to stock bottles.

Suppliers

When ordering stock for the pharmacy, the technician orders from a centralized warehouse the pharmacy owns, from a wholesaler, or directly from the manufacturer. Medications, devices, and other pharmacy supplies are available from various sources.

- **Prime vendors** are large distributors of various medications and retail products to pharmacies. A contract outlining the cost, delivery dates, return policies, and payment schedule is made between the pharmacy and the distributor, usually requiring the pharmacy to order medications through their specific company. Even with the percentage fee that is added for this type of supplier, there can be a substantial savings to the pharmacy. Examples of prime vendors include AmerisourceBergen, McKesson, Total Pharmacy Supply, and Cardinal Health. Advantages of the prime vendor agreement are lower costs and emergency delivery services.

- **Wholesalers** are companies that stock a variety of drug manufacturers' medications and normally have a just-in-time turnaround for ordered drugs. This means that drugs ordered today will arrive tomorrow. This type of ordering is very useful in pharmacies where space is limited for overstock items or the medication is needed by the next day. A percentage fee is added onto the shipments, but the additional fees can be offset by ordering in bulk, resulting in a substantial savings overall. Examples of wholesalers include HD Smith, Anda, and Cardinal Health.

- **Direct manufacturer ordering** may be used under certain circumstances. For example, a group of pharmacies may join a group purchasing organization that contracts with the manufacturer for better pricing. The contract is usually based on the quantity ordered and includes specific return policies and conditions. Other reasons might arise for directly ordering from manufacturers; for example, the wholesaler and/or prime vendor may not stock the drug; the drug may not be available from the normal source at the time of ordering; or the medication may be available only to select patients who meet certain treatment parameters (eg, FDA regulations or investigational protocols). In such cases the manufacturer records and verifies the information before sending the medication for the specific patient. Examples of drug manufacturers include Abbott Laboratories, Bristol-Myers Squibb, Janssen Pharmaceuticals, and Upsher-Smith Laboratories.

Each of these types of suppliers has pros and cons. As seen in Table 13.3, the benefits of using wholesalers as opposed to dealing directly with the manufacturer differ mostly in the amount of stock that must be ordered and kept as overstock and the difference in cost. The fourth column of Table 13.3 describes factors to consider when ordering medications from a warehouse; in this situation the pharmaceutical company orders high volumes of drugs from the manufacturer and may repackage the medications into more suitable sizes for the

TABLE 13.3

Difference in Ordering From Manufacturers, Wholesalers, and Warehouse Repackaging Plants

Factors to Consider	Manufacturer	Wholesaler/Vendor Repackaging Plant	Warehouse
Supplier cost	No shipping fees	Lower per contract	Lowest cost
Supplier has electronic inventory control mechanism	No	Yes	Yes
Supplier can stock large supplies when ordering	Yes	No	Yes
Supplier provides special delivery service	Varies by manufacturer	Yes	Yes
Supplier handles special orders	Yes	Some special orders must be made through manufacturer	Some special orders must be made through manufacturer

ordering physician. This serves several purposes, such as easier handling, increased productivity, and lower cost. However, large-quantity bottles are hard to handle. They are more likely to be dropped, spilling the contents. Medications may be pre-packaged in smaller, easy-to-handle containers to eliminate the bulkiness of the larger bottles. If the pharmacy warehouse prepackages common dosages, the labeling process is faster. For example, sulfamethoxazole/trimethoprim (Septra, Bactrim) normally is taken twice daily for 10 days or twice daily for 15 days. These tablets are prepackaged in bottles of 20 and 30, eliminating the time it takes to count out the proper amount at the pharmacy counter. The technician must check the label against the prescription to determine the appropriate drug and quantity; then the prescription is ready to be inspected by the pharmacist and dispensed. Finally, because the volume of drugs is much higher than what a typical pharmacy can stock, pharmacies have contracts with these warehouses that save the pharmacy a substantial amount of money. This ultimately keeps the cost lower for the consumer.

Special Considerations

Special considerations apply to a host of drugs ordered by pharmacy, such as controlled substances, investigational drugs, cytotoxic drugs, and hazardous substances. Each of these types of medications requires special ordering, inventory, storage, handling, and return documentation. The DEA requires special forms to be completed for ordering, transferring, and returning schedule II controlled substances.

Investigational drugs typically have documentation that must be completed and returned to the manufacturer each time a medication is dispensed. These drugs are stored and inventoried separately. Cytotoxic drugs do not need special documentation, but they should be handled with great care and placed in a safety cabinet according to the manufacturer's guidelines. Certain cytotoxic agents must be refrigerated and should be clearly marked to separate them from other agents. Most pharmacies stock certain chemicals that are considered hazardous. You must know where the **Safety Data Sheets (SDSs)** of your pharmacy are located in case of a spill. Agents such as phenol should be stored behind

cabinet doors to protect individuals from accidentally knocking the bottle off a shelf and inhaling the toxic fumes or coming in contact with the agent.

Although many of the guidelines can be found in each pharmacy's policies and procedures manual, it is the responsibility of the pharmacy technician to be aware of these guidelines and of federal and state regulations. This requires continuous effort to ensure that the regulations that apply to your pharmacy are updated to reflect the current requirements. Patients rely on the knowledge of the pharmacy technician, which is why competencies in the area of billing and inventory are extremely important in the daily functions of pharmacy.

Do You Remember These Key Points?

- Why pharmacy formularies are important
- The major types of insurance and the differences among them
- The differences among government-managed insurance programs
- The parts of a health insurance card
- The necessary information patients must provide to the pharmacy for billing prescriptions to third parties
- The steps involved in billing insurance companies
- The types of problems that often arise when processing insurance claims
- The importance of the National Drug Code and how to decipher it
- The responsibilities of a pharmacy technician concerning stock levels and ordering stock for the pharmacy
- Common types of automated dispensing systems and pharmacy settings in which they are used
- The steps that should be followed when receiving stock
- Reasons for returning stock to the manufacturer or supplier
- Who issues recalls and how they are addressed
- How to return expired or recalled stock
- The importance of storing stock at the appropriate temperature

Scenario Follow-Up

Brian is now the new level 3 technician. He is proud of this accomplishment and plans to continue to look for ways to improve his working environment. He understands that this new position includes more responsibility, and he welcomes the challenge. With his positive attitude and willingness to step up as a leader, Brian has a bright and exciting future in the pharmacy technician field.

Review Questions

Multiple Choice Questions

1. Which of the following is responsible for developing the formulary used by an institution?
   A. State board of pharmacy
   B. Pharmacy and therapeutics committee
   C. US Food and Drug Administration
   D. All of the above

2. Medicare is a government-managed insurance program that covers all of the following *except:*
   A. Senior citizens
   B. Patients using dialysis
   C. Children
   D. People who are disabled

3. Medicaid covers all of the following *except:*
   A. People who are disabled
   B. People with a low income
   C. Women who are pregnant
   D. Single working people with above-average income

4. Which health plan covers in-network provider visits only?
   A. A medical group that is covered under Medicare
   B. Preferred provider organization (PPO)
   C. Health maintenance organization (HMO)
   D. Point-of-service plan (POS)

5. Which regulatory body can issue a drug recall?
   A. FDA
   B. HMO
   C. DEA
   D. PPO

6. Insurance claims that are transmitted electronically to the insurance provider are called:
   A. E-mail claims
   B. NDC claims
   C. Adjudicated claims
   D. Copay claims

7. Various types of agents ordered for a pharmacy may include:
   A. Formulary drugs
   B. Hazardous substances
   C. Cytotoxic drugs
   D. All of the above

8. Which program makes prescription drugs available through private insurance plans?
   A. Medicare Part A
   B. Medicare Part B
   C. Medicare Part C
   D. Medicare Part D

9. An inventory system that automatically orders stock as it is used is called:
   A. Pyxis
   B. POS
   C. Omnicell
   D. Baker Cell

10. When a workers' compensation claim arrives at the pharmacy, the technician must:
    A. Obtain permission from a government agency at a later time
    B. Obtain information from the patient's human resources department
    C. Collect payment from the patient, who then will be reimbursed by the insurance company
    D. Wait until payment is made by the insurance company before releasing the medication

Technician's Corner

Amber is working as a pharmacy technician in a busy retail pharmacy. A patient brings in a prescription for Pegasys, a drug used to treat hepatitis C. When Amber tries to process the medication using the customer's third-party billing information, she gets the rejection code for "prior authorization required." How should Amber handle this situation? What should she do first?

Amber should first discuss with the patient first that the drug will not be available today for pickup because it will require additional paperwork to be completed by the physician. She will then contact the physician for an interim solution and follow up from there.

Bibliography

Biden-Harris Administration Issues Final Guidance to Help People with Medicare Prescription Drug Coverage Manage Prescription Drug Costs. Available at: http://HHS.gov.

CBS News. *U.S. Prescription Drug Spending Drops for First Time in 58 Years*. May 9, 2013.

Medical Plans Offer More Help to Quit Smoking. *Purdue Today*; February 1, 2008. Available at: http://www.purdue.edu/uns/insidepurdue/2008/080201_Cessation.html.

The Medicare Resource Center. *A Brief History of Medicare in America*. Available at: https://www.medicareresources.org/basic-medicare-information/brief-history-of-medicare/.

Websites Referenced

Available at: http://www.medicare.gov.
Available at: http://www.ConsumerReports.org.
Available at: http://www.Webmd.com.
Available at: http://www.drugtopics.com.
Available at: https://www.benefits.gov.
Available at: http://www.nlm.nih.gov.

Available at: http://www.fda.gov.

Available at: http://www.texmed.org.

Drug Recalls | FDA. Available at: http://www.prescriptiondrugre-call.com/.

Available at: http://www.purdue.edu/uns/insidepurdue/2008/080201_Cessation.html.

Affordable Care Act (ACA). Available at: https://www.healthcare.gov/glossary/affordable-care-act/.

Centers for Medicare and Medicaid Services. *Medicare Program General Information*. Available at: https://www.cms.gov/Medicare/Medicare-General-Information/MedicareGenInfo/index.html.

Medicaid.Gov. *Keeping America Healthy. Medicaid Benefits*. Available at: https://www.medicaid.gov/medicaid/program-information/medicaid-and-chip-enrollment-data/report-highlights/index.html.

Medicare. *Medicare.Gov: State Pharmaceutical Assistance Programs*. Available at: http://www.medicare.gov/pharmaceutical-assistance-program/state-programs.aspx.

Military.Com Benefits. *TRICARE Eligibility*. Available at: http://www.military.com/benefits/tricare/tricare-eligibility.html?comp=7000022779075&rank=1.

US Department of Justice, Drug Enforcement Administration, Office of Diversion Control. *National Take-Back Initiative*. Take Back Day. Available at: http://dea.gov.

US Department of Veteran Affairs. *CHAMPVA Frequently Asked Questions*. Available at: https://www.va.gov/health-care/family-caregiver-benefits/champva/.

US Food and Drug Administration. *About the Center for Drug Evaluation and Research*. Available at: https://www.fda.gov/drugs.

US Food and Drug Administration. *Enforcement Reports*. Available at: http://www.fda.gov/Safety/Recalls/EnforcementReports/default.htm.

US Food and Drug Administration. *National Drug Code Directory*. Available at: http://www.fda.gov/Drugs/InformationOnDrugs/ucm142438.htm.

WalletHub. *States With the Most and Least Medicaid Coverage*. Available at: https://wallethub.com/edu/states-with-the-most-and-least-medicaid-coverage/71573.

CHAPTER 14

Medication Safety and Error Prevention

Karen Davis

1. List the five patient rights of medication safety and give an example of each.
2. Describe what constitutes an error.
3. Differentiate among the various types of medication errors.
4. Explain the various causes of medication errors and why errors occur.
5. Explain the necessity of reporting medication errors and list the organizations or groups that track and report medication errors.
6. Identify safety strategies pharmacies, pharmacists, and pharmacy technicians can use to reduce medication errors.
7. List and describe four automated systems and explain how they prevent errors.
8. Discuss patient dose-specific orders, *United States Pharmacopeia* <797> regulations, and the role a medication safety leader can play in reducing errors.
9. Discuss quality assurance practices and risk management guidelines used in the pharmacy.
10. Describe the roles that training and education play in the reduction of medication errors.

Academy of Managed Care Pharmacy (AMCP) Organization of managed care professionals who strive to support the appropriate use of medications

American Society of Health-System Pharmacists (ASHP) An association of pharmacists, pharmacy students, and technicians practicing in hospitals and health care systems, including home health care; ASHP has a long history of advocating for patient safety and establishing best practices to improve medication use

Automated dispensing system (ADS) Electronic system used to dispense medications

Institute for Healthcare Improvement (IHI) A nonprofit organization committed to the improvement of health care by promoting promising concepts through safety, efficiency, and other patient-centered goals

Institute for Safe Medication Practices (ISMP) A nonprofit organization devoted entirely to promoting safe medication use and preventing medication errors; it gathers information on drug errors and suggests new, safer standards to avoid such errors

Medication error Any preventable event that may cause or lead to inappropriate medication use or patient harm

Medication error prevention Methods used by pharmacy, medicine, nursing, and other allied health professionals to prevent medication errors

MedMARx A national Internet-accessible database that hospitals and health care systems use to track adverse drug reactions and medication errors

MedWatch A program established by the US Food and Drug Administration (FDA) for reporting drug and medical product safety alerts and label changes; the program also provides a voluntary adverse event reporting system for medications, medical products, and devices

National Coordinating Council for Medication Error Reporting and Prevention (NCCMERP) Founded by the United States Pharmacopeia, this is an independent council of more than 25 organizations gathered to address interdisciplinary causes of medication errors and strategies for prevention

Pharmacy Technician Certification Board (PTCB) An organization that offers national certification for pharmacy technicians in the United States

Risk evaluation and mitigation strategy (REMS) A strategy for managing a known or potential serious risk associated with a drug or biological product

Society for the Education of Pharmacy Technicians (SEPhT) A national pharmacy technician organization that promotes the education and training of pharmacy technicians; it provides links to medication safety and quality practices for technicians

United States Pharmacopeial (USP) Convention An independent organization that strives to ensure the quality, safety, and benefit of medicines and dietary supplements by setting standards and certification processes

◎ Scenario

Jonathan is an experienced technician at a large municipal hospital pharmacy. He began his career after graduating from a 2-year technician training program. He is certified by the Pharmacy Technician Certification Board (PTCB) and works full-time as an inpatient technician. He has been asked by the pharmacy director to participate on a committee looking into medication errors. What types of issues do you think the committee will address? How can Jonathan prepare for this new assignment?

Drug errors are unacceptable in any situation involving medical treatment or medications, but the reality is that they will never disappear. It is a human trait that people make mistakes. At times, errors may not be realized before they cause harm. When discussing drug errors, it is important to note that not all errors are harmful and not all are caused by the pharmacy. In this chapter, the types and incidence of errors are discussed, and specific cases that unfortunately caused harm are presented. An attempt is made to identify the common causes of many drug errors and ultimately the ways in which they can be avoided. Other topics discussed in this chapter include the process of drug error reporting (ie, when errors should be reported and who should be contacted) and the importance of helping patients learn to take responsibility for their own medical treatment, including their medications.

Pharmacy technicians are at the forefront in the effort to prevent drug errors; ironically, they also can cause errors relatively easily. Many technicians have relied on the pharmacist to catch their mistakes, but this is not the correct approach to preventing medication errors. Anyone can make a mistake, including pharmacists, physicians, and nurses.

It takes a team working together to prevent medication errors. The knowledge requirements for technicians are increasing, along with their additional responsibilities. Today's pharmacy techs must understand their scope of practice and strive to meet the highest standard.

Overview

Patient safety is a major concern for public health care. Pharmacy technicians' education and training organizations, along with medication safety entities, must work to prevent errors at every level of care. Even if an error occurs in the pharmacy and never reaches the patient, it is still an error and must be evaluated. Understanding why an error occurred and creating ways to prevent any future incidents is an ongoing part of the technician's day.

According to the US Food and Drug Administration (FDA), there are more than 400,000 drug-related injuries that happen in the hospital setting because of medication errors. According to the **AMCP (Academy of Managed Care Pharmacy),** the cost to Americans is at least $3.5 billion dollars a year.

The FDA receives more than 100,000 reports every year that are related to medication errors.

With the influx of immigrants in recent years, drugs are becoming more readily available from outside the United States, and according to the World Health Organization (WHO), almost 1% medicines available in the world are counterfeit.

Many organizations track and encourage reporting to alert the public and health care providers best practices to prevent errors in the future. **The Institute for Safe Medication Practices (ISMP)** publishes a list of high-alert medications, which are drugs with a heightened risk for causing significant patient harm when used in error. According to the ISMP, some medications considered "high alert" in connection with errors are insulin, opioids and opiates, methotrexate, warfarin, and potassium chloride (KCl) injections (Box 14.1).

Five Rights of Medication Safety

There are five basic rights involving medication safety. Pharmacy personnel and other health care professionals are expected to adhere to these guidelines to avoid medication errors.

Effective patient care results from the concentrated efforts of the entire pharmacy team. Every patient is entitled to expect the highest standard of accuracy with regard to his or her medication. This accuracy standard is expressed in the following rights and examples.

1. The Right Patient
   - Always make certain the patient identification information is correct.

BOX 14.1   High-Alert Medications

Acute Care Settings

- Epinephrine, subcutaneous
- Epoprostenol (Flolan), IV
- Insulin U-500 (special emphasis)[a]
- Magnesium sulfate injection
- Methotrexate, oral, nononcologic use
- Nitroprusside sodium for injection
- Opium tincture
- Oxytocin, IV
- Potassium chloride injection concentrate
- Potassium phosphates injection
- Promethazine, IV
- Vasopressin, IV or intraosseous

Community and Ambulatory Health Care Settings

- Carbamazepine
- Chloral hydrate liquid, for sedation of children
- Heparin, including unfractionated and low-molecular-weight heparin
- Metformin
- Methotrexate, nononcologic use
- Midazolam liquid, for sedation of children
- Propylthiouracil
- Warfarin

[a]All forms of insulin, subcutaneous and IV, are considered a class of high-alert medications. Insulin U500 has been singled out for special emphasis to bring attention to the need for distinct strategies to prevent the types of errors that occur with this concentrated form of insulin.

IV, Intravenous.

From the Institute for Safe Medication Practices. ISMP list of high-alert medications in acute care settings and ISMP list of high-alert medications in community/ambulatory health care. *https://www.ismp.org/tools/highalertmedication Lists.asp.* Report medication errors or near misses to the ISMP Medication Errors Reporting Program (MERP) at 1-800-FAILSAF(E) or online at *http:// www.ismp.org.*

2. The Right Medication
   - Verify that the medication is exactly what the physician ordered.
   - Is it brand name or generic?
3. The Right Dose
   - Verify how many doses or tablets are to be taken per day.
   - How long is the patient to continue on the medication?
4. The Right Route
   - Should it be swallowed or chewed?
   - Can it be crushed or broken in half?
   - Is it for injection or to be taken orally?
5. The Right Time
   - What time of day should the medication be taken?
   - Is it taken after or before meals?
   - Is it given at bedtime?

Each pharmacy should incorporate checking these rights into the procedural guidelines of their organization as one of the safety goals of the medication process.

What Constitutes an Error?

An error is any type of preventable event that may cause or lead to inappropriate medication use or patient harm. Patients themselves cause many drug errors when taking their own medications at home. They may take their medications at the wrong time, in the wrong amount, in the wrong combination, or with an improper administration technique. It is difficult to know how many drug errors occur at home because they typically are not reported to anyone and may continue to occur unless recognized by the physician or pharmacist or, even worse, manifested by an adverse drug event (ADE) or adverse drug reaction (ADR). These types of situations are part of the drug error dilemma and are taken very seriously by all involved in patient care. An error can involve prescription or over-the-counter (OTC) medications and can be committed by both experienced and inexperienced staff. The **American Society of Health-System Pharmacists (ASHP)** and the **National Coordinating Council for Medication Error Reporting and Prevention (NCCMERP)**, frequently referred to simply as MERP, outline the most common types of errors that may occur (Tables 14.1 and 14.2).

Types of Medication Errors

Medication errors can be broken down into three main categories: prescribing errors, dispensing errors, and administration errors.

Examples of prescribing errors may include the following:
- Incorrect strength of a medication
- Quantity and refill information omitted
- Route of administration not specified
- Illegible handwriting

Examples of dispensing errors may include the following:
- Incorrect prescription interpretation
- Incorrect calculations
- Incorrect drug utilization evaluation
- Sound-alike or look-alike drug errors

Examples of administration errors may include the following:
- Ear medications being placed in the eye
- Oral medications given intravenously
- Intravenous (IV) syringes used to measure oral medications
- Failure to document medication administration records accurately

Physicians' handwriting has long been known for its illegibility, which means that reading drug names, strengths, and dosages can be very problematic. An alternative to a handwritten prescription is a new technology called *e-prescribing.* Prescriptions can be sent by computer or mobile device directly to the pharmacy, where they can be easily and quickly interpreted. Several software programs facilitate e-prescribing. Although e-prescribing has been implemented in various medical institutions and physicians' offices, many physicians still write their orders by hand on prescription pads or order sheets. It is the responsibility of the pharmacy and nurses to interpret these prescriptions correctly.

Case scenario examples show the possible progression of an ultimate drug error.

TABLE 14.1
Types of Medication Errors

Error	Description
Compliance error	Patient does not adhere to prescribed medication regimen (eg, taking a q8h dose every 6 hours or stopping a medication before scheduled)
Deteriorated drug error	Medication is administered that has expired or the integrity of ingredients has been compromised (eg, storing a drug at room temperature when it should be refrigerated)
Improper dose error	Patient administered a dose that is greater or less than prescribed amount (eg, aspirin 325 mg is given instead of 500 mg)
Monitoring error	Failure to review a prescribed medication for proper regimen, appropriateness (eg, not monitoring patient's response to prescribed medication), detection of problems in dosage (eg, not recognizing side effects from drugs), or failure in using laboratory results to correctly adjust dose
Omission error	Failure to administer an ordered dose to a patient before next dose is due, without an apparent reason for omission or appropriate documentation (eg, nurse forgets to give a dose to patient)
Prescribing error	Prescriber orders a medication that is incorrect (eg, incorrect usage, dosage form, route, concentration, rate of infusion) or is selected incorrectly based on indications or contraindications (allergies, existing condition); medication reaches patient
Unauthorized drug error	Medication administered to a patient from an unauthorized prescriber; physician not licensed in that state or not an authorized prescriber
Wrong administration	Drug is given using wrong procedure or technique (eg, giving an intramuscular [IM] dose as an intravenous [IV] dose or placing an ophthalmic solution in wrong eye)
Wrong dosage form	Medication administered in a dosage form other than what was ordered (eg, capsule for tablet, ointment for cream)
Wrong drug preparation	Drug is incorrectly formulated (eg, wrong calculations or wrong solution used for reconstitution) or manipulated (eg, break in aseptic technique), and medication is administered to patient
Wrong time error	Medication administered outside scheduled time frame; if facility allows plus or minus 30 min, dose is given outside of this variance (each facility sets an acceptable time frame for variances)

From American Society of Health-System Pharmacists. Medication misadventures—guidelines. ASHP guidelines for preventing medication errors in hospitals: types of medication errors. *https://www.ashp.org/-/media/assets/policy-guidelines/docs/guidelines/preventing-medication-errors-hospitals.ashx.*

TABLE 14.2
Medication Error Reporting and Prevention Categories

Category	Definition	Type of Resulting Error
A	Circumstances that have potential for causing errors	No error
B	Error occurred but did not reach patient	Error, no harm
C	Error reached patient but did not cause harm	Error, no harm
D	Error reached patient, did not cause harm, but needed monitoring or intervention to prove no harm resulted	Error, no harm
E	Error occurred that may have contributed to or resulted in temporary harm to patient and patient required intervention	Error, harm
F	Error occurred that may have contributed to or resulted in temporary harm to patient and resulted in monitoring or hospitalization	Error, harm
G	Error occurred that may have contributed to or resulted in temporary or permanent harm to patient	Error, harm
H	Error occurred that may have contributed to or resulted in harm to patient and required hospitalization to sustain life	Error, harm
I	Error occurred that may have contributed to or resulted in patient's death	Error, death

Data from Agency for Healthcare Research and Quality (AHRQ). Categories of medication error classification. *https://www.ahrq.gov/patient-safety/resources/match/matchtab6.html.*

Scenario 1: Misinterpretation of Physician's Orders

A prescription arrives in the pharmacy for digoxin 0.125 mg; because of the illegibility of the physician's handwriting, it is transcribed inaccurately as 0.25 mg. The wrong medication strength is sent to the floor, where the nurse gives the patient the wrong dose.

Scenario 2: Missed Dose

A medication order arrives in the pharmacy and is processed correctly and sent to the patient. The nurse pulls the correct drug and dose but forgets to give it to the patient; therefore the patient misses a dose. Whether the nurse forgets to give the dose or the patient (at home) forgets to take the medication, this constitutes a medication error.

Scenario 3: Wrong Patient

A medication order arrives in the pharmacy and is processed and sent to the floor correctly, but the nurse gives the drug to the wrong patient.

Scenario 4: Adverse Effect

A patient takes an OTC drug along with a prescription drug, which results in an adverse or toxic effect because of a drug-drug interaction.

Scenario 5: Noncompliance

A patient obtains his or her prescription at the local pharmacy and begins to take the medication; the prescription instructs the patient to take daily for 30 days. After 1 week the patient feels much better and stops taking the medication.

Responsibility for Errors

Unfortunately, the first response to an error is normally to blame rather than to explain the reasons behind such an occurrence. All health care workers are at risk for being found guilty of errors that are considered negligence according to federal and state laws. The case of a medical error reported in Colorado (Case Study 1) identifies the complexity of a drug error. Two cases that were highly publicized across the country (Case Studies 2 and 3) clearly illustrate the need for well-educated and trained technicians.

Case Study 1

Police charged three nurses with negligent homicide after an infant's death from a fatal overdose of potassium chloride (KCl). A subsequent analysis uncovered a chain of numerous errors from the time of prescription to the time of injection. The police did not charge the physician who wrote the cryptic prescription or the pharmacist who misread the dosage.

Case Study 2

The Ohio State Board of Pharmacy revoked the license of a staff pharmacist at Rainbow Baby's and Children's Hospital in Cleveland after Emily, a 2-year-old patient, died as a result of a sodium overdose in a chemotherapy solution (Emily

Jerry Foundation, n.d.). The board concluded that the pharmacist did not follow proper hospital procedures for the supervision of a pharmacy technician who prepared the solution. No disciplinary action was taken against the technician because Ohio does not license or register pharmacy technicians. The technician resigned in the aftermath of the incident. William Winsley, RPh, MS, executive director of the board, stated that both the pharmacist and the technician were experienced and had prepared intravenous and chemotherapy solutions many times. However, he said, "The pharmacist failed to adequately check the technician's work." The supervising pharmacist who failed to notice the technician's mistake lost his state license and pleaded no contest to involuntary manslaughter; he was sentenced to 6 months in jail and 6 months of house arrest. In 2009 Emily's Law was signed by the governor of Ohio. This act requires all pharmacy technicians in the state to be of legal age, to have a high school diploma or equivalent, to pass a state and federal background check, and to pass a certifying competency examination approved by the board of pharmacy before being awarded technician status. The National Pharmacy Technician Association (NPTA) supports the legislation as a model for national and state standards. US Representative Steve LaTourette proposed Emily's Act for congressional approval on March 1, 2009, but it was rejected.

Case Study 3

In March 2010 ABC News *(http://www.abcnews.go.com, 2010)* reported that a Florida appeals court had ordered Walgreens to pay a $25.8 million judgment for an error made by Janelle Banks* (Patel and Ross, 2009). Ms. Banks was a teenage pharmacy technician who had no formal training and had previously worked at a movie theater popping popcorn. In court she testified that she typed in "ten milligrams" on the prescription when it should have been "one milligram." As a result of this error, Beth Hippely received a dosage of her blood thinner medication that was 10 times too much. She suffered a massive stroke.

Where Errors Are Made

Medication errors can occur in many different settings, including hospitals, clinics, pharmacies, physicians' offices, and even patients' homes. These errors may be intentional or unintentional and often go undetected. Box 14.2 presents a list of common causes of medication errors compiled by the ASHP.

Although errors are made in many different settings, they most often are reported in community and institutional pharmacies, such as hospitals. MERP tracks errors and their causes and has created a list of five recommendations for avoiding errors specifically in nonhospital settings.

---

*Florida no longer allows on-the-job training. Effective January 1, 2011, any individual who wants to work as a pharmacy technician in the state of Florida has to register with the Florida Board of Pharmacy. To register with the Florida Board of Pharmacy, an applicant has to submit a Pharmacy Technician Registration Application and proof of completion of a board-approved pharmacy technician training program.

Why Errors Occur

It is human nature to make errors; humans are not perfect. A person can look at the name and strength of a drug yet fail to register the correct information, substituting unintended information in its place. Errors can result from focusing on more than one task at a time. People tend to filter out information even under normal circumstances. Think about the following examples of errors in everyday life and note whether any have ever happened to you:

- You pick up the phone to call a specific person and you call someone else instead.
- You leave to drive to school and you start to drive to work.
- You read the words on a page of a textbook, and although you read each word correctly, you do not remember what you have just read.
- You reach for the correct spice on the kitchen shelf and you grab the wrong one because it is similar in size, shape, color, or labeling.

Even the most highly skilled person occasionally makes errors. You know what you want to do, but your mind changes its focus and you follow the wrong information. This type of "automatic behavior" plays a role in the occurrence of errors. In addition, when repetitive actions are carried out daily, it is easy to become complacent and lose focus on the task at hand.

Both treating patients and supplying medications accurately are critical responsibilities, and it is expected that errors will be avoided. All health care workers strive to avoid errors on a daily basis. However, various situations and circumstances often hinder this effort. The following are some examples of the daily obstructions encountered by pharmacy personnel:

- Stress as a result of the fast-paced environment and the increase in the number of prescriptions processed daily
- Stress related to difficulties encountered during the insurance online adjudication process
- Noise in the workplace that distracts focus from the medication ordered
- Multitasking—doing two or more things at once (eg, answering the phone and checking medications at the same time)—can distract attention from the order
- Medication names that sound alike
- Medications that look similar (eg, colors, shapes, sizes, or a similar area where they are stored)
- Labels that look similar because of the same color and/or lettering
- Labels that are difficult to read because of small print
- Prescriptions with illegible handwriting
- Excessive workload

Stress

Many studies have shown that over the past few decades, Americans' stress levels have been increasing. Job stress has been identified as a major source of stress for adults. Excessive pressure and demands placed on individuals at work can cause them to feel overwhelmed and unable to perform at their best. This is when errors can occur.

In pharmacies, shortages in personnel and an increasing demand for services contribute to workplace stress. Eventually, this stress can translate into higher occurrences of errors and lower job satisfaction. Some stressors include dealing with angry patients or customers, rude health care personnel, high prescription volumes, employees calling in sick, inadequate supplies or stock, and insurance processing complications. Stress affects everyone, including the pharmacist, pharmacy technician, and other pharmacy personnel. Stress reduction goals should be addressed on a regular basis. Open and honest communication should be used when discussing workplace stressors. Placing blame should be avoided.

Distraction

One of the major causes of medication errors is distractions and can account for many errors. A typical pharmacy environment is full of many types of noise. Sounds such as telephones, machines, intercoms, cell phones, and voices are considered normal. However, an overly noisy workplace can cause distractions, affecting concentration on the task at hand, which could result in medication errors.

Talking or laughing among employees during the prescription filling process can be disruptive and may seem uncaring or unprofessional to the customers or patients. The noise or vibration of a text message can be equally distracting. Most organizations have restrictions on cell phone use and texting at work. We are all very aware of how dangerous texting and driving can be. However, sending and receiving text messages at work can be just as dangerous. Anything that takes the focus away from accurately filling a patient's prescription should be avoided. Every pharmacy employee should be aware of the company policy regarding cell phone use. Patient and staff safety is always the goal. Standards governing the appropriate sound environment should be reviewed with new employees and updated regularly.

Case Study

Hanna worked at a pharmaceutical plant as a packaging technician. She was responsible for making sure the pills were distributed into the correct bottles using the appropriate machines. During her lunch she was texting her boyfriend about their upcoming trip. After lunch she brought her cell phone back into the production area in case her boyfriend needed to text her about the trip. She knew this was against policy, but everyone broke the rule occasionally.

About an hour into her shift, her phone vibrated. When she went to answer it, she dropped it on the conveyor belt. She knew it would jam up the machine and halt the production line, so she reached to stop it. Her hand got caught, and she lost two fingers.

Case Study Follow-Up

1. How could Hanna have avoided this accident?
2. Is there ever an excuse to break the safety rules?

Texting distracts from the job at hand. It is the responsibility of each pharmacy professional to respect the safety guidelines and adhere to company policy.

Multitasking

Skerrett (2012) states that multitasking can increase the chance of making mistakes and hinder problem solving and creativity. With increasingly more health care professionals using electronic devices at work, the temptation to multitask is great. Often errors occur when one task is interrupted by some other device. Everyone needs to be aware of the distractions that come with the use of new technologies. Focusing on one task at a time, giving your full attention before moving on, helps ensure patient safety.

Case Study

An older man with dementia was admitted to the hospital. One of his physicians decided to increase the dose of warfarin he was taking. The next day, the physician decided to reevaluate the warfarin regimen to see whether it was even necessary. He gave the order to temporarily stop the blood thinner to a resident to submit. As the resident was completing the new order in the computerized order entry system, she was interrupted by a text message from a friend and failed to complete the temporary stop on the warfarin. As a result, the man's blood became so thin he needed open heart surgery to save his life.

Case Study Follow-Up Remember to always finish one task before going on to the next task. Text messages can wait. Numerous distractions may arise during any particular work shift. It is the technician's responsibility to be 100% focused on patient safety and accuracy.

Look-Alike, Sound-Alike Drugs

Each year, in an effort to reduce confusion between drug names that look alike or sound alike (LASA), the FDA reviews approximately 300 drug names before they are allowed to enter the market. Approximately one-third of the names that companies propose are rejected. To test these drug names, the FDA enlists the help of about 120 FDA health professionals. This group simulates real-life drug order situations. In addition, the FDA has created a computer program to detect similar names.

◉ Scenario Checkup 14.1

Jonathan is training a newly hired technician today. He is very excited to share his knowledge with his co-worker. Their first task is to scan and put up the medications that arrived from the wholesaler. Jonathan takes time to explain the hospital policy on look-alike, sound-alike (LASA) drugs. He shows her the posted list of commonly confused drug names and describes how the tall man lettering works. Why does a new employee need this information if the pharmacist has the last check to verify accuracy?

Risk Evaluation and Mitigation Strategies

The decision to approve a new drug always includes the question, "Do the benefits outweigh the risks for the patient?" Manufacturers and the FDA are continually evaluating these risks and benefits throughout the entire life cycle of a drug. Traditionally, these risks have been communicated by the manufacturer's package insert. However, in some cases the FDA and/or the manufacturer determine that the risks are significant enough to require additional product labeling to ensure patient safety. In these cases, a **risk evaluation and mitigation strategy (REMS)** is recommended to ensure that benefits outweigh the risks.

The implementation of REMS in the pharmacy workplace is unique to each practice setting. Pharmacists provide education to patients on the benefits and risks of REM medications. Pharmacy technicians are involved with keeping a list of REM medications requiring MedGuides for dispensing and any medications that require REM components, in addition to a MedGuide. Medication Guides are paper handouts that address issues specific to particular drugs and drug classes. They contain FDA-approved information designed to help patients avoid serious adverse events. The list can be found at *https://dailymed.nlm.nih.gov/dailymed/drugInfo.cfm?setid=b074f950-246a-41f0-aedf-32f38998a4b1*.

Pharmacy technicians can identify medications requiring MedGuides by looking for the indication in bold lettering on the stock bottle or box or by looking for a red or yellow symbol. Some pharmacies have a special symbol that prints out with the label for REMS medications. MedGuides can be printed directly from the FDA website.

Look-Alike Drug Names and Tall Man Lettering

The ISMP and The Joint Commission (TJC) promote the use of tall man lettering as one means of reducing confusion between similar drug names. Tall man lettering uses mixed case letters to draw attention to the dissimilarities in look-alike drug names, as in the following examples:

buPROPion—busPIRone
clomiPHENE—clomiPRAMINE
cycloSPORINE—cycloSERINE

DAUNOrubicin—DOXOrubicin
glipiZIDE—glyBURIDE
hydrALAZINE—hydrOXYzine
medroxyPROGESTERone—methylPREDNISolone—
    methylTESTOSTERone
niCARdipine—NIFEdipine
predniSONE—prednisoLONE
sulfADIAZINE—sulfiSOXAZOLE

A complete list of look-alike drug names is available on the ISMP website *(http://www.ismp.org/Tools/tallmanletters.pdf)*.

Case Study

An elderly male patient underwent a coronary arterial bypass and was recovering from anesthesia in the cardiac intensive care unit. He showed mild metabolic acidosis (condition in which too much acid is present in the body fluids) as a result of hypothermia. Sodium bicarbonate was to be given intravenously slowly. A few seconds after injection, the patient's heart stopped. Cardiac resuscitation was initiated, and the patient was revived successfully with an intravenous bolus injection of adrenaline, calcium, and sodium bicarbonate.

When the event was analyzed, it was noted that five broken ampules of potassium chloride (KCl) were found lying on the patient's medication table. The staff attending the patient had given 50 mL (100 mEq) of KCl instead of 50 mL (50 mEq) of sodium bicarbonate. It was determined that the error occurred because of the similar color of the labels of sodium bicarbonate and KCl. The ampules for both drugs were from the same pharmaceutical company; they were both packaged in 10-mL ampules with a red label, and the two medications were kept on the same shelf, side by side. Use of different-sized ampules kept in different places could have prevented this type of look-alike medication error.

Drug Labeling

Drug companies are urged to make changes in the labeling of any type of medication that can be confusing or misinterpreted. The use of color coding, tall man lettering, and boldface lettering can help make drug selection errors less likely. For example, using tall man lettering helps differentiate the drug hydrOXYzine from the drug hydrALAzine. Changes to drug stocking include placing "Name Alert" stickers on the bins containing problematic LASA drugs or placing the bins in different areas of the pharmacy to reduce the possibility of pulling the wrong drug. Drug companies have been encouraged to name their new drugs differently from other medications to help reduce confusion.

Case Study

A woman undergoing a radiology procedure was mistakenly given an injection of chlorhexidine, a skin cleansing agent. She was supposed to have received an injection of contrast dye. The two solutions were in similar, unlabeled containers. The mistake was irreversible, and the patient died.

Case Study Follow-Up The pharmacy could have implemented procedures to clearly label all containers and train the personnel to never use an unlabeled bottle.

Excessive Workload

Many pharmacists and pharmacy technicians think their excessive workloads are a threat to the public's safety. The demands of processing hundreds of prescriptions in a 10- to 12-hour shift are increasing the risks for error. Many pharmacy employees complain of few or no breaks, no time to eat lunch or dinner, and very little time to go to the bathroom when needed. Several state boards of pharmacy (BOPs), such as the Iowa BOP and the Oregon BOP, are beginning to address this issue and develop strategies to combat these problems. In March 2013 the Iowa BOP received the following recommendations from its patient safety task force *(https://www.nodakpharmacy.com/pdfs/20MaierMillerPatientSafetyExecSummaryIa.pdf)*:

- Require the pharmacy to provide sufficient personnel to prevent fatigue, distractions, or conditions that interfere with a pharmacist's ability to practice safely.
- Require the pharmacy to provide opportunities for rest periods and meal breaks.
- Require the pharmacy to provide adequate time for a pharmacist to complete professional duties and responsibilities.
- Prohibit introduction of external factors (eg, productivity quotas or programs such as time limits) that interfere with the pharmacist's ability to provide appropriate professional services.

Case Study

A part-time pharmacy technician at a Walgreens in Florida mistakenly labeled a prescription for methadone with the instruction to take "as needed" (Hodges, 2011). The instruction was supposed to read "Take four 10-mg tablets twice daily." The patient took 22 pills over the course of a day and a half, nearly twice as many as prescribed. His wife found him dead, his body curled on the floor of the shower stall. The pharmacy filled 380 prescriptions that day. No one had offered the patient any counseling.

Case Study Follow-Up It is important to give each patient the opportunity to discuss the medication regimen with the pharmacist. Patient safety is of the utmost importance, and we should never be too busy to ask patients whether they have any questions. If the technician would have made sure the patient understood the instruction by having the patient discuss it with the pharmacist, this tragedy might have been prevented.

Drug Interactions as a Source of Error

Drug interactions are another source of errors in the pharmacy. The probability of drug-drug interactions is increased in seniors and severely ill patients because of the multiple medications they often receive. Seniors may have multiple conditions that are treated concurrently. In addition to the changes in metabolism that occur with aging, taking similar drugs that have the same side effects may increase the risk for and/or severity of adverse effects. Table 14.3 lists examples of drugs that should not be given concurrently.

TABLE 14.3
Examples of Drug-Drug Interactions

Drug	Drug	Result of Drug Interaction
Angiotensin-converting enzyme (ACE) inhibitors	Spironolactone	Increased serum potassium levels
Ciprofloxacin	Multivitamin with minerals	Decreased effect of ciprofloxacin because minerals in multivitamins can decrease antibiotic absorption if taken at the same time
Digoxin	Verapamil and amiodarone	Digoxin toxicity
Theophylline	Quinolones	Theophylline toxicity

TABLE 14.4
Examples of Warfarin Interactions With Drugs, Supplements, and Foods

Product	Product of Interaction	Interaction Result
Drugs		
Warfarin	Aspirin	Possible increased risk for bleeding
Warfarin	Phenytoin	Increased phenytoin or warfarin levels
Warfarin	Quinolones	Increased chance of bleeding
Warfarin	Sulfa drugs	Increased chance of bleeding
Warfarin	Cimetidine	Increased chance of bleeding
Warfarin	Heparin	Increased chance of bleeding
Warfarin	Amiodarone	Increased chance of bleeding
Warfarin	Nonsteroidal antiinflammatory drugs (NSAIDs)	Increased chance of bleeding
Supplements		
Warfarin	*Ginkgo biloba*	Increased chance of bleeding
Warfarin	Vitamin K	Decreased activity of warfarin
Warfarin	Garlic	Increased chance of bleeding
Warfarin	Ginseng	Decreased activity of warfarin
Warfarin	St. John's wort	Decreased activity of warfarin
Foods		
Warfarin	Broccoli and other green vegetables or foods high in vitamin K	Decreased effect of warfarin
Warfarin	Soybean and canola oils	Altered effect of warfarin
Warfarin	Cranberry juice	Altered effect of warfarin

Warfarin Interactions

Anticoagulants, such as warfarin, have the potential for many interactions with drugs, food, and dietary or herbal supplements. Certain warfarin interactions can be deadly. Warfarin is given to prevent clots that can cause strokes or heart attacks; the prothrombin time (PT) and the international normalized ratio (INR) must be maintained at a specific level to ensure that blood clots do not form and that the patient does not bleed internally. Regular blood tests are performed to check the PT/INR level of patients taking warfarin. Examples of common warfarin interactions are shown in Table 14.4. Although warfarin has several drug-drug and drug-food interactions, many other drugs also have the potential to cause severe interactions.

Errors in the Pharmacy

No one wants to make an error, but when it does happen, negative feelings and assumptions may emerge. For example, it may seem that the person who made the mistake is careless, lazy, or untrained. Suspension or termination is a frightening event to consider; the reality that a patient suffered as a result of an error is horrible. Additional fears are the legal ramifications of lawsuits and possible public humiliation. All of these fears are in the back of the technician's mind, along with the constant need to maintain the workflow.

In fact, a pharmacy can fill 1000 prescriptions correctly, but if one error occurs, the pharmacy management will likely counsel the technician and pharmacist to "be more careful," thus placing the blame on these employees specifically. This fear of being reprimanded adds to the stress on the pharmacy staff. Many times no action is taken to review the overall process of how the mistake occurred.

Many pharmacy organizations and entities, such as MedWatch, TJC, ISMP, MERP, and others, have recognized the need to study errors in a much different light. First, the need for open error reporting without fear of retaliation is essential if the root causes of errors are to be revealed. Pharmacy staff members need to know that they will not be punished; instead, the error will be examined and new strategies may be established that make it more difficult for errors to occur. It is important to have tools that can be used for error prevention. Even then, human factor errors will occur, but the goal is to reduce them as much as possible through the knowledge of how they occur. **MedWatch** and other error-reporting agencies encourage reporting of all types of errors by both health care workers and the public. A MedWatch report can be accessed on the Internet, which makes it a simple way to report an error. (See Fig. 2.4 for an example of a MedWatch form.)

Although drug errors do not necessarily cause dire consequences for all patients, in many instances they do. In these cases, the only adequate outcome is to identify the causes of the error and establish safeguards that prevent the error from recurring. For grieving family and friends, this is of little help, and for the person or persons responsible, this is a life-changing event that can result in loss of license, penalty fines, and, in certain instances, incarceration. Examples of various errors are listed in the following sections.

Errors Related to Patient Care

Health Care–Associated Infections

Health care–associated infections (HAIs) have plagued hospitals for decades. It is estimated that at any given time, 1 in 20 inpatients has an infection related to hospital care. Most HAIs involve urinary tract infections, surgical site infections, bloodstream infections, and pneumonia. All hospitals and other institutions have infection control specialists who are responsible for training both staff members and patients as part of the investigation of all cases of HAI. However, the training from institution to institution varies widely. Using Universal Precautions (eg, hand washing) is a necessity in all institutions.

Home Health Care Errors

Many patients are discharged home with instructions for self-administration of medications or with the help of visiting nurses. This is due to rising costs associated with hospital stays. According to the 2011 IMS National Health Perspectives, home health represented a $2.8 billion retail channel for pharmaceuticals. In 2010 the Medicare Payment Advisory Commission (MedPAC) reported payments for home health totaled $19.4 billion. The home infusion industry has grown over the past few years and accounts for $9 billion to $11 billion annually.

Receiving care in the home carries the risk for improper dosing and contamination of IV sets that may ultimately cause infections. Many elderly patients and patients with disabilities do not have coverage for infusion sets and supplies because Medicare covers only the cost of medication. Self-dosing errors can increase the risk for an adverse effect. Patients may try to use medical supplies intended for single use more than once to try to save money; poor aseptic technique may increase the risk for infection.

Age-Related Errors

Medication Errors and the Elderly

More people are living into their 80s and beyond. Life expectancy in the United States has risen from 49 years (1900) to 79 years in the past century. By 2050, approximately 33% of the US population will be over age 55 and 20% will be over age 65. Individuals over age 80 will be the fastest growing segment of the population for the next 40 years. This is due to several reasons, including increased activity, better diets, and improved health care. Medication plays an important role in the longevity of people with various conditions, such as osteoporosis, cardiovascular disease, and diabetes. It is estimated that nearly half of all Americans aged 55 or older take some type of prescription drugs, and about 40% take OTC medications. Many seniors mix medications on a daily basis, and as the number of medications increases, so does the possibility of drug-drug interactions. People tend to think that any medication purchased over the counter is safe. This is a misconception, especially when these agents are mixed with prescription medications. Consideration also must be given to drug-food interactions.

Medical Errors and Pediatric Patients

Most emergency department (ED) cases relating to pediatric patients and medication (more than 66%) are due to overdosing of prescription and OTC medications. Most overdoses are primarily a result of failure to store medications in a secure area out of reach of children. In the United States alone, more than 71,000 children under age 19 are taken to the ED for unintentional overdoses of drugs kept at home. Toddlers (2-year-olds) were most likely to experience poisoning.

Pictograms and the use of plain language have been shown to reduce the possibility of parents dosing their children inappropriately. Pictograms are standardized graphics (pictures) that depict such things as how to take medication, how to store medication, and when to take medication (Fig. 14.1). Many parents in the United States have problems reading and understanding dosage instructions because of low reading levels or poor understanding of the English language. This is more prevalent in multicultural areas where English is a second language. In a study conducted in an urban public hospital ED, a control group (standard labeling information) and an intervention group (using pictograms and plain language) were studied. Both were given standard instructions by the medical staff. Results showed that parent nonadherence was lower in the intervention group (9.3%) than in the control group (38%).

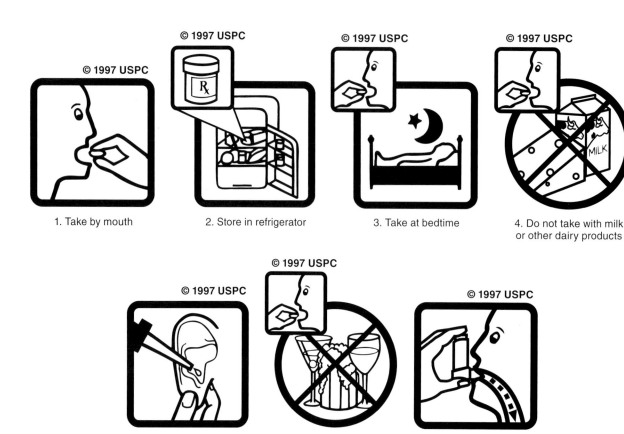

FIG. 14.1 Medication pictograms. (Courtesy US Pharmacopeial Convention.)

1. Take by mouth

2. Store in refrigerator

3. Take at bedtime

4. Do not take with milk or other dairy products

5. Place drops in ear

6. Do not drink alcohol while taking this medicine

7. Inhaler

FDA committees have also suggested the use of new labeling on certain OTC medications to ensure that parents receive proper advice before administering medications to young children. New labels read, "Do not dose children under the age of 4 years." In addition, the new labels state that a physician should be consulted for children ages 4 to 6 years. This has changed from the previous guidelines of not dosing children under 2 years of age. It is hoped that these changes in labeling (voluntarily made by manufacturers) will reduce the number of parents who administer incorrect doses or dose their children at the wrong time. In some cases parents do not use the medication for its intended purpose.

Children and infants are also at risk for drug errors in the hospital; incorrect dosing is the most commonly reported error. Dosing errors include computation errors in dosage and dosing intervals. Children vary in weight, body surface area, and organ system maturity; all of these factors affect their ability both to metabolize and excrete medication. In addition, not many standardized dosing regimens are available for children, which increases the probability of drug errors. Various causes have been identified for errors in the hospital; for example, failure to follow the procedure or protocol, miscommunication, inaccurate or omitted transcription, improper documentation, incorrect calculations, drug distribution system error, computer entry error, and lack of system safeguards.

⊙ Scenario Checkup 14.2

Jonathan is continuing to train Jennifer, the new employee. He explains to her the process for reporting medication errors in the pharmacy. Jennifer has recently read about several cases in which the technician was involved in a fatal medication error. What are some of the reasons technicians fail to report their mistakes? What are the possible consequences if errors go unreported?

Medication Errors That Involve Allergies

Although many people are aware of the medications to which they are allergic, many allergic reactions cannot be avoided before drug administration.

Allergic reactions are not always medication errors; however, many people can have an allergic reaction as a result of the physician failing to document or review the patient's allergies before prescribing medications. In one study of more than 50 patients hospitalized because of allergic reactions to medications, contributing factors to the allergic events were reported and included the following:

- Physician was not aware of allergy (41%).
- Physician did not think allergy was real (5%).
- Physician was aware of allergy but thought the benefit outweighed the risk (4%).
- Physician was not aware that the agent was in the same class of drugs (3%).

The primary reasons for allergy-related prescribing errors included workload and failure to review the patient's drug history and profile. However, on most occasions the physician was alerted about the allergies by a nurse or a pharmacist; most errors were prevented by pharmacists.

Parenteral Errors

The most frightening errors are those that take effect quickly and may not be easily reversed. This is the case with parenteral medications. Several cases of heparin and insulin overdoses have occurred. Heparin is of great concern because it is common to flush IV lines with heparin-lock solutions, which may be confused with similarly sized and labeled vials of much more concentrated heparin solutions (Fig. 14.2). In the hospital, many floors keep several different concentrations of heparin, and the labels can be confusing because they are similar in appearance. KCl solutions are also problematic. In several cases, patients have died from the administration of concentrated KCl injections by personnel who misunderstood the labeling; concentrated KCl should *never* be given undiluted. As a result of these errors, concentrated KCl has been pulled from nursing floors and is strictly regulated by the pharmacy, yet errors can still occur.

Other considerations are important when administering parenteral medications. Pharmacy technicians need to be aware of the range of normal dosages, and if an ordered dose is suspect, they must alert the pharmacist immediately. For example, if a patient with diabetes has orders for several IV medications, which are normally prepared in dextrose, this order should be suspect because of the patient's diabetic condition. The physician may not want the medication prepared in dextrose but instead may wish to use normal saline.

Sustained-Released Dosage Form Errors

The clear advantage of sustained-released (SR) medications is the ability of the patient to take his or her medication once daily rather than several times a day. This improves patient compliance and can ultimately result in better health. Directions that the dosage is in SR form are usually printed below the drug name on the manufacturer's label. If an SR medication is given in place of a regular dose, adverse effects can occur, including death. In addition, if a patient is receiving

nourishment through a feeding tube and an SR dose is crushed, it becomes an immediate release (IR) dose that is much higher in strength and can result in an adverse reaction. Many errors occur because of suffixes on drug products that are not clearly understood. According to a report from the ISMP, suffixes such as LA, CR, CD, ER, XL, and SR on drug products do not provide a clear meaning to indicate release properties or dosing frequency. The *United States Pharmacopeia* defines two categories of modified-release formulations: delayed release and extended release. Delayed release denotes a formulation that has a coating to delay release of the drug until the product has passed through the stomach. Extended release denotes any formulation designed to deliver the dose over a longer interval than an IR product of the same drug. Because of the confusion of suffixes (ie, the choice of a wrong suffix, the use of an unclear suffix, or the omission of a proper suffix during prescribing or dispensing), one form of drug may be given in place of the proper drug product.

Necessity of Reporting Errors

Pharmacist's Daily Routine

Most pharmacies are located in the retail setting, and most pharmacists are overworked on a daily basis. Many pharmacies fill as many as 300 to 400 prescriptions a day; the workload also includes addressing discrepancies in orders and counseling patients. In addition, pharmacists must check the work of technicians.

The limited time that a rushed pharmacist has to check technicians' work adds to the potential for errors. Another potentially dangerous situation arises when the same pharmacists and technicians work together for a long time. After pharmacists have worked many years with the same technicians, a bond of trust may develop, and pharmacists may become complacent about checking the technicians' work, either not checking it at all or just quickly scanning the completed order.

Computerized Prescription Order Entry

Many new systems are available that can help reduce errors. Many physicians use e-prescribing from the physician's office to the pharmacy or computerized physician order entry (CPOE) by the prescriber in institutional settings. The idea behind this type of ordering (ie, electronic ordering) is that it circumvents having to decipher poor handwriting because orders are sent by computer directly to the pharmacy. However, many physicians and institutions have not yet accepted this type of ordering. It should be noted that even when the CPOE system is used, errors can still be made; selecting the wrong drug or dose from drop-down menus is still possible. In addition, introducing new technology often results in the introduction of new types of possible errors. More insurance companies and government-funded plans are pressuring physicians to use e-prescribing to be eligible for bonus payments. However, adoption of the technology can be costly, and in some cases state or federal laws have not allowed for full adoption of e-prescribing in all circumstances (eg, allowing

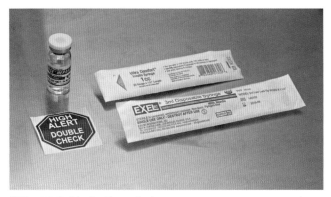

FIG. 14.2 Medications that are more error prone may have specific stickers as recommended by the Institute for Safe Medication Practices.

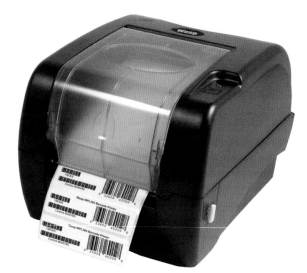

FIG. 14.3 WPL305 desktop bar code printer. (Courtesy Wasp Barcode Technologies.)

the prescription of controlled substances). Data transmission standards must be agreed on and adhered to by all technologies to ensure proper communication between devices and computer databases.

In hospitals and other inpatient institutions, the use of CPOE is becoming more popular, along with bar coding methods (Fig. 14.3). Bar codes provide the following three forms of identification of a drug:

1. National Drug Code
2. Lot number of the drug
3. Expiration date of the drug

Although the overall risk for errors is reduced by the use of CPOE, these systems are not 100% error free. Concerns have arisen about the lack of evaluation of their effectiveness because many different types are marketed. Potential dangers in certain CPOE systems include the facts that the computerized software does not recognize discrepancies in prescribing between the outpatient medication regimen and the hospital treatment plan, and many systems do not require prescribers to address computer alerts.

Other concerns pertaining to CPOE systems include ordering and administration problems (eg, misidentification of patients and patient variables, such as height and weight) and mismatching of drug orders to chemotherapy protocols or miscalculations.

The problems with these systems are due to the newness of the technology. It takes time to address the flaws, which may be why many hospitals are slow to implement these systems. It is very time-consuming to electronically connect all the necessary personnel and still ensure that patient confidentiality is maintained. In addition, it takes time to understand new steps introduced into the health care professional's workflow. For example, after seeing their patients, physicians can sit at a computer or use a handheld device to enter new or changed orders and send them directly to the pharmacy. Nurses may also enter additional nursing notes that are documented in the system.

Tech Note!

Pharmacy employees need to know they will not be punished; instead, the error will be examined and new strategies will be established to ensure that errors are reduced in the future. It is important to have an error prevention plan in place. The goal is to reduce mistakes as much as possible using the knowledge of how they occur.

Reporting Errors

The most important aspect of dealing with errors is the reporting process. In years past, the most common response to an error was to place blame on the person who caused it and then tell the person to be more careful. This type of response was found to be nonproductive because most people will not report errors if they know they will be reprimanded. In addition, "trying to be more careful" does not give the person the tools necessary to avoid further errors. Therefore an emphasis on finding the causes of mistakes and ways to reduce errors has been found to be more productive. For this reason, the tracking systems in place do not target blame but rather focus more on how the error occurred. Thus the reasons an error occurred can be examined and constructive changes can be made and tracked. Examples of organizations that track medication errors in this way are listed in Box 14.3.

The ISMP tracks drug errors and works toward reducing them through MERP. MERP can be accessed on the Internet at *https://www.ismp.org/orderforms/reporterrortoismp.asp*, where health care workers can report errors, near-errors, or hazardous conditions in the workplace. When reporting incidents, questions concerning how the error was discovered and recommendations for preventing recurrence of the error are included in the report (an error report form can be found at *https://www.ismp.org/form/cmerp-form*). Confusion over LASA or similar packaging can cause errors. Other specific incidents or errors to be reported include the following:

- Administering the wrong:
  - Drug, dose, strength, route, or dosage form or using the wrong route of administration

BOX 14.3 Organizations That Track Medication Errors

- FDA MedWatch
- Food and Drug Administration (FDA) Adverse Event Reporting System (FAERS)
- Institute for Safe Medication Practices (ISMP)
- National Academy of Medicine
- National Coordinating Council for Medication Error Reporting and Prevention (NCCMERP)
- The Joint Commission (TJC)
- US FDA and Centers for Disease Control and Prevention (CDC)
- *United States Pharmacopeia* (USP) Medication Errors Reporting Program and MedMARx

- Errors in:
  - Dispensing medications
  - Monitoring medications
  - Performing calculations
  - Preparing medications
  - Prescribing medications
  - Transcribing medications
  MERP recommendations include the following:
- *Medication error understanding:* Improves the collection, classification, and analysis of data linked to types, causes, and sources of error and the impact of errors on patients. Tracking medication errors in a systematic manner and prioritizing reduction activities are also included.
- *Medication error reporting:* Increases awareness of reporting systems available, such as MERP, **MedMARx,** and MedWatch (FDA). These programs maintain a classification system that identifies types of errors; the data obtained can then be used to analyze and report error statistics.
- *Medication error prevention:* With continuous research and reporting, areas can be identified in which changes can be made to prevent future errors. This includes distinctive packaging, labeling, and nomenclature for drugs that are at high risk for errors.

Reporting can be done anonymously and voluntarily without fear of retribution. MERP institute reviews all medication error reports, attempts to understand the reason or reasons for errors, and works toward producing initiatives to educate health care workers and improve medication safety. The following five guidelines are used to share information with health care professionals about potentially dangerous events:

1. Knowledge
2. Analysis (the evaluation of data)
3. Education
   - Providing confidential consulting services to health care systems to proactively evaluate medication systems
   - Educational programs that include:
     - Teleconferences on medications and issues
     - Patient resources (eg, posters, pamphlets, videos, books)
     - High-alert drugs (newsletter) and potentially dangerous abbreviations
4. Cooperation
   - Working with other entities:
     - Health care institutions
     - Health care practitioners
     - Legislative and regulatory bodies
     - Pharmaceutical industry
     - Regulatory and accrediting agencies
5. Communication
   - Bringing information to:
     - Consumers
     - Employers
     - Health care providers
   - Providing a voluntary reporting program

In 2012 the ISMP launched the National Vaccine Error Reporting Program (ISMP VERP) to capture the unique causes and consequences of vaccine-related errors. Health care practitioners from all areas can report a vaccine error by logging onto the website *http://verp.ismp.org.* All reports submitted to this website are shared with the FDA. Errors in vaccine administration are common, but few data are available as to why they occur. It is hoped that this new reporting system will produce valuable data in the fight to reduce errors.

Tech Note!

One area of concern is the use of abbreviations. Many have been misinterpreted, which has resulted in drug errors. The Institute for Safe Medication Practices (ISMP) has provided a list of terms to be avoided (see Table 5.2); they recommend that the term be spelled out completely.

TJC is another organization that helps institutions implement safety standards to reduce errors. TJC's five areas (each having 10 criteria) for ensuring patient safety are summarized as follows:

1. *Leadership process and accountability:* The leadership structure, individual accountability, policies and procedures (in all areas), and the managing of daily operations are identified. The institution is compliant with all laws and regulations. Leaders are educated about quality and are actively involved in setting quality and safety priorities. Leaders and managers collaborate on quality and patient safety activities (eg, patient assessments, medication use systems). The organization provides a mechanism based on the safety of the patient, as it relates to any type of drug research and/or organ transplantation that may take place, through data collection, analysis, and improvement.
2. *Competent and capable workforce:* Personnel files contain the credentials of all employees (eg, education, training, licensure, work history, and copies of evaluations). Personnel job descriptions match the worker's credentials. Proper training is given in areas including cardiopulmonary resuscitation (CPR), basic life support (BLS), infection prevention, and safety. Staff health and safety standards are met, and accurate patient records are reviewed and transferred to the appropriate unit or nurse. The credentials, licensure, education, training, and competence of physicians are reviewed. Nurses' ability to provide appropriate patient services, based on their competence, licensure, training, and education, is reviewed. The credentials of other health professionals are reviewed. Health care students in the institution are adequately monitored, supervised, and oriented to patient safety.
3. *Safe environment for staff and patients:* The institution has regular safety inspections of the building's environment (eg, broken furniture, faulty equipment, and missing signs) and ensures fire safety measures (ie, must work properly, exits not blocked). Water quality and electrical sources required 24 hours a day, 7 days a week work properly; alternative source plans are in place to ensure the safety of patients. All biomedical equipment and biohazardous materials are properly used and maintained. Education, training, and

certification (if applicable) of employees in infection prevention and control is ensured, including proper disposal of needles and infectious wastes. A hand hygiene program with documented guidelines is followed. Reduction of HAIs is achieved through proper implementation of a hand hygiene program and barrier techniques (eg, gloves, masks, eye protection).

4. *Clinical care of patients:* The patient's identification is checked before medication, blood products, treatments, or procedures are administered. Patients understand the risks, treatments, and procedures before giving consent. Medical and nursing assessments are documented in the patient's record in a reasonable time frame so that treatment can take place as soon as possible. Laboratory and diagnostic services are available, reliable, and safe. Consent forms are completed for all treatments and/or procedures. Patient education and training are provided so that patients can participate in their own care (eg, granting consent during hospitalization and learning proper medication use after discharge). All services (eg, surgery, anesthesia, postsurgical unit) are appropriate to the patient's needs.

5. *Improving quality and safety:* An adverse event reporting system is in place, and the system is analyzed. Changes are made to increase patient safety based on causes of adverse events; these include medication errors, unanticipated death of a patient, surgery on the wrong patient or body part, and patient falls. High-risk patients are monitored (eg, immunosuppressed, comatose, emergency care patients). Patient and staff satisfaction is monitored in the facility for improvement purposes. A complaint process is in place for both patients and family members. Staff members understand how to improve processes by participating in improvement activities. Clinical outcomes are monitored and improved if necessary. Quality and safety information is communicated to staff members (eg, through newsletters, reports, and posters) to improve patient safety.

A primary responsibility of TJC is to review documentation that tracks progress in each of these areas. For a comprehensive outline of the five safety standards, visit the website *http://www.jointcommission.org.*

Strategies for Reducing Errors

As we have learned, many factors contribute to medication errors. Each pharmacy should develop a system designed to strengthen its medication management practices and help reduce the number of preventable medication errors. The ISMP has launched the 2014–2015 Targeted Medication Safety Best Practices for Hospitals to help identify and reduce medication errors that recur despite repeated warnings. These best practices provide strategies for error prevention and target a group of six key safety issues.

ISMP's 2014–2015 targeted medication safety best practices for hospitals are as follows:

BEST PRACTICE 1: Dispense vincristine (and other vinca alkaloids) in a minibag of a compatible solution and not in a syringe.

BEST PRACTICE 2
  a. Use a weekly dosage regimen default for oral methotrexate. If the prescription is changed to a daily regimen, require a hard stop verification of an appropriate oncologic indication.
  b. Provide patient education by a pharmacist for all weekly oral methotrexate discharge orders.

BEST PRACTICE 3: Measure and express patient weights in metric units only. Ensure that scales used for weighing patients are set and measure only in metric units.

BEST PRACTICE 4: Ensure that all oral liquids that are not commercially available as unit dose are dispensed by the pharmacy in an oral syringe.

BEST PRACTICE 5: Purchase oral liquid dosing devices (oral syringes/cups/droppers) that display only the metric scale.

BEST PRACTICE 6: Eliminate glacial acetic acid from all areas of the hospital.

Common Pharmacy Technology

Bar Codes

Another part of the medication safety plan for hospitals involves the use of bar coding technology (see Fig. 14.3). Bar codes provide the following three forms of identification of a drug:

1. National Drug Code
2. Lot number of the drug
3. Expiration date of the drug

Although electronic communication among physician, pharmacy, and nursing reduces the number of errors, the system does have some problems. For example, if the nurse scans an alternative dose strength (eg, two 5-mg tablets are substituted for one 10-mg tablet), the system reads this as an error. The nurse must then override the computer to administer the medication.

◎ Scenario Checkup 14.3

Today Jonathan is restocking the ROBOT-Rx. The regular robot filler is out sick. Jonathan has been cross-trained in many positions. His supervisors consider him a very valuable employee. Jennifer is still shadowing Jonathan during her orientation process. She has heard that sometimes these automated machines take the place of technicians, eliminating certain jobs. Is this a true statement? What are the advantages and disadvantages of automation in the pharmacy?

Robot-Rx Machines

Large robotic machines have been used for many years in some hospitals. Patient medication records are read by the machine through the use of bar coding; the appropriate medication's bar code is scanned from the package and then matched to the electronic medication administration record (E-MAR). Once the bar code has been verified, the machine (Fig. 14.4) pulls from a rack of prepackaged unit dose medications stored in the unit. The medications are placed in a patient envelope and are delivered to the appropriate floor. These large fillers are expensive and require a large area to function.

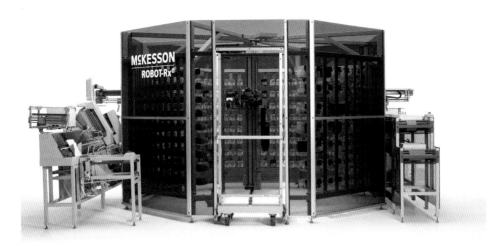

FIG. 14.4 ROBOT-Rx machine. (Image courtesy Omnicell Inc.)

Hospital Pharmacy Automated Dispensing System Machines

Automated dispensing system (ADS) machines have been used for years in hospitals and institutions. ADS machines store unit-dosed medications and nursing supplies to be accessed by nurses on patient floors. The pharmacy receives an order and enters it into the ADS computer, which then allows the nurse to access the medication using the patient's name. These systems work effectively if the medication in the drawer is correct; if the wrong medication is loaded into the drawer and the nurse fails to catch the mistake, an error can occur. However, coupling this system with bar coding greatly reduces the risk for errors. Each cubicle has an attached bar code that identifies the medication; when the technician attempts to fill the cubicle, he or she must match the bar code on the cubicle to the bar code on the medication. The nurse can then use the bar code to match the drug to the patient.

Another type of automated dispensing machine is the MedCarousel. The MedCarousel is a vertical, automated storage and retrieval system for medications in hospital pharmacies. MedCarousel automates medication dispensing and inventory control with its rotating shelves, pick-to-light technology, and forced compliance bar code scanning process (Fig. 14.5).

Community Pharmacy Automated Dispensing Systems

For many years ADS machines have been used in community pharmacies. They are available in many different sizes to accommodate the prescription load. Barcoding is used to verify that the correct dosage is dispensed to the correct patient. The following three main types of ADS are used in community pharmacies:

- *Tabletop automatic pill counters* (eg, model KL20 by Kirby Lester [Fig. 14.6]): These devices are used for counting and verifying every order. The device instructs the technician to first scan the patient's prescription label and then to scan the bottle of medication to ensure a match (of medication, dosage, and quantity to be dispensed). The

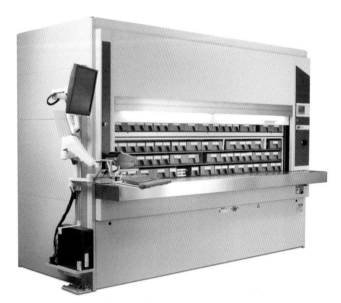

FIG. 14.5 Omnicell's MedCarousel. (Image courtesy Omnicell Inc.)

device's touch screen displays a picture of the medication and specific information about the drug. The tablets or capsules are poured into a hopper and are counted electronically. The device estimates the correct vial size (in drams) to use. The medication is then dispensed into a tray, and the technician pours its contents into a vial. A technician can fill a typical prescription with a KL20 device in 3 to 6 seconds.

- *Large wall units that use cassettes* (eg, Baker Cell systems): The number of cassettes is limited only by the wall space available, and each cassette holds an assortment of preloaded medications. Again, the bar code on the prescription label is scanned, and the appropriate amount is then dispensed. The pharmacist then scans the bottle for a final check. A screen displays the correct appearance of the medication, along with specific information on the drug.

- *Robot technology* (eg, the SP 200 System by ScriptPro [Fig. 14.7]): This system is a fully automated robotic prescription dispensing system. It accepts prescription dispensing instructions from pharmacy computers

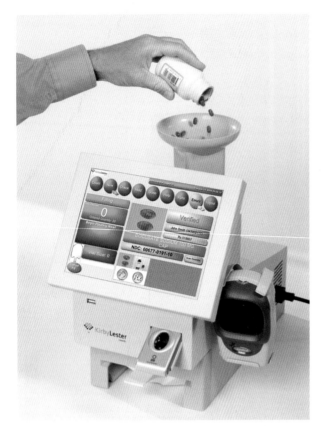

FIG. 14.6 KL20. (Courtesy Kirby Lester.)

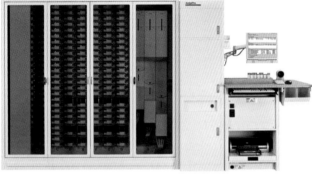

FIG. 14.7 SP 200 robotic prescription dispensing system. (Courtesy ScriptPro.)

and delivers filled and labeled vials at a rate of up to 100 prescriptions per hour.

Many types of community pharmacy ADS and software programs are available, although they are very expensive and require training to use. More pharmacies use these systems so that they can fill more prescriptions in less time and concurrently reduce errors.

● Technician Profile

Mark is a level 2 technician at a large hospital. He has worked in the pharmacy for 8 years. When the pharmacy management began installing robots to help fill patient medications, he was among the first to apply for the new position of robot filler. Mark received extensive

training on how to load these million-dollar machines and how to keep them running smoothly. The automated systems allowed the pharmacy to fill more orders in less time and reduce errors. Mark's position requires an individual who is technologically savvy, has an eye for detail, and is a problem solver. Machines break down, and glitches occur on a regular basis. It is the filler's job to know how to get the operation back on track. Mark reports directly to the pharmacy manager and works with each department to maintain adequate supplies and timely delivery of medications.

Patient Dose-Specific Orders

In the past, when patients required a large amount of liquids over a 24-hour period, a bulk bottle was placed in the patient's drawer. Also, if the liquid was not available in unit dose form, it was sent in bulk form. The nurse poured the proper amount per the MAR and used the liquid until the bottle was empty. The nurse then sent a refill request to the pharmacy. The bottles were sometimes labeled with just the patient's name and room number. Because specific dosing instructions were not noted on the bottle, there was an increased likelihood that the nurse might dose the liquid medication inappropriately. Also, opening and closing lids can increase the risk for contamination of a medication. The pharmacy must have control over each dose to ensure accuracy. TJC requires hospitals and institutions to prepackage all liquid doses in oral syringes or containers. Each dose is prepared by the technician and is labeled with the patient's name, medical record number, and room number. In addition, the name of the drug, dose, strength, and time of administration are indicated on each dose. In this way, each dose is strictly controlled by the pharmacy. Automated robots can also fill and label doses, reducing the time needed by a technician to fill daily doses.

United States Pharmacopeia <797> Regulations

One of the regulations established by *United States Pharmacopeia (USP) Convention* <797> addresses the problem of contamination of any type of sterile product. The adoption of USP <797> has been one of the most dramatic changes for any pharmacy that prepares sterile products, such as IV solutions and other parenteral medications. Because of the new regulations, many pharmacies are contracting their sterile preparations to companies that specialize in this area and have met all guidelines of USP <797>. Chapter 12 lists specifics of USP <797> regulations.

Medication safety is the responsibility of all pharmacy personnel. For any safety system to succeed, there must be an effective leader at the helm. ASHP has identified this role as the medication safety leader. This person is most often a pharmacist and is looked to as an expert on safe medication use. The medication safety leader usually reports to the risk management department or senior administrator; these individuals lead the team in developing strategies for reducing errors.

To reduce errors, pharmacists can do the following:

- Check prescriptions carefully and thoroughly.
- Initial checked prescriptions.
- Document all clarifications made to any orders.
- Visually check the product in the bottle.
- Counsel all patients with new prescriptions.
- Report all errors or adverse events.

To reduce errors, pharmacy technicians can do the following:

- Refer any questions regarding illegible handwriting or ambiguous orders to the pharmacist immediately.
- Triple-count controlled substances.
- Double-check dosage calculations with the pharmacist.
- Keep the work area free of clutter.
- Always keep the prescription and the label together during the filling process.
- Check the drug three times: when removing the medication from the stock, after placing the medication in the prescription bottle, and before returning the medication bottle to the stock.
- Observe and report to the pharmacist any pertinent OTC purchases made by patients.

To reduce errors, pharmacies can do the following:

- Use automated filling systems.
- Scan the original prescription.
- Use electronic prescribing.
- Keep high-alert medications in a separate location in the pharmacy.
- Maintain accurate, up-to-date patient profiles that include OTC and herbal medications.
- Designate a medication safety leader.
- Continually review medication safety policies and procedures, especially with new staff members.
- Encourage error reporting by employees, focusing on change, not punishment.

Medication Reconciliation

Medication reconciliation is another strategy to prevent patient harm. Strong reconciliation practices can play an important role in the reduction of medication-related events. The **Institute for Healthcare Improvement (IHI)** has defined medication reconciliation as the process of identifying the most up-to-date list of all the medications a patient is currently taking. The IHI reported that more than 50% of all errors in hospitals are due to poor communication of medication orders. The necessary information required to clearly analyze a patient's needs includes the following:

- Name of drug
- Dosage
- Frequency
- Route of administration

Reconciliation needs to be performed in all pharmacy settings, although each type of pharmacy must develop its own specific strategies. In all settings, it is important to compare the current list of medications with the patient's electronic profile or any other medication history available. This should include the patient's profile in a community setting or in the institutional setting at the time of admission, at the time of any transfer within the facility, after surgeries, and at the time

of discharge. The goal is to ensure that the patient is given the proper medications at all points and understands the importance of medication adherence. Intervention and counseling should also include lifestyle choices and the long-term benefits of wellness and disease management through prevention. Continuous monitoring of the patient's medications can help errors be identified promptly. The steps involved in completing a medication reconciliation are shown in Procedure 14.1.

Reconciliation involves several parties: the patient, physician, nurse, and pharmacist and technician. Orders must be rewritten each time the patient is transferred to or from the intensive care unit or returns from surgery. In the past, physicians would sometimes write "resume previous medications." This allowed misinterpretation of the medications being dosed. It was much easier to lose track of the medications the patient was taking. This resulted in ADRs and possible harm to the patient. TJC has since prohibited the use of these "blanket orders." At each point throughout the course of treatment, the previous medications must be compared with the current orders. Normally, facilities use a reconciliation form (Fig. 14.8)

Procedure 14.1

Medication Reconciliation

Goal

To understand the steps required to complete a medication reconciliation form (the goal is to ensure that the patient is given the correct medication at all points as he or she moves through the health care system).

Equipment and Supplies

- Medication reconciliation form

Procedural Steps[a]

1. *Verification:* Obtain the patient's medication history and other medical information. This includes all medications, over-the-counter drugs, and herbal remedies.
   PURPOSE: It is critical to have the patient medication history to prevent any drug interactions, contraindications, or therapeutic duplications.
2. *Clarification:* Make sure the medications and dosages are appropriate for the patient. The current physician's orders are compared with the patient's medication list.
   PURPOSE: It is important to clarify the medications are within the acceptable dosage range for the patient; otherwise the patient may be harmed.
3. *Reconciliation:* Clinical decisions are made based on the comparison between the two drug lists. Resolving any observed discrepancies or errors through documentation and direct communication is the final step.
   PURPOSE: This is done to ensure the patient receives the optimum care and no drug interactions or therapeutic duplications of medications are overlooked.

[a]These steps are usually performed by a nurse and may be reviewed by the physician, another nurse, pharmacist, or trained pharmacy technician.

MEDICATION RECONCILIATION FORM

ADMISSION / POINT OF ENTRY RECONCILIATION
▪ The first nurse to interview the patient should initiate completion of this form. Additional nurses and clinicians may continue to use the same form for the same patient.
▪ Circle all sources of information:　　Patient　Caregiver　Rx bottle　EMS　Primary provider　Other:_____

ALLERGIES AND ADVERSE DRUG REACTIONS : _____

ACTIVE MEDICATION LIST			Date of Admission / Point of Entry:				RECONCILIATION
List below all medications patient was taking at time of admission. *(Dosing information REQUIRED, if available.)*							Continue on Admission?
Medication Name	Dose	Route	Frequency	Last Dose (Date/Time)	Date	Initials	Circle **Y** (yes) *or* **N** (no)*
1.							Y　N
2.							Y　N
3.							Y　N
4.							Y　N
5.							Y　N
6.							Y　N
7.							Y　N
8.							Y　N
9.							Y　N
10.							Y　N
11.							Y　N
12.							Y　N
13.							Y　N
14.							Y　N
15.							Y　N
OTC Medications, Herbals, etc.							
							Y　N
							Y　N
							Y　N
							Y　N

*If order to be discontinued, see Admitting Note for comments.

Medication list recorded by RN/MD/PA/NP/LPN/RPh							
Initials	Print Name/Stamp	Signature	Date	Initials	Print Name/Stamp	Signature	Date

Reconciling Prescriber (MD/PA/NP/CNM)			
Print Name/Stamp	Signature	Title	Date

TRANSFER RECONCILIATION	DISCHARGE RECONCILIATION
▪ See Physician Orders for active medication orders upon transfer. ▪ See Medication Administration Record for last dose given.	▪ See Patient Discharge Plan for list of medications patient should continue after discharge. ▪ Discharge plan should include stopped medications.
Reconciling Prescriber (Provide name, date, signature.)	**Reconciling Prescriber (Provide name, date, signature.)**

☐　Check here if multiple pages needed. Please indicate: Page ____ of ____

Pilot Number 2/06

FIG. 14.8 Example of a reconciliation form.

that can be viewed by the entire health care team. In addition, at the time of discharge, the community pharmacy must perform reconciliation. Finally, the patient must be informed about the current instructions compared with any previous instructions. Many resources are available to help pharmacies develop a strong medication reconciliation program. Some examples are given in the website list at the end of the chapter.

> ### Tech Note!
>
> Always include all medications, including over-the-counter (OTC) and herbal products on the medication reconciliation report because they have side effects and interactions. Patients will often forget or not consider them as "medications" when reporting because they are thinking only about prescriptions. A good practice is to ask for "any medications they are taking" and remind them of OTC and herbal products.

Quality Assurance Practices and Risk Management

Quality assurance is most important when preparing medications, and factors such as workflow, physical environment, equipment, and working conditions can affect the accuracy of the daily tasks performed.

Good practices are essential to prevent errors. These quality assurance measures include the following:

- Avoid or question abbreviations that are uncommon or on TJC's "do not use" list.
- Double count opioids.
- Keep the prescription, bulk bottle, and filled bottle together for verification.
- Use a leading zero.
- Write legibly and neatly.
- Keep areas specific to the task; for example, prescriptions already verified by the pharmacists as "ready" should be separated from the "prescriptions to be prepared or filled."
- Use different storage and/or shelving and posted warning signs for LASA or special medications.
- Use technology such as bar code scanning to verify bar code numbers.
- Inspect fire extinguishers and first aid kits.
- Routinely clean facilities.

Risk Management

In addition to good practices, there are reporting systems, physical factors, and equipment considerations that can prevent errors. Programs such as MedWatch, FDA Adverse Event Reporting System (FAERS), VAERS, and MERP and even recalls are designed to report, alert, or track errors in an effort to prevent future occurrences.

> ### Tech Note!
>
> Often the technician is the first to identify an error, and without reporting or responding with a preventive way to stop the event from happening, the errors will continue to occur. Never be afraid to report for fear of punishment.

Institutional documentation, in the form of policies and procedures, is also a way to prevent errors. These documents are often reports and follow-up discussions of ways to improve processes and may change procedures that may have resulted in errors. Physical environment factors, such as specific task areas (workflow), use and locations of first aid or fire safety equipment, running hot and cold water, eye wash stations, and traffic control, can eliminate errors. Personnel should be aware of the physical environment and policies that control the areas or equipment.

Good working equipment such as laminar flow hoods, scales, hot plates, and even counting trays can affect the quality of the work being performed in the pharmacy; for instance, scales and balances must be calibrated periodically to ensure the most accurate measurement. Laminar air flow hoods must be inspected and cleaned periodically to prevent microorganism growth and subsequent patient infections because of product contamination. Other risk management practices and guidelines can include policies for needle recapping, use of sharps containers, and using safety data sheet (SDS) information.

Knowing communication routes inside the organization and being cross-trained also can be beneficial to technicians in preventing errors. Often teams are designated to review errors, and as a technician, there is much input that you can provide in planning and evaluating daily work. Being multiskilled and recognizing possible improvements in a process are invaluable for more efficient work and safer patient care.

> ### Tech Note!
>
> As a new hire in a pharmacy, it is your responsibility to review the policies and procedures of the facility. These will outline safety policies, employee and employer responsibilities, and other organizational procedures related to everyday practices.

Other Considerations

Other conditions that can help reduce errors when filling prescriptions include using good lighting to clearly read the label and checking the drug against the prescription. Also, filling protocol systems must be reviewed and altered if they can potentially cause an error. Reducing the fear and anxiety of reporting errors should be implemented in all medical settings. Each prescription should be checked several times to ensure that it is correct. Physicians should use the metric system when writing doses. In the future, all prescriptions should be electronic rather than written because this greatly improves clarity. Software systems must be improved to aid the pharmacy in identifying potential problems with dosing regimens.

Training and Education

One of the best ways to reduce errors is through training and education. Many states do not have standardized examinations or use the national examination to pretest technicians. Some states do not even fingerprint or conduct a background check on pharmacy technicians. Many schools with pharmacy technician programs are not accredited and do not have standards of learning. Many large pharmacies train their own employees to become technicians. The Pharmacy Technician Certification Board (PTCB) and ASHP have worked toward implementing training standards, and organizations such as the **Society for the Education of Pharmacy Technicians (SEPhT)** promote education and training before and after certification. In addition to obtaining certification, it is important for the technician to consistently self-educate through staff meetings, continuing education, and journal reports.

Beyond certification and continuous training, technicians should always check each prescription three times throughout the filling process. If anything about the prescription seems unclear or confusing, the pharmacist should be notified immediately. There are also specialty certifications offered for certified pharmacy technicians such as Medication History through PTCB that can prepare technicians for advanced roles in medication reconciliation processes.

Conclusion

There are no simple solutions for preventing medication mistakes. However, through consistent monitoring and evaluation, the number of errors can be greatly reduced. The technician must approach each action taken in the pharmacy and other medication settings as requiring 100% commitment to the goal of perfection. Accurate interpretation of drugs and drug orders can mean the difference between life and death to a patient. Reporting drug errors can help instigate a change in the current protocol of a pharmacy that can prevent further errors of the same type. Technicians play an integral part in helping to identify and prevent errors. Participating in risk management and quality assurance programs or teams allows the technician to participate in the improvement processes on a daily basis. Knowing the guidelines for physical environments, safety, and equipment requirements should be aligned with good work practices and proper training.

Although the electronic software and hardware systems in pharmacies, institutions, physicians' offices, and clinics help reduce errors, these systems can malfunction. The ability to catch mistakes before they occur will always be the responsibility of the personnel involved in the prescribing, filling, and dosing of medications. For this reason, it is imperative that every health care worker view drug error prevention as a priority. Only through continuous

education and training can errors be controlled, now and in the future. A summary of practices that can be used to reduce the occurrence of medication errors is presented in Box 14.4.

BOX 14.4 Methods for Avoiding Errors in the Pharmacy

- Altering system factors (eg, clutter, lighting, workflow, distractions, interruptions, poorly designed procedures, stress, fear of reporting errors)
- Automatic dispensing system (ADS) machines
- Barcoding
- Color coding
- Computerized physician order entry (CPOE) systems
- Education
- Medication name alerts
- Medication reconciliation
- Patient dose-specific repackaging
- Pharmacy robots
- Software systems used for identification
- Tall man lettering
- Training

Do You Remember These Key Points?

- The five patient rights
- What constitutes an error
- Different types of medication errors
- The main causes of drug errors
- Where to report an adverse drug event
- The organization or groups that track and report medication errors
- The quality assurance and risk management strategies that pharmacies, pharmacists, and pharmacy technicians can use to reduce medication errors
- The types of automated systems used to reduce drug errors
- How CPOE can reduce the number of confusing drug orders
- The role of training and education in reducing medication errors

---

Scenario Follow-Up

Jonathan finishes training Jennifer and congratulates her on a job well done. He feels confident that she will work to prevent errors and promote patient safety. He understands the importance of education and knowledge in the quest to eliminate medication errors. Because of the implementation of the tech-check-tech system, he has come to realize that he plays an important role in maintaining high standards for order accuracy and patient care. He is proud of the trust his pharmacists have in his abilities, and he is determined to do his best at all times.

Multiple Choice Questions

1. Which of the following is *not* an example of a medication error?
   A. Giving the patient a medication intended for someone else
   B. Giving a chewable tablet instead of a liquid at the patient's request
   C. Giving a generic medication when the physician prescribed a brand name medication and signed "no substitutions"
   D. Giving a nitroglycerin patch when the intended route was nitroglycerin sublingual
2. What is the first step a pharmacy technician should take on detecting a medication error?
   A. Notify the patient.
   B. Notify the physician.
   C. Alert the pharmacist.
   D. Alert the lead pharmacy technician.
3. REMS is a strategy used to manage known and potential serious risks of a drug or biological product. The FDA requires REMS to ensure that the benefits of a drug outweigh its risks. What does the acronym REMS stand for?
   A. Registered emergency medication system
   B. Risk evaluation and mitigation strategy
   C. Risk event monitoring strategy
   D. Registered emergency monitoring system
4. Which of the following does the Institute for Safe Medication Practices (ISMP) consider to be a high-alert medication?
   A. IV oxytocin
   B. IM oxytocin
   C. Oral OxyContin
   D. All of the above
5. When dispensing medication, it is critical to remember the five rights of medication safety. What are the five rights?
   A. Right name, right date of birth, right address, right medication, right route
   B. Right quantity, right refills, right time, right date, right patient
   C. Right patient, right route, right time, right quantity, right dose
   D. Right patient, right time, right route, right dose, right medication
6. Which strategy to reduce errors would label bupropion and buspirone as buPROPion and busPIRone on the pharmacy shelf?
   A. Strategic inventory management (SIM)
   B. Tall man lettering
   C. Risk evaluation and mitigation strategy (REMS)
   D. Inventory bar coding strategy (IBS)
7. Which of the following are used in error reporting?
   A. MERP
   B. REMS
   C. ADS
   D. All of the above
8. All of the following are examples of risk management initiatives except:
   A. Using a sharps container
   B. Using the SDS sheets to verify chemical components
   C. Recapping needles using the one-handed method
   D. Double counting opioids
9. Which of the following is *not* an ADS?
   A. Kirby Lester
   B. ROBOT-Rx
   C. CPOE
   D. MedCarousel
10. Which organization oversees MedWatch?
    A. ISMP
    B. ASHP
    C. TJC
    D. FDA

◼ Technician's Corner

What is your opinion of the criminalization of medication errors? Read the article by Jesse Vivian, "Criminalization of Medication Errors," at the website *http://www.uspharmacist. com/content/d/pharmacy%20law/c/16572/*. Discuss with your classmates and instructor what you think is the proper punishment for technicians and pharmacists who are involved in medication errors. Research your state laws on this topic and any cases that have recently been brought before your state board of pharmacy.

References

Anderson P. Preventing high-alert medication errors in hospital patients. May 2015. Available at: https://www.americannursetoday.com/preventing-high-alert-medication-errors/.

Emily Jerry Foundation. Emily's story. Available at: https://emilyjerryfoundation.org/emilys-story/.

Hodges DW. Walgreens pharmacy lawsuit for medication errors. Available at: http://www.pharmacyerrorlawfirm.com/news/walgreens-pharmacy-lawsuit-for-medication-errors20110914.cfm.

Skerrett PJ. Multitasking: a medical and mental hazard (blog post). *Harvard Health Blog*; 2012. Available at: http://www.health.harvard.edu/blog/multitasking-a-medical-and-mental-hazard-201201074063.

Tariq RA, Vashisht R, Sinha A, et al. Medication dispensing errors and prevention. [Updated 2023 Feb 26]. In: *StatPearls [Internet]*. Treasure Island, FL: StatPearls Publishing; 2023. Available at: https://www.ncbi.nlm.nih.gov/books/NBK519065/ is not included in the bibliography.

Bibliography

Aesynt. MedCarousel: increases accuracy and efficiency of medication dispensing and inventory management; 2013. Available at: http://aesynt.com/medcarousel.

American Society of Hospital Pharmacies. Guidelines on preventing medication errors in hospitals. Available at: https://www.ashp.org/-/media/assets/policy-guidelines/docs/guidelines/preventing-medication-errors-hospitals.ashx.

Anderson P, Anthony L. *Home Infusion Enhances Specialty Pharmaceutical Distribution.* Pharmaceutical Commerce; 2012. Available at: pharmaceuticalcommerce.com.

Arthur D, Cacchione J, Farrell B, et al. Health forum: hospital-acquired infections—leadership challenges. Panel discussion. *Hosp Health Netw.* 2008;82:56.

Ballantyne C. Mystery solved: polo ponies probably died of selenium overdose | Scientific American.

Bates DW. Sustained-release preparations and medication errors. *J Gen Intern Med.* 2002;17:657. Available at: http://www.ncbi.nlm.nih.gov/pmc/articles/PMC1495086/.

Binder L. The shocking truth about medication errors. Forbes (blog post); 2013. Available at: http://www.forbes.com/sites/leahbinder/2013/09/03/the-shocking-truth-about-medication-errors/.

Centers for Disease Control and Prevention. Get smart for healthcare.

Drug Shortages the Worst in 30 Years, ISMP Reports. Available at: https://www.pharmacytimes.com

Hendrick B. Sleep apnea, daytime sleepiness: risky combo. WebMD Health News; 2011.

Hodes RJ. *Fiscal Year 2014 Budget Request: Statement for the Record. Senate Subcommittee on Labor–HHS–Education Appropriations.* Department of Health and Human Services and National Institutes of Health; 2013. Available at: https://www.nih.gov/sites/default/files/institutes/olpa/20130515-senate-testimony-hodes.pdf.

Institute of Medicine. To err is human: building a safer health system. 1999. Available at: https://qualitysafety.bmj.com/content/qhc/15/3/174.full.pdf.

Institute for Safe Medication Practices. Examination of fatal error supports system-based approach to safety. 2010. Available at: https://www.ismp.org/sites/default/files/attachments/2019-01/PR20100316.pdf.

Institute for Safe Medication Practices. ISMP launches new vaccine error reporting program. 2012. Available at: https://www.ismp.org/error-reporting-programs

Institute for Safe Medication Practices. ISMP survey shows prescription time guarantees may lead to errors. 2012.

Institute for Safe Medication Practices. ISMP releases Top 10 list of medication errors and hazards in 2020. *Reac Wkly.* 2021;1844(1):7.

Lifshin L, Nimmo C. Developing and maintaining up-to-date training for pharmacy technicians. *Am J Health Syst Pharm.* 2001;58(11):968-970. Available at: https://doi.org/10.1093/ajhp/58.11.968.

The Merck Manual Home Health Handbook. *Drug errors.*

Mizner JJ. *Pharmacy Technician Certification Examination.* 3rd ed. St. Louis: Elsevier; 2014.

National Association of Boards of Pharmacy. United States Pharmacopeial Convention joins anti-counterfeiting campaign. 2013. Available at: https://nabp.pharmacy/news/news-releases/united-states-pharmacopeial-convention-joins-anti-counterfeiting-campaign/.

National Coordinating Council for Medication Error Reporting and Prevention. Council recommendations: recommendations to reduce medication errors associated with verbal medication orders and prescriptions. 2006. Available at: https://www.nccmerp.org/recommendations-reduce-medication-errors-associated-verbalmedication-orders-and-prescriptions.

National Coordinating Council for Medication Error Reporting and Prevention. Moving into the second decade: developing recommendations and offering tools. 2010. Available at: https://www.nccmerp.org/sites/default/files/fifteen_year_report.pdf.

National League for Nursing. Medication errors injure 1.5 million people and cost billions of dollars annually; report offers comprehensive strategies for reducing drug-related mistakes (press release). Available at: https://www.nln.org/detail-pages/news/2006/08/04/Medication-Errors-Injure-1-5-Million-People-and-Cost-Billions-of-Dollars-Annually.

Pharmacy mistake blamed for heparin overdoses at Texas hospital. Drug Topics: Voice of the Pharmacist; 2011. Available at: https://www.drugtopics.com/view/pharmacy-mistake-blamed-heparin-overdoses-texas-hospital.

Radwan C. Pharmacy technicians face states' scrutiny, regulation. *Drug Topics: Voice of the Pharmacist.* Available at: https://www.drugtopics.com/view/pharmacy-technicians-face-states-scrutiny-regulation.

Reckmann MH, Westbrook JI, Koh Y, et al. Does computerized provider order entry reduce prescribing errors for hospital inpatients? A systematic review. *J Am Med Inform Assoc.* 2009;16:613. doi:10.1197/jMI.M3050.

Rybolt B. CVS will pay $650,000 to resolve prescription medication errors in N.J. *N.J.com* (blog post); 2013. Available at: http://blog.nj.com/independentpress_impact/print.html?entry=/2013/02/cvs_nj_division_of_consumer_af.html.

Vivian JC. Criminalization of medication errors. *US Pharm.* 2009;34:66. Available at: http://www.uspharmacist.com/content/d/pharmacy%20law/c/16572/.

West D, Hastings J, Earley A. *An Economic Justification of the Use of Dispensing Technologies in Independent Community Pharmacies.* National Community Pharmacists Association; 2001. Available at: http://www.ncpafoundation.org/downloads/asset_upload_file169_7723.pdf.

Websites Referenced

2014–2015 Targeted medication safety best practices for hospitals. Available at: http://www.ismp.org/tools/bestpractices/default.aspx.

Florida Board of Pharmacy. Registered pharmacy technician requirements. Available at: http://floridaspharmacy.gov/licensing/registered-pharmacy-technician/.

FreeCE.com. Pharmaceutical education consultants. Medication error prevention. A guide for pharmacists. Available at: http://www.freece.com/freece/CECatalog_Details.aspx?ID=c3800910-420b-4d15-9b55-2e2a065bd29d.

Institute for the Ages. Demographic transition facts. Available at: http://www.institutefortheages.org/facts-on-aging/.

Institute for Healthcare Improvement. New thinking on medication reconciliation; 2008. Available at: https://www.ihi.org/insights/new-thinking-medication-reconciliation.

Institute for Healthcare Improvement. How to guide: prevent adverse drug events (medication reconciliation). Available at: https://oregonpatientsafety.org/tools-and-best-practices/healthcare-associated-infections-m6tkj-bpg2n-fh4g9-nxdmb-36yx5-fnjt8-8ss8l.

Medication errors statistics 2024 | SingleCare

What is Managed Care Pharmacy? AMCP.org.

CHAPTER 15

Pharmacy Operations Management and Workflow

Karen Davis

1. List common areas in a community pharmacy setting, discuss the general layout of a community pharmacy setting, and describe the role of a pharmacy technician in a community pharmacy setting.
2. Describe the general layout and various areas of an institutional pharmacy setting and the role of a pharmacy technician in an institutional pharmacy setting.
3. Identify ways to improve efficiency techniques.
4. Discuss three main goals for all pharmacies.

TERMS AND DEFINITIONS

American Society of Health-System Pharmacists (ASHP) An association of pharmacists, pharmacy students, and technicians practicing in hospitals and health care systems, including home health care; ASHP has a long history of advocating for patient safety and establishing best practices to improve medication use

Automated dispensing system (ADS) Electronic system used to dispense medications

Medication error Any preventable event that may cause or lead to inappropriate medication use or patient harm

Pharmacy Technician Certification Board (PTCB) An organization that offers national certification for pharmacy technicians in the United States

Quality assurance (QA) Establishing systems for ensuring quality of a product

Quality control (QC) The use of established systems to ensure quality of a product

⊙ Scenario

Jerry is an experienced technician at a busy hospital pharmacy. He began his career after graduating from an ASHP/ACPE-accredited technician training program. He is certified by the PTCB and works full time as a technician. He has been asked by the pharmacy director to participate on a department committee looking into making the pharmacy more organized, efficient, and profitable. He is to report his findings regarding his automation supply area. What types of issues do you think the committee will address? How can Jerry prepare for this new assignment?

It takes a team working together to keep a pharmacy and health care organization running smoothly and efficiently. The

layout, equipment placement, arrangement, responsibilities of team members, and standard operating procedures (SOPs) all factor into the way a pharmacy operates. Changes in roles of both pharmacists and technicians are changing the way a pharmacy manages daily tasks and patient care. The knowledge requirements for technicians are increasing, and with that comes additional leadership, advanced opportunities, and legal responsibilities. To meet the demands of a patient's overall wellness, today's pharmacy technicians must understand their place not just in the pharmacy but also in the overall health care system. The health care team members must work together to deliver the highest standard of efficiency and patient safety.

Overview

Each pharmacy setting has specific tasks, and technicians provide distributive functions and supportive clinical roles. With the role of pharmacists becoming more clinical, this requires more pharmacists to be available for direct patient interaction and counseling, so this leaves more of the daily activities to the technician, and workflow practices, organization, and knowledge are key to providing the best and safest services for the patient. The **American Society of Health-System Pharmacists (ASHP)** Pharmacy Practice Model Initiative has a significant focus of "advancing the health and well-being of patients" and maintains optimizing the role of technicians is critical to this goal. Technician education, regulation, and basic knowledge levels are key to providing safe patient care and efficiency in providing those services required to keep up with the increasing complexity of health care and declining reimbursement. Pharmacists and technicians must work as a well-organized team and integrate pharmacy, wellness, and disease prevention services with other health care providers. The ASHP and **Pharmacy Technician Certification Board (PTCB)** held a joint meeting in February 2018. The future of the pharmacy technician profession, an emphasis on leadership, advanced or specialty roles, and requirements to practice were discussed.

The more knowledgeable and professional technicians become, the better patient care will become. Pharmacy workflow and operations require an understanding of the various practice settings, a technician's role in each setting, and how the department and other health care team members work together to provide quality patient care.

Community Pharmacy

Efficiency and quality not only depend on the personnel's knowledge base but also the actual layout and space of a practice setting (Fig. 15.1). The state boards of pharmacy require physical standards such as a sink with hot and cold running water, appropriate lighting, and minimum amounts of space. In *community settings* there are common areas such as the following:

- Automated long-term care equipment (blister card or strip packaging)
- Compounding area
- Counseling area or room
- Counter space for inventory check-in and processing
- Data entry and/or filling stations
- Drive-thru window
- Durable and nondurable equipment
- Front counter (register) with intake and pickup window areas
- Offices for billing or physician calls
- Reconstitution area (pediatric medications)
- Stock (inventory)
- Storefront (over the counter [OTC]) and miscellaneous products shelving

The layout should incorporate a design that provides the most efficient use of workspace and allows workflow to run smoothly (Figs. 15.2 and 15.3). For instance, the technician

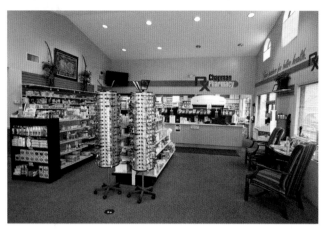

FIG. 15.1 Overall community pharmacy layout.

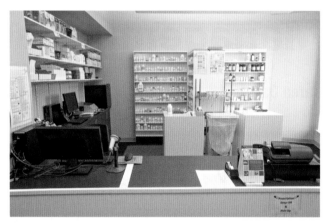

FIG. 15.2 Community pharmacy view.

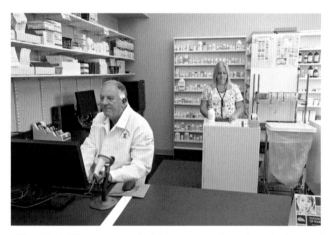

FIG. 15.3 Pharmacy technicians are assigned to designated spots for efficient workflow.

assigned to the *front counter* (register) area or the storefront area (Fig. 15.4) should not be the same person assigned to handle all the incoming phone calls. Customer focus should be priority for the phone person, and distractions can lead to confusion and possible errors. Other duties for this technician might include the drive-thru window, overflow of calls to assist staff working on processing orders, or delivery drivers and mail.

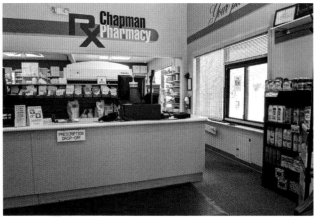

FIG. 15.4 The front counter area at the pharmacy. A technician would work areas for pickup or drive-thru.

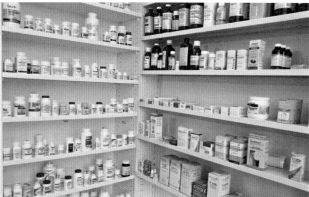

FIG. 15.5 A small section with "fast-moving" items is often located near the front dispensing area for easy and fast access to common medications.

The placement of equipment and use of space in the front counter area are important. The computer screen should always be directed away from the customer, and phone calls should be screened. A technician working in this area should be able to reach the pickup or ready prescriptions and drop-off area within a few steps. This is also a last opportunity to check for accuracy of prescriptions and verify patient information. When working directly with a customer, use good nonverbal and verbal communication (see Chapter 4) to provide quality care. Checking a birth date or spelling of a name can prevent an error at the time of pickup or drop-off. When dropping off a prescription for filling, the technician must ensure the correct patient demographic information such as address, birth date, and any payment or insurance information is readily available to avoid delays or additional work. If there are notes or messages from phone contact, illegible writing can also cause an error if the technician does not take the time to write correctly and provide the note appropriately. Workflow will run smoother if problems are identified early or additional information needed is provided to the pharmacy team.

The *data entry area* and *stocking areas* are usually together. To increase efficiency, a shelving section may be designated as "fast movers" and contain medications that are most frequently prescribed. This allows less walking or movement when preparing prescriptions from the data entry to the filling process (Fig. 15.5). If automation is involved, the machine may include these fast movers as part of their inventory. The choice of medications can be adjusted at different times of the year, such as for flu or allergy season. This section must be organized and kept clean at all times. Phone calls from third-party vendors, customers, and physicians should be handled with utmost privacy in this area. Conversations should never be overheard by customers in the store or at the front counter. Fixtures should include a counter with computers for data entry and possibly one designated for ordering, refill requests, drug look-up, or physician calls. Technicians should be assigned to different roles *within* this area, such as the following:

- Bagging finished prescriptions
- Bulk medications ready to be returned to shelf
- Counting or pouring
- Insurance rejects or refill requests
- New prescription entry
- Physician calls or questions

This area may include scanning technology that also connects with the automated counter, if being used. Automation can be found in most community settings and is an integral part of distribution. The filling and data entry areas may have the machine within it, and inventory is maintained as items are depleted and at the end of the day. Technicians often manage this equipment, and they are assigned to just this task of keeping the inventory replenished. In a busy pharmacy, there is a constant need to restock canisters and monitor counting machines (Fig. 15.6).

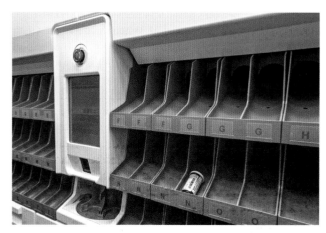

FIG. 15.6 Automated counters are monitored carefully.

The flow of this area must work well, and all personnel should understand each role. Beginning with data entry, the entire process must be organized and allow for interruptions to the process such as insufficient inventory or a problem that requires a physician call. For instance, there should be waiting bins or a filing system to identify prescriptions that require additional attention. Workflow interruptions should not stop the pharmacy from performing the required daily tasks for other customers.

There should be a designated pharmacist checking area to provide a clean and organized way to check final products. It should be close to the bagging area and verification and counseling window to increase efficiency. Finished products should be bagged and maintained in a "pickup" or "will call" area that is accessible to front counter and drive-thru window personnel.

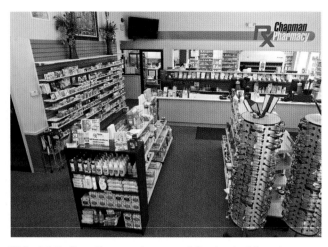

FIG. 15.7 Over-the-counter area at the front of the pharmacy.

> ### ■ Tech Note!
>
> A designated area for "ready-to-check prescriptions" should contain a stock bottle and a prescription for the pharmacist's review. This is important for verification of product National Drug Code and visual inspection at the time of checking. Baskets are often used and color-coded to identify customers waiting or returning, specialty situations, or urgent/priority.

To better understand pharmacy workflow and the technician's role in day-to-day activities, case studies are provided in this chapter. These give scenarios or examples of activities in the pharmacy settings for you to analyze. As you read through them, think about methods you would use to improve a task or solve a problem. As a technician, you are an integral part of the pharmacy team, and your input is valuable in enhancing patient safety and quality of work.

Case Study 1

The regular front counter technician has gone to lunch and a customer requests a pickup. The fill-in technician looks in the section designated for "pickup" and does not see the medications. She checks the back counter data entry area and sees some counted medication with a stock bottle in a basket with the person's name on it. She bags it and provides the customer with the medication. When the data entry technician returns, she asks what happened to the medication. There was another medication to go with it that was waiting for a call from the physician, and then it needed a final pharmacist check.

The *storefront* or *over-the-counter area* is a critical area and often is set up for customers to shop on their own with minimal assistance (Fig. 15.7). Some smaller independent pharmacies have miscellaneous items for sale or offer gifts and baskets, flowers, jewelry, or additional products.

Customers may approach the front counter with questions regarding instructions from a physician or have questions about treatment options. Workflow and organization are important considerations because having a technician leave

the pickup area or the drive-thru window to assist a customer at the front counter can cause a backup if the customer requires a lengthy discussion. There should be a backup and plan in place to accommodate such a situation. Another technician should be prepared to either assist or take over the area left unattended.

Case Study 2

A customer requires some assistance with crutches, and the front counter person, who is also working the drive-thru window, leaves to go out front without telling anyone. Two other customers walk in and a drive-thru customer pulls up. The technician in the processing area does not realize she should be out front, and customers start becoming upset. The customers complain, and it takes a pharmacist and two technicians from behind the counter to wait on the customers and clear out the backup. If the front counter technician had told someone she needed to leave her area or asked someone else to help, the confusion and delay could have been avoided.

Reconstitution or *compounding areas* are often included in today's community practice areas and can sometimes act independently of the retail section (Fig. 15.8). Technicians may be assigned to this area and rotate to the "front" periodically. The inventory

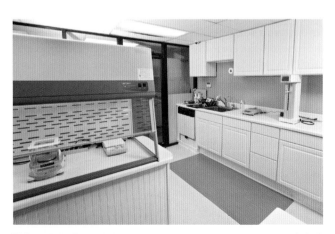

FIG. 15.8 One of the areas pharmacy technicians work in is the compounding area.

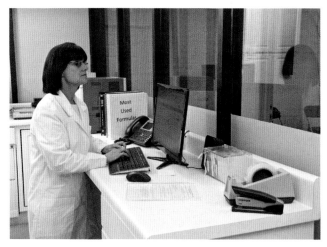

FIG. 15.9 Compounding area roles include keeping data entry, billing, and documentation.

and layout vary somewhat because the process of compounding consists of bulk medications and various measuring equipment (refer to Chapter 11). Movement still needs to be kept to a minimum; counters are standing height, and technicians operate independently from the regular prescription processing in the front. Roles may include data entry, billing, inventory and ordering, preparation of compounds, delivery assignment, and documentation (Fig. 15.9). Workflow starts with obtaining an order, either brought in by a customer or provided by phone by a health care provider. Data entry and preparation may be done by the same personnel, or there may be a separate area or preparation room, depending on the size of the facility. Once the compound is ready and verified by a pharmacist, it is either delivered or possibly picked up. Coordination with the ordering technician in other areas such as durable medical equipment or front section will ensure efficient handling of inventory and keep all required areas stocked.

Tech Note!

The order is usually sent at the close of business, and all departments add their needs to a single order. Often there is a "want book" or designated computer set on the wholesaler's website, and as an item is used, another is entered to replace it. As the designated technician, it is your job to ensure that any items in your area that are out or needed are ordered or provided to the ordering technician. Follow your facility's procedure to avoid mistakes or additional costs.

Counseling and *pickup areas* are the last sections of the pharmacy area that a customer sees. Counseling may be performed only by a pharmacist, but to keep the workflow efficient, a technician can play a valuable role in identifying these customers and inform the pharmacist that a customer is waiting or offer to relieve the pharmacist to enable him or her to spend one-on-one time with the customer. When a customer picks up a prescription, always ask an open-ended question, such as "What are you allergic to?" rather than "Are you allergic to

anything?" An open-ended question requires more than a "yes or no" answer and can prevent **medication errors.**

To accommodate the increased number of patients who are elderly and the increased number of patients with more complicated disease states, pharmacies often include a section for *long-term care packaging* in their practice. This section may also include automation for packaging either in 30-day blister cards or strip packaging (Fig. 15.10). Medications are put into individual pouches that list the medications and identify each one by color, size, and shape. The directions are provided on the pouch and the strip is continuous for a 30-day supply for each patient. Verification is performed by a laser check system, and a 30-day supply of breakfast, lunch, and dinner medications is prepared and placed in a box for delivery (see Fig. 15.10). Patient compliance is enhanced significantly because each pouch holds all the medications for that dose time, which eliminates transferring to a pill box or taking from an open bottle of loose pills. The strip packaging process is performed by a machine with canisters of medications that are filled from bulk medication bottles (Fig. 15.11). A technician maintains inventory and operation of orders that

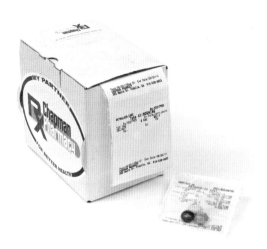

FIG. 15.10 Example of 30-day box for delivery of a patient's strip-packaged medications.

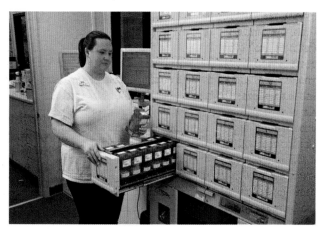

FIG. 15.11 Canister refill for automated filling packaging machine.

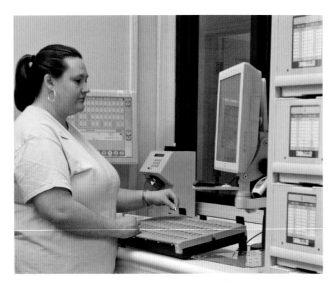

FIG. 15.12 Some special trays are filled by hand.

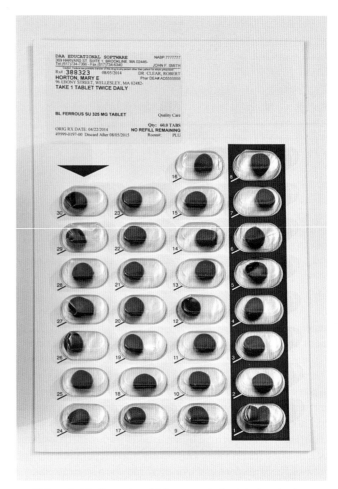

FIG. 15.13 Completed blister pack for 30-day dosing.

are filled monthly as batches and delivered. For certain medications, such as vitamins, there is a special tray that is filled by hand (Fig. 15.12). The right setup is critical; this area is usually not very big, and it demands detail-oriented technicians. Inventory must be monitored, and any special medications that are housed outside the automated cabinet must be available for filling when a batch is due. Deliveries are set up on batch schedules, and coordination is performed directly with drivers and outside facilities.

Blister package cards are also used for patients in assisted living or long-term care facilities. The cards contain blisters or bubbles that hold doses of medications. Each bubble is individual and punched out when the dose is due to be taken (Fig. 15.13). This packaging area usually has several technicians and its own pharmacist, and it is separate from the front operations in the retail pharmacy setting. The pharmacy may have contracts with facilities or organizations and separate delivery schedules for each. Workflow generally uses computers for data entry and several stations for packaging. There is a section within this area where verification is completed by the pharmacist, and technicians divide out the packages for delivery drivers or mail. There also may be separate spaces for packaging liquids and solids within the packaging areas. Inventory should be maintained daily and either ordered or shared with the main pharmacy as one order.

Tech Note!

Remember: Each area requires different, specific packaging, so precise information for ordering is important. For instance, medications in bulk using 1000-count containers would be appropriate for blister packaging or for filling canisters in automated machines, but for front counter dispensing area stock, 100-count containers might be more suitable.

Case Study 3

Tomorrow will be a busy day, because the batch for the 15th of the month will be due. The technician prepared and filled the canisters to full capacity the night before. However, she forgot to special order a medication that has to be hand-filled for one of the patients at a nursing home. The driver must leave with the batch early in the morning because he has a 50-mile radius to cover before the end of the day. She will have to order or borrow the medication and call to see whether the patient has enough of the medication for one more day. In addition, the driver will have to travel 35 miles tomorrow to deliver the single medication that was left out of the patient's order. If the technician had followed the procedure for ordering, this could have been avoided. It is costly to the pharmacy and inconvenient for the patient and caregivers.

Durable and Nondurable Medical Equipment Area

Many chain and independent pharmacies are now including medical equipment services and delivery to customers. As the population of elderly people increases, with many patients remaining in their homes and using in-home care, the demand is increasing for durable medical equipment (DME) such as beds, walkers, wheelchairs, and respiratory equipment. Technicians need a basic understanding of this equipment and other nondurable products such as those for wound

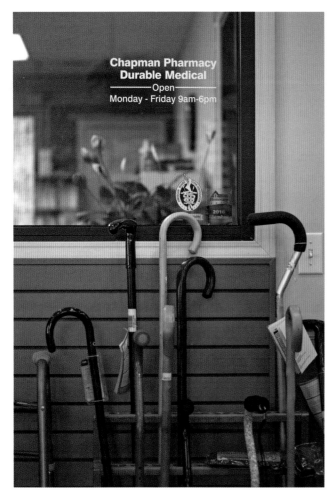

Durable medical equipment (DME) office area.

care, ostomy, diabetes, cancer, and other treatment-related items. Physicians may call in to a direct line or order these supplies in the DME department; these supplies often require delivery, setup, and third-party billing.

Also in the DME area are technicians who perform data entry and phone calls, dedicated insurance billers, and additional personnel for direct customer care and gathering of supplies. Technicians in the DME area must follow a workflow process and coordinate with the other areas to ensure that (1) deliveries are made on time and (2) the DME delivery includes any and all medications that were also ordered (Fig. 15.14). The DME area should be located near the front counter and dispensing area, and there must be communication among all three areas. If equipment and prescriptions for the same patient are being processed, the assembly of all the items should be coordinated so the delivery or pickup is of maximum convenience for the customer and provides the highest quality of patient care.

Case Study 4

You are working in the DME area of a busy local pharmacy. The technician working up front informs you that a customer dropped off a medication prescription for her mother and has left to take the patient home. The customer requested delivery later in the afternoon between 3 and 6 pm and stated that

the physician will call in an order for some wound care supplies that should go to the patient. Once the order is called in, you will need to ensure that the driver knows to include the prescriptions along with the wound care supplies in the delivery. How would you do this? How does proper workflow and area setup help or hurt in this scenario?

Institutional Pharmacy

Workflow and management in the institutional setting varies because of the associated daily activities and critical tasks. The main department itself is generally located in the central hospital with satellites located in areas such as critical care, operating room (OR)/surgery or recovery, the emergency department, and the neonatal nursery. These satellite pharmacies will usually have their own technician and pharmacist who work in that area directly with that health care team. Hospital pharmacies also may have an outpatient department where daily operations perform as a community pharmacy. In addition, there may be a specialty chemotherapy pharmacy where technicians prepare sterile cancer drugs.

The main dispensing pharmacy will be separated into areas such as the following:
- **Automated dispensing system (ADS)** area (Pyxis, SureMed)
- Computerized physician order entry (CPOE), order entry (desks with pharmacists) area
- Emergency or disaster medication supply room
- Filling area with pickup window and pneumatic tube
- Intravenous (IV) room
- Inventory area and storeroom
- Opioids area
- OR tray and crash cart restocking
- Repackaging area (bulk to unit dose [UD])
- Stocking area for nonclinical area for other departments such as central supply or emergency medical services (EMS)

The layout of a hospital pharmacy usually consists of a large room divided by counters or partitions with some offices included. The *CPOE area* is a bank of desks that should be located in a quiet zone where data entry and phone calls between pharmacists and other health care workers either inside or outside the facility can occur with minimum interruptions. This is where orders are scanned or faxed to the pharmacy and processed for filling or supply in an automated dispensing cabinet (ADC) (see Chapter 9).

If the order is for a medication that needs to be in an ADC on the floor, the technicians in the *automated dispensing area* will perform the next step in the workflow (Fig. 15.15). Each medication kept in the ADC must be individually packaged, and if stock is insufficient on the floor, a technician must deliver it to the cabinet. Medications are entered from orders sent from the floor. Once a label has been printed, the technician chooses the stock, counts out the amount, and packages the medication in unit doses. If the medication has to be repackaged from bulk stock, the technician may work with another area to get this accomplished. Deliveries are done continually and in batches that are set up by the department. The hospital maintains a formulary of stocked items in the cabinets, and if

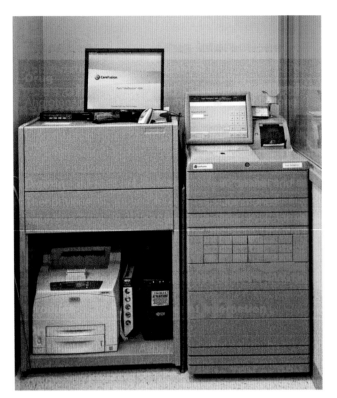

FIG. 15.15 Sample automatic dispensing system (Pyxis).

the drug ordered is a specialty medication or not appropriate for filling a pocket, a different process is followed. The automated dispensing area should be open, well lit, and close to the stock shelves and the CPOE area to allow for less motion for filling and questions if required. Communication may include: "That needs to go up to CCU now, the ADC is out and it's a stat dose!" There are several technicians and possibly multiple pharmacists dedicated to this area because batch deliveries and one-at-a-time orders are constant throughout a 24-hour period.

The other similar area may be located close to the automated dispensing area, and the *window pickup* or *pneumatic tube area*. Once an order is entered in the CPOE area, if the medication is not appropriate for the stock of a cabinet, a label will print, and technicians in this area will fill the order manually. The shelves with stock may be in a square layout or in a cabinet form with bins. Medications are single or UD and set out for final check before delivery or pickup. This area should be small and compact so that personnel save motion from the printer to the shelves and close to the CPOE area for questions or special instructions—for instance, "The nurse is on the way to pick that up," or "Send it in the pneumatic tube, it's stat!" As a technician, you must coordinate with other departments such as IV or narcotics areas. Medications may be ordered that have to be prepared simultaneously, with you filling an order or restocking for an ACD. If a medication you are working on needs to be delivered, you may need to check with another department to ensure that all components can be taken at the same time. This area may have its own pharmacist dedicated to verification of orders being picked up or tubed and technicians for processing and quick deliveries.

Case Study 5

You are working in the filling area today, and the pharmacist entering an order gets your attention to say, "Pull that label for the IV for Mr. Jones, please. The nurse will pick that up in 10 minutes and it needs to go with the other medications I filled." You pull the medication labels and start to fill them and forget about the IV medication. When the nurse comes, you hand her the medication bags prepared, and she asks about the IV medication. What should you have done differently to ensure more efficiency in your area?

Another area critical to dispensing is the *narcotics area*. Medications in this area require special attention and storage, and workflow should be in a minimal or low-flow traffic area and, again, quiet. Technicians are assigned to this area and work within it on a daily basis. It may be a specialty or advanced technician opportunity because it entails additional knowledge and increased responsibility. Controlled medications are stored in an automated system with computer inventory tracking, and the technician(s) are responsible for preparing singles and batches for delivery. A pharmacist is usually assigned to this area because it is busy and requires constant attention.

Another busy packaging area that relates to all the other supply areas must coordinate well because the medications required for automated dispensing systems must be in UD or single packaging. All medications are not made available from the manufacturer in this way, so this requires packaging by technicians and subsequent stocking to the area where they are needed. The *repackaging area* is a busy hub, with medication storage in bulk form (eg, units of 100–1000 tablets). There should be large counter spaces to work with computers and printers for preparing labels. This area may be located alongside the other dispensing areas so that communication for needs for delivery or stocking can be accommodated in a timely manner. This area will be covered by several technicians, with pharmacists for verification dedicated to this process.

Tech Note!

Bar coding and National Drug Code technology are key to ensuring quality and accuracy. From the patient's electronic medication administration record to the actual cabinet (pocket) entry, the medication can be tracked and errors and diversion can be averted (see Chapter 9).

The *IV room* is a unique area that requires special training and procedures. Guidelines established by the ASHP and *United States Pharmacopeia* (USP) <797> publish the layout, equipment, maintenance, training, and all procedures related to preparing these medications. This area is isolated with walls or additional rooms and is considered a no-flow traffic area. Only authorized personnel may enter and leave, and technicians and pharmacists must be dressed appropriately (see Chapter 12). A technician who needs to communicate with personnel inside this area should use caution to enter only authorized spaces and use an intercom or phones. Inventory for this area is maintained separately by technicians working within, and overflow is kept in the storeroom or on outside shelving.

In addition to stocking the cabinets on the nursing floors, the main pharmacy stocks supplies for other departments or satellites, such as OR/surgery and trays for code carts or EMS. Some *nonclinical stocking* or *outside areas*, such as central supply and EMS, will also be stocked by the pharmacy, and this inventory may be kept in the back in the main shelving or overflow area or can have a dedicated space within the dispensing area. Depending on the size of the facility, technicians and a pharmacist may work in this section, which will be close to other dispensing areas. If this stock is only maintained in the back main storage shelving, any technician may pull items needed as requests are made. This area may be located off of the main dispensing area but close to an outside entry because EMS will bring in boxes used on a call that need medications replaced. OR/surgery maintains trays with procedural medications, one for each case, which have to be maintained by the main pharmacy. Staff will drop off trays or carts and pick up fully stocked replacements. The technicians in this area restock the trays and carts left for replenishment. Inventory for these medications is different and usually shelved in its own sections. Code drugs, for instance, which are packaged with ready-to-inject syringes and bags of IV fluids, are items normally kept in EMS boxes and code carts.

Another common area kept in a hospital's main pharmacy is for *emergency* or *disaster medications*. A hospital may often house a special section for the community in case of disaster and a technician may be dedicated to this area. The inventory is maintained separately and consists of antibiotics, maintenance medications, and other items such as batteries that would be necessary for the public in an emergency situation.

All of the areas must coordinate items required for ordering with the *inventory* technician or department. The inventory area may be a section within the storeroom or near the stock area with computers and phones. Technicians are dedicated to this area for daily control of inventory, pricing and negotiation, and formulary control. If items are needed throughout the department, the inventory area must know what is needed to be efficient in providing the medications needed for patients. Computerized systems with bar coding, National Drug Code (NDC) tracking, and other automated technology increase productivity.

Improving Efficiency Techniques

When proper workflow and management are put into place, a pharmacy can provide high-quality and safe patient care while minimizing time and expenses. Layout of facilities, use of educated and trained technicians, and standards of practice established provide a solid foundation for success. Any breakdown in the system or workflow can start to snowball and the pharmacy process can begin to deteriorate. In addition, if workflow is interrupted constantly or there is a lack of attention to processes, errors can occur.

Every pharmacy has three main goals: to provide medications accurately and efficiently, provide high-quality and safe patient care, and maintain a sustainable business. With the

added duties for pharmacy such as immunizations, wellness clinics, and medication therapy management, having a system that flows allows the pharmacist to spend more time with each patient. Technicians are a key to keeping the production system running and organized. Simple things such as proper use of workspace and employing trained individuals can allow the time needed for patients to receive that individual touch.

Getting Started

Establishing a baseline or a starting point is key, and it is the first step in creating a **quality assurance** (**QA**) process. Identifying a problem and its cause will then lead to ways to improve or change a process if needed. Unless all the components of why an error occurred are known, unnecessary decisions may be made and the problem may remain uncorrected. **Quality control** (**QC**) is taking those established plans and discussions and making them into activities that prevent an error or make a process better. Participating in department committees and being observant in the day-to-day activities is a great way to continue to improve the workflow. As a technician, you see the daily management of the workplace and can help identify what does and does not seem to work. Brainstorming ideas and regular meetings with key personnel allow an organization to establish standards of practice and develop a quality plan that can lead to improved safety and efficiency. Using a quality assurance process to ensure practices and daily tasks should be monitored by SOPs and established by setting goals, making observations, performing evaluations, and obtaining staff feedback. As a technician, participating in the development of procedures can improve your department's quality and workflow.

Some ideas for the community setting include the following:

- Keep movement to a minimum to save time and unnecessary steps. Align work areas to flow with the order of processes that must be completed (Fig. 15.16). For instance, space used for the drive-thru window and the pickup/will call area should be close to the final verification station and front counter. Keep fast movers on a front shelf by themselves, close to the dispensing (working) counter area in the community pharmacy. Review inventory levels monthly and keep fewer of those used quickly. This will produce less clutter on shelves and increase the ease of picking medications to count or pour. Perform a monthly check of medications for expired or unused medications and return them for credit. This saves money and reduces the chance for errors when choosing possibly expired bulk medications to process.
- Use automation and technology to assist in error prevention, efficiency, and accuracy. Bar code identification and NDC/scan verification can shorten the time to process orders, improve inventory control, and reduce medication errors. Technicians should rotate through workstations to ensure cross-training and enable callouts, lunches, and breaks. If each person can fill in, the workflow is able to continue to run smoothly. Maintain a designated area or computer for ordering and a quiet (away from front) area with a computer for physician and insurance calls.

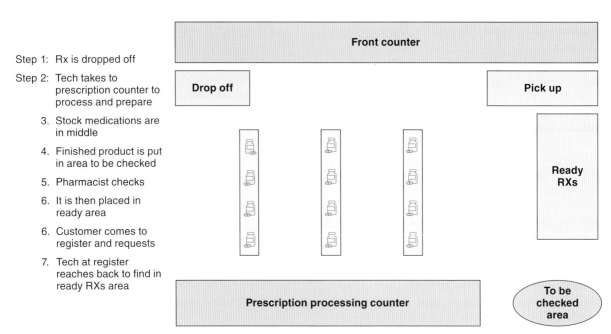

Step 1: Rx is dropped off

Step 2: Tech takes to prescription counter to process and prepare

3. Stock medications are in middle

4. Finished product is put in area to be checked

5. Pharmacist checks

6. It is then placed in ready area

6. Customer comes to register and requests

7. Tech at register reaches back to find in ready RXs area

FIG. 15.16 Example of flow of a community pharmacy.

- Reduce interruptions in workflow by placing technicians in areas appropriate to their level of training and keep movement and distractions to a minimum. For instance, the technician counting new prescriptions or managing the drive-thru window should not be answering refill station phone calls or handling insurance rejections.
- Always try to assign technicians to tasks that match their knowledge and experience. If one technician is great with customers and another is reluctant or shy about interacting with people, match them to appropriate tasks or consider having the reluctant technician train by shadowing a peer.
- Take the time to train the staff. Each member needs to understand their role, and even with automation, there is still a need for a strong team to keep things running smoothly.

Ideas for an institutional setting include the following:

- Cross-train technicians within the department to accommodate callouts, lunch breaks, or short staffing. Technicians should have a basic knowledge of all operations within the department to minimize workflow interruptions when key people are missing from areas. Arrange work areas and the flow of orders to match typical hospital tasks. Place the supplying areas close to inventory shelving and CPOE stations. Consider assigning a separate area for phone calls and disruptive conversation. Keep talking to a minimum and areas of low traffic out of main aisles or station areas. Technicians should be stationed as near as possible to their work area. The technician responsible for answering the window bell should not sit at a desk at the back of the department.
- Community pharmacists' roles have become more clinical, and pharmacy services include opportunities such as medication management, immunizations, medication adherence, and counseling for overall wellness and disease

management. Institutional pharmacists' roles include more clinical trials and research, laboratory value evaluation, admission and discharge planning and reviews, and risk management and evaluation of therapies (Risk Evaluation and Mitigation Strategy [REMS] and error prevention). For these additional and more clinical roles to be performed, the workflow and management of a facility or pharmacy must include SOP and workflow processes tailored to enable high-quality and efficient work to be performed.

- The workforce of tomorrow requires high-quality, trained, and knowledgeable technicians. Providing high-quality and safe patient care, disease prevention, and wellness management requires a staff and business model of efficiency and proper workflow. Management through commonsense practices and sensible changes can lead to a better work atmosphere and more profitable organization. With understanding of how to use resources to improve workflow and management, today's technician has many opportunities in leadership and advanced and specialty roles.

Do You Remember These Key Points?

- Common areas found in institutional and community settings
- Common roles of community technicians in both settings
- Why it is important to consider workflow for efficiency and patient safety
- Best practices to minimize errors in both community and institutional practices
- The difference in quality control and quality assurance
- Benefits associated with being knowledgeable and incorporating best practices for technicians and the future

Scenario Follow-Up

Jerry prepared for the meeting by researching and observing what happens daily in the department. He started by reviewing the layout of his area. The CPOE area and automated supply area were not close to each other. The dedicated space for his dispensing area was lacking counter space and was cramped for the personnel within it. Technicians answering phones were loud, and communication was nearly impossible with outside areas, which caused distractions. The committee evaluated his findings and decided to remodel and place the CPOE and dispensing area next to each other. One technician in his area would answer phones and relay information between the CPOE and his area. In addition, shelving for related medications and more counter (working) space would be added.

Review Questions

Multiple Choice Questions

1. Which of the following is *not* an example of a pharmacy preventable error?
   A. Giving the patient a medication intended for someone else
   B. Giving a sublingual tablet instead of a liquid at the patient's request
   C. Giving a generic medication when the physician prescribed a brand name medication and signed "no substitutions"
   D. Patient taking more medication than was prescribed on the prescription label

2. What is the most appropriate first step a pharmacy technician should take when establishing a quality assurance program for high-alert medication storage in the department?
   A. Participate in departmental discussions or meetings
   B. Change the workflow pattern immediately
   C. Establish a baseline or starting point
   D. Order new labels for the bins

3. Once an order has been entered into the system and a label is created, all of these areas can be next in the workflow process *except* the:
   A. Repackaging area
   B. IV area
   C. CPOE area
   D. Narcotics area

4. A walk-in customer has requested her medications to be packaged in 30-day strip packaging and delivered to her home. What area would this task be completed in?
   A. Long-term care packaging area
   B. Compounding area
   C. Reconstitution area
   D. Data entry area

5. Participating in discussion groups to find better ways to manage a process after an event would be part of which of the following?
   A. QA
   B. QC
   C. SOP
   D. CPOE

6. EMS boxes would be filled and maintained in which area?
   A. Disaster stock area
   B. Repackaging area
   C. DME area
   D. Nonclinical area

7. The type of stock or inventory packaging for automated dispensing cabinets (ADC) in a hospital could be in any of the following *except:*
   A. Unit dose tablets
   B. Bulk bottles
   C. Unit dose liquids
   D. Blister cards

8. Considering the workflow management and layout of a typical community pharmacy, which of the following positions would be the *best* choice for the technician assigned to the drive-thru window?
   A. Front counter technician
   B. Long-term care or repackaging technician
   C. Technician assigned to refills and physician call line
   D. Data entry technician

9. The most appropriate place for the dedicated physician call line in a community pharmacy would be:
   A. In the OTC area
   B. At the front counter
   C. In the compounding area
   D. In the data entry/filling area

10. Which of the following is *not* an example of DME?
    A. Bed
    B. Walker
    C. Wheelchair
    D. Prescription paste for a wound

Technician's Corner

Joe works in a busy community pharmacy and is scheduled to go to lunch at noon. His position this week is taking care of the e-scripts that come through. He is supposed to be relieved by Sally, but she has only worked the e-script station a few times. He is worried about this but does not want to say anything to the pharmacist on duty. He has noticed this has caused problems before and thinks there needs to be a better match/schedule to the station duties for lunches, but he did not say anything at the last department's improvement meeting. He leaves and comes back to a prescription backup for the rest of the day. It takes the whole team to catch up, and several customers were told they would have to come back tomorrow. If you were in charge of scheduling for lunch relief, what would you do differently?

Bibliography

American Society of Health-System Pharmacists. ASHP long range vision for work force in hospitals and health systems. *Am J Health Syst Pharm.* 2007;64:1320-1330.

American Society of Health-System Pharmacists. *Pharmacy Practice Model Initiative Overview.* Available at: https://www.ashp.org/Pharmacy-Practice/PAI/About-PAI-2030.

Ehlert D. *Six Tips to Boost Pharmacy Efficiency*. 2013. Available at: https://www.drugtopics.com/view/six-tips-boost-pharmacy-efficiency.

Grove D. Pharmacy workflow: improving efficiency. *Pharmacy Times*. 2015. Available at: https://www.pharmacytimes.com/view/pharmacy-work-flow-improving-efficiency

Mizner JJ. *Pharmacy Technician Certification Examination*. 3rd ed. St. Louis: Elsevier; 2014.

Smart Retailing. *Five Ways to Improve Your Pharmacy's Workflow and Efficiency*. Available at: https://join.healthmart.com/business-and-operations/5-ways-improve-pharmacys-efficiency/.

Websites Referenced

Grove D. *Pharmacy Workflow: Improving Efficiency*. Available at: http://www.pharmacytimes.com/publications/directions-in-pharmacy/2015/may2015.

PBA Health.com. *How to Improve Pharmacy Workflow in 6 Steps*.

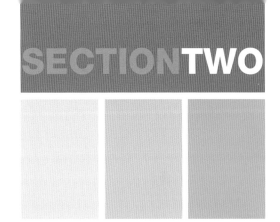

Pharmacology and Medications

16 Drug Classifications, 351

17 Therapeutic Agents for the Nervous System, 363

18 Therapeutic Agents for the Endocrine System, 397

19 Therapeutic Agents for the Musculoskeletal System, 425

20 Therapeutic Agents for the Cardiovascular System, 447

21 Therapeutic Agents for the Respiratory System, 478

22 Therapeutic Agents for the Gastrointestinal System, 503

23 Therapeutic Agents for the Renal System, 525

24 Therapeutic Agents for the Reproductive System, 545

25 Therapeutic Agents for the Immune System, 575

26 Therapeutic Agents for Eyes, Ears, Nose, and Throat, 598

27 Therapeutic Agents for the Dermatologic System, 622

28 Therapeutic Agents for the Hematologic System, 643

29 Over-the-Counter Medications, 661

30 Complementary and Alternative Medicine, 672

CHAPTER 16

Drug Classifications

Tony Guerra

OBJECTIVES	
	1. Differentiate between generic and trade (brand) names. Define generic prefixes, suffixes, and infixes.
	2. Contrast tall man lettering with generic name stems.
	3. Identify drugs from the Institute for Safe Medication Practices confused drug names list.
	4. Demonstrate basic knowledge of anatomy and physiology relating to pharmacokinetics (what the body does to drugs) and pharmacodynamics (how drugs affect the body).
	5. Discuss therapeutic agents and primary medication classes for each pathophysiologic system.
	6. Classify medications using drug schedules under the Controlled Substances Act.

TERMS AND DEFINITIONS

Adrenal Above + kidney, gland above the kidney

Anemic Not + blood condition, red blood cell deficiency

Arthritis Joint + inflammation, inflammation/stiffness of the joints

Cardiovascular Heart + vessel + relating to, relating to the heart and blood vessels

Esophagitis Esophagus + inflammation, inflammation of the esophagus

Gastroesophageal Stomach + esophagus + relating to, relating to the stomach and esophagus

Hypercholesterolemia High + cholesterol + blood condition, excess cholesterol in the blood

Hyperplasia High + formation, organ enlargement

Hypertension High + pressure, high blood pressure

Infix A meaningful stem in a generic name in the middle of the word (eg, methylprednisolone)

International Nonproprietary Name (INN) A generic name

Musculoskeletal Muscle + skeleton, relating to muscles and skeleton

Nephropathy Kidney + disease, disease of the kidneys

Nonsteroidal antiinflammatory drug (NSAID) Drug, such as ibuprofen, used to reduce pain and decrease fever

Osteoarthritis Bone + joint + inflammation, bone, and joint inflammation

Osteoporosis Bone + passage + condition, thinning of bones

Pharmacodynamics How the drug affects the body

Pharmacokinetics How the body affects the drug

Pneumonia Lung + condition, inflamed lung from bacteria or viruses

Polyneuropathy Many + nerve + disease, peripheral nerve degeneration

Prefix Meaningful stem in a generic name at the beginning of the word (eg, cefdinir)

RAAS Renin-angiotensin-aldosterone system, helps regulate blood pressure

Renal Kidney + relating to, relating to the kidneys

Rhinitis Nose + inflammation, inflammation of the nasal mucous membranes

Schizophrenia Split + mind + condition, a mental condition that breaks between thoughts

Stem A meaningful group of letters in a generic name that allows one to classify the medication by those letters

Suffix A meaningful stem in a generic name at the end of the word (eg, penicillin)

Tall man lettering Parts of generic and brand name medications that are in ALL CAPS; meant to distinguish the drug from a look-alike or sound-alike medication

United States Adopted Names Council (USANC) The body that makes decisions on drug names

Classifying Drugs

There are many ways we can classify drugs, and the easiest way to learn the different types of classifications is to see examples. By looking at ways we categorize or group drugs in the chapters that follow, the more we can learn about how agencies come to make specific drug names and where we might run into the potential for mistakes. This chapter is not comprehensive; instead, it gives you an idea of what is ahead. Think of it as an orientation to the language of pharmacology. We start with generic and brand (trade) medication names.

Brand Versus Generic Versus Chemical Names

A brand name is a proprietary name, one that separates it from its competition (eg, Advil and Motrin are both brand names for generic ibuprofen). Generic medication names, sometimes called **International Nonproprietary Names (INNs)**, generally make classification easy by looking at their **stem** in the prefix, infix, or suffix position that has meaning. This meaning might allude to a classification by the following:
- Therapeutic class
- Chemical structure
- Receptor affected
- Neurotransmitter affected

For example, ibu*profen* and keto*profen* are both **nonsteroidal antiinflammatory drugs (NSAIDs)**. Not all generic names have this advantage, but many do. In this chapter, we will look at how the **United States Adopted Names Council (USANC)** works to standardize generic medication names as they relate to their classification. We will review the medication classifications in the same order as they appear in this book, starting with drugs for the nervous, musculoskeletal, and cardiovascular systems, and so on. Let's first look at what the terms prefix, infix, and suffix mean.

Prefix A medication that has a meaningful prefix, such as *pred*nisolone (a corticosteroid) or *cef*uroxime (a cephalosporin antibiotic), provides us with a hint at the drug classification at the beginning of the drug name. We then know when we see *pred*nisone and *cef*dinir that these drugs are a corticosteroid and cephalosporin antibiotic, respectively.

Suffix A medication that has a meaningful suffix, such as amoxi*cillin* (a penicillin antibiotic), or ateno*lol* (a beta-blocker), has its hint at the end of the drug name. This way, when we see ampi*cillin* and metop*rolol*, we know these are a penicillin antibiotic and beta-blocker, respectively.

Infix Rarely, the meaningful part is in the middle, as in methyl*pred*nisolone.

By going through common prefixes, suffixes, and infixes, we can better understand the drug classification before we even look up its function. These will be covered by chapter order starting with the nervous system.

Health professionals rarely use chemical names because of how long and complicated they can be. For example, it is a lot easier to say Tylenol (brand name) or acetaminophen (generic name) than it is to say N-acetyl-para-aminophenol. The same is true with Motrin (brand name) or ibuprofen (generic name) rather than (RS)-2-(4-(2-methyl propyl)phenyl) propanoic acid. A chemical name is meant to describe every molecule in a medication ingredient.

Tall Man Lettering in Brand and Generic Medications Versus the Use of Generic Prefixes, Suffixes, and Infixes

Tall man lettering provides a way to distinguish drugs that have similar letters or sounds. The Institute for Safe Medication Practices publishes a List of Confused Drug Names (*https://www.ismp.org/recommendations/confused-drug-names-list*) that provides a side-by-side indication of which letters should be "tall" to distinguish the medication from another. A possible confusion that can come from this system is in looking at drug class prefixes, infixes, and suffixes for nonproprietary medications as similar to tall man lettering; these systems are distinct but can inadvertently overlap. The purpose of this section is to clarify the two discrete systems. In this book, the generic name stems will appear in *italics* and tall man letters will appear as ALL CAPS.

The Tall Man Letters Can Be Identical to the Generic Name Stem

The generic antidiabetic drug metformin (Glucophage) and antibiotic metronidazole (Flagyl) have three similar letters, m-e-t. The tall man letters in metFORMIN vs. metroNIDAZOLE are identical to the generic name stems in met*formin* and metro*nidazole*.

TABLE 16.1
Tall Man Letters Versus Generic Name Stems

Tall Man Letters	Tall Man Letters	Generic Name Stem	Generic Name Stem
metFORMIN	metroNIDAZOLE	met*formin*	metro*nidazole*
ALPRAZolam	clonazepam	alpr*azolam*	clon*azepam*
NexIUM	NexAVAR	Only generics	Only generics

The Tall Man Letters Can Be Different From the Generic Name Stem

The tall man letters for the antianxiety drugs alprazolam (Xanax) and clonazepam (Klonopin) look like ALPRAZolam and clonazePAM. However, the generic name stems are – azolam and –azepam. Therefore alpr*azolam* and clon*azepam* are in the same benzodiazepine therapeutic class. We will cover this class in more detail later in the book.

Tall Man Letters Intentionally Appear in Brand Names, but Generic Name Stems Do Not

The brand name of an acid reducer, Nexium, which contains generic omeprazole, would appear as NexIUM in tall man letters to distinguish it from the anticancer drug NexAVAR (Table 16.1).

As you learn the generic name stems in the rest of this chapter, you will see how it is, in many ways, a shortcut to know what particular drugs are for therapeutically. You will still be responsible for tall man letters on the licensing examination. Again, my recommendation is that until you have a good understanding of how prefixes, infixes, and suffixes work, you should commit the List of Confused Drug Names to memory.

Medication Characteristics

Effectiveness is whether a drug has provided a patient response that we intended. Did the headache go away, or did it get worse? Does the headache sometimes go away? Would the headache go away with or without the medicine? If a medication is effective, we might consider using it. If the drug is not effective, there is little point in using it, especially because there might be adverse effects.

Safety is a second important characteristic. Although we might think that if a drug is not safe, we will not use it, there must be context. Before systemic antifungals—medicines that fight fungal infections inside the body—came along, there was a dire prognosis for a person who contracted this infection. When we talk about safety, we are determining the level at which we see harmful effects. Chemotherapy, for example, often generates an increased infection risk. A medication as conventional as aspirin can cause a bleeding risk. Ultimately, we weigh the risks against the benefits.

Selectivity is the last important characteristic. When someone is drinking a soda with caffeine, for example, they are hoping to stay alert. However, their heart rate might go up, and they might become shaky or jittery. The caffeine is not selective for just wakefulness. However, some medications, such as antibiotics, only kill bacteria and do not hurt the human. This distinction is an excellent use of selectivity, allowing for better safety than a medicine that could harm the human and the bacteria.

Drug Trials

It is nice to have a foundational understanding of what drug companies do to bring medication to the market. It generally takes a long time, but there are steps and aspects common to these trials. A double-blinded randomized controlled trial is one of the best ways to know whether a novel treatment is effective.

The company compares the new medication against either no medicine or another medication to determine whether this novel drug provides an advantage. *Controls* are those volunteers selected to use no medication or another medication because they are "controlling" for error.

Randomization is the act of choosing people for the group with active medication or inactive medication. By both randomizing the sample and providing for a control group, we can honestly know whether it is the medication or just chance that caused the drug effect.

The subjects and researchers can be blinded. When subjects are "blinded," they do not know whether they are receiving active drug or the placebo. If both the subjects and researchers are blinded, we call this *double-blinded*. This setup avoids personal bias in the trial and allows us to be confident that the medication is effective. We do not want the people involved in the trial to use their judgment to decide how they think the drug affected their condition.

Four Phases of Drug Testing

Before a new drug can go on the market, the medication must go through phases so the researchers can know the medicine's effect on the body.

Phase I: This phase tests how the drug affects healthy volunteers, and scientists look at the metabolism of the drug and pharmacokinetics—how the body affects the drug—and pharmacodynamics—how the drug affects the body.

Phase II: Scientists try different doses on patients to see which is the ideal dose for the condition.

Phase III: Researchers are now testing whether the drug is safe and effective in patients.

Phase IV: After the medication enters the market, the company needs to track any issues that come up in the broader population. This follow-up is also known as postmarketing surveillance.

Anatomy, Physiology, Pharmacology, Pharmacodynamics, and Pharmacokinetics

Each of the following chapters will begin with a review of anatomy and physiology that is especially important for that section. This introductory chapter reviews two important terms and how anatomy and physiology relate to them. Pharmacology (pharmaco- + -logy) is the combination of "drug" and "study of," just as kinesiology (kinesio- + -logy) college majors combine "movement" and "study of."

Pharmacokinetics: ADME

When someone uses an oral medicine, for example, it can go through four stages: absorption, distribution, metabolism, and excretion. We sometimes call this the ADME mnemonic using the first letter of each function. Although this is not the case for all drugs, ADME provides an excellent framework for **pharmacokinetics.**

First, the body can absorb the medication. Whereas most would think the *absorption* happens in the stomach, it is usually the *small intestine* with the small finger-like villi that provides the space for absorption. We talked about routes of medication administration earlier in the book; now we are looking at why we would choose one or the other because of pharmacokinetics. When we give a drug by a parenteral route, outside of the gastrointestinal system, we can have that drug absorbed right away. An intravenous (IV) administration might be the best choice for an emergency. On the other hand, if we are looking for convenience, it is the enteral or oral route that is best for the patient. As we start looking at individual medicines, we can look at which enteral medication might work best.

If the drug needs to pass through the stomach, it will likely have an enteric coating so it does not dissolve or become inactivated before it reaches the intestine. The coating can also protect the stomach from the drug. Aspirin can cause gastric ulcers, for example.

Sustained-release preparations have the advantage of allowing the patient to take the medication only once or a few times a day. For example, someone who wakes up in the middle of the night as an insomniac would want medicine that lasts a bit longer in the bloodstream. As we go through the medication classes, ask yourself, "How fast and/or how long does the patient need this medication to work?"

Second, there is a *distribution* of the drug by the *blood*. Once the medication goes into the body, it needs to get to the tissues to have its best effect. However, there are barriers to distribution such as the blood-brain barrier or the placenta. The blood-brain barrier is meant to keep toxic substances out; however, sometimes it also keeps out medications. In an ideal world, we could replace dopamine directly in patients with Parkinson disease. Still, because of the blood-brain barrier, we must use levodopa, something that can cross the blood-brain barrier and must then be converted to dopamine. This obstacle results in less medicine arriving in the brain. The placenta is a barrier meant to protect the fetus from harm.

The *liver* generally *metabolizes* the medication to an active form, an inactive form, or a different form altogether. When drugs are administered orally, they are absorbed from the gastrointestinal tract and transported to the liver to undergo the first-pass effect. Because this first-pass effect can inactivate many medications, we would administer those parenterally so that they are not transported to the liver. Another example of

a medication that avoids the first-pass effect is sublingual (under the tongue) nitroglycerin. When nitroglycerin is administered sublingually, it readily absorbs into the bloodstream.

Some medications induce (speed up) metabolism. Other medications inhibit (slow down) metabolism. Drugs that increase the rate of metabolism are called inducers. Drugs that slow the rate of metabolism are called inhibitors. If the metabolism of a drug is induced, it means it will be broken down quicker, and the dose would need to be increased to have the same effect. If a drug's metabolism is inhibited or slowed down, that can lead to drug accumulation, which can increase toxicity and adverse effects.

Finally, the body *excretes* the drug, typically through the kidneys in the urine. However, there are other ways that drugs can move outside the body. A drug can leave the body through sweat, saliva, bile, or breast milk or through the lungs by exhaling air. An important metric we can look at with excretion is half-life. Most medications are not given in a single dose; rather, we give multiple doses over time. The half-life is the time it takes for half or 50% of the drug concentration to leave the body. So, if the half-life is long, we give fewer doses. If the half-life is short, we might need to give many doses. Another aspect of a half-life has to do with determining how long a medicine takes to reach a steady-state or plateau in the blood. Usually, it takes around four half-lives to reach this steady state. With azithromycin (Zithromax), an antibiotic, however, we use what is called a loading dose. The first dose is twice the regular daily dose to keep concentrations higher in the blood as the first half-life hits.

As we go through the therapeutic categories, we will see that one of these four processes is usually the most important. For example, if someone is having an asthma attack, it is vital to make sure the absorption happens quickly in the lungs. Instead of using a tablet, which would absorb slowly, we could use an inhaler such as albuterol (ProAir HFA) to deliver the medicine rapidly. These four principles—absorption, distribution, metabolism, and excretion—all play a part in determining how a medication will work (Fig. 16.1). Because measuring the drug concentration at the target (eg, lungs) is so difficult, we often measure ability or draw plasma drug levels. For example, if we see the patient improves in tests meant to measure breathing, we know the lung medicine is working. If we draw plasma drug levels, we are looking to see whether it falls within the therapeutic range. There is a direct correlation between toxicity and effect and the plasma concentration. The therapeutic range refers to the range of plasma levels that are present when a drug is effective without producing toxic effects.

Pharmacodynamics

In contrast, **pharmacodynamics** is how the drug affects the body. With pharmacodynamics, we often go to a much smaller scale, to that of the individual neuron, for example. We want to understand neurotransmitters better; they can deliver the message that certain body functions need to happen. For instance, when serotonin and norepinephrine, two neurotransmitters, hit receptors, they can elevate mood.

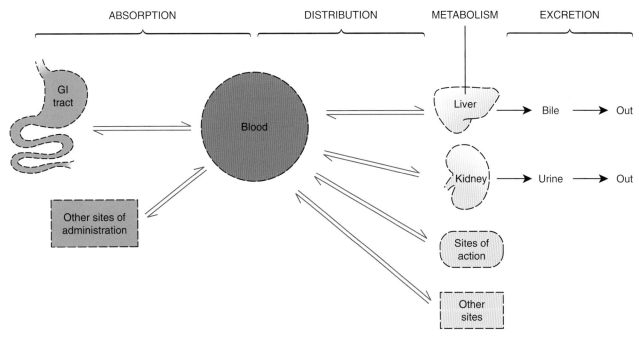

ABSORPTION   DISTRIBUTION   METABOLISM   EXCRETION

GI tract

Blood

Other sites of administration

Liver → Bile → Out

Kidney → Urine → Out

Sites of action

Other sites

FIG. 16.1 The four pharmacokinetic principles and corresponding anatomical structures.

Or when a drug blocks a beta-1 receptor, we can lower heart rate. By mimicking or copying what the body typically does with neurotransmitters, we can frequently reverse the process in many disease states through our understanding of pharmacodynamics.

Often, there is a dose-response relationship that allows us to individualize drugs for patients based on the desired outcome. In other words, a larger dose can increase the response but to a point. That point is the maximum efficacy. The maximum efficacy is the greatest effect a drug can produce. For example, morphine has a greater maximum efficacy in treating pain than acetaminophen or ibuprofen. That means that morphine can treat more intense pain than those over-the-counter (OTC) analgesics.

Relative potency is a measurement of how much of a drug the prescriber needs to elicit an effect. A patient might take 800 mg of ibuprofen (Motrin) or 15 mg of meloxicam (Mobic) as an analgesic for severe arthritis pain. They each can provide about the same amount of pain relief. However, the relative potency of a medication that only needs 15 mg is higher than that of a medicine that needs 800 mg. But the strength or effect is the same. So, a higher milligram strength does not necessarily mean it is stronger.

Drugs and Receptors

A drug is often intended to reach a certain target called a *receptor*. This is a special chemical binding site where the drug acts. If the drug fits the receptor well, like a key into a lock, it might have an excellent effect. Still, the receptor might fit and have no effect. The key fitting in the lock and wanting to be there in the first place is *affinity*. Affinity is the strength of attraction between the receptor and the drug. The second aspect is intrinsic activity. If the receptor fits and has an effect, there is intrinsic activity. If the effect is strong, we say

there is significant intrinsic activity. If the effect is weak, we similarly say there is weak intrinsic activity. Often a drug is simply mimicking a molecule the body already has but may be in short supply. We call these neurotransmitters and hormones that the body makes endogenous substances.

Agonists and Antagonists

When a medication activates a receptor, we call this an agonist. An agonist has a strong effect on a receptor activating it. For example, a breathing rescue inhaler albuterol (ProAir HFA) works as an agonist to open the lungs and airways. We also can have an antagonist that binds to the receptor but has no intrinsic activity. It gets in the way of the body's response. For example, a beta-blocker such as atenolol (Tenormin) reduces heart rate by blocking the sites to increase heart rate. The important take-home point is that whether a drug works as an agonist or antagonist, both have therapeutic effects, or those that make the patient feel better. In one case, we can open the airways with an agonist, and in another, we can lower heart rate and blood pressure with an antagonist.

Therapeutic Index

An important way to know whether a medication is safe and effective is to look at the therapeutic index. When researchers test the drug, they determine the ED_{50} and TD_{50}. An ED_{50} is the effective dose at which 50% of patients have the desired outcome. For example, a dose of ibuprofen (Motrin) relieving pain could be an example of an ED_{50} outcome. However, there might also be a TD_{50}, the toxic dose at which 50% of patients on that same ibuprofen experience gastrointestinal issues. If the ED_{50} and TD_{50} are very close together—that is, the doses are similar in having a good effect and toxicity—we call this a narrow therapeutic index, and this drug is more dangerous. We must monitor that effect more closely and would likely order that drug prescription only so the prescriber could watch the patient carefully. If the two numbers are far apart, that drug is safer because the effective and toxic doses are not close together. A drug with a wide therapeutic index like this might be safe for OTC use.

Drug Interactions

Because many patients use more than one drug at a time, we must be mindful of those drug interactions. There are three things that a drug can do with another drug. It can intensify the effect, reduce the effect, or have no effect at all. For example, if a patient takes albuterol (ProAir HFA), a drug to open the airway, and propranolol, a drug to reduce heart rate, there is a problem. Propranolol blocks receptors not only in the heart but also in the lungs. It blocks some of what the albuterol is trying to accomplish. On the other hand, we can add clavulanic acid to amoxicillin, a penicillin antibiotic. It protects the amoxicillin from bacterial enzymes called beta-lactamases, making amoxicillin effective against more infections. Either way, we must look at medications together to ensure that we are aware of the drug interactions and protect the patient. We also must watch out for drug-food interactions. Something as simple as drinking milk with cereal can get in the way of a drug having its best effect. Ciprofloxacin (Cipro), an antibiotic, binds (chelates) with calcium ions in the milk. We would need to separate this drug and food so the patient has the best outcome.

Other Drug Effects

A side effect is an effect of the drug we do not want at the standard dose. For example, diphenhydramine (Benadryl) is a common allergy medication. At normal doses, it can make a patient drowsy; this is the side effect. However, we sometimes use this side effect as a therapeutic effect. If a patient has trouble sleeping, there are medicines that combine acetaminophen (Tylenol) and diphenhydramine (Benadryl) to relieve pain and insomnia.

Iatrogenic effects are those caused by a medical treatment. For example, a patient on an antipsychotic may develop symptoms that look a lot like Parkinson disease. *Teratogenic* effects are birth defects caused by medicines. We avoid many medicines in pregnancy because we want to avoid teratogenic effects. *Carcinogenic* effects are those that produce or cause cancer. Ranitidine was removed from the market because of a concern about carcinogenic effects. The –genic ending of these words means "causing."

Tachyphylaxis is a rapid build of the body's defenses to a drug; this is a problem with nitro-containing products, so we must give them quite often. With a placebo effect, patients have an effect from what they think is a drug, yet there is no active ingredient. In a clinical trial, a group with a placebo and an active drug might both experience therapeutic outcomes. The key to knowing how well the drug works is seeing what is happening over and above that placebo effect.

Therapeutic Agents for the Nervous System (Chapter 17)

The nervous system is comprehensive, and it is easiest to provide some examples of drug class types and in which stems appear. We will go into a little more detail about neurotransmitters here because they are so significant with these medicines.

Myasthenia Gravis

Pyrido*stigmine* (Mestinon) has the stem –stigmine, which refers to cholinesterase inhibitors. These drugs increase the neurotransmitter acetylcholine within the synaptic cleft of specific neurons. Myasthenia gravis causes antibodies to bind and antagonize acetylcholine receptors, reducing access to the neurotransmitter. By increasing the neurotransmitter acetylcholine, we help reduce the harmful antibody effect.

Polyneuropathy

Dul*oxetine* (Cymbalta), a serotonin-norepinephrine reuptake inhibitor (SNRI) has the –oxetine stem. This stem is also in flu*oxetine* for depression, a selective serotonin reuptake inhibitor (SSRI). The stem is also in atom*oxetine* (Strattera), a nonstimulant for attention-deficit/hyperactivity disorder (ADHD). Usually, dul*oxetine* treats depression but can be used for **polyneuropathy** also. *Gab*apentin (Neurontin) has a prefix, gab–, and is similar in structure to gamma-aminobutyric acid (GABA) but does not precisely affect GABA receptors. Its mechanism of action is unclear, but its ability to help with polyneuropathy is certain.

Epilepsy

In generic carbamaze*pine* (Tegretol), the –pine stem relates to the structure of the drug, indicating that it has a three-ring backbone. Unfortunately, this stem tells us little about its therapeutic purpose. However, in pheny*toin*, we have a particular stem, –toin, that provides information that it is primarily for seizures.

Anxiety

The –azepam and –azolam stems appear on many benzodiazepines that provide anxiety relief. Examples include lor*azepam* (Ativan) and clon*azepam* (Klonopin), and alpr*azolam* (Xanax) and mid*azolam* (Versed). Some practitioners use benzodiazepines for epilepsy as well.

Parkinson Disease

With the combination drug carbidopa/levodopa (Sinemet), the –dopa stem refers to dopamine receptor agonists. The levels of dopamine in the brain in patients with Parkinson disease are much lower than in those without the condition. This combination medicine works to reduce the disease's effects. Note that only levo*dopa* acts as a dopamine agonist; carbidopa simply reduces levo*dopa*'s degradation.

Migraine

In suma*triptan* (Imitrex), we name the drug class after the –triptan stem, calling the group "triptans." This triptans shortcut is much easier to say than "serotonin receptor agonist," which indicates the mechanism of action. A related product is ele*triptan* (Relpax).

Depression

Many types of medications are available for depression, and often the drug name will indicate either that it is a particular class of drugs working on specific neurotransmitters such as serotonin or norepinephrine or that a medicine has a certain shape.

The sertraline (Zoloft) stem –traline indicates an SSRI, and these medications are first-line treatment for depression and various anxiety disorders. Some other SSRIs have the -*oxetine* stem, such as flu*oxetine* and par*oxetine*. Be careful; despite sharing the same stem, dul*oxetine* is a serotonin-norepinephrine reuptake inhibitor (SNRI). Venlafaxine (Effexor XR) has the –faxine stem, which suggests that it inhibits the reuptake of serotonin *and* norepinephrine (SNRI) in the central nervous system. The –triptyline stem in amitriptyline (Elavil) relates to its three-ring structure and antidepressant classification.

Schizophrenia

We divide the medications for **schizophrenia** into the first and second generations. Haloperidol represents the first generation and has specific properties that are different from those of the second generation. The second-generation drugs (also called *atypical antipsychotics*) might have similar endings. Olanzapine (Zyprexa) and clozapine (Clozaril) or ari*piprazole* (Abilify) and brex*piprazole* (Rexulti) share suffixes.

Therapeutic Agents for the Endocrine System (Chapter 18)

Addison Disease

We often use mineralocorticoid medications such as fludro*cort*isone and hydro*cort*isone (Cortef) for conditions such as Addison disease, a deficiency in the **adrenal** gland hormone cortisol. Although the medicines end in the same letters, the stem is not as readily apparent as just "cort." Note this is an infix; the drug stem is in the interior of the medication name.

Diabetes

Although there are many oral medications for diabetes, it is often clear which those are by seeing either gli or gly in the generic name, with the "g-l" alluding to glucose, the elevated sugar in patients with diabetes. In looking at these medication names, we can see patterns that help us classify them as drugs specific for diabetes. The –formin stem in met*formin* (Glucophage) does not have the gli or gly, but from the brand name you can see this drug will eat (phage) excess glucose. The thiazolidinedione pio*glitazone* (Actos), for example, has the glitazone stem with gli inside it. The longer complete stem refers to the thiazolidinedione class. The sulfonylureas *gli*mepiride (Amaryl), *gli*pizide (Glucotrol), and *gly*buride all have gli or gly in the names. Nate*glinide* (Starlix) and repa-*glinide* (Prandin) have the –glinide stem, indicating that they are meglitinide antidiabetics. Similarly, the dipeptidyl peptidase-4 (DPP-4) inhibitors sita*gliptin* (Januvia) and saxa*gliptin*

(Onglyza) both have the –gliptin stem. Understandably, health providers often call these "glinides" and "gliptins," respectively.

The sodium-glucose luminal cotransporter-2 (SGLT2) inhibitors dapa*gliflozin* (Farxiga), empa*gliflozin* (Jardiance), and cana*gliflozin* (Invokana) all have the -gliflozin stem. Currently, the only glucagon-like peptide-1 (GLP-1) receptor agonist available orally is sema*glutide* (Rybelsus), which contains the –glutide stem. The newest drug approved for type 2 diabetes, and the first in its class, is terzepa*tide* (Mounjaro), which acts as both a GLP-1 receptor agonist and a glucose-dependent insulinotropic polypeptide (GIP).

Therapeutic Agents for the Musculoskeletal System (Chapter 19)

Nonopioid Analgesic

Acetaminophen stands as an essential drug that we classify by what it is not—something for pain that is nonopioid. In general, we use acetaminophen for **musculoskeletal** pain, **osteoarthritis,** headache, and fever. Many prescriptions and OTC products contain acetaminophen (Tylenol).

Nonsteroidal Antiinflammatory Drugs

Aspirin (Ecotrin) provides relief from headache, fever, and mild pain. New guidelines specify that only prescribers should recommend it in low doses for thromboembolism prophylaxis. Like acetaminophen, it predates many generic stems, but its chemical name has the "sal," indicating salicylate from acetylsalicylic acid. Shorter-acting ibu*profen* (Advil, Motrin) has the –profen stem, showing its relationship to the nonsteroidal antiinflammatory drug (NSAID) class. Although naproxen (Naprosyn) lacks a similar stem, it is nonetheless a critical longer-acting NSAID. Cele*coxib*, with the –coxib stem, is the cyclooxygenase-2 (COX-2)-specific inhibitor.

Salicylates, such as aspirin, should be avoided in children under the age of 18 with suspected viral infections because there is an increased risk for Reye syndrome. One should avoid NSAIDs in all children younger than 6 months of age.

Opioid Analgesics

Although not a stem, many of the opioid analgesics share similar spellings and are morphine derivatives. Examples include hydrocodone with acetaminophen and oxycodone with acetaminophen (Percocet), which relieve moderate to severe pain.

Bisphosphonates

Some drugs for **osteoporosis** have clear suffixes such as alen-*dronate* (Fosamax) and iban*dronate* (Boniva). Although there are many more medications discussed in the musculoskeletal chapter, the takeaway is that many related medicines have identical and meaningful stems, as do ibandronate and alendronate.

Therapeutic Agents for the Cardiovascular System (Chapter 20)

The **cardiovascular** system's medications are often newer and have many drugs with helpful stems. For example, some relate to the renin-angiotensin-aldosterone system (RAAS) and others to the beta-adrenergic blockade.

Angiotensin-Converting Enzyme Inhibitors

Generic lisino*pril* is part of a class of drugs (angiotensin-converting enzyme inhibitors [ACEIs]) that block an essential enzyme in the RAAS. By blocking this enzyme, the body is less able to vasoconstrict and increase blood pressure. Often, we call lisino*pril* (Zestril, Prinivil) or benaze*pril* (Lotensin) by their stem name, "prils." They help with **hypertension** and other conditions.

Angiotensin II Receptor Blockers

Drugs such as lo*sartan* (Cozaar) and val*sartan* (Diovan) block the receptor where the potent vasoconstrictor enzyme angiotensin II would generally work (angiotensin II receptor blockers [ARBs]). By doing this, some vessels cannot vasoconstrict, resulting in decreased blood pressure. Besides hypertension, we can use these for stroke or diabetic **nephropathy** prevention. As with the prils, we sometimes call these drugs by their endings as "sartans."

Beta-Blockers

There are many beta-1 receptors in the heart, and by blocking them, we can reduce hypertension. Both propran*olol* and metopr*olol* (Toprol XL) have the −olol beta-blocker stem. What the stem does not tell you is that propran*olol* is a first-generation beta-blocker and affects both beta-1 and beta-2 receptors. This beta-2 blockade might affect patients with asthma because there are beta-2 receptors in the lungs that, if blocked, can lead to bronchoconstriction. Metopr*olol* is beta-1 selective, meaning it works only on the heart, and prescribers would prefer this for patients with asthma. Although they have many indications, beta-blockers are generally prescribed for heart failure and atrial fibrillation.

Statins

Drugs such as lo*vastatin* and ator*vastatin* (Lipitor) carry the −statin stem. This stem indicates that they are 3-hydroxy-3-methylglutaryl-coenzyme A (HMG-CoA) reductase inhibitors. This medication class lowers bad cholesterol, the low-density lipoproteins (LDLs). They also include the substem "va" to differentiate them from a medication such as nystatin, which is an antifungal agent. As with other classes, we often call these lipid-lowering drugs "statins."

Statins are a primary preventative for atherosclerotic cardiovascular disease (ASCVD). Health professionals evaluate patients on their preexisting risk factors for experiencing a future major cardiac event using the 10-year ASCVD Risk Estimator. This score dictates the intensity of statin regimen, high or moderate intensity, that will lower cholesterol levels sufficiently. Moderate-intensity statins include lovastatin 40 mg, pravastatin 40 to 80 mg, and atorvastatin 10 to 20 mg. High-intensity statins include atorvastatin doses greater than 40 mg and rosuvastatin greater than 20 mg. Most, but not all, of these medications are best taken in the evening at the time of greatest cholesterol synthesis.

PCSK9 Inhibitors

Newer drugs such as alirocu*mab* (Praluent) and evolocu*mab* (Repatha) have the monoclonal antibody stem −mab. Some of the interior substems have meaning as well, such as the "cu," which is why these two have the same endings. The drugs are for high cholesterol resulting from heterozygous familial **hypercholesterolemia** (HeFH) and are very expensive.

Therapeutic Agents for the Respiratory System (Chapter 21)

Allergy, Cold, and Cough

Although there are dozens of different medications in the allergy, cough, and cold aisle, there are relatively few active ingredients. We classify the medicines as first- and second-generation antihistamines, decongestants, antitussives (anticough), and expectorants. Drugs for pain and fever, such as nonopioid analgesics and NSAIDs, are discussed in a previous section. First-generation antihistamines, which generally cause drowsiness, include generic brompheniramine and chlorpheniramine. We might see them in combination with other drugs and diphenhydramine (Benadryl Allergy). Second-generation drugs such as lor*atadine* (Claritin), cetirizine (Zyrtec Allergy), and fexofenadine (Allegra Allergy 12 Hour) generally do not cause sedation. These antihistamines help with a runny nose and other allergy symptoms. Decongestants such as OTC phenylephrine (Neo-Synephrine Cold + Allergy Regular Strength Spray) and behind-the-counter pseudoephedrine (Sudafed) clear up clogged sinuses. The OTC dextrometh*orphan*, the DM in Robitussin Cough + Congestion DM or Mucinex DM, stops cough. The expectorant guaifenesin helps clear mucus. Although there are stems in lor*atadine* and dextrometh*orphan*, these are not as helpful because there are not many other drugs with identical stems we often use that are just like them.

Bronchodilators and Antiinflammatory Drugs for Asthma

Asthma is a condition of bronchoconstriction and inflammation. The −terol ending in short-acting albu*terol* (ProAir HFA) or long-acting salme*terol* in Advair HFA indicates a beta-2 receptor agonist that opens bronchioles. Although fluticasone in Advair HFA and budesonide in Symbicort have a similar "s-o-n" component, these are not true stems, although it may hint that these are corticosteroids for lung inflammation. The important takeaway is that many medications for asthma have consistent spellings helping us classify.

Drugs for Pneumonia

Antibacterials often have drug endings that make them easier to classify as well. For example, many macrolide antibiotics, such as azithromycin (Zithromax), might end in −thromycin. Although drugs that end in just −mycin are from a specific bacterial strain, it does not tell you that a drug is necessarily a particular type of antibiotic. We see azithromycin used for **pneumonia**, community-acquired pneumonia, and various bacterial infections. Ciproflixacin (Cipro) also has a stem indicating it is part of the fluoroquinolone class. This –floxacin ending is also in levofloxacin and others. Amoxicillin is a penicillin-class antibiotic. This is currently a first-line treatment for uncomplicated outpatient community-acquired pneumonia (CAP). In patients with a penicillin allergy, doxycycline, a tetracycline antibiotic, is the first-line CAP treatment.

Therapeutic Agents for the Gastrointestinal System (Chapter 22)

Histamine-2 Antagonists (–tidine)

Histamine-2 (H$_2$) antagonists bind to H$_2$ receptor sites, reducing acid secretion. They are for **gastroesophageal** reflux disease (GERD), erosive **esophagitis,** gastric ulcer, and duodenal ulcer treatment. Some can be found as OTC products for heartburn and indigestion. Common medications include famotidine (Pepcid), nizatidine (Axid), and cimetidine (Tagamet HB 200). Note that each medication ends in the same "t-i-d-i-n-e," –tidine. Be careful, because the H$_1$ blockers help with allergies and some end with –atadine, a very similar ending.

Proton Pump Inhibitors (–prazole)

Proton pump inhibitors (PPIs) mainly treat GERD and peptic ulcers and are generally dosed once daily. OTC products include esomeprazole (Nexium 24HR), lansoprazole (Prevacid 24HR), omeprazole (Prilosec OTC), and omeprazole/sodium bicarbonate (Zegerid OTC). Be careful, because there are the antipsychotic medications aripiprazole (Aricept) and brexpiprazole (Rexulti) that have the –piprazole stem signifying a type of antipsychotic. These look-alike endings may result in confusion.

Monoclonal Antibodies (–mab)

Many new medications are monoclonal antibodies, which often take the –mab suffix, which stands for *monoclonal antibody*. These have a very complex naming structure that we will briefly discuss with infliximab (Remicade), a gastrointestinal medication for Crohn disease, ulcerative colitis, and rheumatoid arthritis. This drug inhibits the proinflammatory cytokine tumor necrosis factor-alpha (TNF-α) to reduce the inflammatory response.

Therapeutic Agents for the Renal System (Chapter 23)

Diuretics

One of the most important classes of drugs for issues with the **renal** system includes diuretic medications. Two very common classifications include those for thiazide and loop diuretics. A thiazide diuretic works at the distal convoluted tubule, a little further away from the glomerulus than the loop diuretic, so it does not cause as much diuresis. We can recognize some thiazide diuretics by their –thiazide ending, as in hydrochlorothiazide. We will often see a combination pill consisting of an ACEI or an ARB and a thiazide diuretic for hypertension. With loop diuretics, we may see a –semide

suffix as in furosemide (Lasix). Furosemide is generally for conditions that require more diuresis or have more edema, such as congestive heart failure.

Therapeutic Agents for the Reproductive System (Chapter 24)

Oral contraceptives contain either progestin only or some form of estrogen-progestin combination. The stems in these medications differentiate them.

Progestins and Estrogens

Etonogestrel (Nexplanon), a hormonal implant under the skin, levonorgestrel (Mirena), the intrauterine device (IUD), and medroxyprogesterone acetate (Depo-Vera), the injectable, all share the "-gest" stem for progesterone. These forms of birth control contain progesterone only. An oral combination contraceptive with estrogen and progestin might also include ethinyl estradiol, the "estr-" signifying the estrogen component.

Benign Prostatic Hyperplasia

Benign prostatic **hyperplasia** is an enlarged but not cancerous prostate. Drugs such as finasteride (Proscar) and dutasteride (Avodart) block testosterone conversion to a more active androgen, dihydrotestosterone, which causes cell growth. The –steride stem helps classify the drugs as 5-alpha reductase inhibitors.

Additionally, alpha-1 blockers help relieve symptoms of benign prostatic hyperplasia by relaxing the muscle surrounding the bladder and prostate improving urine flow. These medications often end in –azosin; for example, doxazosin, terazosin, and prazosin. Tamsulosin has a slightly different ending.

Viral

A drug such as acyclovir (Zovirax) or valacyclovir (Valtrex) has the –cyclovir stem. The –vir is the suffix indicating an antiviral agent. The –cyclovir entirety is more specific to these medications, which help treat herpesvirus. Similarly, we also see the –vir stem in antivirals for human immunodeficiency virus (HIV) or hepatitis. There are too many to list in this introductory chapter, but we go over them in detail in later chapters.

Therapeutic Agents for the Immune System (Chapter 25)

Two relevant groups of medicines we talk about in this chapter include those that suppress the immune system to combat autoimmune disorders and vaccines.

Rheumatoid Arthritis

A condition such as rheumatoid **arthritis** (RA) affects the joints and manifests as an immune condition. Within the treatment regimens for RA, we have nonbiological medications, such as methotrexate (Trexall), and biological medications, which often end in –mab, for monoclonal antibody, such as adalimumab (Humira). We saw earlier that infliximab (Remicade) had an "m-a-b" ending. When talking about drug classification, although it is useful information that a drug is a monoclonal antibody, this does not necessarily help us know the pathophysiologic disease that the drug affects.

Vaccines

Vaccines protect against bacteria and viruses. Often, we separate the vaccine classes by separating those that are preventive against bacteria, such as the pneumococcal vaccine (Prevnar 20), or those against viruses, such as the human papillomavirus (HPV) vaccine (Gardasil). Vaccines may also be classified as live (attenuated) vaccines—such as measles, mumps, and rubella (MMR); varicella; and rotavirus—and inactivated vaccines, such as the seasonal influenza vaccine. Live (attenuated) vaccines contain a weakened bacteria or virus and allow for long-term immunity, whereas inactivated vaccines contain the dead bacteria or virus and require frequent supplemental, or "booster," vaccinations.

Therapeutic Agents for Eyes, Ears, Nose, and Throat (Chapter 26)

Ophthalmic Preparations

Many of the medications we discussed can come in ophthalmic forms as a sterile product. For example, *pred*nisolone ophthalmic (Pred Forte) has the same stem as oral *pred*nisone, another corticosteroid. Flurbi*profen* and keto*profen* (Acular) have the same –profen stem as ibuprofen, letting us know that all are NSAIDs. Betax*olol* (Betoptic S) and carte*olol* are both beta-blockers for open-angle glaucoma when used in the eye and have the same –olol ending as oral beta-blockers.

Allergic Rhinitis

For allergic **rhinitis**, an inflammation in the nose, we can recognize triamcinolone (Nasacort Allergy 24HR) and fluticasone (Flonase Allergy Relief). Although they do not have proper stems, the "lone" and "sone" often hint toward a corticosteroid for inflammation. The utility of stems extends far past just oral drugs.

Therapeutic Agents for the Dermatologic System (Chapter 27)

Sometimes we will use oral medications to treat topical conditions that come from systemic causes. An example includes diphenhydramine (Benadryl Allergy) for hives, itching, or rash. Or we can give the patient a tetracycline antibiotic such as doxy*cycline* (Doryx) or mino*cycline* (Minocin) for acne. Patients can use these with or without additional topical products. Note that the –cycline stem helps us know that these drugs are tetracycline antibiotics.

Therapeutic Agents for the Hematologic System (Chapter 28)

Ferrous sulfate (OTC) is one medication for patients who are **anemic**, who do not have enough iron in their bodies. Because there are many salt forms, it can be confusing for patients who are typically looking for a certain amount of ferrous sulfate. Usually, there is an equivalency on the back of the box to help the patient. Ferrous or iron products are

often classified as minerals rather than as medications and are usually OTC products. Antiplatelets, such as aspirin and clopido*grel* (Plavix), prevent platelets from clumping together to form a clot in the blood for patient with a history of stroke or heart attack. Similarly, anticoagulants prevent clot formation but through a different mechanism. These "blood thinners" include oral medications, such as war*farin*, api*xaban* (Eliquis), riva*roxaban* (Xarelto), and injectable medications, such as enoxa*parin* (Lovenox) and heparin.

Drug Classifications by Drug Enforcement Administration Schedules I, II, III, IV, and V

Another way we classify drugs is to use the drug schedules under the Controlled Substances Act (CSA). The numbers, in Roman numerals from I to V (1–5), go from most likely to cause harm and abuse to least likely. Here we will provide only a summary of what a medication in each class would look like.

Schedule I

There is no currently accepted medical use for medications in US Drug Enforcement Administration (DEA) schedule I, and possession of many is illegal. Examples include drugs such as heroin and ecstasy. Marijuana varies in its schedule based on individual state laws.

Schedule II

Schedule II controlled substances are medications which have significant opportunity for abuse because of potential for psychological or physical dependence. Examples include hydrocodone/acetaminophen, oxycodone/acetaminophen (Percocet), or fentanyl.

Schedule III

The schedule system is a relative one: III is more hazardous than IV but less hazardous than II. Drugs in this class include certain dosages of acetaminophen with codeine.

Schedule IV

Many anxiolytic medications, such as benzodiazepines, fall into schedule IV. Again, these medications fall somewhere between schedule III and V. Medications include di*azepam* (Valium) or lor*azepam* (Ativan).

Schedule V

Although not without the potential for abuse, that potential in this class is limited. Most of the medications include liquid cough preparations. An example of this group of drugs is guaifenesin/codeine (Cheratussin AC).

Do You Remember These Key Points?

- Stem value within drug names
- Primary medication classes in each pathophysiologic system
- Differences among prefixes, suffixes, and infixes

- Conventional medication stems in generic names
- Generic and trade names for the drugs discussed in this chapter
- General differences between brand (trade) and generic names

Review Questions

Multiple Choice Questions

1. _____ is what we call a meaningful stem at the end of a generic medication name.
   A. Prefix
   B. Suffix
   C. Infix
   D. Substem

2. A medication that has the –profen stem could be classified as the acronym _____.
   A. NSAID
   B. DMARD
   C. ARB
   D. ACEI

3. At the end of a loop diuretic's generic name, we might see the suffix:
   A. –pril
   B. –olol
   C. –semide
   D. –sartan

4. Which medication class that has both ophthalmic and oral preparations ends with –olol?
   A. Angiotensin-converting enzyme inhibitors
   B. HMG-CoA reductase inhibitors for cholesterol
   C. Alpha-blockers
   D. Beta-blockers

5. What is the brand name for the antidiabetic metformin that relates to what it does to glucose?
   A. Prandin
   B. Actos
   C. Glucophage
   D. Lasix

6. _____ is a disease with a deficiency in the production of cortisol.
   A. Addison
   B. Parkinson
   C. Diabetes
   D. Hypothyroid

7. Which medication is approved for the treatment of benign prostatic hyperplasia?
   A. Dutasteride
   B. Metoprolol
   C. Ketoprofen
   D. Furosemide

8. Which medication(s) is/are associated with the opening of the lungs or bronchodilation?
   A. Hydrochlorothiazide
   B. Atenolol
   C. Alirocumab
   D. Albuterol

9. If a medication stem ends in –mab, what do we likely know about it?
   A. It is a monoclonal antibody.
   B. It is always an antiinflammatory drug.
   C. It is always an anticholesterol drug.
   D. It is always a beta-blocker.

10. Which drug cannot be used in the eye?
    A. Betaxolol
    B. Ketoprofen
    C. Prednisolone
    D. Evolocumab

11. If a patient is on a medication that ends in –triptan, what does the patient likely have?
    A. Migraines
    B. Hypertension
    C. Edema
    D. Diabetes

12. _____ is associated with the DEA schedule that is most likely to cause dependence and abuse but is still legal to prescribe.
    A. Schedule I
    B. Schedule II
    C. Schedule III
    D. Schedule IV

13. Which drug ending would indicate the drug works on the renin-angiotensin-aldosterone system (RAAS) to lower blood pressure?
    A. –glitazone
    B. –olol
    C. –pril
    D. –statin

14. Which antidepressant drug stem refers to the number of rings in the chemical structure?
    A. –triptyline
    B. –traline
    C. –faxine
    D. –oxetine

15. If a prescriber gives a progestin-only contraceptive, we might expect which four letters in the generic drug name?
    A. olol
    B. pril
    C. estr
    D. gest

Technician's Corner

Although the –olol tells us that a medication might be a beta-blocker, it does not tell us to which generation it belongs. Look up beta-blocker generations and outline the difference between the first, second, and third generations as it relates to affecting beta-1 and beta-2 receptors and vasodilation. Use generic propranolol as first, metoprolol as second, and carvedilol as the third generation.

Bibliography

Clinical Pharmacology Online. Available at: https://www.clinicalkey.com/pharmacology/.

Guerra T. *How to Pronounce Drug Names: A Visual Approach to Preventing Medication Errors*. Raleigh, NC: Print; 2016.

Guerra T. *Memorizing Pharmacology: A Relaxed Approach*. Raleigh, NC: Print; 2016.

US Drug Enforcement Agency. *Drug Scheduling*. Available at: https://www.dea.gov/drug-information/drug-scheduling.

US National Library of Medicine. *Generic Name Stems—Drug Information Portal*. Available at: https://druginfo.nlm.nih.gov/drugportal/jsp/drugportal/DrugNameGenericStems.jsp.

Therapeutic Agents for the Nervous System

Tony Guerra

TERMS AND DEFINITIONS

Alzheimer disease (AD) A progressive form of dementia that affects memory, thinking, and behavior; eponym named after German neurologist Alois Alzheimer

Attention-deficit/hyperactivity disorder (ADHD) A physiologic brain disorder that affects the ability to engage in quiet, passive activities or to focus one's attention; attributable to a neurotransmitter imbalance

Autonomic nervous system (ANS) The nervous system branch that carries out "automatic" body functions; it includes the sympathetic and parasympathetic systems

Blood-brain barrier (BBB) A brain barrier that results from unique permeability characteristics of capillaries that supply brain cells; the capillaries prevent specific solutes or chemicals from passing from the blood to the brain

Bradykinesia Delayed + movement + condition of, slowed movement

Brainstem A section of the brain consisting of the medulla oblongata, pons, and midbrain, which connect the forebrain and cerebrum to the spinal cord

Central nervous system (CNS) Consists of the brain and spinal cord; it coordinates sensory and motor body function control

Cerebellum Hindbrain, a structure posterior to the pons and medulla oblongata responsible for posture, balance, and voluntary muscle movement

Cerebrospinal fluid (CSF) Brain + spine + pertaining to, continually produced and absorbed clear, watery fluid that flows in the brain ventricles around the brain surface and spinal cord

Epilepsy A brain disorder marked by repeated seizures over time

Extrapyramidal symptoms (EPS) Often result from taking antipsychotic medications and include parkinsonism, dystonia, and tremors

Hemorrhagic stroke A stroke caused by a brain blood vessel rupture

Homeostasis Similar + still, the body's tendency to maintain stability, as with body temperature

Insomnia Not + sleep + condition of, difficulty falling or staying asleep

Ischemic stroke Stop + blood + condition of, a stroke caused by a brain blood vessel blockage

Multiple sclerosis (MS) Harden + condition of, an autoimmune disorder that affects CNS nerves; it leads to hindered motor function

Myasthenia gravis Muscle + weakness + condition of + grave/severe, a neuromuscular disorder leading to skeletal muscle weakness

Neuron The nervous system's basic building block and cell

Parasympathetic nervous system (PSNS) An autonomic nervous system division that functions during rest

Parkinson disease (PD) A movement disorder with the classic symptoms of tremor, rigidity, bradykinesia, and postural instability, an eponym for English physician James Parkinson

Peripheral nervous system (PNS) The nervous system division outside the brain and spinal cord

Polyneuropathy Many + nerve + disease, a neurologic disorder that occurs when many nerves malfunction; it may include painful neuropathy

Psychosis Mind + a state of disease, a mental illness characterized by loss of contact with reality. Psychosis may be a genuine mental illness, the result of an underlying medical condition (eg, dementia, drug withdrawal syndromes), or induced by medications, recreational drugs, or poisons

Schizophrenia Split + mind + condition of, a disorder characterized by inappropriate emotions and unrealistic thinking

Smoking cessation To discontinue tobacco smoking, to quit smoking

Somatic nervous system The motor neurons of the peripheral nervous system that control voluntary actions of the skeletal muscles and provide sensory input (touch, hearing, sight)

Sympathetic nervous system (SNS) An autonomic nervous system division that activates during stress; the "fight-or-flight" response

Tardive dyskinesia (TD) Late + bad + movement, a type of dyskinesia (unwanted, involuntary rhythmic movements) recognized as a potential side effect of dopamine antagonists (eg, phenothiazines, metoclopramide); the symptoms may continue even after the offending drug is discontinued

Select Common Drugs for Conditions of the Nervous System

Trade Name	Generic Name	Pronunciation
Alzheimer Disease		
Aricept	donepezil	(doh-**neh**-puh-zil)
Exelon	rivastigmine	(ri-va-**stig**-meen)
Namenda	memantine	(meh-**man**-teen)
Razadyne	galantamine	(gal-**an**-ta-meen)
Anxiety Disorders		
Ativan	lorazepam	(lor-**a**-zuh-pam)
BuSpar[a]	buspirone	(byoo-**spye**-rone)
Serax[a]	oxazepam	(ox-**a**-zuh-pam)
Valium	diazepam	(dye-**az**-uh-pam)
Xanax	alprazolam	(al-pra-**zuh**-lam)
Attention-Deficit/Hyperactivity Disorder (ADHD)		
Adderall	amphetamine/dextroamphetamine	(am-**fet**-uh-meen/**dex**-troe-am-**fet**-uh-meen)
Dexedrine	dextroamphetamine	(dex-troe-am-**fet**-uh-meen)
Focalin	dexmethylphenidate	(dex-meth-il-**fen**-ih-date)
Qelbree	viloxazine	(vil-**ox**-uh-zeen)
Ritalin	methylphenidate	(meth-il-**fen**-ih-date)
Strattera	atomoxetine	(**a**-tuh-**mox**-uh-teen)
Vyvanse	lisdexamfetamine	(lis-**dex**-am-**fet**-uh-meen)

Trade Name	Generic Name	Pronunciation
Bipolar Disorder		
Depakote	valproic acid	(val-**pro**-ik **a**-sid)
Eskalith[a]	lithium	(**lith**-e-um)
Geodon	ziprasidone	(zi-**pray**-sih-done)
Lamictal	lamotrigine	(la-**moe**-truh-jeen)
Risperdal	risperidone	(ris-**per**-uh-done)
Seroquel	quetiapine	(kwe-**tye**-uh-peen)
Zyprexa	olanzapine	(oh-lan-**zuh**-peen)
Depression		
Celexa	citalopram	(sih-**tal**-uh-pram)
Cymbalta	duloxetine	(du-**lox**-uh-teen)
Effexor XR	venlafaxine	(**ven**-luh-fax-een)
Elavil[a]	amitriptyline	(am-uh-**trip**-tuh-leen)
Lexapro	escitalopram	(**es**-sih-**tal**-uh-pram)
Pamelor	nortriptyline	(nor-**trip**-tuh-leen)
Paxil	paroxetine	(pa-**rox**-uh-teen)
Pristiq	desvenlafaxine	(des-**ven**-luh-**fax**-een)
Prozac	fluoxetine	(floo-**ox**-uh-teen)
Tofranil	imipramine	(im-**ip**-ruh-meen)
Wellbutrin XL	bupropion	(bew-**pro**-pe-on)
Zoloft	sertraline	(**sir**-truh-leen)
Epilepsy		
Depakote	divalproex sodium	(di-val-**pro**-ex so-de-um)
Dilantin	phenytoin	(**fen**-i-toyn)
Gabitril	tiagabine	(tye-**ag**-uh-been)
Keppra	levetiracetam	(**lee**-ve-ti-**ruh**-se-tam)
Lamictal	lamotrigine	(la-**mow**-truh-jeen)
Tegretol	carbamazepine	(kar-ba-**maz**-uh-peen)
Topamax	topiramate	(toe-**pir**-uh-mate)
Trileptal	oxcarbazepine	(**ox**-kar-**baz**-uh-peen)
Insomnia		
Ambien	zolpidem	(zole-**pih**-dem)
Benadryl Allergy	diphenhydramine	(**dye**-fen-**hye**-dra-meen)
Halcion	triazolam	(try-**az**-uh-lam)
Lunesta	eszopiclone	(es-zoe-**pik**-lone)
Restoril	temazepam	(tem-**az**-uh-pam)
Rozerem	ramelteon	(ra-**mel**-tee-on)
Sonata	zaleplon	(**zal**-e-plon)
Unisom SleepGels	diphenhydramine	(dai-fuhn-**hai**-druh-meen)
Migraine Headache		
Axert	almotriptan	(**al**-mo-**trip**-tan)
Frova	frovatriptan	(fro-vuh-**trip**-tan)
Imitrex	sumatriptan	(**soo**-muh-**trip**-tan)
Maxalt	rizatriptan	(**rye**-zuh-**trip**-tan)
Nurtec	rimegepant	(ri-meh-**juh**-pant)
Relpax	eletriptan	(el-uh-**trip**-tan)
Ubrelvy	ubrogepant	(you-broe-**juh**-pant)
Zomig	zolmitriptan	(**zol**-mi-**trip**-tan)

Continued

Select Common Drugs for Conditions of the Nervous System—cont'd

Trade Name	Generic Name	Pronunciation
Multiple Sclerosis		
Ampyra	dalfampridine	(dal-**fam**-pri-**deen**)
Avonex, Rebif	interferon beta-1a	(in-tur-**fear**-on **bay**-ta won ay)
Betaseron	interferon beta-1b	(in-tur-**fear**-on **bay**-ta won bee)
Copaxone	glatiramer	(gla-**tir**-uh-mer)
Gilenya	fingolimod	(fin-**gol**-ih-mod)
Novantrone[a]	mitoxantrone	(mye-toe-**zan**-trone)
Tysabri	natalizumab	(na-ta-**liz**-yoo-mab)
Myasthenia Gravis		
Imuran	azathioprine	(ay-za-**thye**-oh-preen)
Mestinon	pyridostigmine	(pie-rid-o-**stig**-meen)
Parkinson Disease		
Azilect	rasagiline	(ras-**aj**-il-een)
Comtan	entacapone	(en-**tak**-a-pone)
Mirapex	pramipexole	(pram-ih-**pex**-ole)
Neupro	rotigotine	(row-**tig**-oh-teen)
Requip[a]	ropinirole	(row-**pin**-ih-role)
Sinemet	levodopa/carbidopa	(**lee**-vo-**doe**-puh/**car**-bih-**doe**-puh)
Symmetrel[a]	amantadine	(ah-**man**-tuh-deen)
Zelapar	selegiline	(se-**le**-juh-leen)
Peripheral Neuropathy		
Cymbalta	duloxetine	(du-**lox**-uh-teen)
Effexor XR	venlafaxine	(**ven**-luh-fax-een)
Neurontin	gabapentin	(**ga**-buh-**pen**-tin)
Zostrix[a]	capsaicin	(cap-**say**-sin)
Schizophrenia		
Abilify	aripiprazole	(**ar**-ih-**pip**-ruh-zole)
Fanapt	iloperidone	(**eye**-loe-**per**-ih-done)
Geodon	ziprasidone	(zi-**pray**-sih-done)
Haldol[a]	haloperidol	(**hal**-oh-**pear**-uh-dol)
Invega	paliperidone	(pal-ee-**per**-i-done)
Latuda	lurasidone	(loo-**ras**-i-done)
Risperdal	risperidone	(ris-**per**-ih-done)
Seroquel	quetiapine	(kwe-**tye**-uh-peen)
Zyprexa	olanzapine	(oh-lan-**zuh**-peen)

[a]Brand discontinued; now available only as generic.

Nervous System Introduction

The nervous system is a complex structure responsible for controlling and coordinating numerous body functions, including conscious and unconscious activities. Nerves enable the body to perform involuntarily activities, such as regulating heartbeat, digesting a meal, or interpreting visual signals. The nervous system's complexity becomes more accessible as we describe the divisions and specific functions. This chapter begins with common medical terminology and an overview of the nervous system's main branches and roles. Studying the nervous system leads to understanding how medications work on the system. This chapter discusses select nervous system conditions and the common medications used to treat them.

The nervous system coordinates the body's actions. It enables us to interact with our environment. Our nerves allow us to detect and respond to stimuli (changes within or outside our body). The nervous system maintains **homeostasis**, an

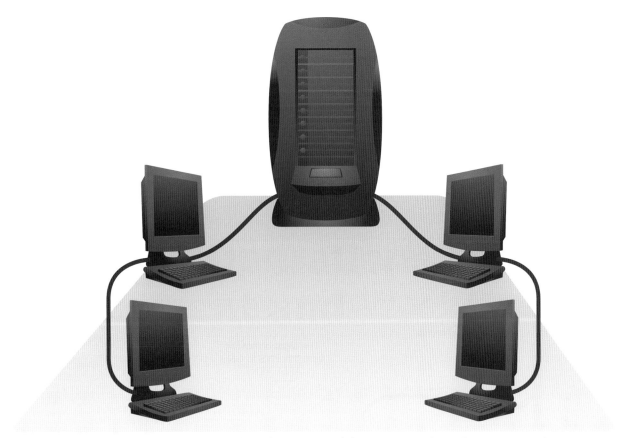

FIG. 17.1 The nervous system is analogous to a mainframe computer (central nervous system) that communicates with other computers farther away (peripheral nervous system).

equilibrium. It is analogous to a complex, mainframe computer system. The nerves work like the Internet with many connections. The mainframe (central nervous system) connects to computers (target sites) that interpret the signals. Likewise, the computer extensions can send messages to the mainframe computer, where they can be interpreted and the body can respond (Fig. 17.1).

The brain, the brainstem, and the spinal cord form the **central nervous system (CNS).** The **peripheral nervous system (PNS)** is outside the CNS and includes afferent (sensory) and efferent (motor) branches. The afferent (sensory) division transmits impulses from the body's organs and tissues to the CNS. The CNS then interprets those signals. The efferent (motor) division then relays the interpreted impulses to appropriate organs to trigger an effect. We further divide the efferent system into the **somatic nervous system** and the autonomic nervous system (ANS). The somatic system relays motor impulses to skeletal muscles, and the autonomic system transmits motor impulses to smooth muscle (eg, the muscle surrounding the blood vessels), cardiac muscle (ie, the heart), and glandular tissue. The ANS has two main branches: the sympathetic nervous system (SNS) and the parasympathetic nervous system (PSNS), described later in the chapter.

Although the nervous system has many divisions, we consider the components as one organ system (Fig. 17.2). We begin by discussing the fundamental nerve cell, the neuron.

Tech Note!

The nervous system includes the CNS and PNS. The CNS is the brain, brainstem, and spinal cord. The PNS carries messages from the body to the CNS for interpretation. The brain and spinal cord relay messages outward to the body, where they trigger an effect. We divide the PNS into the somatic and autonomic divisions.

Neurons

The **neuron** is the smallest unit of the nervous system. Billions of neurons run through our bodies carrying messages back and forth. Neurons have four main sections: the cell body, the dendrite, the axon, and the nerve terminal (Fig. 17.3). As neurons branch, they form a network of relay stations allowing nerve impulses to travel from one neuron to another via small gaps called *synapses*. The dendrites are extensions that receive electrical impulses from the previous neuron's nerve terminal. The cell body processes the electrical message before it enters the axon. Special insulation called a *myelin sheath* covers many axons. The covering consists of phospholipids and proteins and accelerates impulse conduction (see Fig. 17.3).

Nerve Transmission

Chemical message conduction from one neuron to another causes three basic cell membrane changes: polarization,

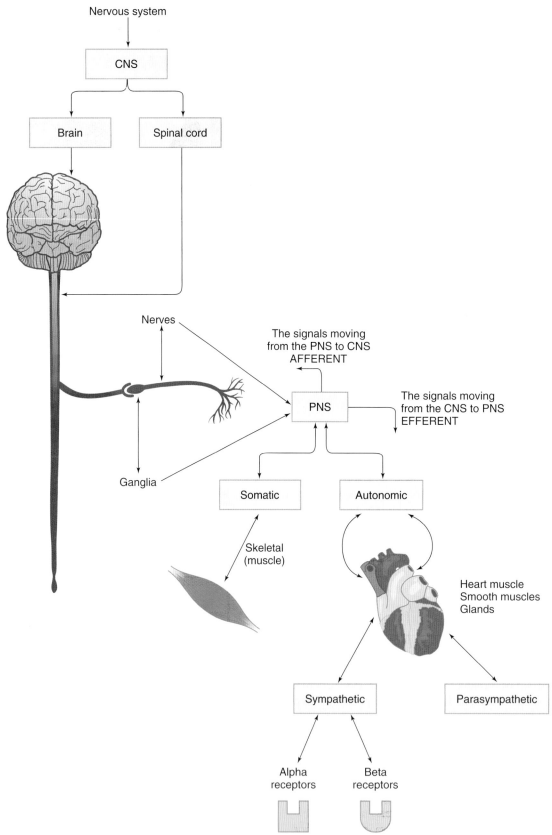

FIG. 17.2 Divisions of the nervous system include the somatic and autonomic branches. The somatic division sends and receives impulses to and from the muscles, and the autonomic system regulates both the sympathetic and the parasympathetic systems. *CNS,* Central nervous system; *PNS,* peripheral nervous system.

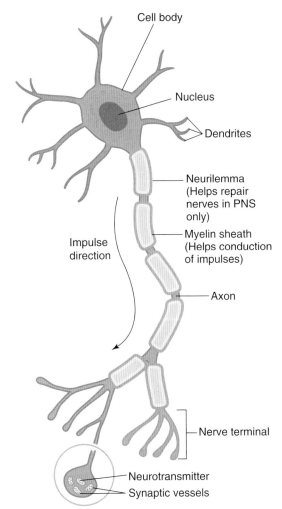

Cell body

Nucleus

Dendrites

Neurilemma
(Helps repair
nerves in PNS
only)

Myelin sheath
(Helps conduction
of impulses)

Impulse
direction

Axon

Nerve terminal

Neurotransmitter
Synaptic vessels

FIG. 17.3 Neuron. Impulses travel down the axon into the nerve terminal, where they are released into the synaptic space between each neuron. Impulses then are transmitted to the following neuron by the dendrites, which extend out of the cell body. The spaces between segments of the myelin sheath are known as the *nodes of Ranvier. PNS,* Peripheral nervous system.

depolarization, and repolarization. When the cell is in a resting state, there is an overall negative charge inside the neuron that consists of potassium ions (positive cations) and chloride ions (negative anions). The neuron's outside is positive with the sodium cation. Now, the cell is polarized and waiting for excitation. When a neurotransmitter activates the cell membrane, an influx of sodium ions occurs, changing the negative charge inside the cell to a positive charge. We call this *depolarization.* The cell restores the resting state by allowing the inside positive charges (potassium ions) to escape. To transition back to the resting state, the cell actively transports sodium back outside and allows potassium to reenter. The cell repolarizes, bringing it full circle and back to the resting stage (Fig. 17.4).

What is a neurotransmitter? Neurotransmitters are chemicals located in and released by neurons. They provide impulses emitted and sent from one nerve cell to another. Neurotransmitters can excite or inhibit other nerve cells or

body tissues. The nervous system uses neurotransmitters to communicate messages. They work by binding to receptors that they specifically activate like a lock and key, triggering a response (Fig. 17.5). There are many more neurotransmitters than we will discuss in this and the following chapters. Note that brain and peripheral neurotransmitter impairment can cause various physical and mental disorders discussed in this chapter.

Central Nervous System

The CNS includes the spinal cord, brainstem, and brain. The following sections outline the CNS's primary functions.

Brain

The brain has several sections. The most extensive brain area is the cerebral cortex that has gray matter lying over white matter. Gray matter includes neuron cell bodies and dendrites. This area is where most neuronal activity happens. Language, memory, and cognitive functions occur in the gray matter. The white matter consists of bundles of nerve fibers. It functions to communicate between other areas of the cerebral cortex and brain. We divide the cerebral cortex into the left and right hemispheres (*hemi* means half). The two halves communicate through the corpus callosum (bundles of axons). We further divide the two hemispheres into four different lobes with specific roles:

1. *Frontal lobe:* Controls motor function, parts of speech, emotions, problem solving, reasoning, and planning
2. *Parietal lobe:* Important in orientation, recognition, sensation, and understanding language
3. *Occipital lobe:* Important in controlling perception and interpretation related to vision
4. *Temporal lobe:* Important in receiving and integrating auditory stimuli and regulating emotion, personality, and behavior

The **brainstem** connects the brain to the spinal cord and has three main areas: the midbrain, pons, and medulla oblongata. These three areas link to many nerves in the brain (Fig. 17.6). The thalamus is above the brainstem. The thalamus serves as a relay station that transmits messages between the brain and spinal cord. It sends messages to the proper area in the cerebral cortex. At the back of the brain, near the brainstem, is the **cerebellum**. This many-folded brain section carries responsibility for precise movements, such as maintaining balance, posture, and coordination.

When we discuss drugs that treat neurologic disorders, we must include the **blood-brain barrier (BBB)**. The BBB prevents certain molecules and substances (eg, bacteria) from entering. However, if an infection happens, the barrier may block some treatments. In addition, some small viruses easily pass through. Viruses can attach to immune cells that cross into the brain. Certain properties make medicines more or less likely to cross the BBB. Small lipophilic "fat-loving" molecules pass readily through the BBB, for example.

Spinal Cord

The spinal cord inside the vertebral column (Fig. 17.7) serves as a path from the brain to the PNS. Vertebrae protect the

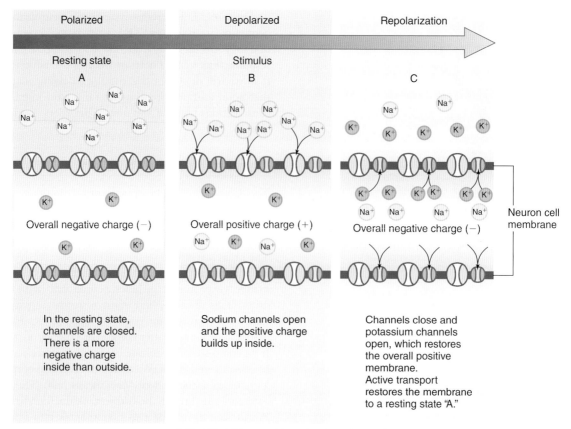

FIG. 17.4 Neuronal impulse transfer cycle.

Polarized

Resting state
A

Overall negative charge (−)

In the resting state, channels are closed. There is a more negative charge inside than outside.

Depolarized

Stimulus
B

Overall positive charge (+)

Sodium channels open and the positive charge builds up inside.

Repolarization

C

Overall negative charge (−)

Neuron cell membrane

Channels close and potassium channels open, which restores the overall positive membrane. Active transport restores the membrane to a resting state "A."

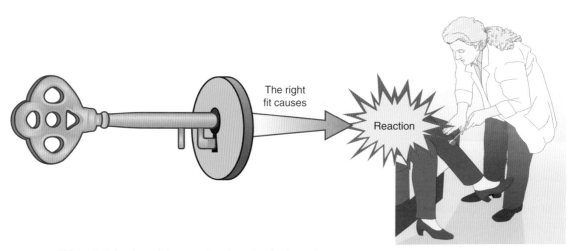

The right fit causes

Reaction

FIG. 17.5 Lock-and-key mechanism. As the knee is tapped, impulses are sent to and from the brain. The neurotransmitters affect specific receptors that are interpreted. The reaction sent via neurotransmitters is to jerk the knee.

spinal nerves. Within the vertebrae, an inner gray matter houses many nerve cells, and an outer white matter contains nerve fibers. The meninges, a thin connective tissue covering, separates and protects the brain and spinal cord from the skull and spinal column's bony structures. A watery liquid called **cerebrospinal fluid** (**CSF**) cushions the brain and spinal cord.

Tech Note!

The brain's nerves crisscross. The brain's left side controls the right side of the body. Therefore patients with stroke can lose the ability to move parts of the body on the opposite side.

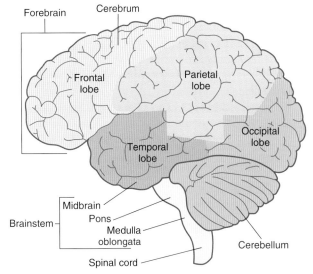

FIG. 17.6 Lobes of the brain, cerebellum, and brainstem, which are all part of the central nervous system.

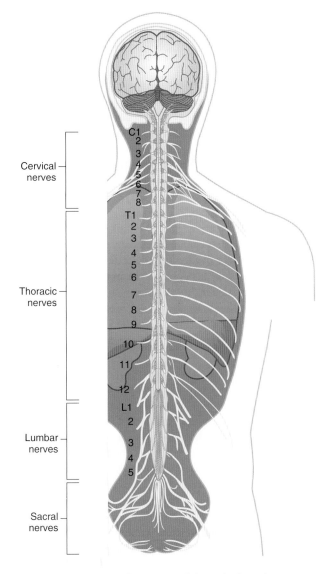

FIG. 17.7 Segments of the spinal cord.

Cranial Nerves

Twelve pairs of cranial nerves originate from the brain (Fig. 17.8). These nerves, designated by Roman numerals, have specific functions. The numerals represent the fibers' location from the brain's front to back. Most nerves have sensory and motor fibers; three sets have sensory fibers only. Table 17.1 lists the primary functions of the cranial nerve sets, nerves I to XII.

Peripheral Nervous System

The PNS is divided into the autonomic and somatic systems. Each system has specific roles. We describe them in the following sections.

Autonomic System

The ANS controls automatic functions. Automatic functions include unconscious heartbeat and breathing. We further subdivide the ANS into two main branches: the SNS and PSNS (see Fig. 17.2). These regulate organs, tissues, and blood vessels (Fig. 17.9).

Tech Note!

The autonomic system is an involuntary branch of the PNS. The autonomic system has two divisions, the sympathetic and parasympathetic. Stress causes the sympathetic system to release the neurotransmitter norepinephrine. The parasympathetic system releases acetylcholine when we are at rest.

Sympathetic Nervous System

The **sympathetic nervous system (SNS)** responds to stressful situations; it is the "fight-or-flight" response. During this stress response, the SNS shuts down the body's nonessential systems. It redirects energy to other areas such as the muscular system. The SNS also sends impulses to various organs and tissues for other emotional situations such as anxiety. A new job interview may cause sweaty palms, increased heart rate, and quick and shallow breathing, a by-product of the sympathetic reaction. As part of the ANS, the SNS response is an instinctive or autonomic reaction.

The main neurotransmitters of the SNS are norepinephrine and epinephrine. Four main receptor types respond to these neurotransmitters. Peripheral blood vessels, the heart, and the eyes have alpha-1 receptors. We primarily find alpha-2 receptors on smooth muscle. Primarily, beta-1 receptors are in the heart muscle, and beta-2 receptors are in the respiratory system, blood vessels, and elsewhere in the body. Drugs that mimic natural SNS neurotransmitters are *sympathomimetics* or *adrenergics*. *Sympatholytics* block drug action; we name them after the specific receptor they inhibit (eg, beta-blockers). Table 17.2 lists the effects of receptor activation with a sympathomimetic.

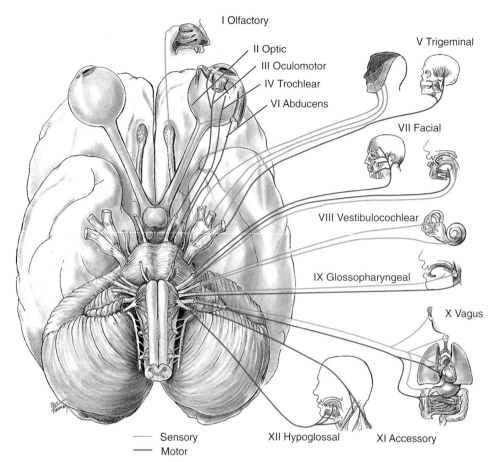

I Olfactory

II Optic
III Oculomotor
IV Trochlear
VI Abducens

V Trigeminal

VII Facial

VIII Vestibulocochlear

IX Glossopharyngeal

X Vagus

—— Sensory
—— Motor

XII Hypoglossal   XI Accessory

FIG. 17.8 Cranial nerves. (From Applegate E. *The Anatomy and Physiology Learning System*. 4th ed. St. Louis: Saunders; 2010.)

Parasympathetic Nervous System

We think of the **parasympathetic nervous system (PSNS)** as the SNS's opposite or counterbalance. The PSNS activates the digestive system. This function includes secreting acidic juices, increasing peristalsis, and inducing pancreatic insulin release. The PSNS works while we rest. The sympathetic system can override the PSNS during intensely stressful periods.

The main PSNS neurotransmitter is acetylcholine (ACh). ACh is important in both the CNS and the PNS. Two cholinergic agent types (agents that activate the PSNS) may either mimic ACh or stop its destruction by acetylcholinesterase, an enzyme. *Parasympathomimetics* are cholinergic drugs that mimic the PSNS. *Anticholinergics* inhibit cholinergic reactions or block receptors. Parasympathetic receptors, which respond to ACh, are on smooth and cardiac muscle cells and in other body areas (see Fig. 17.9).

Somatic System

The somatic system is a nerve network that relays messages from outside the body to the CNS and returns messages. The somatic system includes the spinal and cranial nerves. This system regulates motor nerves that control voluntary skeletal muscle actions and sensory receptor impulses. Receptor sites sense stimuli, including smell, taste, touch, and hearing.

Conditions of the Nervous System and Their Treatments

Nervous system dysfunction produces many conditions. Because so many disorders and diseases can affect the brain and nervous system, we discuss only a sample of the major indications and medications to treat them.

Diseases and Conditions of the Peripheral Nervous System

Myasthenia Gravis

Myasthenia gravis is a rare autoimmune disorder that affects electrical impulse transmission from the CNS to the body's muscles. This results in musculoskeletal weakness affecting the throat muscles, eyes and eyelids, and voluntarily facial movement muscles. Less commonly, the disease can affect other areas. Vocal and visual difficulties may occur, and eyelid drooping is common. Muscles fatigue easily and take longer to recover. Without treatment, this chronic disease worsens over time. Antiacetylcholine receptor (nicotinic receptor) antibody production diminishes the signals from nerves to muscles. This leads to characteristic muscle fatigue in myasthenia gravis (Fig. 17.10). Diagnostic tests can confirm the disease, including a blood test that detects ACh receptor antibodies.

TABLE 17.1
Primary Functions of the Cranial Nerves

Cranial Nerve Number	Cranial Nerve Name	Function
I	Olfactory	Associated with smell. Mucous membranes in the nose transmit information to a region in the cerebral cortex, which processes and then sends a response to the sensory information.
II	Optic	Associated with vision. The optic nerves receive an image that is captured by the retina. These messages travel via the optic nerve through the thalamus to the visual cortex, where they are processed.
III	Oculomotor	Oculomotor muscles are involved in the movement of specific regions of the eye and eyelid.
IV	Trochlear	The trochlear nerves control another area of the eye involved in eye movement.
V	Trigeminal	Located in the brainstem; provides sensation to the face, scalp, nasal mucous membranes, mouth, and eyes. It is also responsible for sensation in the skin and muscles of the jaw.
VI	Abducens	Another cranial nerve involved in eye movement.
VII	Facial	Involved in the sensation of taste in the front of the tongue. Linked to face and head muscles; results in facial expressions.
VIII	Vestibulocochlear	Linked to the inner ear (hearing) and responsible for the sense of balance.
IX	Glossopharyngeal	Linked to sinus, back of the tongue, soft palate, parotid gland, and reflexive control of the heart. Also plays a role in swallowing.
X	Vagus	It extends from the brainstem through the neck and then through the chest and abdominal cavity. Involved in functions such as swallowing, breathing, speaking, heartbeat, and digestion. Linked to other nerves, receiving messages from the ear, pharynx, esophagus, chest, and abdominal area.
XI	Spinal accessory	Composed of two divisions. The cranial branch controls the muscles of the pharynx, larynx, and palate, contributing to swallowing and movement of the digestive tract. The spinal branch is involved in muscle movement of the upper shoulders, head, and neck.
XII	Hypoglossal	The hypoglossal nerve controls the muscles of the tongue.

Prognosis

Patients with myasthenia gravis may lead a relatively normal life. Some patients experience remission in which medications can be stopped. There is no cure for myasthenia gravis except in cases caused by a thymus tumor (15% of cases).

Non-Drug Treatment

Surgery can remove the thymus (thymectomy) containing a tumor. Plasmapheresis is how we can remove antibodies from the patient's blood and replace them with intravenous healthy immune globulins (antibodies).

Drug Treatments

Drug treatments for myasthenia gravis include agents that increase the ACh at the neuromuscular junction and suppress the immune system. Anticholinesterase medications (eg, pyridostigmine) frequently treat myasthenia gravis. These drugs inhibit ACh destruction by acetylcholinesterase. They improve neuronal transmission and increase muscle strength. Side effects may include overstimulation of the PSNS, resulting in nausea, vomiting, diarrhea, and severe abdominal pain. Immunosuppressant drugs (eg, azathioprine, cyclosporine, or prednisone) may slow disease progression by reducing the formation of antiacetylcholine receptor antibodies. Azathioprine is an off-label use for patients who remain symptomatic on pyridostigmine.

GENERIC NAME: pyridostigmine

TRADE NAME: Mestinon

INDICATION: Myasthenia gravis

ROUTES OF ADMINISTRATION: Oral; injection

COMMON ADULT DOSAGE: *Oral:* 60–1500 mg/day in divided doses

MECHANISM OF ACTION: Inhibits acetylcholinesterase to potentiate acetylcholine's action

SIDE EFFECTS: Dizziness, headache, diarrhea, flatulence

AUXILIARY LABEL: Take with food or milk

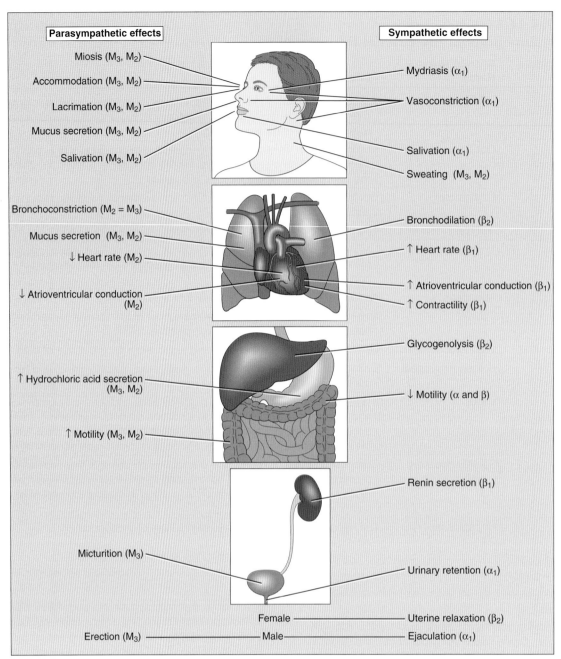

FIG. 17.9 Autonomic nervous system effects on organs.(From Brenner GM, Stevens C. *Pharmacology*. 4th ed. Philadelphia: Saunders; 2014.)

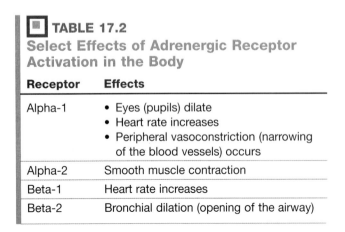

◼ TABLE 17.2
Select Effects of Adrenergic Receptor Activation in the Body

Receptor	Effects
Alpha-1	• Eyes (pupils) dilate • Heart rate increases • Peripheral vasoconstriction (narrowing of the blood vessels) occurs
Alpha-2	Smooth muscle contraction
Beta-1	Heart rate increases
Beta-2	Bronchial dilation (opening of the airway)

GENERIC NAME: azathioprine

TRADE NAME: Imuran

INDICATION: Autoimmune disease

ROUTE OF ADMINISTRATION: Oral; intravenous for renal transplantation only

COMMON ADULT DOSAGE: 1–3 mg/kg/dose per day

MECHANISM OF ACTION: Inhibits antiacetylcholine receptor antibody production

SIDE EFFECTS: Nausea, vomiting, increased risk for infection

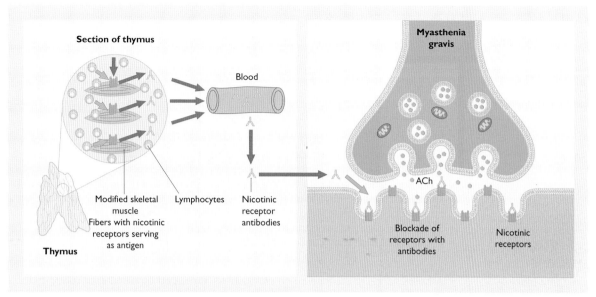

FIG. 17.10 Postulated source of antigen and antibody production in myasthenia gravis. *ACh,* Acetylcholine. (From Page CP, Hoffman B, Curtis M, et al. *Integrated Pharmacology.* 3rd ed. Philadelphia: Mosby; 2006.)

Polyneuropathy

Polyneuropathy manifests as a distal loss of sensation, burning, or weakness, depending on the involved nerves. Polyneuropathy has many causes. These include diabetes mellitus, alcohol abuse, human immunodeficiency virus (HIV) infection, and certain medications' adverse effects, among others. Diabetic neuropathy is a common form. Scientists think nerve damage, secondary to metabolic, vascular, and hormonal factors, is the root cause. Diabetic neuropathy prevention through blood glucose management is the cornerstone treatment for symptoms of diabetic polyneuropathy (which often involves the feet) and can include numbness to tingling to pain in the feet.

Prognosis

Polyneuropathies slowly progress over time. As noted under Drug Treatments, many polyneuropathies (eg, painful diabetic polyneuropathy) are treatment resistant. In other cases, the condition self-limits or symptoms may spontaneously improve.

Non-Drug Treatment

Transcutaneous electrical nerve stimulation (TENS) provides some benefit with painful diabetic polyneuropathy. Daily foot inspections help prevent ulceration, infection, and amputation.

Drug Treatments

Painful diabetic polyneuropathy is difficult to treat. People often try multiple therapies before they find a drug or combination that works well. Drugs used for painful diabetic polyneuropathy include antidepressant agents (eg, duloxetine, venlafaxine, and amitriptyline), anticonvulsants (eg, gabapentin and pregabalin), opioid pain medications (eg, oxycodone and tramadol), anesthetic medications (eg, lidocaine), and over-the-counter (OTC) medicines (eg, capsaicin creams). Providers should dose gabapentin renally when a patient has a creatinine clearance (CrCl) less than 79 mL/min.

GENERIC NAME: duloxetine
TRADE NAME: Cymbalta
INDICATION: Diabetic neuropathy
ROUTE OF ADMINISTRATION: Oral
COMMON ADULT DOSAGE: 60 mg daily
MECHANISM OF ACTION: Inhibits the reuptake of both serotonin and norepinephrine, thus increasing the neurotransmitter availability
SIDE EFFECTS: Dizziness, increased blood pressure, headache
AUXILIARY LABEL: Administer without regard to meals

GENERIC NAME: gabapentin[a]
TRADE NAME: Neurontin
INDICATION: Neuropathic pain
ROUTE OF ADMINISTRATION: Oral
COMMON ADULT DOSAGE: 900–1800 mg/day in divided doses, titrated up
MECHANISM OF ACTION: Increases the gamma-aminobutyric acid (GABA) response (GABA is the primary inhibitory neurotransmitter in the CNS)
SIDE EFFECTS: Fatigue, peripheral edema
AUXILIARY LABEL: Administer without regard to meals

[a] Now regulated as a Schedule V controlled substance in certain states.

■ TABLE 17.3
Types of Seizures

Type	Description
Partial Seizures	
Simple focal motor type	• Involves stiffening or jerking in one extremity followed by a tingling sensation in the same area. • Consciousness is not normally lost, although the seizure may progress to a generalized seizure.
Simple focal nonmotor type	• Involves perceptual distortion, including hallucinations.
Complex focal type	• Effects vary and may include purposeless behavior. • The patient experiences an aura immediately before the seizure begins that may include a pungent smell, nausea, a dreamy sensation, an unusual taste, or a visual disturbance. • Behavior changes may include glassy stare, picking at one's clothing, aimless wandering, lip-smacking or lip-chewing motions, and unintelligible speech. • Symptoms may last seconds to 20 min. • Mental confusion may continue after a seizure.
Generalized Seizures	
Absence (petit mal)	• A brief change in the level of consciousness, indicated by blinking or rolling of the eyes, a blank stare, and slight mouth movements. • Patient retains posture. • Seizures normally last no longer than 10 sec, although they may often repeat throughout the day. • Most often affects children.
Akinetic seizure	• General loss of postural tone and temporary loss of consciousness; also known as *drop attack;* often occurs in children.
Myoclonic (bilateral massive epileptic myoclonus)	• Brief, involuntary muscular jerks of the body or extremities.
Status epilepticus	• A continuous seizure that can occur in all types of seizures and may be accompanied by a loss of consciousness and respiratory distress; a life-threatening event. • May occur as a result of abrupt withdrawal of anticonvulsant medications, head trauma, encephalopathy, or septicemia caused by meningitis.
Tonic-clonic (grand mal)	• Typically starts with a loud cry attributable to air rushing from the lungs through the vocal cords; the patient falls to the ground and loses consciousness, and the body stiffens and then alternates between spasms and relaxation phases.

GENERIC NAME: capsaicin cream

TRADE NAME: Zostrix[a]

INDICATION: Diabetic polyneuropathy

ROUTE OF ADMINISTRATION: Topical

COMMON ADULT DOSAGE: Apply to the affected area 3 or 4 times daily

MECHANISM OF ACTION: Depletion of substance P in peripheral sensory neurons; substance P is the primary chemical mediator of pain impulses from the periphery to the CNS

SIDE EFFECTS: Skin irritation (burning, stinging, and itching)

AUXILIARY LABEL: Avoid contact with eyes and mucous membranes

[a] Brand discontinued; now available only as generic.

Diseases and Conditions of the Central Nervous System

Epilepsy

Epilepsy is a seizure disorder marked by hyperexcitability in some brain nerve cells. The two main types are focal (previously referred to as "partial") and generalized seizures. Focal seizures affect only one brain hemisphere and may cause relatively mild symptoms. Generalized seizures affect both hemispheres. These vary in intensity, ranging from absence seizures (the least violent) to longer, more intense tonic-clonic seizures. Children with epilepsy often have absence seizures. This causes them to stare into the distance for a time. In grand mal seizures, also known as *tonic-clonic seizures,* the person loses consciousness and falls to the ground. Periods of widespread muscle spasms (tonic phase) alternate with muscle relaxation periods (clonic phase). Injuries can occur, depending on where and when the seizure takes place. The seizing person will not remember the episode. Table 17.3 outlines various seizure types.

Prognosis

Epilepsy has no known cure, but many persons with epilepsy live relatively normal lives with drug treatment or surgical intervention. Social stigmas with this condition can cause embarrassment and frustration. Women must consult a doctor about seizure medication risks and pregnancy.

TABLE 17.4
Select Anticonvulsants for the Treatment of Epilepsy

Generic Name	Trade Name	Common Adult Oral Dosage Range
carbamazepine	Tegretol, Tegretol XR	800–1200 mg/day
divalproex sodium	Depakote, Depakote ER	30–60 mg/kg/day
ethosuximide	Zarontin	500–1500 mg/day
lacosamide	Vimpat	200–400 mg/day
lamotrigine	Lamictal	100–400 mg/day
levetiracetam	Keppra	1000–3000 mg/day
oxcarbazepine	Trileptal	600–2400 mg/day
phenytoin	Dilantin	300–400 mg/day up to 400 mg/day
tiagabine	Gabitril	32–56 mg/day
topiramate	Topamax	50–400 mg/day
vigabatrin	Sabril	1000–3000 mg/day
zonisamide	Zonegran	100–600 mg/day

Non-Drug Treatment

If medication does not control seizures, surgery can remove brain lesions. However, surgery is not always effective.

Drug Treatments

The prescriber may use monotherapy (one drug) or polytherapy (more than one drug). Anticonvulsants (Table 17.4) can reduce seizure frequency. Anticonvulsants prevent abnormal CNS impulses and inhibit one or more ions involved in nerve conduction. These include sodium, calcium, or potassium. Drug interactions are common with the anticonvulsants. Avoid anticonvulsants where possible in patients who are pregnant or are expecting to become pregnant. Several of these medications are teratogenic, such as carbamazepine, phenytoin, and valproic acid. Pharmacy technicians and pharmacists should look out for drug interaction warnings when processing anticonvulsant prescriptions. Benzodiazepines (discussed with anxiety treatment) also treat epilepsy.

Most seizures that last 2 minutes or less do not require treatment. However, those seizures that have a duration greater than 5 minutes transition to a medical emergency. For example, status epilepticus without treatment, generally with a benzodiazepine, can cause permanent brain damage. Common benzodiazepines include diazepam (Valium), midazolam (Versed), and lorazepam (Ativan). For emergencies, IV administration provides the fastest onset of action, but sometimes intramuscular midazolam is a better choice. Intranasal and buccal midazolam can be alternatives for children. Diazepam has IV and rectal forms in addition to oral, whereas lorazepam only has IV and oral forms. Generally, the pharmacy team will educate parents, guardians, and the pediatric patients themselves, if old enough, about emergency rescue medications.

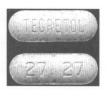

GENERIC NAME: carbamazepine

TRADE NAME: Tegretol, Tegretol-XR

INDICATION: Generalized tonic-clonic, partial seizures

ROUTE OF ADMINISTRATION: Oral

COMMON ADULT DOSAGE: 800–1200 mg/day in divided doses, titrated up

MECHANISM OF ACTION: Blocks sodium channels, inhibiting repetitive firing of neurons

SIDE EFFECTS: Dizziness, drowsiness, dry mouth, headache

AUXILIARY LABELS:
- May cause dizziness or drowsiness
- Take with food
- Do not stop taking abruptly

GENERIC NAME: phenytoin

TRADE NAME: Dilantin, Phenytek

INDICATION: Partial seizures, tonic-clonic seizures, status epilepticus

ROUTES OF ADMINISTRATION: Oral; injection

COMMON ADULT DOSAGE: *IV:* 5–7 mg/kg/day. *Oral:* 300–400 mg/day, up to 400 mg/day for maintenance

MECHANISM OF ACTION: Decreases the seizure threshold through effects on sodium channels

SIDE EFFECTS: Dizziness, insomnia, nausea, vomiting, headache

AUXILIARY LABEL: Do not stop taking abruptly

GENERIC NAME: ethosuximide

TRADE NAME: Zarontin

INDICATION: Absence seizures

ROUTE OF ADMINISTRATION: Oral

COMMON ADULT DOSAGE: 250 mg twice daily initially, titrated up to 1.5 g given in two divided doses

MECHANISM OF ACTION: Treats seizures through effects on calcium channels

SIDE EFFECTS: Drowsiness, nausea, vomiting, headache

AUXILIARY LABELS:
- May cause dizziness or drowsiness
- Do not stop taking abruptly

GENERIC NAME: diazepam (C-IV)

TRADE NAMES: Valium, Diastat Rectal Gel

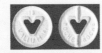

INDICATIONS: Status epilepticus, intermittent treatment of generalized tonic-clonic seizures

ROUTES OF ADMINISTRATION: Oral; rectal gel; injection

COMMON ADULT DOSAGE: *Oral:* 2–10 mg 2–4 times daily. *IV:* 0.15–0.2 mg/kg (max 10 mg), may repeat once. *Rectal:* 0.2–0.5 mg/kg (max 20 mg)

MECHANISM OF ACTION: Benzodiazepine (binds to benzodiazepine receptor and activates GABA inhibitory response)

SIDE EFFECTS: Drowsiness

AUXILIARY LABELS:
- May cause dizziness or drowsiness
- For rectal use only (Diastat Rectal Gel)
- Do not stop taking abruptly
- Do not drink alcohol
- *Caution:* Federal law prohibits the transfer of this drug to any person other than the patient for whom it was prescribed

Alzheimer Disease

Alzheimer disease (AD) is a progressive condition associated with memory loss, confusion, impaired judgment, personality changes, disorientation, and loss of language skills. AD is most common in elderly patients but may occur in younger adults. Multiple dementia (progressive conditions of deteriorating cognitive function) types exist. However, AD is the most common, accounting for 50% to 70% of cases. People with AD have decreased brain ACh production. Acetylcholinesterase inhibitors prevent ACh destruction.

The three major AD categories include early stage, midstage, and late stage. Not all patients experience the onset and progression of AD similarly. However, disease progression classification can help the family and doctor monitor the disease severity. Additionally, seven specific stages describe AD's progression (Table 17.5).

Prognosis

Medications slow AD progression in some cases; however, no treatments stop the progression completely. AD affects individuals differently. Normal function deterioration, such as difficulty swallowing, the inability to move, and the absence of communicative or cognitive skills, occurs in late-stage AD.

Non-Drug Treatment

In addition to drugs to help slow AD progression, individuals may need skilled care for later stages. Education helps patients, families, and friends understand AD and provides realistic treatment expectations. If patients continue in activities that strengthen critical thinking and problem solving, it can help the patient "use it"

rather than "lose it." Active thought reinforces and generates new brain synapses to slow cognition decline and a healthy diet maintains brain health, as well.

Drug Treatment

The US Food and Drug Administration (FDA) approved two drug classes for AD: acetylcholinesterase inhibitors (which prevent ACh breakdown) and memantine (Table 17.6). Drug treatment may delay disease progression but does not typically improve memory or other AD symptoms.

In 2021, the FDA approved aducanumab (Aduhelm) for AD treatment. Aduhelm does not restore lost memories or cognitive function; rather, it targets protein clumps—beta-amyloid plaques—which are toxic to brain cells. Administration is intravenous once monthly.

In 2023, **Lecanemab (Leqembi)** also gained FDA approval for AD and removes amyloid plaques more quickly than Aduhelm, with fewer side effects. The patient receives the medication intravenously every 2 weeks.

Parkinson Disease

Parkinson disease (PD) is a progressive basal ganglia disorder associated with the loss or deficiency of dopamine, a neurotransmitter. The basal ganglia are a group of cells in the medulla of the cerebrum. It regulates skeletal muscle activity and body movement. The overall degeneration of dopamine-producing neurons instigates PD symptoms (Fig. 17.11). Because PD is progressive, symptom severity becomes more pronounced over time. We remember PD hallmark symptoms with the TRAP acronym. It stands for *t*remor, *r*igidity, *a*kinesia (or **bradykinesia**), and *p*ostural instability. Over time, physical movement slows in patients with PD and they can become wheelchair bound. Other problems, such as swallowing and speech difficulties, constipation, and cognitive impairment, also come with PD. Scientists have linked PD's development to genetics and environmental influences, though the ultimate cause is unknown.

Prognosis

PD's course varies by patient. Typically, it is a slow, progressive disorder. Many people can live somewhat normally with medications, exercise, and good health maintenance. However, as the disease progresses, its management becomes increasingly difficult.

Non-Drug Treatment

Non-drug treatments include lifestyle interventions, various therapies, and surgery. As mentioned previously, PD is a disease that leads to slowing of movement. Accordingly, activity is important for patients with PD to maintain functionality. Working with physical therapy, occupational therapy, and speech therapy can help maintain activities of daily living, movement, and speech. For individuals with advanced disease unable to control symptoms with medical therapy, surgeons

TABLE 17.5
Stages Associated With Alzheimer Disease

Stage	Symptom	Description
1	No impairment or normal functioning	• Normal function; the person does not show signs or symptoms of the disease.
2	Very mild decline	• Earliest signs of AD. • A person is aware of memory loss; forgets familiar words and the location of common household items. • No signs of AD seen at physician's examination and within the family unit or friends.
3	Mild cognitive decline	• Signs appear as problems of memory loss continue. • May not be able to remember names of people; reads less because of a decrease in memory retention; loses more items, including those that are valuable; and exhibits a decline in planning or organizational skills. • Presence of disease becomes measurable in a clinical/medical interview.
4	Moderate cognitive decline	• Mild or early-stage AD; deficiencies become evident as the condition progresses. • Decreased knowledge of recent occasions or current events in the world; cannot perform tasks related to more complex cognitive functions, such as managing finances, planning dinner functions, or performing mathematical calculations (eg, counting backward by 7s). • A person suffers reduced memory of personal history and may become withdrawn from individuals and group situations.
5	Moderately severe cognitive decline	• Moderate or mild-stage AD; may include major gaps in memory and in daily activities. • A person may not remember a home address or phone number, may not remember the day of week or month of the year, and has trouble performing basic math manipulations (counting backward by 2s). • Still, the person knows their own name and names of immediate family members; does not require assistance with functions such as eating or using the toilet.
6	Severe cognitive decline	• Moderately severe or mid-stage AD. • Characterized by significant personality changes (eg, becomes suspicious of caretakers, hallucinates), exhibits wandering behavior, occasionally forgets names of family members, cannot dress self or go to the toilet (increasing episodes of incontinence). • May experience a disruption in the sleep-wake cycle and may begin repetitive behaviors such as hand-wringing or shredding tissues.
7	Very severe cognitive decline	• Severe or late-stage AD, the last stage of AD. • A person loses the ability to speak, control movements, or respond to the environment. • Eventually may lose the ability to feed self, use the toilet, walk without assistance, or sit without support. • May not be able to smile or hold head up, and as reflexes continue to decline, muscles become rigid, and swallowing is impaired

Although this is a guide to the stages of AD, not all individuals show these signs in this order, and the rate at which AD progresses varies from person to person.
AD, Alzheimer disease.

TABLE 17.6
Select Medications for the Treatment of Alzheimer Disease

Generic Name	Trade Name	Common Dosage Range	Common Side Effects
Acetylcholinesterase Inhibitors			
donepezil	Aricept	5–23 mg daily	• Gastrointestinal side effects • Slowed heart rate • Weight loss
galantamine	Razadyne	*Immediate-release:* 8–12 mg/bid *Extended-release:* 16–24 mg once daily	
rivastigmine	Exelon	*Oral:* 1.5–6 mg by mouth bid *Patch:* 9.5–13.3 mg/24 hr	
***N*-Methyl-D-aspartate Receptor Antagonist**			
memantine	Namenda	*Immediate-release:* 10 mg bid (start at 5 mg/day and titrate weekly until up to 10 mg bid) *Extended-release:* 14–28 mg once daily (start at 7 mg/day and titrate up to 28 mg/day)	• Dizziness • Fatigue • Headache

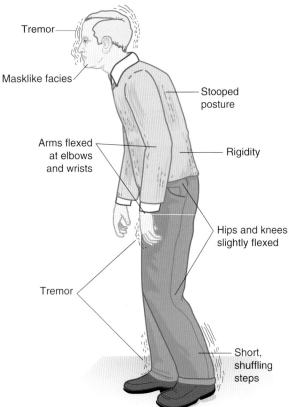

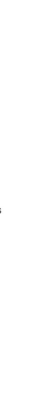

FIG. 17.11 Symptoms and signs of Parkinson disease.

Tremor

Masklike facies

Stooped posture

Arms flexed at elbows and wrists

Rigidity

Hips and knees slightly flexed

Tremor

Short, shuffling steps

can perform deep brain stimulation (DMS). The surgeon inserts electrodes into brain areas to improve motor (movement) symptoms.

Drug Treatment

Several medications treat PD motor symptoms (Table 17.7). Levodopa/carbidopa is the gold standard treatment, although different medication regimens can work. PD can be difficult to differentiate clinically from other movement disorders, so the administration of PD medications (eg, levodopa/carbidopa) may assist in disease diagnosis. Patients may experience the on/off phenomenon, in which symptoms may worsen toward the end of a dose. To optimize entacapone (Comtan), the dose of levodopa may need to be decreased. Benztropine and trihexyphenidyl are on the American Geriatrics Society (AGS) Beers Criteria, and patients 65 years or older should not take them.

Tech Note!

People with PD are in tune with medication needs. Many doctors allow patients with PD to dose their medications according to daily symptoms. Therefore patients with PD may have a less regimented course of treatment than others.

GENERIC NAME: levodopa/carbidopa

TRADE NAMES: Sinemet, Sinemet CR

INDICATION: Parkinson disease

ROUTE OF ADMINISTRATION: Oral

COMMON ADULT DOSAGE: Doses individualized, based on the patient's needs

MECHANISM OF ACTION: Levodopa converts to dopamine and helps manage PD's motor symptoms. Carbidopa prevents the peripheral conversion of levodopa so more levodopa can penetrate the CNS

SIDE EFFECTS: Nausea, dizziness, hallucinations, dyskinesia (excessive, uncontrolled movements)

AUXILIARY LABEL: May cause dizziness or drowsiness

GENERIC NAME: pramipexole

TRADE NAMES: Mirapex, Mirapex XL

INDICATIONS: Parkinson disease, restless legs syndrome

ROUTE OF ADMINISTRATION: Oral

COMMON ADULT DOSAGE: 1.5–4.5 mg/day in divided doses normally three times daily

MECHANISM OF ACTION: Dopamine agonist (mimics the actions of dopamine)

SIDE EFFECTS: Nausea, peripheral edema, hallucinations, compulsive behavior

AUXILIARY LABEL: May cause dizziness or drowsiness

GENERIC NAME: rotigotine

TRADE NAME: Neupro

INDICATIONS: Parkinson disease (PD; drug can be used with other antiparkinsonian agents), restless legs syndrome

ROUTE OF ADMINISTRATION: Transdermal patch

COMMON ADULT DOSAGE: 4- to 8-mg patch daily for maintenance, 2-mg patch for initial dosing in early-stage PD

MECHANISM OF ACTION: Dopamine agonist (mimics the actions of dopamine)

SIDE EFFECTS: Nausea, peripheral edema, hallucinations, compulsive behavior, application site irritation

AUXILIARY LABEL: May cause dizziness or drowsiness

Multiple Sclerosis

Multiple sclerosis (MS) is a chronic neurologic condition. It affects the myelin sheath's integrity on neurons in the CNS.

TABLE 17.7
Select Medications for the Treatment of Parkinson Disease

Generic Name	Trade Name	Common Dosage Range	Common Side Effects
Levodopa/Carbidopa			
Levodopa is converted to dopamine in the central nervous system (CNS), which helps manage the motor symptoms of Parkinson disease (PD); carbidopa blocks the peripheral conversion of levodopa to dopamine so that it can reach the CNS			
levodopa/carbidopa	Sinemet, Sinemet CR	25/100 mg 3–4 times daily titrated to effect; dosage and frequency can vary significantly based on individual needs	• Confusion • Dizziness • Dyskinesia • Hallucinations • Nausea
Dopamine Agonists			
Dopamine agonists mimic the actions of dopamine in the CNS to help treat the motor symptoms of PD			
pramipexole	Mirapex	0.5–1.5 mg tid	• Compulsive behavior • Hallucinations • Nausea • Peripheral edema • Vomiting
	Mirapex XL	0.375–4.5 mg once daily	
ropinirole	Requip[a]	0.75–24 mg day tid	
	Requip XL[a]	2–24 mg once daily	
rotigotine	Neupro	4–8 mg/24 hr (this drug is a patch; start at 2 mg/24 hr, the minimum effective dose is 4 mg)	
Amantadine			
Amantadine may increase dopamine availability in the CNS; it also may help because of its anticholinergic effects			
amantadine	Symmetrel[a]	100–400 mg/day in divided doses	• Nausea • Peripheral edema • Vomiting
Catechol-*O*-Methyltransferase (COMT) Inhibitors			
Prevents the peripheral conversion of levodopa by the enzyme COMT			
entacapone	Comtan	200 mg with each dose of levodopa/carbidopa, max dose of 1600 mg/day	• Abdominal pain • Diarrhea • Dry mouth • Red discoloration of body fluids
tolcapone	Tasmar	100–200 mg tid	
Monoamine Oxidase-B Inhibitors (MAO$_B$-I)			
Inhibition of MAO-B decreases the metabolism of dopamine in the CNS			
rasagiline	Azilect	0.5–1 mg/day	• Dizziness • Headache • Insomnia • Nausea
selegiline	Eldepryl	5 mg bid	
	Zelapar	1.25–2.5 mg/day in the morning	
Anticholinergics			
Anticholinergic activity reduces the excessive cholinergic activity present in PD			
benztropine	Cogentin[a]	1–2 mg at bedtime	• Blurred vision • Confusion • Constipation • Dry mouth • Urinary retention
trihexyphenidyl	Artane[a]	5–15 mg/day to 6–10 mg/day in divided doses	

[a]Brand discontinued; now available only as generic.

Myelin covers the axonal portion of neurons and helps facilitate proper nerve transmission. MS is an autoimmune disorder in which the immune system breaks down the myelin sheath (Fig. 17.12). After immune system damage, sclerotic (hard) tissue replaces the myelin sheaths. Electrical impulses cannot pass from one neuron to another effectively, which leads to impaired movements and other neurologic deficits. The MS course can vary; therefore a series of MS "types" (Table 17.8) help describe the clinical course. Symptoms range from mild to severe and may include muscle weakness, abnormal sensations such as numbness or tingling over parts of the body, vision changes, and loss of coordination.

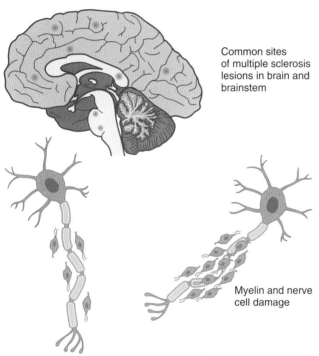

Common sites of multiple sclerosis lesions in brain and brainstem

Myelin and nerve cell damage

FIG. 17.12 Multiple sclerosis lesions in the brain and brainstem.

Prognosis

The prognosis depends largely on the disease pattern and MS severity. Patients with frequent attacks initially or who are older than age 40 before symptoms occur tend to have a poor prognosis.

Non-Drug Treatment

Physical and occupational therapy can help patients recover and maintain functionality in the long term and after attacks. Maximizing strength and balance helps prevent falls and other potential problems.

Drug Treatment

Disease-modifying immunotherapy (eg, interferon use) slows and minimizes disease progression. Symptomatic short-term antiinflammatory corticosteroid treatment can manage flare-ups. Dalfampridine can improve walking in people with MS. Significant medications include those to treat fatigue, spasticity, tremors, pain, depression, and other conditions common with patients with MS.

GENERIC NAME: interferon beta-1a

TRADE NAME: Avonex

INDICATION: Multiple sclerosis

ROUTE OF ADMINISTRATION: Intramuscular (IM) injection

COMMON ADULT DOSAGE: 30 mcg every week

MECHANISM OF ACTION: Inhibits proinflammatory mediator production responsible for triggering autoimmune reactions in MS

SIDE EFFECTS: Dizziness, headache, stomach pain, runny/stuffy nose, depression

AUXILIARY LABELS:
- For intramuscular use only
- May cause dizziness
- Refrigerate

▪ TABLE 17.8
Disease Patterns or "Types" of Multiple Sclerosis

Pattern	Description
Primary progressive MS	Individuals diagnosed with this type of MS have slowly worsening neurologic functions from the onset of the disease. There are no distinct relapses or remissions. Approximately 10% of people with MS have this pattern.
Progressive relapsing MS	People with this type of MS experience a steadily worsening disease from the onset of the condition, along with episodes of deteriorating neurologic functions with each attack. A recovery period may or may not occur, and there are no remission periods.
Relapsing-remitting MS	Individuals with this type of MS experience attacks (ie, flare-ups or relapses) of worsening neurologic function. The flare-ups can be followed by periods of complete recovery (remission). This is the most common type of MS, affecting approximately 85% of patients with MS. Most patients eventually enter a secondary progressive phase.
Secondary progressive MS	In people with this type of MS, the disease worsens more steadily, with or without occasional flare-ups, recovery periods, or plateaus. Many people with this type of MS develop this pattern after an initial period of relapsing-remitting MS.

MS, Multiple sclerosis.

GENERIC NAME: interferon beta-1a

TRADE NAME: Rebif

INDICATION: Multiple sclerosis

ROUTE OF ADMINISTRATION: Subcutaneous injection

COMMON ADULT DOSAGE: 22 or 44 mcg three times weekly; doses should be separated by at least 48 hours

MECHANISM OF ACTION: Inhibits proinflammatory mediator production responsible for triggering autoimmune reactions in MS

SIDE EFFECTS: Headache, weakness or muscle pain, insomnia, injection site reactions, depression

AUXILIARY LABELS:
- For subcutaneous use only
- Refrigerate

■ Tech Note!

Interferon agents should be used cautiously in people with depression.

GENERIC NAME: interferon beta-1b

TRADE NAME: Betaseron

INDICATION: Multiple sclerosis

ROUTE OF ADMINISTRATION: Subcutaneous injection

COMMON ADULT DOSAGE: 0.25 mg every other day

MECHANISM OF ACTION: Inhibits proinflammatory mediator production responsible for triggering autoimmune reactions in MS

SIDE EFFECTS: Headache, weakness or muscle pain, insomnia, injection site reactions, depression

AUXILIARY LABELS:
- For subcutaneous use only
- Refrigerate

GENERIC NAME: glatiramer

TRADE NAME: Copaxone

INDICATION: Multiple sclerosis

ROUTE OF ADMINISTRATION: Subcutaneous injection

COMMON ADULT DOSAGE: 20 mg once daily or 40 mg 3 times per week administered at least 48 hours apart

MECHANISM OF ACTION: Modifies immune processes responsible for MS; the exact mechanism is unknown

SIDE EFFECTS: Injection site edema, rash, infection

AUXILIARY LABELS:
- For subcutaneous use only
- Refrigerate

GENERIC NAME: dalfampridine

TRADE NAME: Ampyra

INDICATION: For improved walking in people with multiple sclerosis (MS)

ROUTE OF ADMINISTRATION: Oral

COMMON ADULT DOSAGE: 10 mg twice daily

MECHANISM OF ACTION: Potassium channel blocker; mechanism of its benefit in MS is unknown

SIDE EFFECTS: Insomnia, constipation, dizziness, headache, seizures

AUXILIARY LABEL: Do not divide, crush, chew, or dissolve tablets

---

Migraine Headache

Migraine headaches are episodic. Severe headaches frequently cause nausea and/or light and sound sensitivity. Migraine triggers vary from one person to the next. They can range from hormonal changes (eg, before menstruation, during pregnancy, and with contraceptive use) to foods, stress, bright lights, and other environmental changes. In some cases, there is no identifiable cause. Drugs may influence migraine frequency and severity. Serotonin agonists (drugs that activate serotonin receptors) frequently treat migraines. Migraine headaches are common and affect about 12% of the population.

Prognosis

No cure exists for migraines. Some medicines work for an active migraine (some are listed in the following drug monographs), and other treatments prevent migraines (prophylactic therapy). Finding the right drug or combination to control migraines often eludes prescribers. However, once found, migraines will interfere less with the patient's lifestyle.

Non-Drug Treatment

Non-drug treatment includes preventive measures (ie, avoidance of triggers) and after-exercise regimens. Headache diaries help identify triggers.

Drug Treatments

For mild to moderate migraines, the first line of treatment involves nonsteroidal antiinflammatory drugs (NSAIDs) or combination analgesics. For patients unresponsive to NSAIDs, migraine-specific agents, such as triptans, may work. Some triptans (eg, sumatriptan) come in nonoral formulations because nausea and vomiting can accompany a migraine. Newer agents for moderate-to-severe migraines are called calcitonin gene-related peptide (CGRP) antagonists. For example, ubrogepant (Ubrelvy) and rimegepant (Nurtec) block CGRP, which is released in the brain during headaches. Those with frequent migraines can use prophylactic agents. These include certain blood pressure medications such as beta-blockers and calcium channel blockers, antidepressants including tricyclic antidepressants (TCAs), selective serotonin reuptake inhibitors (SSRIs), and the anticonvulsant topiramate and some CGRP antibodies. Individual therapies may come as monotherapy or polytherapy, with opioids reserved for severe cases.

GENERIC NAME: sumatriptan

TRADE NAME: Imitrex, Imitrex Nasal

INDICATION: Migraine

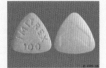

ROUTES OF ADMINISTRATION:
Oral; nasal spray; subcutaneous injection

COMMON ADULT DOSAGE: *Oral:* 25–100 mg at the onset of migraine; dose may be repeated in 2 hours if necessary (not to exceed 200 mg). *Nasal spray:* 1 spray (5–20 mg) into nostril; may repeat in 2 hours (alternate nostrils) × 1 (max 40 mg/24 hr). *Subcutaneous injection:* 1–6 mg; dose may be repeated if necessary but must wait at least 1 hour (max 12 mg/24 hr)

MECHANISM OF ACTION: Binds serotonin receptors, leading to inhibited vasodilation and inflammation

SIDE EFFECTS: Dizziness, nausea, tiredness

AUXILIARY LABELS:
• May cause dizziness or drowsiness
• Take with water

GENERIC NAME: eletriptan

TRADE NAME: Relpax

INDICATION: Migraine

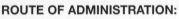

ROUTE OF ADMINISTRATION:
Oral

COMMON ADULT DOSAGE: 20- to 40-mg initial dose, may repeat the dose in 2 hours if needed (max 80 mg/24 hr)

MECHANISM OF ACTION: Binds serotonin receptors, leading to inhibited vasodilation and inflammation

SIDE EFFECTS: Dizziness, nausea, tiredness

AUXILIARY LABELS:
• May cause dizziness or drowsiness
• Take with water

GENERIC NAME: Ubrogepant

TRADE NAME: Ubrelvy

INDICATION: Migraine

ROUTE OF ADMINISTRATION: Oral

COMMON ADULT DOSAGE: 50–100 mg as a single dose, may repeat dose after 2 hours if needed (max 200 mg/24 hr)

MECHANISM OF ACTION: Blocks calcitonin gene-related peptide (CGRP) peptide

SIDE EFFECTS: Nausea, somnolence

AUXILIARY LABEL: May cause dizziness or drowsiness

Stroke

A stroke is an arterial blockage or hemorrhage (ie, a **hemorrhagic stroke**) blocking blood to the brain. Strokes have several causes, but most cases are **ischemic strokes.** This decrease of blood flow to the brain happens when a clot blocks the blood vessel or the vessel becomes too narrow. This blockage or restriction deprives the brain of oxygen, and brain cells can die. Although the disruption is specific to the vascular system, it also affects the nervous system and its function (see Chapter 20 for a detailed discussion of medications to prevent strokes and heart attacks). Damage severity depends on the blockage size and how much it harms brain tissue. Effects range from limb weakness to paralysis on one side of the body to loss of the ability to speak. The most common symptoms of stroke include severe headache, dizziness, visual difficulties, loss of balance, and difficulty moving one side of the body. Weakness in facial muscles can cause difficulty speaking.

Prognosis

The prognosis depends on the severity of damage to the brain. A critical factor includes the time that elapses before treatment begins. If a patient or caregiver suspects a stroke, it is important to call 911 and begin immediate treatment. Quick treatment may reduce long-term symptoms. Some patients never fully recover, but a strong support system can help the patient with daily activities.

Non-Drug Treatment

Patients often require extensive physical and/or speech therapy. This may take place in a rehabilitation hospital, an outpatient center, or the home. Support groups frequently help the survivor cope with emotional stresses.

Drug Treatment

Antithrombotic medications ("clot busters") limit potential brain damage. This is why patients with an ischemic stroke who present to the emergency department quickly have better prognoses. Hemorrhagic strokes may require neurosurgery. Most ischemic stroke treatment aims to prevent future strokes. Treatment includes medications that prevent blood from forming blockages to drugs that control cholesterol levels. Chapter 20 presents a detailed description of preventive agents for stroke and heart attack.

Other Conditions Associated With the Nervous System

Depression

The World Health Organization (WHO) lists major depression among the most burdensome diseases in the world. In the United States the lifetime prevalence of major depression is approximately 16%. This incidence increases in those with chronic medical conditions such as diabetes and heart disease. Depression types range in severity from minor to major depression with thoughts of suicide. Other depression types include postpartum depression (after pregnancy) and seasonal affective disorder (SAD; depression during the winter months). Major depression can be very difficult to treat. It hinders a person's ability to function normally and hinders activities such as sleeping, eating, working, studying, and forms of enjoyment. Many times depression coincides with a serious illness or anxiety disorder.

Depression medications increase brain levels of neurotransmitters. Under normal circumstances, neurotransmitters stimulate the brain as they are released and are then reabsorbed by the brain cells. The enzyme *monoamine oxidase* (MAO) breaks some of these down. Because people with depression may lack adequate levels of neurotransmitters, antidepressants work to increase neurotransmitters available in the brain.

Prognosis

Psychotherapy and/or antidepressant medications help many patients. The prognosis largely depends on depression severity and the patient's support systems. Both short- and long-term treatment options exist.

Non-Drug Treatment

Psychotherapy can help short- or long-term depression. Support groups and other social-based therapies can also help. Other treatment forms include behavioral and cognitive therapy. Doctors reserve electroconvulsive therapy for severe cases of ongoing depression unrelieved by medications or therapy. For seasonal depression, light treatment can alleviate symptoms.

Drug Treatments

Selective serotonin reuptake inhibitors (SSRIs), serotonin and norepinephrine reuptake inhibitors (SNRIs), TCAs, and monoamine oxidase inhibitors (MAOIs) form the mainstays of therapy. These agents help increase brain levels of serotonin and norepinephrine. Antidepressants have variable effects of efficacy and side effects. A serious side effect common to antidepressants is increased suicidal thinking and behavior in children, adolescents, and young adults with major depressive disorder. MAOIs also have many side effects and drug and food interactions. Antidepressants (TCAs, SSRIs, and SNRIs) increase fall risk in patients older than 65 and are on the Beers Criteria list. Table 17.9 presents a description of select antidepressants.

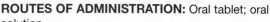

GENERIC NAME: sertraline

TRADE NAME: Zoloft

INDICATIONS: Depression, obsessive-compulsive disorder, panic disorder, posttraumatic stress disorder, social anxiety disorder

ROUTES OF ADMINISTRATION: Oral tablet; oral solution

COMMON ADULT DOSAGE: 50–200 mg once daily

MECHANISM OF ACTION: Selective serotonin reuptake inhibitor (increases the amount of serotonin available in the CNS)

SIDE EFFECTS: Insomnia, dizziness, drowsiness, sexual dysfunction, headache, constipation

AUXILIARY LABEL: Do not drink alcohol

GENERIC NAME: venlafaxine

TRADE NAME: Effexor,[a] Effexor XR

INDICATION: Depression, anxiety disorder

ROUTE OF ADMINISTRATION: Oral

COMMON ADULT DOSAGE: *Effexor*[a]*:* 75–225 mg/day (max 375 mg). *Effexor XR:* 75–225 mg/day (max dose 225 mg)

MECHANISM OF ACTION: Serotonin and norepinephrine reuptake inhibitor (increases the amount of serotonin and norepinephrine available in the CNS)

SIDE EFFECTS: Dry mouth, increased blood pressure, dizziness, drowsiness

AUXILIARY LABELS:
- May cause dizziness and drowsiness
- Do not drink alcohol

[a] Brand discontinued; now available only as generic.

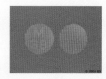

GENERIC NAME: amitriptyline

TRADE NAME: Elavil[a]

INDICATION: Depression

ROUTE OF ADMINISTRATION: Oral

COMMON ADULT DOSAGE: 25–300 mg daily

MECHANISM OF ACTION: Tricyclic antidepressant (increases the amount of serotonin and norepinephrine available in the CNS)

SIDE EFFECTS: Drowsiness, dry mouth, blurred vision, dizziness

AUXILIARY LABELS:
- May cause dizziness and drowsiness
- Take with food
- Do not drink alcohol

[a] Brand discontinued; now available only as generic.

◼ TABLE 17.9
Select Medications for the Treatment of Depression

Generic Name	Brand Name	Common Dosage Range	Common Side Effects
Selective Serotonin Reuptake Inhibitors (SSRIs)			
SSRIs increase the amount of serotonin available in the CNS			
citalopram	Celexa	20–40 mg/day	• Dizziness
escitalopram	Lexapro	10–20 mg/day	• Gastrointestinal side effects
fluoxetine	Prozac	20–80 mg/day	• Headache
paroxetine	Paxil	20–50 mg/day	• Increased risk for suicidal thinking and behavior in children, adolescents, and
	Paxil CR	25–62.5 mg/day	young adults with major depressive disorder
sertraline	Zoloft	50–200 mg/day	• Sleep disturbances
			• Weight gain
Serotonin Norepinephrine Reuptake Inhibitors (SNRIs)			
SNRIs increase the amount of serotonin and norepinephrine available in the CNS			
desvenlafaxine	Pristiq	50 mg/day	• Same as SSRIs
duloxetine	Cymbalta	30–60 mg/day	
venlafaxine	Effexor[a]	75–225 mg/day in divided doses, max 375 mg/day	
	Effexor XR	75–225 mg once daily, max 225 mg/day	
Tricyclic Antidepressants (TCAs)			
TCAs primarily increase the availability of norepinephrine and serotonin in the CNS			
amitriptyline	Elavil[a]	25–300 mg daily in single or divided doses	• Anticholinergic side effects
			• Drowsiness
doxepin	Sinequan[a]	150–300 mg at bedtime	• Sedation
nortriptyline	Pamelor	50–150 mg at bedtime; may give in divided doses in elderly patients	• Suicidal ideation
			• Weight gain
Monoamine Oxidase Inhibitors (MAOIs)			
Inhibition of the MAO enzyme leads to an increased availability of neurotransmitters such as norepinephrine and dopamine; many drug interactions			
phenelzine	Nardil	45–90 mg daily in divided doses	• Confusion
			• Constipation
			• Drowsiness
			• Hypertensive crisis
			• Orthostatic hypotension
Bupropion			
Bupropion increases the availability of dopamine in the CNS			
bupropion	Wellbutrin[a]	100 mg three times a day; Max 450 mg/day	• Dizziness
	Wellbutrin SR	150 mg twice a day: Max 450 mg/day	• Headache
	Wellbutrin XL	150 mg in the morning; Max 450 mg/day	• Increased seizure risk
	Aplenzin	174–348 mg/day	• Insomnia
	Zyban for smoking cessation	300 mg/day in divided doses	• Mood instability
Trazodone			
Trazodone increases the availability of serotonin in the CNS			
trazodone	Desyrel[a]	150–400 mg/day in divided doses	• Confusion
			• Dizziness
			• Drowsiness
			• Orthostatic hypotension

TABLE 17.9

Select Medications for the Treatment of Depression—cont'd

Generic Name	Brand Name	Common Dosage Range	Common Side Effects
Vilazodone			
Vilazodone increases the availability of serotonin in the CNS and is a 5-hydroxytryptamine receptor partial agonist			
vilazodone	Viibryd	10–40 mg/day	• Abnormal dreams • Dizziness • Drowsiness • Fatigue • Insomnia

[a]Brand discontinued; now available only as generic.

CNS, Central nervous system.

GENERIC NAME: Bupropion

TRADE NAMES: Wellbutrin,[a] Wellbutrin SR, Wellbutrin XL

INDICATIONS: Depression, seasonal affective disorder, nicotine withdrawal

ROUTE OF ADMINISTRATION: Oral

COMMON ADULT DOSAGE: *Wellbutrin:* 100 mg three times a day; max 450 mg/day. *Wellbutrin SR:* 150 mg twice a day; max 450 mg/day. *Wellbutrin XL:* 150 mg in the morning; max 450 mg/day

MECHANISM OF ACTION: Miscellaneous antidepressant, increases the amount of dopamine available in the CNS

SIDE EFFECTS: Dizziness, drowsiness, hallucinations, seizures

AUXILIARY LABEL: May cause dizziness and drowsiness

SPECIAL NOTE: Another form of bupropion, Zyban, is used for smoking cessation; although the Zyban brand name has been discontinued, some providers still refer to bupropion in this way.

[a] Brand discontinued; now available only as generic.

Anxiety Disorders

Unease and fear characterize anxiety, and these are normal physiologic reactions. It becomes problematic when it interferes with daily personal and social interactions. It may elicit panic attacks or compulsive behaviors. Anxiety can be expressed as a feeling of fear or dread, with symptoms ranging from a rapid heart rate to trembling. We divide anxiety disorders into several different types. These range from panic disorders, such as post-traumatic stress disorder (PTSD) and phobias, to personality disorders, such as obsessive-compulsive disorder (OCD). Some anxiety disorder types include the following:

- *Generalized anxiety disorder (GAD):* In GAD a person experiences constant anxiety and worries continuously about common life problems (eg, money or relationships) over a period of 6 months or longer.

- *Social anxiety disorder:* Also referred to as *social phobia,* a person experiences constant anxiety and extreme fear around others. The person with social anxiety disorder attempts to avoid public situations and people. The avoidance stems from overwhelming fears of being humiliated, being judged, and feeling uncomfortable. The condition disrupts the person's normal daily activities.

- *Panic disorder:* An anxiety disorder that includes panic attacks. Situation events can trigger these attacks. During a panic attack, the person experiences severe apprehension, fear, and terror, in addition to physical complaints, such as dizziness, heart palpitations, or shakiness. Severe panic disorders can lead to phobias and PTSD.

- *PTSD:* This condition follows traumatic or terrifying incidents. Sights, sounds, and even smells can prompt flashbacks, nightmares, and constant memories. Soldiers returning from war are a common group suffering from PTSD. Other people who may suffer from PTSD include victims of rape, those exposed to violence, and those diagnosed with a life-threatening medical illness. PTSD symptoms can occur any time after the precipitating event.

- *Phobias:* Phobias are marked by an irrational, persistent fear of situations, people, or things. The person with a phobia experiences several symptoms, including a rapid heart rate, shortness of breath, and trembling. Treatment ranges from psychotherapy to antianxiety medications.

Prognosis

With proper diagnosis and treatment, including medication and ongoing therapy, people with anxiety disorders can live relatively normal lives.

Non-Drug Treatments

Most people require psychotherapy and behavioral therapy, which can help the individual learn to resist urges, compulsions, or other triggers that cause an abnormal response.

Drug Treatments

Primary medications used include antianxiety agents (eg, benzodiazepines) and SSRIs.

GENERIC NAME: alprazolam
(Schedule IV [C-IV])

TRADE NAMES: Xanax, Xanax XR

INDICATION: Anxiety disorders

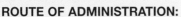

ROUTE OF ADMINISTRATION:
Oral

COMMON ADULT DOSAGE: *Xanax:* 0.25–0.5 mg
3 times daily; max 4 mg/day in divided doses. Xanax
XR: 3–6 mg daily

MECHANISM OF ACTION: Binds benzodiazepine
receptors leading to CNS depression

SIDE EFFECTS: Drowsiness, dizziness,
dry mouth

AUXILIARY LABELS:
- May cause dizziness and drowsiness
- Avoid alcohol
- *Caution:* Federal law prohibits the transfer of this
  drug to any person other than the patient for whom it
  was prescribed

■ Tech Note!

All benzodiazepine medications are schedule intravenous
medications.

GENERIC NAME: buspirone

TRADE NAME: BuSpar[a]

INDICATION: Anxiety disorders

ROUTE OF ADMINISTRATION:
Oral

COMMON ADULT DOSAGE: 7.5–30 mg twice daily.
Initial: 7.5 mg twice daily; *usual:* 20–30 mg/day in
divided doses

MECHANISM OF ACTION: Not well understood but
suppresses serotonergic activity while enhancing
noradrenergic and dopaminergic activity. The net
effect is an improvement in anxiety symptoms

SIDE EFFECTS: Drowsiness, dizziness, nausea

AUXILIARY LABEL: May cause dizziness and
drowsiness

[a] Brand discontinued; now available only as generic.

Bipolar Disorder

Patients with bipolar disorder may experience excessive
mood swings that range from manic (high) to depressive (low)
states. Specific symptoms of mania include agitation, hyper-
activity, inflated self-esteem, risky or reckless behavior, and
decreased sleep. The depression phase can include fatigue,
loss of self-esteem, suicidal thoughts, social withdrawal from
family and friends, and eating and sleeping disturbances. The
goal is to stabilize mood and minimize wide-ranging fluctuations from mania and depression.

Prognosis

With proper medications, patients may find their bipolar
symptoms under control. A problem with medication
compliance with patients with bipolar disorder is that
they feel better (manic stage). A strong support system
helps maintain appropriate continuing treatment.

Non-Drug Treatment

Psychotherapy helps with the depressive phase. For
those whose depressive state resists control by medications, electroconvulsive therapy may be an alternative
treatment form.

Drug Treatment

Treatment primarily involves mood-stabilizing drugs (eg,
lithium) and anticonvulsants (eg, carbamazepine, divalproex, lamotrigine). Although we do not understand the
complete mechanism for lithium, it may alter behavior by
enhancing the serotonin and norepinephrine uptake by
nerve cells. This sets lithium apart from other psychiatric
drugs because it does not cause major CNS changes
such as sedation, feelings of euphoria, or depression.

GENERIC NAME: lithium

TRADE NAME: Eskalith[a]

INDICATION: Bipolar disorder

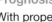

ROUTE OF ADMINISTRATION:
Oral

COMMON ADULT DOSAGE: 900–1800 mg/day in
3 or 4 doses (immediate-release); doses vary based
on laboratory results of serum lithium levels

MECHANISM OF ACTION: Mechanism is unknown,
but efficacy is thought to be due to effects on
neurotransmitters such as serotonin

SIDE EFFECTS: Dizziness, drowsiness, tremor,
nausea, vomiting, diarrhea

AUXILIARY LABELS:
- May cause dizziness and drowsiness
- Take with food or milk

[a] Brand discontinued; now available only as generic.

GENERIC NAME: cariprazine

TRADE NAME: Vraylar

INDICATIONS: Bipolar disorder,
schizophrenia

ROUTE OF ADMINISTRATION: Oral

COMMON ADULT DOSAGES: *Bipolar disorder and
schizophrenia:* Initial dose is 1.5 mg once daily, may
increase to 3 mg once daily; max 6 mg once daily

MECHANISM OF ACTION: Partial agonist for
dopamine D2 and D3

SIDE EFFECTS: Possible **extrapyramidal symptoms
(EPSs),** drowsiness, headache, indigestion

AUXILIARY LABEL: May cause drowsiness,
especially with alcohol

Schizophrenia

Schizophrenia is a psychiatric disorder involving chronic or episodic **psychosis.** It may cause impaired social and occupational functioning. It is among the most socially and economically disabling medical conditions, according to the WHO. Individuals with schizophrenia commonly exhibit both positive and negative symptoms. Positive symptoms can include hallucinations, delusions, and disorganized speech. Negative symptoms can include depressed mood and impairments in attention, memory, and high-level functioning. The schizophrenia diagnosis comes from the presence of symptoms in addition to the diminished social function and/or occupational dysfunction for at least 6 months.

Although schizophrenia's exact cause is unknown, the disorder may have a strong genetic component. Several environmental risk factors may contribute: living in an urban area, immigration, experiencing obstetric complications, and a birth date in late winter to early spring, a reflection of influenza virus exposure during neural development. Additionally, patients with schizophrenia have higher rates of other psychiatric disorders, such as depression, anxiety disorders, and substance abuse, relative to those without schizophrenia.

The symptoms include involuntary movement of the facial muscles, tongue, jaw, and head. If these symptoms appear, the medication must be stopped immediately because these effects can be irreversible. Side effects that mimic Parkinson disease motions also may occur. Antipsychotic medications block dopamine's effects, causing drug-induced parkinsonism. Some antipsychotic medications, especially the atypicals, cause weight gain and an increased incidence of type 2 diabetes. Prescribers may give long-acting antipsychotics, depot preparations, monthly. These depot agents, which may have a slower onset (24–72 hours after injection) and longer duration of action (average of 3–4 weeks), can help with the management of chronic schizophrenia. Examples of antipsychotic medications are discussed in the drug monographs on the pages that follow.

As noted previously, persons with schizophrenia may have a higher risk for other psychiatric disorders. Accordingly, additional medications may include the following:

- *Antianxiety medications:* Benzodiazepines, such as clonazepam (Klonopin) and diazepam (Valium), may help reduce anxiety and nervousness.
- *Anticonvulsant medications:* Antiepileptics, such as carbamazepine (Tegretol) and valproate (Depakote), can stabilize and reduce symptoms during a relapse.
- *Antidepressants:* Various SSRIs (eg, sertraline [Zoloft] or citalopram [Celexa]) or TCAs (eg, nortriptyline [Pamelor]) can treat depressive symptoms.

Prognosis

Although some studies show treatment resistance, certain subsets of patients with schizophrenia can achieve good outcomes with symptoms, employment, and function. The treatment goal is to minimize symptoms and maximize functionality and independence.

Non-Drug Treatments

Both professional counseling and a strong support system are keys to the success of treatment. However, drug therapy remains critical to managing positive and negative disease symptoms.

Drug Treatments

Drug treatments focus on eliminating symptoms, improving quality of life, and allowing the patient to live productively. Treatment options reflect the phases of schizophrenia: acute, stabilizing, maintenance, or recovery. Often prescribers try various medications and/or strengths of agents before finding the most effective combination. This is because patients respond differently to medications. We categorize antipsychotic agents as first generation (sometimes called "typical") and second generation ("atypical" antipsychotics). A particularly devastating adverse reaction that can occur while taking antipsychotics is **tardive dyskinesia (TD).**

GENERIC NAME: haloperidol

TRADE NAME: Haldol[a]

INDICATIONS: Schizophrenia, acute psychosis

ROUTES OF ADMINISTRATION: Oral; solution for injection; suspension for injection (long-acting)

COMMON ADULT DOSAGE: Dosage can vary depending on individual and dosage form. *Oral:* 5–20 mg/day (max 100 mg/day); *IM:* haloperidol decanoate (long-lasting suspension): 10–15 times the daily oral dosage (max 450 mg); *IM:* haloperidol lactate (prompt-acting): 2–5 mg, subsequent doses may be administered as often as every hour if needed (max depends on clinical response and tolerability)

MECHANISM OF ACTION: First-generation antipsychotic (blocks dopamine receptors)

SIDE EFFECTS: Extrapyramidal symptoms, drowsiness, confusion, tardive dyskinesia

AUXILIARY LABEL: May cause dizziness and drowsiness

[a] Brand discontinued; now available only as generic.

GENERIC NAME: clozapine

TRADE NAMES: Clozaril, FazaClo

INDICATION: Schizophrenia

ROUTE OF ADMINISTRATION: Oral

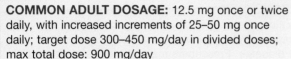

COMMON ADULT DOSAGE: 12.5 mg once or twice daily, with increased increments of 25–50 mg once daily; target dose 300–450 mg/day in divided doses; max total dose: 900 mg/day

MECHANISM OF ACTION: Second-generation antipsychotic (blocks dopamine receptors)

SIDE EFFECTS: Hematologic effects, drowsiness, dizziness, headache, extrapyramidal symptoms

AUXILIARY LABELS:
• May cause dizziness and drowsiness
• Take with or without food
• Do not drink alcohol

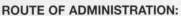
Tech Note!

Clozapine has a risk for hematologic effects, including agranulocytosis. Therefore clozapine is available only through a monitoring and distribution system to ensure that patients receive appropriate blood monitoring.

GENERIC NAME: olanzapine

TRADE NAMES: Zyprexa, Zyprexa Zydis, Zyprexa Relprevv

INDICATIONS: Schizophrenia, agitation

ROUTES OF ADMINISTRATION: Oral; intramuscular (IM) injection

COMMON ADULT DOSAGE: *Oral:* 5–20 mg daily. *IM injection:* 150–300 mg every 2 weeks or 300–405 mg every 4 weeks (max 300 mg every 2 weeks or 405 mg every 4 weeks)

MECHANISM OF ACTION: Second-generation antipsychotic (blocks dopamine receptors)

SIDE EFFECTS: Drowsiness, weight gain, headache, dizziness, extrapyramidal symptoms

AUXILIARY LABELS:
• May cause dizziness and drowsiness
• Do not swallow; let dissolve in the mouth (orally disintegrating tablet [ODT] form)
• Do not drink alcohol

GENERIC NAME: risperidone

TRADE NAMES: Risperdal, Risperdal Consta

INDICATION: Schizophrenia

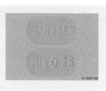

ROUTES OF ADMINISTRATION: Oral; IM injection

COMMON ADULT DOSAGES: *Oral:* 2–8 mg daily. *IM injection:* 12.5–50 mg every 2 weeks

MECHANISM OF ACTION: Second-generation antipsychotic (blocks dopamine receptors)

SIDE EFFECTS: Drowsiness, weight gain, headache, dizziness, extrapyramidal symptoms

AUXILIARY LABELS:
• May cause dizziness or drowsiness
• Do not swallow; let dissolve in the mouth (orally disintegrating tablet form)
• Do not drink alcohol

GENERIC NAME: aripiprazole

TRADE NAMES: Abilify, Abilify Maintena

INDICATIONS: Schizophrenia, agitation, depression, bipolar disorder

ROUTE OF ADMINISTRATION: Oral; IM injection

COMMON ADULT DOSAGE: *Oral:* 10–15 mg once daily; max 30 mg daily. *IM injection:* 400 mg once a month

MECHANISM OF ACTION: Second-generation antipsychotic (blocks dopamine receptors)

SIDE EFFECTS: Drowsiness, weight gain, headache, dizziness, extrapyramidal symptoms

AUXILIARY LABELS:
• May cause dizziness or drowsiness
• Do not drink alcohol

GENERIC NAME: brexpiprazole

TRADE NAME: Rexulti

INDICATIONS: Depression, schizophrenia

ROUTE OF ADMINISTRATION: Oral

COMMON ADULT DOSAGES: *Depression:* initial dose is 0.5–1 mg once daily, titrate up to 2 mg/day; max 3 mg/day. *Schizophrenia:* initial dose is 1 mg once daily, titrate up to 4 mg/day; max 4 mg/day

MECHANISM OF ACTION: Partial agonist for dopamine/serotonin-dopamine activity modulator

SIDE EFFECTS: Weight gain, possible extrapyramidal symptoms, drowsiness, headache

AUXILIARY LABELS:
• May cause drowsiness, especially with alcohol
• May cause weight gain

GENERIC NAME: ziprasidone

TRADE NAME: Geodon

INDICATIONS: Schizophrenia, agitation, bipolar disorder

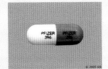

ROUTES OF ADMINISTRATION: Oral; IM injection

COMMON ADULT DOSAGES: *Oral:* 40–100 mg twice daily for schizophrenia and 40–80 mg twice daily for bipolar disorder. *IM injection:* 10 mg every 2 hours or 20 mg every 4 hours (max 40 mg/day)

MECHANISM OF ACTION: Second-generation antipsychotic (blocks dopamine receptors)

SIDE EFFECTS: Drowsiness, weight gain, headache, dizziness, extrapyramidal symptoms

AUXILIARY LABELS:
- May cause dizziness or drowsiness
- Do not drink alcohol

Insomnia

Patients with **insomnia** have impaired daytime functioning because of difficulty falling asleep or difficulty maintaining sleep, or they experience poor-quality sleep. A person is considered to have insomnia when all three of the following factors are present:

- The person reports difficulty falling asleep or maintaining sleep or waking too early.
- Sleep difficulty occurs even though the person has adequate opportunity to sleep.
- The impairment in sleep causes difficulties in daytime functioning.

Insomnia is a common medical complaint. An estimated 30% to 50% of the population has insomnia. Sleeping difficulties may need treatment depending on the frequency and the impact of sleep loss on daily functioning. Insomnia can affect all age groups, but prevalence increases with age. It is more common in women than in men. Insomnia causes range from stress, sleep interruptions, and pain. Medications may cause insomnia and present an important consideration for pharmacists when counseling patients about OTC antiinsomnia agents. Various illnesses also affect sleep patterns and sleep quality; these include sleep apnea, acid reflux disease, PD, and AD. Ideally, the health care professional can diagnose and correct the root cause.

Prognosis

Many patients find effective treatment through risk factor modification, adopting good sleep hygiene, or medication use.

Non-Drug Treatment

The most effective insomnia treatment is cognitive-behavioral therapy for insomnia (CBT-I), which reduces insomnia symptoms by implementing cognitive and lifestyle changes. This therapy aims to optimize sleep hygiene such as regular exercise, a consistent sleep schedule, and avoiding alcohol and caffeine during certain times of the day. Other factors such as keeping the bedroom quiet and an ambient temperature can also help. Relaxation therapy techniques, such as dimming lights, listening to soft music, and meditating before retiring, can also help.

Drug Treatment

Many over-the-counter (OTC) drugs provide relief from transient insomnia episodes. Antihistamines form the mainstay of OTC treatment. Diphenhydramine and doxylamine produce sedation as a welcome side effect in these patients. However, OTC treatment should be short term. Chronic insomnia needs to be evaluated by a clinician. The clinician will perform a sleep analysis to evaluate the patient's quality of sleep or identify any other issues and determine the appropriate therapy. Pharmacists do not recommend OTC sleep products containing diphenhydramine (eg, Tylenol PM) for the elderly because they may cause confusion and increase the risk of falls.

Insomnia medications fall into four categories by mechanism of actions:

1. Benzodiazepine receptor agonists (including benzodiazepines and nonbenzodiazepines)
2. Dual orexin receptor antagonists
3. Melatonin receptor agonists
4. Sedating antidepressants

These medications may work alone, but it is best to employ them in combination with the previously mentioned non-drug treatments. The elderly must demonstrate extreme caution and not combine OTC sleeping agents with prescription medications. Temazepam, eszopiclone, and zolpidem are on the Beers Criteria list. Ramelteon, a melatonin receptor agonist, works to induce sleep onset in a similar manner to melatonin. A newer medication and drug class for treating insomnia is suvorexant (Belsomra), which is a dual orexin receptor antagonist. The medicine is a US Drug Enforcement Agency Schedule IV controlled substance. The orexin system stimulates wakefulness, so blocking orexin receptors type 1 and type 2 might help patients sleep. Examples of antiinsomnia medications are in Table 17.10.

Tech Note!

Manufacturers first marketed nonbenzodiazepines in the United States as not having the same side effects as benzodiazepines. However, they can produce many of the same side effects.

TABLE 17.10
Select Medications Approved for the Treatment of Insomnia

Generic Name	Brand Name	Common Dosage Range	Common Side Effects
Benzodiazepines			
flurazepam	Dalmane[a]	15–30 mg at bedtime	• Amnesia • Confusion • Dizziness • Drowsiness • Fatigue
temazepam	Restoril	7.5–30 mg at bedtime	
triazolam	Halcion	0.125–0.5 mg at bedtime	
Nonbenzodiazepine Hypnotics			
eszopiclone	Lunesta	1–3 mg at bedtime	• Amnesia • Confusion • Dizziness • Drowsiness • Fatigue
zaleplon	Sonata	5–20 mg at bedtime	
zolpidem	Ambien	5–10 mg at bedtime	
	Ambien CR	6.25–12.5 mg at bedtime	
	Edluar	5–10 mg SL at bedtime	
	Intermezzo	1.75–3.5 mg SL once nightly for middle-of-the-night awakening	
	Zolpimist	1–2 sprays (5–10 mg) PO at bedtime	
Melatonin Receptor Agonists			
melatonin[b]	Melatonin	0.3–6 mg at bedtime	• Abdominal pain • Dizziness • Drowsiness • Nightmares
ramelteon	Rozerem	8 mg within 30 min of bedtime	• Dizziness • Drowsiness • Fatigue • Rebound insomnia
Dual Orexin Receptor Antagonist			
suvorexant	Belsomra	10 mg once nightly, max 20 mg/day	• Blurry vision • Dizziness
Antihistamines			
diphenhydramine[b]	Benadryl Allergy	12.5–50 mg at bedtime	• Confusion • Dizziness • Drowsiness • Dry mouth
diphenhydramine[b]	Unisom SleepGels	25 mg at bedtime	

[a]Brand discontinued; now available only as generic.
[b]Available over the counter.
PO, Orally; *SL,* sublingually.

GENERIC NAME: temazepam (C-IV)

TRADE NAME: Restoril

INDICATION: Insomnia

ROUTE OF ADMINISTRATION: Oral

COMMON ADULT DOSAGE: 15–30 mg at bedtime

MECHANISM OF ACTION: Binds benzodiazepine receptors, leading to CNS depression

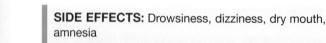

SIDE EFFECTS: Drowsiness, dizziness, dry mouth, amnesia

AUXILIARY LABELS:
• May cause dizziness and drowsiness
• Do not drink alcohol
• *Caution:* Federal law prohibits the transfer of this drug to any person other than the patient for whom it was prescribed

GENERIC NAME: eszopiclone
(C-IV)

TRADE NAME: Lunesta

INDICATION: Insomnia

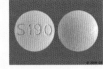

ROUTE OF ADMINISTRATION:
Oral

COMMON ADULT DOSAGE: 1–3 mg at bedtime

MECHANISM OF ACTION: Modulates the GABA system of the CNS, leading to sedation

SIDE EFFECTS: Drowsiness, dizziness, headache, amnesia

AUXILIARY LABELS:
• May cause dizziness and drowsiness
• Do not drink alcohol
• *Caution:* Federal law prohibits the transfer of this drug to any person other than the patient for whom it was prescribed

---

GENERIC NAME: zolpidem (C-IV)

TRADE NAMES: Ambien, Ambien CR, Zolpimist, Edluar, Intermezzo

INDICATION: Insomnia

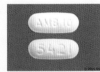

ROUTE OF ADMINISTRATION:
Various oral dosage forms

COMMON ADULT DOSAGES: *Immediate release:* 5–10 mg at bedtime. *Controlled release:* 6.25–12.5 mg at bedtime

MECHANISM OF ACTION: Modulates the GABA system of the CNS, leading to sedation

SIDE EFFECTS: Drowsiness, dizziness, confusion, fatigue, amnesia

AUXILIARY LABELS:
• May cause dizziness and drowsiness
• Do not drink alcohol
• *Caution:* Federal law prohibits the transfer of this drug to any person other than the patient for whom it was prescribed

---

GENERIC NAME: Ramelteon

TRADE NAMES: Rozerem

INDICATION: Insomnia

ROUTE OF ADMINISTRATION: Oral

COMMON ADULT DOSAGES: 8 mg once daily administered, as needed, within 30 minutes of bedtime (Max: 8 mg/day)

MECHANISM OF ACTION: Potent agonist of melatonin receptors, inducing sleepiness

SIDE EFFECTS: Drowsiness, dizziness, fatigue

AUXILIARY LABEL: May cause dizziness and drowsiness

Tech Note!

Ramelteon, for sleep, may be confused with Remeron, an antidepressant.

GENERIC NAME: suvorexant

TRADE NAME: Belsomra

INDICATION: Insomnia

ROUTE OF ADMINISTRATION:
Oral

COMMON ADULT DOSAGE: 10 mg once nightly (max 20 mg/day)

MECHANISM OF ACTION: Antagonizes receptors for orexin-A and orexin-B, which are neuropeptides that promote wakefulness and appetite

SIDE EFFECTS: Headache, dizziness, somnolence, increased risk for suicide

AUXILIARY LABELS:
• May cause dizziness/blurred vision, dizziness, and drowsiness increased with alcohol
• Take right before bed

Attention-Deficit/Hyperactivity Disorder

Attention-deficit/hyperactivity disorder (**ADHD**) is a physiologic brain disorder in which a person struggles to focus his or her attention or to engage in quiet, passive-type behavior, or both. Boys are three times as likely as girls to warrant an ADHD diagnosis, which affects 3% to 5% of school-age children. The symptoms and signs include impulsive, explosive, or irritable behavior. Although intelligence is unaffected, work performance in school is sporadic because of a lack of focus. Older children or adults describe symptoms of distraction by irrelevant thoughts, sounds, or sights. Daydreaming also presents an obstacle to a person's ability to meet deadlines, keep track of school or work materials, and finish assignments.

Prognosis
With proper treatment and understanding, the outlook for a normal productive life with ADHD is very good.

Non-Drug Treatment
Education is important to understanding ADHD. This may involve parents, teachers, and therapists, in addition to the patient and physician. Treatment varies, depending on the child's symptoms and ability to function at home and at school. Behavior modification, coaching, and supportive psychotherapy can help the patient cope. To develop a treatment plan, health professionals urge parents to understand the many professionals available to treat the condition.

Drug Treatment
In certain cases, medications help (Table 17.11). Stimulants and atomoxetine are the most commonly used

Select Medications for the Treatment of Attention-Deficit/Hyperactivity Disorder

Generic Name	Trade Name	Dosage Forms	Notes
amphetamine/ dextroamphetamine (C-II)	Adderall	• Tablets	• Do not crush, chew, or divide
	Adderall XR, Mydayis	• Capsules	• The capsule may be opened and sprinkled onto food, such as applesauce
atomoxetine	Strattera	• Capsules	• May be taken with or without food • May be discontinued without tapering dose • The capsule should not be opened
dexmethylphenidate (C-II)	Focalin	• Tablets	• Do not crush, chew, or divide
	Focalin XR	• Capsules	• The capsule may be opened and sprinkled onto food, such as applesauce
dextroamphetamine (C-II)	Dexedrine, ProCentra Solution	• Oral solution • Spansules (capsules) • Tablets	• Do not crush, chew, or divide tablets or spansules
lisdexamfetamine (C-II)	Vyvanse	• Capsules • Chewable tablets	• Capsule can be opened and entire contents dissolved in a glass of water • Do not divide the dose
methylphenidate (C-II)	Concerta	• ER tablets	• Do not crush, chew, or divide tablets
	Daytrana	• Transdermal patch	• Apply topically once daily in the morning; remove after 9 hours
	Metadate CD	• ER capsules	• The capsule may be opened and sprinkled onto food, such as applesauce
	Metadate ER	• ER tablets	• Do not crush, chew, or divide tablets
	Methylin (discontinued)	• Trade name chewable tablets (Methylin) have been discontinued; generic version is still available • Oral solution	
	Ritalin	• Tablets	• Do not crush, chew, or divide tablets

ER, Extended release.

drugs. Common CNS stimulants include methylphenidate (Ritalin) and amphetamines such as dextroamphetamine (Dexedrine). Those agents are Schedule II (C-II) controlled substances. Patients can develop physical dependence—a continued, pathologic need to take the medication. In 2022, viloxazine (Qelbree), a nonstimulant medication, was approved for ADHD treatment in individuals 6 years and older.

GENERIC NAME:
methylphenidate (C-II)
SELECT TRADE NAMES:
Adhansia XR, Aptensio XR, Concerta, Cotempla XR-ODT, Daytrana, Jornay PM, Metadate CD, Metadate ER, Methylin, QuilliChew ER, Quillivant XR, Ritalin, Ritalin LA
INDICATION: ADHD

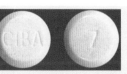

ROUTES OF ADMINISTRATION: Oral; transdermal patch

COMMON DOSAGE: Dosages vary, depending on the dosage form and patient's age

MECHANISM OF ACTION: The ADHD mechanism is not clear. It may stem from modulation of serotonin effects in the brain via changes in dopamine transport

SIDE EFFECTS: Dizziness, drowsiness, headache, loss of appetite, nausea, nervousness, trouble sleeping

AUXILIARY LABELS:
- May cause dizziness and drowsiness
- Do not drink alcohol
- Do not take MAOIs while using this medication
- Do not stop the medication abruptly
- *Caution:* Federal law prohibits the transfer of this drug to any person other than the patient for whom it was prescribed.

GENERIC NAME: Viloxazine

TRADE NAME: Qelbree

INDICATION: ADHD

ROUTE OF ADMINISTRATION: Oral

COMMON ADULT DOSAGE: 200 mg once daily (initial); may titrate up 200 mg increments weekly to a max dose of 600 mg once daily

MECHANISM OF ACTION: Increases levels of norepinephrine in the brain

SIDE EFFECTS: Drowsiness, decreased appetite, nausea, vomiting

BLACK BOX WARNING: May increase risk of suicidal thoughts and behaviors

AUXILIARY LABEL: May cause dizziness or drowsiness

Smoking Cessation

Smoking cessation is a difficult process that the pharmacy staff may be involved with, including recommending OTC products or providing counseling and follow-up with prescription products. Prescribers can employ the antidepressant bupropion or the medication varenicline (Chantix) to help patients quit.

Prognosis

Although some smokers may quit on their own, they often require counseling or to work through repeated attempts

Non-Drug Treatment

Non-drug treatment might involve replacing nicotine products with chewing gum or tying quitting to important goals, such as living longer and healthier for the family.

Drug Treatment

Nicotine replacement therapy is one option, as are the medications bupropion and varenicline (Chantix). If a patient is currently taking theophylline, warfarin, or insulin, smoking cessation may alter the pharmacokinetic properties of those medications. Although the initial therapy might be expensive, reducing the cost of cigarettes or other nicotine products can readily make up the difference.

GENERIC NAME: varenicline

TRADE NAME: Chantix

INDICATION: Smoking cessation

ROUTE OF ADMINISTRATION: Oral

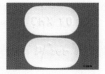

COMMON ADULT DOSAGES: Begin 1 week before quit date. *Initial dosage:* days 1–3: 0.5 mg once daily; days 4–7: 0.5 mg twice daily; day 8 and on: 1 mg twice daily. Treatment is for 12 or 24 weeks

MECHANISM OF ACTION: Partial activity at nicotinic receptors, prevents nicotine from binding to those receptors

SIDE EFFECTS: Nausea, vomiting, headache, insomnia

AUXILIARY LABELS:
- May cause nausea/vomiting
- Limit alcohol while on this medication
- May cause headache

Do You Remember These Key Points?

- Names of the major components and divisions of the nervous system and their functions
- The primary symptoms of the various neurologic conditions associated with the nervous system discussed
- Medications used to treat the various nervous system conditions discussed
- The generic and trade names for the drugs discussed in this chapter
- The appropriate auxiliary labels that should be used when filling prescriptions for drugs discussed in this chapter

Review Questions

Multiple Choice Questions

1. Neurons include each of the following components *except:*
   A. Dendrites
   B. Cell body
   C. Nerve terminals
   D. Amino acids

2. Which of the following is a rare autoimmune disorder that affects the transmission of electrical impulses from the central nervous system to muscles throughout the body?
   A. Myasthenia gravis
   B. Alzheimer disease
   C. Parkinson disease
   D. Multiple sclerosis

3. We divide the autonomic nervous system into the _____ and _____.
   A. Parasympathetic nervous system; sympathetic nervous system
   B. Parasympathetic nervous system; somatic nervous system
   C. Peripheral nervous system; somatic nervous system
   D. Central nervous system; sympathetic nervous system

4. The part of the brain that controls memory, reason, and language skills is the:
   A. Medulla oblongata
   B. Cerebellum
   C. Cerebral cortex
   D. Brainstem

5. _____ generally affect the sympathetic system, whereas _____ affect the parasympathetic system.
   A. Cholinergics, anticholinergics
   B. Cholinergics, adrenergics
   C. Adrenergics, antiadrenergics
   D. Adrenergics, cholinergics

6. Which of the following medications is a dopamine agonist?
   A. Rasagiline
   B. Benztropine
   C. Rotigotine
   D. Amantadine

7. Which of the following medications for Alzheimer disease is available as a patch?
   A. Donepezil
   B. Memantine
   C. Galantamine
   D. Rivastigmine

8. The illness that is marked by extremes in elevated and depressed moods is defined as:
   A. Schizophrenia
   B. Bipolar disorder
   C. Depression
   D. All of the above

9. An important auxiliary label to include on a benzodiazepine bottle would be:
   A. Take in the morning
   B. Take on an empty stomach
   C. May cause dizziness and drowsiness
   D. Take as directed

10. Which medication class should we use cautiously with patients who are depressed?
    A. Dopamine agonists
    B. Interferons
    C. SSRIs
    D. Antipsychotics

11. SSRIs inhibit the reuptake of which of the following neurotransmitters?
    A. Norepinephrine
    B. Epinephrine
    C. Serotonin
    D. Dopamine

12. Which of the following is *not* a classic symptom of Parkinson disease?
    A. Tremor
    B. Rigidity
    C. Postural instability
    D. Diarrhea

13. Which of the following is *not* used to treat insomnia?
    A. Trazodone
    B. Zolpidem
    C. Dexmethylphenidate
    D. Diphenhydramine

14. Sumatriptan (Imitrex) is available in which of the following dosage forms for the treatment of migraines?
    A. Tablet
    B. Injection
    C. Nasal spray
    D. All of the above

15. Which of the following conditions is *not* considered an anxiety disorder?
    A. PTSD
    B. Phobia
    C. OCD
    D. Schizophrenia

■ Technician's Corner

Using a drug reference resource, look up a medication from each of the SSRI, SNRI, TCA, and MAOI antidepressant medication classes and familiarize yourself with the types of medical conditions they are used to treat in addition to depression.

Bibliography

American Geriatrics Society 2019 Updated AGS Beers Criteria® for potentially inappropriate medication use in older adults. *J Am Geriatr Soc*. 2019;67(4):674-694. doi:10.1111/jgs.15767.

Applegate E. *The Anatomy and Physiology Learning System*. 4th ed. St. Louis: Saunders; 2010.

Clinical Pharmacology Online. Available at: https://www.clinicalkey.com/pharmacology/

Damjanov I. *Pathology for the Health Professions*. 4th ed. St. Louis: Saunders; 2011.

Fishback JL. *Pathology*. 3rd ed. Philadelphia: Mosby; 2005.

Huether SE. *Understanding Pathophysiology*. 5th ed. St. Louis: Mosby; 2012.

Scanlon V, Sanders T. *Essentials of Anatomy and Physiology*. 5th ed. Philadelphia: FA Davis; 2007.

Solomon EP. *Introduction to Human Anatomy and Physiology*. 3rd ed. St. Louis: Saunders; 2009.

Thibodeau G, Patton K. *Structure and Function of the Body*. 13th ed. St. Louis: Mosby; 2007.

Thibodeau G, Patton K. *Anatomy and Physiology*. 8th ed. St. Louis: Mosby; 2012.

CHAPTER 18

Therapeutic Agents for the Endocrine System

Tony Guerra

1. Name the major endocrine glands of the body.
2. Describe the locations and functions of the endocrine glands discussed.
3. List the primary symptoms of conditions associated with dysfunction of the principal endocrine glands discussed. In addition, (a) recognize drugs used to treat the endocrine conditions discussed, (b) write the generic and trade names for the medications discussed in this chapter, and (c) list appropriate auxiliary labels when filling prescriptions for drugs discussed in this chapter.

Acromegaly Extremity + enlargement, a condition caused by excessive growth hormone production during adulthood

Addison disease A condition resulting in decreased levels of adrenocortical hormones (eg, mineralocorticoids and glucocorticoids), which causes symptoms such as muscle weakness and weight loss; eponym named after Thomas Addison, a British physician

Adrenal cortex Near + kidney + husk, a portion of the adrenal gland that secretes steroids, including mineralocorticoids, glucocorticoids, and sex steroids

Adrenal medulla Near + kidney + middle, an inner part of the adrenal gland that synthesizes and secretes the catecholamines norepinephrine and epinephrine

Aldosterone The principal mineralocorticoid in the body that maintains sodium and potassium homeostasis by stimulating the kidneys to conserve sodium and excrete potassium

Body mass index (BMI) A measure of body fat based on height and weight of a patient

Calcitonin A thyroid hormone that helps regulate blood concentrations of calcium and phosphate and promotes the formation of bone

Catecholamines Hormones produced in the brainstem, nervous system, and adrenal glands that help the body respond to stress and prepare the body for the "fight-or-flight" response; they are important in regulating heart rate, blood pressure, and nervous system functions

Comorbidity A concomitant, but not necessarily related, medical condition existing simultaneously with another condition

Cretinism A condition in which the development of the brain and body is inhibited by a congenital lack of thyroid hormone secretion

Dwarfism A condition characterized by a growth hormone deficiency during adolescence, resulting in short stature and decreased organ size

Endocrine glands Internal + secrete, glands that produce hormones that enter the bloodstream to reach their target or act at target sites near the area of hormone release

Endocrinologist A physician who specializes in the treatment of conditions of the endocrine system

397

Exocrine glands External + secrete, glands that produce hormones sent to the target organ or tissue via a tube or duct outside the body

Exophthalmos External + eyeball, an eyeball prominence (protrusion) from the orbit; increased thyroid hormone is a common cause of bilateral presentation

Gastroparesis Stomach + paralysis + condition of, delayed gastric emptying

Gigantism Giant + condition of, a condition of excessive growth hormone production during childhood or adolescence that results in excessive height and body tissue growth

Glucometer Glucose + measuring instrument, a device used to test blood sugar levels in patients with diabetes mellitus (DM)

Goiter A condition in which the thyroid gland is enlarged because of a lack of iodine; it can be either a simple goiter or a toxic goiter (ie, resulting from a tumor)

Graves disease A condition caused by thyroid hormone hypersecretion; symptoms include diffuse goiter, exophthalmos, and skin changes; an eponym for Irish physician Robert James Graves

Homeostasis Similar + still + condition of, the equilibrium pertaining to the balance of fluid levels, pH level, osmotic pressures, and concentrations of various substances

Hormones Chemical substances produced and secreted by an endocrine duct into the bloodstream that result in a physiological response at a specific target tissue

Hyperglycemia High + sugar + condition, elevated concentration of glucose in the blood

Hypertension High + pressure + condition, elevated blood pressure

Hyperthyroidism High 1 shield (shape of the thyroid gland) + condition, excessive secretion of thyroid hormone

Hypocalcemia Low + calcium + condition, low concentration of calcium in the blood

Hypoglycemia Low + sugar + condition, excessively low concentration of glucose in the blood

Hypokalemia Low + potassium + condition, low concentration of potassium in the blood

Hypopituitary dwarfism Short stature caused by a deficiency in growth hormone during childhood

Insulin resistance Island + compound (comes from the "islands" that produce insulin), the resistance of body tissues (skeletal muscle and fat) to insulin effects; insulin resistance is associated with the development of type 2 diabetes mellitus

Myxedema Mucus + swelling, a condition associated with a decrease in overall adult thyroid function; also known as hypothyroidism

Oogenesis Egg + birth, production or development of an egg

Orthostatic hypotension Straight + stand and low + pressure, low blood pressure that occurs on standing

Ovulation Egg + discharge, the release of an egg from the ovary

Pancreas An endocrine gland that produces both insulin and glucagon

Parenteral Outside + intestine, a term indicating administration of a substance by a route other than by mouth

Peripheral neuropathy Outside + boundary and nerve + disease, damage to nerves of the peripheral nervous system

Thyroxine (T$_4$) A thyroid hormone derived from tyrosine (amino acid) that influences the metabolic rate

Triiodothyronine (T$_3$) A thyroid hormone that helps regulate growth and development and controls metabolism and body temperature; it is mainly produced through the metabolism of thyroxine

Type 1 diabetes mellitus (T1DM) A form of diabetes mellitus associated with an absolute deficiency of insulin production by the pancreas; people with T1DM require insulin therapy

Type 2 diabetes mellitus (T2DM) A form of diabetes mellitus associated with insulin resistance and a relative deficiency of insulin; people with T2DM can be treated with oral therapies, noninsulin injectable medications, and insulin

Vasopressin Another term used for antidiuretic hormone (ADH)

Common Drugs for Conditions of the Endocrine System

Trade Name	Generic Name	Pronunciation
Agent to Treat Acromegaly and Gigantism		
Sandostatin	octreotide	(ok-**tree**-oh-tide)
Agents to Treat Addison Disease		
Cortef	hydrocortisone	(hye-droe-**kor**-ti-sone)
Deltasone[a]	prednisone	(**pred**-ni-zone)
	fludrocortisone acetate	(floo-**droe**-kor-ti-sone ah-sih-tate)

Trade Name	Generic Name	Pronunciation
Medrol	methylprednisolone	(**meth**-il-pred-**nis**-uh-lone)
Orapred, Millipred	prednisolone	(pred-**nis**-oh-lone)
Solu-Medrol	methylprednisolone sodium succinate	(**meth**-il-pred-**nis**-uh-lone **so**-dee-um **suck**-sin-ate)

Agents to Treat Cushing Syndrome

Lysodren	mitotane	(**mih**-tuh-tane)
Metopirone	metyrapone	(me-**teer**-uh-pone)

Agents to Treat Diabetes Insipidus

DDAVP	desmopressin acetate	(**dez**-mo-**pres**-in ah-sih-tate)
Pitressin,[a] Vasostrict	vasopressin	(**vay**-soe-**pres**-in)

Agents to Treat Hyperparathyroidism

Hectorol	doxercalciferol	(dock-sir-kal-**sih**-fer-all)
Rocaltrol	calcitriol	(**kal**-si-**trye**-ole)
Sensipar	cinacalcet	(sin-ah-**cal**-set)
Zemplar	paricalcitol	(par-ih-**cal**-sih-tahl)

Agents to Treat Hyperthyroidism

	propylthiouracil	(pro-pull-thigh-oh-**yoor**-uh-sill)
Tapazole	methimazole	(meth-**em**-uh-zoll)

Agents to Treat Hypothyroidism

Armour Thyroid, Nature-Throid, NP Thyroid	desiccated thyroid	(**des**-eh-kate-ed **thigh**-roid)
Cytomel, Triostat	liothyronine	(lie-oh-**thigh**-row-neen)
Synthroid, Euthyrox, Levoxyl, Tirosint, Tirosint-SOL,[a] Unithroid	levothyroxine	(lee-vo-**thigh**-rox-een)

Agent to Treat Syndrome of Inappropriate Antidiuretic Hormone Secretion (SIADH)

Declomycin[a]	demeclocycline	(**dem**-e-kloe-**sye**-kleen)

Insulin to Treat Diabetes Mellitus

Rapid-Acting Agents

Apidra	insulin glulisine	(**in**-su-lin **gloo**-lis-een)
Humalog, Admelog	insulin lispro	(**in**-su-lin **lis**-pro)
NovoLog, Fiasp, Fiasp FlexTouch, Fiasp PenFill	insulin aspart	(**in**-su-lin **as**-part)

Short-Acting Agents

Humulin R, Novolin R	regular insulin	(**reg**-yoo-lar **in**-su-lin)

Intermediate-Acting Agents

Humulin N, Novolin N	isophane insulin (NPH)	(**eye**-soe-fane **in**-su-lin)

Long-Acting Agents

Lantus, Basaglar KwikPen, Toujeo Max SoloSTAR, Toujeo SoloSTAR	insulin glargine	(**in**-su-lin **glar**-jeen)
Levemir	insulin detemir	(**in**-su-lin **de**-te-mir)

Oral Antidiabetic Agents to Treat Type 2 Diabetes Mellitus (T2DM)

Biguanides

Glucophage, Fortamet, Glucophage XR	metformin	(met-**four**-men)

Alpha-Glucosidase Inhibitors

Glyset	miglitol	(**mig**-li-tol)
Precose	acarbose	(**ay**-car-bose)

Meglitinides

Prandin	repaglinide	(re-**pag**-lih-nide)
Starlix	nateglinide	(na-**teg**-lih-nide)

Sulfonylureas

Amaryl	glimepiride	(gly-**mep**-ir-ide)

Continued

Trade Name	Generic Name	Pronunciation
Glucotrol	glipizide	(**glip**-eh-zyed)
Micronase,ª DiaBeta,ª Glynase PresTab	glyburide	(**glye**-burr-eyed)
Thiazolidinedione		
Actos	pioglitazone	(pye-oh-**glit**-uh-zone)
DPP-4 Inhibitors		
Januvia	sitagliptin	(**sih**-tuh-**glip**-tin)
Nesina	alogliptin	(**al**-oh-**glip**-tin)
Onglyza	saxagliptin	(**sax**-a-**glip**-tin)
Tradjenta	linagliptin	(**lin**-a-**glip**-tin)
Incretin Mimetics		
Bydureon (discontinued)	exenatide suspension (discontinued)	(ex-**en**-a-tide)
Bydureon BCise	exenatide auto-injector	(ex-**en**-a-tide)
Byetta	exenatide	(ex-**en**-a-tide)
Ozempic	semaglutide (injection)	(**sem**-a-**gloo**-tide)
Rybelsus	semaglutide (oral)	(**sem**-a-**gloo**-tide)
Victoza, Saxenda	liraglutide	(**lir**-a-**gloo**-tide)
Glucagon-Like Peptide 1 Receptor Agonist/Glucose-Dependent Insulinotropic Polypeptide Combo		
Mounjaro	tirzepatide (injection)	(ter-**zep**-a-tide)
SGLT-2 Inhibitors		
Farxiga	dapagliflozin	(dap-a-**glif**-loh-zin)
Invokana	canagliflozin	(kan-uh-**glif**-loh-zin)
Jardiance	empagliflozin	(em-pa-**glif**-loh-zin)

ªBrand discontinued; now available only as generic.

The endocrine system produces and secretes **hormones** from various glands. The Greek word *hormon* means "that which sets in motion." Hormones activate specific target cells and organs to elicit a response. The body produces different hormone types in different glands. **Endocrinologists** are physicians who specialize in the study of glands and hormones. In this chapter, we discuss the location and function of the body's major glands and hormones. We will discuss major conditions affecting the endocrine system, along with the medications used to treat them. All medication dosages listed are based on adult dosage unless otherwise stated.

Anatomy of the Endocrine System

Fig. 18.1 illustrates the major endocrine glands. As shown in the illustration, three glands are located in the head: the pituitary gland, hypothalamus, and pineal gland. The pituitary gland produces hormones that affect other glands and specific organs and regulates the thyroid gland, adrenal cortex, and gonads (ovaries and testes). The hypothalamus, located above the pituitary gland, secretes hormones that regulate hormone secretion by the pituitary gland. The pineal gland, located behind and below the hypothalamus, partially controls circadian rhythms, sleep-wake patterns, and other body functions, primarily through the production of melatonin, a hormone.

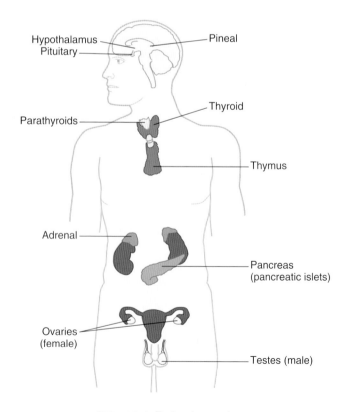

FIG. 18.1 Endocrine anatomy.

At the base of the neck, the thyroid gland produces three hormones that affect metabolism: **thyroxine (T_4), triiodothyronine (T_3),** and **calcitonin.** The parathyroid glands, positioned slightly behind and above the thyroid gland, secrete a hormone called parathyroid hormone (PTH), which helps maintain adequate calcium levels. Located lower in the chest is the thymus, which secretes hormones that play an essential role in the immune system. The two adrenal glands are in the abdominal area, one gland positioned above each kidney. The adrenal glands secrete specific hormones (epinephrine and norepinephrine) linked to the stress responses of the body.

The largest endocrine gland is the **pancreas** and is responsible for producing and secreting hormones from groupings of cells. These "islets of Langerhans" contain alpha cells that produce glucagon and beta cells that produce insulin. Gonads produce sex hormones. In women, the ovaries secrete hormones such as estrogen and progesterone, and in men the primary hormone secreted from the testes is testosterone. A detailed discussion of sex hormones is presented in Chapter 24.

Description of Hormones and Glands

Hormones are responsible for many different human functions, including emotions. Hormone action is classified by the distance the hormone travels. Autocrine hormones act on the same cell from which they are secreted; for example, interleukin-2 stimulates T cells (part of the immune system). Endocrine hormones, in contrast, influence cells that are farther away. The endocrine hormones are the focus of this chapter.

Glands have two mechanisms of action, endocrine or exocrine. Hormones produced by **endocrine glands** either enter the bloodstream to reach their target site or act at target sites near the site of hormone release. Hormones produced by **exocrine glands** are sent to the target organ or tissue via a tube or duct. The sweat glands' duct is an example, secreting outside to the skin's surface. Because of this difference, endocrine glands do not have ducts.

Structure and Function of Hormones

Endocrine system hormones are classified as proteins, steroids, and amines (Fig. 18.2). Proteins include insulin, growth hormone (GH), and calcitonin. Steroids include cortisol and aldosterone from the adrenal cortex, estrogen and progesterone from the ovaries, and testosterone from the testes. The hormones thyroxine, epinephrine, and norepinephrine are examples of amines.

A feedback system maintains hormone levels in a healthy range. The mechanism resembles that of a home thermostat. Hormones can be considered specialized keys that unlock specific doors. When the key enters the lock, a reaction takes place. As the hormone travels through the body, it only reacts with keyholes it fits. **Homeostasis** is disrupted if glands secrete too much or too little hormone; instead, a delicate balance must be maintained to produce the correct response. Accordingly, many hormones are regulated by sensitive "feedback loops" that control the hormone amount produced by any given gland (see the following section, Mechanism of Action). Table 18.1 provides a list of endocrine glands, the hormones they produce, and the general hormone functions. If a gland produces too much or too little hormone, various endocrine conditions may result. Hormones perform many functions, including the following:

- Maintain homeostasis (ie, maintain normal physiologic limits by increasing and decreasing blood glucose levels for energy use)
- Prepare the body for an emergency (ie, instigate the "fight-or-flight" reaction)
- Participate in the development of the reproductive system (ie, cause sexual maturity and reproductive functions such as menstruation and pregnancy)

Mechanism of Action

Receptor sites for hormones are inside and outside of cells. Protein hormones fit into receptor sites outside cells, whereas steroid hormones enter into and attach to receptor sites inside the cell. Both mechanisms cause a reaction. The following three signaling pathways influence the endocrine system and the production of hormones:

1. Negative feedback is the primary regulatory mechanism for maintaining homeostasis. In negative feedback, a stimulus results in actions that reduce the stimulus. Fig. 18.3 provides an example of a negative feedback loop. In this example, an increase in thyroid hormones (T_3 and T_4) above normal levels signals the anterior pituitary gland to reduce the production of thyroid-stimulating

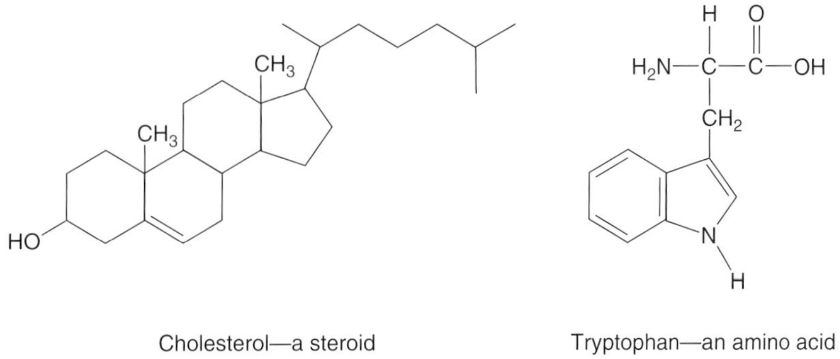

Cholesterol—a steroid

Tryptophan—an amino acid

FIG. 18.2 Structures of a steroid and an amino acid.

Select Endocrine Glands, Hormones, and Their Functions

Hormone	Target Tissue	Function
Adrenal Glands		
Aldosterone	Kidneys	Regulates salt/water balance
Cortisol	Many tissue targets	Regulates metabolism of proteins, fats, and carbohydrates
Epinephrine	Skeletal muscle, heart, blood vessels, liver	Stimulates the sympathetic nervous system
Norepinephrine	Skeletal muscle, heart, blood vessels, liver	Stimulates the sympathetic nervous system
Ovaries		
Estrogens	Many tissue targets	Regulates menstrual cycle; develops and maintains female sex characteristics
Progesterone	Uterus, breast	Stimulates development of the uterine lining
Pancreas		
Glucagon	Liver, adipose (fat) tissue	Increases levels of glucose in the blood
Insulin	Many tissue targets	Facilitates glucose uptake into the tissues, stimulates glycogen production, and stimulates fat storage
Parathyroid Glands		
Parathyroid hormone (PTH)	Bone, kidneys, and digestive tract	Increases calcium levels by stimulating calcium release from bone, stimulating calcium resorption by the kidneys, and increasing calcium absorption from the intestines
Pineal Gland		
Melatonin	Hypothalamus	Influences sleep-wake cycles
Pituitary Gland		
Adrenocorticotropic hormone (ACTH)	Adrenal cortex	Stimulates secretion of adrenocortical hormones
Antidiuretic hormone (ADH)	Kidneys	Stimulates reabsorption of water (conserves water)
Follicle-stimulating hormone (FSH)	Gonads	Stimulates gonad growth and function
Growth hormone (GH)	Many tissue targets	Regulates growth of muscles, bones, and tissues
Luteinizing hormone (LH)	Gonads	Stimulates gonad growth and function
Oxytocin	Uterus and mammary glands	Stimulates uterine contractions during birth and milk ejection into the mammary ducts
Thyroid-stimulating hormone (TSH)	Thyroid gland	Promotes secretion of hormones from the thyroid gland
Testes		
Testosterone	Many tissue targets	Influences sex-related characteristics in males and promotes sperm production
Thyroid Gland		
Calcitonin	Bone	Regulates calcium levels by inhibiting calcium release from bone
Thyroid hormones (T_4 and T_3)	Many tissue targets	Affects metabolism

hormone (TSH). In essence, thyroid hormones can limit their production by this negative feedback mechanism.

2. Positive feedback may also occur; however, in positive feedback, a stimulus results in actions that further increase the stimulus. For example, during labor, specific hormones are released that promote the continued release of more hormones until a result is achieved; contractions result in the birth of a baby.

3. The third response system is via the nervous system. Stressful situations can alter the production and secretion of specific hormones that, when released, prepare the body for the situation. For example, if a person is in

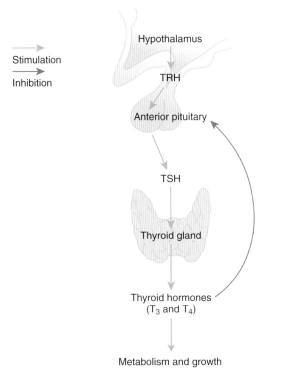

Stimulation

Inhibition

Hypothalamus

TRH

Anterior pituitary

TSH

Thyroid gland

Thyroid hormones
(T_3 and T_4)

Metabolism and growth

FIG. 18.3 Regulation of thyroid hormone secretion by negative feedback. T_3, Triiodothyronine; T_4, thyroxine; *TRH*, thyrotropin-releasing hormone; *TSH,* thyroid-stimulating hormone. (From Solomon EP. *Introduction to Human Anatomy and Physiology.* 3rd ed. St. Louis: Saunders; 2009.)

an emergency, the body requires more energy; therefore hormones such as epinephrine may be released, giving the body an extra boost of energy.

Functions of the Endocrine Glands

Hypothalamus

In the brain, below the thalamus, the hypothalamus is a small organ that links the nervous system to the endocrine system. The hypothalamus stimulates the pituitary gland by neuronal impulses and directly or indirectly regulates most endocrine activity. The hypothalamus plays a crucial role in the regulation of several functions, such as water balance, metabolism of fat and carbohydrates, body temperature, appetite, and emotions. In addition, this organ produces releasing or inhibiting hormones that regulate the anterior pituitary gland. Hormones from the hypothalamus are also sent to the pituitary gland, where they are both stored and secreted.

Pituitary Gland

The pituitary gland is analogous to the control tower of the endocrine system. As noted previously, the pituitary gland is situated close to the hypothalamus. It regulates the release of many hormones from the pituitary gland. As shown in Fig. 18.4, the gland is composed of two portions, the anterior and posterior lobes. Although small, the anterior lobe synthesizes hormones that stimulate many different organs. Table 18.1

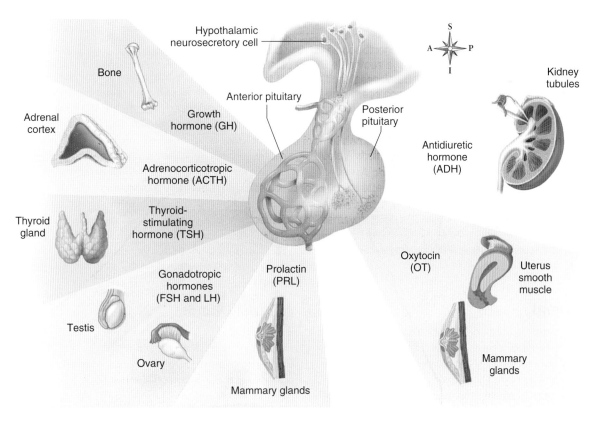

FIG. 18.4 The pituitary gland is suspended from the hypothalamus by a stalk of neural tissue. (From Patton KT, Thibodeau GA. *The Human Body in Health and Disease.* 6th ed. St. Louis: Elsevier; 2014.)

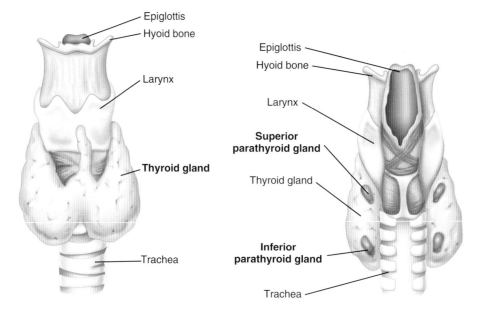

FIG. 18.5 Thyroid and parathyroid glands. (From Thibodeau GA, Patton KT. *Anatomy and Physiology*. 8th ed. St. Louis: Mosby; 2012.)

summarizes the various hormones secreted from the pituitary gland, their target tissues, and their functions. Two hormones, oxytocin and antidiuretic hormone (ADH), are stored in the posterior portion of the pituitary gland. Oxytocin stimulates uterine contractions and cervical dilation during birth and lactation, and ADH (also known as **vasopressin**) affects the kidneys, cardiovascular system, and central nervous system. This entire pituitary system is regulated by negative feedback control from the nervous system (specifically the hypothalamus) and the levels of other hormones.

Pineal Gland

The pineal gland produces and secretes melatonin. Melatonin is a hormone that facilitates sleep onset and influences biological rhythms and the start of sexual maturity. The gland is affected by retinal responses to light, with exposure to light-suppressing melatonin secretion.

> **Tech Note!**
>
> Melatonin is available as an over-the-counter product to help with insomnia.

Thyroid Gland

The thyroid gland is located at the base of the neck (Fig. 18.5). As mentioned previously, this gland is responsible for producing and secreting three hormones: T_4, T_3, and calcitonin. Iodine is necessary for the thyroid gland to synthesize T_4 and T_3; each hormone is named to indicate the number of iodine atoms in its structure. T_4 and T_3 are essential in regulating the rate of metabolism of proteins, fats (lipids), and sugars (carbohydrates) throughout the body; therefore they play an important role in the growth and homeostasis of

the body. Calcitonin plays an active role in the regulation of calcium levels. Calcium is the primary mineral found in bones. Calcium is also vital for the proper functioning of muscle contractions, nerve impulses, and blood clotting. Three different hormones—calcitonin, vitamin D, and PTH—maintain a constant level. The function of calcitonin, specifically, is to inhibit the removal of calcium from bone.

Parathyroid Glands

Located behind the thyroid gland are the parathyroid glands (see Fig. 18.5). The parathyroid organ has two sets of secreting glands. These glands are the primary regulators of calcium levels in the blood through PTH release. PTH increases calcium levels by stimulating calcium release from the bones and by stimulating calcium reabsorption by kidneys. PTH also activates vitamin D to increase the calcium absorbed from the intestine. The parathyroid glands are regulated by the calcium concentration in the blood and bodily fluids (Fig. 18.6). When calcium levels are higher than usual in the blood, it inhibits parathyroid glands and slows PTH release. When calcium levels in the blood fall, however, more PTH is released. In this way, the negative feedback mechanism regulates PTH.

Adrenal Glands

The adrenal glands are located directly on top of each of the two kidneys (Fig. 18.7). Each adrenal gland consists of a central portion, known as the **adrenal medulla,** and an outer region called the **adrenal cortex.** The adrenal glands are essential in helping the body cope with stress (Fig. 18.8). The adrenal medulla synthesizes and secretes the **catecholamines** norepinephrine and epinephrine. These hormones are stored in the adrenal medulla until activated by the sympathetic nervous system (see Chapter 17 for a description of

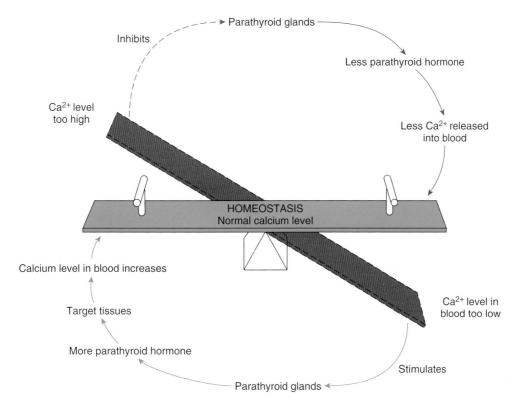

FIG. 18.6 Calcium regulation by negative feedback. (From Solomon EP. *Introduction to Human Anatomy and Physiology*. 3rd ed. St. Louis: Saunders; 2009.)

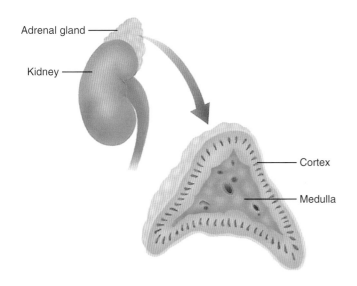

FIG. 18.7 The paired adrenal glands are small, yellow masses of tissues that lie in contact with the upper ends of the kidneys. Each gland consists of a central medulla and an outer cortex. (From Solomon EP. *Introduction to Human Anatomy and Physiology*. 3rd ed. St. Louis: Saunders; 2009.)

the nervous system). For instance, when the body encounters a stressful situation, it prepares itself for fight or flight, depending on the situation, through the sympathetic nervous system. When the sympathetic nervous system activates, the heart rate increases and blood vessels dilate to allow more blood to reach skeletal muscles and to increase blood flow to

the brain. Stored glucose is released into the bloodstream to fuel the body's increased metabolic rate. Approximately 70% to 80% of the released catecholamines are epinephrine, and norepinephrine represents 20% to 30%.

Tech Note!

Norepinephrine is the same substance that neurons in the central nervous system secrete.

The adrenal gland cortex produces three types of hormones: glucocorticoids, mineralocorticoids, and sex hormones (ie, androgens or estrogens). Glucocorticoids, such as cortisol, affect lipid, carbohydrate, and protein metabolism. They increase glucose levels, reduce inflammation, and increase the capacity to cope with stressful situations. Mineralocorticoids are crucial for regulating the body's salt and water balance. The body's principal mineralocorticoid is aldosterone, which maintains sodium and potassium homeostasis by stimulating the kidneys to conserve sodium and excrete potassium. The adrenal cortex also secretes small amounts of both androgens and estrogens in both men and women.

Pancreas

The pancreas is the largest endocrine system organ (Fig. 18.9). It carries out both endocrine and exocrine functions. The pancreatic exocrine function is to secrete digestive

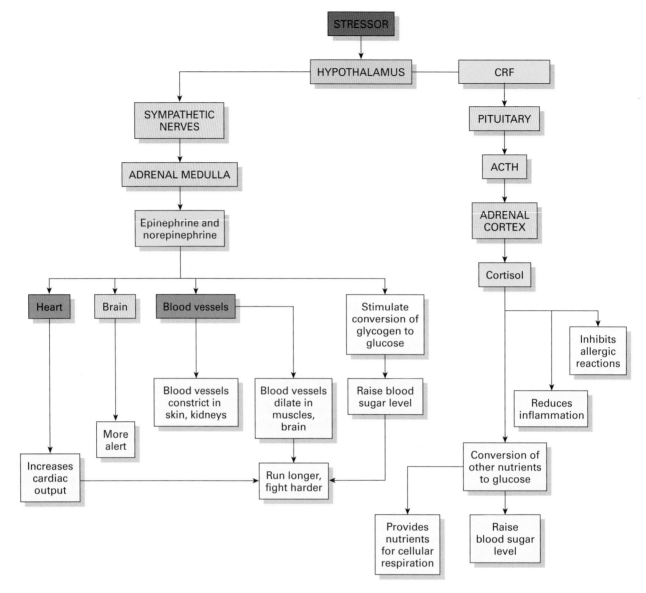

FIG. 18.8 The adrenal medulla and the adrenal cortex both play essential roles in helping the body cope with stress. *ACTH,* Adrenocorticotropic hormone; *CRF,* corticotropin-releasing factor. (From Solomon EP. *Introduction to Human Anatomy and Physiology.* 3rd ed. St. Louis: Saunders; 2009.)

enzymes into the small intestine. The pancreatic endocrine function maintains energy homeostasis throughout the body by regulating blood glucose (sugar) levels. The gland primarily accomplishes this by secreting both glucagon and insulin from cells in the islets of Langerhans. Low blood glucose levels stimulate glucagon secretion. This hormone triggers the liver to release stored glucose. When the blood glucose concentration is high, in contrast, insulin enters the bloodstream. This hormone targets tissues such as the liver, muscle, and adipose tissues to take up glucose from the bloodstream, where it can be used as energy or stored for later use as glycogen. Because glucagon and insulin have opposite actions on blood glucose levels, they work together to maintain glucose homeostasis (Fig. 18.10).

Ovaries

The two female ovaries produce (**oogenesis**) and secrete one or, rarely, two eggs or more (**ovulation**) each month. Located on either side of the uterus (Fig. 18.11), the ovaries sit above the uterus and are close to the fallopian tubes, which connect the two organs. Although ovulation begins at puberty, it is not possible to become pregnant until the menstrual cycle begins. The ability to have children ends as the levels of the responsible hormones (eg, estrogen) decline until the ovarian cycle stops. The ovaries secrete the hormones estrogen and progesterone; the ovaries are the primary source of estrogen in women. The function of estrogen is the development of the breasts and genitals. It also regulates the menstrual cycle, which prepares the female for pregnancy. The anterior

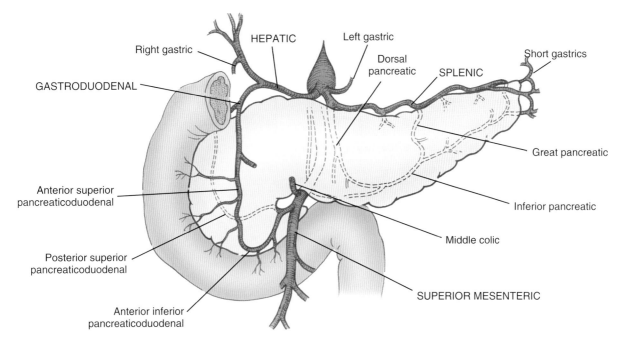

FIG. 18.9 Pancreas. (From Rothrock JC. *Alexander's Care of the Patient in Surgery*. 15th ed. St. Louis: Mosby; 2015.)

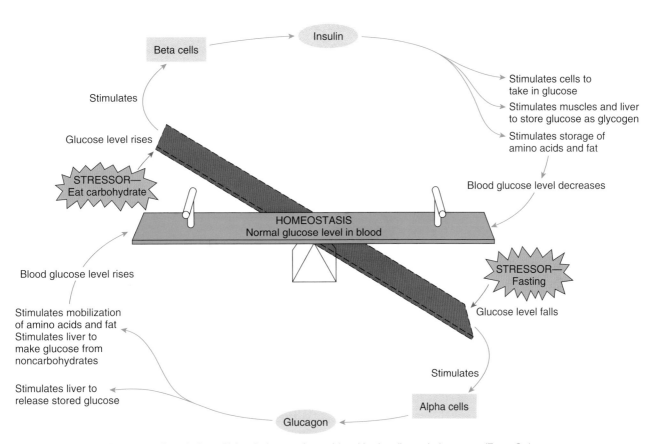

FIG. 18.10 Regulation of blood glucose (sugar) level by insulin and glucagon. (From Solomon EP. *Introduction to Human Anatomy and Physiology*. 3rd ed. St. Louis: Saunders; 2009.)

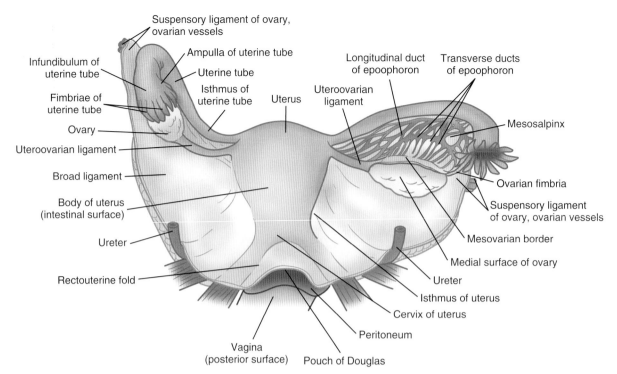

FIG. 18.11 Ovaries. (From Rothrock JC. *Alexander's Care of the Patient in Surgery*. 13th ed. St. Louis: Mosby; 2007.)

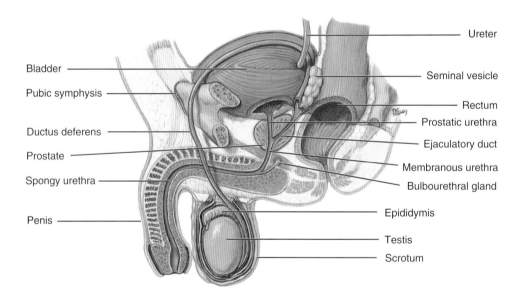

FIG. 18.12 Testes. (From Applegate E. *The Anatomy and Physiology Learning System*. 4th ed. St. Louis: Saunders; 2010.)

pituitary gland releases follicle-stimulating hormone (FSH), which triggers estrogen levels to increase, which in turn causes the secretion of luteinizing hormone (LH), another pituitary hormone. The combination of these two hormones triggers the cascade of events leading to ovulation.

Testes

The testes produce and secrete sperm (spermatogenesis). The testes are in the scrotum (Fig. 18.12). Sperm production begins before the age of puberty and decreases with age, although most men produce sperm throughout their lifetime. FSH is released as puberty begins, causing the stored, immature sperm cells to divide and mature. The production of testosterone in the testes is responsible for the growth of adjacent organs, such as the prostate gland, seminal vesicles, and vas deferens. Testosterone is also responsible for secondary sex characteristics, such as changes in voice pitch as a boy enters puberty and increased muscle development. A detailed discussion of sex hormones and reproductive health is presented in Chapter 24.

Conditions of the Endocrine System and Their Treatments

Many endocrine system conditions result from too much or too little glandular hormone production. Because hormones are critical to the functions of other tissues and organs, diseases of the endocrine system can have a variety of effects throughout the body. Table 18.2 lists select conditions and/or illnesses associated with a defect in the endocrine system. As noted previously, conditions related to reproduction are covered in Chapter 24.

Conditions of the Pituitary Gland and Hypothalamus and Their Treatments

Syndrome of Inappropriate Antidiuretic Hormone Secretion

Syndrome of inappropriate antidiuretic hormone secretion (SIADH) is a disease of the posterior pituitary gland characterized by inappropriately high levels of secretion of ADH (vasopressin). ADH is produced in the hypothalamus and stored in the posterior pituitary gland, and, when needed, it is released into the bloodstream. SIADH is most commonly associated with tumors that secrete ADH, but it also can be due to brain injury or infections. SIADH is associated with increases in total body water secondary to increased water reabsorption by the kidneys, which also leads to hyponatremia (low sodium levels).

◼ TABLE 18.2
Summary of Select Conditions Associated With the Endocrine System

Disease/Condition	Cause	Clinical Conditions/Characteristics
Conditions Associated With the Pituitary Gland		
Syndrome of inappropriate antidiuretic hormone secretion (SIADH)	↑ Antidiuretic hormone (ADH)	• ↑ Total body water • Hyponatremia
Diabetes insipidus	↓ ADH	• Dehydration • Polyuria (frequent urination) • Thirst
Hypersecretion of growth hormone (GH)	↑ GH	• Acromegaly • Gigantism
Hypopituitarism	Absence or deficiency of some or all pituitary hormones	• Panhypopituitarism • Hypopituitary dwarfism
Conditions Associated With the Thyroid Gland		
Hyperthyroidism	↑ Thyroid hormone (TH)	• Goiter • Graves disease
Hypothyroidism	↓ TH	• Cretinism • Myxedema
Conditions Associated With the Parathyroid Glands		
Hyperparathyroidism	↑ Parathyroid hormone (PTH)	• Hypercalcemia
Hypoparathyroidism	↓ PTH	• Hypocalcemia
Conditions Associated With the Adrenal Glands		
Addison disease (primary adrenal insufficiency)	↓ Corticosteroids ↓ Mineralocorticoids ↑ ACTH	• Fatigue • Nausea • Syncope • Weight loss
Cushing disease; Cushing syndrome	↓ Adrenocorticotropic hormone (ACTH)	• Acne • Flushing of the face • Thinning of the hair • Weight gain
Hyperaldosteronism	↑ Aldosterone	• Hypertension • Hypokalemia
Conditions Associated With the Pancreas		
Gestational diabetes	Insulin resistance during pregnancy	• Hyperglycemia
Type 1 diabetes mellitus (T1DM)	Absolute insulin deficiency	• Hyperglycemia
Type 2 diabetes mellitus (T2DM)	Insulin resistance + relative insulin deficiency	• Hyperglycemia

Prognosis

Symptoms typically resolve after treatment and correction of excess fluid and hyponatremia.

Non-drug treatment

Because infections and other underlying conditions can cause the syndrome of inappropriate antidiuretic hormone secretion (SIADH), it is crucial to address the primary reason contributing to its development. With a resolution of hyponatremia, symptoms of hyponatremia can resolve after about 3 days of treatment.

Drug treatment

Emergency treatment of severe hyponatremia with hypertonic saline and fluid restriction is critical. Demeclocycline can be used to treat resistant or chronic SIADH. Demeclocycline works by causing tubules in the kidney to develop resistance to the effects of ADH.

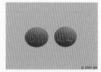

GENERIC NAME: demeclocycline

TRADE NAME: Declomycin[a]

INDICATION: Off-label treatment of syndrome of inappropriate antidiuretic hormone secretion

ROUTE OF ADMINISTRATION: Oral

COMMON ADULT DOSAGE: 600 mg/day given in 2 or 4 divided doses

MECHANISM OF ACTION: Causes the renal tubules to develop resistance to antidiuretic hormone

SIDE EFFECTS: Gastrointestinal upset

AUXILIARY LABEL: Take on an empty stomach with plenty of fluids

[a]Brand discontinued; now available only as generic.

Diabetes Insipidus

Diabetes insipidus is a rare disorder caused by ADH (vasopressin) deficiency. Causes of this condition include brain tumors or infection of the meninges (meningitis) or brain (encephalitis) and hemorrhage in or around the pituitary gland. Kidneys that do not typically respond to the hormone cause the same type of condition and symptoms; this condition is known as *nephrogenic diabetes insipidus.* Symptoms of diabetes insipidus include excessive thirst, frequent urination (polyuria), and dehydration. It is important to note that diabetes insipidus is not the same as diabetes mellitus (DM) (discussed later).

Prognosis

Overall, the prognosis for diabetes insipidus is good, depending on the type and severity. Once controlled, there are no limitations on activity or diet, including the intake of water.

Non-drug treatment

Treatment includes keeping a daily weight record and drinking enough water to prevent dehydration. A person should wear a medical identification bracelet indicating his or her condition and prescribed medications.

Drug treatment

Vasopressin and desmopressin acetate (synthetic forms of antidiuretic hormone [ADH]) are typically prescribed to treat diabetes insipidus. Agents that can stimulate the production of ADH (eg, chlorpropamide) also may be used.

Hypopituitarism

Hypopituitarism (includes panhypopituitarism and dwarfism) involves a range of dysfunctions from the absence of selective pituitary hormones to complete hormone dysfunction. Accordingly, the hypopituitarism signs and symptoms vary and depend on the affected hormones.

Partial or total failure of all anterior pituitary hormone (corticotropin, TSH, LH, FSH, GH, and prolactin) secretion in addition to the posterior pituitary hormone ADH characterizes panhypopituitarism. Partial hypopituitarism and complete hypopituitarism occur in both adults and children. Pediatric GH deficiency may result in hypoglycemia and short stature, resulting in **hypopituitary dwarfism.** Corticotropin deficiency affects normal protein, carbohydrate, and lipid metabolism, resulting in **hypoglycemia,** fatigue, progressive emaciation (weight loss), and death.

Treatments include the following:
- Partial or total hypophysectomy (surgery)
- Radiation treatments
- Chemical agents

Signs and symptoms develop slowly and vary depending on the condition's severity. In adults, impotence, infertility, decreased libido, diabetes insipidus, hypothyroidism, and adrenocortical insufficiency may follow. An interruption in growth or puberty onset may happen in children. Dwarfism is not apparent at birth but appears during the first 3 to 6 months.

Prognosis

The prognosis for hypopituitarism in children is good with early diagnosis and treatment. Symptoms may be controlled or stopped.

Non-drug treatment

A tumor may require surgery, although the patient may still need lifelong medication.

Drug treatment

Treatment of pituitary hypofunction is directed at the underlying cause and hormone replacement. The child's age determines the hormones involved in replacement therapy. In adrenocorticotropic hormone deficiency, the prescriber may use hydrocortisone or prednisone. With thyroid-stimulating hormone deficiency, she may prescribe L-thyroxine. Dosing depends on the patient's age. For gonadotropin deficiency, steroid replacement therapy begins at puberty. Growth hormone replacement therapy may be prescribed in childhood through puberty.

Irregular Secretion of Growth Hormone

Gigantism and acromegaly are two rare, progressive conditions that involve increased GH levels. Tumors can cause pituitary gland hyperfunction. In children, this is called **gigantism.** The bones elongate, resulting in heights as high as almost 9 feet. If the condition arises after puberty, it is called **acromegaly.** Symptoms involve increased head, tongue, nose, hands, foot, and toe size (Fig. 18.13).

Prognosis

Patients with gigantism often have cardiovascular and respiratory complications, are susceptible to diabetes mellitus, and have increased colon cancer risk.

Non-drug treatment

Treatment may involve tumor or growth removal that is causing excessive growth hormone (GH) secretion, although bone growth preceding removal is irreversible. Radiation therapy is another option.

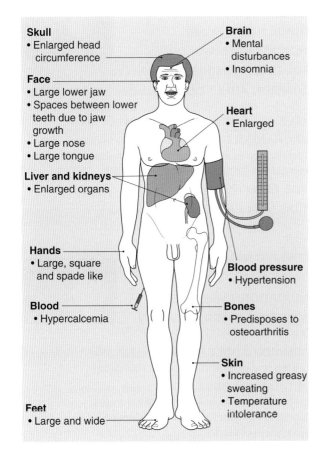

Skull
• Enlarged head circumference

Face
• Large lower jaw
• Spaces between lower teeth due to jaw growth
• Large nose
• Large tongue

Liver and kidneys
• Enlarged organs

Hands
• Large, square and spade like

Blood
• Hypercalcemia

Feet
• Large and wide

Brain
• Mental disturbances
• Insomnia

Heart
• Enlarged

Blood pressure
• Hypertension

Bones
• Predisposes to osteoarthritis

Skin
• Increased greasy sweating
• Temperature intolerance

FIG. 18.13 Features of acromegaly. (From Fishback JL. *Pathology*. 3rd ed. Philadelphia: Mosby; 2005.)

Drug treatment

The treatment goal includes shrinking the pituitary mass, restoring secretory patterns and serum levels to normal, and retaining normal pituitary secretion of other hormones to prevent a recurrence. Currently, octreotide, a somatostatin analog, is the most common pharmacological treatment for GH excess in children and adults. Other agents (eg, lanreotide, pegvisomant, bromocriptine, and cabergoline) may also treat gigantism and acromegaly.

GENERIC NAME: octreotide

TRADE NAME: Sandostatin

INDICATION: Acromegaly

ROUTE OF ADMINISTRATION: Subcutaneous injection

COMMON ADULT DOSAGE: *Initial:* 50 mcg three times daily; most common effective dose is 100–500 mcg three times daily

MECHANISM OF ACTION: Acts as a somatostatin analog to reduce the secretion of pituitary hormones, including growth hormone

SIDE EFFECTS: Gastrointestinal upset, injection site reactions

AUXILIARY LABEL: Administer subcutaneously

In contrast to gigantism, **dwarfism** comes from diminished GH stimulation or production. These patients have short stature and decreased organ size relative to an average adult. There are multiple types and causes of dwarfism, but the primary treatment usually involves somatropin (Humatrope), a once-daily subcutaneous injection that acts like GH in the body. Often, patients continue this therapy even after puberty to maintain a steady GH amount.

GENERIC NAME: somatropin

TRADE NAME: Humatrope

INDICATION: Growth hormone deficiency

ROUTE OF ADMINISTRATION: Subcutaneous injection

COMMON ADULT DOSAGE: Varies depending on weight and severity of disease; max of 0.0125 mg/kg/day

MECHANISM OF ACTION: Acts directly on growth hormone receptors to increase tissue growth, bone growth, and metabolism

SIDE EFFECTS: Edema, injection site reactions, arthralgia, hypothyroidism

AUXILIARY LABEL: Administer subcutaneously

Conditions of the Thyroid Gland and Their Treatment

Hyperthyroidism

Thyrotoxicosis results from increased thyroid hormones. **Hyperthyroidism** is a specific form of thyrotoxicosis secondary to thyroid gland hormone oversecretion. Common diseases that cause hyperthyroidism include Graves disease and toxic multinodular goiter. **Graves disease** is the most common hyperthyroidism cause. It is an autoimmune disorder. The body manufactures antibodies to TSH receptors, leading to an increase in the production of T_4 and T_3. The most common Graves disease symptoms include diffuse thyroid enlargement (goiter); inflammation; ocular orbital tissue enlargement, causing the eyes to bulge, a condition known as **exophthalmos;** and thickening of the skin over the lower legs (Fig. 18.14). Graves disease appears more frequently in women. It happens in less than 1% of the population in the United States.

A **goiter** makes the neck appear enlarged. A nonmalignant tumor or nodules in or on the thyroid gland from excess thyroid hormone production form the root cause (see Fig. 18.14). Goiters are painless. They range in size from barely discernible to grapefruit size. Prescribers usually do not treat small goiters because many resolve on their own. If the goiter continues to grow, medications are an option. Surgery often only happens with medication treatment failure.

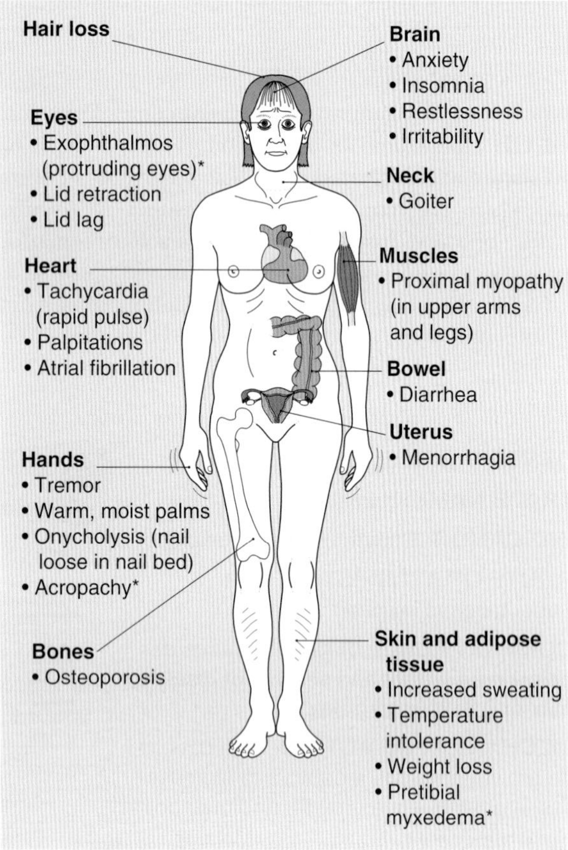

Viruses are another potential hyperthyroidism cause, with the excessive amounts of T_3 and T_4 disappearing after the infection resolves. Hyperthyroidism has various causes but similar symptoms.

Prognosis

Treatments are available for all common hyperthyroidism types; thus the outlook is good.

Non-drug treatment

With tumors, treatment can include surgery or radiation and can destroy part of the thyroid gland.

Drug treatment

For Graves disease, initial therapy with a beta-blocker can ameliorate some hyperthyroidism symptoms, such as palpitations, increased heart rate (tachycardia), tremors, anxiety, and heat intolerance. Antithyroid agents, such as methimazole and propylthiouracil (PTU), can interfere with the thyroid gland's ability to produce hormone. In the United States the most common treatment is radioactive iodine, which destroys thyroid gland cells. Remember that radioactive iodine to destroy the thyroid gland will result in hypothyroidism that requires thyroid supplementation.

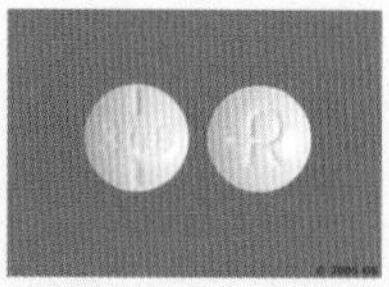

FIG. 18.14 Features of thyrotoxicosis. *Triad found in a patient with Graves disease. (From Fishback JL. *Pathology*. 3rd ed. Philadelphia: Mosby; 2005.)

GENERIC NAME: propylthiouracil (PTU)

TRADE NAME: None

INDICATION: Hyperthyroidism

ROUTE OF ADMINISTRATION: Oral

COMMON ADULT DOSAGE: *Initial:* 300–400 mg/day in divided doses (initial dosage); *maintenance:* 100–150 mg/day in 3 divided doses

MECHANISM OF ACTION: Directly interferes with the first step in thyroid hormone synthesis, leading to a decrease in thyroid hormone production

SIDE EFFECTS: Nausea, headache, urticarial rash

AUXILIARY LABEL: Take as directed

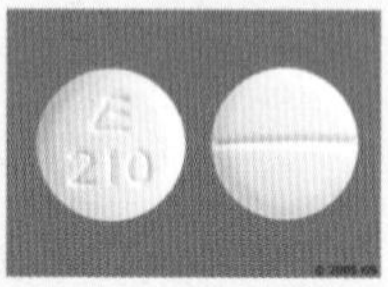

GENERIC NAME: methimazole

TRADE NAME: Tapazole

INDICATION: Hyperthyroidism

ROUTE OF ADMINISTRATION: Oral

COMMON ADULT DOSAGE: *Initial:* 15–60 mg/day in divided doses; *maintenance:* 5–15 mg/day

MECHANISM OF ACTION: Directly interferes with the first step in thyroid hormone synthesis, leading to a decrease in thyroid hormone production

SIDE EFFECTS: Fever, rash, itching

AUXILIARY LABEL: Take as directed

Hypothyroidism

When the thyroid gland does not secrete sufficient levels of T_3 and T_4, a condition called *hypothyroidism* develops. Primary hypothyroidism may be caused by congenital defects, defective thyroid hormone production, and thyroid tissue loss after surgical or radioactive treatment for hyperthyroidism. Hypothyroidism resulting from a congenital deficiency, or *thyroid dysgenesis*, affects the growth and nervous system development of the child's body. If discovered late, this condition will stunt the child's growth (dwarfism) and may produce **cretinism.** Once diagnosed, lifelong thyroid medication therapy is initiated. Any previous mental damage is irreversible.

A lack of dietary iodine can cause a thyroid hormone production deficiency as iodine is a necessary component in the synthesis of T_3 and T_4. Hypothyroidism caused by iodine deficiency is uncommon in developed nations because salt contains added iodine. Therefore patients with hypothyroidism rarely need iodine supplementation. Thyroid gland inflammation, also known as *thyroiditis,* is an autoimmune condition. Thyroiditis happens in about 1 in 20 women after childbirth. This thyroid problem causes little, if any, gland enlargement. Instead, it is usually temporary and resolves within a few months. Later, however, the thyroid gland may not produce enough hormones, resulting in chronic hypothyroidism.

Hypothyroidism is common, and women over 35 are most commonly affected. Symptoms include increased sensitivity to cold, brittle fingernails, constipation, unexplained weight gain, and other issues (Fig. 18.15). Hypothyroidism results in overall energy decrease and a lack of mental alertness. It can also be associated with **myxedema.** Symptoms include skin that appears puffy and waxy. The patient may have dramatic mental status changes with a severe condition such as myxedema coma (Fig. 18.16).

Prognosis

Without treatment, hypothyroidism symptoms may progress, although the condition is not usually life-threatening. When treated appropriately, patients do quite well.

Non-drug treatment

Hypothyroidism caused by tumors benefits from surgical tumor removal. In thyroiditis, surgery may be necessary to remove all or part of the thyroid gland.

Drug treatment

Most patients with hypothyroidism do not have tumors and do well with hormone replacement therapy. Thyroid hormone replacement is lifelong with a daily dose, usually of levothyroxine, thyroid hormone, T_4. Levothyroxine has specific administration instructions because it has many drug interactions. Patients should take levothyroxine with a full glass of water each morning on an empty stomach, waiting 30 minutes before taking any other medications.

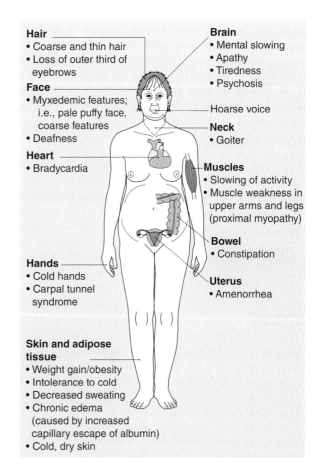

FIG. 18.15 Features of hypothyroidism in the adult. (From Fishback JL. *Pathology*. 3rd ed. Philadelphia: Mosby; 2005.)

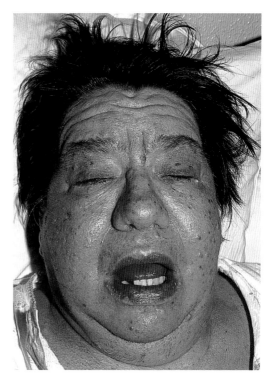

FIG. 18.16 Myxedema. (From Bolognia: Dermatology, ed 2, 2008, Mosby.)

GENERIC NAME: desiccated thyroid (combined T$_4$–T$_3$ product)

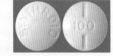

TRADE NAMES: Armour Thyroid

INDICATIONS: Hypothyroidism, goiter

ROUTE OF ADMINISTRATION: Oral

COMMON ADULT DOSAGE: *Initial:* 30 mg/day up to 180 mg/day; *maintenance:* 60–120 mg once daily

MECHANISM OF ACTION: Supplements missing thyroid hormone to normal (euthyroid) levels

SIDE EFFECTS: No significant side effects if the correct dosage is taken

AUXILIARY LABELS:
- Take as directed
- Take with water on an empty stomach

GENERIC NAME: levothyroxine sodium (T$_4$)

TRADE NAMES: Synthroid, Levothroid,[a] Levoxyl, Tirosint, Unithroid

INDICATION: Hypothyroidism

ROUTE OF ADMINISTRATION: Oral

COMMON ADULT DOSAGE: 50–200 mcg once daily

MECHANISM OF ACTION: Supplements missing thyroid hormone to normal (euthyroid) levels

SIDE EFFECTS: No significant effects if the correct dosage is taken

AUXILIARY LABELS:
- Take as directed
- Take with water on an empty stomach

[a]Brand discontinued; now available only as generic.

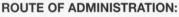

GENERIC NAME: liothyronine sodium (T$_3$)

TRADE NAMES: Cytomel, Triostat

INDICATION: Hypothyroidism

ROUTE OF ADMINISTRATION: Oral

COMMON ADULT DOSAGE: 25–75 mcg once daily

MECHANISM OF ACTION: Supplements missing thyroid hormone to normal (euthyroid) levels

SIDE EFFECTS: No significant effects if the correct dosage is taken

AUXILIARY LABELS:
- Take as directed
- Take with water on an empty stomach

█ Tech Note!

Liothyronine (T$_3$) is sometimes used off-label to augment antidepressant therapy in patients who have not had an adequate response to antidepressant therapy.

Conditions of the Parathyroid Glands and Their Treatment

Hyperparathyroidism

Hyperparathyroidism stems from increased PTH secretion in the bloodstream and can come from one or more of the four parathyroid glands, generally the result of a benign tumor. Another related condition is secondary hyperparathyroidism, in which parathyroid glands compensate for chronic **hypocalcemia** (low blood calcium) resulting from renal failure or poor calcium absorption. These two hyperparathyroidism forms both display increased calcium levels. The increased PTH levels promote calcium release from bones into the bloodstream leading to bone weakening and an increased fracture incidence. In addition, elevated blood calcium levels cause calcium salt buildup in the kidneys, sometimes causing kidney stones. Other hypercalcemia effects include muscle weakness, lethargy, and heart conduction changes.

Prognosis

The hyperparathyroidism prognosis depends on timely diagnosis. In some cases, after removing all or part of the affected gland, functioning may return to normal. Other patients may need to monitor their calcium intake for life. For those with renal failure, continuous dialysis may be necessary until the patient receives a kidney transplant.

Non-drug treatment

Treatment depends on the underlying cause. If hyperparathyroidism is due to a tumor, surgical removal may be necessary. In addition, the removal of several parathyroid glands may be needed. If improper kidney function is the cause, transplantation or dialysis may be required to limit the disease process. Other treatments may include reducing calcium levels by increasing fluid intake and/or restricting dietary calcium intake.

Drug treatment

Hyperparathyroidism has many medication options, although some are unlabeled uses. Osteoporosis medications have been used for hyperparathyroidism, such as the bisphosphonates, raloxifene, and estrogen/progestin therapy (a detailed discussion of these agents is in Chapter 19). Other medications, such as the calcimimetics and vitamin D analogs, suppress parathyroid hormone (PTH) or counteract hyperparathyroidism effects at the PTH receptor.

GENERIC NAME: calcitriol

TRADE NAMES: Calcijex,ᵃ Rocaltrol

INDICATIONS: Hyperparathyroidism, hypocalcemia

ROUTES OF ADMINISTRATION: Oral; intravenous (IV)

COMMON ADULT DOSAGES: *Oral:* 0.25–1 mcg daily; *IV:* 1–2 mcg three times weekly

MECHANISM OF ACTION: Calcitriol is another name for the active form of vitamin D, which is vital in maintaining calcium balance and regulating parathyroid hormone levels

SIDE EFFECTS: Hypercalcemia

AUXILIARY LABEL: Protect from light

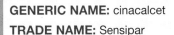

ᵃBrand discontinued; now available only as generic.

GENERIC NAME: doxercalciferol

TRADE NAME: Hectorol

INDICATIONS: Hyperparathyroidism

ROUTES OF ADMINISTRATION: Oral; intravenous

COMMON ADULT DOSAGE: *Oral:* 1–3.5 mcg daily

MECHANISM OF ACTION: Doxercalciferol is metabolized in the liver to active vitamin D, which is essential in maintaining calcium balance and regulating parathyroid hormone levels

SIDE EFFECTS: Hypercalcemia

AUXILIARY LABEL: Take with or without food

GENERIC NAME: paricalcitol

TRADE NAME: Zemplar

INDICATION: Hyperparathyroidism

ROUTES OF ADMINISTRATION: Oral; intravenous

COMMON ADULT DOSAGES: *Oral:* 1–2 mcg/day or 2–4 mcg three times per week

MECHANISM OF ACTION: Inhibits parathyroid hormone secretion

SIDE EFFECTS: Hypercalcemia

AUXILIARY LABEL: Take with or without food

GENERIC NAME: cinacalcet

TRADE NAME: Sensipar

INDICATIONS: Hyperparathyroidism, hypercalcemia

ROUTE OF ADMINISTRATION: Oral

COMMON ADULT DOSAGE: 30–180 mg/day in divided doses

MECHANISM OF ACTION: Mimics calcium at calcium-sensing receptors on the parathyroid gland, leading to a reduction in parathyroid hormone secretion

SIDE EFFECTS: Gastrointestinal symptoms

AUXILIARY LABEL: Take with food

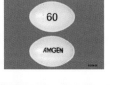

Hypoparathyroidism

Parathyroid gland malfunctioning can cause hypoparathyroidism. Hypoparathyroidism is often due to damage to the parathyroid glands during thyroid surgery. The result is hypocalcemia, which, in turn, reduces vitamin D levels. Symptoms include muscle spasms, irregular heart contractions, and alteration of normal nerve conduction.

Prognosis

The prognosis for hypoparathyroidism is good with long-term replacement therapy.

Non-drug treatment

The only non-drug treatment for hypoparathyroidism is supplemental medication administration with calcium and vitamin D.

Drug treatment

Treatment is directed at correcting hypocalcemia. Acute treatment can involve **parenteral** administration of calcium, with long-term treatment involving calcium and vitamin D supplements. Chapter 19 presents a detailed discussion of calcium and vitamin D supplements.

Conditions of the Adrenal Glands and Their Treatment

Each adrenal gland has two parts, a cortex and medulla. Adrenal cortex disorders range from steroid overproduction to underproduction. The three steroid types produced include mineralocorticoids, glucocorticoids, and sex steroids. A decrease in steroid secretion affects sodium, potassium, and chloride levels and can alter carbohydrate metabolism or cause sexual problems (discussed in Chapter 24).

Cushing Disease

Cushing disease is a condition of excessive ACTH secretion from the anterior pituitary gland. It is more common in

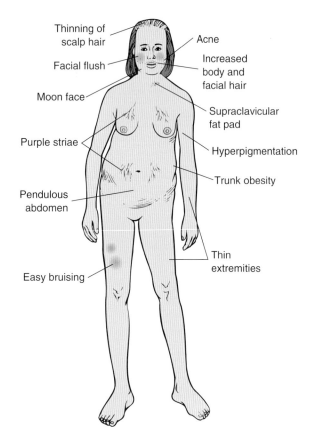

Thinning of
scalp hair

Acne

Facial flush

Increased
body and
facial hair

Moon face

Supraclavicular
fat pad

Purple striae

Hyperpigmentation

Trunk obesity

Pendulous
abdomen

Thin
extremities

Easy bruising

FIG. 18.17 Symptoms of Cushing disease. (From McCance KL, Huether SE. *Pathophysiology: The Biological Basis for Disease in Adults and Children*. 7th ed. St. Louis: Elsevier; 2014.)

adults, is two to three times more common in women, and is an uncommon disorder of too much cortisol, regardless of cause. Cushing syndrome is the most common complication of Cushing disease. As cortisol releases from the adrenal glands, symptoms develop that can include weight gain, facial flushing, thinning hair, and acne (Fig. 18.17). Other symptoms include overall weakness, fatigue, and slow-healing injuries.

In approximately 70% of Cushing syndrome cases, the cause is corticotropin overproduction. Three causes associated with excess corticotropin production include corticotropin hypersecretion from pituitary glands, the presence of a corticotropin-releasing tumor in another organ, or overmedication with corticosteroids (eg, transplant recipients, people with rheumatoid arthritis, and individuals with severe asthma who must take corticosteroids as part of their treatment).

Prognosis

After the removal of a nonmalignant tumor, patients with Cushing disease have a good prognosis. For patients taking corticosteroids for inflammatory conditions, the disadvantages must be weighed against treatment benefits.

Non-drug treatment

Adrenal gland tumors that cause Cushing syndrome also require surgery. After tumor excision, medication

may be necessary. Patients with Cushing disease require either surgical tumor removal or radiation therapy.

Drug treatment

If the condition continues after surgery, patients with Cushing syndrome may require drug therapy (eg, mitotane or metyrapone) that reduces cortisol levels.

Hyperaldosteronism

Hyperaldosteronism is an issue of excessive **aldosterone** secretion by the adrenal glands. Aldosterone promotes the excretion of potassium and the retention of sodium and water. Hyperaldosteronism can be primary or secondary. Primary hyperaldosteronism is due to an adrenal cortex abnormality, whereas secondary hyperaldosteronism is caused by a stimulus outside the adrenal glands. **Hypertension** (high blood pressure) and **hypokalemia** (low blood potassium) are the primary hyperaldosteronism hallmarks.

Prognosis

The prognosis for hyperaldosteronism is good after the identification and treatment of the underlying cause and management of hypertension and hypokalemia.

Non-drug treatment

If an aldosterone-secreting tumor is present, surgical removal is required.

Drug treatment

Drug therapy for hypertension management and the use of potassium supplements to rectify any existing hypokalemia are required.

Addison Disease

Addison disease, which is associated with inadequate corticosteroid and mineralocorticoid synthesis and elevated serum ACTH, is a rare hormonal disorder caused by cortisol deficiency. In approximately 70% of patients with Addison disease, the autoimmune disease causes adrenal cortex dysfunction. Symptoms begin gradually and include fatigue, weight loss, nausea, and syncope (fainting).

Prognosis

Depending on the cause of Addison disease, it is possible to correct the cortisol levels, although the replacement therapy must be taken for the patient's lifetime. If left untreated, Addison disease can be life-threatening.

Non-drug treatment

Surgery may be indicated for tumor removal. In addition, the patient may need to balance both potassium and sodium intake in the daily diet. Monitoring daily weight and recording daily intake and output of fluids also may be required.

Drug treatment

Treatment consists of replacement therapy with oral glucocorticoids and mineralocorticoids.

Tech Note!

Long-term corticosteroid treatment can lead to hyperglycemia and the development of type 2 diabetes mellitus.

Mineralocorticoid

GENERIC NAME: fludrocortisone acetate

INDICATION: Addison disease

ROUTE OF ADMINISTRATION: Oral

COMMON ADULT DOSAGE: *Initial:* 0.1 mg/day, 0.1 mg three times weekly, or 0.2 mg/day

MECHANISM OF ACTION: Mimics the actions of aldosterone

SIDE EFFECTS: Gastrointestinal (GI) upset, edema, hypertension

AUXILIARY LABEL: Take with food to minimize GI upset

Glucocorticoids

GENERIC NAME: hydrocortisone

TRADE NAME: Cortef

INDICATIONS: Addison disease, inflammation

ROUTE OF ADMINISTRATION: Oral

COMMON ADULT DOSAGE: *Addison disease:* 25–30 mg/day in divided doses. *Corticosteroid responsive conditions:* 20–240 mg/day in divided doses.

MECHANISMS OF ACTION: Antiinflammatory, antipruritic, and vasoconstrictive effects

SIDE EFFECTS: Gastrointestinal upset, hyperglycemia, increased risk for fracture

AUXILIARY LABEL: Take with food

SPECIAL NOTE: Additional dosage forms include the following injectables: hydrocortisone acetate and hydrocortisone sodium succinate (eg, A-Hydrocort, Solu-Cortef). Dosages vary depending on the condition treated and the individual's response.

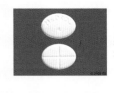

GENERIC NAME: methylprednisolone

TRADE NAME: Medrol

INDICATIONS: Inflammation, Addison disease

ROUTE OF ADMINISTRATION: Oral

COMMON ADULT DOSAGE: 4–48 mg/day in divided doses

MECHANISMS OF ACTION: Antiinflammatory, antipruritic, and vasoconstrictive effects

SIDE EFFECTS: Gastrointestinal upset, hyperglycemia, increased risk for fracture

AUXILIARY LABEL: Take with food

SPECIAL NOTE: Methylprednisolone dose packs are available in 21-tablet sets and are commonly dispensed to slowly taper the patient off the medication or to a maintenance level of continued medication

---

GENERIC NAME: methylprednisolone sodium succinate

TRADE NAME: Solu-Medrol

INDICATIONS: Addison disease, inflammation

ROUTES OF ADMINISTRATION: Intramuscular (IM); intravenous (IV)

COMMON ADULT DOSAGE: *IM or IV:* 10–250 mg every 4–6 hours for up to 48 hours

MECHANISMS OF ACTION: Antiinflammatory, antipruritic, and vasoconstrictive effects

SIDE EFFECTS: Gastrointestinal upset, hyperglycemia, osteoporosis, cataracts, Cushing syndrome

---

GENERIC NAME: prednisolone

INDICATIONS: Addison disease, inflammation

ROUTE OF ADMINISTRATION: Oral

COMMON ADULT DOSAGE: 5–60 mg once daily

MECHANISMS OF ACTION: Antiinflammatory, antipruritic, and vasoconstrictive effects

SIDE EFFECTS: Gastrointestinal upset, hyperglycemia, osteoporosis, cataracts, Cushing syndrome

AUXILIARY LABEL: Take with food

SPECIAL NOTE: Syrup must be measured in calibrated dose cup, oral syringe, or measuring spoon

GENERIC NAME: prednisone

INDICATIONS: Addison disease, inflammation

ROUTE OF ADMINISTRATION: Oral

COMMON ADULT DOSAGES: 5–60 mg/day

MECHANISMS OF ACTION: Antiinflammatory, antipruritic, and vasoconstrictive effects

SIDE EFFECTS: Gastrointestinal upset, hyperglycemia, osteoporosis, cataracts, Cushing syndrome

AUXILIARY LABEL: Take with food

Conditions Affecting the Adrenal Medulla

Most adrenal medulla conditions result from tumor growth. The primary tumor types that affect the adrenal medulla are pheochromocytomas. Pheochromocytomas continually secrete catecholamines, which can result in hypertension. With surgical removal, hypertension resolves, and the patient's prognosis is generally good. Medical therapy typically stabilizes the blood pressure before, during, and after surgery.

Endocrine Conditions of the Pancreas and Their Treatments

The pancreas is responsible for insulin and glucagon production and release. Insulin is essential in the transportation of glucose into the cell. The cell then uses it for energy or stores it as glycogen. Insulin also stimulates protein synthesis and releases fatty acids from adipose (fat) tissue. The condition associated with **hyperglycemia,** or a blood glucose increase, is known as *diabetes mellitus.*

Diabetes Mellitus

Diabetes mellitus (DM) is a chronic endocrine disease associated with hyperglycemia. The two most common types are **type 1 diabetes mellitus (T1DM)** and **type 2 diabetes mellitus (T2DM).** Estimates show that 26 million of the US population live with DM, 7 million of whom are unaware they have the disease.

Type 1 diabetes mellitus T1DM is caused by the destruction of or a defect in the beta cells of the pancreas. This results in an inability of the pancreas to synthesize and secrete insulin, leading to an absolute insulin deficiency in people with T1DM. Because people with T1DM cannot produce insulin, they must use exogenous insulin. The classic hyperglycemia symptoms that can lead to a T1DM diagnosis include polyuria (frequent urination), polydipsia (excessive thirst), and polyphagia (excessive appetite). Glucose loss by urination can cause dehydration, weight loss, fatigue, and extreme hunger.

Type 2 diabetes mellitus Most patients with diabetes have T2DM. T1DM is an absolute deficiency of insulin, whereas T2DM is due to **insulin resistance,** or a decreased ability of tissues to respond to insulin. Insulin resistance increases with obesity; therefore most patients with T2DM are overweight or obese. T2DM commonly affects adults; however, obesity in children has resulted in more children with T2DM. Because of the T2DM insulin resistance, the pancreatic beta cells have to work harder to produce insulin to compensate for insulin resistance and keep blood sugars normal. Over time, the beta cells begin to fail, and a person with type 2 diabetes produces less insulin. These patients have to take insulin injections to manage their blood sugar.

T2DM is a metabolic disease with several **comorbidities.** Conditions commonly associated with T2DM include the following:

- Obesity
- Lack of physical activity
- Hypertension (high blood pressure)
- History of gestational DM
- Older than age 45 years
- Strong family history of T2DM
- Hyperlipidemia (elevated cholesterol levels)

Gestational diabetes mellitus Gestational diabetes mellitus (GDM) occurs in women during pregnancy, and blood glucose levels usually return to normal after childbirth. GDM is associated only with pregnancy; weight gain and an increase in the estrogen concentrations and placental hormones, which antagonize insulin, are the two precipitating factors. The effects may last only through the pregnancy period, although the condition must be treated through diet and possibly medications. Poor GDM management can lead to pregnancy complications and health problems for the child after birth. Some patients with gestational diabetes will have risk factors to develop T2DM later in life. For more information on gestational diabetes, visit the website *https://www.diabetes.org/diabetes/gestational-diabetes.*

Prognosis

With proper diabetes mellitus (DM) treatment and management, a person can lead a healthy life. Thorough education regarding lifestyle, medications, and monitoring is essential to optimizing treatment outcomes.

People with DM are at risk for many complications. Uncontrolled DM can affect both life quality and longevity. Some complications associated with DM include the following:

- Macrovascular disease (cardiac disease, including risk for heart attack and stroke)
- Erectile dysfunction (impotence)
- **Gastroparesis**
- Increased infections of the skin (feet), urinary tract (UTIs), and vagina (vaginitis)
- Nephropathy (kidney disease)
- **Orthostatic hypotension**
- **Peripheral neuropathy**
- Retinopathy (eye disease)

Non-drug treatment

An important first-line treatment for patients with DM are lifestyle changes, including increased physical activity and a healthy diet. This can help maintain blood glucose levels and lead to weight loss (which may help reduce insulin resistance in people with type 2 diabetes mellitus [T2DM]). Many people with DM can benefit from the help of a dietitian. Daily foot checks are also important to monitor for infection or ulceration.

Drug treatments

A variety of medications are available for DM. For type 1 diabetes mellitus (T1DM), patients require insulin. Synthetic human insulin products produced in laboratories are the primary (and essential) treatment option for T1DM. Most patients with T2DM use oral agents and non-insulin injectables as first-line therapy. If patients cannot tolerate the medicine or blood glucose levels remain elevated, patients will require insulin. Many patients with T2DM ultimately will require insulin therapy, particularly as their disease progresses and their beta cells lose the ability to produce insulin. The main categories of insulin used therapeutically are rapid- and short-acting, intermediate-acting, long-acting, and mixed-acting insulin. These categories describe how fast and how long insulin products work. Table 18.3 provides an overview of available single insulin products, and Table 18.4 lists available premixed insulin products. Insulin products differ in the onset of action (how fast they work) and duration of action (how long they work). Great care should be taken when dispensing insulin products to ensure accurate prescription filling, sufficient counseling, and adequate patient understanding. Many products have similar names and are available in similar doses but with very different onsets and durations of action.

People with T2DM often use oral agents and non-insulin injectable medications to manage blood glucose levels. The list in Table 18.5 provides examples of non-insulin agents that can manage T2DM. Of note, the injectable pramlintide can help T1DM or T2DM. Because many new agents emerge, technicians should stay abreast of the various agents.

Combination agents Because many patients with T2DM require multiple medications, combination products provide an easier path to daily compliance. Table 18.6 provides a list of combination T2DM oral products.

Novel drug agents Two products approved to treat diabetes include insulin glargine (Toujeo) and inhaled insulin (Afrezza). Toujeo consists of long-acting insulin that contains the same active ingredient as Lantus. However, Toujeo is three times as concentrated as Lantus (300 units/mL to 100 units/mL, respectively) and is more effective at controlling blood sugar during sleep. Typically, only small dosage adjustments are necessary when converting from Lantus to Toujeo treatment.

Another insulin therapy product is the inhaled insulin Afrezza. The insulin is the same as that in Humulin, but it is inhaled rather than injected. The US Food and Drug Administration (FDA) approved it in 2014 as an alternative for patients with diabetes who did not want to inject insulin. However, Afrezza has gained little popularity in the US market. Patients must demonstrate their ability to breathe in a full dose through regular lung testing. Smokers and those with COPD are generally not considered for this dosage form. Even with good lung function, the patient must use injectable, long-acting insulin in combination with Afrezza. Patients hoping to avoid daily injections will still have to inject once daily.

Sodium-glucose luminal cotransporter-2 (SGLT-2) inhibitors and glucagon-like peptide-1 (GLP-1) receptor agonists, incretin mimetics, are two newer agent classes for diabetes. Dapa*gliflozin* (Farxiga), empa*gliflozin* (Jardiance), and cana*gliflozin* (Invokana) are examples of oral SGLT-2 inhibitors. At the time of this writing, there is a single oral GLP-1 receptor agonist: semaglutide (Rybelsus). Otherwise, all other GLP-1 receptor agonists are injectables. A first-in-its-class medication, tirzepa*tide* (Mounjaro), acts as both a glucagon-like peptide-1 (GLP-1) receptor agonist and a glucose-dependent insulinotropic polypeptide (GIP) to treat diabetes.

Obesity

In the United States, many people continue to struggle with obesity. The Centers for Disease Control and Prevention (CDC) reports that more than one-third (36.5%) of US adults, or 78 million people, are obese, and nearly 13 million children (16.9%) aged 2 to 13 years are also considered obese *(https://www.cdc.gov/nchs/data/databriefs/db219.pdf)*. Being overweight can increase the risk for major chronic health problems, including high blood pressure, heart disease, stroke, diabetes, and more.

Prognosis

Currently, an obesity diagnosis is based mainly on an individual's **body mass index (BMI).** A person with a BMI of 30 or higher is considered obese. However, BMI readings alone do not correctly reflect a person's health. For example, a bodybuilder with considerable muscle mass may be in great shape but have a BMI over 30 for his or her height. The results also do not translate well with children and teens. Because BMI results can vary widely, it is always best to consult a health care professional to determine a healthy weight target and strategies to reduce body fat safely.

Non-drug treatments

As with diabetes prevention, a healthy diet and active lifestyle are excellent long-term strategies to manage weight. It is especially important to avoid foods high in added sugar, sodium, and saturated fats. A dietitian or nutritionist can be a great resource. Gradually increasing the amount of moderate physical activity per day also helps weight loss. It is best to consult a health care professional before beginning a new routine.

Surgery is considered for the most severe cases of obesity. A surgeon can reduce the stomach size by removing part of the stomach or by tying a gastric band around the stomach to reduce its volume. A smaller stomach volume causes the patient to eat less because a feeling of fullness (satiety) occurs more quickly. These types of surgeries can affect vitamin and nutrient absorption and possibly medication absorption.

TABLE 18.3
Select Available Single-Insulin Products for the Treatment of Diabetes Mellitus

Generic Name	Trade Name	Availability	Onset of Action	Duration of Action
Rapid-Acting Insulin Products				
Insulin lispro	Humalog	• 3- and 10-mL vials	lispro 5–15 min aspart 12–18 min glulisine 12–30 min	lispro 4–6 hours aspart 3–5 hours glulisine 3–4 hours
	Humalog	• 5 (3-mL) cartridges		
	KwikPen	• 5 (3-mL) prefilled pens		
Insulin aspart	NovoLog	• 10-mL vial		
	NovoLog PenFill	• 5 (3-mL) cartridges		
	FlexPen	• 5 (3-mL) prefilled pens		
Insulin glulisine	Apidra	• 10-mL vials		
		• 5 (3-mL) cartridges		
	Apidra SoloSTAR	• 5 (3-mL) prefilled pens		
Short-Acting Insulin Products				
Regular human insulin	Humulin R	• 3- and 10-mL vials	0.5–1 hours	6–10 hours
	Humulin R KwikPen	• 5 (3-mL) prefilled pens		
	Novolin R ReliOn	• 10-mL vial		
Intermediate-Acting Insulin Products				
NPH insulin (Humulin N)	Humulin N Humulin KwikPen	• 3- and 10-mL vials • 5 (3-mL) prefilled pens	1–2 hours	10–16 hours
	Novolin N Novolin N FlexPen ReliOn	• 10-mL vial • 5 (3-mL) prefilled pens		
Long-Acting Insulin Products				
Insulin detemir	Levemir	• 10-mL vial	3–4 hours	14–24 hours
	Levemir FlexPen	• 5 (3-mL) prefilled pens		
Insulin glargine	Lantus	• 10-mL vial • 5 (3-mL) cartridges	2–4 hours	~24 hours
	Lantus SoloSTAR	• 5 (3-mL) prefilled pens		

TABLE 18.4
Select Available Premixed Insulin Products[a]

Generic Name	Trade Name
Insulin lispro protamine + insulin lispro	• Humalog Mix 50/50 • Humalog Mix 50/50 KwikPen • Humalog Mix 75/25 • Humalog Mix 75/25 KwikPen
Insulin aspart prot- amine + insulin aspart	• NovoLog Mix 70/30 • NovoLog Mix 70/30 FlexPen
NPH insulin + regular human insulin	• Humulin 70/30 • Humulin 70/30 Pen • Novolin 70/30

[a]The fractions listed in premixed insulins (eg, 70/30) indicate the ratio of long-acting insulin to rapid- or short-acting insulin.

Drug treatments

Some drug treatments are approved for people diagnosed with obesity who are already exercising and eating a reduced-calorie diet. These drugs are not intended to replace proper diet and exercise. These obesity medications either reduce fat absorption in the intestines (eg, orlistat [Xenical or Alli]) or reduce the feeling of hunger by acting on the hypothalamus, the brain's satiety center. When discussing obesity management with patients with diabetes, the 2020 ADA Guidelines state: When choosing glucose-lowering medications for patients with type 2 diabetes who are overweight or obese, consider a medication's effect on weight. They also write that liraglutide (Victoza) is an FDA-approved medication for weight management that can help with both weight management and blood sugar control.

In 2022, the FDA approved tirzepatide (Mounjaro) for the treatment of type 2 diabetes. However, Mounjaro exhibited weight loss benefits and found an off-label use for patients without diabetes for obesity alone as well. Because

TABLE 18.5

Noninsulin Medications for the Treatment of Diabetes Mellitus

Generic Name	Trade Name	Common Dosage Range	Labeling, Storage, Miscellaneous Information	Common Side Effects
Insulin Sensitizers				
Biguanide				
metformin	Glucophage Riomet	500–2550 mg 1–3 times daily (max 2550 mg/day)	• First-line treatment for T2DM • Take PO with food	• Alterations in taste • Diarrhea • Flatulence • GI upset • Nausea
metformin XR	Glucophage XR	500–2000 mg once daily with an evening meal		
metformin XR	Fortamet	500–2500 mg once daily with the evening meal (max 2500 mg/day)		
metformin XR	Glumetza	500–2000 mg once daily with the evening meal (max 2000 mg/day)		
Thiazolidinedione				
pioglitazone	Actos	15–45 mg once daily (max 45 mg/day)	• Take with or without food	• Fluid retention • Weight gain
Insulin Secretagogues				
Sulfonylureas				
glimepiride	Amaryl	1–8 mg once daily (max 8 mg/day)	• Take PO with first main meals	• GI upset • Hypoglycemia • Weight gain
glipizide	Glucotrol	5–40 mg once or twice daily (max 40 mg/day)		
glipizide XL	Glucotrol XL	5–20 mg once daily (max 20 mg/day)		
glyburide		1.25–20 mg once or twice daily with the first meal of the day (max 20 mg/day)		
micronized glyburide	Glynase PresTab	0.75–12 mg once or twice daily with the first meal of the day (max 12 mg/day)		
Meglitinides				
nateglinide	Starlix	60–120 mg PO 3 times daily before meals (max 360 mg/day)	• Take PO within 30 min of the start of a meal	• Hypoglycemia • Weight gain
repaglinide	Prandin	0.5–4 mg PO 2–4 times daily before meals (max 16 mg/day)		
acarbose	Precose	25–100 mg PO 3 times daily with meals (max 150 mg/day if bodyweight 60 kg; max 300 mg/day if bodyweight >60 kg)	• Take PO with food	• Flatulence • GI upset • Weight loss
miglitol	Glyset	25–100 mg PO 3 times daily with meals (max 300 mg/day)		
Dipeptidyl Peptidase-4 (DPP-4) Inhibitor				
sitagliptin	Januvia	50–100 mg PO once daily (max 100 mg/day)	• Take PO in combination with other oral agents	• GI upset • Headache • Sinusitis
saxagliptin	Onglyza	2.5–5 mg once daily (max 5 mg/day)		
linagliptin	Tradjenta	5 mg daily		
alogliptin	Nesina	25 mg PO once daily		
Sodium-Glucose Cotransporter 2 (SGLT2) Inhibitors				
canagliflozin	Invokana	100–300 mg PO once daily (max 300 mg/day)	• Not recommended if eGFR <45 mL/min per 1.73 m^2	• Genital fungal infections • Increased urination • Orthostasis
dapagliflozin	Farxiga	5–10 mg PO once daily (max 10 mg/day)	• Not recommended if eGFR <60 mL/min per 1.73 m^2	
empagliflozin	Jardiance	10–25 mg PO once daily (max 25 mg/day)	• Not recommended if eGFR 45 mL/min per 1.73 m^2	

Continued

Noninsulin Medications for the Treatment of Diabetes Mellitus—cont'd

Generic Name	Trade Name	Common Dosage Range	Labeling, Storage, Miscellaneous Information	Common Side Effects
Glucagon-Like Peptide 1 Receptor Agonist				
exenatide	Byetta	5–10 mcg subcut twice a day	• Take doses within 1 hour of meals • Take in combination with other oral agents	• Hypoglycemia • Nausea/vomiting • Weight loss
exenatide suspension	Bydureon BCise	2 mg subcut once weekly	• Take once weekly	
liraglutide	Victoza	0.6–1.8 mg subcut daily	• Take once daily without regard to meals	
Semaglutide	Ozempic	0.25–2 mg subcut weekly	• take once weekly	
	Rybelsus	3 mg PO for first 30 days 7–14 mg by mouth once dose established	• oral formulations taken daily	
Glucagon-Like Peptide 1 Receptor Agonist/Glucose-Dependent Insulinotropic Polypeptide Combo				
Tirzepatide	Mounjaro	2.5–15 mg subcut weekly	• take once weekly	
Synthetic Amylin Analog				
pramlintide	Symlin	15–120 mcg subcut immediately before large meals (max 120 mcg/dose)	• Can be used in both T2DM and T1DM • Only for use in patients with DM using meal-time insulin	• GI upset • Hypoglycemia

DM, Diabetes mellitus; *eGFR,* estimated glomerular filtration rate; *GI,* gastrointestinal; *PO,* orally; *subcut,* subcutaneously; *T1DM,* type 1 diabetes mellitus; *T2DM,* type 2 diabetes mellitus.

■ TABLE 18.6

Combination Oral Agents for the Treatment of Type 2 Diabetes Mellitus

Generic Name	Trade Name
alogliptin–metformin	Kazano
alogliptin–pioglitazone	Oseni
glipizide–metformin	Metaglip[a]
glyburide–metformin	Glucovance
linagliptin–metformin	Jentadueto
pioglitazone–glimepiride	Duetact
pioglitazone–metformin	ACTOplus Met, ACTOplus Met XR
repaglinide–metformin	PrandiMet
saxagliptin–metformin	Kombiglyze XR
sitagliptin–metformin	Janumet

[a]Brand discontinued; now available only as generic.

Mounjaro activates both the glucose-dependent insulinotropic polypeptide (GIP) and glucagon-like peptide-1 (GLP-1) receptors, it promotes insulin production from the pancreas and slow gastric emptying. This action increases the time a patient feels satiated after meals. This gastric emptying delay leads to lower calorie intake and weight loss.

GENERIC NAME: orlistat

TRADE NAME: Xenical

INDICATION: Obesity management, used with a reduced-calorie diet

ROUTE OF ADMINISTRATION: Oral

COMMON ADULT DOSAGE: 120 mg three times a day (with each meal)

MECHANISM OF ACTION: Inhibits pancreatic lipases, preventing fat from breaking down and being absorbed in the small intestine

SIDE EFFECTS: Abdominal pain, increased frequency of defecation

AUXILIARY LABELS:
• Take with food
• Do not take with multivitamins

GENERIC NAME: phentermine/topiramate

TRADE NAME: Qsymia

INDICATION: Patients with obesity and at least one weight-related condition (hypertension, diabetes, etc.)

ROUTE OF ADMINISTRATION: Oral

COMMON ADULT DOSAGE: *Initial:* Phentermine 3.75 mg/topiramate 23 mg for 14 days, then phentermine 7.5 mg/topiramate 46 mg once daily for 12 weeks. After 12 weeks, evaluate weight loss. If 3% of body weight has not been lost, can titrate up to phentermine 11.25 mg/topiramate 69 mg daily for 14 days and then to phentermine 15 mg/topiramate 92 mg for 12 weeks

MECHANISM OF ACTION: *Phentermine:* Reduces appetite by increasing the release of catecholamines from the hypothalamus. *Topiramate:* Mechanisms unknown from weight management

SIDE EFFECTS: Constipation, dry mouth, dizziness, seizures

AUXILIARY LABELS:
- Do not discontinue unless directed by your physician
- May cause dizziness/blurred vision
- Do not drink alcohol while on this medication

GENERIC NAME: Tirzepatide

TRADE NAME: Mounjaro

INDICATIONS:
FDA approved: Type 2 diabetes
Off-label: Weight management

ROUTE OF ADMINISTRATION: Subcutaneous injection

COMMON ADULT DOSAGE: Start with 2.5 mg once weekly for 4 weeks. Increase the dose as tolerated every 4 weeks, up to a maximum of 15 mg per week

MECHANISM OF ACTION: GIP and GLP-1 receptor agonists

SIDE EFFECTS: Decreased appetite, diarrhea, nausea, indigestion

AUXILIARY LABEL: For subcutaneous injection only

Tech Note!

Mounjaro currently has no generic equivalent, and the brand-name medicine can be very expensive, even with insurance. Often its off-label use in weight management causes insurance companies to deny claims. They will look to the pharmacy team to help them find solutions.

Blood glucose meters Health professionals ask people with diabetes to monitor their blood glucose levels with a **glucometer** by taking a drop of blood using a small needle called a lancet. Although the finger is the most common location for blood sampling, some meters allow blood to be taken from the forearm, thigh, or fleshy part of the hand (this is known as *alternative site testing*). The blood is placed on a test strip that is inserted into the glucometer. Glucometers digitally display the current blood glucose level. A wide range of blood glucose meters are available, including meters with large font size for people with poor eyesight and even glucometers that talk to the user.

Regardless of the type of meter chosen, it is vital to keep the meter clean and the test strips in proper condition.

Wearable devices Newer electronic devices attached to patients' skin connect to mobile devices and provide less invasive ways of monitoring blood glucose. These are not discussed in detail but deserve note.

Do You Remember These Key Points?

- Names of the major endocrine glands of the body
- The locations and functions of the endocrine glands discussed
- The primary symptoms of the various endocrine conditions discussed
- Medications used to treat the different endocrine conditions discussed
- The generic and trade names for the drugs discussed in this chapter
- The appropriate auxiliary labels that should be used when filling prescriptions for medications discussed in this chapter

Review Questions

Multiple Choice Questions

1. Three glands located in the brain are the:
   A. Pineal, pituitary, and pancreas
   B. Hypothalamus, pituitary, and pineal
   C. Pituitary, exocrine, and endocrine
   D. None of the above
2. The islets of Langerhans are found in which gland?
   A. Pineal
   B. Thalamus
   C. Pancreas
   D. Adrenal
3. The condition that affects children suffering from hypothyroidism is known as:
   A. Aphasia
   B. Cretinism
   C. Myxedema
   D. None of the above
4. Glimepiride is used to treat:
   A. Type 2 diabetes
   B. Type 1 diabetes
   C. Both type 1 and type 2 diabetes
   D. None of the above
5. Which combination drug does not have metformin as the main ingredient?
   A. ACTOplus Met
   B. Duetact
   C. Glucovance
   D. Metaglip

6. Vasopressin is another term for which of the following hormones?
   A. Antidiuretic hormone
   B. Calcitonin
   C. Follicle-stimulating hormone
   D. Growth hormone
7. Sandostatin (octreotide) is used to treat which of the following conditions?
   A. Acromegaly
   B. Type 2 diabetes mellitus
   C. Cretinism
   D. Hyperparathyroidism
8. Graves disease is the most common cause of:
   A. Hypothyroidism
   B. Hypopituitarism
   C. Hypergonadism
   D. Hyperthyroidism
9. Levothyroxine is the drug of choice to treat which of the following conditions?
   A. Hyperthyroidism
   B. Diabetes mellitus
   C. Hypoparathyroidism
   D. Hypothyroidism
10. Cushing disease is caused by excessive secretion of:
    A. Antidiuretic hormone
    B. Adrenocorticotropic hormone
    C. Follicle-stimulating hormone
    D. Growth hormone
11. Hyperaldosteronism is associated with which of the following?
    A. Hypertension
    B. Hyperkalemia
    C. Both A and B
    D. None of the above
12. Insulin can be used to treat which of the following?
    A. Type 1 diabetes mellitus
    B. Type 2 diabetes mellitus
    C. Gestational diabetes
    D. All of the above
13. Which of the following is primarily considered a mineralocorticoid?
    A. Methylprednisolone
    B. Hydrocortisone
    C. Prednisone
    D. Fludrocortisone acetate

14. Which of the following is considered the first-line agent for the treatment of type 2 diabetes mellitus?
    A. Metformin
    B. Glipizide
    C. Pioglitazone
    D. Insulin
15. Which of the following hormones is not secreted by the pituitary gland?
    A. Antidiuretic hormone
    B. Insulin
    C. Follicle-stimulating hormone
    D. Growth hormone

■ Technician's Corner

Using a drug reference book or online drug resource, determine which agents in Table 18.5 are associated with causing hypoglycemia (low blood sugar).

Bibliography

Applegate E. *The Anatomy and Physiology Learning System*. 4th ed. St. Louis: Saunders; 2010.

Damjanov I. *Pathology for the Health Professions*. 4th ed. St. Louis: Saunders; 2011.

ElSayed NA, Aleppo G, Aroda VR, et al. Introduction and methodology: introduction and methodology: standards of care in diabetes—2023. *Diabetes Care*. 2022;46:S1-S4. Available at: https://diabetesjournals.org/care/issue/46/Supplement_1.

Fishback JL. *Pathology*. 3rd ed. Philadelphia: Mosby; 2005.

Huether SE. *Understanding Pathophysiology*. 5th ed. St. Louis: Mosby; 2012.

Scanlon V, Sanders T. *Essentials of Anatomy and Physiology*. 5th ed. Philadelphia: FA Davis; 2007.

Solomon EP. *Introduction to Human Anatomy and Physiology*. 3rd ed. St. Louis: Saunders; 2009.

Thibodeau GA, Patton K. *Structure and Function of the Body*. 13th ed. St. Louis: Mosby; 2007.

Thibodeau GA, Patton KT. *Anatomy and Physiology*. 8th ed. St. Louis: Mosby; 2012.

Websites Referenced

Clinical Pharmacology Online. Elsevier. Available at: https://www.clinicalkey.com/pharmacology/login.

Therapeutic Agents for the Musculoskeletal System

Tony Guerra

1. Describe the major components of the musculoskeletal system.
2. List the primary symptoms of conditions associated with the musculoskeletal system. In addition, (a) recognize drugs used to treat the conditions associated with the musculoskeletal system, (b) write the generic and trade names for the drugs discussed in this chapter, and (c) list appropriate auxiliary labels when filling prescriptions for medicines discussed in this chapter.

Analgesic Without + pain, a drug that relieves pain

Antipyretic Against + fire (fever), a drug that prevents or reduces fever

Arthroplasty Joint + molded, surgical reconstruction or replacement of a joint

Bone fracture A break or rupture of a bone

Bone marrow A fatty network of connective tissue that fills the cavities of bones

Cancellous bone A meshwork of spongy bone typically found at the core of vertebral bones in the spine and the ends of long bones; also called spongy bone

Compact bone Rigid bone, which makes up most of the skeleton; also known as cortical bone

Cyclooxygenase (COX) Circle + oxygen + enzyme, either of two related enzymes that control prostaglandin production

Euphoria Well + state of being, feeling or state of intense excitement and happiness

Fascicle A bundle such as muscle fibers

Gout A painful form of arthritis characterized by defective metabolism of uric acid

Ligament A fibrous connective tissue that connects to bones

Miosis Smaller + condition, constriction of the pupil of the eye

Motor nerve A nerve carrying impulses from the brain or spinal cord to a muscle or gland

Muscle fiber Muscle cell

Neuromuscular junction Nerve + muscle, the junction between a nerve fiber and the muscle it supplies

Opioid analgesic An analgesic medication that activates opioid receptors

Osteoarthritis (OA) Bone + joint + inflammation, degeneration of joint cartilage and the underlying bone

Osteoporosis Bone + porous + condition, a medical condition in which the bones become brittle and fragile from loss of bone density and poor microarchitecture

Prostaglandin A mediator responsible for the features of inflammation, such as swelling, pain, stiffness, redness, and warmth

(Bone) Resorption Removal of osseous tissue by osteoclasts

Reye syndrome A life-threatening metabolic disorder of uncertain cause in young children; aspirin use may precipitate the syndrome

Skeletal muscle Muscle that is connected to the skeleton to form part of the mechanical system that moves the limbs and other parts of the body

Skeletal system The hard structure (bones and cartilages) that provides a frame for the body

Spongy bone Meshwork of spongy bone typically found at the core of vertebral bones in the spine and the ends of long bones, also known as cancellous bone

Subchondral bone Bone located below the cartilage, particularly within a joint

Synovium A thin membrane in synovial (freely moving) joints that lines the joint capsule and secretes synovial fluid

Tendon A flexible but inelastic cord of strong fibrous collagen tissue that attaches a muscle to a bone

Uric acid The water-insoluble end product of purine metabolism; deposition of uric acid as crystals in the joints and kidneys causes gout

Common Drugs for Conditions of the Musculoskeletal System

Trade Name	Generic Name	Pronunciation
Salicylate		
Bayer	aspirin	(**ass**-per-in)
Nonsteroidal Antiinflammatory Drugs (NSAIDs)		
Advil, Motrin IB	ibuprofen	(**eye**-bue-**proe**-fen)
Aleve, Naprosyn	naproxen sodium	(nah-**prox**-sin **sow**-dee-um)
Indocin[a]	indomethacin	(in-doe-**meth**-uh-sin)
Lodine[a]	etodolac	(eh-toe-**duh**-lak)
Mobic	meloxicam	(me-**lox**-ih-cam)
Toradol[a]	ketorolac	(**key**-toh-**role**-ak)
Voltaren[a]	diclofenac	(dye-**kloe**-fen-ak)
Cyclooxygenase-2 Inhibitor (COX-2 Inhibitor)		
Celebrex	celecoxib	(**sel**-uh-**kox**-ib)
Opioid Analgesics		
Demerol (C-II)	meperidine	(me-**per**-ih-deen)
Dilaudid (C-II)	hydromorphone	(**hye**-droe-**mor**-fone)
Duragesic[a] (C-II)	fentanyl	(**fen**-tuh-nil)
Lortab, Norco, Vicodin[a] (C-II)	hydrocodone/acetaminophen	(hye-droe-**koe**-done/a-**seet**-uh-**min**-uh-fen)
Percocet (C-II)	oxycodone/acetaminophen	(**ox**-e-koe-done/a-**seet**-uh-**min**-uh-fen)
Tylenol w/Codeine[a] (C-III)	acetaminophen/codeine	(a-**seet**-uh-**min**-uh-phen/**koe**-deen)
Miscellaneous Analgesics		
Nucynta (C-II)	tapentadol	(ta-**pen**-tuh-dol)
Ultram[a] (C-IV)	tramadol	(**tram**-uh-dol)
Osteoporosis Medications		
Actonel	risedronate	(rih-**sed**-ro-nayt)
Boniva	ibandronate	(eye-**ban**-dro-nate)
Evista	raloxifene	(ra-**lox**-ih-feen)
Fosamax	alendronate	(a-**len**-dro-nate)
Prolia	denosumab	(den-**oh**-sue-mab)

Common Drugs for Conditions of the Musculoskeletal System—cont'd

Trade Name	Generic Name	Pronunciation
Gout Medications		
Benuryl[a]	probenecid	(proe-**ben**-uh-sid)
Colcrys	colchicine	(**kol**-chih-seen)
Uloric	febuxostat	(feb-**ux**-oh-stat)
Zyloprim	allopurinol	(al-loh-**pure**-ih-nal)
Skeletal Muscle Relaxants		
Flexeril[a]	cyclobenzaprine	(sye-kloe-**ben**-zuh-preen)
	baclofen	(**bak**-loe-fen)
Robaxin[a]	methocarbamol	(meth-oh-**kar**-buh-mal)
Soma (C-IV)	carisoprodol	(kar-ih-soe-**proe**-dal)
Neuromuscular Blockers		
Nimbex	cisatracurium	(sis-**at**-ra-**kure**-ee-um)
Norcuron[a]	vecuronium	(**veh**-kure-**oh**-nee-um)
Pavulon[a]	pancuronium	(**pan**-kure-**oh**-nee-um)
Tracrium[a]	atracurium	(at-rah-**cure**-ih-um)
Zemuron[a]	rocuronium	(**row**-kure-**oh**-nee-um)

[a]Brand discontinued; now available only as generic.

Anatomy and Physiology of the Skeletal System

The **skeletal system** chiefly provides body support and organ protection. For example, the skull contains and protects the brain and the ribs provide protection for the heart and lungs. Bones also enable movement. **Tendons** attach muscle to bone, which allows bones to work as levers to move and exert muscular forces. **Ligaments** hold bones together at joints allowing bones to articulate at areas such as the knee and elbow (Fig. 19.1).

Long bones, such as the femur in the leg, also contain **bone marrow** (Fig. 19.2). Bone marrow's crucial role comes from the production of blood cells (see Chapter 28). Bones also store important minerals, such as calcium and phosphorus. When blood calcium levels are high, the bones store calcium in cells called osteoblasts. Conversely, when levels are low, osteoclasts remove calcium from the bones. We discuss this important idea later in the osteoporosis section.

The two main types of bone are compact bone and spongy bone. **Compact bone,** also known as *cortical bone*, is dense and found near the bone's surface, where there is the greatest need for strength. **Spongy bone,** on the other hand, is typically on the inner part of bones. Thin strands of bone known as *trabeculae* form the network. The spongy bone (sometimes called **cancellous bone**) is where bone marrow resides (Fig. 19.3).

Anatomy and Physiology of Skeletal Muscle

The body has three types of muscle: skeletal muscle, smooth muscle, and cardiac muscle. This chapter focuses on skeletal muscle. **Skeletal muscles** attach to bones to enable movement such as walking, talking, and chewing food.

It is important to understand how skeletal muscle works to understand best the medicines that work by affecting skeletal muscle contraction. Hundreds to thousands of muscle cells called **muscle fibers** make up skeletal muscle. These fibers, in turn, are grouped into bundles called fascicles. A group of fascicles makes up a muscle (Fig. 19.4). Tiny myofilaments make up *myofibrils* and, in turn, myofibrils make up each muscle fiber. These actin and myosin myofilaments help muscles contract. Actin and myosin muscle filaments ratchet along with one another, causing the filament to shorten (Fig. 19.5). This filament shortening matches the muscle contraction.

So what signals actin and myosin filaments in the skeletal muscle to contract? **Motor nerves** are nerves that carry signals from the central nervous system (CNS) to skeletal muscles, telling them to contract. A given motor nerve can signal one to several hundred muscle fibers. The **neuromuscular junction** is the point where a motor neuron meets and signals the skeletal muscle (Fig. 19.6).

Common Conditions Affecting the Musculoskeletal System

Various musculoskeletal conditions can affect the bones, skeletal muscles, or both. This chapter focuses on common musculoskeletal conditions often found in the ambulatory care setting. We cover other musculoskeletal disorders such as rheumatoid arthritis (RA) separately (see Chapter 25).

Osteoarthritis

Osteoarthritis (OA) is a disease associated with aging that affects articular cartilage, which is the cartilage that lines the

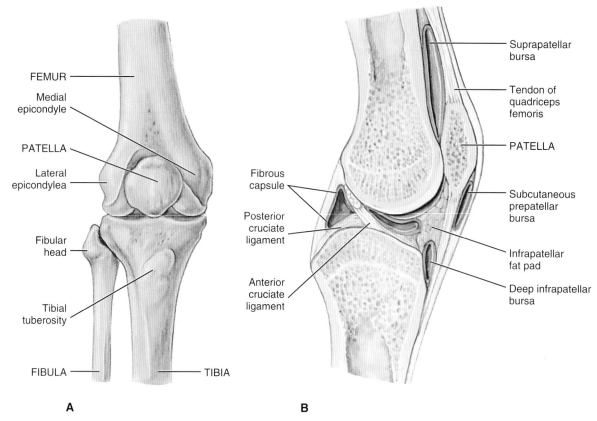

FIG. 19.1 The knee joint is a complex synovial joint. (A) Anterior view of the knee joint. (B) Sagittal section of the knee joint. (From Solomon EP. *Introduction to Human Anatomy and Physiology*. 3rd ed. St. Louis: Saunders; 2009.)

joints (Fig. 19.7). OA is the most common form of joint disease. Risk factors for OA include increasing age, obesity, repetitive joint overuse, and joint trauma. Genetic and environmental causes may also play a role. Advanced age is one of the strongest risk factors associated with OA. In the elderly, it is a major cause of disability and health care costs. X-ray changes of OA of the knee or hip are obvious in most people older than 60 years. The changes in cartilage strength and structure lead to cracking and erosion of cartilage and hypertrophy of **subchondral bone.** Loss of normal cushioning from cartilage upsets the interaction between **synovium,** cartilage, and bone.

OA differs from RA in several important respects. Unlike RA, there is no systemic illness associated with OA. Joint involvement is asymmetrical, with morning stiffness typically lasting less than 30 minutes on rising. OA mainly affects weight-bearing joints such as the hand, foot, knee, hip, and spine. Classic symptoms of OA include pain on joint use and range of motion limits. Short-duration morning joint stiffness is common.

Prognosis

Osteoarthritis (OA) has no known cure. Many treatments can slow disease progression. Although prognoses depend on OA severity, nonpharmacological and pharmacological therapy can help maintain functionality and quality of life.

Non-drug treatment

Treatment of patients with OA should focus on controlling pain and other symptoms to minimize disability and preserve the quality of life. In addition to the education of the patient and family, non-pharmacological interventions should include physical and occupational therapy, regular exercise, and weight loss, if needed. Obesity is an important modifiable risk factor. Surgical options for OA treatment include knee irrigation, arthroscopic lavage, osteotomy, and total joint **arthroplasty.**

Drug treatment

Pharmacological treatment of OA typically relies on the use of analgesics and nonsteroidal antiinflammatory drugs (NSAIDs) at first to reduce pain signals originating from the joints (Fig. 19.8). Acetaminophen is often the first agent recommended for OA pain. Patients can also use oral and topical NSAIDs. There is a risk for increased cardiovascular thrombotic events with NSAIDs. Patients taking chronic oral NSAIDs (as defined by longer than 14 days of treatment) should be evaluated by a provider to assess the need for ulcer prophylaxis. The preventive medications could include a proton pump inhibitor (PPI) such as omeprazole (Prilosec) or a histamine-2 receptor antagonist such as famotidine (Pepcid). The prescriber may choose opioid analgesics for severe pain or corticosteroid injections into the aching joint.

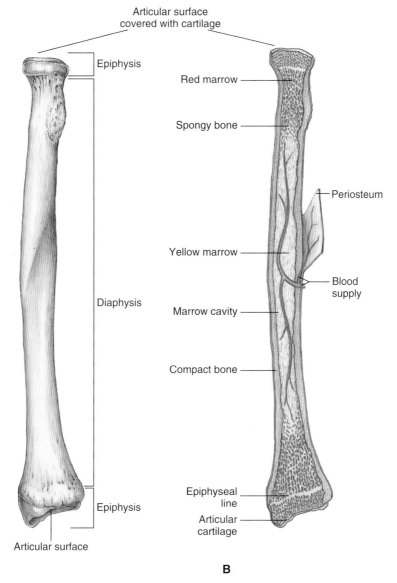

FIG. 19.2 Anatomy of a bone. (A) The structure of a typical long bone. (B) Internal structure of a long bone. (From Solomon EP. *Introduction to Human Anatomy and Physiology*. 3rd ed. St. Louis: Saunders; 2009.)

Naloxone (Narcan) is now available without a prescription for those using opioids and those at risk for overdose. Senna is the recommended laxative for opioid-induced constipation. Corticosteroid treatments are for short-term use only because they can damage the joint.

Acetaminophen, nonsteroidal antiinflammatory drugs (NSAIDs), and opioid analgesics provide relief from many pain conditions. We will discuss them here for OA treatment. Students should note the variability of doses for mild, moderate, and severe pain. The prescribing information contains dosing recommendations for other pain disorders and conditions.

Acetaminophen

Acetaminophen, abbreviated APAP in the United States, is both an **analgesic** and **antipyretic.** Unlike aspirin,

acetaminophen lacks peripheral antiinflammatory properties or platelet inhibitory effects. Health providers consider acetaminophen an analgesic of choice for OA. Acetaminophen has fewer hematologic, gastrointestinal (GI) (ulcer), and renal effects than NSAIDs. However, acetaminophen has risks. Acetaminophen misuse is the most common cause of acute liver failure in the United States. Many cases are unintentional because many products contain acetaminophen, making overdose relatively easy. Table 19.1 provides information on acetaminophen and other nonopioid analgesic medications.

■ Tech Note!

Many prescription and over-the-counter (OTC) products contain acetaminophen. Have the pharmacist verify the acetaminophen content of the patient's purchases.

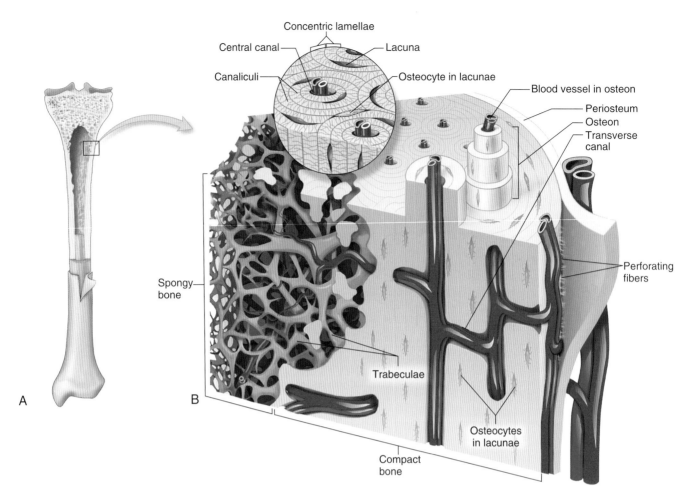

FIG. 19.3 Three-dimensional diagram showing the microscopic structure of bone. (From Patton KT, Thibodeau GA. *The Human Body in Health and Disease*. 6th ed. St. Louis: Elsevier; 2014.)

GENERIC NAME: acetaminophen

TRADE NAME: Tylenol (over the counter [OTC]), Ofirmev (IV)

INDICATIONS: Musculoskeletal pain, osteoarthritis, headache, fever

ROUTES OF ADMINISTRATION: Oral, rectal, intravenous

COMMON ADULT DOSAGE: 500–1000 mg as needed (max 4000 mg/day under the supervision of a health care provider) for most formulations and routes

MECHANISMS OF ACTION: Inhibits cyclooxygenase-1 and cyclooxygenase-2 in the CNS

SIDE EFFECTS: Nausea, vomiting, constipation, liver damage

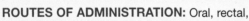

■ Tech Note!

Acetaminophen (Tylenol) is not an antiinflammatory agent. Although it does inhibit cyclooxygenase enzymes and relieves pain and fever, it works in the CNS and does not reduce peripheral inflammation.

Aspirin

Some reported that willow tree bark effectively reduced pain, fever, and inflammation in England in the early 1800s. Other cultures discovered this centuries ago, but in the early 1800s, chemists isolated the active ingredients. Henri Leroux, a French chemist, found a bitter glycoside produced the medicinal bark's properties. This chemical was *salicin*. Chemists can break salicin into glucose (sugar) and salicylic alcohol. Salicylic alcohol can break down into acetylsalicylic acid (ASA). The Bayer Company first marketed this miracle agent in 1899. Bayer called its wonder drug *aspirin*. Other manufacturers have introduced similar medications; however, aspirin remains popular because it is effective and inexpensive.

Aspirin is a useful fever, pain, and inflammation agent. However, parents should avoid giving it to children, especially pediatric patients, with flulike symptoms. Aspirin use in children may cause **Reye syndrome**. This condition may develop after chickenpox or upper respiratory tract viral infection. Reye syndrome may cause vomiting, lethargy, and encephalopathy leading to coma and death.

The maximum dose for aspirin in adults is 4 g/day. An upset stomach is a common side effect. Aspirin effectively inhibits platelet aggregation and can prevent strokes or heart

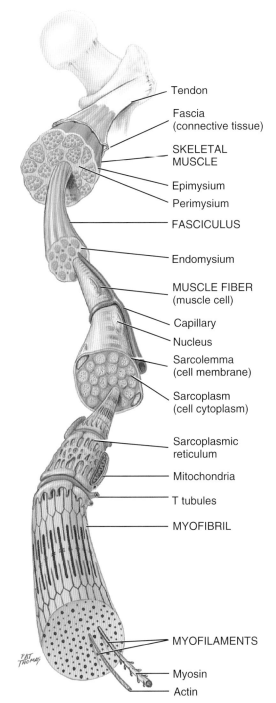

- Tendon
- Fascia (connective tissue)
- SKELETAL MUSCLE
- Epimysium
- Perimysium
- FASCICULUS
- Endomysium
- MUSCLE FIBER (muscle cell)
- Capillary
- Nucleus
- Sarcolemma (cell membrane)
- Sarcoplasm (cell cytoplasm)
- Sarcoplasmic reticulum
- Mitochondria
- T tubules
- MYOFIBRIL
- MYOFILAMENTS
- Myosin
- Actin

FIG. 19.4 Muscle structure. The muscle is attached to bone by a tendon. The muscle is surrounded by a connective tissue covering—the epimysium. The muscle consists of fascicles—bundles of muscle fibers. Each fascicle is wrapped in connective tissue—the perimysium. Individual muscle fibers are surrounded by endomysium. Myofibrils are threadlike structures composed of actin and myosin filaments. One myofibril is magnified and shown in detail to illustrate the filaments. The regular pattern of overlapping filaments gives skeletal and cardiac muscle their striated appearance. (From Applegate E. *The Anatomy and Physiology Learning System*. 4th ed. St. Louis: Elsevier; 2001.)

attacks. Patients with cardiac risk factors (eg, those with diabetes) take aspirin daily. Aspirin can increase bleeding risk, and prescribers should consider this danger. Prescribers should display special care with aspirin and anticoagulants, such as warfarin, to avoid additive bleeding risk (see Chapter 28).

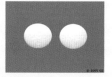

GENERIC NAME: aspirin

TRADE NAME: Bayer Aspirin (OTC)

INDICATIONS: Headache, fever, mild pain, thromboembolism prophylaxis

ROUTE OF ADMINISTRATION: Oral

COMMON ADULT DOSAGE: *For pain:* the typical dosage is 325–650 mg as needed (max of 3.9 g/day). Thromboembolism prophylaxis is 81 mg/day as needed for headache, pain, fever (max 4 g/day); use daily for thromboembolism prophylaxis

MECHANISMS OF ACTION: Inhibits cyclooxygenase-1 and cyclooxygenase-2 enzymes; inhibits platelet aggregation by inhibition of thromboxane-A2

SIDE EFFECTS: Nausea, indigestion, increased bleeding risk

AUXILIARY LABEL: Take with food or milk

▪ Tech Note!

Aspirin's chemical name is acetylsalicylic acid (ASA). This chemical inhibits prostaglandins, thus reducing inflammation, fever, and pain. Many health care providers recommend low-strength 81-mg aspirin for its antiplatelet effects.

Nonsteroidal Antiinflammatory Drugs

Aspirin is a salicylate drug and a prototype for the newer NSAIDs. NSAIDs and aspirin differ slightly chemically, but all have analgesic, antipyretic, and antiinflammatory properties. Naturally occurring and exogenous steroids reduce inflammation by binding to steroid receptors. NSAIDs suppress inflammation by inhibiting the cyclooxygenase (COX) enzyme responsible for **prostaglandin** synthesis.

The **cyclooxygenase (COX)** enzyme takes part in a pathway that synthesizes prostaglandins and other compounds. We find COX in all tissues, where it helps regulate many processes. Cyclooxygenase has two forms, COX-1 and COX-2. COX-1 is present in most tissues and assists with many normal body functions, including protecting gastric mucosa and promoting platelet aggregation. We find COX-2 mainly at sites of tissue injury, where it helps sensitize receptors to pain and mediates inflammation. COX-2 is present in the brain, where it affects fever and pain perception. Therefore COX-1 is an enzyme involved in preserving normal metabolic processes, whereas we associate COX-2 with pain and discomfort.

By inhibiting prostaglandin synthesis, NSAIDs not only suppress inflammation but also help treat pain. Prescribers and patients use NSAIDs for mild to moderate pain and inflammation.

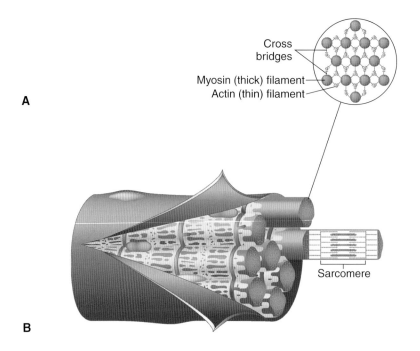

A

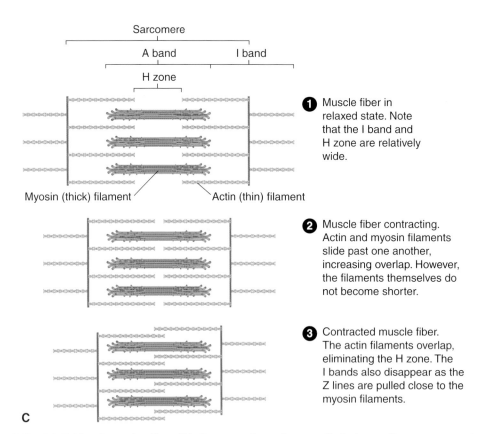

B

Sarcomere

A band | I band

H zone

Myosin (thick) filament   Actin (thin) filament

❶ Muscle fiber in relaxed state. Note that the I band and H zone are relatively wide.

❷ Muscle fiber contracting. Actin and myosin filaments slide past one another, increasing overlap. However, the filaments themselves do not become shorter.

❸ Contracted muscle fiber. The actin filaments overlap, eliminating the H zone. The I bands also disappear as the Z lines are pulled close to the myosin filaments.

C

FIG. 19.5 Muscle contraction. (A) Cross section of a myofibril shows the arrangement of actin and myosin filaments. (B) Part of a muscle fiber showing the location of the filaments. (C) A muscle contracts (shortens) when actin and myosin filaments slide past one another. The amount of overlap between actin and myosin filaments increases. (From Solomon EP. *Introduction to Human Anatomy and Physiology*. 3rd ed. St. Louis: Saunders; 2009.)

Cross bridges
Myosin (thick) filament
Actin (thin) filament

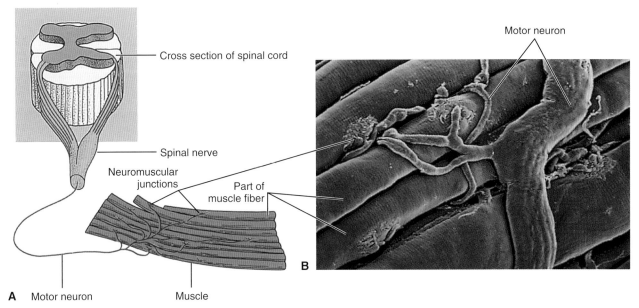

FIG. 19.6 Nerve fibers from a motor nerve transmit impulses to muscle fibers. (A) Each nerve fiber controls many muscle fibers. (B) Scanning electron micrograph of neuromuscular junctions (100×). Note how the motor neuron branches to innervate several muscle fibers. (From Solomon EP. *Introduction to Human Anatomy and Physiology.* 3rd ed. St. Louis: Saunders; 2009.)

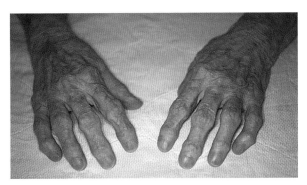

FIG. 19.7 Severe osteoarthritis. (From Swartz M. *Textbook of Physical Diagnosis: History and Examination.* 7th ed. St. Louis: Saunders; 2014.)

NSAIDs also exert an antipyretic effect by acting on the hypothalamus (the body thermostat). Manufacturers created more than 12 prescription NSAIDs. A few are available over the counter (see Chapter 29). Wide variations exist between NSAIDs, even if they belong to the same chemical family (see Table 19.1).

NSAIDs relieve many different conditions and chronic illnesses, such as the following:

- Muscle pain
- RA
- Joint pain (eg, OA)
- Dysmenorrhea

Millions of people use over-the-counter (OTC) and prescription NSAIDs to treat various inflammatory conditions. However, overuse can cause significant problems. NSAIDs can worsen stomach problems, such as gastroesophageal reflux disease (GERD). They can also cause GI ulcers and bleeding. Patients should always take NSAIDs with food to prevent stomach irritation.

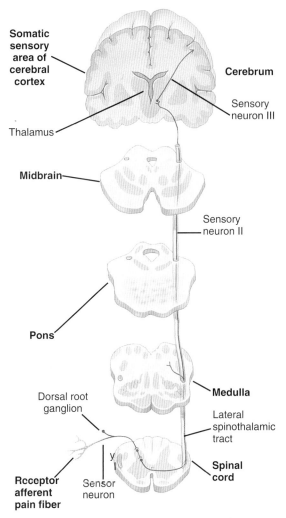

FIG. 19.8 Pain route. (From Potter PA, Perry AG. *Fundamentals of Nursing.* 8th ed. St. Louis: Mosby; 2012.)

TABLE 19.1
Select Nonopioid Analgesic Medications

Generic Name	Trade Name	Common Dosage Range	Common Side Effects	Comments
Acetaminophen (APAP)				
acetaminophen	Tylenol	• *IR:* 500 mg PO 1–2 tablets every 6 hours • *ER:* 650 mg PO 2 tablets every 8 hours	• Nausea • Vomiting • Headache • Liver toxicity	Maximum daily dose of 4000 mg/day under the supervision of a physician
Nonsteroidal Antiinflammatory Drugs (NSAIDs)				
aspirin	Bayer Aspirin, Ecotrin	• 325–650 mg PO every 4 hours or 81 mg PO once daily (max 4 g/day)	• Dyspepsia • Gastrointestinal ulcer • Nausea • Reye syndrome	Antiplatelet effect usually lasts ~4 days
ibuprofen	Advil, Motrin IB	• 200–800 mg PO every 6–8 hours	• Acute renal failure • Dizziness • Fluid retention • Gastrointestinal ulcer • Heartburn • Hypertension • Liver toxicity • Nausea • Rash	
naproxen	Naprosyn	• 250–500 mg PO twice daily		
	EC Naprosyn (delayed-release)	• 375–500 mg PO twice daily		
naproxen sodium	Aleve	• 220–440 mg PO twice daily (max 660 mg/day)		
oxaprozin	Daypro	• 600–1200 mg/day PO		Long duration allows for once-daily dosing
diclofenac	Cataflam[a], Voltaren[a]	• *IR:* 50 mg PO 2 or 3 times daily • *DR:* 75 mg PO twice daily	• Similar to NSAIDs listed above	
	Voltaren XR[a]	• 100 mg PO once or twice daily		
etodolac	Lodine[a]	• 400–500 mg PO twice daily		
	Lodine XL[a]	• 400–1000 mg PO once daily		
indomethacin	Indocin[a]	• 25–50 mg PO 2 or 3 times daily		Rectal suppositories available
	Indocin SR[a]	• 75 mg PO once or twice daily		
nabumetone	Relafen[a]	• 500–1000 mg PO in 1 or 2 doses daily		Long duration allows for once-daily dosing
meloxicam	Mobic	• 7.5–15 mg PO once daily (max 15 mg/day)		
Cyclooxygenase-2 Selective Inhibitor				
celecoxib	Celebrex	• 200 mg/day PO or 100 mg twice daily	• Acute renal failure • Diarrhea • Headache • Hypertension • Nausea • Thrombotic events	Less risk for gastrointestinal ulcer

[a]Brand discontinued; now available only as generic.
DR, Delayed-release; *ER,* extended-release; *IR,* immediate-release; *PO,* orally; *SR,* sustained-release; *XR,* extended-release.

GENERIC NAME: ibuprofen

TRADE NAMES: MOTRIN IB, ADVIL (OTC)

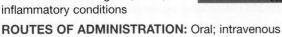

INDICATION: Analgesia, fever, inflammatory conditions

ROUTES OF ADMINISTRATION: Oral; intravenous

COMMON ADULT DOSAGE: 200–800 mg every 6–8 hours (max 3200 mg/day) for either formulation or route

MECHANISM OF ACTION: Inhibits COX-1 and COX-2 enzymes

SIDE EFFECTS: Gastrointestinal ulceration, increased risk for bleeding, increased blood pressure, renal impairment

AUXILIARY LABELS:
- May cause dizziness or drowsiness
- Take with food or milk

GENERIC NAME: naproxen

TRADE NAMES: Aleve (OTC), Naprosyn (Rx)

INDICATIONS: Analgesia, fever, inflammatory conditions

ROUTE OF ADMINISTRATION: Oral

COMMON ADULT DOSAGE: 250–500 mg twice daily (max 1500 mg/day)

MECHANISM OF ACTION: Inhibits COX-1 and COX-2 enzymes

SIDE EFFECTS: Gastrointestinal ulceration, increased risk for bleeding, increased blood pressure, renal impairment

AUXILIARY LABELS:
- May cause dizziness or drowsiness
- Take with food or milk

GENERIC NAME: meloxicam

TRADE NAME: Mobic

INDICATIONS: Osteoarthritis, rheumatoid arthritis

ROUTE OF ADMINISTRATION: Oral

COMMON ADULT DOSAGE: 7.5–15 mg once daily

MECHANISM OF ACTION: Inhibits COX-1 and COX-2 enzymes

SIDE EFFECTS: Gastrointestinal ulceration, increased risk for bleeding, increased blood pressure, renal impairment

AUXILIARY LABELS:
- Shake the suspension well before use
- Take with or without food

Cyclooxygenase-2 Inhibitors

Earlier, we noted cyclooxygenase has COX-1 and COX-2 forms. First-generation NSAIDs inhibit both COX-1 and COX-2 enzymes, which decreases inflammation, pain, and fever. Inhibition of COX-1 enzymes has serious side effects, including gastric ulceration, bleeding, and renal damage. The theory behind COX-2–selective inhibitors is that they could treat pain and inflammation without the risk of nonselective agents that also inhibit COX-1. However, in practice, selective COX-2 inhibition has not reduced NSAID-related side effects as expected. Manufacturers withdrew rofecoxib (Vioxx) and valdecoxib (Bextra) (both COX-2 inhibitors) from the market. There were safety concerns about cardiovascular events. Now health care providers reserve COX-2 inhibitors for patients intolerant of traditional NSAIDs. Celecoxib (Celebrex) is the only COX-2 inhibitor approved for use in the United States.

GENERIC NAME: celecoxib

TRADE NAME: Celebrex

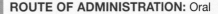

INDICATIONS: Osteoarthritis (OA), rheumatoid arthritis (RA)

ROUTE OF ADMINISTRATION: Oral

COMMON ADULT DOSAGES: *OA:* 200 mg/day or 100 mg twice daily. *RA:* 100–200 mg twice daily

MECHANISM OF ACTION: Selective inhibition of COX-2

SIDE EFFECTS: Nausea, abdominal pain, cardiovascular events

AUXILIARY LABEL: Take with food or milk

Topical Over-the-Counter Pain Relievers

Topical products can help manage OA and muscle strains. Patients widely use products containing menthol and methyl salicylate (eg, Bengay, IcyHot), trolamine salicylate (Aspercreme), camphor plus menthol (Tiger Balm), lidocaine (Salonpas), and diclofenac (Voltaren), a topical NSAID. Patients should only use these products on intact skin, washing hands before and after application.

Opioid Analgesics

Opioid analgesics play a pivotal role in pain management through actions on the brain's opioid receptors. The three main opioid receptor types are mu, kappa, and delta receptors. Analgesia mediates through changes in pain perception at the spinal cord level of the CNS (Fig. 19.9). Clinically effective opioids work as mu-receptor agonists. Most consider morphine the prototypical opioid pain medication. Activation of mu-receptors produces analgesia, **miosis** (pupillary constriction), respiratory depression, **euphoria,** decreased GI motility, and physical dependence. Opioid medications are controlled substances. The US Drug Enforcement Administration (DEA) schedule depends on the agent and formulation. Because opioid prescriptions cause sedation

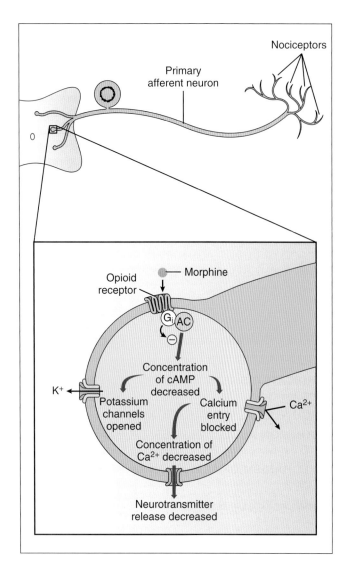

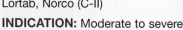
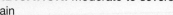

GENERIC NAME: hydrocodone/acetaminophen

TRADE NAMES: Vicodin,[a] Lortab, Norco (C-II)

INDICATION: Moderate to severe pain

ROUTE OF ADMINISTRATION: Oral

COMMON ADULT DOSAGE: 2.5–10 mg of hydrocodone every 4–6 hours as needed for pain

MECHANISMS OF ACTION: Hydrocodone activates opioid receptors; acetaminophen inhibits COX-1 and COX-2

SIDE EFFECTS: Constipation, drowsiness, dependence

AUXILIARY LABELS:
- May cause dizziness or drowsiness
- Avoid alcohol
- *Caution:* Federal law prohibits the transfer of this drug to any person other than the patient for whom it was prescribed.

SPECIAL NOTE: The maximum dose of acetaminophen is 4 g/day.

[a]Brand discontinued; now available only as generic.

FIG. 19.9 Mechanism of opioid action in the spinal cord. *AC,* Adenylate cyclase; *cAMP,* cyclic adenosine monophosphate; G_i, guanine nucleotide binding protein, subunit alpha-1. (From Brenner GM, et al. *Pharmacology.* 4th ed. Philadelphia: Saunders; 2014.)

and respiratory depression, an overdose may be potentially life-threatening.

These opioid analgesics have several important boxed warnings including addiction, abuse, misuse, and respiratory depression. These medications should not be used with central nervous system (CNS) depressants as excessive sedation, confusion, respiratory depression, and death can occur. CNS depressants include alcohol, benzodiazepines, hypnotics, and muscle relaxants, among others. Remind patients to avoid driving or operating heavy equipment or machinery until they know how their bodies react to the opioid dosages.

Opioid antagonists, such as naloxone and naltrexone, can reverse the opioid agonist effects by competing for opioid receptor sites. Table 19.2 provides an overview of select opioid agonists and antagonists.

■ Tech Note!

For combination opioid medications with acetaminophen, it is the acetaminophen that limits the maximum daily amount (3000 mg/day). Some individuals (eg, those with liver disease) may require smaller daily amounts (eg, 2000 mg/day).

GENERIC NAME: oxycodone

TRADE NAME: Roxicodone (C-II)

INDICATION: Moderate to severe pain

ROUTE OF ADMINISTRATION: Oral

COMMON ADULT DOSAGE: 5–15 mg immediate-release (IR) every 4–6 hours as needed initially for opioid-naïve patients, then titrated to effect

MECHANISM OF ACTION: Activation of opioid receptors

SIDE EFFECTS: Constipation, drowsiness, dependence

AUXILIARY LABELS:
- May cause dizziness or drowsiness
- Avoid alcohol
- *Caution:* Federal law prohibits the transfer of this drug to any person other than the patient for whom it was prescribed.

Select Opioid Analgesics and Opioid Receptor Antagonists

Generic Name	Trade Name	Common Starting Dosage Range	Common Side Effects
Opioid Analgesics			
codeine + acetaminophen (C-III)	NA	• 15–60 mg codeine PO every 4–6 hours; max 360 mg codeine/day	• Constipation • Drowsiness • Itchiness (pruritus) • Nausea • Respiratory depression • Vomiting
hydrocodone + acetaminophen (C-II)	Lortab, Norco, Vicodin[a]	• 2.5–10 mg hydrocodone PO every 4–6 hours	
oxycodone (C-II)	Roxicodone, OxyContin (ER)	• *IR:* 5–15 mg PO every 4–6 hours • *ER:* 10 mg PO twice daily	
morphine (C-II)	MS-Contin, Kadian SR	• *IR:* 2.5–10 mg subcut/IM/IV every 2–6 hours, *or* 10–30 mg PO every 4 hours • *ER:* 15–30 mg PO once or twice daily	
hydromorphone (C-II)	Dilaudid	• *IR:* 0.2–1 mg IV every 2–3 hours, *or* 1–2 mg subcut every 2–3 hours, *or* 2–4 mg PO every 4–6 hours • *ER:* 4–8 mg PO every 24 hours	
oxymorphone (C-II)	Opana, Numorphan[a]	• 0.5–1.5 mg IV/IR/subcut every 4–6 hours, *or* 5–10 mg PO every 4–6 hours	
fentanyl (C-II)	Duragesic[a]	• 50–100 mcg IV/subcut every 1–2 hours • *Patch:* 12–25 mcg/hr; change every 72 hours	
methadone (C-II)	Dolophine	• 2.5–10 mg IV/subcut every 8–12 hours, *or* 2.5–10 mg PO every 8–12 hours	
Partial Opioid Agonist			
buprenorphine (C-III)	Buprenex, Subutex[a]	• 0.3 mg IM/IV every 6–8 hours as needed	• Headache • Hypotension • Respiratory depression • Sedation • Sweating
Mixed Opioid Agonists			
nalbuphine	Nubain[a]	• 10 mg IV/IM/subcut every 3–6 hours (max 20 mg/dose for non–opioid-tolerant patients, 160 mg/day)	• Dizziness • Dry mouth • Headache • Nausea • Sedation
Opioid Antagonists (Reversal Agents)			
naloxone	Narcan[a]	• 0.4–2 mg subcut/IM/IV every 2–3 min until reversal (after 10 mg with no reversal, search for other causes)	• Pain • Palpitations • Tremors • Withdrawal symptoms
naltrexone	Vivitrol	• 25–50 mg/day • 380 mg IM once every 4 wk	• Dizziness • Headache • Injection site reaction • Insomnia • Nausea • Syncope

[a]Brand discontinued; now available only as generic.

ER, Extended-release; *IM,* intramuscular; *IV,* intravenous; *PO,* oral; *subcut,* subcutaneous.

GENERIC NAME: fentanyl

TRADE NAMES: Duragesic,[a] Fentora, Onsolis[a], Actiq, Lazanda, Abstral, SUBSYS (C-II)

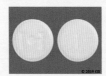

ROUTES OF ADMINISTRATION: Oral; transdermal; intranasal; intravenous; sublingual; transmucosal

INDICATIONS: Moderate to severe pain, general anesthesia

COMMON ADULT DOSAGE: Dosage is highly variable based on the dosage form and baseline opioid use

MECHANISM OF ACTION: Activation of opioid receptors

SIDE EFFECTS: Constipation, drowsiness, dependence

AUXILIARY LABELS:
- May cause dizziness or drowsiness
- Avoid alcohol
- *Caution:* Federal law prohibits the transfer of this drug to any person other than the patient for whom it was prescribed.

[a]Brand discontinued; now available only as generic.

Opioid-Induced Constipation

A common side effect of opioids is constipation. Whether opioids are dosed as needed or scheduled around the clock, all opioids can slow peristalsis resulting in constipation. First-line opioid-induced constipation (OIC) treatment includes stimulant laxatives such as senna and bisacodyl to increase intestinal motility. A stool softener as add-on therapy can help ease difficulty with bowel movements and hard stools. If laxatives are ineffective, other newer options include methylnaltrexone (Relistor) and naloxegol (Movantik), which are antagonists that directly block opioid receptors in the gut, resulting in less constipation.

GENERIC NAME: Methylnaltrexone

TRADE NAME: Relistor

INDICATIONS: Opioid-induced constipation

ROUTE OF ADMINISTRATION: Subcutaneous injection, oral

COMMON ADULT DOSAGE: For OIC with advanced illness: weight-based dose. Administered subcutaneously one dose every other day as needed.

FOR OIC WITH CHRONIC NON-CANCER PAIN: 12 mg subcutaneously once daily or 450 mg by mouth once daily

MECHANISM OF ACTION: Opioid receptor antagonist which blocks opioid receptors in the gut

SIDE EFFECTS: Abdominal pain, flatulence, diarrhea

GENERIC NAME: Naloxegol

TRADE NAME: Movantik

INDICATIONS: Opioid-induced constipation

ROUTE OF ADMINISTRATION: Oral

COMMON ADULT DOSAGE: 25 mg once daily

MECHANISM OF ACTION: Opioid receptor antagonist which blocks opioid receptors in the gut

SIDE EFFECTS: Abdominal pain, flatulence, diarrhea

Osteoporosis

Osteoporosis is a systemic skeletal disease characterized by low bone mass and microarchitectural bone tissue deterioration. These bone changes lead to fragility and possible **bone fracture.** Osteoporosis occurs commonly in postmenopausal women, although osteoporosis in men is a growing public health concern.

The body continually breaks bone down through **resorption** and then rebuilds. Osteoclasts are bone cells that invade the bone surface to erode it. Osteoclasts create a surface cavity. Osteoblasts, bone-forming cells, then fill in the cavity with new bone, which contains collagen and minerals such as calcium and phosphorus. The body couples osteoclast and osteoblast activity and replaces resorbed bone. Osteoporosis happens when bone resorption outpaces the laying down of new bone. Fig. 19.10 depicts this remodeling and shows the mechanism of action by which many osteoporosis drugs work.

Recall that many types of bone form the human skeleton. Cortical bone is relatively dense and compact. Cancellous bone has a lattice network commonly called "spongy" bone and also trabecular bone. Metabolically active cancellous bone is in the vertebrae, ribs, pelvis, and the ends of long bones. Approximately 25% of all trabecular bone turns over annually. In essence, our body forms an entirely new skeleton every 5 to 10 years. When the rate of bone resorption exceeds new bone formation, bone mineral density (BMD) decreases and bone (particularly spongy bone) weakens, becoming prone to fracture. The highest morbidity and mortality come from fractures of the hip and long bones, although fractures can occur anywhere. However, vertebral fractures are the most common and can lead to kyphosis (Fig. 19.11), or a bent-over, stooped posture. The guideline recommendation test to diagnose osteoporosis is the dual-energy x-ray absorptiometry (DEXA) scan. It is an x-ray absorptivity test that measures bone density. Providers recommend the test for women 65 and older and men 70 and older, if a person breaks a bone after age 50, and for women of menopausal age with risk factors, postmenopausal women under age 65 with risk factors, or men age 50 to 69 with risk factors.

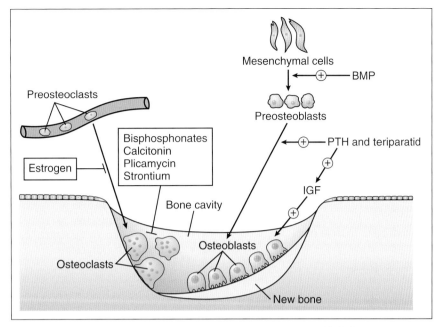

FIG. 19.10 Effects of drugs and hormones on bone remodeling. *BMP,* Bone morphogenetic proteins; *IGF,* insulin-like growth factor; *PTH,* parathyroid hormone. (From Brenner GM, et al. *Pharmacology.* 4th ed. Philadelphia: Saunders; 2014.)

Prognosis

Dietary changes, exercise, and medication can provide an excellent prognosis for osteoporosis. According to the National Osteoporosis Foundation, approximately 10 million people have osteoporosis. Another 34 million may have low bone mass, a precursor of osteoporosis. This condition cost the health care system roughly $19 billion in 2005, and the cost is expected to reach $25.3 billion by 2025.

Non-drug treatments

Primary osteoporosis prevention begins early in life. Recommendations include a healthy lifestyle with physical activity, a healthy diet, and no smoking. Exercise helps increase bone density, as does calcium and vitamin D. Patients can meet calcium needs by drinking milk, eating cheese, or taking calcium supplements.

Drug treatments

Osteoporosis treatment focuses on reducing fracture risk, decreasing bone loss, preserving normal bone remodeling, and preserving the quality of life. Bisphosphonates and raloxifene can prevent and treat osteoporosis. However, bisphosphonates are traditionally first-line therapy with excellent efficacy, administration ease, low cost, and significant safety data. A patient on bisphosphonates should be reassessed after 3 to 5 years of therapy to determine the risk versus benefit of the medication. Denosumab is an alternative to bisphosphonates, but it is not as widely used due to the high cost and subcutaneous administration. Estrogen-based therapies are also alternatives for those who cannot tolerate bisphosphonates or denosumab. Parathyroid hormone

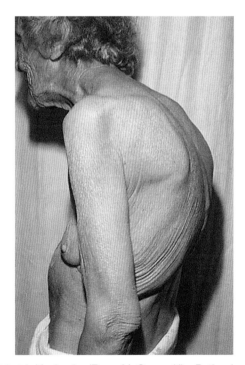

FIG. 19.11 Kyphosis. (From McCance KL. *Pathophysiology: The Biologic Basis for Disease in Adults and Children.* 6th ed. St. Louis: Mosby; 2010.)

analogs are reserved for patients with a very high risk of complication or subsequent fracture as they have a history of several fractures. Calcitonin, due to the risk of cancer with long-term use, is rarely used for this indication. An acceptable intake of vitamin D and calcium is critical in osteoporosis treatment.

Table 19.3 provides a summary of select agents approved for osteoporosis treatment.

GENERIC NAME: alendronate

TRADE NAME: Fosamax

INDICATIONS: Osteoporosis, osteoporosis prophylaxis, Paget disease

ROUTE OF ADMINISTRATION: Oral

COMMON ADULT DOSAGES: 5–10 mg/day or 35–70 mg/week

MECHANISM OF ACTION: Inhibits osteoclast activity to slow bone resorption

SIDE EFFECTS: Abdominal pain, muscle pain, osteonecrosis of the jaw

AUXILIARY LABEL: Take as directed

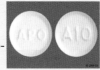

Tech Note!

Patients should take oral bisphosphonate medications on an empty stomach with a full glass of plain water at least 30 to 60 min before eating any food or taking other medications. In addition, patients should remain upright for 30 to 60 min to prevent irritation or esophageal damage.

GENERIC NAME: raloxifene

TRADE NAME: Evista

INDICATIONS: Osteoporosis treatment, osteoporosis prophylaxis

ROUTE OF ADMINISTRATION: Oral

COMMON ADULT DOSAGE: 60 mg/day

MECHANISMS OF ACTION: Selective estrogen receptor modulator (SERM): activates estrogen receptors in some tissues and antagonizes estrogen receptors in other tissues

SIDE EFFECTS: Hot flashes, leg cramps, increased risk for thrombosis

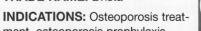
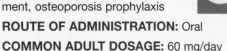

GENERIC NAME: denosumab

TRADE NAME: Prolia

INDICATION: Osteoporosis

ROUTE OF ADMINISTRATION: Subcutaneous

COMMON ADULT DOSAGE: 60 mg subcutaneously every 6 months

MECHANISM OF ACTION: Binds to receptor activator of nuclear factor kappa-B ligand (RANKL), inhibiting osteoclast activation

SIDE EFFECTS: Dizziness/drowsiness, arthralgia, anemia

AUXILIARY LABELS:
- May cause dizziness/drowsiness
- Avoid pregnancy/discontinue use if you become pregnant

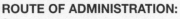
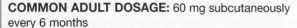

GENERIC NAME: teriparatide

TRADE NAME: Forteo

INDICATION: Osteoporosis

ROUTE OF ADMINISTRATION: Subcutaneous

COMMON ADULT DOSAGE: 20 mcg subcutaneously once daily

MECHANISM OF ACTION: Activates osteoclasts to increase bone density

SIDE EFFECTS: Syncope, arthralgia, angina

AUXILIARY LABELS:
- Rotate injection sites
- May cause drowsiness/dizziness
- Orthostatic hypotension

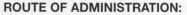

Gout

Gout is a form of arthritis. A **uric acid** buildup in the blood leads to uric acid crystals in the joints, which in turn leads to inflammation and pain (Fig. 19.12). Ninety percent of patients with gout struggle to excrete uric acid, and 10% are overproducers. Acute gout flares are intensely painful inflammatory arthritic attacks that typically involve a single joint but can affect multiple joints.

The overall prevalence of gout is approximately 6 in 1000 in men and 1 in 1000 in women, but prevalence increases with age. Other than hyperuricemia, common risk factors for gout are obesity, hypertension, and renal insufficiency. Alcohol, diuretics, levodopa, and other drugs hinder the renal excretion of uric acid and have been linked to gout. If a patient presents with new-onset or exacerbated gout, a pharmacist should review the medication profile for contributory medications.

Prognosis

The prognosis for gout can be good if health care professionals can identify contributing factors and resolve them to prevent recurrent gout attacks. Medications can both help prevent and treat acute gouty arthritis (Table 19.4).

Non-drug treatment

Various nonpharmacological interventions can reduce the risk for gout attacks. Weight loss, abstaining from alcohol, and adopting a diet low in purines (eg, avoiding meats such as beef, lamb, and pork) can be beneficial.

Drug treatment

Early treatment goals for patients with gout focus on easing the inflammation and pain associated with acute attacks. Therapies include colchicine, NSAIDs, and corticosteroids. Keeping uric acid levels low with uricosuric drugs or xanthine oxidase inhibitors may prevent recurrent attacks. Febuxostat (Uloric) is no

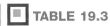 **TABLE 19.3**
Select Medications for the Treatment of Osteoporosis

Generic Name	Trade Name	Common Dosage Range	Common Side Effects
Bisphosphonates			
alendronate	Fosamax	• 5–10 mg/day PO *or* 35–70 mg/w PO	• Abdominal pain • Atrial fibrillation • Atypical femur fractures • Flulike symptoms • Muscle pain • Osteonecrosis of the jaw (ONJ) • Rash
ibandronate	Boniva	• 150 mg/mo PO *or* 3 mg IV bolus every 3 mo	
risedronate	Actonel	• 5 mg/daily PO, *or* 35 mg/wk PO, *or* 150 mg/mo PO	
zoledronic acid	Reclast	• 5 mg IV every 1–2 y	• Bone pain • Fatigue • Injection site reactions • Nausea/vomiting
Calcitonin Hormone Analog			
calcitonin salmon	Miacalcin	• 200 units (1 spray) in one nostril daily, switching nostrils daily • 100 units/day IM/subcut	• Flushing • Nosebleeds • Rhinitis
Selective Estrogen Receptor Modulator (SERM)			
raloxifene	Evista	• 60 mg/day PO	• Hot flashes • Increased risk for clots • Increased triglycerides • Joint pain • Leg cramps
Parathyroid Hormone Analog			
teriparatide	Forteo	• 20 mcg/day subcut for up to 2 y	• Dizziness • Hypercalcemia • Hypercalciuria • Hypotension • Nausea
Monoclonal Antibody			
denosumab	Prolia	• 60 mg subcut once every 6 mo	• Diarrhea • Dizziness • Headache • Vomiting
Supplementation			
vitamin D and calcium	Citracal Maximum Plus D3, Caltrate 600+D	• 1000–1200 mg divided in 2–3 doses of calcium and 400–800 international units of vitamin D by mouth	• Constipation • Kidney stones • Stomach upset

IM, Intramuscular; *IV,* intravenous; *PO,* oral; *subcut,* subcutaneous.

longer recommended because of an increased risk for death versus allopurinol. Rasburicase is an intravenous (IV) agent used in tumor lysis syndrome. Uric acid levels rise precipitously as tumor cells break down from chemotherapeutic treatment. Dosages depend on uric acid levels as 3 mg IV if uric acid is less than 12 mg/dL or 6 mg IV if uric acid is greater than 12 mg/dL. The provider will repeat the uric acid level draw at a designated interval, possibly every 24 hours, then give an added 3-mg IV dose if the uric acid is greater than 7 mg/dL. The US Food and Drug Administration (FDA)–approved dose is 0.2 mg/kg/day up to 5 days.

Other Select Medication Classes That Affect the Musculoskeletal System

Skeletal Muscle Relaxants

Skeletomuscular pain can arise from many causes. Although everyone experiences some distress at one time or another, severe injury or chronic pain may need extra care. Treatments include drug therapies (eg, analgesics, muscle relaxers) and physical therapy (PT) for severe injuries. Surgery may be an alternative if medications and PT prove ineffective in preserving the quality of life and functionality. Prescribers can use skeletal muscle relaxants for musculoskeletal injuries. These medicines reduce muscle tone (Table 19.5).

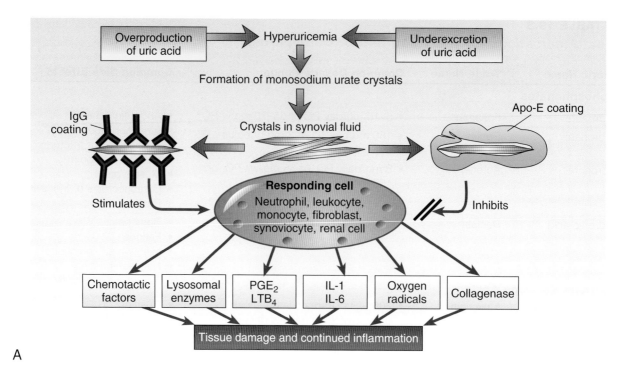

A

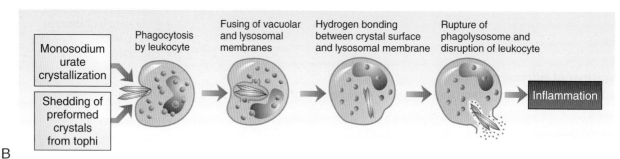

B

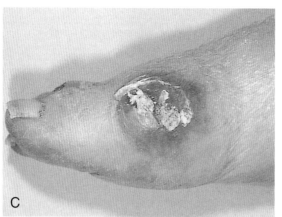

C

FIG. 19.12 Pathogenesis of acute gouty arthritis. (A) Overproduction of uric acid and/or undersecretion of uric acid causes tissue damage and continued inflammation. (B) Monosodium urate crystallization and shedding of preformed crystals from tophi leads to inflammation. (C) Photograph of resultant injury. *Apo-E,* Apolipoprotein E; *IgG,* immunoglobulin G; *IL-1,* interleukin-1; *IL-6,* interleukin-6; *LTB$_4$,* leukotriene B$_4$; *PGE$_2$,* prostaglandin E$_2$. (From McCance KL. *Pathophysiology: The Biologic Basis for Disease in Adults and Children.* 6th ed. St. Louis: Mosby; 2010.)

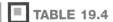

TABLE 19.4
Select Agents for the Treatment of Gout

Generic Name	Trade Name	Common Dosage Range	Common Side Effects
NSAIDs			
ibuprofen	Advil, Motrin IB	• 400–800 mg PO twice daily	• Acute renal failure • Dizziness • Fluid retention • Gastrointestinal ulcer • Hypertension • Nausea
naproxen	Naprosyn	• 500 mg PO twice daily • *During gout attack:* 750 mg once, then 250 mg every 8 hours until the attack subsides	
indomethacin	Indocin[a]	• 50 mg PO 3 times daily *or* 75 mg PO twice daily	
Antigout Agent			
colchicine	Colcrys	• 1.2 mg (2 tabs) PO, then 0.6 mg (1 tab) PO 1 hour later *or* 0.6 mg PO once or twice daily for long-term use to prevent an attack	• Diarrhea • Nausea • Vomiting
Corticosteroids			
prednisone	Deltasone[a]	• 30–40 mg/day PO for 1–2 days, then taper off over 7–10 days	• Fluid retention • High blood pressure • Increased blood sugar
triamcinolone	Kenalog-10 and Kenalog-40	• 10–40 mg INJ (intraarticular); dose depends on joint size	
methylprednisolone	Depo-Medrol	• 4–80 mg INJ (intraarticular); dose depends on joint size	
Xanthine Oxidase Inhibitor			
allopurinol	Zyloprim	• 100–300 mg/day PO (max 800 mg/day); must divide dose if higher than 300 mg	• Diarrhea • Nausea • Rash
febuxostat	Uloric	• 40–80 mg/day PO	
Uricosuric Agent			
probenecid	Benuryl[a]	• 250 mg PO twice daily for 1 wk, then 500 mg PO twice daily (max 2 g/day)	• Dizziness • Flushing • Rash • Stomach upset

[a]Brand discontinued; now available only as generic.

INJ, Injection; *IV,* intravenous; *NSAID,* nonsteroidal antiinflammatory drug; *PO,* oral; *tab,* tablet.

GENERIC NAME: carisoprodol

TRADE NAME: Soma (C-IV)

INDICATION: Musculoskeletal pain

ROUTE OF ADMINISTRATION: Oral

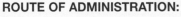

COMMON ADULT DOSAGE: 250–350 mg 3–4 times daily for 2–3 weeks

MECHANISM OF ACTION: Blocks neuronal signaling, leading to muscle relaxation

SIDE EFFECTS: Dizziness, drowsiness, vertigo, headache

AUXILIARY LABELS:
• May cause dizziness or drowsiness
• Avoid alcohol
• *Caution:* Federal law prohibits the transfer of this drug to any person other than the patient for whom it was prescribed.

GENERIC NAME: cyclobenzaprine

TRADE NAMES: Flexeril, Amrix

INDICATION: Muscle spasm

ROUTE OF ADMINISTRATION: Oral

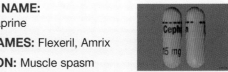

COMMON ADULT DOSAGES: *Immediate release:* 5–10 mg 3 times daily; *extended-release:* 15–30 mg once daily

MECHANISM OF ACTION: Reduces muscle spasm by a direct effect on the CNS

SIDE EFFECTS: Dizziness, drowsiness, blurred vision, dry mouth, constipation

AUXILIARY LABELS:
• May cause dizziness or drowsiness
• Avoid alcohol

TABLE 19.5
Select Skeletal Muscle Relaxants

Generic Name	Trade Name	Common Dosage Range	Common Side Effects
cyclobenzaprine	Flexeril[a]	• *IR:* 5–10 mg PO 3 times daily • *ER:* 15–30 mg PO once daily	• Dizziness • Drowsiness • Dry mouth • Fatigue
methocarbamol	Robaxin[a]	• 1.5 g PO 4 times daily for 2–3 days, then reduce to 4–4.5 g/day divided into 3–6 doses • 1 g IV/IM every 8 hours for no longer than 3 consecutive days	
carisoprodol (C-IV)	Soma	• 250–350 mg 3 times daily and at bedtime (4 doses daily)	
baclofen	Lioresal[a]	• *Initial:* 5 mg PO 3 times daily (max 80 mg/day) • *Usual dose:* 40–80 mg/day	
metaxalone	Skelaxin	• 800 mg PO 3 or 4 times daily	

[a]Brand discontinued; now available only as generic.
ER, Extended-release; *IM,* intramuscular; *IR,* immediate-release; *IV,* intravenous; *PO,* oral.

GENERIC NAME: tizanidine

TRADE NAME: Zanaflex

INDICATION: Spasticity associated with conditions such as multiple sclerosis and spinal cord injury

ROUTE OF ADMINISTRATION: Oral

COMMON ADULT DOSAGE: *Initial:* 2 mg every 6–8 hours; not to exceed 3 doses/day, titrate up as needed (max 36 mg/day)

MECHANISM OF ACTION: Activates central alpha-2 receptors to reduce the spasmodic activity

SIDE EFFECTS: Dizziness, drowsiness, dry mouth

AUXILIARY LABELS:
• May cause dizziness or drowsiness
• Avoid alcohol

■ Tech Note!

Studies have shown the pharmacokinetics of tizanidine capsules and tablets vary enough to cause differences in efficacy and side effects if the patient changes dosage forms. Health care providers should caution patients about potential gaps in clinical outcomes if they switch from one dosage form to another.

Neuromuscular Blockers

Surgeons will use neuromuscular blocking agents with anesthetics for surgery. Neuromuscular blockers relax skeletal muscles to induce paralysis. They help to place the patient on a ventilator and to suppress the patient's spontaneous breathing after a ventilator is in place. We divide the agents into two major categories: depolarizing and nondepolarizing neuromuscular blockers. Depolarizing agents, such as succinylcholine, mimic the effects of the neurotransmitter acetylcholine. By mimicking acetylcholine, succinylcholine competes with acetylcholine for the cholinergic receptors to cause prolonged depolarization. Succinylcholine prolongs depolarization because acetylcholinesterase cannot rapidly degrade succinylcholine. This prolonged depolarization results in skeletal muscle paralysis.

Nondepolarizing agents also compete with acetylcholine but lack agonist activity at receptors. Instead, nondepolarizing agents block receptor activation by acetylcholine and prevent impulse transmission leading to muscle relaxation. The neuromuscular blocker used depends on the needed anesthetic duration (Table 19.6). Additional smaller doses can prolong the blocking agent's action. Pharmacy technicians may be responsible for filling floor stock orders for these medications for the operating room.

▽ Tech Alert!

Remember the following sound-alike, look-alike drugs:
• alendronate, risedronate, ibandronate
• Trandate versus Tridrate

Do You Remember These Key Points?

● Names of the major components of the musculoskeletal system and their functions
● The primary symptoms of the various musculoskeletal conditions discussed
● Medications used to treat the different musculoskeletal conditions discussed
● The generic and trade names for the drugs discussed in this chapter
● The appropriate auxiliary labels that should be used when filling prescriptions for medicines discussed in this chapter

TABLE 19.6
Select Neuromuscular Blocking Agents

Generic Name	Trade Name	Common Dosage Range	Duration
Depolarizing			
succinylcholine	Anectine	• *Initial:* 0.3–1.1 mg/kg IV • *Maintenance:* variable	2–3 min
Nondepolarizing			
atracurium	Tracrium[a]	• *Initial:* 0.4–0.5 mg/kg IV • *Maintenance:* variable	30–60 min
cisatracurium	Nimbex	• *Initial:* 0.15–0.2 mg/kg IV • *Maintenance:* variable	20–35 min
pancuronium	Pavulon[a]	• *Initial:* 0.06–0.1 mg/kg IV • *Maintenance:* variable	2–3 hours
rocuronium	Zemuron[a]	• *Initial:* 0.6–1.2 mg/kg IV • *Maintenance:* variable	30–60 min
vecuronium	Norcuron[a]	• *Initial:* 0.08–0.1 mg/kg IV • *Maintenance:* variable	60–90 min

[a]Brand discontinued; now available only as generic.

IV, Intravenous.

Review Questions

Multiple Choice Questions

1. _____ attach muscles to bones.
    A. Tendons
    B. Muscle fibers
    C. Ligaments
    D. Fascia
2. Acetaminophen (Tylenol) has all of the following pharmacological actions *except:*
    A. Antiinflammatory
    B. Antipyretic
    C. Analgesic
    D. Acetaminophen has all three actions.
3. Celecoxib (Celebrex) selectively inhibits:
    A. COX-1
    B. COX-2
    C. Mu opioid receptors
    D. Kappa opioid receptors
4. _____ are cells that resorb bone.
    A. Osteophytes
    B. Osteoblasts
    C. Osteoclasts
    D. Osteosarcomas
5. _____ is a selective estrogen receptor modulator (SERM) for osteoporosis.
    A. Alendronate
    B. Raloxifene
    C. Denosumab
    D. Calcitonin salmon
6. A doctor can prescribe _____ once weekly.
    A. Alendronate
    B. Raloxifene
    C. Denosumab
    D. Calcitonin salmon

7. _____ is an intranasal dosage form.
    A. Alendronate
    B. Raloxifene
    C. Denosumab
    D. Calcitonin salmon
8. Opioid analgesics cause each of the following side effects *except:*
    A. Miosis
    B. Euphoria
    C. Diarrhea
    D. Respiratory depression
9. A pharmacy technician correctly identifies _____ as a neuromuscular blocker.
    A. Fentanyl
    B. Ibuprofen
    C. Pancuronium
    D. Carisoprodol
10. The maximum recommended daily dose of acetaminophen for people who are otherwise healthy (do not have liver disease) is:
    A. 1000 mg
    B. 2000 mg
    C. 3000 mg (Tylenol recommends 3000 mg/still 4000 mg with FDA)
    D. 8000 mg
11. _____ is a parathyroid hormone analog for severe osteoporosis.
    A. Alendronate
    B. Teriparatide
    C. Denosumab
    D. None of the above
12. Which is a fentanyl dosage form?
    A. Oral
    B. Transdermal

C. Intravenous

   D. All of the above

13. Constipation is a side effect of which drug?

   A. Celecoxib

   B. Oxycodone

   C. Aspirin

   D. Probenecid

14. _____ may precipitate Reye syndrome in children.

   A. Acetaminophen

   B. Ibuprofen

   C. Aspirin

   D. Naproxen

15. Osteoarthritis is considered a/an:

   A. Autoimmune disorder

   B. A degenerative joint disease

   C. An acute allergic reaction

   D. All of the above

■ Technician's Corner

Mary Price presents to the pharmacy and reports having had a recent ultrasound screening examination of her heel to check her bone mineral density. She says that the examination result was abnormal, and she was instructed to speak with her physician about it. Ms. Price is curious about what medications she can take to prevent osteoporosis.

Using a comprehensive drug reference, look up which drugs and/or supplements are used for osteoporosis prophylaxis and familiarize yourself with potential side effects associated with these medications.

Bibliography

Diab DL, Watts NB. Bisphosphonate drug holiday: who, when, and how long. *Ther Adv Musculoskelet Dis*. 2013;5(3):107-111.

McCance KL. *Pathophysiology: The Biologic Basis for Disease in Adults and Children*. 6th ed. St. Louis: Mosby; 2010.

Patton KT, Thibodeau G. *Mosby's Handbook of Anatomy and Physiology*. St. Louis: Mosby; 2000.

Product Information. *CELEBREX(R) Oral Capsules, Celecoxib Oral Capsules*. New York, NY: GD Searle LLC (per FDA); 2016.

Product Information. *ELITEK(R) Intravenous Injection Powder for Solution, Rasburicase Intravenous Injection Powder for Solution*. Bridgewater, NJ: Sanofi-Aventis U.S. LLC (per FDA); 2015.

Solomon EP. *Introduction to Human Anatomy and Physiology*. 3rd ed. St. Louis: Saunders; 2009.

Websites Referenced

Bone Density Test, Osteoporosis Screening & T-score Interpretation. National Osteoporosis Foundation. Available at: https://www.bonehealthandosteoporosis.org/patients/diagnosis-information/bone-density-examtesting/.

CHAPTER 20

Therapeutic Agents for the Cardiovascular System

Tony Guerra

1. Describe the major components of the cardiovascular system.
2. List the primary symptoms of conditions associated with the dysfunction of the cardiovascular system. In addition, (a) recognize drugs used to treat the conditions related to the cardiovascular system discussed in this chapter, (b) write the generic and trade names for the medications discussed in this chapter, and (c) list appropriate auxiliary labels when filling prescriptions for drugs discussed in this chapter.

Aldosterone A steroid hormone secreted by the adrenal cortex that regulates the salt and water balance in the body

Aneurysm Widen + condition, a balloon-like bulge or dilation of an artery resulting from weakening of the arterial wall

Angina Chest pain caused by an inadequate supply of oxygen to the heart muscle

Angiotensin II A peptide hormone that causes vasoconstriction and a subsequent increase in blood pressure

Anticoagulant Against + coagulation, an agent used to prevent the formation of blood clots

Antihyperlipidemics Against + high + lipids + blood condition, a diverse group of pharmaceuticals used in the treatment of hyperlipidemia or excess lipids in the blood

Aorta The great arterial trunk that carries blood from the heart to be distributed to tissues of the body

Arteriosclerosis Artery + hard + condition, a condition characterized by thickening, loss of elasticity (hardening), and calcification of the arterial walls

Artery A vessel that carries oxygenated blood from the heart to the tissues of the body

Atherosclerosis Thick + hard + condition, the process of progressive thickening and hardening of the walls of medium-sized and large arteries as a result of fat deposits on their inner lining, a specific arteriosclerosis

Atrium The entry chamber on both sides of the heart

Blood pressure The pressure of the blood within the arteries

Capillary A tiny vessel that connects the ends of the smallest arteries (arterioles) to the smallest veins (venules), where exchange of nutrients, waste products, oxygen (O_2), and carbon dioxide (CO_2) occurs

Cardiac muscle A type of muscle tissue found only in the heart

Cardiac output (CO) The amount of blood, in liters, the heart pumps through the circulatory system in a minute

Coagulation Solidification or change from a fluid state to a solid state, as in the formation of a blood clot

Coronary artery Either of two arteries that arise from the aorta (one from the left side and one from the right side) and supply the tissues of the heart itself

Diastole The period when the heart is in a state of relaxation and dilation

Dysrhythmias Abnormal or irregular heart rhythms

Embolus A clump of material, often a blood clot, that travels from one part of the body to another and obstructs a blood vessel; an embolus can consist of any material, including bacteria or air

Endocardium Inside + heart, the thin membrane that lines the interior of the heart; the inner layer of the heart wall

Enzyme A protein that accelerates a reaction by reducing the amount of energy required to initiate the reaction

Epicardium Above + heart, the outer layer of the heart wall; the inner layer of the pericardium

Essential hypertension The most common form of hypertension; it occurs in the absence of any evident cause

Fibrates An antihyperlipidemic drug class that primarily lowers triglycerides

Heart failure (HF) A heart that cannot keep up with demand; failure of the heart to pump blood with normal efficiency

Heterozygous familial hypercholesterolemia (HeFH) A genetic disorder based on a gene that encodes LDLR. Very high low-density lipoprotein (LDL) levels within the blood characterize this disorder

High-density lipoprotein (HDL) A blood-plasma lipoprotein composed of a high proportion of protein with little triglyceride and cholesterol and associated with a decreased probability of developing atherosclerosis

Hyperlipidemia High + lipid + blood condition, also known as hypercholesterolemia—a condition marked by an increase in bloodstream cholesterol that can lead to atherosclerosis, or artery hardening

Hypertension High + tension, high blood pressure

Hypotension Low + tension, low blood pressure

Low-density lipoprotein (LDL) A lipid (fat) and protein combined molecule. It is associated with an increased probability of developing atherosclerosis

Low-density lipoprotein receptor (LDLR) A protein found mainly on liver cells that binds to and removes blood LDL

Lumen A channel within a tube (eg, a blood vessel)

Myocardial infarction (MI) Muscle + heart *and* to stuff + into, myocardial tissue death resulting from sudden deprivation of oxygenated blood flow, often a result of a blood clot plugging a coronary artery; also known as a heart attack

Myocardium Muscle + heart, the middle muscular layer of the heart wall; it consists of cardiac muscle tissue

Nicotinic acid A member of the vitamin B complex; also known as niacin

Nitrates A class of drugs used to treat heart conditions, such as angina

Orthostatic hypotension Straight + standing and low + pressure, a temporary, often rapid lowering of blood pressure, usually related to standing up suddenly

PCSK9 An enzyme that binds to and breaks down LDLR (abbreviation for proprotein convertase subtilisin/kexin type 9)

Pericardium Around + heart, a fluid-filled membrane that surrounds the heart; also called the pericardial sac

Peripheral resistance Vascular resistance to the flow of blood in peripheral arterial vessels

Pulmonary artery Lung + of the, one of two vessels formed as terminal branches of the pulmonary trunk; conveys unaerated blood to the lungs

Renin A protein released by the kidney in response to low sodium levels or blood volume

Secondary hypertension Hypertension that results from an underlying identifiable cause

Statin An informal term for 3-hydroxy-3-methylglutaryl-coenzyme A (HMG-CoA) reductase inhibitors referring to the last six letters in the name of each medication name in the class, for example, atorvastatin, simvastatin. Used for the treatment of hyperlipidemia, primarily to lower LDL cholesterol

Stent A tube inserted into a vessel or passageway to keep it open

Stroke The sudden death of brain cells because oxygen deprivation from a blockage (ischemic stroke) or rupture (hemorrhagic stroke) of an artery to the brain impairs blood flow

Syndrome A set of conditions that occur together

Systole The period when the heart is contracting, specifically when the left ventricle of the heart contracts

Tachycardia Fast + heart + condition, a rapid heart rate, usually defined as greater than 100 beats per minute

Thrombin A blood coagulation enzyme from prothrombin; thrombin reacts with fibrinogen and converts it to fibrin, which is essential in the formation of blood clots; thrombin levels are tested by performing a prothrombin time or partial thromboplastin time blood test

Thrombolytic Clot + dissolve, a medication used to break up a thrombus or blood clot

Thrombosis Clot + condition, the formation or presence of a blood clot in a blood vessel

Transient ischemic attack (TIA) A neurologic event in which the signs and symptoms of a stroke appear but resolve within a short time

Triglyceride (TG) The dominant form of body-stored fat consisting of three fatty acid molecules and a molecule of the alcohol glycerol

Vasoconstriction Vessel + narrow, blood vessel narrowing resulting from contraction of the vessel muscular walls

Vasodilation Vessel + widen, blood vessel widening resulting from muscular vessel wall relaxation

Vein A vessel that carries deoxygenated blood to or toward the heart

Vena cava One of the two large veins that carry deoxygenated blood from the upper (superior vena cava) and lower (inferior vena cava) parts of the body to the right atrium of the heart

Ventricle One of the two lower chambers of the heart

Select Common Drugs for Conditions of the Cardiovascular System

Trade Name	Generic Name	Pronunciation
Alpha-Blockers		
Cardura	doxazosin	(dok-**sah**-zoh-sin)
Hytrin	terazosin	(tehr-**ah**-zoh-sin)
Minipress	prazosin	(**prah**-zoh-sin)
Antiarrhythmics		
Betapace, Betapace AF	sotalol	(soe-**tuh**-lol)
Cordarone,[a] Pacerone	amiodarone	(a-mi-**oh**-duh-rone)
Norpace, Norpace CR	disopyramide	(dye-so-**peer**-uh-mide)
Pronestyl,[a] Procanbid[a]	procainamide	(pro-**cane**-uh-mide)
Quinidex[a]	quinidine	(**kwin**-uh-deen)
Rythmol	propafenone	(proe-puh-**feh**-none)
Tikosyn	dofetilide	(doe-**fet**-uh-lide)
Angiotensin-Converting Enzyme Inhibitors (ACEIs)		
Accupril	quinapril	(**kwin**-uh-pril)
Altace	ramipril	(rah-**mih**-pril)
Capoten[a]	captopril	(**cap**-tuh-pril)
Lotensin	benazepril	(ben-**ayz**-uh-pril)
Monopril[a]	fosinopril	(foe-**sin**-uh-pril)
Prinivil, Zestril	lisinopril	(lih-**sin**-uh-pril)
Vasotec	enalapril	(eh-**nal**-uh-pril)
Angiotensin Receptor Blockers (ARBs)		
Atacand	candesartan	(kan-duh-**sar**-tan)
Avapro	irbesartan	(erb-buh-**sar**-tan)
Cozaar	losartan	(low-**sar**-tan)
Diovan	valsartan	(val-**sar**-tan)
Micardis	telmisartan	(tel-meh-**sar**-tan)
Teveten[a]	eprosartan	(eh-pro-**sar**-tan)

Continued

Select Common Drugs for Conditions of the Cardiovascular System—cont'd

Trade Name	Generic Name	Pronunciation
Beta-Blockers (BBs)		
Brevibloc	esmolol	(**es**-muh-lol)
Inderal[a]	propranolol	(pro-**pran**-uh-lol)
Lopressor	metoprolol	(meh-toe-**pruh**-lol)
Tenormin	atenolol	(uh-**ten**-uh-lol)
Trandate	labetalol	(luh-**bay**-tuh-lol)
Visken[a]	pindolol	(**pin**-duh-lol)
Calcium Channel Blockers (CCBs)		
Calan, Isoptin[a]	verapamil	(ver-**ap**-uh-mill)
Cardene[a]	nicardipine	(nye-**kar**-dih-peen)
Cardizem	diltiazem	(dill-**tie**-uh-zem)
Norvasc	amlodipine	(am-**low**-dih-peen)
Plendil[a]	felodipine	(fe-**low**-dih-peen)
Procardia	nifedipine	(nye-**feh**-dih-peen)

Combination Blood Pressure Medications

Combination	Brand Name	Generic Names
ACE inhibitor + Diuretic	Zestoretic	Lisinopril-Hydrochlorothiazide
ARB + Diuretic	Hyzaar	Losartan-Hydrochlorothiazide
	Benicar HCT	Olmesartan-Hydrochlorothiazide
	Diovan HCT	Valsartan-Hydrochlorothiazide
Diuretic combinations	Maxzide, Dyazide	Triamterene-Hydrochlorothiazide

Trade Name	Generic Name	Pronunciation
Anticoagulants		
Coumadin	warfarin	(**war**-fuh-rin)
	heparin	(heh-**puh**-rin)
Direct Thrombin Inhibitor		
Pradaxa	dabigatran	(**da**-bi-**guh**-tran)
Low-Molecular-Weight Heparins		
Fragmin	dalteparin	(**dal**-tuh-**pair**-in)
Lovenox	enoxaparin	(eh-**nox**-uh-**pair**-in)
Antiplatelet Agents		
Aggrenox	aspirin/dipyridamole	(**as**-pih-rin/dye-pehr-**ih**-duh-mole)
Ecotrin	aspirin	(**as**-pih-rin)
Plavix	clopidogrel	(kloh-**pid**-uh-grel)
Nitrates		
Monoket[a]	isosorbide mononitrate	(**eye**-soe-**sor**-bide **mon**-oh-**nye**-trate)
Isordil Titradose	isosorbide dinitrate	(**eye**-soe-**sor**-bide dye-**nye**-trate)
Nitrostat, Tridil[a]	nitroglycerin	(**nye**-troe-**glis**-uh-rin)
Antihyperlipidemic Agents		
Altoprev	lovastatin	(low-**vuh**-stat-in)
Antara, Lipofen, Tricor	fenofibrate	(**fen**-no-**fye**-brate)
Colestid	colestipol	(koe-**les**-tih-pole)
Crestor	rosuvastatin	(row-**soo**-vuh-stat-in)
Lescol	fluvastatin	(**floo**-vuh-stat-in)
Lipitor	atorvastatin	(a-**tor**-vuh-stat-in)
Lopid	gemfibrozil	(gem-**fib**-row-**zil**)
Lovaza	omega-3–acid ethyl esters	(oh-**may**-guh 3 **as**-id **eth**-il **es**-ters)

Trade Name	Generic Name	Pronunciation
Niacor	niacin	(**nye**-uh-sin)
Pravachol	pravastatin	(**pra**-vuh-stat-in)
Questran	cholestyramine	(koe-**les**-teer-uh-meen)
Trilipix, Fibricor	fenofibric acid	(**fen**-oh-fye-**brik** as-id)
Welchol	colesevelam	(**koe**-leh-**sev**-uh-lam)
Zetia	ezetimibe	(eh-**zet**-uh-mibe)
Zocor	simvastatin	(sym-vuh-**stat**-in)
Diuretics		
Aldactone	spironolactone	(spear-**on**-uh-**lak**-tone)
Aquazide H, Hydrocot, Microzide,[a] Zide	hydrochlorothiazide	(hye-droh-klor-oh-**thy**-uh-zide)
Bumex[a]	bumetanide	(byew-**met**-uh-nide)
Demadex	torsemide	(**tore**-seh-mide)
Diamox[a]	acetazolamide	(ah-see-tuh-**zole**-a-mide)
Diuril	chlorothiazide	(klor-oh-**thye**-uh-zide)
Dyrenium	triamterene	(try-**am**-tuh-reen)
Lasix	furosemide	(feur-**oh**-suh-myde)
Thrombolytics		
Activase	alteplase (t-PA)	(**al**-tuh-**place**)
Retavase	reteplase	(reh-**tuh**-place)
TNKase	tenecteplase	(ten-**ek**-tuh-place)

[a]Brand discontinued; now available only as generic.

The cardiovascular system is a network of complex interactions involving the blood, lungs, kidneys, arteries, veins, and heart muscle. We begin with a heart anatomy overview, followed by common conditions affecting the heart. The last section of this chapter discusses treatments available for heart conditions, with an emphasis on medication use. Pharmacy technicians fill many heart medication prescriptions over their careers. It is important to learn basic classification information to assist the pharmacist.

Anatomy of the Heart and Vasculature System

The heart sits in the chest cavity between the lungs. It is a large muscle about the size of a fist that initiates systemic arterial pulse waves, causing blood to circulate throughout the body and supply it with nutrition and oxygen (Fig. 20.1). The heart muscle is called **cardiac muscle. Arteries** are large blood vessels that extend from the heart. These arteries flow into smaller arterioles and ultimately into tiny blood vessels called **capillaries.** The capillaries facilitate oxygen and nutrient exchange with the body's tissues.

A healthy heart beats 60 to 100 times per minute, and connective tissue called the **pericardium** surrounds it. Ligaments anchor it to the chest wall and diaphragm. The heart wall includes three main layers:

1. **Endocardium** (inner layer): The endocardium has a smooth, accordion pleat–like surface, which allows the heart wall to collapse when it contracts.

2. **Myocardium** (middle muscular layer): The myocardium is the heart muscle that contracts to facilitate a heartbeat.

3. **Epicardium** (outer layer): The epicardium is the outer heart wall layer. The coronary arteries that supply the heart with oxygenated blood and the coronary veins that return deoxygenated blood to the heart are in the epicardium.

Oxygenation

The heart has two sides, each of which has two chambers (Fig. 20.2). The first two chambers include the right **atrium** and the right **ventricle.** Blood circulates through the body, exchanging oxygen, nutrients, and other substances in tissues and organs. The blood returns to the heart via two large **veins** called the superior **vena cava** and the inferior vena cava. The superior vena cava transports blood from the upper portion of the body, and the inferior vena cava carries blood from the lower part of the body back to the heart. From the vena cava, blood empties into the right atrium and travels into the right ventricle. During a heartbeat, the right ventricle contracts, expelling blood into the **pulmonary arteries;** the pulmonary arteries carry blood to the lungs, which fully oxygenate the blood from room air (see Chapter 21). Interestingly, the pulmonary arteries carry deoxygenated blood, whereas most arteries carry oxygenated blood. Remember, it is the direction a vessel travels to or from the heart that makes it an artery or vein. The left atrium receives fully oxygenated blood from the lungs via the pulmonary veins. Blood then passes into the left ventricle. The left ventricle

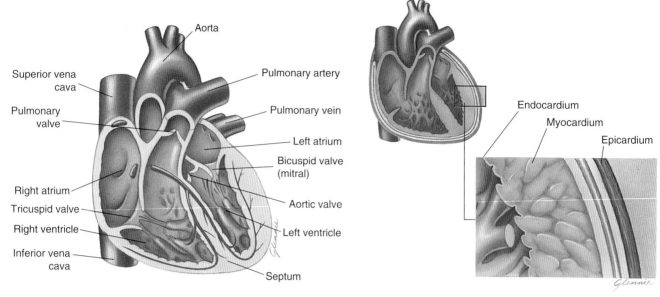

FIG. 20.1 **Anatomy of the heart.** (From Gerdin J. *Health Careers Today*. 5th ed. St. Louis; Mosby; 2012.)

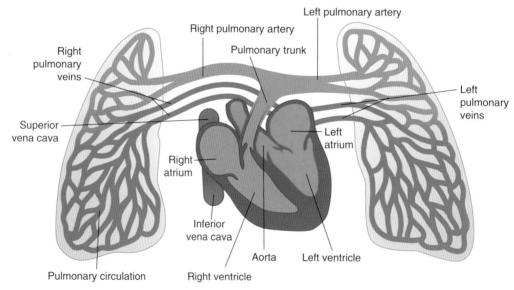

FIG. 20.2 Blood oxygenation.

contracts, expelling the blood through the **aorta** and outward through the vasculature to the body (Fig. 20.3). Although the heart is efficient, it still must be oxygenated, just as other organs are. The main arteries that supply blood to the heart are called the **coronary arteries.**

Cardiac Conduction System

The cardiac conduction system provides the electrical charge that makes the heart pump. This system regulates the heart rate and rhythm. Two nodes, the sinoatrial (SA) node and the atrioventricular (AV) node (Fig. 20.4), initiate and propagate cardiac conduction. The SA node, in the upper right atrium wall, starts the impulse. The signal proceeds down the AV

node in the septum between the right atrium and right ventricle. From the AV node, the impulse continues to the ventricles to initiate a ventricular beat.

The Cardiac Cycle

The *cardiac cycle* is an event series that occurs in one complete heartbeat and has two sequences (Fig. 20.5):

1. **Systole:** The myocardium squeezes blood from the heart chamber into the pulmonary artery or aorta.
2. **Diastole:** Blood refills the chambers (relaxation). During diastole, the atria contract to pack 20% more blood into the ventricles. Most of the body's blood supply is cycled every minute through the heart.

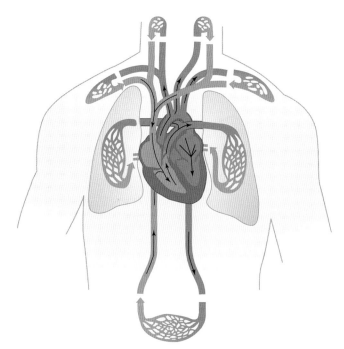

FIG. 20.3 Circulation of blood through the body.

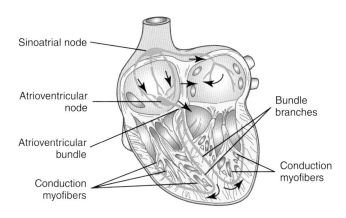

FIG. 20.4 Conduction system of the heart. (From Applegate E. *The Anatomy and Physiology Learning System.* 4th ed. St. Louis: Elsevier; 2001.)

Regulation of the Heart and Vasculature

The parasympathetic and sympathetic branches of the autonomic nervous system have opposite effects on heart rate (see Chapter 17). The parasympathetic nervous system slows the heart. The sympathetic nervous system increases heart rate. In response to exercise or emotional stress, the adrenal glands release norepinephrine and epinephrine to increase heart rate.

Blood pressure is the force exerted by the blood against the inner walls of the blood vessels. The blood flow depends on the heart rate and force of contractions. When the heart works harder to increase **cardiac output (CO),** blood flow increases, causing a rise in blood pressure and vice versa. Blood volume also affects blood flow. For example, blood pressure can fall in a dehydrated patient and blood pressure can rise with excess body fluid. We express blood pressure readings as systolic over diastolic pressure.

Peripheral resistance is resistance to blood flow caused by blood viscosity and the force required to pump blood through vessels. When peripheral resistance increases, blood pressure increases. As the diameter of blood vessels decreases (**vasoconstriction**), peripheral resistance increases. **Vasodilation,** on the other hand, is an increase in blood vessel diameter that results in a peripheral resistance decrease.

Hormones can also regulate blood pressure. In response to low blood pressure, kidneys can release **renin.** This **enzyme** acts on a plasma protein (angiotensinogen), initiating a series of reactions that produce **angiotensin II,** a hormone that causes vasoconstriction. Angiotensin II also works indirectly to maintain blood pressure by signaling the adrenal glands to increase their **aldosterone** output. This hormone raises kidney sodium retention, resulting in greater fluid retention and increased blood volume. This system is the renin-angiotensin-aldosterone system (Fig. 20.6).

Common Medication Classes Used to Treat Cardiac Conditions

Because many different agents treat heart conditions (eg, coronary artery disease [CAD]) and their causes (eg, hypertension and high cholesterol levels), it is vital to understand medication types, mechanisms of action, and possible side effects. Before discussing individual cardiovascular conditions, let us first discuss some standard drug classes for cardiac diseases. Many cardiac drugs work for multiple cardiovascular conditions. The mnemonic "ABCD" (*a*ngiotensin-converting enzyme [ACE] inhibitors, *b*eta-blockers, *c*alcium channel blockers, and *d*iuretics) provides a framework to remember these drug classes. These are the common classifications of agents for heart conditions. This is not necessarily the order in which they are prescribed. Other available classifications are also described in this chapter. Table 20.1 provides an overview of cardiovascular medication classes.

Angiotensin-Converting Enzyme Inhibitors

ACE inhibitors (ACEIs) help reduce blood pressure by dilating arteries. Recall from Fig. 20.6 that ACE converts angiotensin I to angiotensin II, resulting in less vasoconstriction. When blood levels of the enzyme angiotensin II rise, blood vessels narrow; that is, they vasoconstrict in the periphery and kidneys. By using an ACEI to block the conversion of angiotensin I to angiotensin II, the opposite effect, vasodilation, occurs. Vasodilation results in lower blood pressure. As such, the ACEIs' net effect is peripheral vasodilation and blood pressure lowering. However, make sure to avoid using in pregnancy to reduce the chance of congenital disabilities.

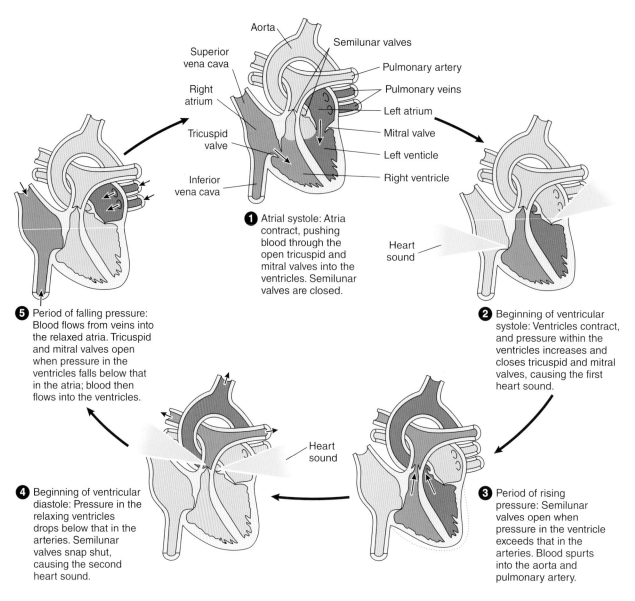

Aorta

Semilunar valves

Superior vena cava

Pulmonary artery

Right atrium

Pulmonary veins

Left atrium

Tricuspid valve

Mitral valve

Left venticle

Inferior vena cava

Right ventricle

1 Atrial systole: Atria contract, pushing blood through the open tricuspid and mitral valves into the ventricles. Semilunar valves are closed.

Heart sound

5 Period of falling pressure: Blood flows from veins into the relaxed atria. Tricuspid and mitral valves open when pressure in the ventricles falls below that in the atria; blood then flows into the ventricles.

2 Beginning of ventricular systole: Ventricles contract, and pressure within the ventricles increases and closes tricuspid and mitral valves, causing the first heart sound.

Heart sound

4 Beginning of ventricular diastole: Pressure in the relaxing ventricles drops below that in the arteries. Semilunar valves snap shut, causing the second heart sound.

3 Period of rising pressure: Semilunar valves open when pressure in the ventricle exceeds that in the arteries. Blood spurts into the aorta and pulmonary artery.

FIG. 20.5 Blood flow through the heart during the cardiac cycle. (From Solomon EP. *Introduction to Human Anatomy and Physiology*. 3rd. ed. Philadelphia: Saunders; 2009.)

◼ Tech Note!

A potential side effect of ACEIs is a characteristic "ACEI cough." This dry, hacking cough does not resolve over time, and providers often switch patients to an alternative class of medications (ARBs).

GENERIC NAME: lisinopril

TRADE NAMES: Prinivil, Zestril

INDICATION: Acute myocardial infarction, heart failure, hypertension

ROUTE OF ADMINISTRATION: Oral

COMMON ADULT DOSAGE: 5–40 mg once daily

MECHANISM OF ACTION: Angiotensin-converting enzyme inhibitor (prevents the conversion of angiotensin I to angiotensin II, thus leading to vasodilation)

SIDE EFFECTS: Dizziness, headache, dry cough

AUXILIARY LABEL: May cause dizziness/drowsiness

GENERIC NAME: benazepril

TRADE NAME: Lotensin

INDICATION: Hypertension, heart failure

ROUTE OF ADMINISTRATION: Oral

COMMON ADULT DOSAGE: 20–80 mg taken in 1 or 2 doses

MECHANISM OF ACTION: Angiotensin-converting enzyme inhibitor (prevents the conversion of angiotensin I to angiotensin II, thus leading to vasodilation)

SIDE EFFECTS: Dizziness, headache, dry cough

AUXILIARY LABEL: May cause dizziness/drowsiness

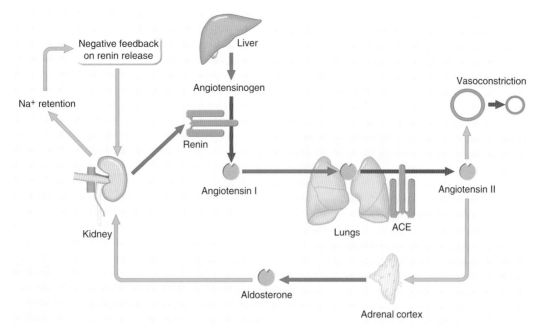

FIG. 20.6 Renin-angiotensin-aldosterone system. *ACE,* Angiotensin-converting enzyme. (From Page C, et al. *Integrated Pharmacology.* 3rd ed. St. Louis: Mosby; 2006.)

◼ TABLE 20.1
Classification of Blood Pressure[a]

Classification	Systolic Pressure (mm Hg)		Diastolic Pressure (mm Hg)
Normal	<120	and	<80
Elevated	120–129	and	<80
Hypertension			
Stage 1 hypertension	130–139	or	80–89
Stage 2 hypertension	>140	or	>90
Hypertensive crisis	>180	and/or	>120

[a]Individuals with SBP and DBP in two categories should be designated to the higher BP category. BP indicates blood pressure (based on an average of two or more occasions).
Whelton PK, et al. 2017 ACC/AHA/AAPA/ABC/ACPM/AGS/APhA/ASH/ASPC/NMA/PCNA Guideline for the Prevention, Detection, Evaluation, and Management of High Blood Pressure in Adults. *J Am Coll Cardiol.* 2018;71(19): e127-e248.

Angiotensin II Receptor Antagonists

Angiotensin II receptor antagonists, also known as *angiotensin II receptor blockers (ARBs),* work by inhibiting the effects of angiotensin II on angiotensin II receptors. The net results are very similar to those of ACEIs, including a reduction in blood pressure as a result of net vasodilation. As with ACEIs, prescribers should avoid them in pregnancy. Caution using with potassium supplements or potassium sparing drugs.

◼ Tech Note!

One of the main clinical differences between ACEIs and ARBs is that ARBs very rarely cause a dry cough as a side effect. In contrast, patients taking ACEIs can experience a dry cough.

GENERIC NAME: losartan

TRADE NAME: Cozaar

INDICATIONS: Hypertension, stroke prophylaxis, proteinuria, diabetic nephropathy

ROUTE OF ADMINISTRATION: Oral

COMMON ADULT DOSAGE: 25–100 mg once daily or twice daily in divided doses

MECHANISM OF ACTION: Antagonizes angiotensin II receptors, blocking the vasoconstrictive effects of angiotensin II

SIDE EFFECTS: Dizziness, nausea, muscle pain

GENERIC NAME: valsartan

TRADE NAME: Diovan

INDICATIONS: Hypertension, heart failure

ROUTE OF ADMINISTRATION: Oral

COMMON ADULT DOSAGE: 80–320 mg once daily

MECHANISM OF ACTION: Antagonizes angiotensin II receptors, blocking the vasoconstrictive effects of angiotensin II

SIDE EFFECTS: Dizziness, nausea, muscle pain

◼ Tech Note!

Generic drug names often provide a clue to the drug class to which they belong. ARBs often end in "-sartan," whereas ACEIs end in "-pril." Beta-blockers typically end in "-olol." These are the United States Adopted Names (USAN) stems in the suffix position for these drug classes.

Entresto

In 2015 the US Food and Drug Administration (FDA) approved Entresto, a combination medication for heart failure (HF). It contains valsartan, an ARB, as well as a new medication named sacubitril. Sacubitril inhibits neprilysin, an enzyme that generally affects endogenous peptides involved with blood pressure.

GENERIC NAME: sacubitril/valsartan

TRADE NAME: Entresto

INDICATION: Heart failure

ROUTE OF ADMINISTRATION: Oral

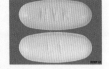

COMMON ADULT DOSAGE: *Initial dosage:* sacubitril 24 mg/valsartan 26 mg–sacubitril 49 mg/valsartan 51 mg twice daily. *Target dosage:* sacubitril 97 mg/valsartan 103 mg twice daily

MECHANISMS OF ACTION: Valsartan is an ARB; sacubitril has vasodilatory effects because of neprilysin inhibition

SIDE EFFECTS: Hypotension, hyperkalemia, dizziness

AUXILIARY LABELS:
- May cause dizziness
- Do not use if pregnant

Renin Inhibitors

Another way to alter the renin-angiotensin-aldosterone system is to use aliskiren (Tekturna). Aliskiren inhibits renin, resulting in many downstream effects, including reduced aldosterone secretion, less water retention, and less vasoconstriction. All of these effects lead to a decrease in blood pressure. Aliskiren is not commonly used in the United States anymore, but when it is, it is often used in conjunction with other blood pressure medications, including amlodipine and hydrochlorothiazide.

GENERIC NAME: aliskiren

TRADE NAME: Tekturna

INDICATION: Hypertension

ROUTE OF ADMINISTRATION: Oral

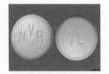

COMMON ADULT DOSAGE: 150 mg once daily, can increase up to 300 mg once daily

MECHANISM OF ACTION: Directly inhibits renin, causing multiple downstream effects to decrease blood pressure

SIDE EFFECTS: Dizziness, headache, hyperkalemia, diarrhea

AUXILIARY LABEL: May cause dizziness/headache

Beta-Blockers

Beta-blockers block both norepinephrine and epinephrine from binding to beta-adrenergic receptors. Blocking these receptors reduces heart rate, which can help lower blood pressure and regulate heartbeat in patients with **tachycardia.** Beta-blockers can act at two sites, the beta-1 and beta-2 receptor sites. Beta-1 receptors are located in the heart, and beta-2 receptors are located in the lungs and arteries. The actions of beta-blocker medications can be specific or nonspecific. Nonspecific agents affect both beta-1 and beta-2 receptors, whereas specific beta-blockers affect only beta-1 receptors in the heart and have weak action in the lungs.

A nonspecific agent, which affects both beta-1 and beta-2 receptors, is unsuitable for patients with asthma because blocking beta-2 receptors in the lungs and bronchi leads to bronchoconstriction (see Chapter 21). For this reason, providers prefer beta-1–selective beta-blockers for treating cardiovascular conditions.

GENERIC NAME: atenolol

TRADE NAME: Tenormin

INDICATIONS: Hypertension, angina, myocardial infarction

ROUTE OF ADMINISTRATION: Oral

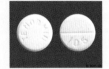

COMMON ADULT DOSAGE: 25–100 mg once daily

MECHANISM OF ACTION: Cardioselective beta-1 receptor blocker

SIDE EFFECTS: Dizziness, drowsiness, fatigue

AUXILIARY LABEL: May cause dizziness/drowsiness

GENERIC NAME: metoprolol tartrate and metoprolol succinate

TRADE NAMES: Lopressor (metoprolol tartrate), Toprol XL (metoprolol succinate)

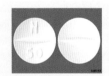

INDICATION: Hypertension, angina, myocardial infarction, heart failure

ROUTES OF ADMINISTRATION: Oral; intravenous

COMMON ADULT DOSAGES: Metoprolol tartrate immediate-release (IR): 50–200 mg twice daily. Metoprolol succinate extended-release (XL): 25–100 mg/day

MECHANISM OF ACTION: Cardioselective beta-1 receptor blocker

SIDE EFFECTS: Dizziness, drowsiness, fatigue

AUXILIARY LABEL: May cause dizziness/drowsiness

GENERIC NAME: propranolol

TRADE NAMES: Inderal LA

INDICATIONS: Hypertension, angina, atrial fibrillation, tremor, migraine prophylaxis

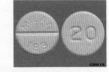

ROUTES OF ADMINISTRATION: Oral; intravenous

COMMON ADULT DOSAGES: *IR for hypertension:* 40–160 mg twice daily. *LA:* 80–160 mg once daily

MECHANISM OF ACTION: Nonselective beta-receptor blocker

SIDE EFFECTS: Dizziness, drowsiness, fatigue

AUXILIARY LABEL: May cause dizziness/drowsiness

Tech Note!

Propranolol is a beta-blocker that readily crosses the blood-brain barrier. Because of this, propranolol is useful for many central nervous system conditions, including migraine prophylaxis and tumor treatment.

Calcium Channel Blockers

Calcium channel blockers (CCBs) reduce the heart muscle and blood vessel calcium influx leading to vascular smooth muscle relaxation, which leads to vasodilation and lower blood pressure. The two main CCB classifications include dihydropyridines and nondihydropyridines. Dihydropyridine CCBs (eg, nifedipine and amlodipine) have a greater effect on the peripheral vasculature and primarily treat high blood pressure. Diltiazem and verapamil, the two currently available nondihydropyridine CCBs, affect the heart in addition to the vasculature and can help with certain dysrhythmias.

Tech Note!

Unlike many other drug classes, not all generic calcium channel blockers are interchangeable with their brand-name counterparts. When substituting a generic calcium channel blocker for a brand-name it is essential to check the Orange Book, provided by the FDA, to choose the correct medication.

GENERIC NAME: diltiazem

TRADE NAMES: Cardizem CD, Cardizem LA, Cardizem SR,[a] Dilacor XR,[a] Tiazac

INDICATIONS: Angina, hypertension, atrial fibrillation

ROUTES OF ADMINISTRATION: Oral; intravenous

COMMON ADULT DOSAGE: Dosage is highly variable, depending on dosage form and condition treated

MECHANISMS OF ACTION: Blocks calcium channels, leading to relaxation of muscle and vasodilation

SIDE EFFECTS: Dizziness, headache, gingival hyperplasia, arrhythmias

AUXILIARY LABEL: May cause dizziness

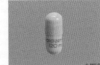

[a]Brand no longer available.

GENERIC NAME: amlodipine

TRADE NAME: Norvasc

INDICATIONS: Hypertension, angina

ROUTE OF ADMINISTRATION: Oral

COMMON ADULT DOSAGE: 5–10 mg once daily

MECHANISMS OF ACTION: Blocks calcium channels, leading to relaxation of muscle and vasodilation

SIDE EFFECTS: Dizziness, drowsiness, peripheral edema

AUXILIARY LABEL: May cause dizziness/drowsiness

Conditions Affecting the Cardiovascular System

Diseases and conditions affecting cardiovascular health include hypertension, HF, hypercholesterolemia, dysrhythmias, and congenital heart disease, among others. Cardiovascular disease is rampant in the United States and other countries. An exhaustive review of cardiovascular diseases is beyond the scope of this chapter; however, the following sections provide an overview of common conditions in both ambulatory and inpatient settings.

Common Conditions

Hypertension

Hypertension, or high blood pressure, affects millions of Americans. This disease gained the moniker "silent killer" because few noticeable signs accompany it. When the cause of hypertension cannot be established, we call it **essential hypertension.** Of those with hypertension, approximately 19 in 20 have essential hypertension, and 1 in 20 has an identifiable cause, such as medications, certain kidney diseases (eg, renal artery stenosis), and diseases of the adrenal glands (eg, Cushing syndrome), to name a few. Hypertension with a known cause is called **secondary hypertension.** Some patients with severe hypertension may have symptoms such as nosebleeds and/or headaches; however, most people are asymptomatic. This lack of symptoms is why blood pressure monitoring is essential. A blood pressure cuff measures blood pressure in millimeters of mercury (mm Hg). Whatever hypertension's cause, the result is that the heart must work harder to pump blood through the vascular system. Four stages of blood pressure have been described (Table 20.2).

Tech Note!

Physicians and pharmacists should inform patients with hypertension that many over-the-counter agents can affect blood pressure. These include nonsteroidal antiinflammatory drugs (NSAIDs), antihistamines, decongestants, and some cold and allergy remedies.

TABLE 20.2
Select Drug Classes Used in the Treatment of Cardiovascular Conditions

Drug Classification	General Use	Generic Name	Trade Name	General Effect
Angiotensin-converting enzyme (ACE) inhibitors	Hypertension	benazepril	Lotensin	Prevent blood vessel constriction
		captopril	Capoten[a]	
		fosinopril	Monopril[a]	
		lisinopril	Prinivil, Zestril	
		moexipril	Univasc[a]	
		ramipril	Altace	
Antiplatelet agents	Thrombosis	aspirin	Ecotrin	Prevent blood clot formation
		clopidogrel	Plavix	
Beta-blockers	Hypertension	acebutolol	Sectral	Reduce workload of the heart
		bisoprolol	Zebeta[a]	
		metoprolol	Lopressor, Toprol XL	
		nadolol	Corgard	
		pindolol	Visken[a]	
Bile acid sequestrants	Hypercholesterolemia	cholestyramine	Prevalite, Questran	Lower cholesterol
		colestipol	Colestid	
Calcium channel blockers	Hypertension	diltiazem	Cardizem CD, Cardizem LA	Increase blood flow and decrease vessel constriction in the heart
		nifedipine	Adalat CC, Procardia XL	
		verapamil	Calan SR, Isoptin[a]	
Diuretics	Hypertension, edema	bumetanide	Bumex[a]	Reduce fluid volume
		chlorothiazide	Diuril	
		furosemide	Lasix	
		hydrochlorothiazide	Esidrex,[a] Microzide	
		metolazone		
		spironolactone	Aldactone	
		triamterene	Dyrenium	
Nitrates	Angina	isosorbide dinitrate	Dilatrate-SR, Isordil Titradose	Relax blood vessels, allowing more blood to reach the heart
		nitroglycerin	Nitrostat, Nitro-Dur[a]	
Statins	Hypercholesterolemia	atorvastatin	Lipitor	Lower cholesterol
		lovastatin	Altoprev	
		pravastatin	Pravachol	
		simvastatin	Zocor	

[a]Brand discontinued; now available only as generic.

Prognosis

With proper diet (and medications, if necessary), hypertension can be effectively controlled.

Non-Drug Treatment

Individuals should have blood pressure measured regularly to identify hypertension early. Some nonpharmacological strategies may help with this condition. Research suggests that even mild hypertension can lead to problems later in life because of the extra work placed on the heart.

Many hypertensive risk factors cannot be changed, such as family history. However, the following lifestyle changes can help manage hypertension:
- Maintaining a healthy weight
- Engaging in regular physical activity
- Avoiding high-sodium foods, such as potato chips, pickles, canned soups, and processed meat (eg, bacon, cold cuts), in addition to table salt
- Increasing daily intake of fruits and vegetables
- Limiting alcohol intake (no more than two drinks per day for men and one per day for women)

- Reducing stress through regular relaxation techniques
- Stopping or avoiding smoking

Drug Treatment

If lifestyle modifications fail, medications may be prescribed. First-line therapy for patients with hypertension usually includes an ACE inhibitor, ARB, calcium channel blockers, or thiazide diuretic. Race and other factors may cause us to prefer a specific drug class. Although we may only use one medication to start, we may need a combination of medications in uncontrolled hypertension. Common combinations include an ACE inhibitor + thiazide diuretic or ARB + thiazide diuretic. Table 20.3 provides information on select agents for hypertension treatment.

Hypertension During Pregnancy

Hypertension during pregnancy is common, and it is divided into four types: chronic hypertension, gestational hypertension, preeclampsia, and preeclampsia superimposed on chronic hypertension. Unfortunately, ACE inhibitors, ARBs, and aliskiren carry a black box warning for birth defects, so they are contraindicated. The patient should discontinue these immediately if a patient is or plans to become pregnant. Medications safe in pregnancy include the beta-blocker labetalol, the calcium channel blocker nifedipine, and an alpha-2 adrenergic agonist methyldopa. The American College of Obstetricians and Gynecologists recommends a blood pressure goal of 120–160 mm Hg systolic and 80–110 mm Hg diastolic for pregnant women.

■ TABLE 20.3
Select Medications Used for the Treatment of Hypertension

Generic Name	Trade Name	Common Dosage Range	Common Side Effects
Angiotensin-Converting Enzyme (ACE) Inhibitors			
benazepril	Lotensin	• 20–80 mg PO once daily or 2 divided doses daily	• Angioedema • Cough • Hyperkalemia • Hypotension
lisinopril	Prinivil, Zestril	• 5–40 mg PO once daily	
captopril	Capoten[a]	• 25 mg PO 2–3 times daily	
ramipril	Altace	• 2.5–20 mg PO once daily or in 2 divided doses daily (max 20 mg/day)	
enalapril	Vasotec	• 2.5–40 mg PO once daily or 2 divided doses daily (max 40 mg/day)	
Beta-Blockers			
nadolol	Corgard	• 40–120 mg PO once a day	• Atrioventricular (AV) block • Bradycardia • Dizziness • Fatigue • Hypotension
metoprolol	Lopressor	• 50–200 mg/day PO or twice daily (max 450 mg/day)	
	Toprol-XL	• 50–200 mg PO once daily (max 400 mg/day)	
atenolol	Tenormin	• 25–100 mg PO once a day (max 100 mg/day)	
propranolol	Inderal[a]	• *IR:* 80–240 mg/day PO divided 2–3 times daily • *LA:* 80–160 mg once daily	
labetalol	Trandate[a]	• 100–400 mg PO twice daily • 20 mg IV push over 2 min	
carvedilol	Coreg CR	• *IR:* 6.25–25 mg PO twice daily • *ER:* 20–80 mg PO once daily (max 80 mg/day)	
Angiotensin Receptor Blockers (ARBs)			
losartan	Cozaar	• 25–100 mg PO once daily or 2 divided doses daily	• Hyperkalemia • Orthostatic hypotension
valsartan	Diovan	• 80–320 mg PO once daily	
olmesartan	Benicar	• 20–40 mg PO once daily	
candesartan	Atacand	• 8–32 mg PO once daily or 2 divided doses daily	
Direct Renin Inhibitor			
aliskiren	Tekturna	• Initially 150 mg PO once daily, may increase to a max of 300 mg/day	• Diarrhea • Hyperkalemia • Rash
Calcium Channel Blockers: Dihydropyridines			
nifedipine	Adalat CC, Procardia XL	• 30–90 mg PO once daily (max 120 mg/day)	• Constipation • Dizziness • Gingival overgrowth • Headache • Peripheral edema
amlodipine	Norvasc	• 5–10 mg PO once daily	
nicardipine	Cardene[a]	• 20–40 mg PO 3 times daily	

Continued

TABLE 20.3
Select Medications Used for the Treatment of Hypertension—cont'd

Generic Name	Trade Name	Common Dosage Range	Common Side Effects
Calcium Channel Blockers: Nondihydropyridines			
diltiazem	Cardizem CD, Cardizem LA	• 180–360 mg PO once daily (max 480–540 mg/day)	• AV block • Bradycardia • Dizziness
verapamil	Calan SR	• *IR:* 80–120 mg 3 times daily (max 480 mg/day) • *ER:* 180–480 mg/day PO divided daily to twice a day (max 480 mg/day)	• Edema • Headache • Pain
Loop Diuretics			
furosemide	Lasix	• 20–80 mg PO once daily or 2 divided doses daily	• Headache • Hypokalemia
bumetanide	Bumex[a]	• 0.5–2mg PO once daily or 2 divided doses daily (max 10 mg/day)	• Hypotension • Weakness
Thiazide Diuretics			
hydrochlorothiazide (HCTZ)	Microzide[a]	• 12.5–50 mg PO once daily or 2 divided doses a day (max 100 mg/day)	• Hyperglycemia • Hypokalemia
chlorothiazide	Diuril	• 500–2000 mg once daily or 2 divided doses daily	• Hyponatremia • Hypotension
metolazone		• 2.5–5 mg PO once daily for hypertension; 2.5–10 mg PO once daily (max 20 mg/day) for edema-associated heart failure	• Photosensitivity
Potassium-Sparing Diuretics			
spironolactone	Aldactone	• 25–100 mg PO once daily day or 2 divided doses daily	• Decreased libido • Gynecomastia • Hyperkalemia
triamterene	Dyrenium	• 50–100 mg PO once daily in single or in 2 divided doses for hypertension; 100–300 mg PO once daily or 2 divided doses daily (max 300 mg/day) for edema	• Hyperkalemia • Hypotension • Muscle cramps
Alpha-1 Receptor Blockers			
doxazosin	Cardura	• 1–16 mg PO once daily (max 16 mg/day)	• Dizziness • Headache
	Cardura XL (extended-release)	• 4 mg PO once daily with breakfast, then titrate upward to 8 mg PO once daily	• Orthostasis • Reflex tachycardia
terazosin	Hytrin	• 1–10 mg PO at bedtime (max 20 mg/day)	
prazosin	Minipress	• *Initial:* 1 mg PO 2 or 3 times daily • *Usual:* 6–15 mg in divided doses	
Alpha-2 Adrenergic Agonists			
methyldopa	Aldomet[a]	• 250–1000 mg/day in 2–3 divided doses	• Dry mouth • Hepatitis
clonidine	Catapres	• *IR:* 0.1–0.4 mg PO twice daily (max 2.4 mg/day)	• Rebound hypertension if withdrawn too fast • Sedation

[a]Brand discontinued; now available only as generic.

ER, Extended-release; *IR,* immediate-release; *IV,* intravenous; *PO,* oral; *prn,* pro re nata, Latin for "as needed."

Hypotension

Hypotension, by definition, is low blood pressure. One of the more common problems that people experience is **orthostatic hypotension.** This lowered blood pressure occurs because a large amount of blood remains in the lower extremities (ankles and feet). When a person stands quickly, the blood returning to the heart decreases considerably, and the body responds by increasing the heartbeat, compensating for the lack of blood flow. This rapid shift in position results in a feeling of lightheadedness. Symptoms of hypotension include syncope (fainting) and/or dizziness. For people who have chronic hypotension, physicians may recommend non-drug therapies and/or may prescribe medication to help increase blood pressure.

Prognosis

With proper medical treatment and lifestyle changes, hypotension can be effectively controlled in most cases.

Non-Drug Treatment

Adjustments in medications may alleviate hypotension resulting from medication use. Increasing salt intake can also raise blood pressure. However, this can be done only if a salt increase does not affect comorbid medical conditions. Drinking more water helps increase bloodstream fluid volume and relieves dehydration. For patients with orthostatic hypotension, moving or standing up slowly can help minimize symptoms. Compression stockings can help prevent blood pooling in the legs.

Drug Treatment

The two most common drugs for postural hypotension are fludrocortisone (which increases blood volume) and midodrine (which raises blood pressure).

■ Tech Note!

Many people who experience hypotension have a disease associated with the development of hypotension, such as Parkinson disease. In addition, many patients who experience hypotension are experiencing a drug side effect.

GENERIC NAME: fludrocortisone

INDICATION: Orthostatic hypotension, Addison disease, adrenocortical insufficiency

ROUTE OF ADMINISTRATION: Oral

COMMON ADULT DOSAGE: 0.1–0.2 mg once daily

MECHANISM OF ACTION: Mimics the actions of aldosterone, leading to sodium and water retention that increases blood pressure

SIDE EFFECTS: Weakness, muscle cramps, osteoporosis, fragile skin

AUXILIARY LABEL: Take with food or milk

GENERIC NAME: midodrine

TRADE NAME: ProAmatine[a]

INDICATION: Orthostatic hypotension

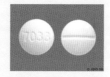

ROUTE OF ADMINISTRATION: Oral

COMMON ADULT DOSAGE: 10 mg three times daily

MECHANISM OF ACTION: Activates alpha-1 receptors in the vasculature, leading to vasoconstriction and an increase in blood pressure

SIDE EFFECTS: Headache, urinary retention, chills

[a]Brand discontinued; now available only as generic.

Hyperlipidemia

Hyperlipidemia (also known as *hypercholesterolemia*) is a bloodstream cholesterol level increase that can lead to **atherosclerosis,** or arterial hardening. Atherosclerosis increases the incidence of angina, heart attack, and **stroke.** When discussing body fats (lipids), it is essential to recognize that cholesterol is only one lipid type, and it performs many vital functions, including steroid hormone and cell membrane synthesis. When people eat high-fat and high-cholesterol foods, they often ingest too much. This excess of cholesterol and fats ends up being stored in fat tissue. In addition to diet, hyperlipidemia may also be inherited. The most widespread genetically associated disorder is familial hypercholesterolemia. Blood tests measure serum levels of different cholesterol forms, such as **low-density lipoproteins (LDLs)** and **high-density lipoproteins (HDLs).** The LDL function is to carry cholesterol to the tissues, where it can lodge in blood vessel walls and contribute to atherosclerosis. HDL, or "good cholesterol," removes cholesterol from the arteries and transports it to the liver. **Triglycerides (TGs),** generally transported throughout the body by LDLs, are linked to the atherosclerosis development. Fig. 20.7 illustrates atherosclerotic plaque development, which is a complex interplay among the vasculature, cholesterol, and immune system cells.

Prognosis

In severe cases, individuals may need bypass surgery or cardiac stenting to relieve atherosclerotic ischemia.

Non-Drug Treatment

By eating a healthy diet and engaging in regular physical activity, many people can lower cholesterol levels. Diet and lifestyle changes (exercise, weight control, and smoking cessation) are a critical initial approach for patients without other major heart disease risk factors. People with significant risk factors for heart disease and stroke (or those with familial hyperlipidemia) can incorporate drug treatments immediately, along with diet and lifestyle changes, to reduce the risk for serious cardiovascular events.

Drug Treatment

Antihyperlipidemic agents include 3-hydroxy-3-methylglutaryl-coenzyme A (HMG-CoA) reductase inhibitors (also known as "statins"), bile acid sequestrants, fibrates, niacin, and ezetimibe (Table 20.4).

The **statins** inhibit an enzyme responsible for one of the first steps in the overall conversion of fats into cholesterol. They raise HDL levels and reduce LDL and TG levels. Therefore these drugs are the most widely used agents for hyperlipidemia treatment in the United States.

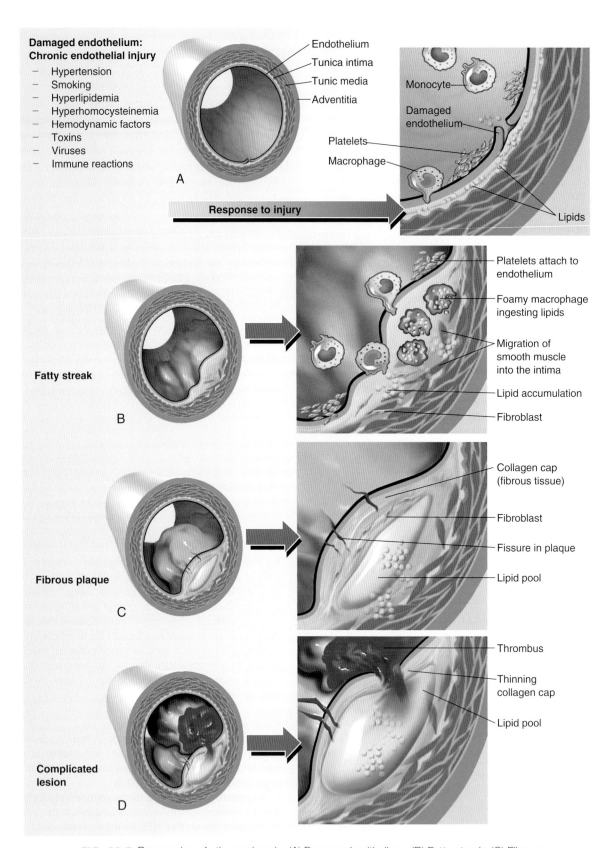

Damaged endothelium:
Chronic endothelial injury
- Hypertension
- Smoking
- Hyperlipidemia
- Hyperhomocysteinemia
- Hemodynamic factors
- Toxins
- Viruses
- Immune reactions

Endothelium
Tunica intima
Tunic media
Adventitia

A

Response to injury

Monocyte
Damaged endothelium
Platelets
Macrophage
Lipids

Fatty streak

B

Platelets attach to endothelium
Foamy macrophage ingesting lipids
Migration of smooth muscle into the intima
Lipid accumulation
Fibroblast

Fibrous plaque

C

Collagen cap (fibrous tissue)
Fibroblast
Fissure in plaque
Lipid pool

Complicated lesion

D

Thrombus
Thinning collagen cap
Lipid pool

FIG. 20.7 Progression of atherosclerosis. (A) Damaged epithelium. (B) Fatty streak. (C) Fibrous plaque. (D) Complicated lesion. (From McCance KL, Huether SE. *Pathophysiology: The Biologic Basis for Disease in Adults and Children*. 7th ed. St. Louis: Elsevier; 2014.)

Select Medications Used for the Treatment of Hyperlipidemia

Generic Name	Trade Name	Common Dosage Range	Common Side Effects
Nicotinic Acid			
niacin[a]	Niacor, Niaspan	• *IR:* 1.5–2 g PO in 3 divided doses daily (max 6 g/day) • *ER:* 1–2 g PO once daily at bedtime	• Dyspepsia • Flushing • Hyperglycemia • Hyperuricemia • Itching
Bile Acid Sequestrants			
cholestyramine	Questran	• 4–8 g PO in 2 divided doses (max 24 g/day)	• Bloating • Constipation • Headache • Upset stomach
colestipol	Colestid	• *Granules:* 5–30 g PO once daily or 2 divided doses daily • *Tablets:* 2–16 g PO once daily or 2–4 divided doses daily	
colesevelam	Welchol	• 3.75 g PO once daily or 1.875 g PO twice daily	
HMG-CoA Reductase Inhibitors (Statins)			
atorvastatin	Lipitor	• 10–80 mg PO once daily	• Headache • Liver toxicity • Muscle pain • Upset stomach
lovastatin	Altoprev	• 10–80 mg PO once daily	
pravastatin	Pravachol	• 10–80 mg PO once daily	
simvastatin	Zocor	• 5–40 mg PO once daily	
rosuvastatin	Crestor	• 5–40 mg PO once daily	
fluvastatin	Lescol	• 20–80 mg/day once daily or 2 divided doses daily	
Fibrates			
gemfibrozil	Lopid	• 600 mg PO twice daily	• Abdominal pain • Diarrhea • Myopathy • Upset stomach
fenofibrate	Lofibra[b]	• 54–160 mg PO once daily	
	Tricor	• 48–145 mg PO once daily	
Cholesterol Absorption Inhibitors			
ezetimibe	Zetia	• 10 mg PO once daily	• Angioedema • Diarrhea • Fatigue • Headache • Upper respiratory infection
PCSK9 Inhibitors			
alirocumab	Praluent	• 75–150 mg subcut once every 2 weeks or 300 mg every 4 weeks	• Primary heterozygous familial hypercholesterol-emia (HeFH)
evolocumab	Repatha	• 140 mg subcut once every 2 weeks or 420 mg every 4 weeks	
Omega-3 Fatty Acids			
fish oil	Lovaza	• 4 g PO once daily or 2 divided doses daily	• Nausea • Prolonged bleeding • Vomiting • Weight gain

[a]Taking 325 mg of aspirin before niacin helps reduce flushing and itching.
[b]Brand discontinued; now available only as generic.
ER, Extended-release; *IR,* immediate-release; *PO,* oral; *subcut,* subcutaneous.

GENERIC NAME: lovastatin

TRADE NAMES: Altoprev

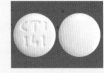

INDICATIONS: Hypercholesterol-emia, myocardial infarction prophylaxis

ROUTE OF ADMINISTRATION: Oral

COMMON ADULT DOSAGES: *Immediate-release:* 10–80 mg/day at bedtime. *Altoprev:* 20–60 mg/day at bedtime

MECHANISM OF ACTION: Inhibits the enzyme HMG-CoA reductase, which is responsible for one of the first steps in the overall conversion of fats into cholesterol

SIDE EFFECTS: Muscle pain, liver toxicity, nausea, constipation

AUXILIARY LABELS:
- Take with meals
- Take in the evening

GENERIC NAME: simvastatin

TRADE NAME: Zocor

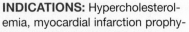

INDICATIONS: Hypercholesterol-emia, myocardial infarction prophy-laxis, stroke prophylaxis

ROUTE OF ADMINISTRATION: Oral

COMMON ADULT DOSAGE: 5–40 mg/day in the evening

MECHANISM OF ACTION: Inhibits the enzyme HMG-CoA reductase, which is responsible for one of the first steps in the overall conversion of fats into cholesterol

SIDE EFFECTS: Muscle pain, liver toxicity, nausea, constipation

AUXILIARY LABELS:
- Take with meals
- Take in the evening

GENERIC NAME: atorvastatin

TRADE NAME: Lipitor

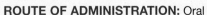

INDICATIONS: Hypercholesterol-emia, myocardial infarction prophy-laxis, stroke prophylaxis

ROUTE OF ADMINISTRATION: Oral

COMMON ADULT DOSAGE: 10–80 mg once daily in the evening

MECHANISM OF ACTION: Inhibits the enzyme HMG-CoA reductase, which is responsible for one of the first steps in the overall conversion of fats into cholesterol

SIDE EFFECTS: Muscle pain, liver toxicity, nausea, constipation

AUXILIARY LABELS:
- Take with meals
- Take in the evening

■ Tech Note!

Statins have many drug interactions including grapefruit, antifungals, antibiotics, and/or calcium channel block-ers. Muscle soreness or weakness is an important ad-verse effect which can develop into rhabdomyolysis and serious muscle injury. Drug interactions can also inten-sify statins' adverse effects. Some statins must be taken in the evening for best results as the body produces most of its cholesterol at nighttime.

Bile acid sequestrants, such as cholestyramine, increase cholesterol loss through the gastrointestinal tract. They do this by binding to gastrointestinal tract bile acids to prevent reabsorption. Because bile acids are made from cholesterol, the loss of bile acids through the feces has a net effect of low-ering cholesterol levels.

GENERIC NAME: cholestyramine

TRADE NAMES: Questran, Questran Light, Prevalite

INDICATION: Hypercholesterolemia

ROUTE OF ADMINISTRATION: Oral (powder)

COMMON ADULT DOSAGE: Initially, 4 g once or twice daily before meals (max 24 g/day in divided doses)

MECHANISM OF ACTION: Binds to bile acids in the gastrointestinal tract, preventing their reabsorption and thus lowering cholesterol levels

SIDE EFFECTS: Constipation, flatulence

AUXILIARY LABELS:
- Take before meals
- Take with plenty of fluids

SPECIAL NOTE: Patients should mix the powder form into 60–180 mL of liquid. Other medications should be taken 4–6 hours apart from cholestyramine to avoid absorption interference.

■ Tech Note!

The bile acid sequestrant colesevelam (Welchol) is ap-proved for hyperlipidemia and type 2 diabetes mellitus treatment. The mechanism of action of colesevelam in helping to lower blood glucose levels is not entirely clear.

Fibrates, such as gemfibrozil and fenofibrate, are less ef-fective at lowering LDL cholesterol but can increase HDL levels and lower TGs. Because of this, they are frequently used in combination with statins in people with persistently low HDL and high TG levels. The exact mechanism by which fibrates affect cholesterol is not known.

GENERIC NAME: gemfibrozil

TRADE NAME: Lopid

INDICATIONS: Hyperlipidemia, hypertriglyceridemia

ROUTE OF ADMINISTRATION: Oral

COMMON ADULT DOSAGE: 600 mg twice daily administered 30 minutes before morning and evening meals

MECHANISM OF ACTION: Exact mechanism is not known

SIDE EFFECTS: Dyspepsia, abdominal pain, diarrhea, liver toxicity

AUXILIARY LABEL: Take with food

GENERIC NAME: ezetimibe

TRADE NAME: Zetia

INDICATION: Hyperlipidemia

ROUTE OF ADMINISTRATION: Oral

COMMON ADULT DOSAGE: 10 mg once daily

MECHANISM OF ACTION: Inhibits the absorption of cholesterol from the GI tract

SIDE EFFECTS: Abdominal pain, fatigue, dizziness, headache

SPECIAL NOTE: Ezetimibe can be given concurrently with statins but should be given at least 2 hours before or 4 hours after a bile acid sequestrant.

Nicotinic acid (niacin) is a B-complex vitamin that reduces LDL and TG levels and increases HDL levels. Although the exact mechanism by which niacin treats hyperlipidemia is unknown, the effect may come from niacin's role as a vitamin. Another niacin effect is cutaneous blood vessel dilation, particularly to the face, neck, and chest. Because of this, the characteristic "niacin flush" can result in headaches, pain, and pruritus.

GENERIC NAME: nicotinic acid

TRADE NAMES: Niacor, Niaspan

INDICATIONS: Hyperlipidemia, hypertriglyceridemia

ROUTE OF ADMINISTRATION: Oral

COMMON ADULT DOSAGES: *Niacor:* 1.5–2 g three times daily with meals. *Niaspan:* 500 mg/day at bedtime initially, then 1–2 g/day at bedtime

MECHANISM OF ACTION: Exact mechanism is not known

SIDE EFFECTS: Photosensitivity, niacin flush

AUXILIARY LABEL: May cause photosensitivity

Tech Note!

"Nonflushing" niacin forms are available for people who experience niacin flush. Aspirin (unless otherwise contraindicated) also can be taken before niacin to help minimize flushing symptoms.

Ezetimibe (Zetia) is an oral medication approved as monotherapy or in combination with statins or fenofibrate for hyperlipidemia. Ezetimibe inhibits gastrointestinal tract cholesterol absorption.

Fish Oil

Fish oils, commonly known as omega-3 fatty acids, can serve as an add-on treatment for lowering high triglycerides. Prescription-strength fish oils, icosapent ethyl (Vascepa), and omega-3 acid ethyl esters (Lovaza) can reduce the risk of stroke and heart attack when combined with statins.

GENERIC NAME: Icosapent ethyl

TRADE NAME: Vascepa

INDICATION: Hypertriglyceridemia

ROUTE OF ADMINISTRATION: Oral

COMMON ADULT DOSAGE: 2 g twice daily

MECHANISM OF ACTION: Thought to reduce the production of triglycerides by the liver

SIDE EFFECTS: Burping, indigestion, altered taste

GENERIC NAME: Omega-3 acid ethyl esters

TRADE NAME: Lovaza

INDICATION: Hypertriglyceridemia

ROUTE OF ADMINISTRATION: Oral

COMMON ADULT DOSAGE: Up to 4 g once daily

MECHANISM OF ACTION: Thought to reduce the production of triglycerides by the liver

SIDE EFFECTS: Burping, indigestion, altered taste

Heterozygous familial hypercholesterolemia (HeFH) is a genetic disorder that results from a defect on chromosome 19 that codes for **low-density lipoprotein receptor (LDLR),** which is a protein found extensively on liver cells that binds to and clears LDL from circulation. Prescribers can use high-dose statins, bile acid sequestrants, or a relatively new medication class called **PCSK9** inhibitors. PCSK9 breaks down LDLR, reducing blood LDL. Currently, two US medications inhibit this enzyme: alirocumab (Praluent) and evolocumab (Repatha). (See Table 20.4 for more PCSK9 inhibitor information.)

GENERIC NAME: alirocumab

TRADE NAME: Praluent

INDICATION: High cholesterol due to heterozygous familial hypercholesterolemia (HeFH)

ROUTE OF ADMINISTRATION: Subcutaneous

COMMON ADULT DOSAGE: 75 mg subcutaneously once every 2 weeks; max 150 mg every 2 weeks or 300 mg every 4 weeks

MECHANISM OF ACTION: Decreases LDLR protein degradation on liver cells, allowing cells to clear LDL from the blood

SIDE EFFECTS: Diarrhea, rash at the injection site

AUXILIARY LABEL: For injection only

GENERIC NAME: evolocumab

TRADE NAME: Repatha

INDICATION: High cholesterol as a result of heterozygous familial hypercholesterolemia (HeFH)

ROUTE OF ADMINISTRATION: Subcutaneous

COMMON ADULT DOSAGES: 140 mg subcutaneously once every 2 weeks, or 420 mg subcutaneously every 4 weeks

MECHANISM OF ACTION: Decreases LDLR protein degradation on liver cells, allowing cells to clear LDL from the blood

SIDE EFFECTS: Upper respiratory tract infection, rash at the injection site

AUXILIARY LABEL: For injection only

Tech Note!

PCSK9 inhibitors are relatively new drugs, they are often extremely expensive and require prior authorization for coverage.

Coronary Artery Disease

Coronary artery disease (CAD) is a condition in which the cardiac arteries do not receive proper oxygenation, often because of arterial narrowing secondary to atherosclerosis. Symptoms can include hypertension, angina pectoris, hyperlipidemia, and myocardial infarction (Fig. 20.8).

Atherosclerosis is a **syndrome** (more than one condition) that affects arterial blood vessels. Inflammation occurs as a result of the lifelong buildup of small plaques, mainly composed of lipids, and the clumping of platelets (see Fig. 20.7). Over time, minor injuries can occur in the vessel wall. When damage occurs to the arterial wall, the body responds by sending macrophages and T lymphocytes to fight the plaques; however, instead of eliminating plaques, these lymphocytes increase the blockage. This cycle continues, potentially causing total blockage of a vessel that can result in a heart attack or stroke. **Arteriosclerosis** is a condition that results from thickening, loss of elasticity (hardening), and calcification of arterial walls. Hypertension, hyperlipidemia, diabetes mellitus, and normal aging all contribute to arteriosclerosis progression. Patients with atherosclerosis often also have arteriosclerosis.

CAD is a leading cause of death in both men and women. This statistic may be partially due to not making lifestyle changes after a first heart attack. With proper medication and lifestyle changes, many people can live with CAD and reduce risk factors for heart attack and stroke. Because CAD blocks blood flow to heart muscle areas, a primary disease symptom is **angina** resulting from a lack of myocardial oxygenation.

Angina Pectoris

Angina pectoris results from a decrease in cardiac blood flow, which causes chest pain or a sense of pressure. The pain varies

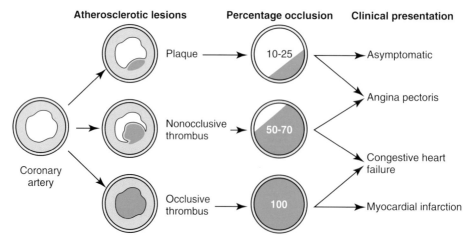

FIG. 20.8 Narrowing of the coronary artery may cause different clinical symptoms, depending on the extent of occlusion and the speed at which it develops. (From Damjanov I. *Pathology for the Health Professions*. 4th ed. Philadelphia: Saunders; 2011.)

from minor to severe. Hardening of the arteries (atherosclerosis), hypertension, and cigarette smoking can decrease blood flow. Environmental and genetic influences can also play a role in acquiring angina (chest pain). The three angina types include the following:

1. Stable angina
2. Variant angina
3. Unstable angina

In classic stable (chronic) angina, the person can experience short ischemic episodes. Patients often describe chest pressure, which they may describe as "an elephant sitting on my chest." This pain can occur in the chest, neck, arms, teeth, and jaw. This anginal form is precipitated by exertion and generally occurs after a set level of physical activity. Many times this anginal attack happens after exercise, excessive activity, or emotional stress, and therefore the episodes are usually predictable.

Variant angina (also called *Prinzmetal* or *vasospastic angina*) may not be related to atherosclerosis; instead, the patient experiences coronary artery spasms that can occur spontaneously. These spasms can narrow the **lumen** (or cavity) of the artery and reduce blood flow to the heart. Variant angina does not necessarily occur after physical exercise or stress and is less predictable than stable angina.

Unstable angina, which may worsen in patients with a known history of anginal attacks, can occur at rest. For people with preexisting angina, unstable angina may develop when symptoms become more severe in pattern compared with the patient's usual symptoms. Unstable angina may be due to atherosclerotic plaque rupture. Because unstable angina may be a sign of an impending heart attack, it requires immediate medical attention.

Prognosis

The angina prognosis depends on the type of angina and the severity of the condition. A history of heart conditions, such as dysrhythmias or heart attacks, also influences the outcome and treatment approach.

Non-Drug Treatment

Modifying behaviors to lessen angina attacks include smoking cessation, stress reduction, weight loss, lowering blood pressure and cholesterol levels, and controlling any underlying conditions (eg, hypertension). Surgical procedures may relieve occlusion in some patients. Angioplasty and coronary artery bypass graft (CABG) (Fig. 20.9) are two surgical procedures that can be used. Angioplasty is the insertion and inflation of a small balloon into the affected area, which removes and/or stabilizes the plaque. In the CABG procedure, a piece of a healthy blood vessel from another part of the body is grafted to bypass the affected heart vessel. Stent placement is another intervention that widens arteries to improve coronary blood flow. A **stent** is a small cylindrical device inserted into the affected artery, providing a framework to hold the artery open. The stent is placed by inserting a catheter through a vein and guiding the stent to the affected site. Stents can be uncoated or coated with a slow-release medication that keeps the artery from clotting and ultimately closing.

Drug Treatment

Nitrates, calcium channel blockers, and beta-blockers commonly treat and prevent angina symptoms. Nitroglycerin is the most frequently prescribed antianginal drug. Many individuals carry nitroglycerin sublingual

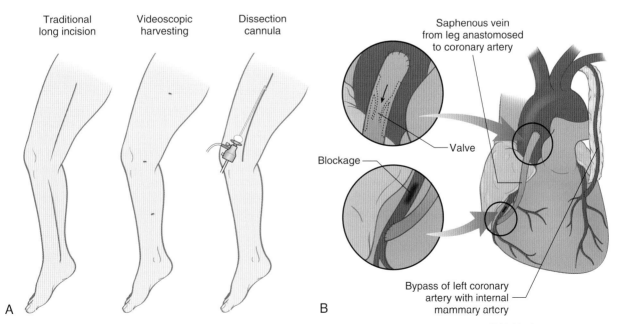

FIG. 20.9 Coronary artery bypass graft surgery. (A) A vein is taken from the leg. (B) Vein is attached to the heart. (From Sole ML, et al. *Introduction to Critical Care Nursing*. 6th ed. Philadelphia: Saunders; 2013.)

TABLE 20.5
Select Common Nitrate Agents

Trade Name	Generic Name	Normal Usage
Tridil	nitroglycerin (NTG) solution for injection	Emergency management of acute angina
NTG in D$_5$W	nitroglycerin + dextrose solution for injection	Emergency management of acute angina
Nitrostat	nitroglycerin (sublingual tablet)	Treatment of acute angina
NitroMist	nitroglycerin (sublingual spray)	Treatment of acute angina
Nitro-Time[a]	nitroglycerin (extended-release capsule)	Routine medication for stable angina
Nitro-Dur,[a] Minitran[a]	nitroglycerin (transdermal patch)	Routine medication for stable angina
Imdur[a]	isosorbide mononitrate	Routine medication for stable angina
	isosorbide dinitrate (sublingual tablet	Treatment of acute angina
Dilatrate SR, Isochron[a]	isosorbide dinitrate (extended-release capsule)	Routine medication for stable angina

[a]Brand discontinued; now available only as generic.

tablets in their pockets or purses in the event of an acute angina attack. Nitroglycerin has many dosage forms, including capsules, topical patches, ointments and creams, and sublingual sprays. The sublingual tablets and injectable forms are used for emergencies.

Nitrates (Table 20.5) are vasodilators; that is, they dilate the arteries to permit an increase of blood flow to the heart muscle. They also reduce heart workload. Isosorbide dinitrate, isosorbide mononitrate, and nitroglycerin are common nitrate agents used for angina treatment. Both isosorbide dinitrate and nitroglycerin come as sublingual tablets, which are effective because of their rapid absorption. Fig. 20.10 shows a common sublingual nitroglycerin prescription order for acute angina attack treatment.

Nitroglycerin sublingual tablets must be kept in a dry area and in the original light-protected glass container to prevent the active agent from deteriorating. Another form for acute relief is translingual nitroglycerin spray. The patient sprays metered doses under the tongue, with a maximum of three sprays in 15 minutes. Sublingual dosages are kept at the patient's bedside in an institution, or constantly with the ambulatory individual, for emergency relief of angina attacks. In the hospital, nitroglycerin is often given by intravenous (IV) infusion for a variety of circumstances, including unstable angina treatment.

Longer acting nitrate dosage forms are available for chronic angina treatment to prevent attacks. Transdermal dosage forms (nitroglycerin) or oral dosage forms (eg, nitroglycerin, isosorbide dinitrate, and isosorbide mononitrate) are available. The nitroglycerin transdermal patches are typically applied once a day in the morning and removed at bedtime to reduce possible medication tolerance.

Other agents commonly used for the chronic treatment of angina include beta-blockers and calcium channel blockers. These reduce heart ischemia by mechanisms different from those of nitrate agents.

Doctor David Gall
1000 Archway
St. Louis, MO
ph: 816-555-5555

Patient name: R. Jones-Lewis
Address: 106 Nutree Way   Date: 1-30-XX
Rx: NTG 0.4mg sl #100
        Take 1 sl q 5 mm x3
        if no relief call 911

                            Dr. Gall
                    Dr. Signature
Refills: 6   DEA # _____

FIG. 20.10 Nitroglycerin sublingual tablet prescription.

Tech Note!

When filling a nitroglycerin sublingual tablet prescription (eg, Nitrostat), never take the tablets out of the manufacturer's amber glass container. The nitroglycerin must be protected from degradation by light. Instead, place the glass container in a larger plastic vial with the prescription label. Package nitroglycerin with a non-childproof cap so people can readily open the vial if experiencing chest pain or a heart attack.

Thrombotic Events

The formation of a vessel clot blocking blood flow is a **thrombosis.** Coagulation (blood clotting) is a normal body function aimed at stopping hemorrhage and starting healing.

Unfortunately, our bodies can also form unwanted blood clots. This clotting can occur because of an overactive clotting mechanism (genetic), can result from narrowing of the arteries (as in people with atherosclerosis), or may be due to prolonged inactivity. An **embolus** (plural, emboli) is a blood clot that has broken away from the thrombus (main clot) and traveled through the body to another area, where it can become lodged and create a blockage. Thrombi and emboli can precipitate myocardial infarction, stroke, or deep vein thrombosis (DVT).

All anticoagulants have the potential to cause significant bleeding and death, garnering them a "high-alert" or "high-risk" classification. Common bleeding due to anticoagulants may include nosebleeds, blood in vomit or stool, and bruising. Serious bleeding events include a gastrointestinal bleed or a life-threatening bleed that may require reversal agents.

Prognosis

If the thrombus/embolus is treated quickly, the prognosis can be good. In some instances, an anticoagulant or low-dose heparin may need to be taken for a prolonged period.

Non-Drug Treatment

Wearing support stockings and standing and walking regularly facilitates circulation in the lower extremities. These are potential nonpharmacological means to minimize clot risk.

Drug Treatment

Depending on clot severity, either an anticoagulant (to prevent clotting) or a thrombolytic agent (to break up or dissolve the clot) can be used. Thrombolytics are given parenterally under the supervision of a physician. These must be used soon after a clot occurs, before the affected organ or tissue is damaged (such as the brain in the case of a stroke). Table 20.6 provides an overview of anticoagulants, antiplatelet agents, and thrombolytics. Clots are formed by fibrin, a protein that holds blood cells together to make a blood clot. Heparin inhibits thrombosis by accelerating the activity of antithrombin III to inactivate thrombin. This impedes the coagulation mechanism. Patients admitted to the hospital with myocardial infarction or stroke may be administered an IV heparin drip to prevent blood coagulation. Heparin is effective and intended for short-term use in a hospital.

GENERIC NAME: heparin

TRADE NAME: Generic only

INDICATIONS: Treatment and prevention of clot formation

ROUTES OF ADMINISTRATION: Injection (intravenous, subcutaneous)

COMMON ADULT DOSAGE: Dosing is highly variable, depending on patient factors and indication

MECHANISM OF ACTION: Inhibits thrombosis by accelerating the activity of antithrombin III to inactivate thrombin

SIDE EFFECTS: Hemorrhage, injection site reactions

Another type of **anticoagulant** is warfarin. Unlike heparin, orally administered warfarin is for long-term use and usually taken once a day. Warfarin interferes with vitamin K–dependent coagulation factor synthesis (II, VII, IX, and X) in the liver. Prothrombin time and international normalized ratio (INR) tests monitor how long it takes blood to form clots while the patient is taking medication. A warfarin overdose can potentially cause life-threatening bleeding. Warfarin interacts with many other prescription medications, over-the-counter products, herbals, and even food. People receiving warfarin often undergo regular monitoring.

Some patients are treated in the hospital and/or discharged to their homes with low-molecular-weight heparin (LMWH), such as enoxaparin, which is administered as a subcutaneous injection (see Table 20.6). The dosage depends on the indication and the patient's weight. LMWHs are frequently "bridge therapy" after orthopedic surgeries while the patient is started on warfarin. Bridge therapy means that an LMWH is used to prevent clot formation until warfarin achieves a therapeutic level.

Tech Note!

Foods such as broccoli contain a large amount of vitamin K, which may counteract the effectiveness of warfarin. Other foods high in vitamin K include liver, brussels sprouts, spinach, Swiss chard, coriander, collards, and cabbage. Patients should try to keep the amount of vitamin K in their diets consistent. For example, people who usually do not eat broccoli and who begin to take warfarin should avoid suddenly consuming large amounts of broccoli (or other vegetables with vitamin K). This diet will counteract warfarin's effectiveness. Consistency is key.

GENERIC NAME: warfarin

TRADE NAMES: Coumadin,[a] Jantoven

INDICATION: Prevention of clot formation

ROUTE OF ADMINISTRATION: Oral

COMMON ADULT DOSAGE: Dosage varies depending on treatment goals and response; a typical starting dose is 2–5 mg/day

MECHANISM OF ACTION: Interferes with the synthesis of vitamin K–dependent coagulation factors to prevent clot formation

SIDE EFFECT: Hemorrhage

AUXILIARY LABEL: Avoid alcohol

[a]Brand no longer available.

TABLE 20.6

Medication Class	Generic Name	Trade Name	Common Adult Dosage
Vitamin K antagonist (VKA)	warfarin	Coumadin	PO; dosage titrated to goal INR
Anticoagulant—heparin	heparin		Varies widely; dosage depends on indication
Low-molecular-weight heparins (LMWHs)	dalteparin	Fragmin	2500–5000 units subcut every 24 h
	enoxaparin	Lovenox	30 mg subcut every 12 hr or 40 mg daily for prophylaxis; dosage for treatment is different
Antiplatelet agents	aspirin/dipyridamole	Aggrenox[a]	1 capsule (25/200 mg) PO twice daily
	aspirin	Ecotrin	81–325 mg PO once daily
	cilostazol		100 mg PO twice daily
	clopidogrel	Plavix	75 mg PO once daily
	prasugrel	Effient	10 mg once daily
	ticagrelor	Brilinta	90 mg PO twice daily
Factor Xa inhibitors	apixaban	Eliquis	2.5–5 mg PO twice daily for set number of days (2–4 wk average)
	fondaparinux	Arixtra	2.5 mg subcut once daily for prophylaxis; dosage for treatment is different
	rivaroxaban	Xarelto	20 mg PO once daily or 15 mg PO twice daily
Direct thrombin inhibitors	argatroban		Titrate to target steady-state aPTT achieved
	bivalirudin	Angiomax	Dosage depends on indication
	dabigatran	Pradaxa	150 g PO twice a day
Glycoprotein IIb/IIIa inhibitors	eptifibatide	Integrilin	180 mcg/kg IV over 1–2 min
	tirofiban	Aggrastat	*Initial:* 25 mcg/kg over 5 min, then 0.15 mcg/kg/min
Thrombolytics	alteplase (t-PA)	Activase	0.9 mg/kg IV infusion over 1 h
	reteplase	Retavase	10 units IV over 2 min with a second dose 30 min later
	tenecteplase	TNKase	*Bolus:* 30–50 mg IV (weight based) over 5 seconds

[a]Brand discontinued; now available only as generic.

aPTT, Activated partial thromboplastin time; *INR,* international normalized ratio; *IV,* intravenous; *PO,* oral; *subcut,* subcutaneous.

Currently, warfarin is widely used for long-term clot prevention for people undergoing surgery or for those with atrial fibrillation. However, other medications, including dabigatran (Pradaxa), apixaban (Eliquis), and rivaroxaban (Xarelto), are rapidly gaining popularity. Apixaban is often preferred to rivaroxaban because of lower major bleed risk.

Dabigatran is a direct thrombin inhibitor. It inhibits thrombin to prevent thrombin-induced platelet aggregation and clot development. Rivaroxaban prevents clotting by inhibiting factor Xa that is a necessary enzyme for clot formation. Both dabigatran and rivaroxaban do not require routine blood monitoring. This gives these medications an advantage over warfarin in anticoagulant therapy. (See Table 20.6 for more information about other anticoagulants.)

GENERIC NAME: dabigatran

TRADE NAME: Pradaxa

INDICATIONS: Stroke prophylaxis, embolism prophylaxis in people with atrial fibrillation

ROUTE OF ADMINISTRATION: Oral

COMMON ADULT DOSAGE: 150 mg twice daily

MECHANISM OF ACTION: Inhibits thrombin to prevent thrombin-induced platelet aggregation and the development of a clot

SIDE EFFECT: Hemorrhage

AUXILIARY LABEL: Do not repackage or store capsules in any other container

Another medication class that reduces clot formation is the antiplatelet class. Drugs in this group include aspirin (Ecotrin), clopidogrel (Plavix), prasugrel (Effient), and ticagrelor (Brilinta), among others. Antiplatelet agents bind directly to platelets, inhibiting aggregation and clot formation. Often, physicians prescribe two antiplatelet agents simultaneously. This regimen conforms to the Dual Antiplatelet Therapy (DAPT) guidelines set by the American College of Cardiology (ACC). A current option is to consider therapy with an oral anticoagulant plus a P2Y12 receptor inhibitor such as clopidogrel *without* aspirin. Studies show this regimen to be superior to DAPT in the primary prevention of patients with increased stroke risk.

One antiplatelet medication in this therapy is often low-dose aspirin (81 mg in the United States). However, in 2019, the American Heart Association/ACC/Heart Rhythm Society updated the guidelines for aspirin use. Traditionally, prescribers would give aspirin to any patient with atherosclerotic cardiovascular disease (ASCVD) risk. The updated guidelines recommend that aspirin should not be used routinely in the primary prevention of ASCVD because of a lack of net benefit. Of particular concern are patients who have an increased bleeding risk from past gastrointestinal bleed or peptic ulcer disease. Other risk factors for bleed include age older than 70, thrombocytopenia, coagulopathy, chronic kidney disease, and concurrent NSAID use. Although guidelines no longer generally recommend aspirin therapy for primary prevention, there are three rules to follow when initiating aspirin therapy for primary prevention:

1. Low-dose aspirin can be considered for the primary prevention of a cardiovascular event in adults with high ASCVD risk scores aged 40 to 60 who are not at increased bleeding risk.
2. Low-dose aspirin should not be administered routinely for the primary prevention of ASCVD in adults older than 60 years.
3. Low-dose aspirin should not be administered for primary prevention at any age who are at an increased bleeding risk.

Like a direct thrombin inhibitor, these medications do not require routine blood monitoring.

GENERIC NAME: clopidogrel

TRADE NAME: Plavix

INDICATIONS: Stroke, CAD, and myocardial infarction prophylaxis; often used in combination with another antiplatelet medication (DAPT)

ROUTE OF ADMINISTRATION: Oral

COMMON ADULT DOSAGE: 75 mg once daily

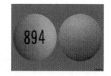

MECHANISM OF ACTION: Binds to platelets and directly inhibits platelet aggregation

SIDE EFFECT: Hemorrhage

AUXILIARY LABEL: Do not discontinue medication unless directed by your health care professional

Myocardial Infarction

If coronary blood flow to a heart area becomes entirely blocked because of a thrombus or embolism, that area of the heart muscle cannot receive necessary oxygen. This blockade results in heart muscle death, a condition known as **myocardial infarction (MI),** also known as a heart attack. Different people experience MI with dissimilar symptoms. One might be unaware that his or her symptoms indicate a heart attack. Depending on the blockage severity, the patient may have an MI from which he or she can recover over time. A massive MI may weaken the heart, resulting in HF or death.

Prognosis

Many people survive a myocardial infarction (MI) because of prompt medical treatment. Several drug classes can manage various conditions. Lifestyle changes can reduce MI recurrence. Some patients are at high risk for heart dysrhythmia, heart failure, or other complications after an MI.

Non-Drug Treatment

The many medications available for patients after an MI have been discussed previously in this chapter. Cardiac rehabilitation, dietary changes, and reduction of risk factors (eg, cessation of smoking) are all critical actions to implement after a heart attack. However, if the patient's MI was severe or if the condition of the coronary arteries is such that the blockages place the patient at high risk, an intervention such as bypass surgery may be necessary (as discussed previously).

Drug Treatment

After an MI, drug treatment goals are to reduce patient mortality (risk for death) and to prevent reinfarction. After an MI, the heart undergoes structural changes. Another major drug therapy goal is to preserve the remaining left ventricular function and avoid heart dysrhythmias and heart failure. Many medications are used, including beta-blockers, angiotensin-converting enzyme inhibitors, statins, aspirin, and other antiplatelet drugs

TABLE 20.7

Select Agents Used in the Treatment of Acute Coronary Syndrome/Myocardial Infarction

Medication Class	Generic Name	Trade Name	Common Dosage Range
Vasodilator/antianginal	nitroglycerin	Nitrostat	• 400 mcg SL or spray every 5 min (max 3 doses)
	isosorbide mononitrate	Imdur[a]	• *IR:* 20 mg PO twice daily • *ER:* 30–60 mg PO once daily in the morning (max 240 mg/dose)
	isosorbide dinitrate	Isordil Titradose	• *IR:* 5–20 mg PO 2 or 3 times daily • *ER:* 40 mg once or twice daily
Opioid	morphine	MS Contin	• 2–8 mg IV every 5–15 min after nitroglycerin
Gas	oxygen	NA	• 2–4 L/min by nasal cannula for first 6 hr
Beta-blocker	metoprolol	Lopressor	• 50–100 mg PO twice daily or 5 mg IV slow push over 2 min (max 15 mg)
Anticoagulant-heparin	heparin		• *For MI:* 60 units/kg IV bolus, then 12 units/kg/hr
Glycoprotein IIb/IIIa inhibitors	eptifibatide	Integrilin	• 180 mcg/kg IV over 1–2 min
	tirofiban	Aggrastat	• *Initial:* 25 mcg/kg over 5 min, then 0.15 mcg/kg/min for 18 h
Thrombolytic	alteplase (t-PA)	Activase	• Varying protocols depending on indication: max 100 mg/total dose
Antiplatelet (in combination with aspirin)	clopidogrel	Plavix	• *Loading dose:* 300 mg PO, then 75 mg PO once daily
	ticagrelor	Brilinta	• *Loading dose:* 180 mg PO, then 90 mg PO twice daily
	prasugrel	Effient	• *Loading dose:* 60 mg PO, then 10 mg once daily

[a]Brand discontinued; now available only as generic.

ER, Extended-release; *IR,* immediate-release; *IV,* intravenous; *PO,* oral; *SL,* sublingual.

(eg, clopidogrel [Plavix]). The treatment depends on the individual patient's history, type of infarction, and previous procedures. Table 20.7 provides an overview of potential treatments during an acute MI and for maintenance post-MI therapy.

Transient Ischemic Attacks and Strokes

Transient ischemic attacks (TIAs) are caused by a short period of reduced oxygenation to the brain, possibly as a result of atherosclerotic cerebrovascular disease. TIAs are similar to strokes, except that TIA duration is much quicker with typically no permanent loss of function. TIAs may last only a few minutes or may occur many times over a day. If an atherosclerotic plaque forms a clot, a thrombus can develop that may obstruct the vessel, causing a stroke. We sometimes refer to TIAs as ministrokes, and they are considered a precursor to a stroke.

The two types of strokes are ischemic (clot) strokes and hemorrhagic (bleeding) strokes. Hemorrhagic strokes occur when weakened vessels, or **aneurysms,** in the brain rupture. When a vessel ruptures, blood flows into areas of the brain, causing damage; additional injury is caused by the lack of oxygenated blood flow to areas of the brain where it is needed. Most of the symptoms of TIAs and strokes may appear rapidly. These include vision or hearing problems, weakness on one or both sides of the body, dizziness, slurred speech, and sudden, severe headache.

Prognosis

As mentioned, a TIA may be a precursor to a stroke. If a patient presents with TIA symptoms, specific diagnostic tests can be performed to determine the likelihood of more TIAs or even an impending stroke. Standard diagnostic tests include computed tomography (CT) and magnetic resonance imaging (MRI) scans.

Non-Drug Treatment

As for other cardiovascular diseases discussed previously, reducing the factors that contribute to the underlying causes is a change that must be made. These changes include smoking cessation, reducing fat and alcohol consumption, weight loss if necessary, engaging in physical activity, and eating a balanced diet. Nonfatal strokes are one of the most common causes of disability, resulting in possible brain damage and the necessity for physical and occupational therapy.

Drug Treatment

TIAs are treated by improving arterial brain blood flow so that a stroke can be avoided. In the case of a TIA, patients may be treated with antiplatelet medication (eg, aspirin) to reduce the risk for clot formation or with anticoagulants (eg, warfarin). Usually, the last resort is carotid artery surgery to remove arterial plaques.

The main agents used to treat an acute ischemic stroke in progress are thrombolytics, such as tissue plasminogen activator (t-PA, Activase), if indicated. Therapy must be given within 3 hours of the onset of the symptoms of the event after the patient has been evaluated to rule out intracranial bleeding (see Table 20.6).

Dysrhythmia

The heart beats in a regular rhythm via special fibers that run throughout the heart. The pacemaker is in the SA node. Many factors influence the efficient operation of the pacemaker, including chemical balance. If an imbalance results from chemicals (eg, electrolytes) or oxygen deprivation, irregular heartbeats, or **dysrhythmias,** can occur. Medications can also cause dysrhythmias. Depending on the severity, acute care may or may not be required. Some patients may require chronic use of drugs to help maintain the heart's normal rhythm.

Prognosis

The outcome depends on location and severity. Dysrhythmias originating in the atrium may ultimately be controlled with medications or other treatment; however, ventricular tachycardia or fibrillation is generally more severe.

Non-Drug Treatment

Identifying the root cause of dysrhythmia is a critical aspect of care. If the dysrhythmia is caused by a medication or identifiable cause, addressing the causative factor should be a primary treatment approach. In severe cases in which medications cannot correct the rhythm, a pacemaker implant may be needed.

Drug Treatment

The medicines used in treating dysrhythmias are called antidysrhythmic or antiarrhythmic agents. Quinidine sulfate, procainamide, amiodarone, sotalol, and verapamil are some common agents used in these situations. Table 20.8 provides select examples of antiarrhythmic medications.

◼ Tech Note!

Serious medication errors can occur because the medication names quinidine and quinine look similar. Quinine is an antimalarial. Quinidine is an antiarrhythmic. These two medications often sit close to each other on the pharmacy shelf and pose a risk for mistakes.

Heart Failure

Heart failure (HF) is a progressive disease in which the heart cannot pump enough blood to meet the body's oxygen and nutrient demands. Several treatments can help patients with HF, but there is no cure. Edema is a characteristic HF component because the kidneys compensate for the lack of blood flow by retaining more fluid. This fluid increases the heart's workload, further weakening it. Eventually, the heart can no longer pump adequately. Many cardiovascular conditions can contribute to HF, including hypertension, MI, and CAD. Other conditions that may cause HF include valvular heart disease, congenital heart defects, cardiomyopathy, and endocarditis. Symptoms of HF include fatigue, shortness of breath during activities of daily living or when lying down, peripheral edema, and pulmonary edema.

Prognosis

We can treat HF in several ways, although certain conditions associated with the onset of HF often cannot be reversed. With medications and lifestyle changes, the life of a patient with HF can significantly improve.

Non-Drug Treatment

Many changes can influence the severity of HF. Such nonpharmacological treatments include reduction of salt intake, cessation of smoking, weight loss, rest and modification of daily activities, and reduction of stress. If a valvular or congenital heart disease is the source of a patient's heart failure, surgery may correct the defects and improve heart function.

Drug Treatment

The goal of these drug treatments is to enhance heart function. Initial therapies without contraindications include ACE inhibitors, ARBs, or angiotensin receptor and neprilysin inhibitors (ARNI), beta-blockers, and loop diuretics. Additional agents include aldosterone receptor antagonists, sodium-glucose cotransporter 2 inhibitors, nitrates, and digoxin (Table 20.9). Digoxin, which is a cardiac glycoside, increases the force of cardiac contraction (inotropic effect). Diuretics can help lower blood pressure and manage HF-associated edema.

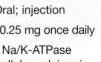

GENERIC NAME: digoxin

TRADE NAME: Lanoxin

INDICATIONS: Heart failure, atrial fibrillation

ROUTES OF ADMINISTRATION: Oral; injection

COMMON ADULT DOSAGE: 0.125–0.25 mg once daily

MECHANISM OF ACTION: Inhibits Na/K-ATPase pump, leading to an increase in intracellular calcium in cardiac muscle, which in turn leads to more forceful heart contractions

SIDE EFFECTS: Nausea, vomiting, diarrhea, dizziness, visual changes (if toxic levels reached)

AUXILIARY LABELS:
- Take as prescribed
- Do not stop taking the medication without consulting a health care professional

Select Agents Used in the Treatment of Arrhythmias

Generic Name	Trade Name	Common Dosage Range[a]	Common Side Effects
sotalol	Betapace, Betapace AF	• 80–160 mg PO twice daily	• Depression • Dizziness • Stomach upset
amiodarone	Cordarone[b], Pacerone	• 150 mg IV over 10 min, then 1 mg/min for 6 h, then 0.5 mg/min • 600–800 mg/day PO in divided doses until 10 g total, then 200–400 mg/day	• Hypotension • Photosensitivity
digoxin	Lanoxin	• 0.125–0.25 mg PO once daily • 2.4–3.6 mcg/kg IV or IM once daily	• Dizziness • Headache • Heart block • Nausea • Visual disturbances
disopyramide	Norpace	• *IR:* 100–200 mg PO every 6 h • *ER:* 200–400 mg PO every 12 h • Max 1600 mg/day	• Constipation • Dry mouth
procainamide	Pronestyl[b], Procanbid[b]	• 50 mg/kg/day IM divided into doses every 3–6 h • 50 mg/min IV repeated prn every 5 min until a total dose of 1 g	• Hypotension • Taste changes
quinidine	Quinidex[b]	• *IR:* 200–300 mg PO every 4–6 hours • *ER:* 300–600 mg PO every 8–12 h	• Diarrhea • Hypotension • Lightheadedness
propafenone	Rythmol, Rythmol SR	• *IR:* 150–300 mg PO every 8 hours • *ER:* 225 mg PO twice daily (max 425 mg/dose every 12 h)	• Bronchospasm • Dizziness • Stomach upset
dofetilide	Tikosyn	• 500 mcg PO twice daily (max 500 mcg twice daily)	• Bradycardia • Dizziness • Hypotension
flecainide	Tambocor[b]	• 100–200 mg PO twice daily	• Blurred vision • Dizziness • Headache
dronedarone	Multaq	• 400 mg PO twice a day	• Bradycardia • Rash • Stomach upset
lidocaine	Xylocaine	• *Bolus:* 1–1.5 mg/kg IV/IO • *Infusion:* 1–4 mg/min IV	• Psychosis • Seizures

[a]Dosing can vary depending on type and severity of arrhythmia.
[b]Brand no longer available.
ER, Extended-release; *IM,* intramuscular; *IO,* intraosseous; *IR,* immediate-release; *IV,* intravenous; *PO,* oral; *prn,* pro re nata, Latin for "as needed."

■ **Tech Note!**

The antidote for a digoxin overdose or symptomatic toxicity is digoxin immune Fab. This agent binds to the digoxin molecule, and the drug is excreted from the body. This treatment must be done in the emergency department, and the antidote is available in injectable form only.

A variety of diuretic agents can help reduce edema in patients with HF. With thiazides and loop diuretics, a vital consideration is potassium loss. For this reason, both classes generally necessitate potassium supplementation, although this is more common with loop diuretics. Potassium-sparing diuretics, such as triamterene and spironolactone, on the other hand, retain potassium. Chapter 23 presents a detailed discussion of diuretics.

TABLE 20.9
Select Agents Used in the Treatment of Heart Failure

Medication Class	Generic Name	Trade Name	Common Dosage Range	Common Side Effects
Acute Heart Failure				
Loop diuretic	furosemide	Lasix	• 10–40 mg PO twice a day	• Headache • Hypokalemia • Hypotension • Weakness
Vasodilators	nitroglycerin	Nitrostat[a]	• 10–20 mcg/min IV infusion, titrate upward to effect (max 200 mcg/min)	• Flushing • Headache • Hypotension • Peripheral edema
	nitroprusside	Nitropress	• 3–4 mcg/kg/min IV: max of 10 mcg/kg/min for 10 min	• Flushing • Hypotension
Adrenergic agonist	dobutamine	Dobutrex[a]	• 2–40 mcg/kg/min IV infusion	• Chest pain • Fever • Headache • Increased blood pressure • Increased heart rate
Phosphodiesterase enzyme inhibitor	milrinone	Primacor[a]	• 0.375–0.75 mcg/kg/min IV infusion	• Chest pain • Headache • Hypotension • Ventricular arrhythmia
Chronic Heart Failure				
ACE inhibitors	benazepril	Lotensin	• 5–20 mg PO daily	• Angioedema • Cough • Hyperkalemia • Hypotension
	lisinopril	Prinivil, Zestril	• 5–40 mg PO once daily	
	captopril	Capoten[a]	• 6.25–50 mg PO three times a day: max 150 mg/day	
	ramipril	Altace	• 1.25–10 mg PO daily: max 10 mg/day	
	enalapril	Vasotec	• 2.5–20 mg by mouth twice a day	
Beta-blockers	metoprolol	Toprol XL	• 12.5–200 mg by mouth daily PO once daily (target 200 mg/day)	• Bradycardia • Dizziness • Fatigue • Hypotension • Nausea
	carvedilol	Coreg, Coreg CR	• 3.125–25 mg PO twice daily • 20–80 mg by mouth each morning: max 80 mg/day	
Loop diuretic	furosemide	Lasix	• 10–40 mg PO twice a day	• Cross-sensitivity to sulfa • Headache • Hypokalemia • Hypotension • Weakness
Thiazide diuretics	hydrochlorothiazide (HCTZ)	Microzide[a]	• 12.5–50 mg PO in 1–2 doses daily (max 100 mg/day)	• Hyperglycemia • Hypokalemia • Hyponatremia • Hypotension • Photosensitivity
	metolazone		• 5–20 mg PO daily	
Cardiac glycoside	digoxin	Lanoxin	• 0.125–0.5 mg PO once daily	• Dizziness • Headache • Mental disturbances • Nausea • Visual disturbances

Continued

TABLE 20.9
Select Agents Used in the Treatment of Heart Failure—cont'd

Medication Class	Generic Name	Trade Name	Common Dosage Range	Common Side Effects
Aldosterone inhibitors	spironolactone	Aldactone	• 12.5–50 mg/day in divided doses one to two times a day (max 50 mg/day)	• Decreased libido • Gynecomastia • Hyperkalemia • Hyponatremia
	eplerenone	Inspra	• 25–50 mg PO once daily (max 50 mg/day)	
Vasodilators	hydralazine	Apresoline[a]	• 25–100 mg PO three times a day (max 300 mg/day); use in combination with isosorbide dinitrate	• Anxiety • Chest pain • Flushing • Rash
	isosorbide dinitrate	Isordil Titradose	• *IR:* 20–40 mg by mouth three times a day (max 120 mg in divided doses); use in combination with hydralazine	• Headache • Hypotension • Lightheadedness

[a]Brand discontinued; now available only as generic.
IV, Intravenous; *PO,* oral.

▽ Tech Alert!

Remember the following sound-alike, look-alike drugs:
• Cardene versus Cardizem
• Cardene SR versus Cardizem SR
• nicardipine versus nifedipine versus nimodipine
• Lotensin versus Lioresal[a]

[a]No longer a branded drug.

Do You Remember These Key Points?

● Names of the major components of the cardiovascular system and their functions
● The primary symptoms of the various cardiovascular conditions discussed
● Medications used to treat the various cardiovascular conditions discussed
● The generic and trade names for the drugs discussed in this chapter
● The appropriate auxiliary labels that should be used when filling prescriptions for drugs discussed in this chapter

Review Questions

Multiple Choice Questions

1. The artery responsible for supplying the heart muscle with oxygen is called the:
   A. Pulmonary artery
   B. Aorta
   C. Coronary artery
   D. Myocardial passageway

2. A cardiac condition in which fluids can build up within tissues is known as:
   A. Myocardial infarction
   B. Angina pectoris
   C. Heart failure
   D. Hypertension

3. Factor(s) that may affect the development of atherosclerosis is/are:
   A. Lifestyle
   B. Family history
   C. Smoking
   D. All of the above

4. In "ACE inhibitors," ACE stands for:
   A. Activating coronary electrical
   B. Altering and converting enzyme
   C. Angiotensin-converting enzyme
   D. Angina-converting enzyme

5. Beta-blockers are effective for cardiac conditions because they work by:
   A. Blocking receptor sites in the heart
   B. Blocking receptor sites in the heart and kidneys
   C. Activating receptor sites in the heart and lungs
   D. Activating receptor sites in the heart and kidneys

6. Which instruction is *not* necessary patient information for taking oral nitroglycerin medications?
   A. Take with food
   B. Keep the medication in the original container
   C. Take as needed for chest pain; maximum three times in 15 minutes; if no relief after the first dose, call 911
   D. Keep the medication out of direct sunlight

7. t-PA is classified as a:
   A. Vasoconstrictor
   B. Vasodilator
   C. Prophylaxis thrombolytic
   D. Thrombolytic

8. The four chambers of the heart are:
   A. Right and left: upper and lower atrium
   B. Right and left: atrium and superior and inferior venae cavae
   C. Right and left: atrium and ventricle
   D. None of the above

9. Which of the following is used to dissolve blood clots?
   A. Heparin
   B. Aspirin
   C. t-PA
   D. Warfarin

10. Which of the following diuretics is associated with hyperkalemia (elevated potassium levels)?
    A. Furosemide
    B. Bumetanide
    C. Hydrochlorothiazide
    D. Spironolactone

11. Fondaparinux (Arixtra) is a(n):
    A. Vitamin K antagonist
    B. Factor Xa inhibitor
    C. LMWH
    D. Direct thrombin inhibitor

12. Nitrostat is a trade name for:
    A. Diltiazem
    B. Verapamil
    C. Atenolol
    D. Nitroglycerin

13. Which of the following is *not* a calcium channel blocker?
    A. Verapamil
    B. Hydrochlorothiazide
    C. Nifedipine
    D. Diltiazem

14. Which of the following is a bile acid sequestrant?
    A. Niacin
    B. Colesevelam
    C. Simvastatin
    D. Fenofibrate

15. Which of the following would be used to treat deep vein thrombosis (DVT)?
    A. Anticoagulants
    B. Thrombolytics
    C. Calcium channel blockers
    D. Both A and B

◻ Technician's Corner

Mrs. Lewis arrives at the pharmacy with several prescriptions. Using a comprehensive drug reference, such as *Drug Facts and Comparisons*, look up the medications listed and determine which conditions may be affecting Mrs. Lewis. Also, classify each of the medications and transcribe the prescription into lay terms as though you were preparing a prescription label.

- Simvastatin 5 mg qd, #30
- Digoxin 0.125 mg qd, #30
- Furosemide 40 mg bid, #60
- Albuterol inhaler 1 to 2 puffs prn SOB, #17g
- Nitroglycerin (NTG) 0.4 mg sl tab prn cp, 1q5min, max 3 tabs over 15 min; call 911 if chest pain unrelieved after first dose, 4/#25s
- Atenolol 25 mg qd, #30

Bibliography

Arnett DK, Blumenthal RS, Albert MA, et al. 2019 ACC/AHA guideline on the primary prevention of cardiovascular disease: a report of the American College of Cardiology/American Heart Association Task Force on Clinical Practice Guidelines. *J Am Coll Cardiol*. 2019;74(10):e177-e232.

Damjanov I. *Pathology for the Health Professions*. 4th ed. St. Louis: Saunders; 2011.

Fishback JL. *Pathology*. 3rd ed. Philadelphia: Mosby; 2005.

Huether S, McCance K. *Understanding Pathophysiology*. 5th ed. St. Louis: Mosby; 2012.

McCance KL. *Pathophysiology: The Biologic Basis for Disease in Adults and Children*. 6th ed. St. Louis: Mosby; 2010.

Page C, Hoffman B, Curtis M, Walker M. *Integrated Pharmacology*. 3rd ed. St. Louis: Mosby; 2006.

Patton KT, Thibodeau GA. *Mosby's Handbook of Anatomy and Physiology*. St. Louis: Mosby; 2000.

Price SA, Wilson LM. *Pathophysiology: Clinical Concepts of Disease Processes*. 6th ed. St. Louis: Mosby; 2003.

Sole ML, Klein D, Moseley M. *Introduction to Critical Care Nursing*. 6th ed. St. Louis: Saunders; 2013.

Solomon EP. *Introduction to Human Anatomy and Physiology*. 3rd ed. St. Louis: Saunders; 2009.

Websites Referenced

Clinical Pharmacology Online. Available at: https://www.clinicalkey.com/pharmacology/.

UpToDate Online. Available at: http://www.uptodate.com.

CHAPTER 21

Therapeutic Agents for the Respiratory System

Tony Guerra

OBJECTIVES

1. Describe the major components of the respiratory system.
2. List the primary symptoms of conditions associated with the dysfunction of the respiratory system. In addition, (a) recognize prescription and over-the-counter drugs used to treat conditions of the lower and upper respiratory systems, (b) write the generic and trade names for the drugs discussed in this chapter, and (c) list appropriate auxiliary labels when filling prescriptions for drugs discussed in this chapter.

TERMS AND DEFINITIONS

Allergen A substance that causes an allergic reaction

Alveoli Tiny air sacs in the lungs where oxygen and carbon dioxide exchange takes place

Anticholinergic Against + acetylcholine, an agent that inhibits the physiologic action of acetylcholine

Antihistamine Against + histamine, a drug or other compound that inhibits the effects of histamine; often used to treat allergies

Antitussive Against + cough, a drug that can decrease the central nervous system coughing reflex

Aspiration To draw a foreign substance into the respiratory tract during inhalation

Bronchi The major lung air passages that diverge from the windpipe

Bronchioles Small branches that divide from the bronchus in the lungs

Cilia Short, microscopic, hairlike structures

Decongestant Remove + congestion, a drug that shrinks the swollen membranes in the nasal cavity, making it easier to breathe

Diaphragm Through + fence, a dome-shaped, muscular partition separating the thorax from the abdomen that plays a major role in breathing

Dyspnea Bad + breathing, difficult or labored breathing

Expectorant A drug that helps remove mucous secretions from the respiratory system; it loosens and thins sputum and bronchial secretions for ease of expectoration

Expiration Out + breath, the act of breathing out; exhalation

Influenza A respiratory tract infection caused by an influenza virus

Inspiration In + breath, the act of breathing in; inhalation

Prophylactic Before + guard, treatment given before an event or exposure to prevent the condition or symptom

Sputum Fluid (mucus) expectorated from the lungs and bronchial tissues

Select Common Drugs for Conditions of the Respiratory System

Trade Name	Generic Name	Pronunciation
Antihistamines		
Allegra Allergy 12 Hour/Allegra Allergy 24 Hour	fexofenadine	(**fex**-oh-**fen**-uh-deen)
Benadryl Allergy	diphenhydramine	(die-fen-**hy**-druh-meen)
Claritin	loratadine	(loh-**rah**-tuh-deen)
Xyzal Allergy 24HR	levocetirizine	(lee-voh-sih-**teer**-uh-zeen)
Zyrtec Allergy	cetirizine	(sih-**teer**-uh-zeen)
Anticholinergics—Oral Inhalers		
Atrovent HFA	ipratropium bromide	(**ip**-ruh-**troe**-pee-um/**bro**-mide)
Spiriva Respimat/Spiriva Handihaler	tiotropium	(tye-oh-**troe**-pee-um)
Incruse Ellipta	umeclidinium	(u-meh-clih-**din**-ee-um)
Mucolytic		
Mucomysta	acetylcysteine	(a-**seet**-ill-**sis**-teen)
Bronchodilators		
Anoro Ellipta	vilanterol/umeclidinium	(vih-**lan**-ter-ol/u-meh-clih-**din**-ee-um)
Foradil Aerolizer^a	formoterol	(for-**moe**-ter-ol)
Proventil HFA, Ventolin HFA	albuterol	(al-bu-**ter**-ol)
Serevent Diskus	salmeterol	(sal-**meh**-ter-ol)
Xopenex HFA	levalbuterol	(leh-val-**byoo**-ter-ol)
Inhaled Corticosteroids		
AeroBid^a	flunisolide	(flew-**nis**-oh-lide)
Beclovent^a	beclomethasone	(beck-low-**meth**-ah-sone)
Flovent Diskus/Flovent HFA	fluticasone	(floo-**tic**-uh-sone)
Pulmicort Flexhaler	budesonide	(byoo-**des**-uh-nide)
Mast Cell Stabilizer		
NasalCrom	cromolyn	(**krom**-uh-lin)
Nasal Corticosteroids		
Flonase Allergy Relief	fluticasone	(floo-**tic**-uh-sone)
Nasacort Allergy 24HR	triamcinolone	(try-am-**sin**-uh-lone)
Nasonex	mometasone	(moe-**met**-uh-sone)
Rhinocort Allergy Spray	budesonide	(byoo-**dess**-uh-nide)
Immunomodulator		
Xolair	omalizumab	(**oh**-muh-**liz**-yoo-mab)
Leukotriene Inhibitors		
Accolate	zafirlukast	(zay-fur-**loo**-cast)
Singulair	montelukast	(mon-teh-**loo**-cast)
Xanthine		
Theo-24	theophylline	(thee-**off**-uh-lin)
Agents to Treat Tuberculosis		
	isoniazid	(eye-**soe**-nye-uh-**zid**)
Rifadin	rifampin	(rif-am-**pin**)
	streptomycin	(strep-**toe**-mye-sin)

^aBrand discontinued; now available only as generic.
HFA, Hydrofluoroalkane.

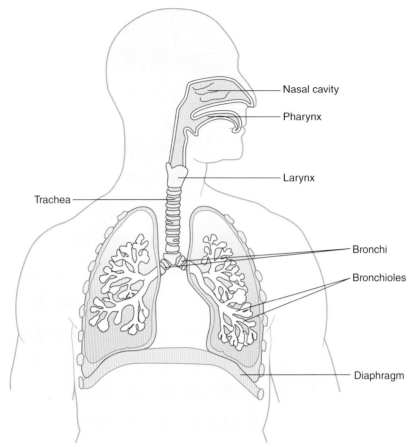

FIG. 21.1 Diagram of the respiratory system.

The lungs and airways play an essential role in the body. The respiratory system has many elements with various functions (Fig. 21.1). For example, the lungs facilitate oxygen absorption during inhalation and carbon dioxide removal during exhalation. The fine nose hairs and bronchial mucosal lining filter and trap dust, microorganisms, and foreign particles. Mucus engulfs these unwanted particles, and then cilia propel the mucus for the throat to swallow. The nose also helps to heat and humidify cold, dry air to our body temperature. This chapter discusses the respiratory system's structure and function, the events during respiration, and conditions and treatments for the respiratory system.

Structure and Function of the Respiratory System

The lungs resemble a large, inverted multibranched tree. The large trunk is the trachea, and the two main branches represent **bronchi** (see Fig. 21.1). The smaller branches are **bronchioles**, and the leaves are the alveolar sacs for gas exchange (Fig. 21.2). We can more easily discuss the system as two parts, the upper and lower respiratory tract. Let's first focus on the upper respiratory tract. The primary roles of the upper respiratory tract are to filter, warm, and moisten the air before it enters the lower respiratory tract.

Upper Respiratory System

The nose and nasal cavities, the pharynx (ie, the throat), and the larynx (ie, the voice box) make up the upper respiratory tract (Fig. 21.3). A mucosal lining covers the inside of the respiratory tract, forming a protective barrier that purifies air by trapping inhaled irritants, including dust and pollens. The nasal septum separates the nasal interior into two distinct cavities. Mucous membranes with microscopic, hairlike structures called **cilia** line these openings. The mucous membrane warms and moistens inhaled air. The nose detects smell and drains tears from the eyes. The respiratory and digestive systems share the pharynx. Food passes into the esophagus, and air flows through the trachea (the *windpipe*). The tonsils, composed of lymphatic tissue (see Chapter 25), sit in the pharynx.

The larynx, or voice box, contains the vocal cords for speech. Women have smaller, nonprotruding larynxes compared with men. This cartilage, visible in men, has another name: the "Adam's apple." The larynx's entrance houses the epiglottis, which is thin, leaf-shaped, and made of elastic cartilage (see Fig. 21.3). It automatically obstructs the trachea, similar to a trapdoor, when swallowing takes place. This keeps food, liquid, and saliva from entering the airway. Choking can happen if food enters the trachea rather than the esophagus.

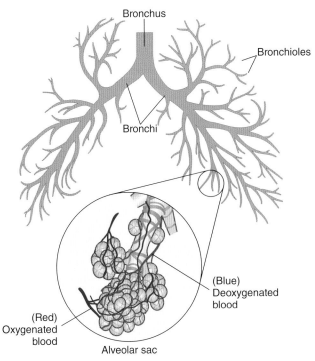

Bronchus

Bronchioles

Bronchi

(Blue)
Deoxygenated
blood

(Red)
Oxygenated
blood

Alveolar sac

FIG. 21.2 Bronchial tree.

> **Tech Note!**
>
> In people who have swallowing difficulties (eg, individuals with Parkinson disease), food, liquids, and medications can make their way into the trachea instead of the esophagus. This is aspiration, which can lead to serious health problems, such as aspiration pneumonia.

Lower Respiratory System

The trachea, bronchial tree, and lungs form the lower respiratory system. Mucous membranes line the trachea (windpipe) and trap airborne particles. The cilia propel the particles upward for swallowing. The trachea branches into the *right bronchus* and *left bronchus*, leading to the right and left lungs, respectively. Rings of cartilage reinforce the trachea so that it does not collapse when the neck bends (see Fig. 21.3).

Two bronchi branch from the trachea. They split, in turn, into smaller bronchi and bronchioles. Bronchioles deliver air through the lungs and into **alveoli**. Respiration occurs in the alveoli as oxygen and carbon dioxide pass between the tiny capillaries surrounding them. Oxygen diffuses from the alveoli into the bloodstream. Carbon dioxide also passes from the blood to the alveoli for exhalation.

The lungs fill the chest cavity, except for the space occupied by the heart and large vessels. Their purposes include ventilation and gas exchange. The lungs have many lobes, three in the right lung and two in the left (Fig. 21.4). The left lung has a surface dent, the *cardiac notch*, to accommodate the apex of the heart. At the base of the chest cavity is a major

respiratory muscle called the **diaphragm**, that enables inspiration and expiration. This large, dome-shaped muscle separates the chest cavity from the abdominal cavity. It contracts and flattens during inspiration, and it relaxes during exhalation. Other muscles support breathing. We will discuss them in the next section.

Respiration

We divide respiration into two distinct phases. **Inspiration** is air movement into the lungs. **Expiration** moves air out. Changes in the size and shape of the chest cavity (or thorax) during respiration change air pressure forcing air into and out of the lungs (Fig. 21.5). As a person actively inhales (inspiration), the diaphragmatic muscles and intercostal muscles contract, and the thoracic cavity expands. The increased chest cavity volume creates pressure inside the lungs that is lower than the atmospheric pressure. Air then flows into the lungs. Expiration, on the other hand, occurs as the chest relaxes, and the thorax returns to its resting size and shape. The compressed thoracic cavity increases the pressure in the thorax and the lungs to expel air. Breathing is involuntary. The body automatically breathes out and inhales without your thought. The respiratory control center, in the medulla in the brainstem, automatically controls the rate and depth of breathing, depending on the body's oxygen needs.

> **Tech Note!**
>
> The average respiratory rate for adults is 12 to 18 breaths/min, whereas a 6- to 12-year-old child's rate is higher at 18 to 30 breaths/min. The infant rate from birth to 1 year can range from 30 to 60 breaths/min.

Breathing rates vary, depending on the size of the person. For example, small children can breathe twice as fast as adults. The typical amount of air expelled from the lungs in a usual exhalation is approximately 500 mL, or 0.5 L, for an average adult. Note, the total lung capacity is more than 5 L of air. The lung's elasticity allows the capacity to vary widely, depending on oxygen needs. Table 21.1 lists common medical terms used to describe different types of breathing dysfunction.

> **Tech Note!**
>
> Some medications can alter respiratory rates. For example, opioids (eg, morphine) can suppress the respiratory rate.

Gas Exchange

Room air contains approximately 21% oxygen, 79% nitrogen, and less than 0.5% carbon dioxide. As we breathe, the lungs exchange inspired oxygen for expired carbon

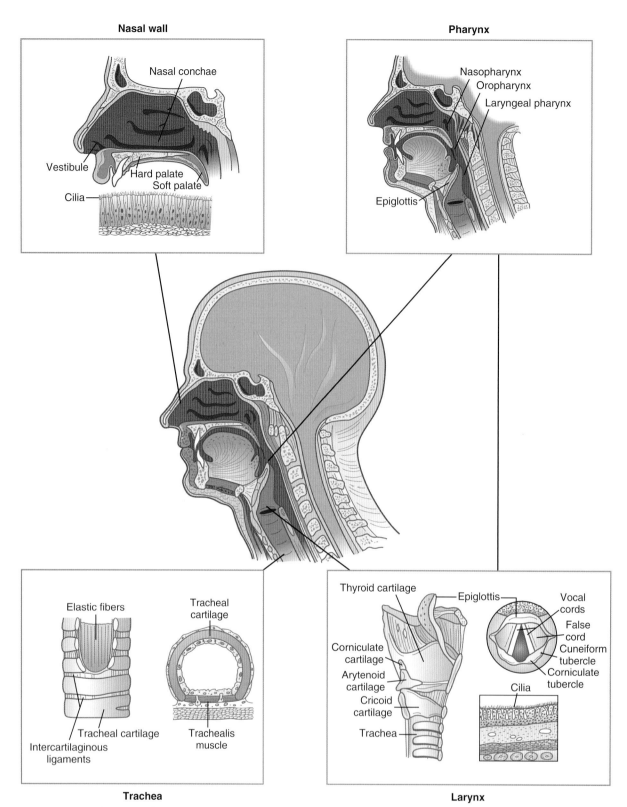

Nasal wall

Nasal conchae

Vestibule

Hard palate

Soft palate

Cilia

Pharynx

Nasopharynx

Oropharynx

Laryngeal pharynx

Epiglottis

Trachea

Elastic fibers

Tracheal cartilage

Tracheal cartilage

Trachealis muscle

Intercartilaginous ligaments

Larynx

Thyroid cartilage

Epiglottis

Vocal cords

False cord

Cuneiform tubercle

Corniculate tubercle

Corniculate cartilage

Arytenoid cartilage

Cricoid cartilage

Trachea

Cilia

FIG. 21.3 Structures of the upper airway. (From McCance KL. *Pathophysiology: The biologic basis for disease in adults and children*. 6th ed. St. Louis: Mosby; 2010.)

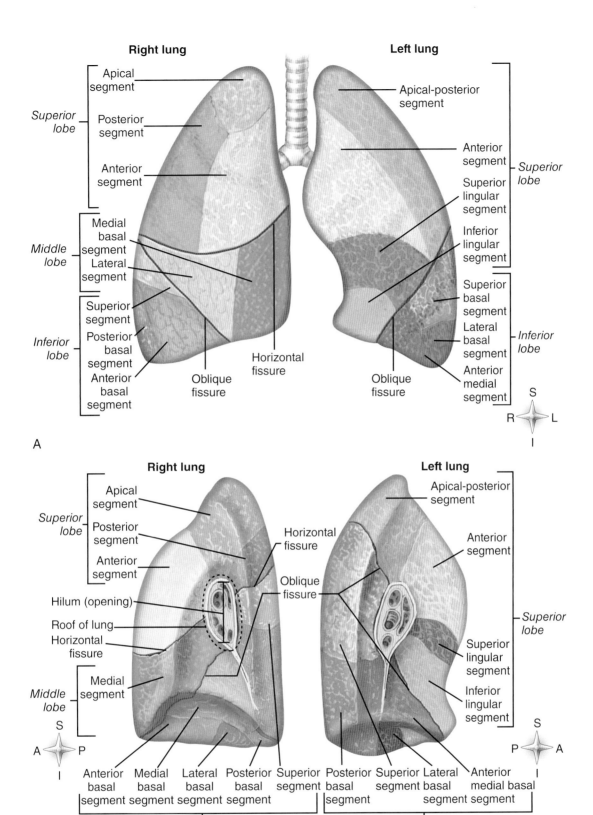

FIG. 21.4 Lobes and segments of the lungs. (A) Anterior view. (B) Posterior view. (From Patton KT, Thibodeau G. *Mosby's Handbook of Anatomy and Physiology*. St. Louis: Mosby; 2000.)

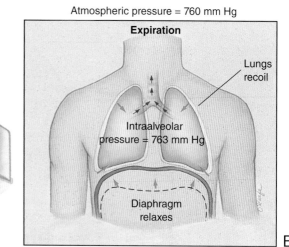

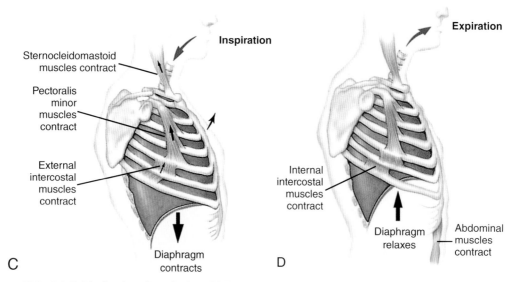

FIG. 21.5 Mechanics of ventilation. (A) Frontal view of inspiration. (B) Frontal view of expiration. (C) Side view of inspiration. (D) Side view of expiration. (From Patton KT, Thibodeau G. *Mosby's Handbook of Anatomy and Physiology*. St. Louis: Mosby; 2000.)

■ TABLE 21.1

Medical Terms Used to Describe Various Types of Breathing Dysfunction

Condition	Description
Apnea	Respiration stops
Bradypnea	Abnormally slow respiratory rate
Cyanosis	Discoloration of the skin (blue-gray) because of lack of oxygenation
Dyspnea	Labored or difficult respiration
Hyperventilation	Deep and rapid respiration
Hypopnea	Shallow breathing and/or abnormally low respiratory rate
Orthopnea	Labored or difficult respiration while lying down
Tachypnea	Rapid respiratory rate

dioxide (waste). From the alveolus, oxygen molecules move across thin membranes into passing red blood cells in nearby vessels. Red blood cells drop off carbon dioxide molecules and recover oxygen molecules. Carbon dioxide molecules move from the lung capillary blood supply into the alveolar sacs and out via expired air. The heart pumps oxygenated red blood cells to tissues and organs (Fig. 21.6).

Respiratory regulation permits the body's adjustment to oxygen supply and carbon dioxide removal. The respiratory center in the medulla oblongata ensures efficiency. The exchange of oxygen and carbon dioxide also keeps blood pH balanced. The body uses some carbon dioxide to make bicarbonate, which maintains the blood pH close to 7.4. Because of carbon dioxide's important role, abnormal respiration may result in acid-base disorders.

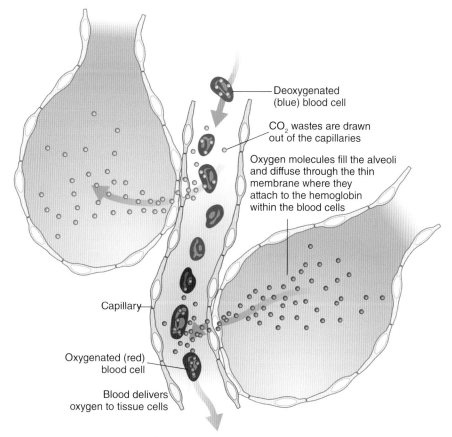

FIG. 21.6 Exchange of oxygen and carbon dioxide.

- Deoxygenated (blue) blood cell
- CO_2 wastes are drawn out of the capillaries
- Oxygen molecules fill the alveoli and diffuse through the thin membrane where they attach to the hemoglobin within the blood cells
- Capillary
- Oxygenated (red) blood cell
- Blood delivers oxygen to tissue cells

Disorders and Conditions of the Respiratory System

Conditions of the Upper Respiratory System

Conditions that affect the respiratory system include genetic, contagious infections, habits (eg, smoking), and environmental factors. Respiratory illness symptoms manifest as abnormal breathing and coughing. Although upper respiratory tract illnesses are diverse, similar types of medications treat most conditions. These drugs include antitussives, analgesics, and antipyretics, among others. For severe conditions (eg, bacterial infection or allergy), a prescriber may choose antibiotics or corticosteroids. Table 21.2 lists common upper respiratory tract conditions, symptoms, and drug class medications. The following sections describe the causes, symptoms, and treatment of common upper respiratory tract disorders. Many symptomatic treatments are available over the counter (OTC) (see Chapter 29 for additional information).

Common Cold

The common cold is the most frequent acute illness in the United States and other industrialized countries. Common symptoms of this mild upper respiratory tract infection include nasal congestion and rhinorrhea (runny nose), sneezing, sore throat, cough, fever, headache, and fatigue. Efforts to reduce the transmission of the common cold usually focus on preventive measures. Good hygiene (eg, hand washing and/or use of hand sanitizers) and proper sneezing techniques help limit viral spread.

Prognosis

The average incidence of the common cold ranges from five to seven episodes per year in preschool children to two or three episodes per year in adults. With rest and time, a cold runs its course. In some individuals, colds can aggravate chronic conditions such as asthma, emphysema, and bronchitis.

Non-Drug Treatment

Drinking plenty of water and getting enough rest are important parts of the non-drug treatment of the common cold. Vaporizers can help relieve worsening night congestion. Gargling with warm saline can help relieve a sore throat.

Drug Treatment

Common cold treatment depends on presenting symptoms as it is often a self-limiting disease caused by various viruses. The treatment is to relieve symptoms and reduce the illnesses duration. Conventional symptomatic treatments include decongestants, antihistamines, antitussives, and expectorants. These are available in various dosage forms, such as liquids, lozenges, nasal sprays, and oral tablets and capsules. The following text

TABLE 21.2
Common Infections of the Upper Respiratory System

Infections	Common Symptoms	Medications for Symptomatic Management
Allergic rhinitis	Stuffy nose, congestion	Antihistamines, nasal corticosteroids, allergy eye drops
Bronchitis (bacterial or viral)[a]	Cough, shortness of breath, fatigue, chest pain	Bronchodilators, analgesics, expectorants, cough suppressants
Common cold (viral)	Stuffy nose, sore throat, sneezing, headache, muscle aches	Decongestants, antihistamines, analgesics
Influenza (viral)[a]	Fever, chills, headache, muscle aches, fatigue, cough	Analgesics, antipyretics, antivirals
Sinusitis	Stuffy nose, headache, congestion	Antihistamines, nasal corticosteroids, analgesics, decongestants
Strep throat (bacterial)	Fever, headache, sore throat	Antibiotics, analgesics, antipyretics

[a]Can affect both the upper and lower respiratory tract.

outlines common agents for symptomatic relief. Some use vitamin C (which has limited data), and others use zinc to help reduce symptoms. Zinc treatments can require 220 mg twice daily. A more detailed OTC product discussion of conventional cold treatments is in Chapter 29. Product selection should aim to relieve troublesome specific symptoms.

Antihistamines alleviate rhinorrhea and sneezing. Their use, especially of first-generation products, causes sedating and mucous membrane drying side effects (eyes, nose, mouth).

GENERIC NAME: diphenhydramine (OTC)

TRADE NAME: Benadryl Allergy

INDICATIONS: Cough, allergic rhinitis, rhinorrhea, insomnia, motion sickness

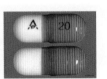

ROUTES OF ADMINISTRATION: Oral; topical; injectable

COMMON ADULT DOSAGE: *Oral dose for the common cold:* 12.5–50 mg every 4–6 hours (not to exceed 300 mg every 24 hours)

MECHANISM OF ACTION: Blocks the effects of histamine at histamine-1 (H$_1$) receptors

SIDE EFFECTS: Drowsiness, dry mouth, dizziness, confusion, urinary retention

Antitussives suppress a cough. Patients with the common cold may have a dry, unproductive cough, and antitussives give symptomatic relief. However, the American College of Chest Physicians recommends against cough suppressants when patients have upper respiratory tract infections. Antitussives are

available by prescription and OTC. Dextromethorphan, a common OTC antitussive, has abuse potential at high doses from its ability to induce hallucinations and euphoria. Prescription antitussives can contain codeine, which, in concentrations of less than 200 mg per 100 mL, are US Drug Enforcement Agency Schedule V controlled substances.

GENERIC NAME: dextromethorphan (OTC)

TRADE NAME: Delsym, Robitussin[a]

INDICATION: Cough

ROUTE OF ADMINISTRATION: Oral

COMMON ADULT DOSAGE: *IR:* 10–20 mg every 4 hours or 30 mg every 6–8 hours; *ER:* 60 mg every 12 hours or 120 mg every 24 hours (max 120 mg/24 hr)

MECHANISM OF ACTION: Thought to suppress the cough center in the medulla of the brain

SIDE EFFECTS: Drowsiness, dizziness, fatigue

[a] Brand no longer available.

GENERIC NAME: promethazine/codeine

TRADE NAME: Phenergan with codeine (C-V)[a]

INDICATIONS: Cough, the common cold

ROUTE OF ADMINISTRATION: Oral

COMMON ADULT DOSAGE: 5 mL (promethazine 6.25 mg/codeine 10 mg) every 4–6 hours, not to exceed 30 mL (promethazine 37.5 mg/codeine 60 mg) in 24 hours

MECHANISMS OF ACTION: Codeine suppresses the cough center in the medulla, and promethazine primarily antagonizes H$_1$ receptors

SIDE EFFECTS: Constipation, drowsiness, respiratory depression

AUXILIARY LABELS:
- May cause drowsiness
- May cause dizziness
- *Caution:* Federal law prohibits the transfer of this drug to any person other than the patient for whom it was prescribed

ª Brand discontinued; now available only as generic.

Expectorants such as guaifenesin break up thick mucus lung and bronchial secretions for easy removal through coughing. Pharmacists should counsel patients to increase fluid intake, which helps thin mucus.

GENERIC NAME: guaifenesin (OTC)

TRADE NAME: Mucinex

INDICATIONS: Cough, congestion

ROUTE OF ADMINISTRATION: Oral

COMMON ADULT DOSAGES: 200–400 mg (10–20 mL) every 4 hours (max 2400 mg/day); extended-release dosing, 600–1200 mg every 12 hours (max 2400 mg/day)

MECHANISM OF ACTION: Increases the ability to clear phlegm and bronchial secretions by reducing their viscosity

SIDE EFFECTS: Diarrhea, drowsiness, dizziness, headache

Decongestants affect the adrenergic receptors of the vascular smooth muscle, leading to constriction of blood vessels and a decrease in mucus production. Many decongestants are available as OTC products. Hypertensive patients should avoid these.

GENERIC NAME: pseudoephedrine

TRADE NAME: Sudafed 12 Hour, Sudafed 24 Hour

INDICATIONS: Nasal congestion, common cold, allergic rhinitis

ROUTES OF ADMINISTRATION: Oral

COMMON ADULT DOSAGES: *IR:* 60 mg every 4–6 hours; *ER:* 120 mg every 12 hours or 240 mg every 24 hours (max 240 mg/24 hr)

MECHANISM OF ACTION: Adrenergic agonist activates alpha- and beta-adrenergic receptors, leading to vasoconstriction to reduce nasal congestion

SIDE EFFECTS: Increased blood pressure, insomnia, restlessness

SPECIAL NOTE: Law enforcement now regulates pseudoephedrine sales because of its role in making

the street drug methamphetamine. Pharmacies keep pseudoephedrine containing products behind the counter (BTC) and patients must present photo identification to purchase them. States have daily and monthly maximums for pseudoephedrine sales to a single person.

GENERIC NAME: phenylephrine (OTC)

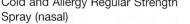

TRADE NAMES: Sudafed PE Congestion (oral); Neo-Synephrine Cold and Allergy Regular Strength Spray (nasal)

INDICATION: Nasal congestion

ROUTES OF ADMINISTRATION: Oral; intranasal

COMMON ADULT DOSAGES: *Oral:* 10 mg every 4 hours as needed for 7 days or less (max 60 mg/24 hr). *Intranasal:* 2–3 sprays in each nostril no more than every 4 hours for 3 days or less

MECHANISM OF ACTION: Adrenergic agonist that activates alpha- and beta-adrenergic receptors, leading to vasoconstriction to reduce nasal congestion

SIDE EFFECTS: Dizziness, insomnia, increased blood pressure, rebound congestion

---

Tech Note!

Many decongestants can worsen nasal congestion with *rebound congestion* if patients use them for more than 3 consecutive days. OTC nasal inhaler medications that can have this effect include oxymetazoline (Afrin) and phenylephrine (Neo-Synephrine).

Cromolyn sodium is a synthetic compound manufacturers hoped was an improved bronchodilator. Although it lacks bronchodilating properties, cromolyn inhibits antigen-induced bronchospasm. Cromolyn therefore works as a **prophylactic** agent for asthma and a nasal preparation for seasonal allergic rhinitis and nasal congestion. Some evidence suggests that cromolyn may improve symptoms of the common cold.

GENERIC NAME: cromolyn sodium

TRADE NAMES: NasalCrom (nasal) available OTC, Opticromª (ophthalmic), Gastrocrom (oral)

INDICATIONS: Asthma prophylaxis, seasonal allergic rhinitis, nasal congestion

ROUTES OF ADMINISTRATION: Intranasal; inhaled; ophthalmic; oral

COMMON ADULT DOSAGE: *Intranasal:* 1 spray into each nostril 3 or 4 times daily

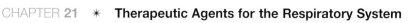

MECHANISM OF ACTION: Inhibits degranulation of mast cells of the immune system, preventing the release of histamine and inhibiting inflammation

SIDE EFFECTS: Sneezing, nasal irritation

AUXILIARY LABEL: Nasal formulations: Shake well

 ᵃ Brand no longer available.

Allergies

An allergy is an abnormal response of the immune system to an unrecognized, typically harmless substance. This response does not occur in all people and varies widely. In certain people, the allergic reaction can be severe to life-threatening. Types of **allergens** vary widely and include pollens, animal dander, foods, medications, chemicals, or environmental pollutants. Allergies are one of the most common types of respiratory problems, experienced by approximately 50 million US residents. Symptoms and reactions include rash, hives, itching, and nasal congestion. Severe reactions can cause stomach pain, vomiting, wheezing, shortness of breath (SOB), hypotension (low blood pressure), swelling of the throat, and anaphylactic shock if left untreated.

Prognosis

Health professionals can control most allergic symptoms through medication. Allergy shots can lessen symptoms in patients with identifiable allergens.

Non-Drug Treatment

Avoiding specific allergens is the best way to prevent an allergic reaction. If a reaction occurs, the allergic type and severity determine pharmacological or non-drug treatment. For allergic reactions caused by allergens in the home, removing the allergen is an excellent first step. Using a humidifier and/or air purifier may lessen the concentrations of an airborne allergen. Providers should document trigger foods and medications in the individual's medical record and pharmacy profile. In some instances, wristbands should list life-threatening allergies. Face masks or staying indoors during high pollen days can also help.

Drug Treatments

Many of the medications used for allergies mimic those used to treat the common cold. Allergy medications include oral, intranasal, ophthalmic, and topical antihistamines and/or decongestants (Table 21.3). Many allergy medications are available OTC. First-generation older antihistamines (eg, diphenhydramine) cause drowsiness. Newer second-generation drugs may have a mild sedative effect or cause no sedation (see Chapter 29). Loratadine (Claritin) and fexofenadine (Allegra) are considered nondrowsy, and cetirizine (Zyrtec) exhibits some sedative effects. Oral corticosteroids, intranasal or respiratory corticosteroids, leukotriene inhibitors, and epinephrine may require a prescription. In life-threatening cases, injectable epinephrine can open the airways.

■ Tech Note!

Patients with allergy or cold-induced nasal congestion can opt for a combination product with an antihistamine and a decongestant. If a product has a hyphen D after the name, for example, Allegra-D or Claritin-D, the product contains the D, decongestant, pseudoephedrine. As mentioned earlier, these products require photo ID for purchase.

■ TABLE 21.3
Select Prescription Medications for the Treatment of Allergies

Generic Name	Trade Name	Common Dosage Range	Common Side Effects
Intranasal Corticosteroids			
beclomethasone	Beconase AQ, Qnasl	• 1 or 2 sprays in each nostril twice daily	• Cough
budesonide	Rhinocort Allergy Spray	• 1 spray in each nostril once daily	• Headache
flunisolide		• 2 sprays in each nostril twice daily	• Nasal burning
fluticasone	Flonase Allergy Relief	• 2 sprays in each nostril once daily *or* • 1 spray in each nostril twice daily	• Nasal dryness
mometasone	Nasonex	• 2 sprays in each nostril once daily	
triamcinolone	Nasacort Allergy 24HR	• 2 sprays in each nostril once daily	
Antihistamines			
desloratadine	Clarinex	• 5 mg once daily	• Cough
fexofenadine	Allegra Allergy 12 Hour	• 60 mg twice daily	• Dizziness
	Allegra Allergy 24 Hour	• 180 mg once daily	
levocetirizine	Xyzal Allergy 24HR	• 2.5–5 mg once daily	
olopatadine	Patanase	• 2 sprays in each nostril twice daily	
triprolidine	Histex	• 2.5 mg every 4–6 hours	

GENERIC NAME: fexofenadine

TRADE NAME: Allegra Allergy 12 Hour, Allegra Allergy 24 Hour

INDICATION: Allergic rhinitis, urticaria

ROUTE OF ADMINISTRATION: Oral

COMMON ADULT DOSAGE: 60 mg twice daily or 180 mg/day

MECHANISM OF ACTION: Selective H₁ receptor blocker

SIDE EFFECTS: Headache, vomiting, dizziness, fatigue

AUXILIARY LABEL: Take with water

GENERIC NAME: desloratadine

TRADE NAME: Clarinex

INDICATIONS: Allergic rhinitis, urticaria, pruritus

ROUTE OF ADMINISTRATION: Oral

COMMON ADULT DOSAGE: 5 mg once daily

MECHANISM OF ACTION: Selective H₁ receptor blocker

SIDE EFFECTS: Headache, dry mouth, fatigue, dizziness

AUXILIARY LABEL: Do not crush or chew the tablet

Rhinitis

Rhinitis is an irritation and inflammation of the mucous membranes lining the nasal passage. Several different factors, including colds, influenza, allergens (as described previously), air pollution, or strong odors (eg, perfume, chemicals, or even certain medications), cause it. Rhinitis is either acute (eg, colds or flu) or chronic (eg, continuous or seasonal exposure to allergens). Common symptoms include runny and itchy nose, sneezing, congestion, and postnasal drip. Postnasal drip comes from mucus accumulating in the back of the nose and throat. Drinking fluids thins the postnasal drip mucus and helps with expectoration. Additional symptoms may include coughing, runny or watery eyes, and headache.

Prognosis

Rhinitis caused by colds or the flu usually is short-lived, subsiding over several days. Chronic rhinitis continues through allergy season and may require prolonged treatment.

Non-Drug Treatments

OTC saline irrigation products can treat cold or flu virus rhinitis. Saline can help relieve postnasal drip symptoms. For rhinitis from allergen exposures, symptomatic relief can come from air purifiers or humidifiers, cotton bedding, closed windows during pollen season, and avoiding live indoor plants depending on allergy type. Bathe allergy-causing animals often to minimize dander shedding.

Drug Treatments

In addition to rhinitis treatments (eg, decongestants and antihistamines), corticosteroid nasal sprays, such as beclomethasone, flunisolide, budesonide, mometasone, and fluticasone, can reduce sinus inflammation. With nasal decongestants, patients should not use them beyond 3 days because rebound congestion can occur 3 to 5 days after starting the medication.

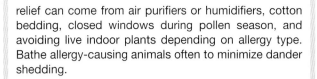

GENERIC NAME: triamcinolone

TRADE NAME: Nasacort Allergy 24HR (available OTC)

INDICATION: Allergic rhinitis

ROUTE OF ADMINISTRATION: Intranasal

COMMON ADULT DOSAGE: 2 sprays into each nostril once daily

MECHANISM OF ACTION: Corticosteroid produces antiinflammatory and vasoconstrictive effects that help treat rhinitis symptoms

SIDE EFFECTS: Dry mouth, nasal dryness, cough, nasal irritation

AUXILIARY LABEL: Shake well before use

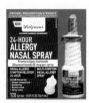

GENERIC NAME: fluticasone

TRADE NAME: Flonase Allergy Relief

INDICATION: Allergic rhinitis

ROUTE OF ADMINISTRATION: Intranasal

COMMON ADULT DOSAGE: 1 or 2 sprays into each nostril once daily

MECHANISM OF ACTION: Corticosteroid produces antiinflammatory and vasoconstrictive effects that help treat rhinitis symptoms

SIDE EFFECTS: Headache, nosebleed, cough, nasal irritation

AUXILIARY LABEL: Shake well before use

Influenza

A severe viral respiratory illness is the flu, or **influenza** (Fig. 21.7). Influenza infects the respiratory system, including the nose, throat, bronchial tubes, and lungs. Influenza causes millions of dollars of lost wages and health care costs each year. In young children have developing organs, elderly have degrading organ function, and immunocompromised have suppressed function, it can be deadly.

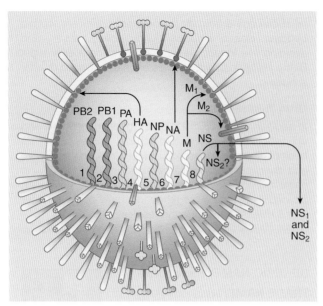

FIG. 21.7 Influenza. (From Goldman M. *Procedures in Cosmetic Dermatology Series: Photodynamic Therapy.* 2nd ed. St. Louis: Saunders; 2008.)

Prognosis

With proper treatment, most people recover from influenza. However, older, younger, and immunocompromised populations are at risk and may have a slow recovery or even die. Getting a flu vaccine each year is the best way to avoid or lessen the risk for contracting influenza.

Non-Drug Treatment

Usually, the best remedy is bed rest and drinking plenty of fluids.

Drug Treatment

For severe influenza, a prescriber may give antivirals at early onset (usually within 48 hours) to help shorten the course or lessen illness severity. Health providers may give antivirals prophylactically on exposure to somebody with the virus (Table 21.4). However, some influenza strains resist antiviral medications. Providers give vaccines during the peak flu season. Chapter 25 presents a detailed vaccine discussion.

■ Tech Note!

Antibiotics, usually a word that means *antibacterial,* are not suitable for treatment of *viral infections* such as colds and influenza. Prescribing antibiotics for viral infections contributes to the development of resistant bacterial strains.

Conditions of the Lower Respiratory System

Conditions and disorders of the lower respiratory tract originate from the lungs but can also affect the upper respiratory system.

Asthma

Asthma is a chronic inflammatory condition that affects the airways. It is one of several obstructive lung diseases that share some clinical characteristics of chronic obstructive pulmonary disease (COPD), which is described later (Fig. 21.8). The classic asthma signs include intermittent **dyspnea** (SOB), cough, and wheezing. In asthma, the muscles around the bronchioles contract, narrowing the air passages. Besides

■ TABLE 21.4
Select Agents for the Treatment and/or Prophylaxis of Influenza

Generic Name	Trade Name	Common Dosage Range	Indications
Adamantane Antivirals			
amantadine[a]		• Influenza A virus infection: 200 mg/day in 1–2 doses • Influenza prophylaxis: 200 mg/day in 1–2 doses; begin as soon as possible after exposure and continue for at least 10 days	• Influenza A virus infection • Influenza prophylaxis • Parkinson disease
rimantadine	Flumadine	• Influenza A virus infection: 100 mg twice daily • Influenza prophylaxis: 100 mg twice daily	• Influenza A virus infection • Influenza prophylaxis
Neuraminidase Inhibitors			
oseltamivir	Tamiflu	• Influenza A or B virus infection: 75 mg twice daily for 5 days • Influenza prophylaxis: 75 mg daily for 7–10 days to 6 wk (immunocompromised)	• Influenza A virus infection • Influenza B virus infection • Influenza prophylaxis
zanamivir	Relenza Diskhaler	• Influenza A or B virus infection: 10 mg (2 oral inhalations) twice daily for 5 days • Influenza prophylaxis: 10 mg (2 oral inhalations) once daily for 28 days	• Influenza A virus infection • Influenza B virus infection • Influenza prophylaxis

[a]No longer recommended by the Centers for Disease Control and Prevention for treatment and prophylaxis of influenza A due to high levels of amantadine resistance.

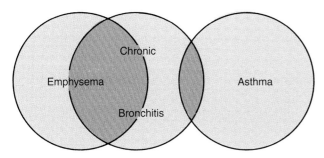

FIG. 21.8 Interrelationship between the disease entities making up COPD. (From Price SA, Wilson LM. *Pathophysiology: Clinical Concepts of Disease Processes*. 6th ed. St. Louis: Mosby; 2003.)

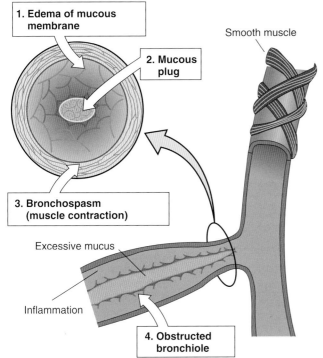

FIG. 21.9 Asthma obstruction. (From Moscou K, Snipe K. *Pharmacology for Pharmacy Technicians*. 2nd ed. St. Louis: Mosby; 2013.)

resisting air flow, mucous edema worsens the condition (Fig. 21.9). These pathologic changes lead to the characteristic crackling and wheezing sounds heard during an asthma attack. Because asthma is an inflammatory disease, specific triggers can cause inflammation of the airways, leading to the mucus production and bronchiole constriction previously mentioned. The most common triggers of asthma attacks are exposure to allergens, such as animals or environmental irritants, and exercise and stress.

Prognosis

The prognosis for this disease is highly dependent on the severity of the individual's asthma. Prophylactic and rescue agents can effectively manage the condition.

Non-Drug Treatments

Asthma management begins with patient education to avoid allergens and irritants that trigger asthmatic attacks. Calming techniques can help patients relax during an asthma attack.

Drug Treatments

Prescribers generally use two medication categories for asthma: those for prophylaxis (or maintenance) and those for acute attacks (abortive therapies) (Table 21.5). Health providers often treat with metered dose inhalers (MDIs). Patients should learn how to use them properly so they obtain the correct medication dosage (Fig. 21.10).

Tech Note!

Patients might use spacers (a generic term) with certain inhalers. Spacers are manufactured tubes that attach to inhalers with a one-way valve. This allows patients to inhale, not exhale, into the device. That mechanism allows more active drug to reach the lungs. Spacers help patients who may lack the dexterity to actuate their inhalers. Some respiratory medications come as dry powder inhalers (DPIs). These do not require patients to time their inhalation.

Corticosteroids Corticosteroids act as antiinflammatory medications and lessen bronchial tube swelling. Many inhalers were given twice daily, but newer inhalers such as fluticasone/vilanterol (Breo Ellipta) require only once-daily dosing. Inhaled corticosteroids (ICSs), in combination with long-acting beta-agonists (LABAs), are the most effective treatment to prevent severe asthma exacerbation in patients with chronic asthma, as shown in the Salmeterol Multicenter Asthma Research Trial (SMART). Inhaled corticosteroids can cause thrush or candidiasis, a type of fungal infections. Health providers should remind patients to rinse their mouth with water to avoid this infection or dysphonia, a voice hoarseness.

GENERIC NAME: budesonide

TRADE NAME: Pulmicort Flexhaler

INDICATION: Asthma prophylaxis (maintenance therapy)

ROUTE OF ADMINISTRATION: Inhalation

COMMON ADULT DOSAGE: Twice daily

MECHANISM OF ACTION: Antiinflammatory actions to reduce inflammation in the airway

SIDE EFFECTS: Bronchospasm, cough, oral candida infection

AUXILIARY LABELS:
• Shake well
• Take as directed

TABLE 21.5

Select Common Agents Used in the Treatment of Asthma and/or Chronic Obstructive Pulmonary Disease

Generic Name	Trade Name	Indications	Common Side Effects
Inhaled Corticosteroids			
Exert antiinflammatory actions to reduce inflammation in the airways			
beclomethasone	Qvar Redihaler	Asthma	• Cough • Dry mouth • Thrush
budesonide	Pulmicort Flexhaler, Pulmicort Respules	Asthma	
fluticasone	Flovent Diskus, Flovent HFA	Asthma	
Short-Acting Beta-Agonists			
Activate beta-2 receptors in the lung, leading to relaxation of the bronchial smooth muscle, in turn leading to bronchodilation and an increase in bronchial air flow			
albuterol beta-2 selective	ProAir HFA, Ventolin HFA, Proventil HFA, VoSpire ER[a]	Asthma, acute bronchospasm	• Cough • Dizziness • Headache • Insomnia • Nervousness • Tremor
levalbuterol beta-2 selective	Xopenex, Xopenex HFA	Asthma, acute bronchospasm	
Long-Acting Beta-Agonists			
Activate beta-2 receptors in the lung, leading to relaxation of the bronchial smooth muscle, in turn leading to bronchodilation and an increase in bronchial air flow			
arformoterol beta-2 selective	Brovana	COPD	• Cough • Headache • Upper respiratory tract infection
formoterol beta-2 selective	Perforomist	Asthma, COPD	
salmeterol beta-2 selective	Serevent Diskus	Asthma, COPD	
Inhaled Anticholinergics			
Block the effects of acetylcholine, leading to bronchial smooth muscle relaxation			
ipratropium	Atrovent HFA	Bronchospasm prophylaxis, COPD	• Dizziness • Drowsiness • Nausea • Vomiting
tiotropium	Spiriva Handihaler and Spiriva Respimat	Bronchospasm prophylaxis, COPD	
Methylxanthines			
Relax the smooth muscle of the bronchial airways and pulmonary blood vessels			
theophylline	Elixophyllin, Theochron[a], Theo-24	Asthma, asthma prophylaxis, COPD	• Dizziness • Insomnia • Nausea • Seizures • Vomiting
Leukotriene Receptor Antagonists			
Inhibit the effects of leukotrienes to reduce bronchial smooth muscle contraction, airway edema, and mucus formation			
montelukast	Singulair	Asthma, bronchospasm prophylaxis	• Fatigue • Headache • Heartburn • Nausea
zafirlukast	Accolate	Asthma, bronchospasm prophylaxis	
Phosphodiesterase-4 Inhibitor			
Inhibits the enzyme PDE4, an effect that is thought to reduce inflammation			
roflumilast	Daliresp	COPD	• Anxiety • Diarrhea • Insomnia • Nausea

Generic Name	Trade Name	Indications	Common Side Effects
Anti-IgE Antibody			
Blocks the inflammatory effects of IgE			
omalizumab	Xolair	Asthma	• Hypersensitivity reactions • Injection site reactions • Rash
Mast Cell Stabilizer			
Inhibits degranulation of mast cells of the immune system, preventing the release of histamine and inhibiting inflammation			
cromolyn sodium	Gastrocrom, NasalCrom	Asthma, bronchospasm prophylaxis	• Cough • Headache • Throat irritation
Mucolytic Agent			
Reduces the viscosity of mucus secreted in the lungs and aids in the removal of these secretions through coughing and/or drainage			
acetylcysteine	Acetadote, Cetylev[a], Mucomyst[b]	COPD	• Airway irritation • Drowsiness • Fever
Combination Products			
albuterol/ipratropium	Combivent Respimat, DuoNeb	COPD	
budesonide/formoterol	Symbicort	Asthma, COPD	
formoterol/mometasone	Dulera	Asthma	
fluticasone/salmeterol	Advair Diskus, Advair HFA	Asthma, COPD	

[a]Brand no longer available.
[b]Canada only.
COPD, Chronic obstructive pulmonary disease; *HFA,* hydrofluoroalkane; *IgE,* immunoglobulin E; *PDE4,* phosphodiesterase-4.

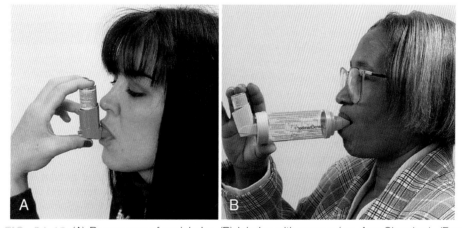

FIG. 21.10 (A) Proper use of an inhaler. (B) Inhaler with spacer (eg, AeroChamber). (From Elkin MK, Perry AG, Potter PA. *Nursing Interventions and Clinical Skills.* 4th ed. St. Louis: Elsevier; 2007.)

GENERIC NAME: fluticasone propionate

TRADE NAMES: Flovent HFA, Flovent Diskus

INDICATION: Asthma prophylaxis (maintenance therapy)

ROUTE OF ADMINISTRATION: Inhalation

COMMON ADULT DOSAGE: *Flovent HFA:* 88 mcg (2 sprays) twice daily. *Flovent Diskus:* 100 mcg twice daily

MECHANISM OF ACTION: Antiinflammatory actions to reduce inflammation in the airway

SIDE EFFECTS: Bronchospasm, cough

AUXILIARY LABELS:
- *Flovent HFA:* Shake well
- Take as directed
- Rinse mouth after each use

GENERIC NAME: salmeterol

TRADE NAME: Serevent Diskus

INDICATION: Asthma maintenance

ROUTE OF ADMINISTRATION: Inhalation

COMMON ADULT DOSAGE: 50 mcg (1 inhalation) twice daily

MECHANISM OF ACTION: Activation of lung beta-2 receptors leads to bronchial smooth muscle relaxation and ensuing bronchodilation, which increases bronchial air flow

SIDE EFFECTS: Headache, cough, upper respiratory tract infection

AUXILIARY LABELS:
- Use as directed
- Not a rescue inhaler for asthma attacks

Long-acting beta-agonists Airways contain beta-receptors. After medications activate these receptors, the smooth muscle surrounding the airways relaxes and opens the airways. Many patients with asthma find relief from maintenance medications such as ICSs and LABAs. Before SMART, prescribers gave beta-2–selective agonists alone. The SMART trial was designed to study possible severe side effects of salmeterol, a LABA widely used to treat asthma. The study began in 1996, hoping to enroll 60,000 patients. However, in 2003, researchers terminated the study prematurely after analyzing the collected data and finding significant rates of increased respiratory-related mortality in patients taking the LABA alone. Patients at the highest risk for adverse effects were those not taking an ICS before beginning the trial.

Salmeterol lost support as monotherapy in asthma treatment. All inhalers that contain salmeterol now must include a "Black Box Warning" that summarizes the SMART study findings. Subsequent studies support the positive therapeutic effects of inhalers that combine a LABA such as salmeterol with an ICS, such as fluticasone. These two active medications, salmeterol and fluticasone, are in the Advair Diskus inhaler. Researchers have not found serious negative hazardous effects while researching the efficacy of these combination inhalers. These LABA-ICS combination inhalers remain the most therapeutically effective treatments for patients with severe, uncontrolled asthma. Note, high doses of beta-agonists may cause tachycardia because of beta-1 receptor stimulation on the heart.

Now, health providers use bronchodilators and antiinflammatories in tandem as a best practice. The Global Initiative for Asthma (GINA) guidelines from 2019 no longer recommend starting with a short-acting beta-agonist (SABA)-only treatment; rather, that all adults and adolescents with asthma should receive ICS-containing controller treatment to reduce the risk for severe exacerbations and control symptoms.

GENERIC NAME: formoterol

TRADE NAME: Perforomist

INDICATION: COPD maintenance

ROUTE OF ADMINISTRATION: Inhalation

COMMON ADULT DOSAGE: 20 mcg (one inhalation) twice daily

MECHANISM OF ACTION: A long-acting beta-2 agonist that causes bronchodilation

SIDE EFFECTS: Cough, headache

AUXILIARY LABELS:
- Do not swallow capsules; only use capsules by inserting into the inhaler
- Not for acute asthma attacks

Tech Note!

Many inhaler devices are available. MDIs move medication into the lungs with a propellant. Although manufacturers previously used chlorofluorocarbons (CFCs) as propellant in MDIs, now they use hydrofluoroalkane (HFA). HFA does not damage the ozone layer. Patients need to coordinate their breath with inhaler activation. Because MDIs propel actuated drug, the drug comes out when actuated. Albuterol inhalers are MDIs. DPIs do not require coordinated patient timing. DPIs often use blisters that are punctured and subsequently inhaled by the patient. Tiotropium (Spiriva HandiHaler) is an example of a DPI.

Leukotriene receptor antagonists (leukotriene inhibitors) Leukotriene inhibitors reduce leukotrienes' inflammatory actions. This mechanism induces bronchial smooth muscle contraction, airway edema, and mucus formation.

GENERIC NAME: montelukast

TRADE NAMES: Singulair, Singulair Chewable Tablet

INDICATIONS: Asthma, allergic rhinitis, bronchospasm prophylaxis

ROUTE OF ADMINISTRATION: Oral

COMMON ADULT DOSAGE: 10 mg once daily in the evening

MECHANISM OF ACTION: Inhibits leukotrienes to reduce bronchial smooth muscle contraction, airway edema, and mucus formation

SIDE EFFECTS: Headache, heartburn, nausea, fatigue

AUXILIARY LABEL: *Chewable tablets:* Chew tablet well before swallowing

Phosphodiesterase-4 (PDE-4) inhibitor PDE-4 inhibitors decrease lung swelling to reduce COPD exacerbations or improve symptoms. Like montelukast (Singulair), this is an oral, not an inhaled, form.

GENERIC NAME: roflumilast

TRADE NAME: Daliresp

INDICATIONS: COPD, chronic bronchitis

ROUTE OF ADMINISTRATION: Oral

COMMON ADULT DOSAGE: 500 mcg once daily

MECHANISM OF ACTION: Inhibits PDE4 to decrease inflammatory cell activity

SIDE EFFECTS: Weight loss, diarrhea, dizziness, nausea, insomnia

AUXILIARY LABELS:
- May cause dizziness
- Not a rescue inhaler

COPD, Chronic obstructive pulmonary disease.

Short-acting beta-agonists As described previously, the beta-2 receptor activation relaxes bronchial smooth muscle, leading to bronchodilation and increased air flow. These short-acting agents, albuterol (ProAir HFA) and levalbuterol (Xopenex HFA), routinely work as "rescue" inhalers. Prescribers can schedule their use regularly or as needed for worsening asthma symptoms. SABAs come as both metered dose inhalers and nebulizer solutions.

GENERIC NAME: albuterol

TRADE NAMES: ProAir HFA, Ventolin HFA

INDICATIONS: Asthma, acute bronchospasm, bronchospasm prophylaxis

ROUTES OF ADMINISTRATION: Inhalation; oral

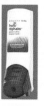

COMMON ADULT DOSAGES: *MDI:* 1 or 2 puffs every 4–6 hours or as needed. *Nebulizer:* 2.5 mg 3 or 4 times daily as needed

MECHANISM OF ACTION: Activates lung beta-2 receptors leading to bronchial smooth muscle relaxation, bronchodilation, and increased bronchial air flow

SIDE EFFECTS: Headache, nervousness, dizziness, insomnia, tremor, cough, tachycardia

AUXILIARY LABELS:
- *Inhalers:* Shake well before using
- May cause dizziness

Anticholinergics Patients widely use ipratropium for asthma. This **anticholinergic** medication blocks acetylcholine's effects and leads to bronchial smooth muscle relaxation. Prescribers can combine ipratropium with albuterol.

GENERIC NAME: ipratropium

TRADE NAMES: Atrovent HFA

INDICATIONS: Bronchospasm prophylaxis, COPD

ROUTES OF ADMINISTRATION: Inhalation

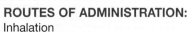

COMMON ADULT DOSAGES: *MDI:* 2 inhalations (17 mcg/spray) 4 times daily (max 12 inhalations). *Nebulizer:* 500 mcg every 6 hours

MECHANISM OF ACTION: Blocks acetylcholine to relax bronchial smooth muscle.

SIDE EFFECTS: Nausea, vomiting, dizziness, drowsiness

AUXILIARY LABEL: May cause dizziness

COPD, Chronic obstructive pulmonary disease.

GENERIC NAME: aclidinium

TRADE NAME: Tudorza Pressair

INDICATIONS: COPD maintenance, bronchospasms

ROUTE OF ADMINISTRATION: Inhalation

COMMON ADULT DOSAGE: 400 mcg (1 inhalation) twice daily

MECHANISM OF ACTION: Inhibits muscarinic receptors, leading to bronchodilation

SIDE EFFECTS: Cough, headache, diarrhea

AUXILIARY LABELS:
- For inhalation only/do not swallow capsules
- Will not stop an acute asthma attack

COPD, Chronic obstructive pulmonary disease.

Chronic Obstructive Pulmonary Disease

COPD comprises a group of chronic pulmonary diseases that restrict air flow. Depending on its characteristics and presentation, asthma sometimes falls into the broad COPD category. A collaboration between the National Institutes of Health (NIH) and the World Health Organization (WHO) resulted in the Global Initiative for Chronic Obstructive Lung Disease (GOLD). The initiative provided prescribers with objective criteria for COPD. This work allowed providers to assess disease severity in individual patients. GOLD classifications factor a ratio of the amount of air a patient can forcefully expire in 1 second versus the total air the patient can expire. As COPD worsens, this ratio generally declines. Within this system, COPD severity comes in four stages. These range from stage I (least severe) to stage IV (most severe). Researchers first published the GOLD classification system in 2001. Physicians at that time noted good outcomes for some stage IV patients, but patients in stage I or II experienced frequent hospital readmissions. The panel

of respiratory experts addressed the inconsistencies with key revisions to GOLD that take into account a patient history of symptoms and exacerbations. The panel also more recently included up-to-date therapeutic and management options for patients with COPD. The three general COPD types include chronic bronchitis, emphysema, and asthma (if the air flow is not entirely reversible). Any long-term lung conditions or exposure to lung irritants that damage the lungs can contribute to COPD development. Emphysema destroys the alveolar walls, leading to lung elasticity loss. Smoking, environmental hazards (eg, asbestos and fiberglass), or, in rare cases, genetic predisposition can lead to COPD. Normal exhalation requires an elastic lung. The affected lungs allow for inhaled air, but the individual cannot exhale all of the air. Fig. 21.11 represents the pathologic findings graphically. This changes within the lung with the various forms of COPD.

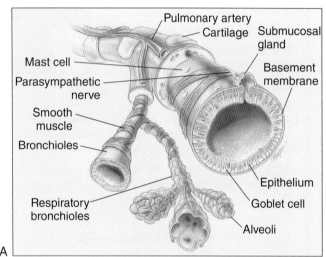
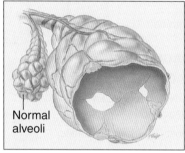
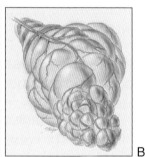
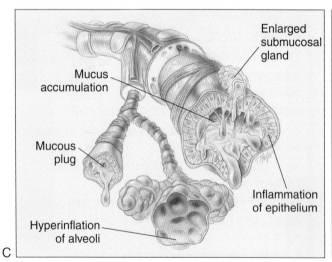
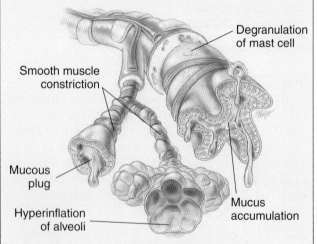

FIG. 21.11 Airway obstruction. (A) The normal lung. (B) Emphysema. (C) Chronic bronchitis. (D) Bronchial asthma. (From Huether S, McCance K. *Understanding Pathophysiology*. 5th ed. St. Louis: Mosby; 2012.)

Prognosis

Chronic obstructive pulmonary disease (COPD) is a chronic condition associated with physical impairment, incapacity, and decreased quality of life. It can lead to death. However, with proper management, patients with COPD can lead productive lives.

Non-Drug Treatment

Smoking cessation is an essential aspect of nondrug therapy. Smoking cessation drug treatments are discussed in Chapter 17. In extreme cases, a lung transplant may be needed to remove parts of the affected lung.

Drug Treatment

Given the interrelationship between asthma and COPD, many asthma medications are also for COPD. A long-acting muscarinic agonist (LAMA) is the mainstay of therapy. If a LAMA alone is not effective, then a LABA may be added. If both are not effective, add triple therapy with an inhaled corticosteroid (ICS). Trelegy is the brand name for a triple therapy inhaler that includes umeclidinium (LAMA), vilanterol (LABA), and fluticasone furoate (ICS). Additional combination product examples for COPD are listed later and in Table 21.5.

GENERIC NAME: fluticasone/salmeterol

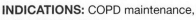

TRADE NAMES: Advair HFA, Advair Diskus (powder), AirDuo RespiClick

INDICATIONS: COPD maintenance, asthma maintenance

ROUTE OF ADMINISTRATION: Inhalation

COMMON ADULT DOSAGES: *Advair MDI:* 2 inhalations twice daily. *Advair Diskus or AirDuo RespiClick:* 1 inhalation twice daily

MECHANISM OF ACTION: Combination product contains an inhaled corticosteroid and long-acting beta-agonist

SIDE EFFECTS: Throat irritation, fungal infection, headache, nausea, dizziness

AUXILIARY LABELS:
- Will not stop an acute asthma attack
- *Advair HFA:* Shake well before use
- *Advair Diskus and AirDuo RespiClick:* Discard 30 days after opening

COPD, Chronic obstructive pulmonary disease.

GENERIC NAME: formoterol/budesonide

TRADE NAME: Symbicort

INDICATIONS: COPD, asthma

ROUTE OF ADMINISTRATION: Inhalation

COMMON ADULT DOSAGE: 2 inhalations twice daily

MECHANISMS OF ACTION: Combination product contains an inhaled corticosteroid and long-acting beta-agonist

SIDE EFFECTS: Throat irritation, fungal infection, headache, nausea, dizziness

AUXILIARY LABELS:
- Shake well before using
- Will not stop an acute asthma attack

COPD, Chronic obstructive pulmonary disease.

GENERIC NAME: umeclidinium/vilanterol

TRADE NAME: Anoro Ellipta

INDICATION: COPD

ROUTE OF ADMINISTRATION: Inhalation

COMMON ADULT DOSAGE: 1 inhalation once daily

MECHANISMS OF ACTION: Combination product contains a long-acting anticholinergic and a long-acting beta-2 agonist

SIDE EFFECTS: Tachycardia, prolonged QT interval, diarrhea, nausea, arthralgia

AUXILIARY LABELS:
- For inhalation only/do not swallow capsules
- Will not stop an acute asthma attack

COPD, Chronic obstructive pulmonary disease.

GENERIC NAME: fluticasone/vilanterol

TRADE NAME: Breo Ellipta

INDICATIONS: COPD, asthma

ROUTE OF ADMINISTRATION: Inhalation

COMMON ADULT DOSAGE: 1 inhalation once daily

MECHANISM OF ACTION: Combination product contains a corticosteroid and a long-acting beta-2 agonist

SIDE EFFECTS: Headache, upper respiratory tract infection, tachycardia

AUXILIARY LABELS:
- Rinse mouth after every use
- For inhalation only/do not swallow capsules
- Will not stop an acute asthma attack

COPD, Chronic obstructive pulmonary disease.

GENERIC NAME: ipratropium/albuterol

TRADE NAMES: Combivent Respimat

INDICATIONS: COPD, bronchospasm

ROUTE OF ADMINISTRATION: Inhalation

COMMON ADULT DOSAGE: *MDI:* 1 inhalation 4 times daily. *Nebulizer:* 1 vial (3 mL) 4 times daily

MECHANISM OF ACTION: Combination product contains an anticholinergic and short-acting beta-agonist

SIDE EFFECTS: Tachycardia, dry mouth, dizziness, insomnia

COPD, Chronic obstructive pulmonary disease.

Pneumonia

Pneumonia is an infection that causes acute lung airway inflammation. This infection can affect one or both lungs and individual lung lobes. Bacteria, viruses, fungi, protozoa, or parasites can cause pneumonia. Aspirating food, fluids, or other foreign substances into the lung can cause *aspiration pneumonia.* After organisms such as bacteria or viruses enter the lung, they multiply. As the body fights the infection, fluid and pus fill the lungs, making breathing difficult. The most causative bacterial organism for community-acquired pneumonia is *Streptococcus pneumoniae.* Older adults are at high risk, especially after an injury that requires them to remain in bed. Patients who are immunocompromised are also at a higher risk for pneumonia development.

Prognosis

Most patients recover from pneumonia with rest, hydration, and appropriate medications. Of those admitted to a hospital, only a fraction die of pneumonia.

Non-Drug Treatment

As noted previously, rest and proper hydration are vital components of non-drug therapy. Avoiding irritants that may compromise breathing (eg, dust, cigarette smoke, allergens) can help with breathing.

Drug Treatment

Prescribers often use antibiotics for bacterial pneumonia or antifungals for fungal infections. Health providers may add bronchodilators and corticosteroids, described previously for asthma and COPD treatment. Bacterial pneumonia pharmacotherapy often depends on the infectious organism, but it is crucial to reinforce patient inhaler technique; antibiotics may be required or systemic corticosteroids.

GENERIC NAME: azithromycin

TRADE NAMES: Zithromax, Z-Pak

INDICATIONS: Pneumonia, community-acquired pneumonia, miscellaneous bacterial infections

ROUTES OF ADMINISTRATION: Oral; intravenous (IV)

COMMON ADULT DOSAGES: *Oral:* 500 mg on day 1, followed by 250 mg once daily on days 2–5; *IV:* 500 mg once daily

MECHANISM OF ACTION: Macrolide antibiotic (inhibits bacterial protein synthesis)

SIDE EFFECTS: Diarrhea, nausea, vomiting, abdominal pain, anorexia

AUXILIARY LABEL: Take until gone

GENERIC NAME: levofloxacin

TRADE NAME: Levaquin[a]

INDICATIONS: Pneumonia, community-acquired pneumonia, miscellaneous bacterial infections

ROUTES OF ADMINISTRATION: Oral; intravenous

COMMON ADULT DOSAGE: 750 mg daily for 5 days, or 500 mg daily for 7–14 days

MECHANISM OF ACTION: Fluoroquinolone antibiotic (inhibits bacterial DNA synthesis)

SIDE EFFECTS: Diarrhea, nausea, vomiting, abdominal pain, dyspepsia, tendinitis

AUXILIARY LABELS:
- Take at least 2 hours before or after any antacid or multivitamin
- Take until gone

[a] Brand no longer available.

Tech Note!

Fluoroquinolone antibiotics, such as levofloxacin (Levaquin), have a boxed warning associating them with an increased risk for tendinitis and tendon rupture.

Tuberculosis

Tuberculosis (TB) is a leading cause of morbidity and mortality worldwide. At one time, TB was the leading cause of death in the United States. TB management can be difficult because the causative organism, *Mycobacterium tuberculosis,* is often drug resistant. Although the bacterium typically infects the lungs to cause TB, it can infect other organs such as the kidneys, brain, and spine. The primary TB treatment goal is to eradicate the bacteria with antibiotics and prevent drug resistance and disease relapse. Because TB is highly contagious, health care workers and other at-risk individuals in health centers often test positive for illness with a tuberculin skin test (also known as a purified protein derivative [PPD] skin test). Fig. 21.12 shows a positive PPD skin test result example. A PPD skin test shows whether a person has developed an *M. tuberculosis* immune response. People test positive if they have an active TB infection, if they were exposed to TB in the past, or if they received the bacille Calmette-Guérin (BCG) vaccine against TB (which is not given in the United States).

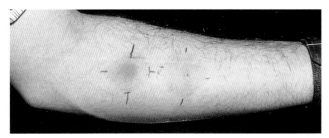

FIG. 21.12 Positive result on a tuberculosis test. (From Zitelli BJ, Davis HW. *Atlas of Pediatric Physical Diagnosis*. 6th ed. Philadelphia: Saunders; 2007.)

Prognosis

Prescribed medications can eradicate tuberculosis (TB). If left untreated, a TB infection can result in morbidity and death.

Non-Drug Treatment

Non-drug treatments cannot be used to cure TB, but good hygiene can help prevent highly contagious TB transmission.

Drug Treatment

Most antituberculin agents are bactericidal and kill *M. tuberculosis* (Table 21.6). These agents work with other medications that last many months. This length of therapy is a reason patient education is critical. Sputum tests can confirm if patients should stop treatment. Although TB medications are effective, many patients do not comply with the long-duration drug regimen. One treatment with the RIPE acronym includes rifampin, isoniazid, pyrazinamide, and ethambutol. Rifampin and isoniazid are given for 6 months, and ethambutol 15 mg/kg/day and pyrazinamide 1000 to 2000 mg/day are given for 2 months each.

GENERIC NAME: isoniazid (INH)

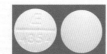

INDICATION: TB infection, TB prophylaxis

ROUTE OF ADMINISTRATION: Oral; injectable

COMMON ADULT DOSAGE: 5 mg/kg (up to 300 mg) once daily for up to 6 months

MECHANISM OF ACTION: Inhibits mycobacterial cell wall synthesis

SIDE EFFECTS: Diarrhea, abdominal pain, nausea, vomiting, hepatitis

AUXILIARY LABELS:
- Take on an empty stomach
- Take as directed

INH, Isoniazid; *TB,* tuberculosis.

◼ TABLE 21.6
Select Medications Used in the Treatment of Tuberculosis

Generic Name	Trade Name	Common Adult Oral Dosages[a]
ethambutol	Myambutol	Once-daily therapy: • 40–55 kg: 800 mg • 56–75 kg: 1200 mg • 76–90 kg: 1600 mg Three-times-weekly DOT: • 40–55 kg: 1200 mg • 56–75 kg: 2000 mg • 76–90 kg: 2400 mg Twice-weekly DOT: • 40–55 kg: 2000 mg • 56–75 kg: 2800 mg • 76–90 kg: 4000 mg
ethionamide	Trecator	15–20 mg/kg PO once daily or in divided doses
isoniazid, INH		5 mg/kg/day IM or PO for up to 6 months
		Three-times-weekly DOT: 15 mg/kg/dose
		Twice-weekly DOT: 15 mg/kg/dose
		Once-weekly DOT: 15 mg/kg/dose
PZA		Once-daily therapy: • 40–55 kg: 1000 mg • 56–75 kg: 1500 mg • 76–90 kg: 2000 mg Three-times-weekly DOT: • 40–55 kg: 1500 mg • 56–75 kg: 2500 mg • 76–90 kg: 3000 mg Twice-weekly DOT: • 40–55 kg: 2000 mg • 56–75 kg: 3000 mg • 76–90 kg: 4000 mg
rifabutin	Mycobutin	5 mg/kg PO once daily as a substitute for rifampin
rifampin	Rifadin	• 10 mg/kg/day (max 600 mg/day) • 600 mg PO or IV once daily
rifapentine	Priftin	600 mg PO twice weekly for 2 months
streptomycin		• Daily therapy: 15 mg/kg/day IM (max 1 g) • Two or three times weekly DOT: 25–30 mg/kg IM (max 1.5 g)

[a]Agents are typically used in combination regimens as a result of drug resistance.
DOT, Direct observed therapy; *IM,* intramuscularly; *INH,* isoniazid; *IV,* intravenously; *PO,* orally; *PZA,* pyrazinamide.

GENERIC NAME: rifampin

TRADE NAME: Rifadin

INDICATIONS: TB infection, meningococcal infection prophylaxis

ROUTES OF ADMINISTRATION: Oral; injectable

COMMON ADULT DOSAGE: 600 mg once daily

MECHANISM OF ACTION: Inhibits bacterial and mycobacterial RNA synthesis

SIDE EFFECTS: Nausea, vomiting, cramps, diarrhea, orange to reddish discoloration of urine and other body fluids

AUXILIARY LABELS:
- Take at least 1 hour before or 2 hours after a meal
- Take as directed

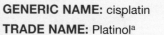

TB, Tuberculosis.

▪ Tech Note!

Rifampin is replete with drug-drug interactions, so it is essential to double-check a patient's medication list. Patients should also watch out for red-orange urine, which is harmless but may be misconstrued as blood in the urine.

Lung Cancer

Lung cancer is the most common cancer worldwide. Lung cancer became the most common cause of cancer deaths in men in the 1950s. It became the leading cause of cancer death in women in the mid-1980s. With reduced smoking rates, death rates from lung cancer have decreased in recent years. Lung cancer refers to malignancies of the airways. Approximately 95% of all lung cancers are classified as either small cell lung cancer (SCLC) or non–small cell lung cancer (NSCLC). This classification fits closely with treatment and prognosis.

Prognosis

As with any cancer, the disease stage, presence of metastases, and other patient-specific factors determine the prognosis for lung cancer.

Non-Drug Treatment

Aside from smoking cessation, doctors can treat lung cancers with radiation and surgical resection for surgical candidates.

Drug Treatment

Chemotherapy is a primary treatment modality for many types and stages of lung cancer. Chemotherapy also plays a role as adjuvant therapy after surgical resection. Various chemotherapeutic agents treat lung carcinomas. Although the treatment is oncologist driven as to specific cancer, pharmacy plays a significant role in side effect management, including nausea, diarrhea, etc.

GENERIC NAME: cisplatin

TRADE NAME: Platinol[a]

INDICATIONS: NSCLC, bladder cancer, mesothelioma, ovarian cancer, testicular cancer

ROUTE OF ADMINISTRATION: Intravenous

COMMON ADULT DOSAGE: Dosage varies based on cancer stage, patient's weight, and combination therapies

MECHANISM OF ACTION: Inhibits DNA synthesis

SIDE EFFECTS: Allergic reactions, ototoxicity, renal toxicity, mouth sores, infection, diarrhea

[a] Brand no longer available.
NSCLC, Non–small cell lung cancer.

GENERIC NAME: vinorelbine

TRADE NAME: Navelbine

INDICATION: NSCLC

ROUTE OF ADMINISTRATION: Intravenous only

COMMON ADULT DOSAGE: Dosage varies based on cancer stage, patient's weight, and combination therapies

MECHANISM OF ACTION: Inhibits cell division by interfering with microtubule formation

SIDE EFFECTS: Myelosuppression, neuropathy, fatigue, alopecia

AUXILIARY LABELS:
- For IV use only
- Fatal if given intrathecally

NSCLC, Non–small cell lung cancer.

Cystic Fibrosis

The cystic fibrosis transmembrane conductance regulator (CFTR) gene has a mutation that results in cystic fibrosis, a hereditary disease. Cells produce significant mucus and sticky secretions. The thick mucus can blockage airways and lungs and the gastrointestinal tract, resulting in labored breathing, complications of the lung, and digestive system damage.

Prognosis

Although treatment can help prevent complications, patients with cystic fibrosis will ultimately need lung transplantation. Unfortunately, cystic fibrosis is a progressive disease that has no cure.

Non-Drug Treatment

Physical therapy, such as a percussion vest, can break up lung mucus and improve respiratory measures. During exhalation, positive expiratory pressure (PEP) therapy can use a mouthpiece to drive out mucus.

Drug Treatment

CFTR modulators are the mainstay of cystic fibrosis treatment. The agent choice depends on the patient's age and specific mutation. CFTR modulators can include ivacaftor (Kalydeco), lumacaftor/ivacaftor (Orkambi), tezacaftor/ivacaftor (Symdeko), and elexacaftor/tezacaftor/ivacaftor and ivacaftor (Trikafta).

GENERIC NAME: Ivacaftor

TRADE NAME: Kalydeco

INDICATION: Cystic fibrosis

ROUTE OF ADMINISTRATION: Oral

COMMON ADULT DOSAGE: 150 mg every 12 hours

MECHANISM OF ACTION: A CFTR modulator that opens CFTR channel to improve the activity of ion and water absorption

SIDE EFFECTS: Headache, nausea, upper respiratory tract infections, cataracts

GENERIC NAME: Elexacaftor/tezacaftor/ivacaftor and ivacaftor

TRADE NAME: Trikafta

INDICATION: Cystic fibrosis

ROUTE OF ADMINISTRATION: Oral

COMMON ADULT DOSAGE: Elexacaftor 100 mg/tezacaftor 50 mg/ivacaftor 75 mg in the morning and 150 mg ivacaftor in the afternoon

MECHANISM OF ACTION: Elexacaftor and tezacaftor: correct CFTR protein's mutation defect Ivacaftor: opens CFTR channel to improve the activity ion and water absorption

SIDE EFFECTS: Headache, nausea, upper respiratory tract infections, cataracts

■ Tech Note!

Remember the following sound-alike, look-alike drugs:
- diphenhydramine versus dicyclomine or dimenhydrinate
- epinephrine versus ephedrine
- Alupent versus Atrovent
- albuterol versus atenolol

Do You Remember These Key Points?

- Names of the major components of the respiratory system and their functions
- The primary symptoms of the various upper and lower respiratory tract conditions discussed

- Medications used to treat the various respiratory conditions discussed
- The generic and trade names for the drugs discussed in this chapter
- The appropriate auxiliary labels that should be used when filling prescriptions for drugs discussed in this chapter

Review Questions

Multiple Choice Questions

1. Lung gas exchange takes place specifically in the:
   A. Brainstem
   B. Brain
   C. Medulla
   D. Alveoli
2. The large dome-shaped muscle that separates the chest cavity from the abdominal cavity is the:
   A. Larynx
   B. Diaphragm
   C. Bronchus
   D. Trachea
3. The main function(s) of the cilia in the upper respiratory tract is/are:
   A. To smell
   B. To catch foreign material
   C. To warm and moisten air molecules
   D. Both A and C
4. Gas exchange functions include all of the following *except:*
   A. Balancing the pH of the body
   B. Oxygenation of the bloodstream
   C. Discarding unused carbon dioxide
   D. Exchanging nitrogen for carbon dioxide
5. Oseltamivir (Tamiflu) is approved to treat:
   A. Influenza
   B. Chronic obstructive pulmonary disease (COPD)
   C. Asthma
   D. Lung cancer
6. COPD describes a group of chronic pulmonary diseases. These include all of the following *except:*
   A. Emphysema
   B. Postnasal drip
   C. Chronic bronchitis
   D. Asthma
7. Albuterol is a/an:
   A. Inhaled corticosteroid
   B. Long-acting beta-agonist
   C. Short-acting beta-agonist
   D. Inhaled anticholinergic
8. The following microorganism causes tuberculosis (TB):
   A. *Mycobacterium tuberculosis*
   B. *Staphylococcus aureus*
   C. *Streptococcus pneumoniae*
   D. *Haemophilus influenzae*
9. We classify dextromethorphan as a/an:
   A. Antitussive
   B. Antihistamine

C. Corticosteroid

D. Mucolytic

10. We divide respiration into two distinct phases: _____, the movement of air into the lungs, and _____, the movement of air out of the lungs.

A. inspiration; expiration

B. expiration; inspiration

C. inspiration; absorption

D. expiration; absorption

11. Which asthma medication class may cause thrush as a side effect?

A. Short-acting beta-agonists

B. Long-acting beta-agonists

C. Inhaled corticosteroids

D. Inhaled anticholinergics

12. What is the brand name for fexofenadine?

A. Nasarel

B. Clarinex

C. Allegra

D. Singulair

13. Which of the following asthma medications is an injectable?

A. Zafirlukast (Accolate)

B. Omalizumab (Xolair)

C. Cromolyn sodium (NasalCrom)

D. Tiotropium (Spiriva)

14. Which of the following is an inhaled anticholinergic for the treatment of COPD?

A. Ipratropium (Atrovent hydrofluoroalkane)

B. Salmeterol (Serevent Diskus)

C. Tiotropium (Spiriva)

D. Both A and C

15. Agents that break up thick lung mucus secretions are called:

A. Mucolytics

B. Antitussives

C. Expectorants

D. Both A and C

■ Technician's Corner

Many conditions of the respiratory tract discussed in this chapter are treated symptomatically with OTC products such as diphenhydramine, guaifenesin, and pseudoephedrine. Using a drug reference, identify key contraindications to these products and patients who should avoid using them.

Bibliography

Damjanov I. *Pathology for the Health Professions*. 4th ed. St. Louis: Saunders; 2011.

Fishback JL. *Pathology*. 3rd ed. Philadelphia: Mosby; 2005.

Global Initiative for Asthma. *Pocket Guide for Asthma Management and Prevention*. Global Initiative for Asthma; 2019.

Goldman M. *Procedures in Cosmetic Dermatology Series: Photodynamic Therapy*. 2nd ed. St. Louis: Saunders; 2008.

McCance KL. *Pathophysiology: The Biologic Basis for Disease in Adults and Children*. 6th ed. St. Louis: Mosby; 2010.

Moscou K, Snipe K. *Pharmacology for Pharmacy Technicians*. 2nd ed. St. Louis: Mosby; 2013.

Patton KT, Thibodeau G. *Mosby's Handbook of Anatomy and Physiology*. St. Louis: Mosby; 2000.

Price SA, Wilson LM. *Pathophysiology: Clinical Concepts of Disease Processes*. 6th ed. St. Louis: Mosby; 2003.

Solomon EP. *Introduction to Human Anatomy and Physiology*. 3rd ed. St. Louis: Saunders; 2009.

Websites Referenced

Clinical Pharmacology Online. Available at: https://www.clinicalkey.com/pharmacology.

Wolters Klewer. UpToDate Online. Available at: www.uptodate.com.

CHAPTER 22

Therapeutic Agents for the Gastrointestinal System

Tony Guerra

OBJECTIVES

1. Describe the major components of the gastrointestinal system.
2. List the primary symptoms of conditions associated with the dysfunction of the gastrointestinal system. In addition, (a) recognize prescription and over-the-counter drugs discussed for the treatment of conditions associated with the gastrointestinal system, (b) write the generic and trade names for the drugs discussed in this chapter, and (c) list appropriate auxiliary labels when filling prescriptions for drugs discussed in this chapter.

TERMS AND DEFINITIONS

Absorption Movement of nutrients, fluids, and medications from the gastrointestinal tract into the bloodstream

Amino acids Molecules that are the building blocks of proteins

Antiemetics Against + vomiting, a drug that prevents or treats nausea and vomiting

Carbohydrates Chemical compounds that contain carbon, hydrogen, and oxygen; examples include sugars, glycogen, starches, and cellulose

Chyme The resulting soupy mixture (semifluid) after food mixes with stomach acids and digestive enzymes

Digestion The mechanical, chemical, and enzymatic action of breaking food into molecules for metabolism

Emesis Vomit + condition, a medical term for vomiting

Excretion Elimination of waste products mainly through stools and urine

Fistulae Permanent abnormal passageways between two organs or between an organ and the outside

Ingestion Taking in food, liquid, or other substances (eg, medications)

Peristalsis Around + place, tubular muscle contraction and relaxation of the esophagus, stomach, and intestines to move substances through the gastrointestinal tract

Surface area Extent of an object's surface in contact with its surroundings

Common Drugs for Conditions of the Gastrointestinal System

Trade Name	Generic Name	Pronunciation
Agents to Treat Gastroesophageal Reflux Disease (GERD)		
AcipHex	rabeprazole	(rah-**beh**-pruh-zole)
Axid	nizatidine	(nye-**zah**-tih-deen)
Dexilant	dexlansoprazole	(dex-**lan**-soe-pruh-zole)
Nexium, Nexium 24HR (OTC)	esomeprazole	(es-o-**meh**-pruh-zole)
Pepcid, Pepcid AC (OTC)	famotidine	(fa-**mo**-tih-deen)
Prevacid, Prevacid 24HR (OTC)	lansoprazole	(lan-**sew**-pruh-zole)
Prilosec, Prilosec OTC (OTC)	omeprazole	(oh-**meh**-pruh-zole)
Protonix	pantoprazole	(pan-**toe**-pruh-zole)
Tagamet HB 200 (OTC)	cimetidine	(sy-**meh**-tih-deen)
Tums	calcium carbonate	(**kal**-see-um **car**-bow-nate)
Zegerid, Zegerid OTC (OTC)	omeprazole/sodium bicarbonate	(oh-**meh**-pruh-zole/**so**-dee-um by-**kar**-buh-nate)
Agents to Treat Constipation		
Amitiza	lubiprostone	(loo-**beh**-pros-tone)
Citrucel	methylcellulose	(meth-ill-**cell**-you-lows)
Colace	docusate sodium	(**dok**-yoo-sate sow-dee-um)
Constulose	lactulose	(**lak**-tyoo-lose)
Dulcolax	bisacodyl	(bih-suh-**coh**-dill)
FiberCon	calcium polycarbophil	(**kal**-cee-uhm **pol**-ee-**kar**-boh-phyl)
Fleet Enema Extra (OTC)	sodium phosphate	(**soe**-dee-um **fos**-fate)
Glycerin, Babylax,[a] Colace Glycerin[a]	glycerin anhydrous	(**glis**-ir-in)
Linzess	linaclotide	(lynn-ah-**cloh**-tide)
Metamucil	psyllium	(**sill**-ee-um)
MiraLAX	polyethylene glycol 3350	(**pol**-ee-**eth**-il-een **glye**-kol)
Phillips' Milk of Magnesia, Maalox[a]	magnesium hydroxide	(mag-**nee**-see-um hye-**drock**-side)
Senokot, Ex-Lax	senna	(**sen**-uh)
Agents to Treat Diarrhea		
Imodium AD	loperamide	(low-**pear**-uh-myde)
Lomotil	diphenoxylate/atropine	(die-fen-**ox**-ih-late/at-row-peen)
Pepto-Bismol	bismuth subsalicylate	(**biz**-muth sub-suh-**lih**-suh-late)
Agents to Treat Severe Diarrhea-Predominant Irritable Bowel Syndrome		
Lotronex	alosetron	(a-**low**-seh-tron)
Agents to Treat Nausea/Vomiting		
Aloxi	palonosetron	(**pal**-oh-**noh**-seh-tron)
Anzemet	dolasetron	(doe-**lah**-seh-tron)
Compro[a]	prochlorperazine	(pro-klor-**pear**-uh-zeen)
Dramamine	dimenhydrinate	(die-men-**hi**-druh-nate)
Dramamine Less Drowsy, Travel Sickness	meclizine	(**meck**-luh-zeen)
Emend	aprepitant	(uh-**preh**-pih-tant)
Emend IV	fosaprepitant	(faw-suh-**preh**-pih-tant)
Kytril[a]	granisetron	(gra-**nih**-seh-tron)
Phenergan	promethazine	(pro-**meth**-uh-zeen)
Reglan	metoclopramide	(meh-tuh-**clow**-prah-myde)
Tigan	trimethobenzamide	(try-meth-oh-**ben**-zuh-mide)
Transderm Scop	scopolamine	(sko-**pole**-luh-meen)
Varubi	rolapitant	(**roh**-luh-pih-tant)
Zofran	ondansetron	(on-**dan**-seh-tron)
Agents to Treat Flatulence		
Children's Mylicon	simethicone	(sih-**meth**-ih-cone)

[a]Brand no longer available.

The digestive tract extends from the mouth to the anus and converts food and fluids for absorption and distribution. Insoluble large materials break down to absorbable smaller substances for energy production and protein synthesis and as enzymes for metabolism. As the body breaks food down, it absorbs nutrients and excretes nonessential remnants. This chapter reviews the anatomy and physiology of the gastrointestinal (GI) tract and discusses medications to treat GI conditions.

Form and Role of the Gastrointestinal System

The GI system carries out four main roles: digestion, absorption, metabolism, and **excretion.** The parasympathetic nervous system (see Chapter 17) directs various "rest and digest" activities of the GI system. This chapter reviews the anatomy and physiology of the stomach, intestinal tract, and other organs important to the GI system, such as the tongue, salivary glands, liver, pancreas, and gallbladder. These auxiliary (also called *ancillary* or *accessory*) organs play important secondary roles in **digestion.**

Anatomy and Physiology of the Gastrointestinal System

Most consider the stomach the primary GI organ; however, digestion begins in the mouth. Fig. 22.1 shows the entire system. The organs discussed in this chapter, in sequence, are the mouth, salivary glands, pharynx, and esophagus for **ingestion** and digestion. The stomach and small intestine follow for digestion and nutrient absorption. The large intestine reabsorbs water and electrolytes and stores feces, and the rectum and anus remove waste. Auxiliary organs perform various supporting roles.

Ingestion

The mouth begins digestion by breaking down food into smaller pieces through chewing. The mouth's three pairs of salivary glands (sublingual, submandibular, and parotid) secrete enzymes and start the food's chemical breakdown. The sublingual and submandibular glands sit below the tongue and jaw, respectively. Each parotid gland rests immediately in front of the ear (Fig. 22.2). The saliva works as an enzyme and moistens the esophagus to help with swallowing. The tongue ensures food travels to the pharynx (ie, the throat) and then the esophagus. **Peristalsis** is involuntary muscle contraction and relaxation, which begins in the esophagus to propel food downward. As the food arrives in the stomach, it enters an acidic environment that further breaks down chemicals in food. Fig. 22.3 shows the pH (a measure of acidity) of the stomach related to other liquids and products.

> **Tech Note!**
>
> The stomach's acidity can affect drug and mineral absorption. Drug interactions can occur between acid-lowering medications (eg, proton pump inhibitors) and medicines that need an acidic stomach environment for proper absorption.

Food activates gastric juice, a combination of hydrochloric acid and various enzymes. The enzymes allow the intestines to absorb the nutrients and chemicals for metabolism. However, the stomach's acid can destroy the medicine. Some medications use a special protective coating. Other medications such as insulin need an injectable form to bypass the acidic

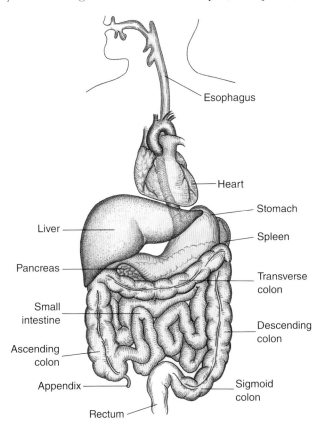

FIG. 22.1 Anatomy of the gastrointestinal system (including the mouth, pharynx, esophagus, stomach, and intestines). (From Potter PA, Perry AG. *Fundamentals of Nursing*. 8th ed. St. Louis: Mosby; 2013.)

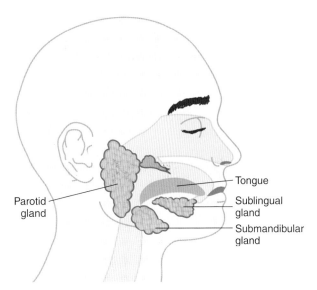

FIG. 22.2 Major glands of the mouth.

pH Scale

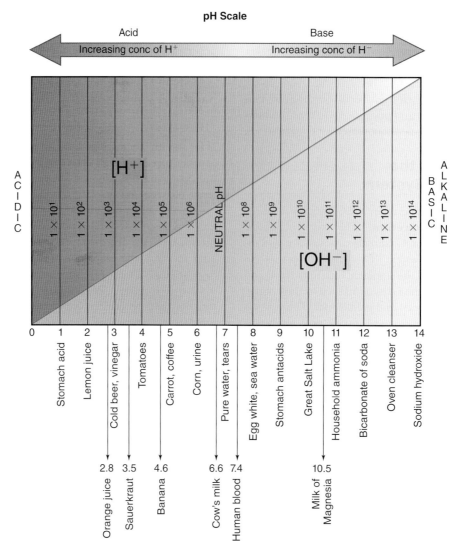

FIG. 22.3 The pH scale ranges from 1 (the most acidic) to 14 (the most basic). The pH of normal human blood is 7.4, approximately the midpoint of the range. *Conc,* Concentration.

stomach. To balance this acidic pH, the inner mucosal lining of the stomach is alkaline for protection.

Several types of stomach muscle aid digestion by churning and mixing the gastric contents (Fig. 22.4). **Chyme** is the semifluid mixture that remains. Chyme exits the stomach and passes through the pyloric sphincter, a muscle that opens into the small intestine for further digestion and nutrient absorption (see Fig. 22.4). The pancreas produces bicarbonate to neutralize the acidic contents as they pass from the stomach to duodenum, the first part of the small intestine.

Absorption

Absorption of nutrients occurs mainly in the small intestine. The vitamins and minerals move through the gut lining. The small intestine's length and multiple folds and villi increase its absorptive **surface area** (Fig. 22.5). Glucose molecules, **amino acids,** and fatty acids absorb and begin to circulate through the bloodstream for delivery to the body's cells. The small intestine, about 6 m long, performs the final digestive steps.

The small intestine has three sections in this order: the duodenum, jejunum, and ileum. The duodenum, about 25 cm long, connects to the liver, gallbladder, and pancreas. The liver and gallbladder unload bile. The pancreas secretes bicarbonate and amylase, lipase, and trypsin—three digestive enzymes. The jejunum, about 2.5 m long, and the ileum (the distal section) about 3.5 m long, follow.

These three sections of the small intestine absorb most of the food and oral drugs. The alkaline intestinal pH allows for proper nutrient absorption. Various enzymes continue to break down starch into sugars (amylase), fats (lipase), and protein (trypsin). Active transport and diffusion move drugs and nutrients into the bloodstream. Each villus (a fingerlike projection; see Fig. 22.5) on the surface of the small intestine has a network of capillaries and fine lymphatic vessels. The villi's epithelial cells carry nutrients and drugs from the lumen into the capillaries. Any undigested or unabsorbed substances pass into the large intestine.

Excretion

The large intestine, only about 1.5 m long, follows the small intestine and absorbs mostly water and electrolytes. The substances moving through this portion of the intestine form solid fecal matter as water and electrolytes reabsorb.

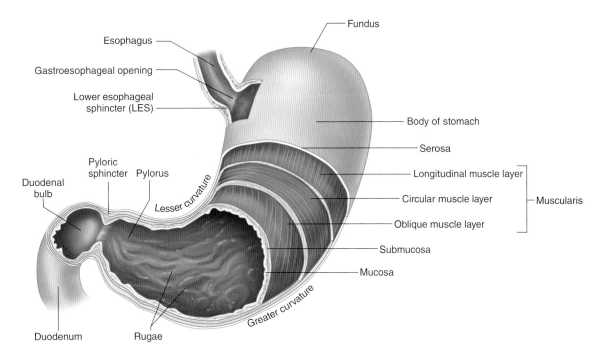

FIG. 22.4 Structure of the stomach. (From Patton KT, Thibodeau GA. *The Human Body in Health and Disease*. 6th ed. St. Louis: Elsevier; 2014.)

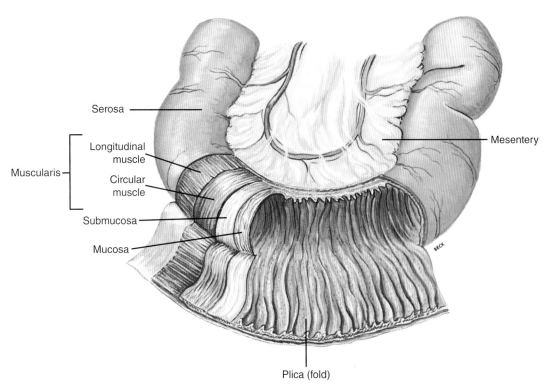

FIG. 22.5 Wall of the small intestine (segment of jejunum). (From Patton KT, Thibodeau GA. *Mosby's Handbook of Anatomy and Physiology*. St. Louis: Mosby; 2000.)

The rectum, the shortest section of the intestinal tract, follows the large intestine and connects to the anal canal. Normal fecal (waste matter) removal takes from 3 to 5 days. In the anal canal, the involuntarily regulated internal anal sphincter controls the urge to defecate. The external anal sphincter, under voluntary control, gives the individual management of the bowels.

Auxiliary Organs

The body converts proteins, **carbohydrates,** and fats from complex molecules to simple molecules. The pancreas, liver, and gallbladder produce enzymes that are carried by ducts to the duodenum to help this action. Trypsin and chymotrypsin from the pancreas break down large proteins into smaller peptides and amino acids. Amylase breaks down large carbohydrates into disaccharides (two sugars). In the duodenum, the body breaks disaccharides (two sugars) into monosaccharides (one sugar) for easy absorption and energy needs. Long carbon chains of fat are difficult to metabolize. Bile, which is produced by the liver and stored in the gall-bladder, helps the body absorb fats and fat-soluble vitamins. *Emulsification* (break up of fat globules) makes fats water soluble, and *lipases* further break them down. Fig. 22.6 provides a visual summary of the GI anatomy and physiology in this section.

Conditions Affecting the Gastrointestinal System

Hyperacidity treatments such as antacids, histamine-2 (H₂) blockers, and proton pump inhibitors (PPIs) help alleviate heartburn, upset stomach, and symptoms of gastroesophageal reflux disease (GERD). Laxatives and antidiarrheals can speed up or slow the passage of contents through the bowels to treat acute or chronic constipation and diarrhea. Immunosuppressants and corticosteroid antiinflammatories serve to treat inflammatory bowel conditions such as Crohn disease and ulcerative colitis. Combinations of antibiotics and acid reducers are used to treat *Helicobacter pylori* organisms often found in gastric and duodenal ulcers.

This chapter focuses on these GI conditions and the drugs that help these disorders.

Conditions Mainly Associated With the Stomach

The acidic stomach fluids can cause upset stomach, indigestion, or heartburn. Antacids such as calcium carbonate and magnesium hydroxide work quickly (a few minutes) to increase gastric pH and relieve occasional dyspepsia (upset stomach) or heartburn. H₂ antagonists, such as famotidine and PPIs, such as esomeprazole and omeprazole, start their work a bit more slowly. However, these drugs need less frequent dosing. Patients can easily access these medications—most are over-the-counter (OTC; see Chapter 29) products. Patients should contact their doctor for persistent GERD or pain that may signal a peptic ulcer.

<table>
<tr><td>■ **Tech Note!**</td></tr>
<tr><td>Antacids may interact with medications and prevent proper absorption. For example, patients taking doxycycline (Doryx) and ciprofloxacin (Cipro) should avoid taking antacids containing calcium, magnesium, or aluminum at the same time. The antacid can chelate (bind to) the antibiotic and reduce its absorption. Changing drug administration times often helps avoid interactions.</td></tr>
</table>

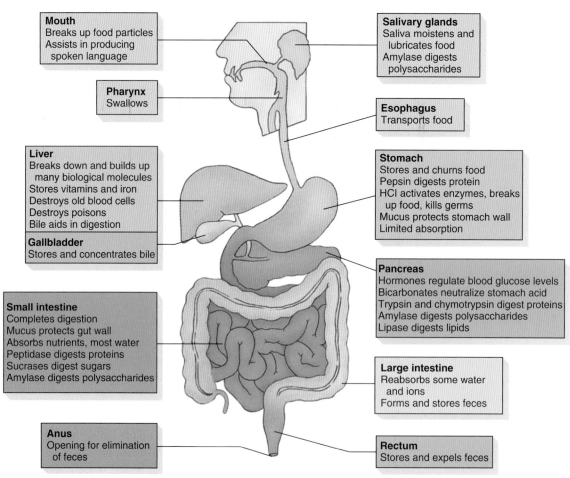

FIG. 22.6 Summary of digestive function. *HCl,* Hydrochloric acid. (From Patton KT, Thibodeau GA. *Mosby's Handbook of Anatomy and Physiology.* St. Louis: Mosby; 2000.)

Gastroesophageal Reflux Disease

GERD can occur when the upper sphincter (opening) at the top of the stomach relaxes. This relaxation allows the stomach's acidic contents to back up into the unprotected esophagus. Patients feel this burning sensation in the chest around the area of the heart, also known as heartburn. The risk for GERD increases with obesity, smoking, and pregnancy.

Prognosis

With medicine and diet changes, patients can fully recover from GERD.

Non-Drug Treatments

Large food amounts trigger significant stomach acid. By reducing portion size, patients can reduce hyperacidity. Another non-drug approach is to raise the head of the bed if the person's GERD symptoms are prominent at bedtime.

Drug Treatments

Besides antacids, H_2 antagonists reduce acidity in reflux disease. Famotidine and cimetidine block H_2 receptors in the stomach's lining. PPIs, such as esomeprazole and omeprazole, inhibit gastric acid production by blocking the final enzymatic reaction before acid secretion. All of these medication classes have OTC alternatives, but some PPIs still need a prescription. PPI use is linked to hypomagnesemia, an increased risk for *Clostridioides difficile* infection, osteoporosis, and increased gastric cancer risk with very long-term use. H_2 receptor antagonists are slowly being transitioned as the mainstay of therapy as more evidence for long-term PPI risk becomes available. Note that ranitidine was removed from the shelves in 2020 after having *N*-nitrosodimethylamine (NDMA) found in its tablets. NDMA is a class B2 carcinogen, which means it might cause cancer in humans. Oral liquid preparations did not have NDMA in them and are reserved for children and those intolerant of other H_2 receptor antagonists. Patients should obtain a formal GERD diagnosis from their prescriber to rule out other disease states and esophageal cancer rather than self-treating.

Antacids Antacids include aluminum carbonate, sodium bicarbonate, calcium carbonate, magnesium hydroxide, and aluminum hydroxide. Each of these generic names is the inorganic molecule's chemical name as well. Antacids neutralize acid and increase the stomach's pH level (ie, make it less acidic) very quickly, providing symptomatic relief in minutes. This speed of action and convenience makes antacids the preferred over-the-counter option for mild and infrequent heartburn symptoms. Pay close attention to antacids' ingredients because some contain aspirin. Patients with a high bleed risk and pediatric patients should avoid aspirin- or salicylate-containing products. Table 22.1 lists examples of single-ingredient antacids, and Table 22.2 provides a list of key antacid combinations to treat stomach conditions.

◼ TABLE 22.1
Select Over-the-Counter Antacid Agents (Single Ingredient)

Active Ingredient	Dosage Form	Strength
Aluminum hydroxide	Oral suspension	320 mg/5 mL
Calcium carbonate (Tums)	Chewable tablets	500 mg
Magnesium hydroxide (Phillips' Milk of Magnesia)	Oral suspension	400 mg/5 mL
	Chewable tablets	311 mg

◼ Tech Note!

Understand the difference between histamine-1 (H_1) and H_2 receptors. H_1 receptors run throughout the body, in smooth muscles, vascular endothelial cells, the heart, and the central nervous system. We call agents that block H_1 receptors and treat allergic reactions *antihistamines*. H_2 receptors remain chiefly in the stomach's parietal cells. We call these H_2 *antagonists*, and these medications treat hyperacidity disorders.

Histamine-2 antagonists H_2 antagonists bind to H_2 receptor sites, reducing acid secretion. The rare side effects of histamine antagonists include drowsiness, headache, and rash. Prescription formulas typically are stronger than OTC formulations. Although most of the prescription agents have standard dosages approved by the US Food and Drug Administration (FDA) for specific medical conditions, many doctors allow patients to take H_2 antagonists as needed for occasional indigestion.

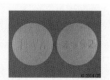

GENERIC NAME: famotidine

TRADE NAMES: Pepcid, Pepcid AC

INDICATIONS: GERD, erosive esophagitis, gastric ulcer, duodenal ulcer treatment and prophylaxis (OTC for heartburn and indigestion)

ROUTES OF ADMINISTRATION: Oral; intravenous (IV)

COMMON ADULT DOSAGES: *Oral Rx for GERD:* 20 mg twice daily. *IV:* Variable depending on indication and setting

MECHANISM OF ACTION: Competitively inhibits histamine binding to H_2 receptors on gastric parietal cells to reduce gastric acid secretion

SIDE EFFECTS: Headache, dizziness, constipation

AUXILIARY LABELS (Rx):
- May cause dizziness and drowsiness
- Suspension: Shake well

GERD, Gastroesophageal reflux disease.

TABLE 22.2
Select Over-the-Counter Combination Antacids

Active Ingredients	Trade Name	Dose Form OTC	Strength of Active Ingredients
AlOH and magnesium carbonate	Gaviscon Extra Strength	Chewable tablets	AlOH 160 mg, magnesium carbonate 105 mg
AlOH and MgOH	Mag-Al[a]; Mylanta[a]	Suspension	AlOH 200 mg + MgOH 200 mg/5 mL
AlOH, MgOH, and simethicone	Almacone[a]	Oral liquid	AlOH 200 mg, MgOH 200 mg, simethicone 20 mg/5 mL
	Maalox Advanced Maximum Strength[a]; Mylanta Maximum Strength	Oral liquid	AlOH 400 mg, MgOH 400 mg, simethicone 40 mg/5 mL
	Mintox Plus	Suspension	AlOH 200 mg, MgOH 200 mg, simethicone 25 mg/5 mL
Sodium bicarbonate, aspirin, and citric acid	Alka-Seltzer	Effervescent tablets	Sodium bicarbonate 1700 mg, aspirin 325 mg, citric acid 1000 mg
Sodium bicarbonate, citric acid, and potassium bicarbonate	Alka-Seltzer Gold	Effervescent tablets	Sodium bicarbonate 1050 mg, citric acid 1000 mg, potassium bicarbonate 344 mg

[a]Brand no longer available.

AlOH, Aluminum hydroxide; *APAP,* acetaminophen; *MgOH,* magnesium hydroxide; *OTC,* over the counter.

Proton pump inhibitors PPIs are used mainly to treat GERD and peptic ulcers. Most agents are a once-daily, delayed-release form. PPIs block gastric acid secretion. Currently, the only PPI products available OTC are esomeprazole (Nexium 24HR), lansoprazole (Prevacid 24HR), omeprazole (Prilosec OTC), and omeprazole/sodium bicarbonate (Zegerid OTC). PPIs inhibit the action of a specific stomach pump blocking gastric acid secretion. Prescribers often turn to PPIs in patients who have failed twice-daily H$_2$ antagonist therapy for GERD treatment, those with erosive esophagitis, or those with frequent or severe symptoms. General PPI dosing is once daily 30 to 60 minutes before the first daily meal.

Table 22.3 provides a summary of select H$_2$ antagonists and PPIs for GERD treatment.

GENERIC NAME: esomeprazole

TRADE NAMES: Nexium, Nexium 24HR

INDICATIONS: GERD, duodenal ulcer, erosive esophagitis, and prophylaxis for NSAID-induced ulcer

ROUTES OF ADMINISTRATION: Oral; IV

COMMON ADULT DOSAGE: Dosage varies, depending on the severity of the condition; a standard dosage is 20 mg once daily

MECHANISM OF ACTION: Prevents gastric acid secretion from parietal cells of the stomach

SIDE EFFECTS: Diarrhea, nausea, headache, stomach pain, increased risk for fractures

AUXILIARY LABELS:
- Take 1 hour before meals on an empty stomach
- Do not crush or chew

GERD, Gastroesophageal reflux disease; *NSAID,* nonsteroidal antiinflammatory drug.

GENERIC NAME: lansoprazole

TRADE NAMES: Prevacid, Prevacid 24HR

INDICATIONS: GERD, duodenal ulcer, gastric ulcer, prophylaxis for NSAID-induced ulcer, erosive esophagitis

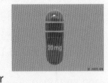

ROUTES OF ADMINISTRATION: Oral; IV

COMMON ADULT DOSAGE: Dosage varies, depending on the severity of the condition; common dosage is 15–30 mg once daily

MECHANISM OF ACTION: Prevents gastric acid secretion from parietal cells of the stomach

SIDE EFFECTS: Diarrhea, nausea, headache, stomach pain, increased fracture risk

AUXILIARY LABELS:
- Take before meals
- Do not crush or chew

GERD, Gastroesophageal reflux disease; *NSAID,* nonsteroidal antiinflammatory drug.

Select Histamine-2 Antagonists and Proton Pump Inhibitors for the Treatment of Gastroesophageal Reflux Disease

Generic Name	Trade Name	Common Dosage Range	Common Side Effects
Histamine-2 Antagonists			
cimetidine	Tagamet HB 200 (OTC)	• 800 mg twice daily	• Constipation
famotidine	Pepcid, Pepcid AC (OTC)	• 20 mg twice daily for up to 6 wk	• Nausea
nizatidine	Axid	• 150 mg twice daily for up to 12 wk	• Abdominal pain
Proton Pump Inhibitors (PPIs)			
dexlansoprazole	Dexilant	• 30 mg once daily for up to 4 wk	• Diarrhea
esomeprazole	Nexium, Nexium 24HR	• 20 mg once daily for up to 4 wk	• Nausea
lansoprazole	Prevacid, Prevacid 24HR (OTC)	• 15–30 mg once daily for up to 8 wk	• Headache
omeprazole	Prilosec, Prilosec (OTC)	• 20 mg once daily for up to 4 wk	• Abdominal pain
omeprazole + sodium bicarbonate	Zegerid	• 20 mg once daily for up to 4 wk	• Increased risk for fractures
pantoprazole	Protonix	• 40 mg once daily for up to 8 wk	
rabeprazole	Aciphex	• 20 mg once daily for up to 4 wk	

GENERIC NAME: omeprazole

TRADE NAMES: Prilosec, Prilosec OTC

INDICATIONS: Gastric ulcer, duodenal ulcer, GERD, erosive esophagitis; OTC for frequent heartburn occurring 2 or more days per week for up to 2 weeks

ROUTE OF ADMINISTRATION: Oral

COMMON ADULT DOSAGES: Dosage varies, depending on the severity of the condition; a standard dosage is 20 mg once daily. *OTC dosage:* 20 mg/day for up to 14 days

MECHANISM OF ACTION: Prevents gastric acid secretion from parietal cells of the stomach

SIDE EFFECTS: Diarrhea, nausea, headache, stomach pain, increased fracture risk

AUXILIARY LABELS (Rx):
• Take before meals
• Do not crush or chew

GERD, Gastroesophageal reflux disease; *OTC,* over the counter.

MECHANISM OF ACTION: Prevents gastric acid secretion from parietal cells of the stomach

SIDE EFFECTS: Diarrhea, nausea, headache, stomach pain, increased fracture risk

AUXILIARY LABEL: Do not crush or chew

GERD, Gastroesophageal reflux disease.

■ **Tech Note!**

Patients often need advice on treating upset stomach and/or heartburn. Pharmacists can suggest a nonprescription alternative or refer the patient to a prescriber for evaluation. Many OTC stomach agents interact with prescription medications.

Peptic Ulcer Disease

Peptic ulcer disease (PUD) is a chronic condition of stomach and/or duodenal ulceration (Fig. 22.7). Occasionally, esophageal ulcers appear. PUD's primary symptoms include abdominal pain relieved by food or antacids. Drugs (eg, NSAIDs) and bacterial infection *(H. pylori)* are leading causes of PUD. They damage the stomach, duodenum, or esophagus by affecting the body's natural defenses. The prescriber will look to differentiate between an NSAID-induced ulcer or a bacterial infection. The patient who takes chronic NSAIDS might need ulcer prophylaxis and education on what to watch for, including signs and symptoms of GI bleeding such as bloody stools, emesis, or GI pain. Patients can get *H. pylori* through food, infected water, or person-to-person contact. Health care providers often treat *H. pylori* with a PPI and two antibiotics to minimize drug resistance and side effects of a single antimicrobial agent.

GENERIC NAME: pantoprazole

TRADE NAME: Protonix

INDICATIONS: GERD, erosive esophagitis

ROUTES OF ADMINISTRATION: Oral; IV

COMMON ADULT DOSAGE: Dosage varies, depending on the severity of the condition; a standard dosage is 40 mg once daily

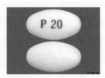

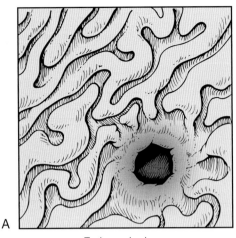

A

Endoscopic view

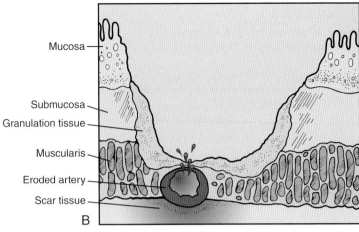

B

Histological cross section

FIG. 22.7 Peptic ulcer. (A) Endoscopic view. (B) Histologic cross section. (From Damjanov I. *Pathology for the Health Professions*. 4th ed. St. Louis: Saunders; 2011.)

Prognosis

Relapse is low with PUD when the patient receives proper treatment. For NSAID-associated ulcers, avoiding future NSAID use helps prevent relapse.

Non-Drug Treatment

Hand washing reduces *Helicobacter pylori* contamination. Avoid long-term NSAID use because they interfere with prostaglandins, which are essential for gastric defenses. Some acid-lowering agents can help prevent ulcers (eg, proton pump inhibitors [PPIs]). Cigarette smoking is an aggressive factor for ulcers, and it increases complications such as ulcer bleeding and perforation. Smoking cessation can help. Health care providers may recommend eating a bland diet, removing aggravating foods, and/or decreasing stress.

Drug Treatments

PUD positive for *H. pylori* needs antibiotic treatment. The bacterium lives in the gastric, duodenal, and rectal lining. Table 22.4 gives a summary of approved *H. pylori*–associated ulcer treatments. Therapy includes multiple agents given with an acid reducer such as a PPI. PPIs reduce stomach acid production to promote peptic ulcer healing and reduces the risk of stomach bleeds. Antacids can relieve acute abdominal pain.

■ TABLE 22.4
First-Line Recommendations for the Treatment of *Helicobacter pylori* Infection

Patient Characteristics	Regimen (Adult Oral Dosage)[a]
Patients who: 1. Are not allergic to penicillin 2. Have not previously received a macrolide antibiotic	10- to 14-day course of: • Standard or double dosage of PPI twice daily • Clarithromycin 500 mg once daily • Amoxicillin 1000 mg once daily
Patients who: 1. Are allergic to penicillin 2. Have not previously received a macrolide or metronidazole or are unable to tolerate bismuth quadruple therapy	10- to 14-day course of: • Standard or double dosage of PPI twice daily • Clarithromycin 500 mg once daily • Metronidazole 500 mg 3 times daily
Patients who: 1. Are allergic to penicillin or have failed one course (above) of *Helicobacter pylori* treatment	10- to 14-day course of: • Bismuth subsalicylate 300 mg 4 times daily • Metronidazole 250–500 mg 4 times daily • Tetracycline 500 mg 4 times daily • Standard dosage PPI twice daily

[a]Dosing recommendations from the American College of Gastroenterology.
PPI, Proton pump inhibitor.
From Chey WD, Leontiadis GI, Howden CW, Moss SF. ACG clinical guideline: treatment of *Helicobacter pylori* infection. *Am J Gastroenterol.* 2017;112(2):212–239.

Conditions Mainly Associated With the Intestines

Two of the most common symptoms affecting the intestinal tract are diarrhea and constipation. Infections caused by bacteria, viruses, and parasites can result in diarrhea. Tumors and other blockages can cause constipation. Patients can often treat diarrhea or constipation with OTC medications. However, some medicines cause diarrhea or constipation. To prevent constipation, many health care providers recommend taking a stool softener such as docusate sodium to patients taking opioids and other constipation-causing medicines. Chronic inflammatory bowel conditions such as ulcerative colitis and Crohn disease can cause diarrhea, but these disorders need aggressive prescription therapy.

After a bowel resection for tumor removal or other reasons, the patient may need to wear an ileostomy or colostomy bag. Ostomy bags attach to the abdomen with adhesive strips. Intestinal contents empty into the bag through the stoma (ostomy opening). Ostomy sites vary depending on the location of the resection in the bowel. Nutrient absorption takes place throughout the intestinal tract; therefore ostomy sites close to the stomach result in fewer absorbed nutrients. Patients with ostomies often need nutrient supplements. A person can live a normal life with an ostomy bag. Specialty pharmacies usually provide ostomy care supplies. Ostomy types include the following:

- *Colostomy:* A surgically created opening (stoma) in the abdominal wall that allows feces to pass from the bowel through the stoma rather than the anus. A colostomy may be temporary or permanent (eg, because cancer of the colon or rectum).

- *Ileostomy:* A surgical opening made through the abdominal wall into the ileum to allow for fecal passage. An ileostomy may be performed in patients with colon cancer, severe or recurrent Crohn disease, or ulcerative colitis.

Another common abdominal condition is excess intestinal gas. This gas causes pain and distention and can be uncomfortable and embarrassing. The intestinal bacteria produce hydrogen and/or methane as a by-product while digesting the foods we eat (sugars, starch, cellulose). OTC agents containing simethicone can treat this condition.

Inflammatory Bowel Disease

Inflammatory bowel disease (IBD) comprises two major disorders: Crohn disease and ulcerative colitis. Although both conditions fall under the umbrella of IBD, Crohn disease and ulcerative colitis have distinct clinical traits that distinguish them (Fig. 22.8). Table 22.5 provides information on select agents to treat these conditions.

Crohn disease Crohn disease is a chronic inflammatory intestinal disease that can cause ulcerations in the small and large intestinal lining. It can also affect parts of the digestive tract. Crohn disease is a close relative of ulcerative colitis. Autoimmune and genetic causes may play roles in the development of the condition, although the cause of Crohn disease is unknown. Symptoms include cramping, tenderness, flatulence, nausea, fever, and diarrhea. Unlike ulcerative colitis, Crohn disease can produce inflammation and ulceration throughout the thickness of the bowel (transmural) that can result in microperforations and **fistulae** in the bowel (Fig. 22.9).

Comparison of the basic features of Crohn disease and ulcerative colitis		
	Crohn disease	**Ulcerative colitis**
Prevalence in United States	~30–50 per 100,000 in United States	~80 per 100,000
Site	Any part of gastrointestinal system but typically terminal ileum	Colon and rectum only
Macroscopic • Disease continuity • Bowel wall • Ulcers	Discontinuous Thickened with strictures and adhesions Deep fissures form basis of fistulae	Continuous Not thickened Flat based; do not extend to submucosa
Microscopic • Pattern of inflammation • Crypt pattern	Transmural Focal Granulomas (in 60% of cases) Little distortion	Mucosal and submucosal Diffuse No granulomas Distorted in long-standing disease; crypt abscesses
Anal lesions	Present in 75%; anal fistulae; ulceration or chronic fissure	Present in <25%
Frequency of fistula	10%–20% of cases	Uncommon
Risk of developing cancer	Slightly increased	Significantly increased

FIG. 22.8 Comparison of the basic features of Crohn disease and ulcerative colitis. *GI,* Gastrointestinal. (From Fishback JL. *Pathology.* 3rd ed. Philadelphia: Mosby; 2005.)

◼ TABLE 22.5
Select Agents for the Treatment of Inflammatory Bowel Disease

Generic Name	Trade Name	Common Side Effects	Comments
5-Aminosalicylates			
mesalamine (5-ASA)	Apriso, Pentasa, Asacol HD, Rowasa, Canasa	• Dizziness • Abdominal pain • Rectal irritation with rectal formulations	• Approved by the FDA for ulcerative colitis • Used off-label for Crohn disease
sulfasalazine	Azulfidine		
balsalazide	Colazal		• FDA-approved for ulcerative colitis
Tumor Necrosis Factor (TNF)-Alpha Inhibitors			
adalimumab	Humira	• Nausea • Infusion/injection site reactions • Increased risk for infection • Diarrhea	• FDA-approved for Crohn disease
certolizumab pegol	Cimzia		
infliximab	Remicade		• FDA-approved for Crohn disease and ulcerative colitis
Alpha-4 Integrin Antagonist			
natalizumab	Tysabri	• Allergic reactions • Increased risk for infection • Rash	• FDA-approved for Crohn disease

FDA, US Food and Drug Administration.

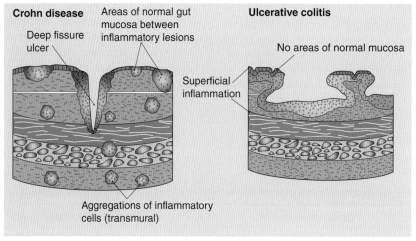

FIG. 22.9 Depth and distribution of lesions in the bowel wall in Crohn disease. (From Fishback JL. *Pathology.* 3rd ed. Philadelphia: Mosby; 2005.)

Prognosis
The prognosis for Crohn disease depends on the severity of the condition. With lifestyle changes and medication, the condition can be adequately controlled.

Non-Drug Treatment
Effective treatment includes lifestyle changes such as physical rest and a restricted diet. Patients should identify trigger foods and avoid them. A weakened patient may need parenteral nutrition to preserve nutritional status while resting the bowels. The health care provider may prescribe vitamin B_{12} injections, supplements, and the removal of dairy products from the diet. Surgery (colectomy with ileostomy) may be necessary to correct bowel perforation, massive hemorrhage, fistulae, or acute intestinal obstruction.

Drug Treatment
Agents such as 5-aminosalicylates (5-ASA), sulfasalazine (Azulfidine), and mesalamine (Asacol) are used to control inflammation in mild-moderate disease. Corticosteroids (eg, prednisone) can have adverse effects with long-term use, so prescribers taper dosages and subsequently discontinue them after a short time to minimize or avoid adverse effects. Immunomodulators such as azathioprine (Imuran) and 6-mercaptopurine (6-mp) provide an alternative if corticosteroids are ineffective or if the condition's severity warrants it. These require

more frequent physician monitoring. Biological agents such as infliximab (Remicade) and adalimumab (Humira) are additional options and are often very expensive. As such, health providers reserve these for severe symptoms or those that do not respond to other measures. Antibiotics combat infections that arise from bacterial overgrowth in the small intestine. Antidiarrheals control diarrhea, and fluid/electrolyte replacements work against dehydration. Although not ideal, many agents are used in a trial-and-error fashion to determine the best choice while minimizing symptoms.

GENERIC NAME: infliximab

TRADE NAME: Remicade

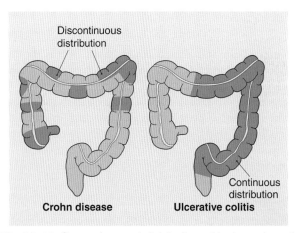

INDICATIONS: Crohn disease, ulcerative colitis, rheumatoid arthritis, psoriasis

ROUTE OF ADMINISTRATION: Intravenous (IV) infusion

COMMON ADULT DOSAGES: 5 mg/kg infused IV and then 2 and 6 weeks later, followed by a maintenance regimen of 5 mg/kg every 6–8 weeks after that depending on indication treated

MECHANISM OF ACTION: Inhibits the proinflammatory cytokine tumor necrosis factor-alpha (TNF-α) to reduce the inflammatory response

SIDE EFFECTS: Nausea, infusion site reactions, increased risk for infection, diarrhea

AUXILIARY LABELS:
- For infusion only
- Keep vials refrigerated before use

SPECIAL NOTE: A doctor or nurse usually gives infliximab in a medical setting. An extra patient information sheet, called a *Medication Guide,* accompanies each infliximab prescription

Ulcerative colitis Ulcerative colitis causes inflammation and sores in the lining of the large intestine or colon. Ulcerative colitis affects only the colon and rectum, whereas Crohn disease can affect the entire GI system (Fig. 22.10). Symptoms of ulcerative colitis include stomach pain, cramps, bloody diarrhea, or bleeding from the rectum. Some patients experience fever, loss of appetite, and weight loss. Ulcerative colitis symptoms can resemble related conditions, and the prescriber should rule out an infection.

Prognosis

The course of ulcerative colitis typically involves intermittent exacerbations alternating with periods of symptomatic remission.

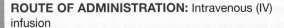

FIG. 22.10 Comparisons of distribution of lesions along the bowel in Crohn disease and ulcerative colitis. (From Fishback JL. *Pathology*. 3rd ed. Philadelphia: Mosby; 2005.)

Non-Drug Treatment

Treatment can include making lifestyle changes, such as adjusting dietary intake to avoid triggers, reducing stress, and maintaining a strong support network. In severe cases, surgery may be necessary.

Drug Treatment

Treatment depends on severity. For mild symptoms, antidiarrheals, corticosteroids, or 5-aminosalicylates provide short-term relief. Corticosteroids and aminosalicylates work for moderate to severe symptoms. Ulcerative colitis medications are often the same as those used to treat Crohn disease (see Table 22.5).

GENERIC NAME: mesalamine (5-aminosalicylates)

TRADE NAME: Asacol HD

INDICATIONS: Mild to moderate ulcerative colitis, Crohn disease

ROUTES OF ADMINISTRATION: Oral; rectal

COMMON ADULT DOSAGES: *Ulcerative colitis—oral tablet (Asacol):* 1.6 g 3 times a day for 6 weeks. *Rectal suppository (Canasa):* 1000 mg suppository given once daily. *Rectal enema (Rowasa):* 4 g (rectal instillation) at bedtime for 3–6 weeks or until remission.

MECHANISM OF ACTION: Inhibits the cyclooxygenase (COX) enzyme to reduce inflammation in the bowel

SIDE EFFECTS: Abdominal pain, nausea, vomiting, rectal irritation with rectal formulas

AUXILIARY LABELS:
- *Oral ER products:* Give whole; do not open, crush, or chew.
- *Suspension enema:* Shake well before using it. For rectal use only.
- *Suppository:* For rectal use only.

Irritable Bowel Syndrome

Patients with irritable bowel syndrome (IBS) have chronic abdominal pain and altered bowel habits. IBS is the most commonly diagnosed GI condition and affects men, women, young patients, and older people. Gastroenterologists list IBS as responsible for 25% to 50% of all referrals to their offices. Abdominal pain associated with IBS can range from mild to debilitating. Altered bowel habits vary from episodic diarrhea, constipation, and alternating diarrhea and constipation.

Prognosis

Although there is no cure for IBS, the prognosis is good with treatment and known trigger avoidance.

Non-Drug Treatment

The primary non-drug treatment includes avoiding specific irritants and triggers, including foods or stress. A high-fiber diet can help control constipation. Foods that may cause IBS symptoms include gas-producing foods, sugarless chewing gum and candy, coffee, and alcohol. Food allergies may play a role in IBS development. Health care providers may evaluate food allergies in patients with severe IBS. Stress management techniques, with regular exercise, can also help.

Drug Treatment

Antispasmodics such as dicyclomine are often given to manage IBS. However, patients who use this agent long term may become dependent on it. Another IBS treatment includes antidiarrheals (eg, diphenoxylate with atropine, loperamide), which slow intestinal movement. Bile acid sequestrants (eg, cholestyramine) can prevent bile acids from stimulating the colon and relieve diarrhea. Alosetron (Lotronex) helps in cases of diarrhea-type IBS that are unresponsive to other medications. Antidepressants or antianxiety agents can relieve depression or anxiety issues that may occur with this condition. Patients with constipation-type IBS may respond to lubiprostone (Amitiza).

GENERIC NAME: dicyclomine

TRADE NAME: Bentyl

INDICATION: Irritable bowel syndrome

ROUTE OF ADMINISTRATION: Oral

COMMON ADULT DOSAGE: 20 mg 4 times daily

MECHANISM OF ACTION: Thought to reduce muscular tone in the GI tract to decrease muscle spasms

SIDE EFFECTS: Drowsiness, dizziness, blurred vision, constipation

AUXILIARY LABELS:
- May be administered without regard to meals
- Avoid alcohol

GENERIC NAME: alosetron

TRADE NAME: Lotronex

INDICATION: Diarrhea–prominent irritable bowel syndrome (IBS)

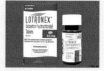

ROUTE OF ADMINISTRATION: Oral

COMMON ADULT DOSAGE: 0.5 mg twice daily for 4 weeks; may be increased to 1 mg twice daily if well tolerated

MECHANISM OF ACTION: Antagonizes serotonin (5-HT3) receptors, which diminishes pain and decreases diarrhea

SIDE EFFECTS: Constipation, drowsiness, headache

AUXILIARY LABEL: Take with a full glass of water

SPECIAL NOTES:
- Prescribers use alosetron in women with IBS for at least 6 months. The manufacturer has not proven effectiveness in men with IBS.
- Infrequent but serious adverse effects with alosetron use include ischemic colitis and severe constipation, which may result in hospitalization and, in rare cases, blood transfusion, surgery, and death.
- The patient must read and sign a patient-physician agreement form before receiving a prescription.

GENERIC NAME: lubiprostone

TRADE NAME: Amitiza

INDICATIONS: Irritable bowel syndrome with constipation in women; idiopathic and opioid-induced constipation

ROUTE OF ADMINISTRATION: Oral

COMMON ADULT DOSAGE: 8–24 mcg twice daily with food and water

MECHANISM OF ACTION: Increases intestinal fluid secretion by activating chloride channels in the GI tract, leading to softer stools and increased motility of the GI tract

SIDE EFFECTS: Nausea, vomiting, headache, diarrhea

AUXILIARY LABEL: Take with food and water

■ Tech Note!

The primary difference between irritable bowel syndrome (IBS) and inflammatory bowel disease is that IBS is not considered a disease, nor does it involve inflammation. IBS is a functional disorder with no known structural cause. Providers must diagnose it through symptomatology.

Diarrhea

Diarrhea is an abnormal increase in the frequency, fluidity, or volume of bowel movements. Abdominal cramping, gas, and general discomfort may accompany it. There are two main types of diarrhea: acute and chronic. The acute type is short term and is often caused by viral and bacterial infections.

In chronic diarrhea, symptoms continue for longer periods, generally lasting 1 month or more. Diarrhea can have many causes, including colon disorders (colitis), GI tumors, metabolic disorders, and infection. In cases of severe infectious diarrhea, the number of bowel movements may reach 20 or more daily. Although treatment depends on the cause, diarrhea is usually treated with antidiarrheal agents.

As diarrhea continues, the patient loses fluids and electrolytes. If fluids and electrolytes are not replenished, death can occur, making diarrhea a significant cause of death worldwide. The most susceptible populations are older adults and young children. Many conditions cause diarrhea; therefore, if OTC agents do not control the symptoms, a provider may need to diagnose the cause for proper treatment. A health care provider should immediately evaluate children younger than 3 years, patients with a fever, and anyone experiencing diarrhea for more than 2 days.

Prognosis

Diarrhea often resolves quickly without treatment. The prognosis largely depends on the underlying cause.

Non-Drug Treatments

Resting and drinking clear fluids (eg, oral rehydrating solutions such as Pedialyte) until diarrhea subsides are commonly suggested to prevent dehydration and electrolyte loss.

Drug Treatments

Several agents, OTC and prescription, can manage diarrhea. OTC medications include FiberCon to increase the solidity of stools and bismuth subsalicylate (Pepto-Bismol), which may turn stools black, which is normal. Several prescription drugs are also available for the treatment of diarrhea (Table 22.6). Agents such as diphenoxylate/atropine (Lomotil) are generally reserved for short-term use because they can become less effective with continued use. Patients experiencing diarrhea for longer than 48 hours should be evaluated for infection.

GENERIC NAME: diphenoxylate/atropine (C-V)

TRADE NAME: Lomotil

INDICATION: Diarrhea

ROUTE OF ADMINISTRATION: Oral

COMMON ADULT DOSAGE: 5 mg 3–4 times daily until control is achieved (max 20 mg/day)

MECHANISM OF ACTION: Slows intestinal motility to treat diarrhea

SIDE EFFECTS: Dry mouth, dizziness, drowsiness, constipation

AUXILIARY LABELS:
- May cause dizziness and drowsiness
- *Caution:* Federal law prohibits the transfer of this drug to any person other than the patient for whom it was prescribed

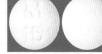

GENERIC NAME: loperamide

TRADE NAME: Imodium AD (OTC)

INDICATION: Diarrhea

ROUTE OF ADMINISTRATION: Oral

COMMON ADULT DOSAGES:
4 mg initially after loose stool, followed by 2 mg after each loose stool (max 16 mg/day for 2 days for an acute episode)

MECHANISM OF ACTION:
Slows GI motility

SIDE EFFECTS:
Dizziness, drowsiness, dry mouth

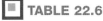 **TABLE 22.6**

Select Agents for the Treatment of Diarrhea

Generic Name	Trade Name	Common Dosage Range	Common Side Effects
diphenoxylate/ atropine (C-V)	Lomotil	• 5 mg 3 or 4 times daily, then reduce the dose as needed (max 20 mg/day)	• Constipation • Dizziness • Drowsiness • Dry mouth
bismuth subsalicylate	Pepto-Bismol (OTC)	• 524 mg every 30–60 min or 1050 mg every 60 min as needed for up to 2 days (max 4200 mg)	• Dark stools • Tongue discoloration
loperamide	Imodium AD (OTC)	• 4 mg initially for loose stool, followed by 2 mg after each loose stool (max 16 mg/day)	• Dizziness • Drowsiness • Dry mouth
psyllium	Metamucil (OTC)	• 2.5–30 g per day in divided doses	• Abdominal pain • Flatulence • Nausea

OTC, Over the counter.

GENERIC NAME: bismuth subsalicylate

TRADE NAME: Pepto-Bismol (OTC)

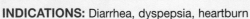

INDICATIONS: Diarrhea, dyspepsia, heartburn

ROUTE OF ADMINISTRATION: Oral

COMMON ADULT DOSAGES: 524 mg every 30–60 minutes or 1050 mg every 60 minutes for up to 2 days (max 4200 mg)

MECHANISM OF ACTION: Antidiarrheal effect is likely from prostaglandin synthesis inhibition

SIDE EFFECTS: Stools may appear grayish-black; tongue discoloration

AUXILIARY LABEL: Use cautiously in those with salicylate allergy

Constipation

Constipation manifests as hard, dry feces or infrequent or irregular bowel movements. Some people have bowel movements once to several times daily, whereas others may usually have them less often. The ease of bowel movement outweighs the frequency in defining constipation. Many people self-treat temporary constipation with dietary changes or OTC agents. However, if symptoms such as weight loss, abdominal pain, or rectal bleeding occur, constipation may indicate a more serious condition. Opioid pain medications (eg, codeine, oxycodone), antidepressants (eg, amitriptyline, imipramine), anticonvulsants (eg, phenytoin, carbamazepine), calcium channel blockers (eg, diltiazem, nifedipine, verapamil), and aluminum-containing antacids can cause constipation.

Prognosis

Patients can manage most cases through dietary or medication changes. Increased physical activity can help. If a tumor is the cause, the patient may require surgery or chemotherapy.

Non-Drug Treatments

Adequate hydration and dietary fiber through fruit and vegetable intake may resolve constipation naturally. Roughage also aids in proper digestion and elimination, and hydration and exercise are both keys to a healthy bowel.

Drug Treatments

First, a prescriber will assess baseline bowel movements as some older patients may go infrequently. They will look for causative agents. Many medicines work for constipation (Table 22.7). Stool softeners pull water and fatty compounds into the intestine to aid in elimination. Hyperosmotic agents work by osmosis, increasing pressure in the bowels by absorbing water, similar to bulk-forming agents. Stimulant laxatives increase intestinal peristalsis in the colon, forcing the contents out. People who take stimulant laxatives regularly may find themselves dependent on them. Therefore prescribers recommend that OTC stimulant laxatives be used only on a short-term basis. Enemas also resolve constipation.

Naloxegol (Movantik), a medication for opioid-induced constipation, moved from the US Drug Enforcement Administration Schedule II status to being available by prescription. Naloxegol is a mu-opioid receptor antagonist without mu-opioid agonist or partial agonist properties. Sennoside (Senokot Regular Strength) is recommended for opioid-induced constipation.

■ Tech Note!

Bowel evacuants are used to empty the intestines before a procedure or surgery. The solutions contain polyethylene glycol and replacement electrolytes because the intestines cannot absorb needed ions from the expelled fecal material. Typically, a patient must drink 2 to 4 L (2000–4000 mL) of a solution within a short time. The patient should stay home after taking the bowel evacuant because it has a rapid onset of action and causes frequent elimination.

Bulk-forming laxatives Bulk-forming agents (eg, psyllium) work by absorbing water from the body to increase the moisture and overall bulk of the stools, allowing for more natural elimination. Their significant advantages include their effectiveness for constipation and diarrhea and safety long term. Health providers may refer to them as "bowel stabilizing" agents. Examples of bulk-forming agents include polycarbophil (FiberCon) and methylcellulose (Citrucel).

GENERIC NAME: psyllium (OTC)

TRADE NAME: Metamucil

INDICATION: Constipation

ROUTE OF ADMINISTRATION: Oral

COMMON ADULT DOSAGE: 2.5–30 g/day in divided doses

MECHANISM OF ACTION: Absorbs liquid into the GI tract, leading to increased bulk of the stool, which helps peristalsis and bowel motility

SIDE EFFECTS: Bloating, gas, abdominal cramping

SPECIAL NOTE: Take with at least 8 oz of fluid to prevent choking

Emollient laxatives (stool softeners) Docusate improves the ability of water in the colon to penetrate, mix with, and soften the feces. Health care providers generally employ stool softeners as a preventive measure rather than as an active constipation treatment. The agents are gentle and effective.

GENERIC NAME: docusate (OTC)

TRADE NAME: Colace

INDICATION: Constipation

ROUTES OF ADMINISTRATION: Oral; rectal (enema)

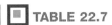

TABLE 22.7
Select Agents for the Treatment of Constipation

Generic Name	Trade Name	Common Adult Dosage	Common Side Effects
Bulk-Forming Laxatives			
methylcellulose	Citrucel (OTC)	• 2 g in 8 oz water 1–3 times daily	• Abdominal pain • Flatulence
psyllium	Metamucil (OTC)	• 2.5–30 g per day in divided doses	• Nausea
Stool Softener (Emollient Laxative)			
docusate	Colace (OTC)	• 50–360 mg daily	• Abdominal pain • Gastrointestinal (GI) cramping
Osmotic Laxatives			
polyethylene glycol	MiraLAX (OTC)	• 17 g of powder in 4–8 oz fluid once daily	• Abdominal pain • Cramping • Flatulence • Nausea
Stimulant Laxatives			
bisacodyl	Dulcolax (OTC)	• 5–15 mg once daily	• Abdominal cramping • GI irritation
senna	Senokot Regular Strength (OTC)	• 17.2–50 mg once or twice daily	• Nausea • Tolerance/dependence
Miscellaneous			
lubiprostone	Amitiza	• 8–24 mcg twice daily with food and water	• Nausea • Vomiting • Headache • Diarrhea
Combination Products			
docusate sodium/ sennosides	Senna Plus (OTC)	• 2 tablets once daily (max 4 tablets twice daily)	• See individual ingredients above
Opioid Antagonist			
naloxegol	Movantik	• 25 mg once daily; if not tolerated, reduce to 12.5 mg	• Abdominal pain, diarrhea, nausea, and vomiting

GI, Gastrointestinal; *OTC,* over the counter.

COMMON ADULT DOSAGE: *Oral:* 50–360 mg once daily or in divided doses

MECHANISM OF ACTION: Stool softener; lowers the feces' surface tension, allowing water and lipids to penetrate the stool

SIDE EFFECTS: GI cramping, abdominal pain

Stimulant laxatives Stimulant laxatives cause the muscles of the small intestine and colon to propel their contents rapidly. They also increase the water content of the feces as the colon reduces absorption or adds secretion of water in the small intestines. Stimulant examples include senna compounds and castor oil.

GENERIC NAME: bisacodyl (OTC)
TRADE NAME: Dulcolax
INDICATION: Constipation

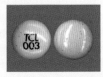

ROUTES OF ADMINISTRATION: Oral; rectal (suppository or enema)

COMMON ADULT DOSAGE: 10 mg orally or rectally once daily as needed

MECHANISM OF ACTION: Increases intestinal motility by irritating the GI mucosa

SIDE EFFECTS: Abdominal pain, dizziness, nausea, perianal irritation (rectal use)

GENERIC NAME: senna (OTC)
TRADE NAME:
Senokot Regular Strength
INDICATION: Constipation (also used for constipation from opioid agents)
ROUTE OF ADMINISTRATION: Oral

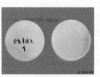

COMMON ADULT DOSAGE: Dosage depends on the preparation

MECHANISM OF ACTION: Increases intestinal motility by irritating the GI mucosa

SIDE EFFECTS: GI irritation, nausea, abdominal cramping

Osmotic laxatives These agents remain in the GI tract and hold water already in the colon to soften the stool. Examples include polyethylene glycol (MiraLAX) and lactulose (Constulose).

GENERIC NAME: polyethylene glycol (OTC)

TRADE NAME: MiraLAX

INDICATION: Constipation

ROUTE OF ADMINISTRATION: Oral

COMMON ADULT DOSAGE: 17 g powder in 4–8 oz fluid once daily

MECHANISM OF ACTION: Osmotic agent binds water and retains it in the stool

SIDE EFFECTS: Abdominal pain, cramping, flatulence, nausea

GENERIC NAME: naloxegol

TRADE NAME: Movantik

INDICATION: Opioid-induced constipation

ROUTE OF ADMINISTRATION: Oral

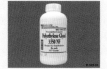

COMMON ADULT DOSAGE: 25 mg once daily; if not tolerated, reduce to 12.5 mg once daily

MECHANISM OF ACTION: Mu-opioid receptor antagonist, specific for the GI tract

SIDE EFFECTS: Abdominal pain, diarrhea, nausea/vomiting

AUXILIARY LABELS:
- Take on an empty stomach
- May cause diarrhea

Flatulence

The nitrogen, carbon dioxide, and methane by-products of microbial breakdown cause flatulence. Sugars (lactose, sorbitol, fructose) and starches (rice, wheat, certain vegetables) pose a problem because they are difficult to digest. People who are lactose intolerant do not have the lactase enzyme in the intestinal lining. This missing enzyme hinders their capacity to metabolize the carbohydrate lactose and results in poor digestion of dairy products.

Poor food absorption allows undigested food to reach bacteria in the small intestine or colon, thus producing flatulence. Symptoms include bloating, discomfort, and pain in the abdomen.

Prognosis

Flatulence is a normal digestive process that can be controlled with proper treatment.

Non-Drug Treatment

Soy products provide an alternative for people with lactose intolerance, who can also take a lactase enzyme supplement. Removing gas-causing triggers can reduce symptoms. For patients with pancreatic insufficiency, specific enzyme replacements can be taken with meals. Beano, an OTC product, contains alpha-D-galactosidase, an enzyme that helps break down vegetable sugars and reduces intestinal gas.

Drug Treatment

Simethicone is available OTC for gas in tablets, chewable tablets, and liquid for children.

GENERIC NAME: simethicone

TRADE NAMES: Gas-X, Phazyme (OTC)

INDICATION: For the relief of gas and abdominal distention caused by gas

ROUTE OF ADMINISTRATION: Oral

COMMON ADULT DOSAGE: 40–125 mg 4 times daily after meals and at bedtime as needed (max 500 mg/day)

MECHANISM OF ACTION: Reduces the surface tension of gas bubbles; prevents gas pockets

SIDE EFFECTS: None reported

Miscellaneous Conditions of the Gastrointestinal System

Nausea and Vomiting

Emesis is a synonym for vomiting. The medulla oblongata controls this violent reaction. Smell, pain, medication, motion sickness (from the inner ear), and emotions can activate the chemoreceptor trigger zone (CTZ). When activated, chemical signals travel via the nervous system to the vomit center, which relays the message to the stomach. The muscles of the diaphragm, stomach, esophagus, and salivary glands work in concert to vomit. Nausea and/or vomiting is often an isolated event. Other causes include food or drug poisoning, alcohol overconsumption, pregnancy, or a postsurgical reaction to anesthesia. Patients undergoing chemotherapy may contend with extreme nausea and vomiting as the agents activate the CTZ, causing emesis.

Prognosis

Untreated vomiting causes severe dehydration and electrolyte disturbances, including potassium, sodium, and alkalosis. Emesis is a symptom, not a disease. Treating the underlying condition normally relieves emesis.

Non-Drug Treatments

To prevent the transfer of infectious causes of vomiting, avoid undercooked foods and wash your hands before eating. If nausea occurs, eating a soda cracker or toast can sometimes help. Dehydration can occur with repeated vomiting. Replacing lost liquids and electrolytes becomes critical.

Drug Treatments

Drugs for vomiting are called **antiemetics.** Most require a prescription, but a simple sugar formula, a phosphorated carbohydrate solution (Emetrol), is available OTC. Prescription medications include anticholinergics, antidopaminergics, H_1 antihistamines, cannabinoids (dronabinol), corticosteroids (dexamethasone, methylprednisolone), and benzodiazepines (lorazepam). Agents for anticipatory chemotherapy emesis (before it happens) include corticosteroids, serotonin antagonists, and benzodiazepines. The doxylamine/pyridoxine combination (Diclegis) contains a first-generation sedating antihistamine with a B vitamin. Prescribers weigh risks, benefits, and appropriateness when deciding on an agent.

GENERIC NAME: doxylamine succinate and pyridoxine hydrochloride

TRADE NAME: Diclegis

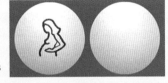

INDICATION:
Nausea and vomiting of pregnancy (NVP)

ROUTE OF ADMINISTRATION: Oral

COMMON ADULT DOSAGE: *NVP:* 2 tablets (10 mg of doxylamine and pyridoxine per tablet) at bedtime; max 4 tablets/day

MECHANISMS OF ACTION: *Doxylamine,* H_1 receptor blocker (antihistamine). *Pyridoxine,* a form of vitamin B_6. How the combination helps with nausea and vomiting is unknown

SIDE EFFECT: Drowsiness from the doxylamine

AUXILIARY LABELS:
- May cause dizziness/drowsiness
- Swallow whole; do not crush or break
- Take on an empty stomach

GENERIC NAME:
metoclopramide

TRADE NAME: Reglan

INDICATIONS: Nausea and vomiting, gastroparesis

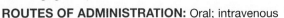

ROUTES OF ADMINISTRATION: Oral; intravenous

COMMON ADULT DOSAGES: *Nonchemotherapeutic dosage:* 5–10 mg before meals and at bedtime as needed. *Chemotherapeutic dosage:* 10 mg in 50 mL of normal saline given over 30 min; administer once before chemotherapy treatment, may repeat every 2 hours for 2 doses, or every 3 hours for 3 doses

MECHANISM OF ACTION: Antagonism of dopamine receptors in the CTZ

SIDE EFFECTS: Diarrhea, drowsiness, fatigue, parkinsonism

AUXILIARY LABEL: May cause dizziness and drowsiness

CTZ, Chemoreceptor trigger zone.

Tech Note!

Patients with Parkinson disease should not use metoclopramide because it blocks dopamine receptors in the brain. Metoclopramide has a boxed warning regarding tardive dyskinesia (a movement disorder) because of its effect on dopamine receptors.

GENERIC NAME: prochlorperazine

TRADE NAME: Compro[a]

INDICATIONS: Nausea and vomiting

ROUTES OF ADMINISTRATION:
Oral; intravenous (IV) or intramuscular (IM); rectal

COMMON ADULT DOSAGES: *Oral or IM:* 5–10 mg 3 or 4 times daily as needed (max 40 mg/day). *IV:* 2.5–10 mg every 3 or 4 hours (max 10 mg/dose or 40 mg/day); *rectal:* 25 mg every 12 hours

MECHANISM OF ACTION: Blocks dopamine receptors in the mesolimbic system

SIDE EFFECTS: Dizziness, drowsiness, dry mouth, extrapyramidal side effects

AUXILIARY LABEL: May cause dizziness and drowsiness

[a] Brand no longer available.

GENERIC NAME: ondansetron

TRADE NAMES: Zofran, Zofran ODT, Zuplenz

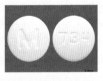

INDICATION: Nausea and vomiting (including chemotherapy-induced)

ROUTES OF ADMINISTRATION: Oral; intravenous (IV)

COMMON ADULT DOSAGES: *Oral:* 8 mg twice daily. *IV:* 8 mg or 0.15 mg/kg (max 16 mg/dose) infused over 15 min beginning 30 minutes before the initiation of chemotherapy

MECHANISM OF ACTION: Blocks serotonin (5-HT3) receptors in the chemoreceptor trigger zone

SIDE EFFECTS: Fever, headache, constipation, diarrhea

AUXILIARY LABEL: Take as directed

GENERIC NAME: meclizine

TRADE NAMES: Dramamine Less Drowsy, Travel Sickness (OTC)

INDICATIONS: Motion sickness, vertigo

ROUTE OF ADMINISTRATION: Oral

COMMON ADULT DOSAGE: 25–50 mg 1 hour before exposure to the stimulus, repeating every 24 hours if needed

MECHANISMS OF ACTION: H_1 receptor antagonist; anticholinergic

SIDE EFFECTS: Dizziness, drowsiness, dry mouth, blurred vision

AUXILIARY LABEL: May cause drowsiness, use care when operating a car or dangerous machinery

Colorectal Cancer

Colorectal cancer (CRC) is a relatively common form of cancer, and it has a high mortality rate. Although this rate has decreased, CRC remains the fourth most common cause of cancer-related death worldwide. Early symptoms of CRC include abdominal pain, a change in bowel habits, blood in the stool, weakness, anemia, and weight loss.

Prognosis
The pathologic stage of colorectal cancer (CRC) at the time of diagnosis is the best indicator of the long-term prognosis; therefore early detection is ideal for a good prognosis.

Non-Drug Treatments
Health care providers consider surgery the only cure for localized CRC. Surgery can remove cancers localized to the wall of the colon and/or rectum wall and/or regional lymph nodes. Unfortunately, some cases are inoperable.

Drug Treatments
Many chemotherapeutic agents are used to treat CRC.

GENERIC NAME: bevacizumab

TRADE NAME: Avastin

INDICATIONS: Colorectal cancer, non–small cell lung cancer, renal cell cancer

ROUTE OF ADMINISTRATION: Intravenous

COMMON ADULT DOSAGE: Dosage varies based on cancer, stage, patient weight, and combination therapies used

MECHANISM OF ACTION: Binds vascular endothelial growth factor (VEGF) to decrease the formation of new blood vessels to the tumor

SIDE EFFECTS: Allergic reactions, mouth sores, infection, chest pain

---

GENERIC NAME: irinotecan

TRADE NAME: Camptosar

INDICATION: Colorectal cancer

ROUTE OF ADMINISTRATION: Intravenous

COMMON ADULT DOSAGE: Dosage varies by weight and other combination chemotherapeutic agents used

MECHANISM OF ACTION: Inhibits DNA synthesis

SIDE EFFECTS: Anemia, alopecia, cholinergic syndrome, mouth sores, infection, diarrhea

---

GENERIC NAME: oxaliplatin

INDICATION: Colorectal cancer

ROUTE OF ADMINISTRATION: Intravenous

COMMON ADULT DOSAGE: Dosage varies based on cancer stage, patient weight, and combination therapies used

MECHANISM OF ACTION: Inhibits DNA synthesis

SIDE EFFECTS: Peripheral neuropathy, fatigue, nausea, anemia, infection, diarrhea

Pancreatic Cancer

Pancreatic cancer is the third deadliest form according to 2022 data from the National Cancer Institute. Risk factors include a pancreatic cancer family history, smoking, long-term, uncontrolled diabetes, chronic pancreatitis, and obesity.

Prognosis
Pancreatic cancer, with a 7% 5-year survival rate, is often considered fatal because providers generally uncover the disease in its later stages.

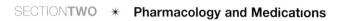

Non-Drug Treatments

Surgery to remove all cancer cells can cure pancreatic cancer, but it is not always appropriate.

Drug Treatments

Various chemotherapeutic agents can work to treat pancreatic cancer.

GENERIC NAME: gemcitabine

TRADE NAME: Infugem

INDICATIONS: Pancreatic cancer, breast cancer, non–small cell lung cancer, ovarian cancer

ROUTE OF ADMINISTRATION: Intravenous

COMMON ADULT DOSAGE: Dosage varies based on the patient's weight and other concomitant therapies

MECHANISM OF ACTION: An antimetabolite that inhibits DNA synthesis

SIDE EFFECTS: Peripheral edema, flu-like symptoms, dyspnea

AUXILIARY LABEL: For IV use only

▽ Tech Alert!

Remember these sound-alike, look-alike drugs:
- Cimetidine versus simethicone
- Hydroxyzine versus hydralazine
- Prevacid versus Pravachol or Prinivil
- Metoclopramide versus metolazone
- Ranitidine versus amantadine
- Zantac versus Zofran

Do You Remember These Key Points?

- Names of the major organs of the GI system and their functions
- Primary symptoms of the various GI conditions discussed
- Medications used to treat the different GI conditions discussed
- Generic and trade names for the drugs discussed in this chapter
- Appropriate auxiliary labels that should be used when filling prescriptions for medicines discussed in this chapter

Review Questions

Multiple Choice Questions

1. The primary gastrointestinal system functions include all of the following *except:*
   A. Digestion
   B. Absorption
   C. Secretion
   D. All of the above are GI functions

2. The small intestine does not include the ____.
   A. Duodenum
   B. Jejunum
   C. Colon
   D. Ileum

3. The _____ makes bile and the ____ stores it.
   A. Gallbladder; liver
   B. Liver; gallbladder
   C. Gallbladder; pancreas
   D. Liver; pancreas

4. Only ___ is a proton pump inhibitor.
   A. Ranitidine
   B. Omeprazole
   C. Sucralfate
   D. Aluminum hydroxide

5. Dicyclomine (Bentyl) helps patients with ___.
   A. Constipation
   B. Ulcerative colitis
   C. Irritable bowel syndrome
   D. None of the above

6. A patient with gastroesophageal reflux disease may receive which of the following medications?
   A. Calcium carbonate
   B. Famotidine
   C. Omeprazole
   D. All of the above

7. Which diarrhea medication is a C-V controlled substance?
   A. Loperamide (Imodium)
   B. Bismuth subsalicylate (Pepto-Bismol)
   C. Atropine/diphenoxylate (Lomotil)
   D. None of the above

8. Which of the following is OTC?
   A. Protonix
   B. AcipHex
   C. Prevacid 24HR
   D. Asacol

9. Two autoimmune disorders are:
   A. Diarrhea and constipation
   B. Ulcerative colitis and irritable bowel syndrome
   C. Irritable bowel syndrome and diarrhea
   D. Ulcerative colitis and Crohn disease

10. *Helicobacter pylori* is commonly present in ___.
    A. Peptic ulcer disease
    B. Crohn disease
    C. Ulcerative colitis
    D. GERD

11. An important treatment target for ___ is the chemoreceptor trigger zone.
    A. Nausea and vomiting
    B. Inflammatory bowel disease
    C. PUD
    D. IBS

12. Which of the following treats flatulence?
    A. Bismuth subsalicylate
    B. Simethicone
    C. Loperamide
    D. Famotidine

13. Colorectal cancer is currently the _____ most common cause of cancer-related death in the world.
    A. Second
    B. Third
    C. Fourth
    D. Fifth
14. Which of the following is a "stool softener"?
    A. Senna
    B. Docusate
    C. Omeprazole
    D. Psyllium
15. Which of the following manages vertigo or dizziness?
    A. Pepto-Bismol
    B. Meclizine
    C. Docusate sodium
    D. Esomeprazole

◼ Technician's Corner

A patient fills a prescription for codeine 30 mg; take one to two tablets every 4 to 6 hours as needed for pain. The quantity indicates #100.

● What over-the-counter medication might a doctor prescribe or pharmacist suggest? Why?
  A patient tests positive for *H. pylori*. The doctor prescribes:
● Clarithromycin
● Omeprazole
● Metronidazole

What strengths and doses are appropriate? How long should the patient take the medications? How does the doctor determine a stop date?

Bibliography

American Geriatrics Society Beers Criteria Update Expert Panel. American Geriatrics Society 2019 updated AGS Beers Criteria® for potentially inappropriate medication use in older adults. *J Am Geriatr Soc*. 2019;67(4):674-694.

Damjanov I. *Pathology for the Health Professions*. 4th ed. St. Louis: Saunders; 2011.

Fishback JL. *Pathology*. 3rd ed. Philadelphia: Mosby; 2005.

Institute for Safe Medication Practices. Safety Briefs. *ISMP Medication Safety Alert. Community/Ambulatory Care Edition*. 2018; 17(3):1-4.

Patton KT, Thibodeau GA. *Mosby's Handbook of Anatomy and Physiology*. St. Louis: Mosby; 2000.

Potter PA, Perry AG. *Fundamentals of Nursing*. 8th ed. St. Louis: Mosby; 2013.

Solomon EP. *Introduction to Human Anatomy and Physiology*. 3rd ed. St. Louis: Saunders; 2009.

Suzuki Y, Iida M, Ito H, et al. 2.4 g mesalamine (Asacol 400 mg tablet) once daily is as effective as three times daily in maintenance of remission in ulcerative colitis: a randomized, noninferiority, multi-center trial. *Inflamm Bowel Dis*. 2017;23(5): 822-832.

Websites Referenced

Clinical Pharmacology Online. Available at: https://www.clinicalkey.com/pharmacology/.

UpToDate Online. Available at: www.uptodate.com.

CHAPTER 23

Therapeutic Agents for the Renal System

Tony Guerra

OBJECTIVES

1. Describe the major components of the renal and urologic systems.
2. List the primary symptoms of conditions associated with the dysfunction of both the renal and the urologic systems. In addition, (a) recognize prescription and over-the-counter drugs used to treat the conditions associated with the renal and urologic systems as discussed in this chapter, (b) write the generic and trade names for the drugs discussed in this chapter, and (c) list appropriate auxiliary labels when filling prescriptions for the drugs discussed for the treatment of conditions associated with the renal and urologic systems.

TERMS AND DEFINITIONS

Acidosis Acid + condition, an increase in the blood's acidity, resulting from the accumulation of acid or loss of bicarbonate; the blood's pH is lower

Alkalosis Base + condition, an increase in the blood's alkalinity, resulting from the accumulation of alkali or reduction of acid content; the blood's pH is higher

Anions Anode + ion, negatively charged ions

Cations Cathode + ions, positively charged ions

Chronic kidney disease (CKD) A condition that reduces the kidneys' ability to function properly

Collecting duct A series of tubules in the kidneys that connect the nephrons to the ureter

Dialysate The fluid into which material passes by way of the membrane in dialysis

Dialysis The passage of a solute through a semipermeable membrane to remove toxic materials and to maintain fluid, electrolyte, and pH levels when the kidneys malfunction

Diuretic An agent that increases urine output and excretion of water

Edema An excess of watery fluid in the cavities or tissues of the body

Erythropoietin Red + create + proteins, a hormone that kidneys secrete that increases the rate of red blood cell production

Interstitial space Small, narrow spaces between tissues

Ions Atoms or molecules with a net electrical charge (positive or negative)

Lithotripsy Stone + rubbing, a treatment with ultrasound shock waves to break kidney stones into small particles

Micturition Urination

Nephron The filtering unit of the kidneys

Nosocomial infection An infection that originates in the hospital or institutional setting

Osmosis Push + condition, the diffusion of water from low-solute concentrations to higher solute concentrations across a semipermeable membrane

Peritonitis Peritoneum + inflammation, an inflammation of the peritoneum, typically caused by a bacterial infection

Plasma The colorless fluid portion of the blood

Renal artery One of the pair of arteries that branch from the abdominal aorta; each kidney has one renal artery

Renal vein The vein in which filtered blood from the kidneys is sent back into the body's circulatory system; each kidney has one renal vein

Renin An enzyme secreted by and stored in the kidneys that promotes production of the protein angiotensin

Stress incontinence Involuntary emission of urine when the pressure in the abdomen suddenly increases

Tubular reabsorption The conservation of protein, glucose, bicarbonate, and water from the glomerular filtrate by the tubules

Tubular secretion A function of the nephron in which ions, toxins, and water are secreted into the collecting duct to be excreted

Ureteroscopy Ureter + viewing, an examination of the upper urinary tract, usually performed with an endoscope passed through the urethra

Urethritis Urethra + inflammation, an inflammation of the urethra

Urge incontinence Urinary incontinence because of involuntary bladder contractions that result in an urgent need to urinate

Urinary acidification The conversion of urine to a more acidic content

Urolithiasis Urinary + stone + condition, solid mineral deposits that form stones in the urinary tract

Common Drugs for Conditions of the Renal and Urinary Systems

Trade Name	Generic Name	Pronunciation
Loop Diuretics		
Bumex[a]	bumetanide	(byew-**meh**-tuh-nide)
Demadex	torsemide	(**tore**-seh-myde)
Edecrin	ethacrynic acid	(eth-a-**krin**-ik **as**-id)
Lasix	furosemide	(fyoor-**oh**-suh-myde)
Osmotic Diuretic		
Osmitrol	mannitol	(**man**-uh-tall)
Potassium-Sparing Diuretics		
Aldactone	spironolactone	(spir-own-oh-**lak**-tone)
Dyrenium	triamterene	(try-**am**-tur-een)
Inspra	eplerenone	(eh-**pler**-uh-nown)
Midamor[a]	amiloride	(ah-**mill**-or-ide)
Thiazide and Thiazide-Like Diuretics		
Microzide[a]	hydrochlorothiazide	(hye-droe-klor-oh-**thy**-uh-zide)
Thalitone[a]	chlorthalidone	(klor-**thal**-ah-doan)
Zaroxolyn[a]	metolazone	(me-**toe**-luh-zone)
Agents to Treat Chronic Kidney Disease		
Common Phosphorus-Binding Agents		
PhosLo	calcium acetate	(**kal**-see-uhm **ass**-uh-tate)
Renagel, Renvela	sevelamer	(se-**vel**-a-mer)
Hematopoietic Agents (to Treat Anemia in Chronic Renal Failure)		
Aranesp	darbepoetin alfa	(dar-beh-**poh**-ee-tin **al**-fuh)

Common Drugs for Conditions of the Renal and Urinary System—cont'd

Trade Name	Generic Name	Pronunciation
Epogen, Procrit	epoetin alfa	(ee-**poh**-ee-tin **al**-fuh)
Iron Supplement		
Feosol[a]	ferrous sulfate	(fair-**us** sul-**fate**)
Ferretts Iron	ferrous fumarate	(fair-**us fue**-mer-ate)
Vitamin D Analog		
Calciferol	ergocalciferol	(**ur**-go-kal-**sih**-fer-all)
Rocaltrol	calcitriol	(**kal**-sih-**trye**-ol)
Antibiotics to Treat Urinary Tract Infections		
Bactrim	sulfamethoxazole/trimethoprim	(sul-fuh-meth-**ox**-a-zole/trye-**meth**-oh-prim)
Cipro	ciprofloxacin	(sip-roe-**flox**-uh-sin)
Keflex	cephalexin	(cef-uh-**lex**-in)
Macrobid	nitrofurantoin	(**nye**-troe-fue-**ran**-toin)
Monurol	fosfomycin	(**fos**-fuh-my-cin)
Agents to Treat Overactive Bladder		
Detrol	tolterodine	(tol-**ter**-uh-deen)
Ditropan, Oxytrol, Gelnique	oxybutynin	(**ox**-ee-**bue**-tih-nin)
Enablex	darifenacin	(dar-eh-**fen**-uh-sin)
Sanctura[a]	trospium chloride	(trose-**pee**-um **klor**-ide)
Toviaz	fesoterodine	(**fes**-oh-**ter**-oh-deen)
VESIcare	solifenacin succinate	(sol-ih-**fen**-uh-sin **suhk**-suh-neyt)

[a] Brand discontinued; now available only as generic.

The kidneys are the major organs of the renal and urinary systems. The kidneys maintain the chemical composition of electrolytes, fluids, and tissues in the body. This role includes acid-base balance, preservation of normal blood pressure, and production of hormones such as the active form of vitamin D, renin, and erythropoietin. This chapter discusses the location and function of the renal and urologic systems with an overview of common conditions and treatments.

Anatomy and Physiology of the Renal and Urologic Systems

The kidneys are inside the upper abdominal cavity, with one kidney on each side of the vertebral column (Fig. 23.1). The right kidney is a little lower than the left because the liver is directly above it. These two organs are shaped like a kidney bean, with a small indentation called the *hilus*. The kidney filters blood as it enters the kidneys at the hilus from the **renal artery** (Fig. 23.2) and reabsorbs important **ions** such as sodium and chloride. The **renal vein** and ureter leave the kidney at the hilus. The renal vein returns blood to the body after the kidney filters it. The ureters carry wastes removed from the blood to the bladder, which stores the waste for excretion as urine (see Fig. 23.1).

The bladder resembles a holding tank that can expand, depending on the volume of urine it contains. When the bladder becomes full, we feel the urge to urinate. The body eliminates urine through the urethra, a short tube leading from the bladder to the outside of the body.

Function of the Kidneys

The kidneys play a crucial role and regulate many bodily processes. The body is constantly developing waste products as by-products of normal metabolism by active tissues (eg, muscles) and from digesting food. Ultimately the kidneys filter the blood and remove these wastes. The cleansed blood and other vital components, such as proteins, return to the body. Waste products filtered out of the blood by the kidneys enter the urinary system to be excreted in the urine.

Excretion is one of the four major important pharmacokinetic (drug movement) or body functions. These four functions are:

1. *Absorption:* The intake of liquids, solids, and gases into the body
2. *Distribution:* How chemicals, nutrients, and drugs move throughout the body to their target organs and tissues
3. *Metabolism:* The chemical changes and reactions in the body system; metabolism includes anabolism (building-up processes) and catabolism (breaking-down processes)
4. *Excretion:* The elimination of chemicals and substances from the body system

Normal urinary output for an adult is 1 to 2 L/day. The liver produces urea that ends up in the urine. Urea is a form of nitrogen that the body converts to ammonia, which causes

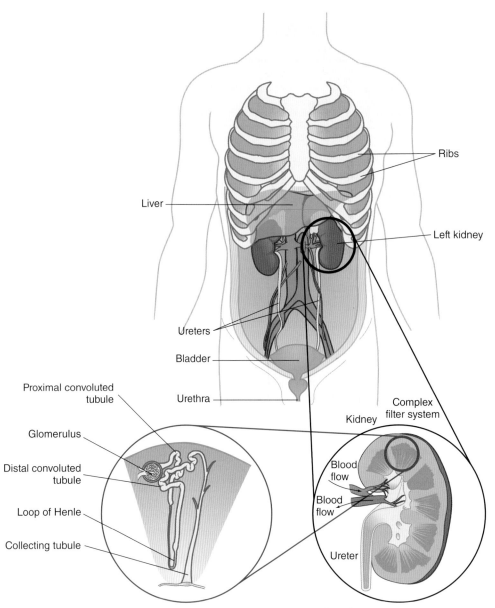

FIG. 23.1 Anatomy of the urinary tract and nephrons.

the characteristic urine smell. Another important kidney function is balancing fluids and electrolytes. The kidneys balance ions in the blood and eliminate excess ions through urinary excretion. The filtered fluid, referred to as *filtrate*, contains water, ions (eg, sodium, potassium, chloride), glucose (sugar), and small proteins. If electrolyte concentrations fall out of balance because the kidneys cannot filter appropriately, conditions such as metabolic acidosis or **alkalosis** can develop. **Acidosis** is an excess of free hydrogen ions (H^+) in the body fluids. Alkalosis is the retention of bicarbonate (HCO_3^-) or excessive loss of hydrogen ions. Although the kidneys are only about fist size, they filter about 45 gallons of blood daily.

Nephron Function

The functional unit of the kidney is the **nephron.** Nephrons regulate fluids, solutes, and wastes in the body. Each kidney

contains millions of microscopic nephrons (Fig. 23.3). Each nephron is shaped like an inverted pyramid, and its tubules have many twists and turns. The nephrons actively filter blood 24 hours a day. The following list systematically describes the filtering process as the blood flow enters the kidney (see Fig. 23.3):

1. The renal artery enters the kidney and divides into progressively smaller vessels until it becomes the afferent arterioles. Blood then passes from the afferent arterioles into a cluster of capillaries called the *glomerulus.* A double-layered epithelial cup that resembles a baseball glove surrounds each glomerulus; this structure is called the *Bowman capsule.*

2. Blood cells, platelets, and large proteins cannot pass through glomerular capillaries into the Bowman capsule; only plasma can. **Plasma,** mostly water, is the blood's liquid component. However, some plasma components (eg, albumin and antibodies) are too large to leave the

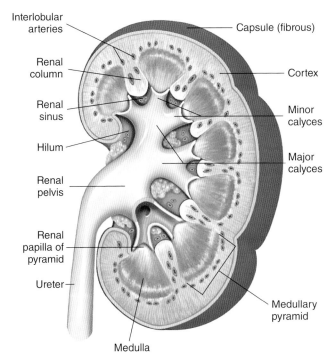

FIG. 23.2 Kidney structure. (From McCance KL. *Pathophysiology: The Biologic Basis for Disease in Adults and Children.* 6th ed. St. Louis: Mosby; 2010.)

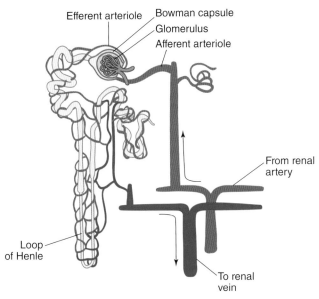

FIG. 23.3 Nephron anatomy.

capillaries. Other plasma components include toxins, which may accumulate in the blood. These are often small, leave the capillaries, and easily enter the Bowman capsule.

3. The Bowman capsule filtrate travels down the descending tubule (the *proximal convoluted tubule*), makes a U-turn through the *loop of Henle*, and returns up the ascending tubule (called the *distal convoluted tubule* [DCT]).

4. As the filtrate passes through the nephron tubules, various nutrients, water, and important chemical ions (eg, sodium,

chloride, and potassium) are pulled out of the filtrate (ie, reabsorbed) and returned to the plasma to be used by the body. At the same time, other ions in the tubules (eg, those in excess) are excreted.

5. The filtrate, now called urine, travels from the nephrons to the **collecting ducts.**

6. The collecting ducts empty directly into the ureter.

7. The ureter extends from the hilus of each kidney directly to the bladder.

8. The bladder empties the urine into the urethra for elimination.

■ Tech Note!

Sodium is an important electrolyte that helps conduct nerve impulses and balance body fluids. Kidney reabsorption regulates sodium content.

Tubular Reabsorption

An important nephron function is **tubular reabsorption.** The nephron-produced filtrate contains water, ions, glucose, and other molecules small enough to pass through the glomerulus. The urine excretes some filtrate molecules. Glucose (sugar), water, sodium, chloride, and amino acids may remain. The nephrons can reabsorb small molecules to reenter the plasma. This process takes place at various points along the proximal convoluted tubule, DCT, and loop of Henle (Fig. 23.4). The fact that pressure is highest near the glomerulus is important in understanding the diuretic mechanism of action.

Tubular reabsorption enables the kidneys to carry out another important function: regulation of acid-base balance. Two mechanisms affect ion balance. The first is the exchange of sodium ions from the tubules for hydrogen ions. As sodium accumulates outside of the proximal convoluted tubules, it creates an osmotic gradient and water molecules move toward the higher sodium concentration to equilibrate the concentration. The water molecule movement is **osmosis** (Fig. 23.5). The overall effect is a decrease in excreted water. Ion exchange also takes place in the DCT. As sodium ions exit the DCT, they are exchanged for potassium ions. The loop of Henle has a different transport mechanism, called *active transport* (see Fig. 23.4). Instead of ion exchange, there is a one-way uptake of sodium and chloride. These ions return to the circulatory system. Overall, the body resorbs most renal system sodium.

Tubular Secretion

Tubular secretion is another major function throughout the nephrons. The collecting duct secretes various ions, toxins, and water. First, the nephron excretes toxins, water-soluble molecules, and excess or unnecessary chemicals (including some medications). The second secretive function allows the kidneys to regulate the blood pH through **urinary acidification** to a pH of 4 to 5, whereas blood pH is about 7.4.

As the nephron takes in hydrogen ions, they combine with other molecules to produce bicarbonate. Bicarbonate enters the bloodstream as a buffer, where it regulates the overall

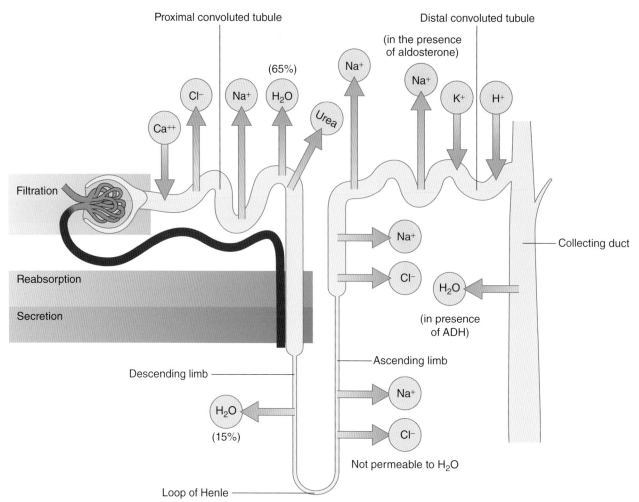

Proximal convoluted tubule

Distal convoluted tubule

(in the presence of aldosterone)

(65%)

Filtration

Reabsorption

Secretion

Collecting duct

(in presence of ADH)

Ascending limb

Descending limb

Not permeable to H₂O

Loop of Henle

(15%)

FIG. 23.4 Tubular reabsorption and secretion. *ADH,* Antidiuretic hormone.

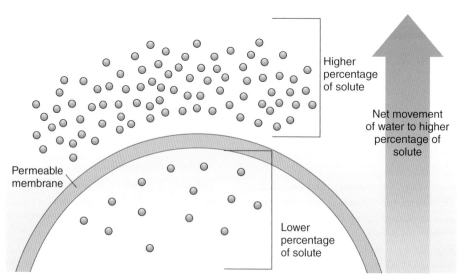

Higher percentage of solute

Net movement of water to higher percentage of solute

Permeable membrane

Lower percentage of solute

FIG. 23.5 Osmotic gradient: the smaller water molecules gravitate toward the highly concentrated sodium ions.

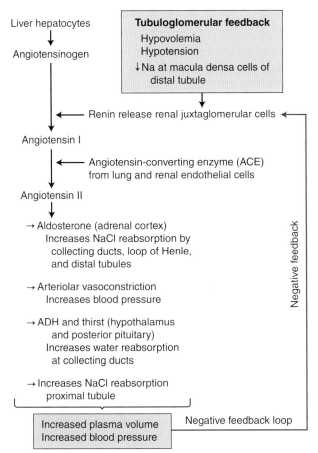

Tubuloglomerular feedback
Hypovolemia
Hypotension
↓Na at macula densa cells of distal tubule

Liver hepatocytes

Angiotensinogen

Renin release renal juxtaglomerular cells

Angiotensin I

Angiotensin-converting enzyme (ACE) from lung and renal endothelial cells

Angiotensin II

→ Aldosterone (adrenal cortex)
  Increases NaCl reabsorption by collecting ducts, loop of Henle, and distal tubules

→ Arteriolar vasoconstriction
  Increases blood pressure

→ ADH and thirst (hypothalamus and posterior pituitary)
  Increases water reabsorption at collecting ducts

→ Increases NaCl reabsorption proximal tubule

Negative feedback

Increased plasma volume
Increased blood pressure

Negative feedback loop

FIG. 23.6 Renin-angiotensin-aldosterone system. (From McCance KL. *Pathophysiology: The Biologic Basis for Disease in Adults and Children*. 6th ed. St. Louis: Mosby; 2010.)

body pH to maintain homeostasis. Buffers can bind hydrogen to create basic environments or release hydrogen for acidic environments, balancing blood pH. In other words, acids can release hydrogen ions, whereas bases can remove hydrogen ions by binding to them. Tubules take up the extra hydrogen ions to excrete them.

The kidneys produce **renin,** an enzyme that maintains body water balance. Stressors, especially fluid loss, prompt the kidneys to secrete renin. The renin enters the bloodstream, transforms angiotensinogen into angiotensin I, and circulates throughout the system. The liver transforms angiotensin I to angiotensin II. Angiotensin II activates the adrenal cortex, which excretes aldosterone, a hormone. Aldosterone circulates back to the kidneys, where it activates the kidneys to increase fluid reabsorption (Fig. 23.6). This activation increases body fluid volume to raise blood pressure and protect against dehydration.

Importance of Electrolytes

Kidneys maintain homeostasis by balancing electrolyte levels. An understanding of ion function is foundational to understanding the importance of kidney function.
Cations:
- *Calcium (Ca^{2+}):* Bone and teeth formation, cell membrane integrity, cardiac conduction, nerve impulse conduction, muscle contraction, hormone secretion

- *Magnesium (Mg^{2+}):* Aids in cardiac and skeletal muscle excitability, enzyme activities, and neurochemical activities
- *Potassium (K$^+$):* Necessary for glycogen (sugar) deposits in the liver (to maintain blood sugar levels) and skeletal muscles (for energy); aids in nerve impulse and cardiac conduction; helps in contraction in skeletal and smooth muscles
- *Sodium (Na$^+$):* Maintains water balance, nerve impulse transmission, and regulation of acid-base balance; participates in cellular chemical reactions

Anions:
- *Bicarbonate (HCO$_3$):* The most important chemical buffer; essential for proper acid-base balance
- *Chloride (Cl):* The main anion in the transport of sodium, hydrogen, and potassium; essential to acid-base balance
- *Phosphate (PO$_4^{3-}$):* Aids as a buffer to balance acid-base regulation in cells; promotes normal neuromuscular action and participates in carbohydrate metabolism; essential for formation and strength of bones and teeth; also needed for many biochemical pathways (eg, production of energy, cell division)

Conditions Affecting the Renal and Urologic Systems

Many people live with just one kidney, thanks to an efficiency that allows for as little as 20% function for survival. Despite the kidneys' resiliency and efficiency, people need to closely monitor diet, medications, and activities to maintain kidney health. In some cases, dialysis or kidney transplantation may be necessary.

Other conditions that we have not highlighted can include kidney, ureter, bladder, or urethral blockages or infections. If the bladder retains residual urine, an infection can result. Significant water intake helps maintain the system's good health by flushing toxins and other unwanted chemicals.

Common Conditions Associated With the Renal and Urologic Systems

This section describes some of the more common disorders associated with the renal and urologic systems and discusses common medications for their treatment.

Chronic Kidney Disease

Chronic kidney disease (CKD) is the progressive loss of renal function. Diabetes mellitus and uncontrolled hypertension are the most common causes of CKD in adults in the United States. Other CKD potential causes include kidney diseases such as glomerulonephritis, pyelonephritis, and vascular disorders. Kidney function decreases with age resulting in higher CKD incidence in older individuals. As a kidney ages, it is less able to compensate for fluid imbalances. Depending on the disease level, health professionals stratify CKD into five stages based on the glomerular filtration rate (GFR), a measure of kidney filtration (Table 23.1). CKD progression may correlate with common kidney changes.

TABLE 23.1
Stages of Chronic Kidney Disease

Stage	Severity	GFR Range (mL/min)	Symptoms
1	Kidney damage with normal or increased GFR	≥90	Usually absent, mild hypertension
2	Kidney damage with a mild decrease in GFR	60–89	Mild hypertension
3	Moderate decrease in GFR	30–59	Mild hypertension
4	Severe decrease in GFR	15–29	Moderate hypertension, hyperphosphatemia, anemia
5	ESRD	<15	Severe hypertension, hyperphosphatemia, anemia

ESRD, End-stage renal disease; *GFR,* glomerular filtration rate.
From National Kidney Foundation. KDOQI clinical practice guidelines for chronic kidney disease: evaluation, classification, and stratification. Retrieved from *https://www.kidney.org/sites/default/files/docs/ckd_evaluation_classification_stratification.pdf*

TABLE 23.2
Select Systemic Effects of Chronic Kidney Disease

System	Effect
Cardiovascular	Hypertension, heart failure
Endocrine	Hyperparathyroidism, osteomalacia
Gastrointestinal	Nausea, vomiting, gastrointestinal bleeding
Immunologic	Suppressed immunologic responses, increased infection risk
Nervous	Fatigue, peripheral neuropathy
Respiratory	Pulmonary edema, dyspnea

These include glomerular hypertension and hyperfiltration, glomerulosclerosis, and tubule inflammation.

As renal failure progresses, other areas may suffer from waste product effects and a fluid imbalance. Early symptoms include fatigue, headache, shortness of breath (SOB), sudden weight changes, and edema. Signs can progress to include systemic symptoms (Table 23.2). Anemia manifests in advanced CKD because kidneys produce the hormone **erythropoietin.** When kidney function declines, less erythropoietin leads to decreased red blood cell production and anemia.

Prognosis

The gradual kidney function decline in patients with chronic kidney disease (CKD) is often asymptomatic initially but can progress to volume overload, metabolic acidosis, hypertension, anemia, and bone disease. These outcomes may lead to patient morbidity, but not all people with early CKD experience a progressive kidney function loss. Therefore a prognosis may vary. When the disease progresses, however, patients with CKD have an increased risk for cardiovascular disease and death. The risk for death in people with CKD is higher than the risk for progression to dialysis.

Non-Drug Treatment

Dietary management is vital in CKD treatment. Patients should limit the consumption of foods high in phosphate (eg, colas) and dairy products (eg, milk, cheese). For patients with significant edema and/or hypertension, low to moderate sodium intake is important. Protein restriction may help reduce damage to the kidneys.

Dialysis is a procedure that removes waste products from the blood of patients with end-stage renal disease (ESRD). Dialysis compensates for lack of kidney filtration to remove waste products from the blood and balance electrolytes and fluid volume. Two major life-sustaining methods exist, hemodialysis and peritoneal dialysis, each with drawbacks. Negative dialysis aspects include needed extra medications to balance pH and fluids, the inconvenience of being stationary for long dialysis sessions, and that sophisticated machinery cannot perform as efficiently as our kidneys. The pharmacy team has a vital role in timing medications before, during, and after dialysis.

Hemodialysis requires the patient to visit a clinic or hospital for treatment. A vein shunt (needle puncture with a reinforced opening) is used to connect the patient's bloodstream to the dialysis machine. The dialysis machine uses a mechanical filtration system to clean a small but steady stream of blood from the patient's body. Although the length of treatment varies, traditional hemodialysis takes typically 3 hours or longer two or three times weekly.

Peritoneal dialysis is an alternative to hemodialysis. A provider connects the patient's bloodstream to a bag of an osmotic solution and implants a catheter plug into the abdominal cavity for administration to remove the **dialysate.** The osmotic solution (dialysate) flows into the peritoneal cavity. The peritoneal membrane is a thin lining that encases the organs of the abdomen, including the stomach, liver, spleen, and kidneys. The osmotic solution works as the sodium gradient in the kidneys. As the solution fills the cavity, wastes are pulled into the

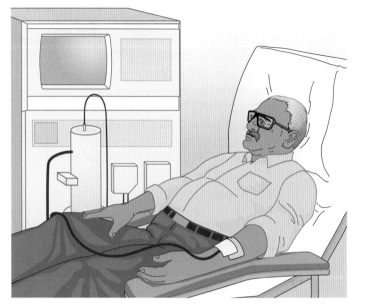

Hemodialysis

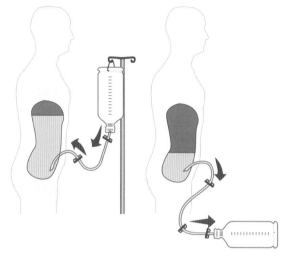

Continuous ambulatory peritoneal dialysis

FIG. 23.7 Two types of dialysis.

solution, where they drain from the cavity into an empty bag attached outside the abdominal wall. This treatment happens several times daily to keep toxin levels to a minimum. Treatment can be done at home or can occur in clinics for patients who cannot afford a home health nurse (Fig. 23.7). Aseptic technique is crucial in this dialysis type to prevent **peritonitis,** an abdominal cavity infection.

Nocturnal hemodialysis allows patients to sleep during treatment. Dialysis is done with a portable peritoneal or hemodialysis machine, 8 to 12 hours nightly. Patients do not have to wait between treatments for toxic buildup, and patients avoid the inconvenient dialysis clinic. If dialysis is done at home, patients must be able to troubleshoot machinery problems. Finally, home health nurses may need to help.

Drug Treatment

Patients on dialysis must watch their fluid and salt intake because electrolyte balance is essential. With any treatment, ion and nutrient loss needs to be supplemented with each dialysis session. The most common ESRD side effect is anemia, for which we use iron and epoetin alfa (Epogen, Procrit). Epoetin alfa may pose a clot risk with a clot that might appear in the access port (atrioventricular [AV] shunt), however. Patients should let their provider know if this happens. Iron supplements increase the oxygen-carrying capacity of red blood cell hemoglobin. Other medications may include vitamin supplements, antihypertensives, and phosphorus-lowering medications such as calcium carbonate, calcium acetate, and sevelamer. Vitamin D supplements compensate for the kidney's inability to synthesize an active form of vitamin D, placing patients with CKD at risk for weak bones.

Patients with CKD are more likely to experience hyperkalemia, which is an elevated potassium level. As kidney function falls its excretion ability diminishes which can exacerbate existing hyperkalemia from potassium-sparing drugs. Hyperkalemia treatments include calcium gluconate, insulin, sodium bicarbonate, and sodium polystyrene sulfonate.

Guidelines now recommend the initiation of an SGLT2 inhibitor in patients with CKD. SGLT2 inhibitors, as introduced in Chapter 18, can lower blood sugar levels in type 2 diabetes. They can also prevent CKD progression and decrease poor renal outcome risks.

GENERIC NAME: ferrous sulfate (over the counter [OTC])

TRADE NAME: None

INDICATION: Iron deficiency anemia

ROUTE OF ADMINISTRATION: Oral

COMMON ADULT DOSAGE: 300 mg (60 mg as elemental iron) 1–3 times daily for 4 weeks

MECHANISM OF ACTION: Increases blood iron concentrations to increase red blood cell production

SIDE EFFECTS: Constipation, black stools

GENERIC NAME: epoetin alfa

TRADE NAMES: Epogen, Procrit

INDICATION: Anemia with hemoglobin less than 10 g/dL as a result of CKD

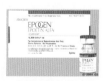

ROUTES OF ADMINISTRATION: Subcutaneous (subcut); intravenous (IV)

COMMON ADULT DOSAGE: 50–100 units/kg subcut (IV preferred if on hemodialysis) 3 times; reduce dose if hemoglobin approaches or exceeds 11 g/dL

MECHANISM OF ACTION: Stimulates red blood cell production and mimics endogenous erythropoietin action

SIDE EFFECTS: Hypertension, headache, injection site reactions, rash

AUXILIARY LABELS:
- Refrigerate
- Do not shake
- Protect from light

GENERIC NAME: darbepoetin alfa

TRADE NAME: Aranesp

INDICATION: Anemia with hemoglobin less than 10 g/dL as a result of CKD

ROUTES OF ADMINISTRATION: Subcutaneous (subcut); intravenous (IV)

COMMON ADULT DOSAGES: 0.45 mcg/kg subcut (IV if on hemodialysis) once weekly or 0.75 mcg/kg every 2 weeks adjusting doses based on response and hemoglobin; reduce the dose or interrupt treatment if hemoglobin exceeds 11 g/dL

MECHANISMS OF ACTION: Stimulates red blood cell production, mimics the action of endogenous erythropoietin

SIDE EFFECTS: Hypertension, headache, injection site reactions, rash

AUXILIARY LABELS:
- Refrigerate
- Do not shake
- Protect from light

GENERIC NAME: calcium carbonate (OTC)

TRADE NAME: Tums

INDICATION: Hyperphosphatemia

ROUTE OF ADMINISTRATION: Oral

COMMON ADULT DOSAGE: 500–2000 mg 3 times daily with meals; adjusted based on calcium and phosphate levels (max 2000 mg/day)

MECHANISM OF ACTION: Binds to dietary phosphate in the gastrointestinal (GI) tract to inhibit absorption, reducing phosphate levels

SIDE EFFECT: Constipation

GENERIC NAME: calcium acetate (Rx)

TRADE NAME: PhosLo

INDICATION: Hyperphosphatemia

ROUTE OF ADMINISTRATION: Oral

COMMON ADULT DOSAGE: 1334 mg (2 tablets or gel caps) daily with meals initially; adjusted based on calcium and phosphate levels

MECHANISM OF ACTION: Binds to dietary phosphate in the gastrointestinal tract to inhibit its absorption, reducing phosphate levels

SIDE EFFECT: Constipation

AUXILIARY LABELS:
- Protect from moisture
- Take with meals

GENERIC NAME: sevelamer (Rx only)

TRADE NAMES: Renagel, Renvela

INDICATION: Hyperphosphatemia

ROUTE OF ADMINISTRATION: Oral

COMMON ADULT DOSAGE: 800–1600 mg 3 times daily with meals; dosage based on phosphate levels

MECHANISM OF ACTION: Binds to dietary phosphate in the GI tract to inhibit its absorption, reducing phosphate levels

SIDE EFFECTS: Headache, heartburn, diarrhea

AUXILIARY LABELS:
- Protect from moisture
- Take with meals

GENERIC NAME: calcitriol

TRADE NAME: Rocaltrol

INDICATION: Renal osteodystrophy

ROUTES OF ADMINISTRATION: Oral; intravenous (IV)

COMMON ADULT DOSAGES: *Oral:* 0.25–1 mcg/day for most patients; *IV:* 0.5–4 mcg 3 times weekly; based on serum calcium levels and other parameters

MECHANISM OF ACTION: Active form of vitamin D; does not require activation by the kidneys

SIDE EFFECT: Hypercalcemia (elevated calcium levels)

AUXILIARY LABEL: Do not crush or chew

GENERIC NAME: Cinacalcet

TRADE NAME: Sensipar

INDICATION: Renal osteodystrophy/hyperparathyroidism

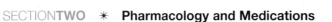

ROUTES OF ADMINISTRATION: Oral; intravenous (IV)

COMMON ADULT DOSAGES: *Oral:* 0.25–1 mcg/day for most patients; *IV:* 0.5–4 mcg 3 times weekly; based on serum calcium levels and other parameters

MECHANISM OF ACTION: A calcimimetic that mimics the actions of calcium. Only used in patients on dialysis

SIDE EFFECT: Hypocalcemia (decreased calcium levels)

AUXILIARY LABEL:
Do not crush or chew

Tech Note!

It is essential to adjust medication dosages for patients with CKD when appropriate. As renal failure progresses, the kidney's ability to eliminate many drugs diminishes. As such, drug accumulation can lead to drug toxicity. These drug dosing recommendations use data such as the estimated creatinine clearance (CrCl) and estimated glomerular filtration rate (eGFR). Information on drug dosing in special populations such as CKD or pregnancy or hepatic disease can be found in the package insert or on DailyMed.

Hypertension and Diabetes in CKD

Hypertension and CKD High blood pressure causes decreased kidney blood flow from peripheral vasoconstriction. Over time, the lack of blood flow can lead to CKD progression. Treatments for patients with CKD and hypertension include angiotensin-converting enzyme inhibitors, angiotensin receptor blockers, nondihydropyridine calcium channel blockers, and diuretics. The addition of an SGLT2 can provide protective benefits to the renal and cardiovascular systems.

Diabetes and CKD The kidneys must work harder to effectively filter excess blood sugar. Long-term uncontrolled diabetes can damage kidney blood vessels, leading to renal failure. Guidelines recommend metformin and an SGLT2 inhibitor for patients with CKD and type 2 diabetes because the combination is found to reduce cardiovascular events such as strokes and heart attacks as well as CKD progression.

Kidney Stones

Kidney stones are small aggregations of material (usually calcium, magnesium, or uric acid salts) that form in the kidney and/or urinary tract. Hundreds of thousands of Americans experience a condition known as **urolithiasis** (kidney stones) annually. Stones can affect anyone but are most common in those aged 20 to 55. The first sign of a kidney stone is pain during urination. Kidney stones can pass naturally through the urine without treatment. Medical treatment helps with difficult stones. In severe cases, kidney stones can block the urinary tract. Blockage symptoms can include fever,

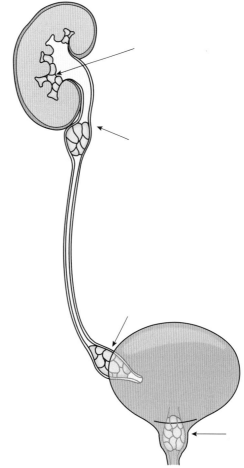

FIG. 23.8 Common locations of kidney stones *(arrows)*. (From Monahan F, Sands J, Neighbors M, Marek J, Green-Nigro C. *Phipps' Medical-Surgical Nursing: Health and Illness Perspectives*. 8th ed. St. Louis: Mosby; 2007.)

vomiting, blood in the urine, and extreme flank, back, and abdominal pain. Different stone types can form at different urinary tract locations (Fig. 23.8).

Prognosis

Patients have several options to prevent and remove kidney stones. Through dietary changes and medication, people can limit future stone development.

Non-Drug Treatment

Small stones may require no treatment or only pain management and fluid intake while the stone passes through the tract. For larger stones, options vary. **Lithotripsy** uses shock waves to break up stones. **Ureteroscopy** is the procedure in which a ureteroscope, a lighted instrument inserted through the urethra, retrieves the stones with a camera and endoscopic instruments. More invasive surgical procedures may retrieve stones based on size and location. Hydration is a necessary treatment that helps flush out small stones and may help prevent future stones. A healthy diet and electrolyte balance reduce the risk.

Drug Treatments

Analgesics, such as over-the-counter (OTC) nonsteroidal antiinflammatory drugs (NSAIDs) and acetaminophen, can relieve mild pain. High-potency opioids are necessary for more severe pain. Calcium channel blockers (CCBs) (eg, nifedipine) and alpha-blockers (eg, tamsulosin) can accelerate the stone's passage. The mechanism of action of CCBs is unclear, but they act on the ureter. Preventive agents include thiazide diuretics and potassium citrate. Agents that prevent uric acid stone formation include allopurinol and potassium citrate.

GENERIC NAME: allopurinol

TRADE NAMES: Zyloprim, Aloprim

INDICATIONS: Kidney stones, gout

ROUTE OF ADMINISTRATION: Oral

COMMON ADULT DOSAGE: 200–300 mg once daily or in divided doses (max 800 mg/day)

MECHANISM OF ACTION: Inhibits the enzyme xanthine oxidase, which blocks the production of uric acid

SIDE EFFECTS: Nausea, vomiting, dyspepsia, rash

AUXILIARY LABELS:

- May cause dizziness/drowsiness
- Take with a full glass of water

GENERIC NAME: potassium citrate

TRADE NAME: Urocit-K

INDICATIONS: Kidney stones, renal tubular acidosis

ROUTE OF ADMINISTRATION: Oral

COMMON ADULT DOSAGE: 10–30 mEq 2 or 3 times daily with meals (max 100 mEq/day)

MECHANISM OF ACTION: Increases urine pH and citrate concentrations in the urine to produce urine that is less likely to lead to stone crystallization

SIDE EFFECTS: Nausea, vomiting, diarrhea, gas

AUXILIARY LABEL: Take with food

Edema

Edema is a buildup of fluid in body tissues. Edema can occur in the extremities (peripheral edema), the lungs (pulmonary edema), and other areas. The body typically stores fluids in the blood and **interstitial spaces** (spaces around cells), but some conditions cause fluids to accumulate in other tissues, leading to edema (Box 23.1). Two general types of peripheral edema include pitting edema and nonpitting edema. When someone applies pressure, indentations, or pitting, can occur (Fig. 23.9). This fluid buildup seems to correlate with high-salt diets and/or heart failure (HF). (Chapter 20 presents

---

BOX 23.1 Select Causes of Edema

Chronic venous insufficiency: Attributable to poor blood flow caused by a weakness in the veins; often seen in older people and people with obesity

Cirrhosis: Chronic hepatic disease characterized by destruction and fibrotic regeneration of hepatic cells

Heart failure: Decreased ability to function properly because of overload; can occur after myocardial infarction or be due to congestive heart failure, cardiomyopathy, or coronary artery disease

High salt intake: Can cause fluids to be retained in cells if kidneys cannot eliminate excess sodium and fluids

Kidney disease: Inability of the kidneys to function properly in the regulation of fluids; a result of hypertension, diabetes, or any condition affecting any part of the renal system

Thrombophlebitis: Inflammation of the veins as a result of clot formation; can be caused by trauma, inactivity, or varicose veins

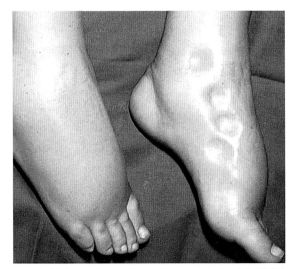

FIG. 23.9 Pitting edema. (From Bloom A, Ireland J, Watkins P. *A Colour Atlas of Diabetes.* 2nd ed. St. Louis: Mosby; 1992.)

a detailed HF–edema discussion.) Nonpitting edema does not leave a skin indentation, and it is more difficult to treat because of the underlying cause.

Prognosis

High altitude, exercise, or medication may cause temporary edema that self-corrects in a few days. In chronic edema, for example, edema secondary to heart failure, medication, and dietary changes may control the issue.

Non-Drug Treatment

Sodium restriction can help manage edema. Elevating the legs above the chest can help move fluid toward the heart to reduce peripheral edema. Support stockings can help deter excess fluid buildup in the legs.

Drug Treatment

Medication-induced edema is not likely to respond to diuretic treatment, but most other causes of edema respond to them. **Diuretic** classes include thiazides, thiazide-like agents and loop, potassium-sparing, carbonic anhydrase inhibitor, and osmotic classes. We will discuss each classification along with drug action and relevant examples. The standard dosage is an adult maintenance dose for edema treatment (Table 23.3). Certain diuretics (eg, loop diuretics, thiazides, and potassium-sparing agents) treat hypertension with blood pressure lowering secondary to reduced blood volume. Kidney function and electrolytes need to be monitored.

■ TABLE 23.3
Select Diuretic Medications

Generic Name	Trade Name	Common Dosage Range	Common Side Effects
Loop Diuretics			
Inhibit sodium and chloride reabsorption in the loop of Henle and on the proximal and distal tubules			
furosemide	Lasix	• *For edema:* 10–80 mg PO/IV once or twice daily (max 600 mg/day)	• Headache • Hypotension • Weakness
bumetanide	Bumex[a]	• 0.5–1 mg PO/IV once or twice daily (max 10 mg/day)	
torsemide	Demadex	• 5–20 mg PO/IV once daily (max 200 mg/day)	
ethacrynic acid	Edecrin	• 50–200 mg/day PO in 1 or 2 divided doses (max 400 mg/day)	
Thiazide-Type Diuretics			
Block reabsorption of sodium and chloride ions, increasing the amount of sodium crossing the distal tubule and thus increasing water excretion through the kidneys			
hydrochlorothiazide (HCTZ)	Microzide[a]	• 12.5–50 mg PO in 1 or 2 doses daily (max 200 mg/day)	• Low blood pressure • Photosensitivity
chlorthalidone	Thalitone[a]	• 12.5–50 mg PO once daily (max 100–200 mg/day)	
metolazone	Zaroxolyn	• 2.5–10 mg PO once daily (max 20 mg/day)	
Potassium-Sparing Diuretics			
Inhibit sodium reabsorption at distal convoluted tubule, cortical collecting tubule, and collecting duct and reduce potassium excretion			
triamterene	Dyrenium	• 50–100 mg PO once or twice daily (max 300 mg/day)	• Low blood pressure • Muscle cramps • Headache
amiloride	Midamor[a]	• 5–10 mg PO once or twice daily (max 20 mg/day)	
Aldosterone Antagonists/Potassium-Sparing Diuretics			
Compete against aldosterone for receptors in the distal renal tubules, which increases sodium and water excretion while retaining potassium			
spironolactone	Aldactone	• 25–200 mg/day PO in 1 or 2 divided doses	• Decreased libido • Diarrhea • Gynecomastia • Hypotension • Nausea • Vomiting
eplerenone	Inspra	• 50 mg PO once or twice daily (max 100 mg/day)	
Carbonic Anhydrase Inhibitors			
Inhibit the reabsorption of bicarbonate in the proximal convoluted tubule and increase the excretion of water, sodium, and potassium			
acetazolamide	Diamox Sequels	• 250–500 mg PO once daily (max 1000 mg/day)	• Flushing • Hyperglycemia • Hypokalemia • Hyponatremia • Hypotension • Metabolic acidosis

[a]Brand discontinued; now available only as generic.
IV, Intravenously; *PO,* orally.

Thiazides and thiazide-like agents Thiazides (eg, hydrochlorothiazide) and thiazide-like diuretics (eg, metolazone) increase urinary excretion of sodium and chloride ions by blocking ionic reabsorption in the DCT. They also lower urinary calcium excretion, increase potassium loss, and necessitate potassium supplementation or a potassium-sparing companion medication. Thiazides also work for hypertension and kidney stone prevention.

GENERIC NAME: hydrochlorothiazide (HCTZ)

TRADE NAME: Microzide[a]

INDICATIONS: Edema, hypertension

ROUTE OF ADMINISTRATION: Oral

COMMON ADULT DOSAGE: 12.5–100 mg once or twice daily

MECHANISM OF ACTION: Increases the excretion of sodium, chloride, and water by inhibiting sodium ion transport across the renal tubules

SIDE EFFECTS: Hypotension, photosensitivity, increased blood sugar, increased uric acid

AUXILIARY LABEL: May cause photosensitivity

---

[a] Brand discontinued; now available only as generic.

▼ **Tech Alert!**

Common side effects for all diuretics include frequent urination. For this reason, patients take them early in the day to avoid nocturia (urination at night).

GENERIC NAME: metolazone

INDICATIONS: Edema, hypertension

ROUTE OF ADMINISTRATION: Oral

COMMON ADULT DOSAGE: 2.5–20 mg/day

MECHANISM OF ACTION: Increases the excretion of chloride, sodium, and water by inhibiting sodium transport across the renal tubule

SIDE EFFECTS: Hypotension, photosensitivity, increased blood sugar, increased uric acid

AUXILIARY LABEL: May cause photosensitivity

Loop diuretics Loop diuretics inhibit reabsorption of sodium and chloride in the proximal convoluted tubule, DCT, and loop of Henle. Because of their intense action, significant potassium leaves with urination. Potassium supplements help maintain potassium levels, and doctors prescribe both concurrently. Patients take loop diuretics early in the day to avoid excessive nocturia.

GENERIC NAME: furosemide

TRADE NAME: Lasix

INDICATIONS: Edema, hypertension, pulmonary edema

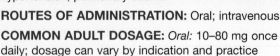

ROUTES OF ADMINISTRATION: Oral; intravenous

COMMON ADULT DOSAGE: *Oral:* 10–80 mg once daily; dosage can vary by indication and practice setting

MECHANISM OF ACTION: Inhibits sodium and chloride resorption in the ascending limb of the loop of Henle

SIDE EFFECTS: Dehydration, low potassium levels, hypotension

AUXILIARY LABELS:
• May cause dizziness
• May cause photosensitivity

Potassium-sparing agents Potassium-sparing agents work primarily in the DCT to inhibit sodium reabsorption and reduce potassium loss. Patients should avoid excess potassium-rich foods and allow their provider to monitor potassium levels regularly.

GENERIC NAME: spironolactone

TRADE NAME: Aldactone

INDICATIONS: Edema, hypertension, heart failure

ROUTE OF ADMINISTRATION: Oral

COMMON ADULT DOSAGE: 25–200 mg/day

MECHANISM OF ACTION: Inhibits the effects of aldosterone on the distal renal tubules

SIDE EFFECTS: Drowsiness, gynecomastia, high potassium levels (hyperkalemia)

AUXILIARY LABEL: May cause dizziness and drowsiness

GENERIC NAME: triamterene

TRADE NAME: Dyrenium

INDICATIONS: Edema, ascites, hypokalemia

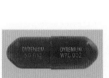

ROUTE OF ADMINISTRATION: Oral

COMMON ADULT DOSAGE: 50–100 mg once or twice daily

MECHANISM OF ACTION: Inhibits sodium-potassium ion exchange in the distal renal tubule, causing diuresis

SIDE EFFECTS: Nausea, headache, fatigue, hyperkalemia

AUXILIARY LABEL: Take with food

Osmotic diuretics Osmotic diuretics inhibit tubular reabsorption of water by increasing the glomerular filtrate's osmolarity. Doctors prescribe them for prophylaxis of low-GFR acute renal failure. The only osmotic agent for edema treatment is mannitol (Osmitrol), which forces kidney urine production in patients with acute kidney failure. The increased urine production helps prevent a progression to CKD and helps eliminate toxic substances. Dosage is based on patient weight. We give the medication intravenously.

> ### ▽ Tech Alert!
>
> Mannitol is available only as an injectable solution, and we should store it at 15°C to 30°C (59°F–86°F). It can crystallize at lower temperatures because of its high sugar content (eg, the solution is supersaturated at room temperature). If mannitol crystallizes, we can place it for short periods in 70°C water and periodically shake it. We cannot warm the vials in a microwave because they may explode.

Urinary Tract Infection

A urinary tract infection (UTI), either bacterial or fungal, may occur in any part of the urinary tract (kidneys, bladder, ureters, or urethra). The most common UTI cause is *Escherichia coli* acquired from the colon. A urethral infection is **urethritis.** *Cystitis* indicates infection/inflammation of the bladder, and *pyelonephritis* is infection/inflammation of the kidney. Once cystitis or pyelonephritis is confirmed, the drug therapy, duration, and dose change. Sexually transmitted diseases (STDs) also cause UTIs. Those with weakened immune systems have a higher risk, as do people with diabetes because of elevated urine glucose levels. Symptoms vary but can include a painful, burning sensation when urinating, fever, lack of urine output, cloudy or bloody urine, nausea and vomiting, and, rarely, confusion.

Prognosis

The prognosis for UTIs is good with proper treatment; recurrent infections may warrant prophylactic therapy.

Non-Drug Treatment

Several precautions can minimize UTI risk. These include wiping from front to back after urination or defecation, making sure the genital area is cleaned both before and after sexual intercourse, and urinating after sexual intercourse.

Drug Treatment

Antimicrobial agents are the primary treatment course for UTIs. Select antibiotics for bacterial infections and other symptomatic management agents are shown in Table 23.4. Antibiotic selection comes from an assessment of the patient's allergies, tolerability, previous antibiotic use, local antibiotic resistance rate, and cost. For symptomatic fungal UTIs, which are much less common than bacterial UTIs, fluconazole (Diflucan) is an available antifungal. Most symptoms resolve after antibiotic therapy begins, but the entire course should be completed to avoid recurrence and resistance. The current emphasis from the Infectious Diseases Society of America (IDSA) is to reduce fluoroquinolone usage in patients because of a risk for tendon rupture. Further, UTIs that are asymptomatic or uncomplicated do not need to be treated, unless the patient is pregnant.

▣ TABLE 23.4
Select Agents for the Treatment of Urinary Tract Infections[a]

Medication Class	Generic Name	Trade Name	Common Dosage Range
Cephalosporin	cephalexin	Keflex	• 500 mg PO twice daily for 7 days
Fluoroquinolone	ciprofloxacin	Cipro	• 250 mg PO twice daily for 3 days
Fluoroquinolone	levofloxacin	Levaquin[b]	• 250 mg PO once daily for 3 days
Nitrofuran antibacterial	nitrofurantoin	Macrobid	• 100 mg PO twice daily for 5 days
Penicillin	amoxicillin/clavulanate	Augmentin	• 875 mg/125 mg PO twice daily for 10 days
Penicillin and aminoglycoside	ampicillin + gentamicin	Omnipen[b] + Garamycin[b]	• 1–2 g ampicillin IV every 6 hr with 1.5 mg/kg gentamicin IV every 8 hr
Sulfonamide	sulfamethoxazole/ trimethoprim	Bactrim DS	• *DS:* 1 tablet (800 mg sulfamethoxazole/160 mg trimethoprim) PO twice daily for 3 days
Urinary analgesic	phenazopyridine	Pyridium	• 200 mg PO 3 times daily after meals as needed (prn) for 2 days
Urinary antispasmodic	flavoxate	Urispas[b]	• 100–200 mg PO 3 or 4 times daily; reduce the dosage as symptoms improve

[a]The treatment of urinary tract infections (UTIs) is tailored to specific organisms when applicable, and the duration and strength of therapy depend on the severity and location of the infection, in addition to the patient's age and history of UTIs.
[b]Brand discontinued; now available only as generic.
IV, Intravenously; *PO,* orally.

GENERIC NAME: nitrofurantoin

TRADE NAMES: Macrobid, Macrodantin

INDICATIONS: UTI, cystitis

ROUTE OF ADMINISTRATION: Oral

COMMON ADULT DOSAGE: 100 mg twice daily for 7 days

MECHANISMS OF ACTION: Inhibits bacterial carbohydrate metabolism and cell wall formation

SIDE EFFECTS: Nausea, diarrhea, abdominal pain, drowsiness

AUXILIARY LABEL: Take until gone

GENERIC NAME: cephalexin

TRADE NAME: Keflex

INDICATIONS: UTI, pneumonia, otitis media, other infections

ROUTE OF ADMINISTRATION: Oral

COMMON ADULT DOSAGE: 500 mg twice daily for 7–14 days

MECHANISM OF ACTION: Inhibits bacterial cell wall synthesis

SIDE EFFECTS: Nausea, vomiting, diarrhea, dizziness

AUXILIARY LABELS:
- May cause dizziness
- Take until gone

Urinary Incontinence

A common condition that affects millions of Americans is incontinence or overactive bladder (OAB), a loss of urinary control. Older adults, especially women, are more prone to this condition. Women with multiple pregnancies may have this condition later in life because of pelvic muscles stretched during childbirth.

Micturition is the medical term to describe urination. Although the bladder can store almost 1 L of fluid, receptors trigger when the bladder is about half full, and the urge to urinate begins. Even after urinating, a small amount of urine (about 100 mL) remains in the bladder. When a person coughs or sneezes, it can force the bladder to release a small amount of urine. This condition is called **stress incontinence.** Weight gain can intensify this condition. **Urge incontinence** is involuntary urination resulting from sudden, uncontrollable impulses to urinate. Urge incontinence can come from decreased bladder capacity, infection, or irritation. Increased fluid intake, including alcohol or caffeine ingestion, can increase the risk. One essential step in helping patients with urinary incontinence is ensuring that their medications are not the cause.

Prognosis

Doctors can treat overactive bladder (OAB) effectively with nonpharmacological or pharmacological means and, if necessary, surgery.

Non-Drug Treatment

The most common incontinence nondrug therapy is pelvic muscle (Kegel) exercises. This exercise involves pelvic floor muscle strengthening. The patient tightens the muscles around the pelvis as he or she would hold urine. The typical exercise regimen includes three sets of 8 to 12 slow-velocity contractions held for 6 to 8 seconds each. Patients perform these exercises 3 or 4 times per week and continue for 15 to 20 weeks.

Drug Treatment

Anticholinergic medications can manage urge incontinence (Table 23.5), but there are some newer medications on the market with different mechanisms of action. Anticholinergics are dangerous in the elderly. Mirabegron (Myrbetriq) is a beta-3 adrenergic agonist that increases bladder capacity but is expensive. Vibegron (Gemtesa) is a drug similar to mirabegron with less hypertensive effects and fewer drug interactions. Note, anticholinergics often cause side effects such as dry mouth. A drug such as mirabegron, which works on the sympathetic nervous system, may cause hypertension if the patient takes higher or toxic doses. It might seem strange to hear of Botox OAB treatment, but the mechanism of action correlates to improved results. Trospium and tolterodine seem to be the most effective; oxybutynin is available as a patch for convenience.

GENERIC NAME: oxybutynin

TRADE NAMES: Ditropan, Ditropan XL, Oxytrol (patch), Gelnique (topical gel), Oxytrol for Women (OTC Patch)

INDICATION: Overactive bladder

ROUTES OF ADMINISTRATION: Oral; transdermal

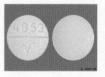

▣ TABLE 23.5
Select Antimuscarinic Medications[a] for the Treatment of Urinary Incontinence

Generic Name	Trade Name	Common Dosage Range	Common Side Effects
darifenacin	Enablex	• 7.5–15 mg PO once daily	• Confusion • Constipation • Dry mouth
fesoterodine	Toviaz	• 4–8 mg PO once daily	• Confusion • Constipation • Dry mouth • Increased heart rate
oxybutynin	Ditropan	• 5 mg PO 2–4 times daily	• Confusion • Constipation • Dry mouth (highest incidence with overactive bladder [OAB] medications)
	Ditropan XL (extended-release)	• 5–30 mg PO once daily	
	Gelnique (gel formulation)	• 3% or 10%; apply correct gel content once daily to thigh, abdomen, or shoulder	
	Oxytrol for Women (transdermal patch)	• *Patch:* 3.9 mg/day applied twice a week	
solifenacin	VESIcare	• 5–10 mg PO once daily	• Confusion • Constipation • Dry mouth
tolterodine	Detrol	• 2 mg PO twice daily	• Confusion • Constipation • Dry mouth
	Detrol LA (extended-release)	• 4 mg PO once daily	
trospium	Sanctura[b]	• 20 mg PO twice daily, 1 hr before meals	• Confusion • Constipation • Dry mouth
	Sanctura XR[b]	• 60 mg PO once daily, 1 hr before a meal	

[a]Antimuscarinics inhibit the action of acetylcholine on smooth muscle, creating an antispasmodic effect.
[b]Brand discontinued; now available only as generic.

COMMON ADULT DOSAGES: *Tablet:* 5 mg 2 or 3 times daily; *extended-release tablets:* 5–30 mg once daily; *patch:* apply a patch every 3–4 days; *gel:* apply 1 packet topically once daily

MECHANISM OF ACTION: Relaxes bladder smooth muscle

SIDE EFFECTS: Dizziness, drowsiness, confusion, blurred vision, dry mouth, constipation

AUXILIARY LABELS:
• May cause dizziness/drowsiness
• Ditropan XL: Do not crush, break, or chew
• Transdermal patch or gel: For topical use only

GENERIC NAME: tolterodine

TRADE NAMES: Detrol, Detrol LA

INDICATIONS: Overactive bladder, urinary urgency

ROUTE OF ADMINISTRATION: Oral

COMMON ADULT DOSAGES: *Detrol:* 1 to 2 mg twice daily. *Detrol LA:* 2 to 4 mg once daily

MECHANISM OF ACTION: Relaxes bladder smooth muscle

SIDE EFFECTS: Dizziness, drowsiness, confusion, blurred vision, dry mouth, constipation

AUXILIARY LABELS:
• May cause dizziness
• Detrol LA: Do not crush, break, or chew

GENERIC NAME: trospium

TRADE NAMES: Sanctura,[a] Sanctura XR[a]

INDICATION: Overactive bladder

ROUTE OF ADMINISTRATION: Oral

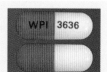

COMMON ADULT DOSAGES: *Immediate release:* 20 mg twice daily; *XR:* 60 mg once daily in the morning

MECHANISM OF ACTION: Antimuscarinic; relaxes smooth muscle within the bladder

SIDE EFFECTS: Constipation, xerostomia (dry mouth), headache

AUXILIARY LABELS:
• May cause dizziness/blurred vision
• May cause headache
• Take on an empty stomach

[a] Brand discontinued; now available only as generic.

GENERIC NAME: darifenacin

TRADE NAME: Enablex

INDICATION: Overactive bladder

ROUTE OF ADMINISTRATION: Oral

COMMON ADULT DOSAGE: 7.5 mg once daily; may increase to 15 mg once daily

MECHANISM OF ACTION: Antimuscarinic; relaxes smooth muscles in the bladder

SIDE EFFECTS: Constipation, xerostomia (dry mouth), headache

AUXILIARY LABELS:
- May cause dizziness/blurred vision
- May cause headache

GENERIC NAME: solifenacin

TRADE NAME: VESIcare

INDICATION: Overactive bladder

ROUTE OF ADMINISTRATION: Oral

COMMON ADULT DOSAGE: 5 mg once daily; may increase to 10 mg/day

MECHANISM OF ACTION: Antimuscarinic; relaxes bladder smooth muscles

SIDE EFFECTS: Constipation, xerostomia (dry mouth), prolonged QT interval

AUXILIARY LABEL: May cause dizziness/blurred vision

GENERIC NAME: fesoterodine

TRADE NAME: Toviaz

INDICATION: Overactive bladder

ROUTE OF ADMINISTRATION: Oral

COMMON ADULT DOSAGE: 4 mg once daily; may increase to 8 mg once daily

MECHANISM OF ACTION: Antimuscarinic; relaxes smooth muscles in the bladder

SIDE EFFECTS: Constipation, xerostomia (dry mouth), headache, dry eyes

AUXILIARY LABEL: May cause dizziness/blurred vision

GENERIC NAME: mirabegron

TRADE NAME: Myrbetriq

INDICATION: Overactive bladder

ROUTE OF ADMINISTRATION: Oral

COMMON ADULT DOSAGE: 25 mg once daily; may increase to 50 mg once daily

MECHANISM OF ACTION: Beta-3 adrenergic agonist; increases bladder capacity

SIDE EFFECTS: Hypertension, increased risk of UTI, headache, constipation

AUXILIARY LABELS:
- May cause dizziness/blurred vision
- May cause headache
- Monitor BP while on this medication

UTI, Urinary tract infection.

GENERIC NAME: Vibegron

TRADE NAME: Gemtesa

INDICATION: Overactive bladder

ROUTE OF ADMINISTRATION: Oral

COMMON ADULT DOSAGE: 75 mg once daily

MECHANISM OF ACTION: Selective beta-3 adrenergic agonist; increases bladder capacity

SIDE EFFECTS: Constipation, headache

AUXILIARY LABEL: May cause headache

GENERIC NAME: onabotulinumtoxinA

TRADE NAME: Botox

INDICATION: Overactive bladder, among others

ROUTES OF ADMINISTRATION: Injection, intramuscular (IM)

COMMON ADULT DOSAGE: Twenty 0.5-mL injections (10 units/mL) into detrusor muscle; space injections about 1 cm apart; max 100 units (10 mL) per treatment

MECHANISM OF ACTION: Inhibits acetylcholine release at nerve terminals with temporary bladder smooth muscle paralysis by chemical denervation.

SIDE EFFECTS: Headache, dry eyes, pain at the injection site, dysuria, increased risk of UTI

AUXILIARY LABEL: May cause headache/dizziness

UTI, Urinary tract infection.

▽ **Tech Alert!**

Remember the following sound-alike, look-alike drugs:
- Chlorthalidone versus chlorothiazide
- Bumex versus Buprenex
- Furosemide versus torsemide
- Metolazone versus metoclopramide
- Ditropan versus diazepam

- The anatomy of the renal and urologic systems and the names of their anatomical components
- The primary symptoms of the various conditions associated with the renal and urologic systems
- Medications used to treat the different renal and urologic conditions discussed
- The generic and trade names for the drugs discussed in this chapter
- The appropriate auxiliary labels that should be used when filling prescriptions for medicines discussed in this chapter

Review Questions

Multiple Choice Questions

1. Blood enters the kidneys through the:
   A. Renal fascia
   B. Renal artery
   C. Renal vein
   D. Hilus

2. All of the following are nephron components *except:*
   A. The glomerulus
   B. The urethra
   C. The Bowman capsule
   D. The loop of Henle

3. When taking loop diuretics, prescribers may supplement with ____.
   A. Potassium
   B. Calcium
   C. Multivitamins
   D. All of the above

4. Which of the following is *not* a loop diuretic?
   A. Furosemide
   B. Chlorthalidone
   C. Bumetanide
   D. Torsemide

5. Buffers can prevent:
   A. Large changes in pH
   B. Edema
   C. Renal failure
   D. Blood loss

6. Plasma is a component of:
   A. Buffers
   B. Water
   C. Blood
   D. Dialysis

7. Chronic kidney disease (CKD) has ____ stages.
   A. 3
   B. 4
   C. 5
   D. 6

8. Which of the following is *not* indicated for the treatment of urinary incontinence?
   A. Oxybutynin
   B. Allopurinol
   C. Tolterodine
   D. Trospium chloride

9. Mannitol (Osmitrol) falls into which category?
   A. Loop diuretic
   B. Osmotic diuretic
   C. Thiazide diuretic
   D. Potassium-sparing diuretic

10. Which classifications include diuretics?
    A. Blood formers
    B. Thiazides
    C. Carbonic anhydrase inhibitors
    D. Both B and C

11. Loop diuretics and thiazides:
    A. Have a slow mechanism of action
    B. Cause a loss of potassium
    C. Cause a loss of sodium
    D. Cause fluid retention

12. Prescribers use ____ to treat hyperphosphatemia in CKD.
    A. Sevelamer
    B. Calcitriol
    C. Epoetin alfa
    D. Hydrochlorothiazide

13. Which of the following is a severe infection that raises a risk for peritoneal dialysis if aseptic technique is not used?
    A. Otitis media
    B. UTI
    C. Peritonitis
    D. Cystitis

14. Which of these procedures can be used to treat specific kidney stones?
    A. Lithotripsy
    B. Ureteroscopy
    C. Surgery
    D. All of the above

15. Which of the following is *not* a potassium-sparing agent?
    A. Spironolactone
    B. Furosemide
    C. Amiloride
    D. Both B and C

Technician's Corner

Using a drug information resource, look up the various clinical indications, in addition to edema, that are treated with the diuretics discussed in this chapter.

Bibliography

American Geriatrics Society Beers Criteria Update Expert Panel. American Geriatrics Society 2019 updated AGS Beers Criteria® for potentially inappropriate medication use in older adults. *J Am Geriatr Soc.* 2019;67(4):674-694.

Bloom A, Ireland J, Watkins P. *A Colour Atlas of Diabetes.* 2nd ed. St. Louis: Mosby; 1992.

Damjanov I. *Pathology for the Health Professions.* 4th ed. St. Louis: Saunders; 2011.

Fishback JL. *Pathology*. 3rd ed. Philadelphia: Mosby; 2005.

Gupta K, Hooton TM, Naber KG, et al. International clinical practice guidelines for the treatment of acute uncomplicated cystitis and pyelonephritis in women: a 2010 update by the Infectious Diseases Society of America and the European Society for Microbiology and Infectious Diseases. *Clin Infect Dis*. 2011;52(5): e103-e120.

McCance KL. *Pathophysiology: The Biologic Basis for Disease in Adults and Children*. 6th ed. St. Louis: Mosby; 2010.

Monahan F, Sands J, Neighbors M, Marek J, Green-Nigro C. *Phipps' Medical-Surgical Nursing: Health and Illness Perspectives*. 8th ed. St. Louis: Mosby; 2007.

National Kidney Foundation. *Chronic Kidney Disease 2006: A Guide to Select NKF KDOQI Guidelines and Recommendations*. 2006. Available at: http://www.kidney.org/atoz.

Patton KT, Thibodeau GA. *Mosby's Handbook of Anatomy and Physiology*. St. Louis: Mosby; 2000.

Solomon EP. *Introduction to Human Anatomy and Physiology*. 3rd ed. St. Louis: Saunders; 2009.

Websites Referenced

Clinical Pharmacology Online. Available at: https://www.clinicalkey.com/pharmacology/login.

UpToDate Online. Available at: http://www.uptodate.com.

CHAPTER 24

Therapeutic Agents for the Reproductive System

Tony Guerra

1. Describe the anatomy and physiology of the reproductive system.
2. List the primary signs and symptoms of common conditions associated with the reproductive system. In addition, (a) recognize prescription and over-the-counter drugs used to treat common conditions of the reproductive system discussed in this chapter, (b) write the generic and trade names for the drugs discussed in this chapter, and (c) list appropriate auxiliary labels when filling prescriptions for drugs discussed in this chapter.

Abortifacient Any treatment that causes abortion of a fetus

Androgen Male sex hormone

Benign A condition, tumor, or growth that is not cancerous and therefore will not metastasize (spread)

Benign prostatic hyperplasia (BPH) Enlargement of the prostate

Depot An area of the body where a substance can accumulate or be stored for later distribution

Endometrium Inside + uterus, the mucous membrane lining the inner wall or layer of the uterus

Erectile dysfunction (ED) Inability of a man to maintain an erection sufficient for satisfying sexual activity

Estrogen Any of a group of anabolic sex hormones that promote the development and maintenance of female sexual characteristics

Fallopian tube A narrow tube that connects the ovary to the uterus

Fertilization The process by which a sperm unites with an ovum

Gametes Sex cells, or ova and sperm

Mammary gland The milk-producing gland of women

Menopause Month + stop, cessation of menstruation; a natural phenomenon in which a woman passes from a reproductive state to a nonreproductive state

Menses The time of menstruation

Negative feedback A self-regulating mechanism in which the output of a system has input or control on the process; in this case, the stimulus results in reactions that reduce the effects of the stimulus

Nocturia Night + urine, urination at night

Oocyte (ovum) Egg + cell, the female reproductive germ cell, more commonly known as an egg

Ovaries The female reproductive organs in which ova, or eggs, are produced

Palliative Something that brings relief but does not cure

Pelvic inflammatory disease (PID) Inflammation of the female genital tract, accompanied by fever and lower abdominal pain

Progesterone An anabolic sex hormone that stimulates the uterus to prepare for pregnancy

Prostate A gland surrounding the neck of the bladder in males that produces a fluid component of semen

Sperm (plural, spermatozoa) The male reproductive germ cell

Spermatogenesis Seed + birth, the development of sperm in the testes

Spermicide Seed + kill, an agent that kills sperm

Teratogen Any agent that causes abnormal embryonic or fetal development

Testes The male reproductive organs that produce sperm

Testosterone Testes + hormone, an anabolic sex hormone produced in the testes that stimulates the development of male sexual characteristics

Uterus The organ in the lower abdomen of a woman where gestation of a fetus occurs

Select Common Drugs for Conditions Affecting the Male and Female Reproductive Systems

Trade Name	Generic Name	Pronunciation
Androgens		
Androderm,[a] AndroGel, Depo-Testosterone	testosterone	(tes-**toss**-ter-own)
Methitest	methyltestosterone	(meth-ill-tes-**toss**-ter-own)
Alpha-Adrenergic Blockers		
Flomax	tamsulosin	(tam-**sue**-lo-sin)
Uroxatral	alfuzosin	(al-**fue**-zoe-sin)
5-Alpha-Reductase Inhibitors		
Avodart	dutasteride	(doo-**tah**-ster-ide)
Proscar	finasteride	(fin-**ass**-ter-ide)
Estrogens		
Estrace, Estraderm,[a] Vivelle-Dot, Climara, Evamist, Femring, Depo-Estradiol	estradiol	(ess-truh-**dye**-ol)
Ogen,[a] Ortho-Est	estropipate	(ess-troe-**pih**-pate)
Premarin	conjugated estrogens	(kon-juh-**gat**-ed **ess**-troe-genz)
Prempro, Premphase	conjugated estrogens/medroxyprogesterone	(kon-juh-**gat**-ed **ess**-troe-gens/meh-drox-ee-proe-**jess**-ter-own)
Progestins		
Ortho Micronor, Nora-BE, Camila	norethindrone	(nor-**eth**-in-drone)
Ogestrel[a]	norgestrel/ethinyl estradiol	(nor-**jess**-trel)/**eth**-in-ill ess-tra-**dye**-ol)
Prometrium	progesterone	(pro-**jess**-ter-own)
Provera	medroxyprogesterone	(me-drox-ee-proe-**jess**-ter-own)
Oral Contraceptives		
Monophasic Combinations		
Desogen, Azurette	ethinyl estradiol/desogestrel	(**eth**-in-ill ess-truh-**dye**-ol/des-o-**jess**-trel)
Necon 1/35	ethinyl estradiol/norethindrone	(**eth**-in-ill ess-truh-**dye**-ol/nor-**eth**-in-drone)
Generic only	mestranol/norethindrone	(**mess**-truh-nol/nor-**eth**-in-drone)
Ogestrel	ethinyl estradiol/norgestrel	(**eth**-in-ill ess-truh-**dye**-ol/nor-**jess**-trel)
Ortho Evra Patch	ethinyl estradiol/norelgestromin	(**eth**-in-ill ess-truh-**dye**-ol/nor-el-**jess**-tro-min)
Portia	ethinyl estradiol/levonorgestrel	(**eth**-in-ill ess-truh-**dye**-ol/**lev**-o-nor-**jess**-trel)
Yasmin, Yaz	drospirenone/ethinyl estradiol	(dro-**spih**-reh-nown/**eth**-in-ill ess-tra-dye-ol)
Zovia	ethinyl estradiol/ethynodiol diacetate	(**eth**-in-ill ess-tra-**dye**-ol/eh-the-no-**dye**-ol di-**as**-uh-tate)
Triphasic Combinations		
Enpresse	ethinyl estradiol/levonorgestrel	(**eth**-in-ill ess-tra-**dye**-ol/**lev**-o-nor-**jess**-trel)

Trade Name	Generic Name	Pronunciation
Ortho 7/7/7	ethinyl estradiol/norethindrone	(**eth**-in-ill ess-tra-**dye**-ol/nor-**eth**-in-drone)
Ortho Tri-Cyclen/TriNessa/ Tri-Sprintec	ethinyl estradiol/norgestimate	(**eth**-in-ill ess-truh-**dye**-ol/nor-**jess**-ti-mate)
Long-Acting Contraceptives		
Depo-Provera	medroxyprogesterone	(me-drox-ee-pro-**jess**-ter-own)
Infertility Medications		
Clomid[a]	clomiphene	(**kloe**-mi-feen)
Crinone, Endometrin	progesterone	(pro-**jess**-ter-own)
Follistim AQ	follitropin beta (r-FSH)	(fol-**li**-troe-**pin bet**-ah)
Luveris	lutropin alfa (r-LH)	(lou-**tro**-peen **al**-fa)
Ovidrel	choriogonadotropin alfa (r-HCG)	(kor-ee-oh-**goe**-nad-uh-**troe**-pin **al**-fa)
Emergency Contraceptive		
Plan B, Plan B One-Step, Next Choice[a]	levonorgestrel	(**lev**-o-nor-**jess**-trel)
Agents to Treat Endometriosis		
Lupron Depot	leuprolide	(loo-**pro**-lide)
Synarel	nafarelin	(**naf**-a-rell-in)
Zoladex	goserelin	(**goe**-ser-a-lin)
Agents to Treat Erectile Dysfunction		
Cialis	tadalafil	(tah-**dal**-uh-fill)
Levitra, Staxyn	vardenafil	(var-**den**-uh-fill)
Viagra	sildenafil	(sil-**den**-uh-fil)
Agents to Treat Reproductive System Infections/Sexually Transmitted Diseases		
Flagyl	metronidazole	(met-row-**nih**-duh-zole)
Valtrex	valacyclovir	(val-a-**sye**-kloe-veer)
Zovirax	acyclovir	(a-**sye**-kloe-veer)
Select Agents to Treat Vaginal Fungal Infections		
Diflucan	fluconazole	(floo-**kon**-uh-zole)
Generic only	tioconazole	(**tye**-oh-**kon**-uh-zole)

[a]Brand no longer available.

The male and female reproductive systems operate interdependently with other systems such as the endocrine system (which provides the hormones responsible for the maturation, development, and regulation of the reproductive system) and the urinary system. In men and women, reproductive functions divide among primary, secondary, and accessory organs. The primary reproductive organs are the gonads (ovaries or testes), which produce the **gametes** (sex cells, namely the *ova* and *sperm*). The gonads also secrete hormones that provide male or female gender characteristics. The secondary reproductive organs include structures necessary for transport and sustenance of eggs and sperm and the organs necessary for the growth of the developing fetus in the female. Accessory organs include ducts, glands, and external genitalia. Hormones largely control the reproductive system's functions. **Estrogen** and **testosterone** are present in both men and women, although their effects are somewhat different because of the different concentrations present in each gender (Table 24.1). This chapter reviews the anatomy and physiology of the female and male reproductive systems, select common reproductive conditions in both genders, and treatments for those conditions.

Female Reproductive System

The two **ovaries** in women are responsible for the production (oogenesis) and secretion of one or, in rare cases, two eggs or more (ovulation) each month. Located on either side of the **uterus,** the ovaries sit above the uterus attached to the **fallopian tubes,** which connect the ovary to the uterus (Fig. 24.1). Although ovulation begins at puberty, it is not possible to become pregnant until the menstrual cycle begins. The ability to have children ends as the levels of the responsible hormones (eg, estrogen) decline until the ovarian cycle stops. The ovaries,

TABLE 24.1
Select Hormones Affecting the Reproductive System and Their Functions

Hormone	Sex	Functions
Androgens	Male	• Steroid hormone that stimulates and controls the development and maintenance of male characteristics
	Female	• A precursor to estrogens in women
Follicle-stimulating hormone (FSH)	Female	• Stimulates ovarian follicles, producing many mature gametes (eggs)
	Male	• Maturation of sperm production
Gonadotropin-releasing hormone (GnRH)	Male	• Stimulates luteinizing hormone, which then stimulates gonadal secretion of testosterone, estrogen, and progesterone; sex steroids inhibit secretion of GnRH (negative feedback system)
	Female	• Same as in males
Luteinizing hormone (LH)	Male	• Stimulates secretion of sex steroids from gonads • Stimulates synthesis and secretion of testosterone; this is converted into estrogen
	Female	• Secretion of steroid hormones progesterone and estradiol
Progesterone	Female	• Necessary for maintenance of pregnancy and luteinization of ovarian follicles
	Male	• Not applicable
Testosterone	Male	• Affects production of GnRH • Bone and skeletal muscle growth (affects size and mass) • Responsible for sex drive • Skin changes (thicker skin, acne) • Stimulates growth and maturation of male reproductive organs • Stimulates sperm production • Triggers development of secondary sex characteristics (pubic and facial hair, enhanced hair growth on chest and other areas) • Voice changes
	Female	• Responsible for sex drive

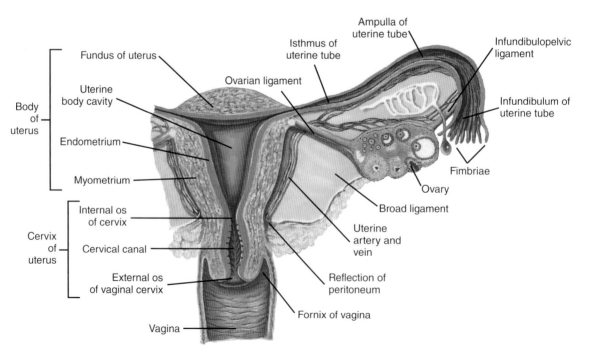

FIG. 24.1 Female pelvic organs. (From Patton KT, Thibodeau GA. *Mosby's Handbook of Anatomy and Physiology*. St. Louis: Mosby; 2000.)

which secrete the hormones estrogen and progesterone, are the primary source of estrogen in women. The function of estrogen includes the development of breasts and genitals and the regulation of the menstrual cycle, which prepares the female for pregnancy. The anterior pituitary gland releases follicle-stimulating hormone (FSH), which triggers estrogen levels to increase; this in turn causes the secretion of luteinizing hormone (LH), another pituitary hormone. The combination of these two hormones triggers the cascade of events that causes ovulation (Fig. 24.2).

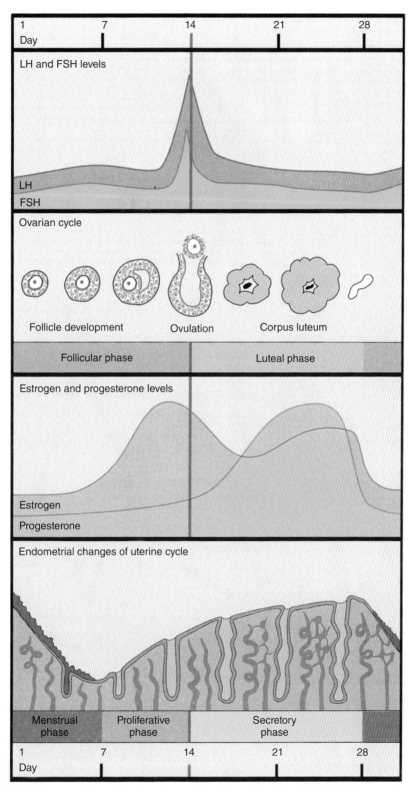

FIG. 24.2 The normal menstrual cycle consists of a proliferative (follicular) phase and a secretory (luteal) phase. *FSH*, Follicle-stimulating hormone; *LH*, luteinizing hormone. (From Damjanov I. *Pathology for the Health Professions*. 4th ed. St. Louis: Saunders; 2011.)

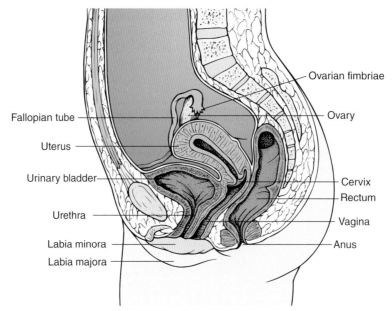

FIG. 24.3 Female reproductive system.

After puberty, the female ovary matures one or more eggs each month. At birth, the female ovary contains all the eggs available for the woman's lifetime. Thus women do not produce viable eggs throughout their lifetime. When an egg is mature, it is gathered by the ovarian fimbriae at the opening to the fallopian tubes. The fimbriae are in constant motion and sweep the egg into the fallopian tube. At ovulation, their activity increases, and currents generated in the peritoneal fluid are created to propel the egg into the fallopian tube. During the next 7 days, the **oocyte (ovum)** moves down the fallopian tube, where it may become fertilized by sperm. Because an ovum is viable only for 24 to 38 hours, **fertilization** usually occurs in the fallopian tube. The fallopian tubes exit into the uterus, which either houses the fertilized ovum or sloughs the ovum and **endometrium** during **menses** if fertilization has not occurred. This cycle begins at puberty and continues until menopause (Fig. 24.3).

Gonadotropin-releasing hormone (GnRH) secreted from the hypothalamus acts on the anterior pituitary gland to secrete FSH and LH, the hormones necessary for ovulation (see Table 24.1). These hormones are controlled by **negative feedback** and are secreted in cycles (Fig. 24.4), unlike the continuous secretion of sex hormones in males (discussed later). The levels of hormones peak when a woman is in her 20s and gradually decline throughout her life.

The **mammary glands** (or breasts) are accessory organs of the female reproductive system. Hormonal secretions regulate breast tissue. At puberty, the estrogen increase stimulates the development of glandular tissue, causing adipose tissue accumulation, and progesterone stimulates the growth of the duct system used during milk production and secretion (Fig. 24.5).

Conditions Affecting the Female Reproductive System

The principal medications that affect the female reproductive system are hormones. Some agents stimulate secretions,

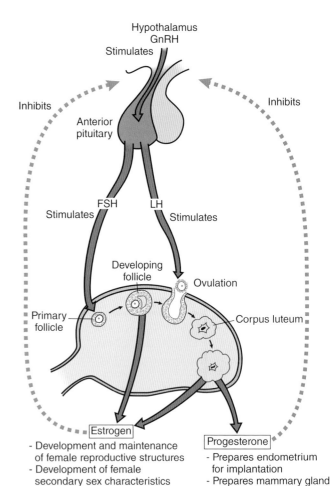

FIG. 24.4 Function of the ovaries in response to hormone stimulation. *FSH,* Follicle-stimulating hormone; *GnRH,* gonadotropin-releasing hormone; *LH,* luteinizing hormone.

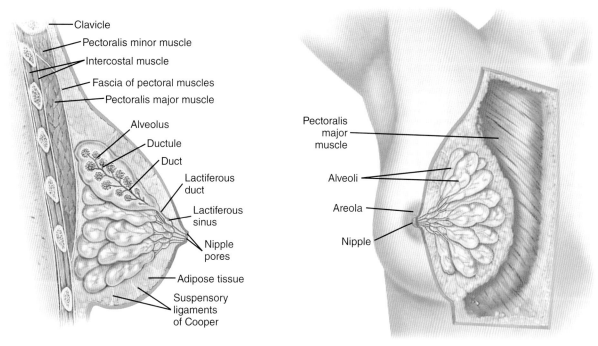

FIG. 24.5 Female breast. (From Patton KT, Thibodeau GA. *Mosby's Handbook of Anatomy and Physiology*. St. Louis: Mosby; 2000.)

whereas others inhibit or counteract the actions of other hormones. Medication therapy for conditions of the reproductive tract can be complicated. Even male hormones are used to treat endometrial or breast cancer, endometriosis, and fibrocystic disease in women. When discussing hormonal therapies, it is important to remember that the hypothalamus cannot distinguish between hormones naturally produced by the body and those administered as medications. Therefore the body reacts to synthetic and naturally occurring hormones similarly. (This chapter discusses male and female sex hormones; Chapter 18 presents a review of other endocrine system hormones.) Table 24.2 provides a summary of hormonal therapies for select female reproductive conditions.

Estrogens are one of the most common forms of medical therapy used for conditions of the female reproductive system. Conditions such as abnormal uterine bleeding can result from hormone imbalance, abnormal ovulation, and even infertility. Box 24.1 presents a summary of select menstrual disorders. In women, estrogens may be used to treat hypogonadism, to increase the possibility of contraception, and to relieve symptoms of menopause (natural or surgical). Estrogens support the development and maintenance of reproductive organs and secondary sex characteristics and have profound influences on the menstrual cycle.

The primary oral estrogen products in use clinically are conjugated estrogens and estradiol. Estrogens are also available in several forms; some forms are unique, such as implants, vaginal inserts, and transdermal systems. The most common forms are oral and injectable preparations (water-based or oil-based). The oil-based injectable estrogen medications, called **depot** medications, are prepared to prolong the medication's action. Transdermal preparations are applied to the skin to provide continuous release of the medication. Drug-laden vaginal rings are pressed into the vaginal canal for the constant release of medicines into the local tissues. Other locally administered estrogens include vaginal inserts and creams that provide absorption of hormones at the site of application. The choice of preparation to be used depends on the reason for use, the benefits versus the risks of treatment, the cost, the reliability of the patient to use it correctly, and convenience. Adverse effects of estrogens in females may include photosensitivity, nausea, vomiting, and bloating. Dysmenorrhea, breast tenderness and enlargement, and increased susceptibility to thrombotic disease are also risks of estrogen treatment.

As mentioned previously, male hormones can be used for treating certain female breast tumors that grow faster in the presence of estrogen. **Androgens** suppress the effects of estrogen, thus preventing rapid growth. For women with endometriosis, androgens can cause suppression of the endometrium and thus prevent the excessive uterine bleeding associated with the disease. Women receiving androgen therapy for prolonged periods can experience amenorrhea or menstrual irregularities. Hot flashes, headaches, sleep disorders, increased libido, vaginitis, and masculinization are also found. Changes in the voice (lowering of the voice) are often permanent. In contrast, other symptoms, such as loss of breast mass, increased facial and body hair, and increased muscle mass may reverse when the testosterone therapy is discontinued.

Progesterone, naturally occurring as progestin, is the female hormone secreted from day 14 through day 28 of the menstrual cycle. This hormone has many functions, including changing the secretions of the cervix and reducing

Select Hormonal Therapies for the Treatment of Certain Female Reproductive Conditions

Generic Name	Trade Name	Common Dosage Range	Common Side Effects
Endometriosis			
Gonadotropin-Releasing Hormone			
leuprolide	Lupron	• 3.75 mg IM once/mo (max 6 mo) or 11.25 mg every 3 mo for 2 doses	• Amenorrhea • Bone density decrease
nafarelin	Synarel	• One 200-mcg spray into one nostril in the morning and into the other nostril in the evening; start between days 2–4 of the cycle (max 4 sprays/day for 6 mo)	• Headaches • Hot flashes • Night sweats • Vaginal atrophy • Vaginitis
goserelin	Zoladex	• 3.6 mg subcut every 28 days for 6 mo	
Androgen			
danazol	Danocrine[a]	• 200–800 mg/day PO in 2 divided doses for 3–6 mo	• Acne • Edema • Eosinophilia • Flushing • Hair loss/growth • Hypertension • Pain
Infertility			
Gonadotropin-Ovulation Stimulator			
menotropins	Menopur	• 150 units subcut daily for first 5 days then adjust based on ultrasound (max 450 units/day for ≤20 days)	• Abdominal pain • Headache • Injection site reaction • Nausea
urofollitropin (FSH)	Bravelle	• 150 units IM/subcut for the first 5 days, then adjust by 75–150 units every 2 days based on ultrasound monitoring (max 450 units/day for <12 days)	• Acne • Breast tenderness • Headache • Hot flashes • Hypertension
choriogonadotropin alfa (r-HCG)	Ovidrel	• 250 mcg subcut given once after the last dose of an FSH agent	• Abdominal pain • Nausea • Ovarian cyst • Pain
lutropin alfa (r-LH)	Luveris	• 75 units subcut daily until adequate follicular development is noted (max 14 days)	• Breast pain • Constipation • Fatigue • Headache • Nausea
Selective Estrogen Receptor Modulator (SERM)—Ovulation Stimulator			
clomiphene	Clomid[a]	• 50 mg PO once daily for 5 days (begin on or about day 5 in the cycle; can be repeated 30 days later if needed)	• Bloating/discomfort • Headache • Hot flashes • Ovarian enlargement • Visual changes
Progestin			
progesterone	Crinone	• 90 mg intravaginal gel applied once or twice daily • 100 mg intravaginal insert 2–3 times daily	• Breast enlargement • Constipation • Depression • Genital discomfort • Headache • Nausea • Nervousness • Somnolence

TABLE 24.2
Select Hormonal Therapies for the Treatment of Certain Female Reproductive Conditions—cont'd

Generic Name	Trade Name	Common Dosage Range	Common Side Effects
Hormone Replacement Therapy			
Estrogen Derivative			
estradiol	Estrace	• 1–2 mg PO once daily (3 wk on, then 1 wk off, cycle)	• Bleeding • Clots • Decreased sex drive • Depression • Edema • Nausea • Swollen breasts • Vomiting
	Vivelle-Dot	• *Patch:* 0.025 mg, replaced twice wkly	
	Estring	• 2 mg intravaginally replacing ring every 90 days	
esterified estrogen	Menest	• 1.25 mg PO daily (3 wk on, then 1 wk off, cycle)	
conjugated estrogens	Premarin	• 0.3 mg PO daily (or cyclically)	
estropipate	Generic only	• 0.75–6 mg/day PO (often cyclically)	
Estrogen and Progestin Combination			
conjugated estrogens (CE) and medroxypro-gesterone (MPA)	Prempro	• 1 tab 0.625 mg CE/5 mg MPA PO once daily	• Changes in weight/appetite • Decreased sex drive • Headache • Nausea • Stomach pain • Swollen breasts
estradiol and levonorgestrel	Climara Pro	• *Patch:* 0.045 mg estradiol/0.015 mg levonorgestrel; replace/apply 1 patch/wk	• Breast pain • Depression • Site reaction • Upper respiratory tract infection • Vaginal bleeding

aBrand no longer available.

FSH, Follicle-stimulating hormone; *PO,* orally; *r-HCG,* recombinant human chorionic gonadotropin; *r-LH,* recombinant luteinizing hormone; *subcut,* subcutaneously.

BOX 24.1   Menstrual Disorders

Amenorrhea: Absence of menstrual periods

Dysmenorrhea: Abdominal pain attributable to menstrual cramping

Hypomenorrhea: Low menstrual flow over a short menstrual period

Menorrhagia: Heavy menstrual flow over a long menstrual period

Oligomenorrhea: Light and infrequent menstrual periods

Polymenorrhea: Frequent menstruation

Premature menopause: Loss of ovarian function before age 40

Premenstrual syndrome: A group of symptoms that occur before the onset of menstruation (eg, bloating, edema, headache, mood swings, and breast discomfort)

uterine contractility. Other actions include stimulating the development of ducts and glands of the breasts in preparation for lactation. Prescribers use synthetic progestins more frequently than natural forms because synthetic forms are more effective. Synthetic forms are either injected or administered orally, and the action of synthetic progestin is prolonged over that of progesterone. We use progestins for treating amenorrhea and abnormal uterine bleeding from hormone imbalances, for contraception, in combination with estrogen hormone replacement therapy (HRT) to prevent endometrial overgrowth if the woman has an intact uterus, and as therapy for renal and endometrial cancer. When combined with oral estrogen, progestin dosages come in milligrams, and the estrogen component is measured in micrograms. Used to treat infertility, progesterone, and progesterone-like products stimulate the development of ova and subsequent ovulation. The side effects associated with progestins include weight gain, stomach pain and cramping, swelling of the face and legs, headaches, mood swings, anxiety, weakness, rashes, acne, and insomnia. Menstrual changes and breast tenderness may occur.

GENERIC NAME: progesterone

TRADE NAMES: Prometrium, Crinone, Endometrin

INDICATIONS: Amenorrhea, abnormal uterine bleeding, infertility, hyperplasia

ROUTES OF ADMINISTRATION: Injectable; vaginal; oral

COMMON ADULT DOSAGE: Varies by indication and dosage form

MECHANISMS OF ACTION: Induces secretory activity in the endometrium in preparation for implantation of a fertilized egg and aids in the maintenance of a pregnancy; suppresses midcycle surge of luteinizing hormone to prevent pregnancy

SIDE EFFECTS: Bloating, breast tenderness, cramping, dizziness, depression, headache

AUXILIARY LABEL: Use as directed

GENERIC NAME: medroxyprogesterone

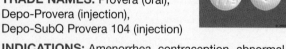

TRADE NAMES: Provera (oral), Depo-Provera (injection), Depo-SubQ Provera 104 (injection)

INDICATIONS: Amenorrhea, contraception, abnormal uterine bleeding, endometrial cancer, endometriosis

ROUTES OF ADMINISTRATION: Oral; injection (IM, subcut)

COMMON ADULT DOSAGES: *Oral:* 5 to 10 mg once daily for 5 to 10 days for amenorrhea and abnormal bleeding. *IM:* 150 mg every 3 months as a contraceptive. *Subcut:* 104 mg subcutaneously every 3 months as a contraceptive or for endometriosis.

MECHANISM OF ACTION: Primary contraceptive effect involves inhibition of gonadotropin secretion to prevent follicular maturation and ovulation

SIDE EFFECTS: Amenorrhea, headache, nervousness, weight gain

AUXILIARY LABEL: Take as directed

IM, Intramuscularly; *Subcut*, subcutaneous.

Common Conditions

The following sections provide specific information on women's health issues, such as female hypogonadism, pelvic inflammatory disease (PID), infertility, contraception, and menopause.

Female Hypogonadism

Female hypogonadism is the lack of estrogen production in the ovaries and is classified as either congenital or acquired. The mechanism of congenital hypogonadism is often from a genetic mutation or unknown. Acquired hypogonadism can result from medications or disease. In childhood, symptoms include a lack of menstruation and breast development and short height. If the condition occurs during puberty, symptoms include loss of menstruation, hot flashes, loss of body hair, and decreased libido. In adult women, hypogonadism can cause infertility and early menopause. Menopause is a natural transition that happens between the ages of 50 and 60 years. The effects of menopause increase the risk for osteoporosis and heart disease after menopause is complete.

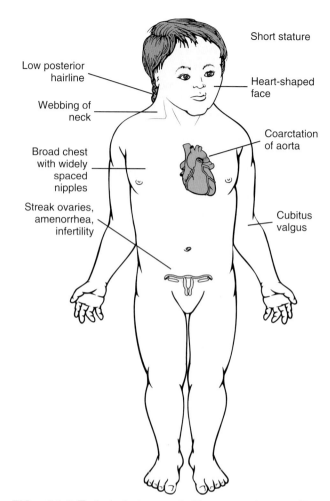

FIG. 24.6 Typical features of Turner syndrome. (From Damjanov I. *Pathology for the Health Professions*. 4th ed. St. Louis: Saunders; 2011.)

A genetic defect causes Turner syndrome, a type of female hypogonadism. Infant symptoms include swollen hands and feet and a wide, webbed neck (Fig. 24.6). In older females, symptoms may include drooping eyelids, absent or incomplete development at puberty (small breasts, scant pubic hair), absence of menstruation, short height, and vaginal dryness. Hormonal therapies can improve the body image of individuals with Turner syndrome, but treatment cannot reverse infertility.

Prognosis

Hormonal therapies can improve body image and fertility in some forms of female hypogonadism, but in all forms of congenital hypogonadism, infertility cannot be reversed.

Non-Drug Treatments

The female reproductive system does not have to function properly to sustain life; still, many women wish to conceive and bear offspring. The only non-drug treatment would come from the prevention of conditions that result in hypogonadism. In addition, maintaining ideal body weight, eating a healthy diet, refraining from smoking, and adhering to an exercise regimen may improve infertility.

Drug Treatments

The treatment goals include focusing on the underlying cause, improving fertility, and preventing or delaying hypogonadism complications. Hormone replacement therapies can diminish hypogonadism symptoms. Estrogen and progestin used for hormone replacement may help ovarian stimulation. Low-dose testosterone may increase sex drive. Estrogen is available in tablet form, topical lotions or gels, or as transdermal patches. Testosterone is available in injectable form, gels, or topical patches (discussed in more detail later). With Turner syndrome, a health professional will typically start estrogen, progestin, and other hormone therapy around puberty to trigger breast and pubic hair growth and ensure proper stature. No treatment restores fertility. See Table 24.2 for select hormone replacement therapies.

Infertility

An infertility treatment evaluation typically begins after 1 year of regular unprotected intercourse in women under age 35 and after 6 months in women over age 35. In many cases, pharmacological treatment can correct anovulation, a cause of infertility. Medications can promote maturation of the ovarian follicle and stimulate ovulation. Endometriosis attributable to PID can obstruct the fallopian tubes. Women with irregular menstrual cycles or no menstruation may also have problems with infertility.

Prognosis

The prognosis for infertility depends on the ages of the partners, the condition's cause, the treatment methods, assisted reproduction techniques, and other factors.

Non-Drug Treatment

Surgery may correct fertility problems originating from structural abnormalities of the fallopian tubes, uterus, or ovaries. Another treatment that may help with infertility is assisted reproductive technology (ART), which uses in vitro fertilization, embryo transfer, and both egg and sperm transfer. The likelihood of success depends on several factors, including the woman's age. In the case of ART, hormonal medications control and direct the ovulation and implantation cycles. Providers may treat male infertility with medication or by using alternative techniques, such as sperm donation.

Drug Treatment

Hormone treatment is the most common treatment for infertility. Most drugs mimic human hormones that trigger ovulation. Doctors can prescribe clomiphene, progesterone, and letrozole as oral medications. Injectable medications include gonadotropins such as follitropin beta injection (Follistim AQ), menotropins (Menopur), and gonadotropin-releasing hormone agonists such as leuprolide (Lupron). Table 24.2 and the following drug monographs present hormonal treatments for female infertility.

Tech Note!

In rare cases, a prescriber will use clomiphene (Clomid) and menotropins (Menopur) for male infertility. Some use these agents off-label for oligospermia (low sperm concentration in the semen).

GENERIC NAME: clomiphene

TRADE NAME: Clomid[a]

INDICATION: Ovulation induction

ROUTE OF ADMINISTRATION: Oral

COMMON ADULT DOSAGE: 50-mg tablet once daily for 5 days (initial cycle therapy)

MECHANISM OF ACTION: Stimulates follicle-stimulating hormone and luteinizing hormone secretion by increasing gonadotropin-releasing hormone levels, leading to ovarian follicle growth with ensuing follicular rupture.

SIDE EFFECTS: Hot flashes, bloating, breast tenderness

AUXILIARY LABEL: Take as directed

[a] Available only in Canada.

GENERIC NAME: menotropin

TRADE NAMES: Menopur, Repronex

INDICATIONS: Hypogonadism, infertility

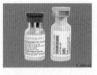

ROUTES OF ADMINISTRATION: Injectable (IM, subcutaneous)

COMMON ADULT DOSAGE: Varies by indication and dosage form

MECHANISM OF ACTION: Contains purified preparations of human follicle-stimulating hormone and luteinizing hormone, which act to stimulate follicle maturation and ovulation in females and spermatogenesis in males.

SIDE EFFECTS: Headache, nausea, diarrhea, abdominal cramping

AUXILIARY LABEL:
Take as directed

IM, Intramuscularly.

GENERIC NAME: Letrozole

TRADE NAME: Femara

INDICATION: Ovulation stimulation

Route Of Administration: Oral

COMMON ADULT DOSAGE: 2.5 mg daily for 5 days, starting on day 3, 4, or 5 following menses

MECHANISM OF ACTION: Decreased estrogen to increase follicle-stimulating hormone and luteinizing hormone

SIDE EFFECTS: Fatigue, dizziness, headache, flushing

GENERIC NAME: Leuprolide

TRADE NAME: Lupron

INDICATION: Off-label use for infertility

ROUTE OF ADMINISTRATION: Injection

COMMON ADULT DOSAGE: The usual dose is 0.1 or 0.2 cc daily as a single injection but this may differ depending on institution's protocol

MECHANISM OF ACTION: Decreased follicle-stimulating hormone and luteinizing hormone to prevents premature egg resulting in lower risk of pregnancy loss

SIDE EFFECTS: Hot flashes, headache, emotional volatility

Contraception

Oral contraceptives Oral contraceptives provide birth control by preventing ovum fertilization through an oral dosage form. Other forms of contraception include vaginal rings, patches, intrauterine devices (IUDs), and injections. Hormonal contraceptives inhibit luteinizing hormone (LH) and follicle-stimulating hormone (FSH) production, preventing ovulation. Beyond contraception, these medications can manage the symptoms and complications of irregular menstrual cycles, dysmenorrhea (menstrual cramps), endometriosis, and acne. Nonpharmacological methods, such as surgery, the rhythm method, and mechanical devices, also work. Of the various birth control methods, oral contraceptives have the highest incidence of side effects. These range from nausea and vomiting to menstrual abnormalities to thrombotic complications. Concurrent cigarette smoking increases the risk for serious cardiovascular effects. Barrier methods have the fewest side effects but may lack the effectiveness of hormone-based medications (Fig. 24.7).

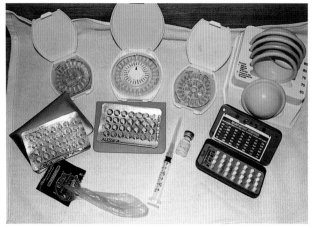

FIG. 24.7 Common contraceptives, including barrier and medicinal methods: condoms, diaphragm, oral contraceptives, and parenteral contraceptives.

Combination oral contraceptives may consist of estrogen and progestin to inhibit ovulation. The progestin-only contraceptives are called "minipills." Providers most frequently prescribe the highly effective combination contraceptives. These combination medications come in monophasic, biphasic, triphasic, and estrophasic formulas. In monophasic regimens, the daily estrogen and progestin dose remains constant throughout the menstrual cycle. In the biphasic regimen, the estrogen dose remains constant but the second half of the cycle's progestin dose increases. Triphasic regimens divide the menstrual cycle into three phases. The progestin amount changes in each phase. The estrophasic cycle has a constant progestin amount, and the estrogen component increases gradually throughout the cycle. The goal of phasic oral contraceptives is to mimic the female's natural cycle while lessening birth control pill side effects.

Oral contraceptive effectiveness largely depends on the woman's adherence to the medication regimen. Usually, a woman will start the medication on the fifth day of the menstrual cycle. She should take the pill at the same time each day for 21 days. If she misses a single dose of a combination oral contraceptive, the chance of ovulation is still small. However, the risk for pregnancy increases with each dose she misses. Have the patient read the contraception package insert for missed dose directions. In general, if she misses one dose, she should take it as soon as she remembers, and she should take the next pill on the regular schedule. This regimen may mean taking two pills in 1 day or in the same dose. If she misses two doses, she should take two tablets on each of the next 2 days. The patient should use a backup barrier contraceptive for 7 days if she misses 5 or more pills or any pills from the first 2 weeks of the cycle.

Some oral contraceptive side effects include nausea, vomiting, mood changes, appetite changes, changes in sex drive, and headaches. Women taking combination oral contraceptives may also experience breast tenderness; however, women taking progestin-only pills do not seem to experience as much breast tenderness or nausea. Some combination oral contraceptive risks include thromboembolism (including myocardial infarction and stroke). These risks increase in smokers. Table 24.3 provides a list of select oral and nonoral contraceptive products.

Most women take oral contraceptive products, but there are other available dosage forms (see Table 24.3). Nonoral products can help individuals who struggle to remember to take their pill daily. Injectable products, for example, can be effective for 3 months. Some nonoral contraceptive dosage forms include the following:

- *Etonogestrel and ethinyl estradiol (NuvaRing):* Similar to the traditional oral contraceptive but administered as a vaginal ring. It can be left in place for up to 3 weeks

TABLE 24.3
Select Contraceptive Products

Medication Class	Generic Name (Progestin)	Trade Name	Common Dosage or Duration
Oral combination (estrogen and progestin) pills	desogestrel	Azurette, Kariva, Desogen	• Taken PO every day about the same time
	drospirenone	Yasmin, Yaz	
	ethynodiol diacetate	Zovia, Kelnor	
	levonorgestrel	Seasonique, Lessina, Portia	
	norethindrone	Brevicon, Necon	
	norethindrone acetate	Junel, LoEstrin, Microgestin	
	norgestimate	Sprintec, Ortho Tri-Cyclen[a]	
	norgestrel	Cryselle, Ogestrel[a]	
Oral progestin only	norethindrone	Ortho Micronor	• Taken PO every day about the same time
Injection (progestin only)	medroxyprogesterone acetate	Depo-SubQ Provera	• Subcut injection every 3 mo
	Depo-Provera		• IM injection every 3 mo
Intrauterine system (progestin only)	levonorgestrel	Mirena	• Effective for 5 y
Transdermal combination (estrogen and progestin) patch	norelgestromin	Xulane	• Apply 1 patch for 3 wk, followed by 1 wk patch free; repeat cycle
Vaginal ring (estrogen and progestin)	etonogestrel	NuvaRing	• Ring remains in vagina for 3 wk and then is removed for 1 wk; user repeats cycle
Implantable device (progestin only)	etonogestrel	Nexplanon	• Effective for 3 y
Emergency oral (progestin only)	levonorgestrel	Next Choice One Dose, Plan B One-Step, React	• 1–2 tablet(s) as soon as possible within 72 hr of intercourse depending on if using single-dose regimen or two-dose regimen

[a]Brand no longer available.

IM, Intramuscularly; *PO*, orally; *subcut*, subcutaneously.

- *Levonorgestrel (Mirena):* Intrauterine device (IUD) that contains only progestin; contraceptive action lasts up to 5 years
- *Norelgestromin (Ortho Evra):* Contraceptive patch applied weekly for 3 weeks, followed by 1 patch-free week.

Tech Note!

The US Food and Drug Administration mandates that oral contraceptives be dispensed with the Patient Package Insert (PPI) or patient information. The PPI should come in the medication's product packaging.

GENERIC NAMES: ethinyl estradiol/norelgestromin

TRADE NAME: Xulane

ROUTE OF ADMINISTRATION: Transdermal patch

COMMON ADULT DOSAGE: *Patch:* Applied weekly for 3 weeks; the fourth week is patch free

MECHANISM OF ACTION: Suppresses the hypothalamic-pituitary system, reducing the secretion of gonadotropin-releasing hormone

SIDE EFFECTS: Nausea, breast tenderness, headache, dizziness, menstrual irregularity

AUXILIARY LABELS:
- Apply topically
- Take as directed

Tech Note!

The current recommendation for contraceptive transdermal patches, such as Ortho Evra, is to apply the patch to the upper arm, back, abdomen, or buttock. The patient should wear the patch for 1 week and then remove it. She should apply a new patch on the same day of the week that the first patch was applied. The fourth week should be patch free.

GENERIC NAME: levonorgestrel intrauterine system

TRADE NAMES: Mirena, Kyleena, Liletta, Skyla

INDICATIONS: Contraception, heavy menstrual bleeding (menorrhagia)

ROUTE OF ADMINISTRATION: Intrauterine

COMMON ADULT DOSAGE: Insert one system into the uterus; each system is effective for 3 (Skyla), 5 (Mirena, Kyleena), or 6 (Liletta) years, at which time a new system can be inserted

MECHANISM OF ACTION: Levonorgestrel in the intrauterine device is thought to contribute to contraception by thickening cervical mucus, inhibiting sperm survival, and altering the endometrium

SIDE EFFECTS: Menstrual irregularities, abdominal pain

Other contraceptive products include **spermicides.** These contraceptives are available as foam, jelly, gel, cream, suppository, and vaginal film. The correct use of a spermicide is essential for contraceptive efficacy. The spermicide must be applied before but no more than 1 hour in advance of sexual intercourse. The customer can purchase spermicides without a prescription and must apply them each time she anticipates intercourse.

Barrier devices are nonpharmacological methods of birth control, although a prescriber will write a prescription for cervical caps and diaphragms to ensure proper fitting. These devices include male and female condoms, cervical caps, and diaphragms. The most common barrier method is the male condom. Male condoms come in latex, polyurethane, and lamb intestine forms. The female condom is a loose-fitting tubular polyurethane pouch with flexible rings at both ends. The diaphragm is a soft rubber cap with a metal spring that fits over the cervix. Before a woman inserts a diaphragm, she should fill it with spermicide to block the cervix completely. The cervical cap, another contraceptive device, is a small cup-shaped barrier that fits directly over the cervical rim. Suction holds it in place.

Medroxyprogesterone acetate (**Depo-Provera**) is an injection that contains progestin only, the synthetic progesterone form. This injection creates a deposit of drug under the skin that has been formulated to slowly release over a 3-month period. Health care professionals provide these injections, which need to be readministered every 12 to 14 weeks.

An emergency form of contraception is the "morning-after pill," which prevents conception and pregnancy after intercourse. Morning-after pills are contraceptives formulated of high-dose progestin only or both estrogen and progestin. The combined emergency contraceptive form is about 75% effective, but the one almost universal side effect is nausea and vomiting. Therefore progestin-only emergency contraception, less likely to cause nausea, is the preferred product. Plan B One-Step contains one or two large doses of levonorgestrel and comes as a single- or two-dose regimen that has to be administered within 72 hours of intercourse.

Progestin-only emergency contraception is more effective than a combined estrogen and progestin regimen, primarily because women tolerate it better. Other emergency options include the ulipristal acetate (Ella) and a copper IUD (Paragard). Ella is a prescription-only oral tablet that should be taken within 120 hours of intercourse. Copper IUDs must be placed by a physician or nurse within 5 days of intercourse and are more effective for a wider group of patients relative to oral formulations. Emergency contraception products pose some risk, and patients should not use them as a regular birth control means.

Mifeprex, or mifepristone (formerly known as RU-486), is more commonly known as the abortion pill. Mifepristone acts as an antiprogestin. Because progesterone is necessary for the establishment and maintenance of pregnancy, mifepristone acts as an antagonist to progesterone and prevents the maintenance of the pregnancy. For safety, this medication must be used within the first 7 weeks of pregnancy. Because of the **abortifacient** effects of the medication, a qualified health care professional in the prescriber's office must administer mifepristone on three separate office visits over 1 to 2 weeks.

Menopause

As previously described, estrogen and progesterone secretion responds to hormones released from the anterior pituitary gland. GnRH (from the hypothalamus) stimulates FSH and LH (from the anterior pituitary gland) to cause the ovaries to secrete estrogen and progesterone. Unlike testosterone in men, these hormones follow cyclical monthly patterns, beginning at puberty and continuing until menopause, when hormone secretion decreases. During perimenopause, the ovaries gradually reduce estrogen production.

Menopause is an age-related natural loss of hormone production. Although this is not a "disease," menopausal symptoms such as hot flashes can lead women to seek HRT.

Prognosis

Uncomfortable, but not life-threatening, the symptoms of menopause can last for many years.

Non-Drug Treatments

Some lifestyle changes that can lessen the symptoms associated with menopause include weight reduction, consuming a healthy diet, smoking cessation, physical activity, and stress reduction techniques. Additionally, some herbal and other naturopathic treatments can help manage menopause.

Drug Treatments

The ovaries produce estradiol as the major natural estrogen. Doctors prescribe estradiol for hormone replacement therapy (HRT) in naturally postmenopausal women or in women who have had their ovaries surgically removed. The regimen usually combines estradiol and progestin for women with an intact uterus. This is because of an increased risk for endometrial overgrowth and the potential risk for endometrial cancer with single therapy. Estrogen alone is appropriate for patients without a uterus.

The use of HRT for menopausal symptoms is controversial. Although effective in treating menopausal symptoms such as hot flashes, mood swings, and night sweats, HRT may increase a woman's risk for developing breast cancer, stroke, blood clots, and heart disease. Understandably, findings confused women and health care professionals, with many women discontinuing HRT or deciding not to initiate HRT. Currently, many practitioners prescribe HRT as short-term therapy to help women with severe menopausal symptoms. HRT initiation takes into account the benefits, risks, family health factors, personal health risks, and preferences of the individual.

Estrogen therapy has many side effects; therefore prescribers use the smallest dose for the shortest time necessary. All estrogens have a Pregnancy Category X rating because they can act as **teratogens.** Teratogenic agents cause congenital disabilities (birth defects) by causing abnormal development of the embryo or fetus during pregnancy. Table 24.2 and the following drug monographs present examples of HRT products.

GENERIC NAME: estradiol

TRADE NAMES: Estrace (oral), Vivelle-Dot, Divigel, EstroGel, Alora, Climara (transdermal), Femring, Vagifem (vaginal), Depo-Estradiol (IM)

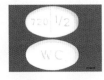

INDICATIONS: Menopausal symptoms, female hypogonadism, osteoporosis prevention, breast/prostate cancer

ROUTES OF ADMINISTRATION: Oral; transdermal (patches, lotions, or gels); vaginal; IM

COMMON ADULT DOSAGE: Varies widely by dosage form and route of delivery

MECHANISM OF ACTION: Supplements estrogen to treat menopausal symptoms associated with a decline in estrogen levels

SIDE EFFECTS: Nausea, vomiting, breast tenderness, dizziness, abnormal vaginal bleeding, thrombotic events

AUXILIARY LABEL: Use as directed

IM, Intramuscularly.

GENERIC NAME: esterified estrogen

TRADE NAME: Menest

INDICATIONS: Menopausal symptoms, female hypogonadism, atrophic vaginitis, breast/prostate cancer

ROUTE OF ADMINISTRATION: Oral

COMMON ADULT DOSAGE: 0.3 to 1.25 mg once daily

MECHANISM OF ACTION: Supplements estrogen to treat menopausal symptoms associated with a decline in estrogen levels

SIDE EFFECTS: Nausea, vomiting, breast tenderness, dizziness, abnormal vaginal bleeding, thrombotic events

AUXILIARY LABEL: Use as directed

GENERIC NAME: conjugated estrogens

TRADE NAME: Premarin

INDICATIONS: Menopausal symptoms, osteoporosis prophylaxis, female hypogonadism, atrophic vaginitis, abnormal uterine bleeding, breast/prostate cancer

ROUTES OF ADMINISTRATION: Oral; vaginal; injectable (IM, IV)

COMMON ADULT DOSAGE: Varies widely by dosage form and route of delivery

MECHANISM OF ACTION: Supplements estrogen to treat menopausal symptoms associated with a decline in estrogen levels

SIDE EFFECTS: Headache, abdominal pain, dizziness, abnormal vaginal bleeding, thrombotic events

AUXILIARY LABEL: Use as directed.

GENERIC NAME: estropipate

TRADE NAME: None

INDICATIONS: Menopausal symptoms, osteoporosis prophylaxis, female hypogonadism, atrophic vaginitis

ROUTE OF ADMINISTRATION: Oral

COMMON ADULT DOSAGE: 0.75 to 9 mg once daily depending on the indication

MECHANISM OF ACTION: Supplements estrogen to treat menopausal symptoms associated with a decline in estrogen levels

SIDE EFFECTS: Nausea, vomiting, breast tenderness, dizziness, abnormal vaginal bleeding, thrombotic events

AUXILIARY LABEL: Take as directed

Pelvic Inflammatory Disease

Pelvic inflammatory disease (PID) is an inflammation of the female reproductive organs. The severe inflammation of the uterine lining, fallopian tubes, or ovaries can cause chronic pain and permanent infertility. Tubal ectopic pregnancy (ie, the egg attaches to and grows in the fallopian tube) occurs 6 to 10 times more often in women with a PID history. Ectopic pregnancy is ordinarily fatal to the fetus and possibly life-threatening to the mother.

PID is usually caused by a sexually transmitted infection (STI), although this is not exclusively the case. An untreated infection of the genital tract may result in PID. Infection duration ranges from days to months. Symptoms include abnormal or increased vaginal discharge, bleeding between periods, painful menstruation, painful urination/bowel movements, fever, painful intercourse, and pain in the upper right abdomen. PID, especially when the patient does not respond to antibiotics, can require hospitalization.

The following are risk factors for PID:

- *History of PID:* Prior episodes of PID, especially those caused by gonorrhea and chlamydia, increase a woman's risk for future PID.
- *Age:* PID occurs most frequently among those 15 to 25 years of age.
- *Multiple sex partners:* Women who have multiple sex partners or whose partner has multiple sex partners have an increased risk for contracting PID.

Prognosis

With a rapid diagnosis, treatment, and prevention methods, the outlook for PID is good. For women with a PID history, the risk for subsequent episodes increases. Prevention is a crucial factor.

Non-Drug Treatments

Barrier contraceptive use, in addition to screening young women and their sexual partners for sexually transmitted diseases (eg, chlamydia), may prevent PID.

Drug Treatments

Specific antimicrobials target the causative microbe (bacteria, protozoa, or fungi). Patients treated at home usually employ oral medications. Treatment for hospitalized patients may include intravenous antibiotic, antiprotozoal, or antifungal therapy. The Centers for Disease Control and Prevention (CDC) recommend various drug combinations for PID. As outlined in Table 24.4, the recommended regimens depend on whether the patient is inside or outside the hospital.

Male Reproductive System

The two **testes** in men (Fig. 24.8) produce and secrete **sperm (spermatogenesis).** The testes are in the scrotum. Sperm production begins before puberty and declines with age, although most men produce sperm throughout their lifetime. The body releases FSH as puberty begins and causes

◼ TABLE 24.4
Select Treatment Regimens for Pelvic Inflammatory Disease

Oral Regimen A[a]

Ceftriaxone 250 mg IM single dose	*plus*	Doxycycline 100 mg PO twice daily for 14 days	*with or without*	Metronidazole 500 mg PO twice daily for 14 days

Oral Regimen B[a]

Cefoxitin 2 g IM single dose and probenecid 1 g PO single dose	*plus*	Doxycycline 100 mg PO twice daily for 14 days	*with or without*	Metronidazole 500 mg PO twice daily for 14 days

Oral Regimen C[a]

Ceftizoxime or cefotaxime 1 g IM as single dose	*plus*	Doxycycline 100 mg PO twice daily for 14 days	*with or without*	Metronidazole 500 mg PO twice daily for 14 days

Parenteral Regimen A[a]

Cefotetan 2 g IV every 12 hr	*or*	Cefoxitin 2 g IV every 6 hr	*plus*	Doxycycline 100 mg PO or IV every 12 hr

Parenteral Regimen B[a]

Clindamycin 900 mg IV every 8 hr	—		*plus*	Gentamicin loading dose IV/IM (2 mg/kg), followed by 1.5 mg/kg every 8 hr

Parenteral A or B to Be Followed With:

Doxycycline 100 mg PO twice daily for 14 days	*or*	Clindamycin 450 mg PO 4 times daily for 14 days

Alternative Parenteral Regimens[a]

Ampicillin/sulbactam (Unasyn) 3 g IV every 6 hr	—		*Plus*	Doxycycline 100 mg PO or IV every 12 hr for 14 days

[a]Regimens are optional so that the physician can determine the best course of treatment.

IM, Intramuscularly; *IV,* intravascularly; *PO,* orally.

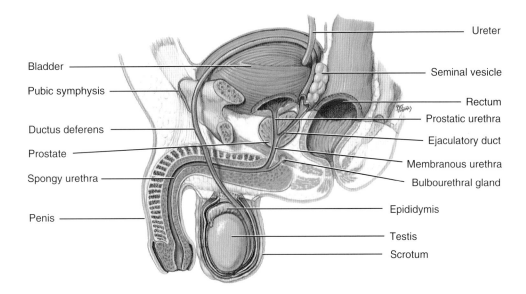

FIG. 24.8 Testes. (From Applegate E. *The Anatomy and Physiology Learning System*. 4th ed. St. Louis: Saunders; 2011.)

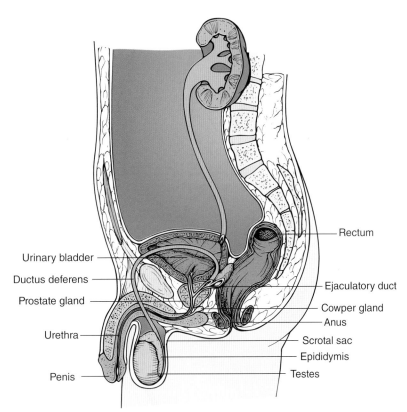

FIG. 24.9 Male reproductive system.

the stored immature sperm cells to divide and mature. Each sperm contains half of the genetic material contributed to a new life during reproduction. The production of testosterone (also from the testes) helps adjacent organs grow: the prostate gland, seminal vesicles, vas deferens, and others. Testosterone also carries responsibility for secondary sex characteristics such as male voice deepening into puberty and increased muscle development. This hormone also affects the differences in the physiques of men and women.

In the man, the reproductive system is closely tied to the urinary system (Fig. 24.9). The urethra passes through the penis, is surrounded by the prostate gland, and is responsible for voiding urine and serving as an exit route for sperm on ejaculation. After sperm form, they mature and the body stores them in the epididymis (a series of tightly coiled tubes wrapped around the back of the testes). They then travel into the vas deferens (a muscular tube that extends from the epididymis to the ejaculatory duct), where peristaltic movements transport the sperm into the ejaculatory duct.

The **prostate** is about the size and shape of a walnut. It encircles part of the urethra, the tube that carries urine out of the bladder and through the penis. Prostate gland secretions both enhance sperm motility and viability and provide a slightly alkaline environment that tolerates the acidic vaginal environment. Sperm and fluids pass through the urethra in the penis for ejaculation during sexual intercourse.

The release of GnRH from the hypothalamus stimulates male sex hormones. GnRH then travels to the anterior pituitary and causes it to secrete LH (also called *interstitial cell–stimulating hormone*) in the male and FSH. Interstitial cell-stimulating hormone then promotes interstitial cell growth in the testes and stimulates testosterone secretion. Testosterone and FSH stimulate spermatogenesis (creation of sperm) in the testicles (Fig. 24.10).

Collectively, **androgens** are male sex hormones. Testosterone is the most abundant androgen. At puberty, androgens stimulate the formation of secondary male characteristics such as increased muscle mass, voice deepening, and facial hair growth. Although females produce testosterone, androgens play a less significant role in female sexual characteristic development and reproductive processes.

Conditions Affecting the Male Reproductive System

Various conditions affect the male reproductive system, and we can identify and treat many conditions. Many medications can cure or mitigate male reproductive system diseases and conditions.

Common Conditions

Male Hypogonadism

Hypogonadism is a condition in which men cannot produce enough testosterone. This condition can occur in the fetus, during puberty, or in adulthood. Underdevelopment of the

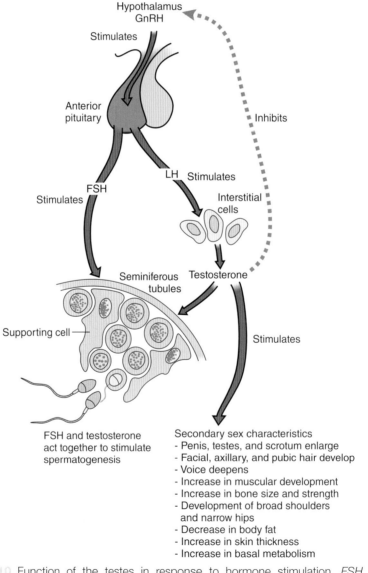

FIG. 24.10 Function of the testes in response to hormone stimulation. *FSH*, Follicle-stimulating hormone; *GnRH*, gonadotropin-releasing hormone; *LH*, luteinizing hormone.

genitals (during fetal development), impaired growth (at puberty), infection (bacterial or viral), or injury to the glands that produce testosterone (tumors or trauma) can cause hypogonadism. Lack of testosterone can cause fatigue, decreased sex drive, and difficulty concentrating.

Prognosis

We can treat male hypogonadism symptoms effectively with testosterone replacement therapy.

Non-Drug Treatment

Stress reduction can minimize anxiety and improve the man's attitude about this condition.

Drug Treatment

Androgens can help treat male hypogonadism or infertility resulting from a low sperm count. Increased secretion of testosterone, follicle-stimulating hormone, and interstitial cell–stimulating hormone can increase sperm count. Different medication delivery systems can promote puberty and secondary sex characteristic development in children with male hypogonadism. Dosage forms include intramuscular, subcutaneous, transdermal, and oral formulations.

Androgens provide a sense of well-being, mental stability, and energy to patients with male hypogonadism. Testosterone provides resistance to fatigue. Originally, natural testosterone came from bull testes. Now manufacturers chemically synthesize it. Because of the abuse potential of androgen products, the US Drug Enforcement Agency placed these products on the Schedule III list of controlled medications. Table 24.5 provides a list of select androgens for the treatment of male hypogonadism. Testosterone is now a popular discussion topic between patient and provider for age-related decreases. Common testosterone adverse effects include male pattern baldness, gynecomastia (increase in breast tissue in males), and acne.

GENERIC NAME:
methyltestosterone (C-III)

TRADE NAMES: Testred, Android, Methitest

INDICATIONS: *Men:* Male hypogonadism, delayed puberty. *Women:* Palliative treatment of metastatic breast cancer

ROUTE OF ADMINISTRATION: Oral

COMMON ADULT DOSAGES: *Males:* 10 to 50 mg/day. *Females:* 50 to 200 mg/day

MECHANISM OF ACTION: Supplements and replaces testosterone

SIDE EFFECTS: Acne, headache, nausea, increased sex drive

AUXILIARY LABELS:
- Use as directed
- *Caution:* Federal law prohibits the transfer of this drug to any person other than the patient for whom it was prescribed

TABLE 24.5
Select Androgen Supplements

Generic Name	Trade Name	Common Dosage Range	Common Side Effects
Androgens			
testosterone	Androderm	• *Patch:* 4 mg placed on skin once daily (replaced for each new patch)	• Acne • Application/injection site reactions • Deep vein thrombosis • Edema • Erections • Hair loss/growth • Hypertension
	AndroGel	• 1% or 1.62% applied once daily in the morning to shoulder/upper arms	
	Depo-Testosterone	• 50–400 mg IM every 2–4 wk	
	Striant SR	• 30-mg buccal tablet PO every 12 hr	
	Testopel	• 150–450 mg pellets implanted in subdermal fat every 3–6 mo	
fluoxymesterone	Androxy	• 5–20 mg PO daily	• Acne • Edema • Hair growth • Priapism • Prostate cancer
Gonadotropin			
human chorionic gonadotropin	Novarel	• 500–1000 units IM 3 times/wk for 3 wk, followed by same dose twice weekly for 3 wk	• Depression • Edema • Headache • Injection site reaction

IM, Intramuscularly; *PO,* orally.

GENERIC NAME: testosterone (C-III)

TRADE NAMES: Androderm,[a] Depo-Testosterone, Fortesta

INDICATIONS: Androgen replacement therapy, male hypogonadism

ROUTES OF ADMINISTRATION: Transdermal, implant, injection, buccal

COMMON ADULT DOSAGES: Varies by indication and dosage form

MECHANISM OF ACTION: Supplements and replaces testosterone

SIDE EFFECTS: Topical irritation, benign prostatic hyperplasia

AUXILIARY LABELS:
- Use as directed
- *Caution:* Federal law prohibits the transfer of this drug to any person other than the patient for whom it was prescribed

[a] Brand no longer available.

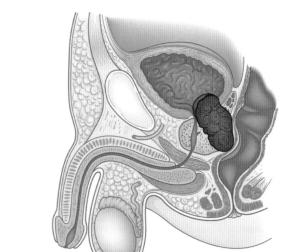

GENERIC NAME: testosterone (C-III)

TRADE NAME: AndroGel

INDICATIONS: Androgen replacement therapy, male hypogonadism

ROUTE OF ADMINISTRATION: Transdermal (gel)

COMMON ADULT DOSAGE: Initially 50 mg of 1% gel applied once daily to skin of upper arms and/or abdomen

MECHANISM OF ACTION: Supplements and replaces testosterone

SIDE EFFECTS: Topical irritation, acne, prostatic disorders

AUXILIARY LABELS:
- Topical
- Use as directed
- *Caution:* Federal law prohibits the transfer of this drug to any person other than the patient for whom it was prescribed

Tech Note!

Secondary exposure of children to testosterone gel products is a concern. Men using this product should cover the application site and not hold small children to avoid testosterone transfer.

Benign Prostatic Hyperplasia

Benign prostatic hyperplasia (BPH) is an enlargement of the prostate gland. The prostate gland is positioned between the bladder and urethra and encircles the urethra.

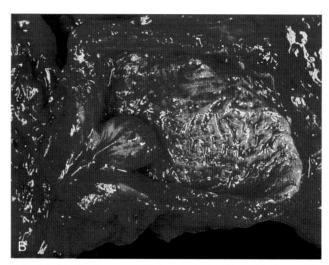

FIG. 24.11 Benign prostatic hyperplasia. (From McCance KL. *Pathophysiology: The Biologic Basis for Disease in Adults and Children*. 6th ed. St. Louis: Mosby; 2010.)

When the prostate enlarges, it makes urination difficult (Fig. 24.11). This condition is **"benign"** because the prostate growth is noncancerous and will not metastasize (spread). BPH occurs in about half of men by age 50. BPH is noncancerous and nonlethal but is a daily disruption. The BPH treatment goals are to relieve symptoms such as urinary hesitancy, urine stream decrease, postvoiding dribbling, urinary frequency, and **nocturia** and to prevent urinary tract infections.

Prognosis

Several treatments effectively lessen benign prostatic hyperplasia (BPH) symptoms. Treatments range from lifestyle changes to medication or surgery. Several procedures may reduce an enlarged prostate gland and relieve BPH symptoms.

Non-Drug Treatment

For mild BPH symptoms, non-drug treatments can reduce the condition's severity. These include avoiding smoking, alcohol, caffeine, and over-the-counter antihistamines and decongestants, in addition to exercising regularly. Surgery is an option for patients unresponsive to medication. The surgeon physically removes excess prostate gland tissue. Low-level radiofrequency waves can also destroy excess prostate tissue as another option.

Drug Treatment

Two primary drug classes help BPH: 5-alpha-reductase inhibitors and alpha-blockers (Table 24.6). 5-Alpha-reductase inhibitors reduce prostate size. It can take up to 6 months to achieve maximum effectiveness. Alpha-blockers act quickly to lessen urinary BPH symptoms, although they do not stop the prostate enlargement process. The two medication classes can work concurrently for the best results.

5-Alpha-reductase inhibitors 5-Alpha-reductase inhibitors block the conversion of testosterone to a more active androgen (5-alpha-dihydrotestosterone [DHT]) that increases the growth of cells, thus reducing the prostate tissue growth. These agents can take several months to reach full effect.

GENERIC NAME: finasteride
TRADE NAME: Proscar
INDICATION: Benign prostatic hyperplasia

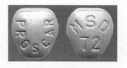

TABLE 24.6
Select Treatments for the Management of Benign Prostatic Hyperplasia

Generic Name	Trade Name	Common Dosage Range	Common Side Effects
5-Alpha-Reductase Inhibitors			
Block the conversion of testosterone to dihydrotestosterone (DHT), which slows prostate growth and can shrink the prostate			
dutasteride	Avodart	• 0.5 mg PO once daily	• Breast tenderness
finasteride	Proscar	• 5 mg PO once daily	• Rash • Sexual dysfunction
Alpha-1 Blockers			
Relax prostate smooth muscle, reducing bladder outlet resistance			
doxazosin	Cardura	• 1 mg PO once daily, then titrate upward to a goal of 4–8 mg PO once daily	• Abnormal ejaculation • Dizziness
	Cardura XL (extended-release)	• 4 mg PO once daily with breakfast, then titrate upward to 8 mg PO once daily	• Headache • Orthostasis • Reflex tachycardia
terazosin	Hytrin	• 1 mg PO at bedtime, then titrate upward prn; most patients need 10 mg (max 20 mg/day)	
alfuzosin	Uroxatral	• 10 mg PO once daily	• Same side effect profile listed above but with less orthostatic hypotension
tamsulosin	Flomax	• 0.4 mg PO once daily 30 min after the same meal each day	
5-Alpha-Reductase Inhibitors/Alpha-1 Blockers			
See mechanisms previously described for 5-alpha-reductase inhibitors and alpha-1 blockers			
dutasteride and tamsulosin	Jalyn	• 1 capsule (0.5 mg dutasteride/0.4 mg tamsulosin) PO once daily 30 min after the same meal each day	• See side effects listed above
Phosphodiesterase Type 5 Inhibitors			
Increase cyclic guanosine monophosphate (cGMP) levels in the vascular smooth muscle cells, promoting relaxation and vasodilation			
tadalafil	Cialis	• 2.5–5 mg PO once daily before intercourse	• Headache • Hypotension • Muscle aches

PO, Orally.

ROUTE OF ADMINISTRATION: Oral

COMMON ADULT DOSAGE: 5 mg once daily

MECHANISM OF ACTION: Blocks the conversion of testosterone to a more active androgen (dihydrotestosterone [DHT]) known to increase the growth of cells

SIDE EFFECTS: Dizziness, erectile dysfunction, ejaculatory dysfunction, decrease in libido

AUXILIARY LABEL: Take as directed

■ Tech Note!

Finasteride is also available in a 1-mg dose under the trade name Propecia for the treatment of male pattern baldness.

GENERIC NAME: dutasteride

TRADE NAME: Avodart

INDICATION: Benign prostatic hyperplasia

ROUTE OF ADMINISTRATION: Oral

COMMON ADULT DOSAGE: 0.5 mg once daily

MECHANISM OF ACTION: Blocks the conversion of testosterone to a more active androgen (dihydrotestosterone [DHT]) that is known to increase the growth of cells

SIDE EFFECTS: Erectile dysfunction, ejaculatory dysfunction, decrease in libido

AUXILIARY LABEL: Take as directed

■ Tech Note!

5-Alpha-reductase inhibitors may cause congenital disabilities; therefore a woman who is pregnant or trying to become pregnant should avoid contact with crushed or broken tablets because the active drug can penetrate through the skin.

GENERIC NAME: terazosin

TRADE NAME: Hytrin

INDICATIONS: Benign prostatic hyperplasia (BPH), hypertension

ROUTE OF ADMINISTRATION: Oral

COMMON ADULT DOSAGE: 1 mg initially at bedtime; then titrate upward to 10 mg once daily (BPH) or 20 mg once daily (hypertension) if needed

MECHANISM OF ACTION: Relaxes smooth muscle tissue in the prostate and the bladder neck by blocking alpha receptors

SIDE EFFECTS: Orthostatic hypotension, dizziness, drowsiness, muscle weakness, blurred vision

AUXILIARY LABELS:
- May cause dizziness/drowsiness
- Do not drive or perform any hazardous tasks until accustomed to side effects

---

GENERIC NAME: tamsulosin

TRADE NAME: Flomax

INDICATION: Benign prostatic hyperplasia

ROUTE OF ADMINISTRATION: Oral

COMMON ADULT DOSAGE: 0.4 mg once daily 30 minutes after the same meal each day; titrate up to 0.8 mg daily after 2 to 4 weeks if needed

MECHANISM OF ACTION: Relaxes smooth muscle tissue in the prostate and the bladder neck by blocking alpha receptors

SIDE EFFECTS: Orthostatic hypotension, dizziness, blurred vision, diarrhea, headache, ejaculation dysfunction, rhinitis

AUXILIARY LABELS:
- May cause dizziness/drowsiness
- Do not drive or perform any hazardous tasks until you know how this drug affects you

---

Alpha-adrenergic blockers Alpha-adrenergic blockers for BPH work selectively to inhibit alpha-1 receptor sites. Some agents (eg, terazosin) are less selective for prostate tissue and more appropriate for hypertension treatment. Agents such as terazosin and doxazosin commonly cause orthostatic hypotension. Patients should take their first dose just before bedtime to avoid becoming lightheaded and falling. Other drugs (eg, tamsulosin) have more targeted activity for prostate tissues. They still pose a risk for orthostatic hypotension, dizziness, and falls. These agents treat BPH symptoms by relaxing prostate smooth muscle tissue and the bladder neck. This mechanism facilitates bladder urine flow.

Erectile Dysfunction

Erectile dysfunction (ED) is the inability of the male to achieve or maintain an erection, commonly referred to as *impotence.* ED is caused by an insufficient amount of blood flowing to the penis rather than a lack of sexual desire. ED ranges from rarely occurring to a chronic problem. As a man ages, the probability of experiencing ED increases. As men age, their risk increases that they will develop prostate conditions and other disease states that affect ED, such as diabetes, atherosclerosis, high blood pressure, and cardiovascular diseases. Additional ED conditions and causes are provided in Table 24.7.

Prognosis

In many cases, erectile dysfunction (ED) occurs only on rare occasions. It does not pose a significant problem or warrant treatment. Persistent ED can signify an underlying problem. When a patient reports ED, the physician should identify any underlying contributing conditions. With proper treatment and lifestyle changes, the frequency of ED episodes may diminish.

Non-Drug Treatments

Lifestyle changes such as lower alcohol intake, smoking cessation, weight loss, and exercise can help if appropriate. Nonpharmacological devices can also help treat ED. Vacuum devices (penis pumps) can increase penile blood flow and initiate an erection. Psychotherapy may also help men overcome anxieties that may contribute to psychogenic ED.

Drug Treatments

In 1998 Pfizer introduced sildenafil (Viagra), a phosphodiesterase inhibitor for ED. Sildenafil research initially targeted lowering blood pressure and treating angina pectoris. Today it is widely used to treat ED. Sildenafil (and other medications in this class) increases blood flow to the penis and causes penile rigidity. Possible side effects of phosphodiesterase inhibitors include headaches, flushing of the skin, gastrointestinal symptoms, nasal congestion, and diarrhea. Other phosphodiesterase inhibitors are tadalafil and vardenafil, all with the -afil ending. Patients taking nitrates should not take sildenafil or related drugs concurrently because of the potential for dangerous decreases in blood pressure that can occur upon combination. Table 24.8 lists select medications for ED. Note that injectable and intraurethral products are available for ED; however, with an oral dosage form available, these options are far less palatable.

Prostate Cancer

Prostate cancer is a condition in which the prostate cells grow uncontrolled and form tumors (Fig. 24.12). This growth blocks the urine flow through the prostate. If left untreated, cancer can metastasize through the body. Genetics may affect the onset. African American men are more likely to develop prostate cancer, as are men who have relatives with prostate cancer. Symptoms include nocturia, dysuria, blood in the urine or semen, painful ejaculation, and pelvic or lower back pain that does not subside. Prostate cancer has four stages; cancer staging provides information to determine the most effective treatment plan.

Prognosis

Although prostate cancer is a severe condition, treatment advancements have improved outcomes for many. Early diagnosis, increased public awareness, and new chemotherapy agents can increase survival rates for patients with prostate cancer.

Non-Drug Treatment

A surgeon can remove the prostate (radical prostatectomy) or testicles (orchidectomy) as treatment. A partial prostate tissue removal (transurethral resection of the prostate [TURP]) may remove some of the cancer. Radiologic treatment can treat recurrent or advanced-stage prostate cancer.

Drug Treatment

The cancer stage determines prostate cancer treatment. Hormone therapy is the most common medical treatment. The hormonal activity can be eradicated or reduced such that cancerous cells stop reproducing.

■ TABLE 24.7
Select Causes of Erectile Dysfunction

Condition or Cause That Leads to ED	Effects
Cigarette smoking	Smoking can worsen atherosclerosis, which increases the possibility of ED
Depression/anxiety	Depression can cause or worsen ED because of stress, anxiety, low self-esteem, fears, guilty feelings
Low testosterone levels	Hypogonadism can lower sex drive and cause ED
Medications	Medications can have side effects that may cause sexual dysfunction, including ED, such as certain beta-blockers, calcium channel blockers, antidepressants, antihypertensive agents, antihistamines, histamine-2 antihistamines, and antiseizure medications
Nerve damage	Injury to nervous system caused by trauma, surgery, or disease
Prostatism	Enlargement of the prostate gland
Prostatitis	Inflammation of the prostate gland
Prostatocystitis	Inflammation of the prostate gland and bladder
Substance abuse	Alcohol leads to atrophy of testes, lowering testosterone levels, other drugs (eg, heroin, cocaine, marijuana) contribute to ED

ED, Erectile dysfunction.

TABLE 24.8
Select Agents for the Treatment of Erectile Dysfunction

Generic Name	Trade Name	Common Dosage Range	Common Side Effects
Phosphodiesterase-5 Inhibitors (PDE-5)			
sildenafil	Viagra	• 50 mg PO once daily 60 min before anticipated sexual activity; max 100/day	• Flushing • Headache • Hypotension • Priapism (lasting longer than 4 hr) • Upset stomach
vardenafil	Levitra, Staxyn	• 10 mg 60 min before anticipated sexual activity	
tadalafil	Cialis	• 5–20 mg PO 30 min before anticipated sexual activity	
Prostaglandin/Vasodilator			
alprostadil	Caverject	• 2.5 mcg intracavernous injection before sexual activity (dose is individualized and based on type/cause of erectile dysfunction, max 60 mcg)	• Headache • Penile pain • Priapism • Scarring (injection) • Urethral burning
	Muse	• 125–250 mcg intraurethral suppository administered prn for erection (max 2/day)	

PO, Orally.

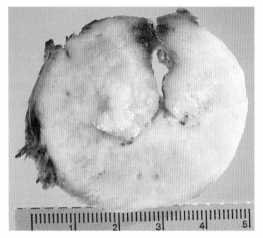

FIG. 24.12 Prostate cancer. (From Kumar V, Cotran RS, Robbins SL. *Basic Pathology*. 7th ed. Philadelphia: Saunders; 2003.)

Antiandrogens and luteinizing hormone–releasing hormone (LHRH) agonists can decrease hormone activity and are the most common agents. These treatments usually begin with stage 2 prostate cancer. Table 24.9 presents examples of these hormonal medications. For advanced prostate cancer forms, doctors can use a variety of chemotherapeutic agents and regimens.

Sexually Transmitted Diseases

Any disease transmitted by sexual intercourse is considered a sexually transmitted disease (STD). Some practitioners use the expression sexually transmitted infection (STI) to indicate that some infections never develop into a disease. Diseases can be transmitted in other ways. For example, patients can spread the human immunodeficiency virus (HIV) by intercourse or needle sharing. Herpesvirus can move from mother to child through childbirth. Pubic lice and scabies can spread from sharing towels or bedding and close contact. Because STDs are embarrassing to some, many do not seek immediate treatment. Additionally, certain STDs (eg, syphilis, herpes) can remain dormant (latent) for long periods. This dormancy results in more transference between partners until the symptoms become more apparent. Even then, many people resist providing the names of those infected.

Bacterial, viral, fungal, and protozoal organisms can cause STDs. If untreated, some STDs can cause irreversible sterility, blindness, and death. Several diseases, including chlamydia, gonorrhea, hepatitis, acquired immunodeficiency syndrome (AIDS), and syphilis, are on the list of Notifiable Infectious Diseases. The law requires medical practitioners to notify the local health department in these cases. The CDC updates this list annually. Table 24.10 presents a list of

TABLE 24.9
Select Hormonal Prostate Cancer Treatments

Type of Hormone Therapy	Generic Name	Trade Name	Effect in Men
Luteinizing hormone–releasing hormone (LHRH)	leuprolide	Lupron Depot	Blocks hormone production in testes
	goserelin	Zoladex	Blocks hormone production in testes
Antiandrogens	flutamide	Eulexin[a]	Blocks effects of testosterone
	nilutamide	Nilandron	Blocks effects of testosterone

[a]Brand discontinued; now available only as generic.

Select Sexually Transmitted Diseases and Potential Treatments

Organism	Infection	Generic Name	Trade Name	Common Dosage Range
Chlamydia trachomatis	Chlamydia	azithromycin	Zithromax	• 1 g PO once
		doxycycline	Vibramycin	• 100 mg PO twice daily for 7 days
		erythromycin	E-Mycin[a]	• 500 mg PO 4 times daily for 7 days
		levofloxacin	Levaquin[a]	• 500 mg PO daily for 7 days
		ofloxacin	Floxin[a]	• 300 mg PO twice daily for 7 days
Neisseria gonorrhoeae	Gonorrhea	ceftriaxone	Rocephin[a]	• 250 mg IM once
		cefixime	Suprax	• 400 mg PO once
		plus azithromycin	Zithromax	• 1 g PO once
Herpes simplex	Genital herpes	acyclovir	Zovirax	• 400 mg PO 3 times daily for 7–10 days
		famciclovir	Famvir[a]	• 250 mg PO 3 times daily for 7–10 days
		valacyclovir	Valtrex	• 1 g PO twice daily for 10 days
Treponema pallidum	Syphilis	benzathine, penicillin G	Bicillin L-A	• 2.4 million units IM once
Trichomonas vaginalis	Trichomoniasis vaginalis	tinidazole	Tindamax	• 2 g PO once
		metronidazole	Flagyl, Metrogel Vaginal	• 2 g PO once
Gardnerella vaginalis	Bacterial vaginitis	metronidazole	Flagyl, Metrogel Vaginal 0.75%	• 500 mg PO twice daily for 7 days • 1 applicatorful (37.5 mg) intravaginally daily for 5 days
		clindamycin	Clindesse	• 1 applicatorful (5 g) intravaginally at bedtime for 7 days
Candida albicans	Vaginal candidiasis	clotrimazole	Gyne-Lotrimin	• 2%: 1 applicatorful intravaginally daily for 3 days • 1%: 1 applicatorful intravaginally daily for 7 days
		fluconazole	Diflucan	• 150 mg PO as a single dose
		miconazole	Monistat-1	• 1200 mg vaginal suppository inserted for 1 day
		terconazole	Terazol	• 0.8% cream: 1 applicatorful (40 mg) intravaginally daily at bedtime for 3 days • 0.4% cream: 1 applicatorful (20 mg) intravaginally for 7 days
		tioconazole	—	• 1 applicatorful (300 mg) intravaginally before bedtime as a single dose

[a]Brand discontinued; now available only as generic.
IM, Intramuscularly; *PO,* orally.

organisms that cause STDs, along with select drugs and dosage forms for their treatment.

STD symptoms vary by disease and infection severity. Chlamydia caused by *Chlamydia trachomatis* can permanently damage a woman's reproductive organs; symptoms may be mild or even absent. Gonorrhea, caused by *Neisseria gonorrhoeae,* may have mild or no symptoms. Both chlamydia and gonorrhea can eventually cause PID in women and epididymitis in men if left untreated. Both are painful conditions that can lead to sterility. Early HIV symptoms typically include fever, headache, fatigue, and rash. As the disease

progresses, increased severity of early symptoms may manifest, along with night sweats, chronic diarrhea, and chills. Genital herpes, which can lie dormant for months, years, or decades, causes small red bumps or blisters or a rash on the genitals. Hepatitis, which infects the liver, can cause fatigue, nausea, vomiting, darkening of the urine, or yellowing of the skin. Many disease symptoms are absent in the early infection stages, making the infection transference more likely. Because infections are typically passed during sexual contact, protection and education are key components to preventing their spread.

Some may mistakenly think that oral birth control or contraceptive gels can protect against STDs, but this is not true. Some vaccines, such as Gardasil, can protect against certain human papillomavirus (HPV) infections but do not protect against all STDs. Research is underway to develop an HIV vaccine; however, at this time, there is no viable vaccine. Because of the wealth of information and misinformation available to the public, patients may become confused about how to remain uninfected. The CDC, US Public Health Department, and each state's public health department print brochures, produce videos, and maintain websites for up-to-date, reliable information. Tables 24.11 and 24.12 provide an overview of select agents used for the treatment of HIV and hepatitis, respectively.

■ TABLE 24.11
Select Agents for the Treatment of Human Immunodeficiency Virus Infection and Acquired Immunodeficiency Syndrome[a]

Generic Name	Trade Name	Abbreviation	Common Dosage Range
Nucleoside Reverse Transcriptase Inhibitors (NRTIs)			
abacavir	Ziagen	ABC	• 300 mg PO twice daily or 600 mg/day

didanosine	Videx, Videx EC	ddl	• *Weight-based EC dosing:*
			  • 25 kg to <60 kg: 250 mg once daily
			  • ≥60 kg: 400 mg once daily

emtricitabine	Emtriva	FTC	• 200 mg PO daily
lamivudine	Epivir	3TC	• 150 mg PO twice daily or • 300 mg/day PO

stavudine	Zerit	D4T	• *Weight-based dosing:*
			  • <60 kg: 30 mg PO twice daily
			  • ≥60 kg: 40 mg PO twice daily

zidovudine	Retrovir	AZT	• 300 mg PO twice daily • 1 mg/kg IV every 4 hr
Nucleotide Reverse Transcriptase Inhibitor (NTRTI)			
tenofovir	Viread	TFV	• 300 mg/day PO
Protease Inhibitors (PIs)			
atazanavir	Reyataz	ATV	• 400 mg/day PO or 300 mg/day PO boosted with RTV 100 mg/day PO
darunavir	Prezista	DRV	• 800 mg/day PO boosted with RTV 100 mg/day PO
fosamprenavir	Lexiva	FPV	• 1400 mg PO twice daily or 1400 mg/day PO boosted with RTV 100–200 mg/day PO
indinavir	Crixivan	IDV	• 800 mg PO every 8 hr
lopinavir and ritonavir	Kaletra	LPV	• 400 mg LPV/100 mg RTV PO twice daily
nelfinavir	Viracept	NFV	• 750 mg PO three times daily or 1250 mg PO twice daily
ritonavir	Norvir	RTV	• "Booster" for other PIs: 100–400 mg/day PO
saquinavir	Invirase	SQV	• 1000 mg PO twice daily boosted with ritonavir 100 mg PO twice daily
tipranavir	Aptivus	TPV	• 500 mg PO twice daily boosted with ritonavir 200 mg twice daily
Non–Nucleoside Reverse Transcriptase Inhibitor (NNRTI)			
efavirenz	Sustiva	EFV	• 600 mg PO once daily
etravirine	Intelence	—	• 200 mg PO twice daily
nevirapine	Viramune	NVP	• 200 mg PO once daily for 14 days, then 200 mg PO twice daily
Fusion Inhibitor			
enfuvirtide	Fuzeon	T-20	• 90 mg subcut twice daily
CCR5 Blocker			
maraviroc	Selzentry	—	• 300 mg PO twice daily
Integrase Inhibitor			
raltegravir	Isentress	—	• 400 mg PO twice daily or 1200 mg once daily

[a]Many of the medications are available in combination formulations, especially the NRTIs.
IV, Intravenously; *PO,* orally; *RTV,* ritonavir; *subcut,* subcutaneously.

TABLE 24.12
Select Agents for the Treatment of Hepatitis B and C

Generic Name	Trade Name	Common Dosage Range	Common Side Effects
Hepatitis B			
Interferon			
interferon alfa-2b	Intron A	• 5 million units/day IM/subcut or 10 million units IM/subcut 3 times/wk for 16 wk	• Depression • Flulike symptoms • Headache • Injection site reactions
interferon alfa-2a pegylated	Pegasys	• 180 mcg subcut once wkly for 48 wk	
Nucleoside Reverse Transcriptase Inhibitors (NRTIs)			
lamivudine	Epivir-HBV	• 100 mg once daily	• Diarrhea • Fatigue • Headache • Nausea • Vomiting
entecavir	Baraclude	• 0.5–1 mg PO once daily	• Fatigue • Headache • Nausea • Vomiting
Nucleotide Reverse Transcriptase Inhibitors (NTRTIs)			
adefovir	Hepsera	• 10 mg PO once daily	• Abdominal pain • Diarrhea • Headache • Hematuria • Weakness
tenofovir	Viread	• 300 mg PO once daily	• Depression • Insomnia • Nausea • Pain • Weakness
Hepatitis C			
Interferon			
interferon alfa-2b	Intron A	• 3 million units IM/subcut 3 times wkly for 18–24 mo	• Depression • Flulike symptoms • Headache • Injection site reactions
interferon alfa-2a pegylated	Pegasys	• 180 mcg subcut once wkly	
interferon alfa-2b pegylated	PegIntron	• 1 mcg/kg subcut once wkly	
Antiviral			
ribavirin	Rebetol	• 800–1400 mg/day PO daily for 24 or 48 wk in combination with pegylated interferons	• Anemia • Fatigue • Headache • Hypotension • Insomnia
Protease Inhibitors			
boceprevir	Generic only	• 800 mg PO 3 times daily (added to PEG-INF + ribavirin after 4 wk of dual therapy)	• Anemia • Fatigue • Insomnia • Nausea • Rash • Taste changes
telaprevir	Generic only	• 1125 mg PO twice daily (added to PEG-INF + ribavirin after 11 wk of dual therapy)	
Combination Products			
ledipasvir	Found in Harvoni	• 1 tablet (ledipasvir 90 mg/sofosbuvir 400 mg) PO once daily	• Dizziness • Fatigue • Headache • Nausea
sofosbuvir			

HBV, Hepatitis B virus; *IM,* intramuscularly; *PEG-IFN,* pegylated interferon; *PO,* orally; *subcut,* subcutaneously.

GENERIC NAME: valacyclovir

TRADE NAME: Valtrex

INDICATIONS: Herpes, varicella

ROUTE OF ADMINISTRATION: Oral

COMMON ADULT DOSAGES: Varies by indication

MECHANISM OF ACTION: Inhibits viral DNA synthesis

SIDE EFFECTS: Headache, nausea, abdominal pain, fatigue

Hepatitis C

Recently drug research has made major breakthroughs for chronic hepatitis C treatment. A disease cure is now possible with certain novel antiviral combinations. Standard hepatitis C therapy previously included ribavirin with interferon alfa. Interferon alfas help activate certain immune cells. The mechanism of action is, however, very unspecific; the activated immune cells attack other virus-infected cells but also tend to attack and destroy healthy uninfected cells. This mechanism causes unwanted side effects and a low success rate. New medications such as ritonavir, ombitasvir, and sofosbuvir have more specific mechanisms of action. They target key enzymes for hepatitis C virus replication, resulting in fewer side effects and a better chance of therapy success. These enzymes include NS3, NS5A, and NS5B.

Two trade name medications for hepatitis C include Viekira Pak and Harvoni. Both medicines have multiple active ingredients combined in a single pill, increasing compliance. Unfortunately, the treatment cost is prohibitive. Patients usually pay between $40,000 and $45,000 for one treatment even after assistance from Medicaid. See Table 24.12 for more information on the latest treatments of hepatitis C.

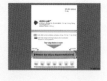

GENERIC NAMES: ombitasvir/paritaprevir/ritonavir/dasabuvir

TRADE NAMES: Viekira Pak, Viekira XR

INDICATION: Hepatitis C

ROUTE OF ADMINISTRATION: Oral

COMMON ADULT DOSAGE: 2 tablets (ombitasvir 12.5 mg/paritaprevir 75 mg/ritonavir 50 mg per tablet) orally once every morning, plus 1 tablet (dasabuvir 250 mg) orally twice daily in the morning and evening for 12 or 24 weeks depending on hepatitis C genotype. Often used in combination with ribavirin

MECHANISM OF ACTION: Combines three direct-acting hepatitis C antiviral agents that disrupt viral replication. Ritonavir is used to increase serum levels of paritaprevir

SIDE EFFECTS: Nausea, insomnia, pruritus, weakness

AUXILIARY LABELS:
- Do not abruptly stop taking this medication
- Take extended-release tablet with food and do not crush

GENERIC NAMES: ledipasvir/sofosbuvir

TRADE NAME: Harvoni

INDICATION: Hepatitis C

ROUTE OF ADMINISTRATION: Oral

COMMON ADULT DOSAGE: *Immediate release:* 1 tablet (ledipasvir 90 mg/sofosbuvir 400 mg per tablet) orally once daily for 12 or 24 weeks depending on hepatitis C genotype

MECHANISMS OF ACTION: Ledipasvir blocks HCV NS5A viral replication protein. Sofosbuvir blocks NS5B RNA-dependent RNA polymerase needed for viral replication. Works as the chain terminator

SIDE EFFECTS: Fatigue, myalgia, headache

AUXILIARY LABEL: Do not abruptly stop taking this medication

▽ Tech Alert!

Remember these sound-alike, look-alike drugs:
- Cardura versus Coumadin and Cardene
- Clomiphene versus clomipramine
- Methyltestosterone versus methylprednisolone
- Provera versus Premarin
- Yasmin versus Yaz

Do You Remember These Key Points?

- Names of the major anatomical components of the male and female reproductive systems and their functions
- The primary signs and symptoms of the various conditions discussed in this chapter
- Medications used to treat the various conditions discussed in this chapter
- The generic and trade names for the drugs discussed in this chapter
- The appropriate auxiliary labels that should be used when filling prescriptions for drugs discussed in this chapter

Review Questions

Multiple Choice Questions

1. The primary female reproductive organs are:
   - **A.** Uterus
   - **B.** Ovaries
   - **C.** Testes
   - **D.** Both A and B

2. Male sex hormones are collectively called:
   A. Estrogens
   B. Androgens
   C. Progestins
   D. Testosterones
3. Testosterone is used to treat which condition?
   A. Hypogonadism in females
   B. Hypogonadism in males
   C. Breast and endometrial cancers in females
   D. Both B and C
4. Estrogens are used to treat which condition?
   A. Menopausal symptoms
   B. Hypogonadism in males
   C. Hypogonadism in females
   D. Both A and C
5. Which medication class is used for the treatment of HIV/AIDS?
   A. Nucleoside reverse transcriptase inhibitors
   B. Protease inhibitors
   C. Nonnucleoside reverse transcriptase inhibitors
   D. All of the above
6. The trade name for tamsulosin is:
   A. Cardura
   B. Uroxatral
   C. Hytrin
   D. Flomax
7. How is clomiphene (Clomid) administered?
   A. Orally
   B. Intramuscularly
   C. Intravaginally
   D. Transdermally
8. Medications used to treat benign prostatic hyperplasia include:
   A. 5-Alpha-reductase inhibitors
   B. Estrogens
   C. Androgens
   D. Alpha-adrenergic blockers
   E. Both A and D
9. Which of the following is *not* a risk factor for pelvic inflammatory disease (PID)?
   A. Age
   B. Multiple sexual partners
   C. History of PID
   D. Hypertension
10. PID can be caused by:
    A. Intrauterine device (IUD) usage
    B. Sexually transmitted diseases (STDs)
    C. Bacterial infection
    D. All of the above
11. Gonorrhea may be treated with:
    A. Azithromycin
    B. Valacyclovir
    C. Acyclovir
    D. Both B and C

12. Interferons (eg, Intron A, Pegasys) are used to treat which infectious disease?
    A. PID
    B. HIV
    C. Hepatitis
    D. Chlamydia
13. Which medication(s) is (are) associated with orthostatic hypotension?
    A. Doxazosin
    B. Finasteride
    C. Dutasteride
    D. All of the above
14. Which product is an intraurethral suppository for the treatment of erectile dysfunction?
    A. Caverject
    B. Muse
    C. Cialis
    D. Viagra
15. Medications and/or devices used to treat erectile dysfunction (ED) include:
    A. Sildenafil, vacuum devices, penile implants
    B. Cialis, Levitra, prostaglandin suppositories
    C. Atenolol, leuprolide, penile implants
    D. Both A and B

■ Technician's Corner

A 55-year-old male patient with diabetes mellitus, hypertension, and coronary artery disease presents a prescription to the pharmacy for sildenafil (Viagra). As the pharmacy technician, you review his medication history and find that he takes the following medications regularly:

- Glucotrol-XL 5 mg/day
- Metformin 500 mg 3 times daily
- Tenormin 50 mg/day
- Lipitor 20 mg q am
- Isordil 10 mg 2 times daily

Using a drug reference resource, answer the following questions:

- Is Viagra safe for dispensing with the previously listed medication history?
- Which of the medications are in the correct dosage?
- Which medications could be given with sildenafil?
- Which are contraindicated with sildenafil, if any?
- What should you, as a pharmacy technician, do if this prescription is presented for dispensing?

Bibliography

Applegate E. *The Anatomy and Physiology Learning System*. 3rd ed. Philadelphia: Saunders; 2006.

Centers for Disease Control and Prevention. Sexually transmitted diseases (STDs). Available at: https://www.cdc.gov/sti/.

Damjanov I. *Pathology for the Health Professions*. 4th ed. St. Louis: Saunders; 2011.

Fishback JL. *Pathology*. 3rd ed. Philadelphia: Mosby; 2005.

Huether S, McCance K. *Understanding Pathophysiology*. 5th ed. St. Louis: Mosby; 2012.

McCance KL. *Pathophysiology: The Biologic Basis for Disease in Adults and Children*. 6th ed. St. Louis: Mosby; 2010.

Page C, Hoffman B, Curtis M, Walker M. *Integrated Pharmacology*. 3rd ed. London: Mosby; 2006.

Patton KT, Thibodeau GA. *Mosby's Handbook of Anatomy and Physiology*. St. Louis: Mosby; 2000.

Price SA, Wilson LM. *Pathophysiology: Clinical Concepts of Disease Processes*. 6th ed. St. Louis: Mosby; 2003.

Solomon EP. *Introduction to Human Anatomy and Physiology*. 3rd ed. St. Louis: Saunders; 2009.

Thibodeau GA, Patton KT. *Anatomy and Physiology*. 8th ed. St. Louis: Mosby; 2012.

Websites Referenced

Clinical Pharmacology Online. Available at: https://www.clinicalkey.com/pharmacology.

UpToDate Online. Available at: www.uptodate.com.

Therapeutic Agents for the Immune System

Tony Guerra

CHAPTER 25

OBJECTIVES

1. Describe the organs and cells of the immune system and their roles.
2. List the primary signs and symptoms of common conditions associated with dysregulation of the immune system. In addition, (a) recognize prescription and over-the-counter drugs used to treat common conditions discussed in this chapter, (b) write the generic and trade names of the drugs discussed in this chapter, and (c) list appropriate auxiliary labels when filling prescriptions for drugs discussed in this chapter.
3. Discuss immunizations and differentiate between various types of vaccines.

TERMS AND DEFINITIONS

Anaphylaxis An extreme, potentially life-threatening allergic reaction

Antibodies Complex molecules (immunoglobulins) made in response to an antigen's presence (eg, a protein of bacteria or other infecting organism) that neutralize a foreign substance's effect

Antigen A substance that prompts antibody production, resulting in an immune response

Antigen-presenting cell (APC) An immune system cell that presents antigens to lymphocytes to activate an immune response

Attenuated A term that describes an altered or weakened live vaccine made from the disease organism against which the vaccine protects

Biological response modifier (BRM) An agent used to modify the body's immune response

Cytokine A protein that signals cells of the immune system

Hashimoto thyroiditis An autoimmune disease leading to hypothyroidism

Hematopoiesis Blood + production, the formation of blood cells

Humoral immunity The immune response mediated by antibodies

Immunity An infection resistance type caused by the body's immune response after exposure to antigens or vaccine administration

Immunization The act of conferring immunity, such as with vaccination

Immunoglobulin An antibody

Inflammation A localized physical condition associated with red, swollen, hot, and often painful tissue

Innate immunity Natural immunity

Juvenile rheumatoid arthritis (JRA) Rheumatoid arthritis that affects children

Leukocyte White + cell, a white blood cell (WBC)

Lymph node A structure that consists of many small, oval nodules that filter lymphatic fluid and fight infection; the site of lymphocyte, monocyte, and plasma cell production

Lymphocyte Lymph + cell, a mononuclear leukocyte found in the blood, lymph, and lymphoid tissues

Monocyte Single + cell, a phagocytic leukocyte

Phagocyte Eating + cell, a cell of the immune system that engulfs cells, debris, and antigens

Plasma cell A cell of the immune system that secretes antibodies

Rheumatoid arthritis (RA) A progressive degenerative and crippling autoimmune joint disease

Spleen A lymphatic organ involved in blood cell production and removal and lymphocyte storage

Systemic Pertaining to the entire organism; "widespread" in contrast to "local"

Systemic lupus erythematosus (SLE) An autoimmune inflammatory disease of connective tissue with variable features, including fever, weakness, fatigue, and other systemic manifestations

Toxoids Vaccines in which toxins have been rendered harmless but still evoke an antigenic response, improving immunity against active toxins at some future date

Transplant rejection An immune response after tissue or organ transplantation

Vaccine A biological preparation that improves immunity to a particular disease by invoking an immune response and a "memory" of the response for future use

Vasodilation Widening of the vasculature, leading to increased blood flow

Virion A virus particle

Virus A microscopic, nonliving organism that replicates exclusively inside the host's cell using parts of the host cell, including DNA, ribosomes, and proteins

Select Vaccines That Affect the Immune System

Vaccine/Drug	Pronunciation
Immune Globulins	
Botulism immune globulin (BIG)	(**bot**-ue-lizm im-**myoon glob**-yoo-lin)
Cytomegalovirus immune globulin (CMV-IG)	(sye-toe-**meg**-a-lo-vye-rus im-**myoon glob**-yoo-lin)
Hepatitis B immune globulin (HBIG)	(hep-ah-**ty**-tiss **B** ih-**myoon glob**-yoo-lin)
Immune globulin G (IgG)	(im-**myoon glob**-yoo-lin)
Rabies immune globulin (RIG)	(**ray**-beez ih-**myoon glob**-yoo-lin)
Respiratory syncytial virus immune globulin (RSV-IG)	(**res**-pih-rah-tory sin-**sih**-shul **vye**-rus ih-**myoon glob**-yoo-lin)
Tetanus immune globulin (TIG)	(**tet**-nus ih-**myoon** glob-yoo-lin)
Vaccinia immune globulin (VIG)	(vax-**in**-ee-uh ih-**myoon glob**-yoo-lin)
Varicella-zoster immune globulin (VZIG)	(var-ih-**sel**-uh-**zos**-ter ih-**myoon glob**-yoo-lin)
Antitoxins	
Botulinum antitoxin	(**bot**-ue-lih-num an-tee-**tok**-sin)
Diphtheria antitoxin	(**dip**-theer-ee-a an-tee-**tok**-sin)
Tetanus antitoxin	(**tet**-n-us an-ti-**tok**-sin)
Vaccines Against Viral Illness	
Avian influenza	(**a**-vee-un in-floo-**en**-za)
Hepatitis A	(hep-uh-**ty**-tiss **A**)
Hepatitis B	(hep-uh-**ty**-tiss **B**)
Herpes zoster (varicella-zoster)	(her-**pees zos**-ter)
Human papillomavirus (HPV)	(hyoo-man **pap**-ih-**loh**-muh-**vye**-rus)
Inactivated influenza virus injectable	(in-**ak**-tih-vay-ted in-**floo-en**-zuh **vye**-rus)
Inactivated poliovirus (IPV)	(in-**ak**-tih-vay-ted **poe**-lee-oh-**vye**-rus)
Intranasal influenza	(in-floo-**en**-za in-**truh**-naz-al)
Japanese encephalitis virus	(**jap**-uh-**neez** en-**cef**-uh-**lye**-tis **vye**-rus)
Measles, mumps, rubella (MMR)	(**mee**-zels, **mumps**, roo-**bel**-uh)
Poliovirus vaccine live oral (OPV)	(**poe**-lee-oh-vye-ris)

Vaccine/Drug	Pronunciation
Rotavirus oral	(**roe**-tuh-vye-ris)
Smallpox (vaccinia)	(**small**-pox)
Varicella (chickenpox)	(var-ih-**sel**-uh)
Yellow fever	(yel-**oh** fee-**ver**)
Vaccines Against Bacterial Illness	
Anthrax vaccine	(**anth**-rax vax-**een**)
Haemophilus influenzae type b Conjugate	(hee-**maw**-fil-us in-floo-**en**-za)
Lyme disease	(**lime** dis-**ease**)
Meningococcal	(meh-**nin**-juh-**kok**-al)
Playg	(**pla**-gwe)
Pneumococcal	(**noo**-moe-**kok**-al)
Typhoid	(**tye**-foid)

Select Immunosuppressive Agents for the Treatment of Autoimmune Disorders and Transplant Rejection

Trade Name[a]	Generic Name	Pronunciation
Azasan, Imuran	azathioprine	(ay-za-**thigh**-oh-preen)
CellCept, Myfortic	mycophenolate	(**mye**-koe-**fen**-uh-late)
Cytoxan[b]	cyclophosphamide	(**sye**-kloe-**fos**-fuh-mide)
Gengraf, Neoral, Sandimmune	cyclosporine	(**sye**-kloe-**spor**-en)
Orthoclone OKT3[b]	muromonab-CD3	(**mue**-roe-**moe**-nab)
Prograf	tacrolimus	(ta-**kroe**-lih-mus)
Rapamune	sirolimus	(sir-**oh**-lih-mus)
Simulect	basiliximab	(bass-ih-**lix**-ih-mab)
Trexall	methotrexate	(meth-oh-**trex**-ate)

[a]Listing of trade names on the same row does not indicate that products are interchangeable in patient treatment regimens.
[b]Brand discontinued; now available only as generic.

Bacterial and viral microbes that cause disease and death have always plagued human beings. In addition to these invaders, the body may need to defend against internal assailants, such as cancer cells or a misdirected attack from the immune system (ie, autoimmune disease). Fortunately, we can better manage autoimmune disorders and morbidity and mortality resulting from infections with vaccine development and immune-modulating medications. This chapter describes the primary immune system functions and discusses the immunization rationale. It also covers autoimmune disorder treatment and transplant rejection.

Although this chapter covers medications to treat common autoimmune diseases, infectious diseases are presented in other, more specific chapters of this textbook. Chapter 26 covers common antibiotics such as amoxicillin, and Chapter 24 (Table 24.10) covers multiple antivirals used to treat sexually transmitted diseases (STDs).

Anatomy and Physiology of the Immune System

The body has a built-in defense mechanism that helps protect it from invading organisms. From birth, a primary body function is to defend against invasion. The lymphatic system produces immune cells and supports the immune system function correctly (Fig. 25.1). The lymphoid organs are sites of residence, proliferation, and differentiation of **lymphocytes** (eg, T cells and B cells) and mononuclear **phagocytes** (eg, macrophages). The many **lymph nodes** contain a large number of lymphocytes, monocytes, and macrophages. Lymphatic veins collect interstitial fluid from tissues and transport it back into the circulatory system as lymph passing through lymph nodes (Fig. 25.2). As lymph passes through lymph nodes, immune cells filter the fluid from debris and microorganisms. In an infection,

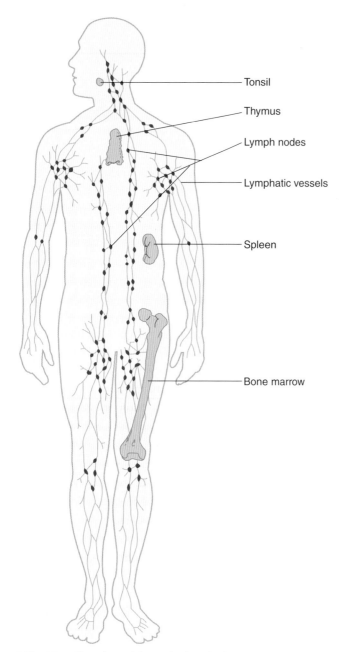

FIG. 25.1 Overview of the major lymphatic organs of the body.

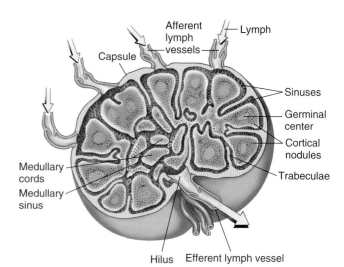

FIG. 25.2 Cross section of a lymph node. Several afferent, valved lymphatics bring lymph to the node. A single efferent lymphatic leaves the node at the hilus. Note that the artery and vein also enter and leave at the hilus. *Arrows* show direction of lymph flow. (From Huether S, McCance K. *Understanding Pathophysiology*. 5th ed. St. Louis: Mosby; 2012.)

Thymus

The thymus is in the upper chest (see Fig. 25.1). The thymus's primary function is to produce and "educate" lymphocytes, which ultimately circulate through lymph nodes and lymphatic tissues and help provide **immunity.** The thymus begins producing these lymphocytes before birth; thus the organ is more massive in childhood than in adulthood.

Spleen

The **spleen** is the largest lymphoid organ and sits on the left side of the upper abdomen. The spleen filters large amounts of blood cells as they reach the end of their life cycle. The spleen is also the primary site for immune responses to blood-borne disease. The spleen has two main areas: red pulp and white pulp (Fig. 25.4). The red pulp contains macrophages and red blood cells that are being removed from circulation. The white pulp contains lymphocytes (T cells and B cells). The spleen contains approximately 25% of all of the body's lymphocytes.

Cells and Mediators of the Immune System

The immune system has many specialized cells (Fig. 25.5). **Leukocytes,** or white blood cells (WBCs), and their functions are described briefly in the following list.

- *Neutrophils:* Neutrophils are the most abundant leukocyte in adults, accounting for approximately 55% of the total leukocyte count. Neutrophils are the first cells to the site of inflammation and act as phagocytes. Phagocytes ingest and destroy other cells (eg, bacteria) and debris. Laboratories test neutrophil cell counts to determine whether a person has an infection.
- *Eosinophils:* In healthy adults, eosinophils account for approximately 1% to 6% of WBCs. Eosinophils fight parasitical infections and form allergic responses.

microbes activate lymphocytes in lymph nodes to fight infection. The bone marrow, thymus, tonsils, and spleen are larger organs of the lymphatic system, each with specific functions.

Bone Marrow

As discussed further in Chapter 28, the bone marrow is essential in immune and hematological system cell production. **Hematopoiesis,** or blood cell production, takes place in the bone marrow. Hematopoiesis is a complicated process involving the differentiation of stem cells in the bone marrow into various immune and hematopoietic cells. These cells carry out different bodily functions (Fig. 25.3). As discussed in Chapter 28, certain medications, *colony-stimulating factors,* can stimulate certain types of cell production that may be low.

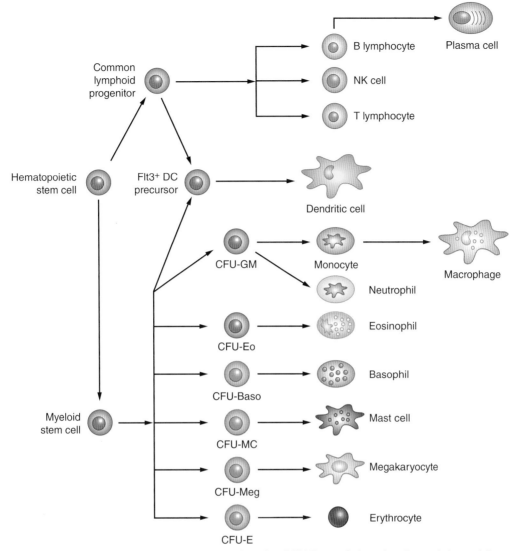

FIG. 25.3 Differentiation of hematopoietic cells. *CFU-Baso,* Colony-forming unit–basophil; *CFU-E,* CFU-erythroid; *CFU-Eo,* CFU-eosinophil; *CFU-GM,* CFU–granulocyte, monocyte; *CFU-MC,* CFU–mast cell; *CFU-Meg,* CFU-megakaryocyte; *DC,* dendritic cell; *NK,* natural killer (cell). (From Huether S, McCance K. *Understanding Pathophysiology.* 5th ed. St. Louis: Mosby; 2012.)

- *Macrophages:* Macrophages are powerful phagocytes important in immune and inflammatory responses. The bone marrow produces immature macrophages, **monocytes,** which migrate to tissues where they mature and fight infections. Macrophages also ingest dead or defective cells. Macrophages additionally act as **antigen-presenting cells (APCs);** this means that when macrophages come in contact with an **antigen** (eg, a bacterium) in the tissues, they migrate to the lymph nodes to signal T and B cells to gear up to fight infection.
- *Mast cells:* Mast cells play various roles in the immune system, including wound healing and pathogenic defense. However, mast cells are best known for their role in allergies and anaphylactic reactions (discussed later). Mast cells contain histamine, which they release during an allergic response.
- *Natural killer (NK) cells:* NK cells are a lymphocyte form that specializes in killing tumor cells and some virus-infected cells as part of the innate immune response. The bone marrow produces NK cells to circulate through the bloodstream.
- *T cells:* T cells, or T lymphocytes, contribute to the adaptive immune response. The thymus produces T cells that remain in the spleen and lymph nodes until they are activated by APCs to attack an invading pathogen.
- *B cells:* B cells, or B lymphocytes, are another critical lymphocyte that acts as an APC. B cells can also differentiate into **plasma cells** that produce **antibodies** against pathogen invaders to help clear infection.

Cytokines are additional mediators that help drive immune responses. **Cytokines,** molecules secreted by a variety of cells (including immune cells), signal inflammation and the immune response activation. Cytokines such as tumor necrosis factor (TNF) and interleukin-1 (IL-1) help drive the inflammatory response (Fig. 25.6). As is discussed

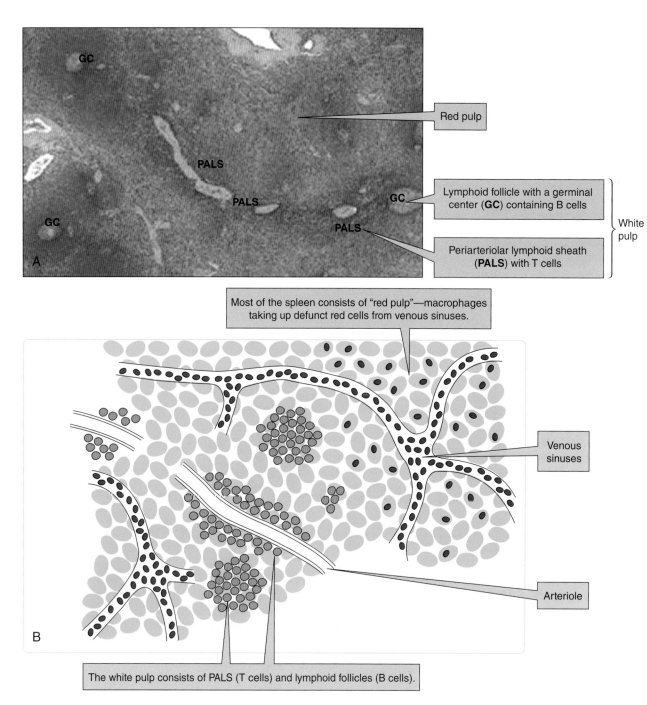

FIG. 25.4 (A) Photomicrograph of spleen specimen. (B) Structures of red pulp and white pulp. (From Nairn R, Helbert M. *Immunology for Medical Students*. 2nd ed. St. Louis: Mosby; 2007.)

later, medications that inhibit cytokine effects can treat conditions of chronic inflammation, such as rheumatoid arthritis (RA).

Types of Immunity

We can divide the immune response into (1) innate immunity and (2) adaptive immunity (Fig. 25.7). **Innate immunity** involves immune system cells that respond rapidly to infection. Phagocytic cells (eg, macrophages and neutrophils) migrate to infection sites and begin to ingest bacteria or other antigens. These cells, in turn, release cytokines to facilitate the inflammatory response to infection. APCs at

the inflammatory site process the antigen for presentation to lymphocytes in the lymph nodes. This preparation helps mount the adaptive immune response.

Many lymphocytes remain in lymph nodes and tissues, waiting to mount an immune response against invading pathogens. The two primary types of lymphocytes are T cells and B cells, described previously. B cells and their products, **immunoglobulins** (antibodies), contribute to **humoral immunity,** also known as *antibody-mediated immunity.* When activated, B cells become plasma cells that produce antibodies specific to an invading antigen. After an immune response, some B cells become memory cells that "remember"

INNATE

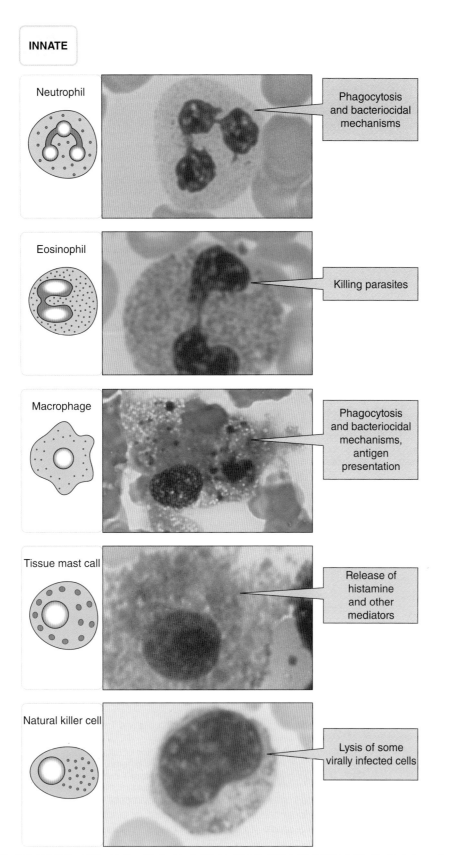

Neutrophil — Phagocytosis and bacteriocidal mechanisms

Eosinophil — Killing parasites

Macrophage — Phagocytosis and bacteriocidal mechanisms, antigen presentation

Tissue mast call — Release of histamine and other mediators

Natural killer cell — Lysis of some virally infected cells

FIG. 25.5 Major cells of the immune system. (From Nairn R, Helbert M. *Immunology for Medical Students*. 2nd ed. St. Louis: Mosby; 2007.)

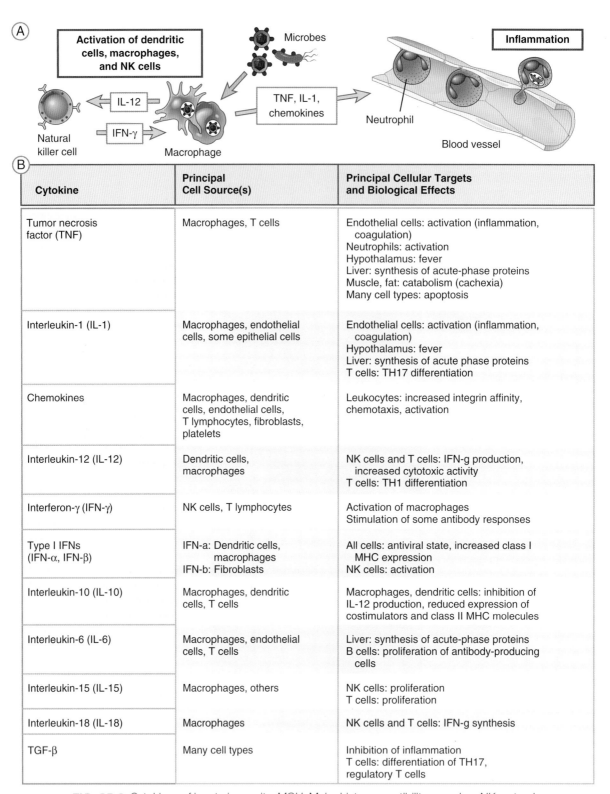

(A)

Activation of dendritic cells, macrophages, and NK cells

Microbes

IL-12

IFN-γ

Natural killer cell

Macrophage

TNF, IL-1, chemokines

Inflammation

Neutrophil

Blood vessel

(B)

Cytokine	Principal Cell Source(s)	Principal Cellular Targets and Biological Effects
Tumor necrosis factor (TNF)	Macrophages, T cells	Endothelial cells: activation (inflammation, coagulation) Neutrophils: activation Hypothalamus: fever Liver: synthesis of acute-phase proteins Muscle, fat: catabolism (cachexia) Many cell types: apoptosis
Interleukin-1 (IL-1)	Macrophages, endothelial cells, some epithelial cells	Endothelial cells: activation (inflammation, coagulation) Hypothalamus: fever Liver: synthesis of acute phase proteins T cells: TH17 differentiation
Chemokines	Macrophages, dendritic cells, endothelial cells, T lymphocytes, fibroblasts, platelets	Leukocytes: increased integrin affinity, chemotaxis, activation
Interleukin-12 (IL-12)	Dendritic cells, macrophages	NK cells and T cells: IFN-g production, increased cytotoxic activity T cells: TH1 differentiation
Interferon-γ (IFN-γ)	NK cells, T lymphocytes	Activation of macrophages Stimulation of some antibody responses
Type I IFNs (IFN-α, IFN-β)	IFN-a: Dendritic cells, macrophages IFN-b: Fibroblasts	All cells: antiviral state, increased class I MHC expression NK cells: activation
Interleukin-10 (IL-10)	Macrophages, dendritic cells, T cells	Macrophages, dendritic cells: inhibition of IL-12 production, reduced expression of costimulators and class II MHC molecules
Interleukin-6 (IL-6)	Macrophages, endothelial cells, T cells	Liver: synthesis of acute-phase proteins B cells: proliferation of antibody-producing cells
Interleukin-15 (IL-15)	Macrophages, others	NK cells: proliferation T cells: proliferation
Interleukin-18 (IL-18)	Macrophages	NK cells and T cells: IFN-g synthesis
TGF-β	Many cell types	Inhibition of inflammation T cells: differentiation of TH17, regulatory T cells

FIG. 25.6 Cytokines of innate immunity. *MCH*, Major histocompatibility complex; *NK*, natural killer (cell). (From Abbas AK, Lichtman AHH. *Basic Immunology Updated Edition: Functions and Disorders of the Immune System*. 4th ed. Philadelphia: Saunders; 2014.)

the invasion for a future date. They can then respond more quickly to a repeat infection. T cells are also in the lymph nodes and remain there until activated by an APC (Fig. 25.8). When enabled, lymph node T cells can divide and expand to form an army of cells to attack and eliminate an invading pathogen. This response can be direct destruction of the attached cell and antigen, or the T cells can release a chemical signal that enlists the help of macrophages to destroy the invading antigen. As with B cells, memory T cells develop. On subsequent exposure to the same antigen, the memory cells produced from the first encounter can rapidly destroy the antigen and prevent disease.

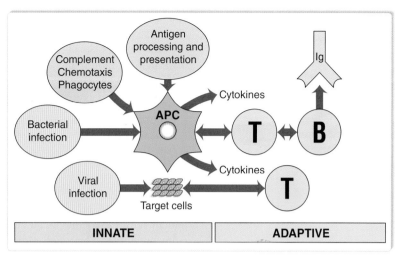

FIG. 25.7 Innate and adaptive immunity. *APC,* Antigen-presenting cell. (From Nairn R, Helbert M. *Immunology for Medical Students.* 2nd ed. St. Louis: Mosby; 2007.)

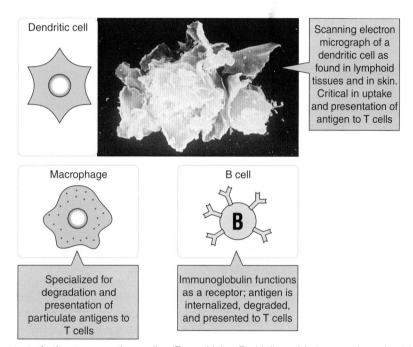

FIG. 25.8 Antigen-presenting cells. (From Nairn R, Helbert M. *Immunology for Medical Students.* 2nd ed. St. Louis: Mosby; 2007.)

The Inflammatory Response

Infection, allergic reactions, or injury can cause **inflammation.** Inflammation is a necessary response to injury. Along with inflammatory swelling, other effects are felt rather than seen. Thousands of years ago, the Romans described inflammatory symptoms such as redness, swelling, heat, pain, and eventual loss of function. The body tries to repair the damage with the help of blood, cells, and natural chemicals. **Vasodilation** occurs during inflammation, allowing more blood to reach the affected area. The increased blood flow creates a warmer area. Edema (buildup of fluids) in the surrounding tissues may develop. Many immune cells previously described migrate to the inflamed area (Fig. 25.9).

The body's cells contain many different chemicals that play a role in inflammation. Each compound has a specific

job. One chemical found in many cells is an enzyme called *cyclooxygenase (COX).* This enzyme produces hormones called *prostaglandins* that are responsible for other chemical reactions that cause inflammation, pain, and increased temperature. Aspirin is one agent that inhibits COX pathways, thereby attenuating the production of prostaglandin. (See Chapter 19 to review other antiinflammatory medications.)

Inflammatory conditions can be either acute or chronic. Acute inflammation characteristically lasts a few days. The body might recover without medications. Chronic inflammation can arise from acute inflammation or injury. Chronic inflammation can occur locally, such as at a cut on the surface of the skin, or **systemically,** throughout the body. When inflammation becomes chronic, the injury site may swell again, and low-grade fever can result. Chronic

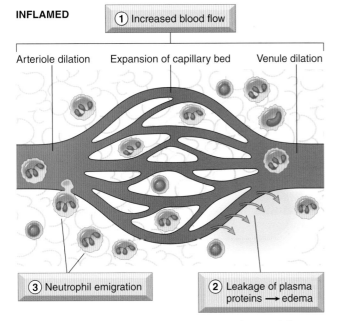

NORMAL

Extracellular matrix

Occasional resident lymphocyte or macrophage

Arteriole

Venule

INFLAMED

① Increased blood flow

Arteriole dilation

Expansion of capillary bed

Venule dilation

③ Neutrophil emigration

② Leakage of plasma proteins → edema

FIG. 25.9 The major local manifestations of acute inflammation. (From Kumar V, Abbas AK. *Robbins and Cotran Pathologic Basis of Disease*. 8th ed. Philadelphia: Saunders; 2010.)

inflammation can cause damage to affected sites or internal organs. As the body heals, it may leave scar tissue. This scar tissue can alter the affected area's physiology. For instance, scarring of the heart can affect its ability to pump or circulate blood. If pelvic inflammatory disease (PID) scars fallopian tubes, a woman may become sterile (see Chapter 24). Inflammation can damage the kidneys to the extent that a person requires dialysis. Pain can accompany inflammation and swelling.

Anaphylaxis

Anaphylaxis is the most severe case of an allergic reaction. It can be deadly without immediate treatment. For most people, allergies are inconvenient but not life-threatening. For others, a reaction can cause airway swelling within minutes. Most people have an allergic reaction to one agent or another in their lifetime, and it may occur more than once. Individuals who know they can experience anaphylactic shock from a bee sting or other allergic reaction should always carry an

epinephrine autoinjector (eg, EpiPen or EpiPen Jr.) in case they are stung or have an allergic exposure. This device is available in packs of two injectors per kit in strengths of 0.15 mg for children and 0.3 mg for adults.

> ### Tech Note!
> For detailed information on EpiPen use, visit this website: *https://www.epipen.com/en/about-epipen-and-generic/how-to-use-epipen.*

Drug Allergy Versus Drug Intolerance

A drug allergy is an allergic response to a drug where the patient may experience facial swelling, hives, rash, or difficulty breathing. This often-rapid reaction can be mild or, more rarely, fatal. A drug intolerance is a negative drug side effect that might result in discontinuation or nonadherence. Differentiating between these effects allows the medical team to choose the appropriate treatment.

A commonly reported drug allergy is to penicillin. Patients with a true penicillin allergy can experience rash, hives, or an anaphylactic-type hypersensitivity reactions. These patients should not use penicillins or related drugs like cephalosporins.

Other patients may report penicillin-caused GI upset, which is a more benign side effect common to antibiotics but is not a true penicillin allergy; rather, it is a drug intolerance. The patient would be tested for a true allergy before trying related medicines. Patients can also find drug intolerance and allergies in response to the inactive ingredients such as preservatives, dyes, egg, gelatin, gluten, and more.

Drug allergies are unpredictable and occur from an overly responsive immune system. Some common drugs, besides penicillin, that are associated with drug allergies include antibiotics such as sulfa drugs and anticonvulsants such as carbamazepine and lamotrigine.

Drug intolerance does not involve the immune system and is somewhat predictable. For example, angiotensin-converting enzyme inhibitors (ACEIs) like lisinopril can cause dry cough. Other common drug intolerance symptoms can include dizziness, drowsiness, nausea, and even vomiting. The prescriber would have to weigh the intolerance against the need for the medication.

Autoimmune Disorders

Although the immune system can efficiently recognize and eliminate invaders, it can sometimes mistake healthy cells for foreign material and mount an immune response against healthy tissues. We refer to this as autoimmunity. There are several autoimmune disorders. Type 1 diabetes mellitus (T1DM; see Chapter 18) is one example. In T1DM, immune system cells attack and destroy the insulin-producing pancreatic beta cells. Therefore patients with T1DM require insulin treatment to manage their blood glucose levels. Other autoimmune disorders include Crohn disease (see Chapter 22), myasthenia gravis (see Chapter 17), and certain dermatological conditions (eg, psoriasis). This chapter discusses the treatment of systemic lupus erythematosus

(SLE), RA, Graves disease, and Hashimoto thyroiditis (also known as *Hashimoto disease*).

In many autoimmune disorder treatments, the therapy aims to suppress the immune system. Medicines known as **biological response modifiers (BRMs)** are targeted therapies that can "turn off" certain immune cells or neutralize cytokines to diminish a destructive inflammatory process. Table 25.1 provides examples of BRMs and other immunomodulating agents for autoimmune disorders, cancer treatments, and organ transplant rejection prevention.

◼ TABLE 25.1

Select Biological Response Modifiers and Immunomodulators for Treatment of Autoimmune Disorders and Transplant Rejection Prophylaxis

Generic Name	Trade Name	Indications[a]	Common Dosage Range[b]	Common Side Effects
Calcineurin Inhibitors				
cyclosporine A	Gengraf, Sandimmune	Transplant rejections Rheumatoid arthritis Severe psoriasis	• 2.5–5 mg/kg/day PO in divided doses twice daily	• Gum hyperplasia • Nephrotoxicity • Neurotoxicity
tacrolimus	Astagraf XL, Prograf, Envarsus XR	Organ rejections	• *Immediate-release oral:* 0.1–0.2 mg/kg/day PO in divided doses twice daily • *IV:* CIVI 0.03–0.05 mg/kg/day	• Headache • Hypertension • Nephrotoxicity • Neurotoxicity • Tremor
Antimetabolites				
mycophenolate mofetil	CellCept, Myfortic	Solid-organ transplant	• 1 g PO/IV twice daily	• Leukopenia • Nausea • Thrombocytopenia • Vomiting
azathioprine	Imuran, Azasan	Renal transplant Rheumatoid arthritis	• *IV/oral:* 1–3 mg/kg/day	• Leukopenia • Nausea • Thrombocytopenia • Vomiting
Rapamycin Inhibitors				
sirolimus	Rapamune	Renal transplant	• 1–15 mg PO once daily	• Anemia • Hypercholesterolemia • Peripheral edema
everolimus	Zortress, Afinitor	Transplant rejection prophylaxis and cancer treatments	• *Cancer:* 10 mg/day PO • *Rejection prophylaxis:* 1 mg twice daily	• Anemia • Fever • Hypercholesterolemia • Peripheral edema • Rash
Oral Disease-Modifying Antirheumatic Drugs (DMARDs)				
methotrexate	Trexall, Otrexup, Rasuvo, Xatmep	Breast cancer Transplant Lymphoma Leukemia Osteosarcoma Psoriasis	• *RA:* 7.5 mg PO once weekly (titrate up to 10–15 mg) (max 20–30 mg/wk)	• Alopecia • Diarrhea • Leukopenia • Nausea • Photosensitivity • Vomiting
sulfasalazine	Azulfidine	Rheumatoid arthritis Ulcerative colitis	• *Maintenance:* 1 g twice daily	• Headache • Nausea • Rash
Glucocorticoids				
prednisone	Deltasone	Acute exacerbations of multiple sclerosis	• 5–200 mg/day PO	• Cushing syndrome • Fluid retention
prednisolone	Orapred	Asthma exacerbations Multiple sclerosis	• 5–200 mg/day PO	• Hyperglycemia • Hypernatremia
dexamethasone	DexPak[a], ZonaCort[a]	Endocrine disorders Asthma exacerbations Multiple sclerosis	• 0.5–30 mg in divided doses	• Hypertension • Myopathy • Osteoporosis

Continued

Select Biological Response Modifiers and Immunomodulators for Treatment of Autoimmune Disorders and Transplant Rejection Prophylaxis—cont'd

Generic Name	Trade Name	Indications[a]	Common Dosage Range[b]	Common Side Effects
Biological Response Modifiers: Tumor Necrosis Factor (TNF)-Alpha Inhibitors				
adalimumab	Humira	Crohn disease Ulcerative colitis Psoriasis Rheumatoid arthritis Ankylosing spondylitis	• *Loading dose*: 80–160 mg • 40 mg subcut every other wk	• Headache • Hematological toxicities • Injection site reactions • Sinusitis
certolizumab pegol	Cimzia	Crohn disease Rheumatoid arthritis Psoriatic arthritis Ankylosing spondylitis	• 400 mg subcut at 0, 2, 4 wk; then 200 mg subcut every other wk or 400 mg every 4 wk	• Arthralgia • Infections • Urinary tract infection • Cancers
etanercept	Enbrel	Rheumatoid arthritis Psoriatic arthritis Ankylosing spondylitis	• 50 mg/wk subcut	• Infections • Injection site reactions • Rhinitis • Cancers
golimumab	Simponi	Psoriasis arthritis Rheumatoid arthritis Ankylosing spondylitis Ulcerative colitis	• 50 mg/mo subcut with methotrexate	• Infections • Injection site reactions • Cancers
infliximab	Remicade, Inflectra, Renflexis	Crohn disease Psoriasis Rheumatoid arthritis Ankylosing spondylitis Ulcerative colitis	• 3–5 mg/kg IV at 0, 2, 6 wk; then every 8 wk	• Abdominal pain • Leukopenia • Nausea • Rash
Biological Response Modifiers: Interleukin Antagonists				
anakinra	Kineret	Rheumatoid arthritis	• 100 mg/day subcut	• Diarrhea • Infections • Injection site reactions • Nausea • Neutropenia
tocilizumab	Actemra	Rheumatoid arthritis Systemic juvenile idiopathic arthritis	• *IV:* 4 mg/kg IV every 4 wk (max 800 mg/infusion) • *Subcut:* 162 mg once wkly (>100 kg) or every other week (<100 kg)	• Diarrhea • Elevated liver enzymes • Hypertension • Neutropenia • Rash • Cancers
basiliximab	Simulect	Solid-organ transplant	• 20 mg IV on postoperative days 0 and 4	• Abdominal pain • Edema • Fever • Hypertension • UTI
Biological Response Modifiers: Lymphocyte-Specific Agents				

abatacept	Orencia	Juvenile idiopathic arthritis
		Rheumatoid arthritis
		Psoriatic arthritis
			• *Subcut:* 125 mg once weekly
			• *IV maintenance dosing:* every 4 wk:
			  <60 kg: 500 mg
			  60–100 kg: 750 mg
			  >100 kg: 1 g
				• Headache
				• Nausea
				• UTI

belatacept	Nulojix	Kidney transplant rejection	• *Initial:* 10 mg/kg on days 1 and 5, end of wk 2, 4, 8, and 12 • *Maintenance:* 5 mg/kg every 4 wk	• Diarrhea • Edema • Electrolyte imbalances • Fever • Infection

Select Biological Response Modifiers and Immunomodulators for Treatment of Autoimmune Disorders and Transplant Rejection Prophylaxis—cont'd

Generic Name	Trade Name	Indications[a]	Common Dosage Range[b]	Common Side Effects
rituximab	Rituxan	Rheumatoid arthritis Many cancers	• 1000 mg IV infusion on days 1 and 15 with methotrexate	• Fatigue • Fever • Infusion reaction • Nausea • Neuropathy • Rash • Tumor lysis syndrome
belimumab	Benlysta	Systemic lupus erythematosus	• *IV:* 10 mg/kg every 2 wk for 3 doses, then every 4 wk • *Subcut:* 200 mg once wkly	• Diarrhea • Infusion reactions • Nausea
glatiramer	Copaxone	Multiple sclerosis	• 20 mg subcut once daily *or* • 40 mg 3 times wkly	• Chest tightness • Dyspnea • Flushing • Pain/itching at injection site
natalizumab	Tysabri	Multiple sclerosis Crohn disease	• 300 mg IV infusion over 1 hr every 4 wk	• Depression • Flulike symptoms • Rash
alemtuzumab	Campath[c]	B-cell and T-cell cancers Leukemias Transplant prophylaxis Multiple sclerosis	• Depends on indication and dosage form	• Fever • Hypotension • Injection site reaction • Nausea • Rash • Vomiting
Interferons				
interferon beta-1b	Betaseron, Extavia	Multiple sclerosis	• 0.0625 mg subcut every other day (target dose 0.25 mg every other day)	• Depression • Flulike symptoms • Injection site reaction
interferon beta-1a	Avonex	Multiple sclerosis	• 30 mcg IM once/wk	• Flulike symptoms • Leukopenia • Nausea
	Rebif	—	• 22 or 44 mcg subcut 3 times wkly	
Biological Response Modifier: Anthracenedione				
Mitoxantrone	None	Multiple sclerosis (MS) Prostate cancer Acute nonlymphocytic leukemias	• *MS:* 12 mg/m^2 IV infusion every 3 mo (max lifetime dose 140 mg/m^2)	• Cardiotoxicity • Diarrhea • Hepatotoxicity • Nausea • Vomiting

CIVI, Continuous intravenous infusion; *IM,* intramuscularly; *IV,* intravenous; *PO,* orally; *subcut,* subcutaneously; *UTI,* urinary tract infection.

[a]Indications listed include both FDA-approved and common off-label uses.

[b]Doses can vary depending on the formulation and indication for use.

[c]Brand discontinued; now available only as generic.

Systemic Lupus Erythematosus

Systemic lupus erythematosus (SLE) is a chronic inflammatory disease that can affect many tissues and organs, including the joints, kidneys, skin, gastrointestinal tract, cardiovascular system, and nervous system. Nearly all patients with SLE can experience various symptoms that are somewhat nonspecific to the condition, such as fatigue, fever, and weight changes. Autoantibody production is an SLE hallmark. Although the condition's exact cause is unknown, a variety of conditions and events have been linked to SLE flares or first symptom occurrence. Such events include pregnancy, severe infections, exposure to ultraviolet light, and surgery.

Prognosis

The clinical course of SLE is highly variable and often associated with periods of remission and chronic or acute symptomatic relapses. As mentioned previously, patients with SLE can experience various symptoms related to an inflammatory involvement of virtually any body organ. The prognosis for any given patient is highly dependent on the level and/or presence of severe organ dysfunction as a result of the inflammatory process associated with SLE. Many markers of disease activity have been described, such as antibody levels, erythrocyte sedimentation rate (a measure of fibrosis), and other inflammatory markers that can help determine the condition's severity and drive treatment decisions.

Non-Drug Treatment

Some nonpharmacological strategies can mitigate SLE flares. Sunscreen minimizes exposure to ultraviolet light. Physical activity may also prove beneficial. Researchers associate cigarette smoking with an increased risk for developing SLE. Smoking cessation may help. Providers should encourage patients to update immunizations before immunosuppressant SLE drug initiation. As with all autoimmune disorders, rest, meditation, and stress avoidance can be helpful for non-drug interventions.

Drug Treatment

The primary goal of SLE treatment is to prevent the progression of organ damage through immune system suppression. Nonsteroidal antiinflammatory drugs (NSAIDs), hydroxychloroquine, glucocorticoids, and immunosuppressive agents can provide some relief, though that may come up to 6 months later. Immunosuppressive agents for SLE management include cyclophosphamide, cyclosporine, tacrolimus, methotrexate, belimumab, azathioprine, with anifrolumab (Saphnelo), a monoclonal antibody, a recent addition approved for moderate to severe SLE.

GENERIC NAME: belimumab

TRADE NAME: Benlysta

INDICATION: Systemic lupus erythematosus

ROUTE OF ADMINISTRATION: Intravenous (IV)

COMMON ADULT DOSAGE: 10 mg/kg IV over 1 hour every 2 weeks for the first 3 doses, then once every 4 weeks

MECHANISM OF ACTION: Inhibits B cells from becoming plasma cells and reduces B cell numbers

SIDE EFFECTS: Increased risk for infection, allergic reactions, infusion-related reactions

---

GENERIC NAME: azathioprine

TRADE NAME: Imuran, Azasan

INDICATIONS: Rheumatoid arthritis, prophylaxis of kidney transplant rejection, systemic lupus erythematosus

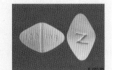

ROUTE OF ADMINISTRATION: Oral; intravenous

COMMON ADULT DOSAGE: *Lupus nephritis (off-label):* 2 mg/kg/day

MECHANISM OF ACTION: Inhibits DNA and RNA synthesis, reducing the formation of immune cells and thus leading to immunosuppression

SIDE EFFECTS: Bone marrow suppression, nausea, vomiting, increased infection risk

AUXILIARY LABEL: Take as directed

GENERIC NAME: hydroxychloroquine

TRADE NAME: Plaquenil

INDICATION: Systemic lupus erythematosus, malaria

ROUTE OF ADMINISTRATION: Oral

COMMON ADULT DOSAGE: 200 to 400 mg daily

MECHANISM OF ACTION: An antimalarial used to suppress autoantibody activity (antibodies present in blood that attack the body's cells)

SIDE EFFECTS: Nausea, diarrhea, retinopathy

Rheumatoid Arthritis

Rheumatoid arthritis (RA) is an autoimmune form of arthritis that is painful and can lead to bone and joint deformation (Fig. 25.10). More women than men have RA, and **juvenile rheumatoid arthritis (JRA)** affects children. In RA, joint inflammation leads to erosion and bone and

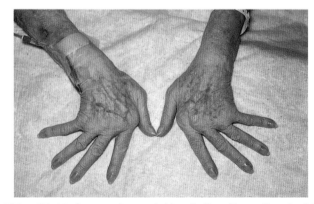

FIG. 25.10 Severe rheumatoid arthritis. (From Swartz M. *Textbook of Physical Diagnosis: History and Examination*. 6th ed. Philadelphia: Saunders; 2009.)

cartilage remodeling. This change makes movement extremely painful. As the disease progresses, joint deformity becomes irreversible. Therefore treatment approaches to RA target both symptomatic management and prevention of joint destruction and disability. Treatment for RA includes physical therapy, medications (antiinflammatories and/or analgesics and disease-modifying antirheumatic drugs [DMARDs]), and diet.

Prognosis

Because rheumatoid arthritis (RA) has no known cure, the only recourse is to slow the progression of this disease, treat the pain associated with the condition, and minimize long-term disability.

Non-Drug Treatment

Treatments include increasing mobility and having the patient obtain psychological counseling if necessary. Physical and occupational therapy can help increase mobility and functionality to maintain independence. Physical activity can also help keep flexibility and joint function.

Drug Treatment

RA medications include nonsteroidal antiinflammatory drugs (NSAIDs), analgesics (nonopioid and opioid), corticosteroids, and disease-modifying antirheumatic drugs (DMARDs). Biological response modifiers (BRMs) are a subcategory of DMARDs that are increasingly being used in early RA to minimize the progression of joint damage. BRMs modify the immune system through inhibition of cytokines and immune cells that contribute to inflammation and cell-mediated joint damage. Examples of DMARDs (including BRMs) are provided in the following monographs and in Table 25.1. For a general review of NSAIDs and other analgesics that are often used in RA, see Chapter 19.

GENERIC NAME: methotrexate

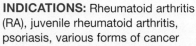

TRADE NAMES: Trexall, Otrexup, Rasuvo, Xatmep

INDICATIONS: Rheumatoid arthritis (RA), juvenile rheumatoid arthritis, psoriasis, various forms of cancer

ROUTES OF ADMINISTRATION: Orally (PO); injectable

COMMON ADULT DOSAGES: *RA:* 7.5 mg PO once weekly or 2.5 mg PO every 12 hours for 3 doses/wk (max 20 mg once weekly)

MECHANISM OF ACTION: Inhibits the dihydrofolate reductase enzyme, inhibiting cell proliferation and leading to immunosuppression

SIDE EFFECTS: Dizziness, fatigue, nausea, mouth ulcers, fever, increased risk for infection

AUXILIARY LABELS:
- Do not take if pregnant
- Avoid alcohol

Tech Note!

Remember that methotrexate is administered once weekly (or every 12 hours for 3 doses). A common pharmacy error is filling methotrexate on a daily schedule. Always check the methotrexate instructions when typing a prescription for this medication.

GENERIC NAME: etanercept

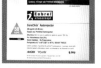

TRADE NAME: Enbrel

INDICATIONS: Rheumatoid arthritis (RA), juvenile rheumatoid arthritis, psoriasis, psoriatic arthritis, ankylosing spondylitis

ROUTE OF ADMINISTRATION: Subcutaneous injection

COMMON ADULT DOSAGE: *RA:* 50 mg/wk

MECHANISM OF ACTION: Inhibits the cytokine tumor necrosis factor, leading to decreased inflammation

SIDE EFFECTS: Diarrhea; injection site reactions; increased infection risk, especially respiratory infection

AUXILIARY LABEL: Dispose of properly

GENERIC NAME: adalimumab

TRADE NAME: Humira

INDICATIONS: Rheumatoid arthritis (RA), juvenile rheumatoid arthritis, Crohn disease, psoriasis, psoriatic arthritis, ulcerative colitis, ankylosing spondylitis

ROUTE OF ADMINISTRATION: Subcutaneous (subcut) injection

COMMON ADULT DOSAGE: *RA:* 40 mg subcut every other week

MECHANISM OF ACTION: Inhibits the cytokine tumor necrosis factor, leading to decreased inflammation

SIDE EFFECTS: Headache, skin rash, injection site reactions, increased infection risk

AUXILIARY LABEL: Dispose of properly

GENERIC NAME: abatacept

TRADE NAME: Orencia

INDICATIONS: Rheumatoid arthritis, juvenile rheumatoid arthritis, psoriasis

ROUTES OF ADMINISTRATION: Injection (intravenous [IV] and subcutaneous [subcut])

COMMON ADULT DOSAGES: *IV:* After the initial IV infusion (<60 kg: 500 mg, 60–100 kg: 750 mg, >100 kg: 1000 mg), repeat IV infusion at 2 weeks and 4 weeks after the initial infusion and every 4 weeks after that; *subcut:* 125 mg/wk subcut

MECHANISM OF ACTION: Inhibits T-cell activation, diminishing T-cell responses

SIDE EFFECTS: Headache, nausea, dizziness, injection site reactions, increased risk for infection

AUXILIARY LABEL: Dispose of properly

Graves Disease

Graves disease is an autoimmune disorder that results in thyroid gland overstimulation leading to hyperthyroidism. In this condition, the immune system produces antibodies that bind to and activate thyroid-stimulating hormone (TSH) receptors in the thyroid gland, leading to an increased release of thyroid hormone. Graves disease is the underlying cause of 50% to 80% of cases of hyperthyroidism. This condition is seen more commonly in women. Various clinical manifestations are associated with Graves disease (Fig. 25.11).

Prognosis

The prognosis for Graves disease can be good if the condition is identified early and the patient receives proper treatment. Although medication, radioactive iodine, and surgical interventions can effectively manage most symptoms, current treatments do not reverse symptoms of infiltrative ophthalmopathy or myxedema.

Non-Drug Treatment

No non-drug treatments are available for Graves disease.

Drug Treatment

Therapy for Graves disease includes antithyroid medications such as propylthiouracil or methimazole, radioactive iodine, or surgery.

GENERIC NAME:
propylthiouracil (PTU)

TRADE NAME: None

INDICATION: Hyperthyroidism

ROUTE OF ADMINISTRATION: Oral

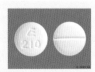

COMMON ADULT DOSAGES: *Initial:* 300–400 mg/day in 3 divided doses; *maintenance:* 100–150 mg/day in 3 divided doses

MECHANISM OF ACTION: Directly interferes with the first step in thyroid hormone synthesis, thus leading to a decrease in thyroid hormone production. Full effect takes 3–4 weeks

SIDE EFFECTS: Nausea, headache, urticaria rash

AUXILIARY LABEL: Take as directed

GENERIC NAME: methimazole

TRADE NAME: Tapazole

INDICATION: Hyperthyroidism

ROUTE OF ADMINISTRATION: Oral

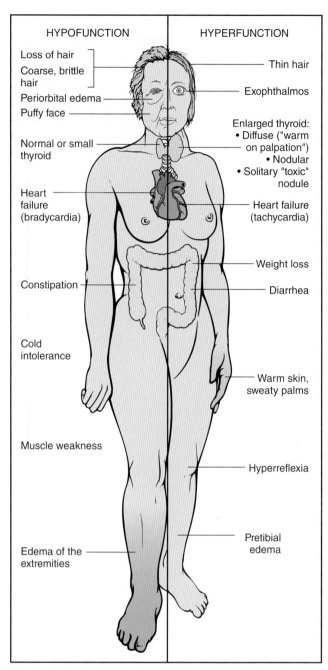

FIG. 25.11 Clinical manifestations of hyperthyroidism and hypothyroidism. (From McCance KL. *Pathophysiology: The Biologic Basis for Disease in Adults and Children.* 6th ed. St. Louis: Mosby; 2010.)

COMMON ADULT DOSAGES: *Initial:* 15–60 mg/day; *maintenance:* 5–15 mg/day. Full effect takes 3–4 weeks

MECHANISM OF ACTION: Directly interferes with the first step in thyroid hormone synthesis, thus leading to a decrease in thyroid hormone production

SIDE EFFECTS: Fever, rash, itching

AUXILIARY LABEL: Take as directed

Hashimoto Thyroiditis

Hashimoto thyroiditis, the most common cause of hypothyroidism in the United States, is characterized by autoimmune-mediated destruction of the thyroid gland. This autoimmune disease is thought to be the result of a combination of genetic and environmental factors; infection, stress, pregnancy, iodine intake, and radiation exposure are known to be possible precipitating factors for Hashimoto's thyroiditis. (See Chapter 18 for a review of symptoms associated with hypothyroidism.)

Prognosis

The prognosis for Hashimoto thyroiditis is good. Treatment involves thyroid supplementation to achieve a euthyroid state.

Non-Drug Treatment

No non-drug treatments are available for Hashimoto thyroiditis.

Drug Treatment

Thyroid hormone replacement agents must be taken for life (1 dose daily) because of the chronic nature of the condition. Physicians often prescribe levothyroxine because of its ease of dosing (ie, it contains one thyroid hormone, thyroxine [T_4]; see Chapter 18 for a detailed discussion of hypothyroidism treatment).

Transplant Rejection

Another use of immunosuppressive agents is in organ transplant rejection management. Because organ transplants involve foreign donated organs, a risk with transplantation is **transplant rejection.** In transplant rejection, the host's immune system recognizes the transplanted organ as foreign and attacks it (Fig. 25.12). To avoid transplant rejection, health providers use immunosuppressive drugs to suppress the immune system and keep the organ viable. Immunosuppressive drugs used in transplant rejection include corticosteroids, antimetabolites, calcineurin inhibitors, rapamycin inhibitors, and belatacept (Nulojix). Table 25.1 provides examples of agents for transplant rejection prophylaxis. Nonpharmacological approaches to preventing infection are critical when immunosuppressive agents are used. Individuals with immunosuppression risk infection when around people who are ill. In some instances, the risk warrants face masks and isolation.

Tech Note!

Immunosuppressive drugs not only have drug interactions, but suppressing the immune system puts patients at risk for infection, so it is doubly important to notify pharmacists of drug-drug interaction alerts.

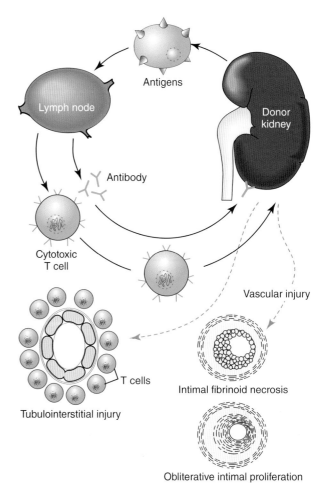

FIG. 25.12 Transplant rejection is antibody mediated, cell mediated, or both. (From Damjanov I. *Pathology for the Health Professions*. 4th ed. Philadelphia: Saunders; 2011.)

GENERIC NAME: sirolimus

TRADE NAME: Rapamune

INDICATION: Prophylaxis of kidney transplant rejection

ROUTE OF ADMINISTRATION: Oral

COMMON ADULT DOSAGES: Dosing depends on patient weight, immunological risk, and trough levels

MECHANISM OF ACTION: Inhibition of T-cell activation and proliferation

SIDE EFFECTS: Hyperlipidemia, hypertension, headache, edema, increased risk for infection

AUXILIARY LABEL: Do not administer with grapefruit juice

GENERIC NAME: belatacept

TRADE NAME: Nulojix

INDICATION: Prophylaxis of kidney transplant rejection

ROUTE OF ADMINISTRATION: Intravenous (IV)

COMMON ADULT DOSAGES: *Maintenance:* 5 mg/kg IV over 30 minutes every 4 weeks

MECHANISM OF ACTION: Blocks the activation of T cells, inhibiting T-cell functions

SIDE EFFECTS: Increased risk for infection, diarrhea, nausea, vomiting, infusion reactions

Immunizations

Historically, thousands of children died from diseases such as measles and mumps or have been physically scarred by the effects of polio. Although children still can contract these diseases today, they are seen less commonly, and death is rare because of the widespread use of **immunizations.** Many **vaccines** are available (Table 25.2).

TABLE 25.2
Vaccines Available in the United States (2017)

Vaccine	Trade Name	Type	Route	Comments
Adenovirus	Adenovirus	Live viral	Oral	Approved for military populations age 17–50 y
Anthrax	BioThrax	Inactivated bacterial	IM	Reserved in the event of a biological warfare emergency
DTaP	Daptacel, Infanrix	Inactivated bacterial	IM	Tetanus and diphtheria toxoids and acellular pertussis vaccine; minimum age 6 wk
DT	Generic	Inactivated bacterial toxoids	IM	Pediatric formulation (through age 6)
DTaP–IPV	Kinrix, Quadracel	Inactivated bacterial and viral	IM	Licensed for fifth (DTaP) and fourth (IPV) booster at 4–6 y
DTaP–Hep B–IPV	Pediarix	Inactivated bacterial and viral	IM	Licensed for doses at 2, 4, and 6 mo (through age 6 y); not licensed for boosters
DTaP–IPV/Hib	Pentacel	Inactivated bacterial and viral	IM	Licensed for 4 doses at 2, 4, 6, and 15–18 mo
Haemophilus influenzae type b (Hib)	PedvaxHIB	Inactivated bacterial	IM	—
	ActHIB	Inactivated bacterial	IM	—
	Hiberix	Inactivated bacterial	IM	Booster only Age range 1–4 y
Hepatitis A (Hep A)	Havrix	Inactivated viral	IM	Pediatric and adult formulations available; minimum age 12 mo
Hepatitis A	Vaqta	Inactivated viral	IM	Pediatric and adult formulations available; minimum age 12 mo
Hepatitis B (Hep B)	Engerix-B	Inactivated viral	IM	3-dose series started at birth; pediatric and adult formulations available
	Recombivax HB	Inactivated viral	IM	Pediatric, adult, and dialysis formulations available; 2 pediatric doses = 1 adult dose
Hepatitis A–hepatitis B	Twinrix	Inactivated viral	IM	Pediatric dose of Hep A + adult dose of Hep B; minimum age 18 y; 3-dose routine series
Herpes zoster (shingles)	Zostavax	Live attenuated viral	Subcut	Licensed for 50 y; recommended to give at 60 y or older
	Shingrix[a]	Nonlive recombinant subunit	IM	Licensed for 50 y
Human papillomavirus (HPV)	Gardasil 9	Inactivated viral	IM	Licensed for males and females 9–26 y
	Cervarix[b]	Inactivated viral	IM	Licensed for females 9–26 y

Vaccine	Trade Name	Type	Route	Comments
Influenza (trivalent, types A and B)	Fluarix	Inactivated viral	IM	Minimum age 3 y
	Fluvirin[b], Flucelvax	Inactivated viral	IM	Minimum age 4 y
	Fluzone	Inactivated viral	IM	Age range, 6 mo–3 y, depending on the amount in a prefilled syringe
	Fluzone high-dose, Fluad	Inactivated viral	IM	Licensed for ≥65 y
	Fluzone Intradermal	Inactivated viral	Intradermal	Age range 18–64 y
	Flublok	Recombinant	IM	Licensed for ≥18 y
	Flulaval	Inactivated viral	IM	Minimum age 6 mo
	Afluria Quadrivalent	Inactivated viral	IM	Minimum age 18 y; nonquadrivalent ≥9 y
	FluMist Quadrivalent	Live attenuated viral	Intranasal	2–49 y
Japanese encephalitis	Ixiaro	Inactivated viral	IM	Licensed for ≥17 y; 2-dose series
Measles-mumps-rubella	M-M-R II	Live attenuated viral	Subcut	Minimum age 12 mo; 2-dose series
Measles-mumps-rubella-varicella	ProQuad	Live attenuated viral	Subcut	Age range 1–12 y; 2-dose series
Meningococcal	Menactra	Inactivated bacterial	IM	Age range 9 mo–55 y
	Menveo	Inactivated bacterial	IM	Age range 2–55 y
	Bexsero, Trumenba	Recombinant proteins	IM	Age range 10–25 y
Pneumococcal	Pneumovax 23	Inactivated bacterial	Subcut or IM	Minimum age 2 y; normally given 1 y after Prevnar 13 regimen
	Prevnar 13	Inactivated bacterial	IM	Age ranges 6 wk through 5 y and ≥50 y
Polio	IPOL	Inactivated viral	Subcut or IM	Trivalent, types 1, 2, 3
Rabies	Imovax Rabies, RabAvert	Inactivated viral	IM	
Rotavirus	RotaTeq, Rotarix	Live viral	Oral	*RotaTeq:* First dose between 6 wk and 14 wk 6 days; complete 3-dose series by 8 mo *Rotarix:* Same as for RotaTeq but in a 2-dose series
Tetanus (reduced), diphtheria (Td)	Tenivac	Inactivated bacterial toxoids	IM	Adult formulation (≥7 y)
Tetanus (reduced), diphtheria (reduced) Pertussis (Tdap)	Boostrix, Adacel	Inactivated bacterial	IM	Tetanus and diphtheria toxoids and pertussis vaccine; minimum age 10 y *Adacel:* Acellular; age range 11–64 y
Tetanus toxoid	(Generic)	Inactivated bacterial toxoid	IM	May be used for adults or children
Typhoid	Typhim Vi	Inactivated bacterial	IM	
	Vivotif Berna	Live attenuated bacterial	Oral	
Vaccinia (smallpox)	ACAM2000	Live attenuated viral	Percutaneous	Minimum age 16 y
Varicella	Varivax	Live attenuated viral	Subcut	Minimum age 12 mo; 2-dose series
Yellow fever	YF-Vax	Live attenuated viral	Subcut	Minimum age 9 mo

[a]From *https://www.gsk.com/en-gb/media/press-releases/shingrix-approved-in-the-us-for-prevention-of-shingles-in-adults-aged-50-and-over/*.
[b]Brand no longer available.

DT, Diphtheria-tetanus; *DTaP–Hep B–IPV,* diphtheria-tetanus-pertussis–hepatitis B–inactivated poliovirus; *DTaP–IPV,* diphtheria-tetanus-pertussis–inactivated poliovirus; *DTaP–IPV/Hib,* diphtheria-tetanus-pertussis–inactivated poliovirus/*Haemophilus influenzae* type b; *IM,* intramuscular; *subcut,* subcutaneous.

When practitioners immunize children and adults, communities are better protected against diseases such as chickenpox, measles, and influenza. People with weakened immune systems, such as older adults, patients undergoing chemotherapy, transplant recipients, and individuals with acquired immunodeficiency syndrome (AIDS), are also at higher risk for developing and even dying from communicable diseases. Another high-risk group includes individuals from countries where immunizations are unavailable. Because children are at high risk for catching and spreading many infectious diseases, a series of immunizations has been recommended to protect children and to promote community health (Table 25.3). In the United States, children cannot register for school unless they have proof of their immunizations or have obtained and filed appropriate medical or religious exemptions. A variety of immunizations are likewise recommended for adults (Table 25.4), such as annual influenza vaccines and herpes zoster vaccines to prevent shingles.

The administration of vaccines results in the development of active acquired immunity. Vaccines can be either live or inactive. Live vaccines must be **attenuated** (weakened) so that they do not cause disease. Once the body manufactures antibodies against the injected antigen, it has long-lasting immunity. With vaccines made from killed or inactive antigens, the risk for infection is lower. The disadvantage of using killed or inactive antigens in a vaccine is that booster shots are needed to maintain a sufficient level of antibodies to prevent disease.

Vaccine Types
Viral Vaccines

Some available vaccines (eg, measles, mumps, rubella [MMR]; oral polio; oral rotavirus; intranasal influenza; smallpox [vaccinia]; and varicella [chickenpox]) contain live **viruses** that have been attenuated before they are given to patients. The **virions** taken are weakened so that they do not cause disease. The attenuated virus may replicate but at a prolonged rate. A person with an active immune system quickly begins to make a full complement of antibodies and antigen-induced reactions that produce immunity. The advantage of live vaccine administration is the durable and complete immunity produced. However,

TABLE 25.3
Centers for Disease Control and Prevention Recommended Immunization Schedule: Birth to 18 Years (2017)

Vaccine	Birth	1 mo	2 mo	4 mo	6 mo	12 mo	15 mo	18 mo	19–23 mo	2–3 y	4–6 y	7–10 y	11–12 y	13–18 y
DTaP	—	—	✓	✓	✓	—		✓	—	—	✓	—	—	—
Tdap	—	—	—	—	—	—	—	—	—	—	—	—	✓	—
Hep A	—	—	—	—	—		✓		—	—	—	—	—	—
Hep B	✓	✓	—			✓			—	—	—	—	—	—
Hib	—	—	✓	✓	✓		✓	—	—	—	—	—	—	—
HPV	—	—	—	—	—	—		—	—	—	—	—	✓	✓
Influenza	—	—	—	—	✓ Recommended yearly									
MCV	—	—	—	—	—		—	—	—	—	—	—	✓	✓
MMR	—	—	—	—	—	✓		—	—	—	✓	—	—	—
PCV	—	—	✓	✓	✓	✓		—	—	—	—	—	—	—
Polio	—	—	✓	✓		✓		—	—	—	✓	—	—	—
Rotavirus	—	—	✓	✓	✓	—	—	—	—	—	—	—	—	—
Varicella	—	—	—	—	—	✓		—	—	—	✓	—	—	—

DTaP, Diphtheria-tetanus-pertussis; *Hep A*, hepatitis A; *Hep B*, hepatitis B; *Hib*, Haemophilus influenzae type b; *HPV*, human papillomavirus; *MCV*, meningococcal vaccine; *MMR*, measles-mumps-rubella; *PCV*, pneumococcal conjugate vaccine.

TABLE 25.4

Centers for Disease Control and Prevention: Recommended Adult Immunization Schedule (2017)

Vaccine	19–26 y	27–49 y	50–59 y	60–64 y	≥65 y
Tdap/Td	✓ Substitute Tdap for Td once, then Td booster every 10 y				
HPV	✓	—	—	—	—
Influenza	✓ Recommended yearly				
MMR	✓			—	—
PCV13	—	—	—	—	✓
PPSV23	—	—	—	—	✓
Varicella	✓ Adults without evidence of immunity to varicella 2 doses 4–8 weeks apart, or a second dose if they have received only 1 dose.				
Zoster	—	—	—	✓	✓

DTaP, Diphtheria-tetanus-pertussis; *PPSV,* pneumococcal polysaccharide vaccine; *Td,* tetanus-diphtheria.

if a person is immunocompromised, live vaccines could carry a risk for disease and other problems. (See the table at the beginning of the chapter, which presents examples of medications that cause immunosuppression; administration of vaccines to patients with immunosuppression should be avoided.)

An inactivated viral vaccine is one in which the virus products are grown in culture, and the virus is then destroyed so that it cannot replicate and cause disease. Although much of the virus is destroyed, the viral capsid proteins (outer shells) remain intact and are easily recognized by the immune system. Because the capsule, or outer shell, of the antigen does not continually reinforce the response needed for the body to resist further attacks, boosters must be given to remind the body to develop antibodies in the immune system.

Bacterial Vaccines

The typhoid vaccine is an example of a live-attenuated bacterial vaccine. Some vaccines are referred to as **toxoids;** these are inactivated bacterial toxins. Although the bacterial cell has been altered so that it cannot cause disease, it still can induce an antibody response in the body.

Many people think that immunizations are not necessary after 18 years of age. However, some vaccines, such as the tetanus toxoid, should be given to adults. Although the tetanus immunizations given to children are combined with diphtheria and pertussis, tetanus booster immunizations should be given every 10 years throughout a person's lifetime. Tetanus is a disease caused by a toxin-secreting bacterium that can be contracted through scrapes and cuts caused by dirty objects.

Tech Note!

The tuberculosis vaccine is routinely administered in many countries, such as the Philippines. Although a vaccine is available for tuberculosis, it is not used in the United States because a tuberculosis vaccine does not guarantee immunity. If a vaccine is given, antibodies are developed against the antigen; therefore all tuberculosis tests would show positive results, and a chest x-ray film would be necessary to rule out active tuberculosis.

A questionnaire helps pharmacists and providers determine vaccine appropriateness. For example, if a patient has a history of severe allergic reactions from a vaccine, an alternative formulation might be dispensed and administered.

Miscellaneous Vaccines

The two most common vaccines are inactivated (killed) and live-attenuated (weakened) vaccines. Other less common types of vaccines are available (Box 25.1). These vaccines are

BOX 25.1 Less Common Vaccines and Their Specific Characteristics

Antiidiotypic vaccines: Antiidiotypic vaccines are a newer type of vaccine based on the use of an antibody that is shaped like the antigen. When the antibody is administered, the body reacts as though it were the antigen. The immune system creates antibodies to fight the disease. In effect, the body is making an antibody against the injected antibody. This second antibody then can be injected to act as the vaccine, and it creates a third antibody. In the future, this method may make it possible to kill deadly viruses such as human immunodeficiency virus (HIV).

Subunit vaccines: Subunit vaccines are small pieces of the genetic code that originate from the disease microbe. These pieces are injected into a bacterium or yeast and then grown. They are harvested and used as a vaccine to stimulate the body to produce an immune response. Because only pieces of the original virion or antigen are used, they do not carry the full extent of immunity provided by a complete antigen. Hepatitis B is a subunit vaccine that is grown in yeast cells and then given as a vaccine.

Acellular and conjugated vaccines: When a vaccine is disassembled or fragmented to isolate specific antigens from entire cells, it is referred to as an *acellular vaccine.* Pertussis is one type of vaccine made in this manner. Bacterial cells that have been altered and mixed with toxoids to increase their overall effectiveness are called *conjugated vaccines* (eg, tetanus and diphtheria).

slightly different in their composition from the usual types. Unfortunately, the only two types of vaccines available are those that protect against viruses and bacterial microbes. Immunizations for diseases caused by a parasite such as malaria and for fungal infections have not been developed to date.

Storage of Vaccines

The CDC guidelines on the storage of vaccines have been established to ensure vaccine effectiveness. Most vaccines should be kept at temperatures between 2°C and 8°C (36°F and 46°F); however, some (eg, varicella vaccine) require freezing until the time of use. Always refer to the storage information for any vaccine product you receive to ensure proper storage and handling.

■ Tech Note!

Follow the manufacturer's instructions on storing vaccines. Vaccines are always kept in either the refrigerator or the freezer at the pharmacy to prevent loss of effectiveness. Never freeze refrigerate-only vaccines because this may compromise their potency and efficacy. A thermometer must be kept in the refrigerator and/or freezer, and the temperature must be documented daily to ensure stability.

Antitoxins and Antivenins

Antitoxins and antivenins are another form of antibody-based therapy that can protect from severe symptoms associated with acute toxins or envenomation. These agents contain antibodies that can neutralize dangerous toxins. For example, stepping on a rusty nail may allow the pathogen *Clostridium tetani* to enter the wound and pass into the bloodstream, where it may develop into a dangerous condition called *tetanus*. Administration of the tetanus antitoxin can protect the individual against this potentially life-threatening condition. Antivenins counteract poison from creatures such as snakes and spiders. Common antitoxins include those for diphtheria, rabies, and botulism. Common antivenins include antivenin for the black widow spider *(Latrodectus mactans)* and Crotalidae polyvalent antivenin against rattlesnake venom.

▼ Tech Alert!

Remember these sound-alike, look-alike drugs:
- Cyclosporine versus cycloserine or cyclophosphamide
- Erlotinib versus gefitinib

Do You Remember These Key Points?

- Names of the major cells and organs that make up the immune system and their functions
- The primary signs and symptoms of the various conditions discussed

- The types of immunizations currently available for children and adults
- Medications used to treat the various conditions discussed in this chapter
- The generic and trade names for the drugs discussed in this chapter
- The appropriate auxiliary labels that should be used when filling prescriptions for drugs discussed in this chapter

---

Review Questions

Multiple Choice Questions

1. Which cells of the immune system produce antibodies?
   A. T cells
   B. Macrophages
   C. Plasma cells
   D. Eosinophils
2. Which lymphoid organ is responsible for the maturation and "education" of T cells?
   A. Lymph nodes
   B. Thymus
   C. Spleen
   D. None of the above
3. Which condition(s) is/are an autoimmune disorder?
   A. Type 1 diabetes mellitus (T1DM)
   B. Systemic lupus erythematosus (SLE)
   C. Rheumatoid arthritis (RA)
   D. All of the above
4. What is the trade name for adalimumab?
   A. Humira
   B. Cimzia
   C. Enbrel
   D. Simponi
5. Vaccines can protect humans against all of the following organisms *except:*
   A. Viruses
   B. Fungi
   C. Bacteria
   D. All of the above
6. The two basic types of immunity are:
   A. Bacterial and viral
   B. Live and inactive
   C. Innate and acquired
   D. Active and passive
7. Vaccines can be altered using which of the following methods?
   A. Attenuated or weakened
   B. Inactivated or killed
   C. Attenuated or activated
   D. A and B
8. When the body comes into contact with a contagious disease, it causes:
   A. Antibodies to be produced
   B. Antigens to be produced
   C. A body rash
   D. No reaction

9. Which of these statements is/are true about toxoids?
   A. Toxoids are bacterial toxins that have been inactivated
   B. All bacterial vaccines are toxoids
   C. Both A and B
   D. None of the above
10. Vaccines composed of small pieces of genetic code harvested from bacteria or yeast are:
   A. Acellular vaccines
   B. Conjugated vaccines
   C. Subunit vaccines
   D. Toxoid vaccines

■ Technician's Corner

Visit the website of the Centers for Disease Control and Prevention at *https://www.cdc.gov/vaccines/schedules/index.html* and review the most recent list of suggested immunizations for children and adults. For conditions with which you are not familiar, review the symptoms and management of that condition.

Bibliography

Abbas AK, Lichtman AHH. *Basic Immunology Updated Edition: Functions and Disorders of the Immune System*. 3rd ed. Philadelphia: Saunders; 2011.

Centers for Disease Control and Prevention (CDC). Immunization Schedules. Available at: www.cdc.gov/vaccines/schedules.

Damjanov I. *Pathology for the Health Professions*. 4th ed. St. Louis: Saunders; 2011.

Fishback JL. *Pathology*. 3rd ed. Philadelphia: Mosby; 2005.

Huether S, McCance K. *Understanding Pathophysiology*. 5th ed. St. Louis: Mosby; 2012.

Kumar V, Abbas AK. *Robbins and Cotran Pathologic Basis of Disease*. 8th ed. Philadelphia: Saunders; 2010.

McCance KL. *Pathophysiology: The Biologic Basis for Disease in Adults and Children*. 6th ed. St. Louis: Mosby; 2010.

Nairn R, Helbert M. *Immunology for Medical Students*. 2nd ed. St. Louis: Mosby; 2007.

Page C, Hoffman B, Curtis M, Walker M. *Integrated Pharmacology*. 3rd ed. London: Mosby; 2006.

Price SA, Wilson LM. *Pathophysiology: Clinical Concepts of Disease Processes*. 6th ed. St. Louis: Mosby; 2003.

Solomon EP. *Introduction to Human Anatomy and Physiology*. 3rd ed. St. Louis: Saunders; 2009.

Thibodeau GA, Patton KT. *Anatomy and Physiology*. 8th ed. St. Louis: Mosby; 2012.

Thompson JM, Farland GK, Hirsch JE, Tucker SM. *Mosby's Clinical Nursing*. 5th ed. St. Louis: Mosby; 2001.

Websites Referenced

UpToDate Online. Available at: www.uptodate.com.

Clinical Pharmacology Online. Available at: https://www.clinicalkey.com/pharmacology/login.

CHAPTER 26

Therapeutic Agents for Eyes, Ears, Nose, and Throat

Tony Guerra

1. Describe the anatomy and physiology of the eyes, ears, nose, and throat.
2. List the primary signs and symptoms of common conditions associated with the eyes, ears, nose, and throat that are discussed in this chapter. In addition, (a) recognize prescription and over-the-counter drugs used to treat common conditions discussed in this chapter, (b) write the generic and trade names for the drugs discussed in this chapter, and (c) list appropriate auxiliary labels when filling prescriptions for drugs discussed in this chapter.

Aqueous humor The fluid found in the anterior chamber of the eye, in front of the lens

Auditory canal A 1-inch segment of the tube that extends from the external ear to the middle ear

Auditory ossicles Hearing + bones, small bones (ossicles) of the middle ear that transmit sound from the eardrum to the inner ear

Auricle The outer projecting portion of the ear

Bactericidal Bacteria + kill, causes bacterial cell death

Bacteriostatic Bacteria + stand still, inhibits bacterial cell growth

Carbonic anhydrase An enzyme that converts carbonic acid into carbon dioxide and water

Cerumen Earwax

Ciliary body The part of the eye that connects the iris to the choroid

Conjunctiva The transparent protective mucous membrane that lines the underside of the eyelid

Cornea The transparent tissue covering the anterior portion of the eye

Eustachian tube A structure in the middle ear that connects with the nasopharynx (throat); it equalizes pressure between the outside air and middle ear and drains mucus

Exudate A mass of cells and fluid that has seeped out of blood vessels as a result of inflammation

Fungicidal Fungi + kill, able to destroy or inhibit the growth of fungi

Glomerulonephritis Acute inflammation of the kidney, typically caused by an immune response

Intraocular pressure (IOP) The pressure exerted by the fluids inside the eyeball

Iris The colored part of the eye seen through the cornea; it consists of smooth muscles that regulate pupil size

Lacrimal fluid The fluid in the eye that cleans and lubricates the eyes

Larynx A hollow muscular organ that forms an air passage to the lungs and holds the vocal cords

Lens Flexible, clear tissue that focuses images

Miosis Contraction of the pupil

Mydriasis Dilation of the pupil

Myopia Nearsightedness

Ophthalmic Eye + pertaining to, pertaining to the eye as in ophthalmic (eye) drops

Orbit The eye socket

Otic Ear + pertaining to, pertaining to the ear as in otic (ear) drops

Ototoxicity Ear + toxicity, toxic effects on the organs of hearing or balance or the auditory nerve

Pharynx The membrane-lined cavity behind the nose and mouth that connects them to the esophagus

Pupil The circular opening in the iris that allows light to enter

Retina The innermost layer of the eye; a complex structure considered part of the central nervous system; the retina contains photoreceptors (rods and cones) that transmit impulses to the optic nerve, in addition to the macula lutea (a yellow spot in the center of the retina)

Rheumatic fever A noncontagious acute fever marked by inflammation and pain in the joints

Sclera The white of the eyes

Sympathomimetic Producing physiological effects resembling those caused by the sympathetic nervous system

Tinnitus Ringing or buzzing in the ears

Tympanic membrane A thin membrane that separates the external ear from the middle ear; also known as the eardrum

Vitreous humor A gel-like substance that fills the posterior cavity of the eye between the lens and retina; it helps maintain the shape of the eye

Select Common Drugs Used for Conditions of the Eye, Ears, Nose, and Throat

Trade Name	Generic Name	Pronunciation
Products for Conditions Affecting the Eye		
Adrenergic Agonists		
Alphagan P	brimonidine	(brih-**moe**-nih-deen)
Afrin	oxymetazoline	(**ox**-ee-**met**-ah-zoe-lin)
Visine Advanced Relief	tetrahydrozoline	(tet-ruh-hye-**droz**-uh-leen)
Mast Cell Stabilizers		
Alocril	nedocromil	(ne-doe-**kroe**-mil)
Alomide	lodoxamide	(low-**dox**-uh-mide)
Opticrom[a]	cromolyn	(**kroe**-moe-lin)
Nonsteroidal Antiinflammatory Drugs (NSAIDs)		
Acular	ketorolac	(**kee**-toe-**role**-ak)
None	flurbiprofen	(**flur**-bih-**pro**-fen)
Voltaren Ophtha[a]	diclofenac	(dye-**kloe**-fen-ak)
Antiinfectives		
Antibiotics		
Ciloxan	ciprofloxacin	(sih-pro-**flox**-uh-sin)
Genoptic, Gentak	gentamicin	(**jen**-tah-**my**-sin)
Ocuflox	ofloxacin	(oh-**flox**-uh-sin)
Tobrex	tobramycin	(**toe**-bruh-**my**-sin)
Vigamox, Moxeza	moxifloxacin	(mox-ee-**flox**-uh-sin)
Zymaxld	gatifloxacin	(gat-ih-**flox**-uh-sin)

Continued

Select Common Drugs Used for Conditions of the Eye, Ears, Nose, and Throat—cont'd

Trade Name	Generic Name	Pronunciation
Antifungal		
Natacyn	natamycin	(**na**-tuh-**my**-sin)
Antiviral		
Viroptic	trifluridine	(try-**floor**-ih-dean)
Beta-Adrenergic Blocking Agents		
Betagan	levobunolol	(lee-voe-**byoo**-noe-lol)
Betoptic-S	betaxolol	(be-**tax**-uh-lol)
None	carteolol	(**car**-tee-uh-lol)
None	metipranolol	(me-ti-**pran**-uh-lol)
Timoptic, Betimol, Istalol	timolol	(**tim**-uh-lol)
Carbonic Anhydrase Inhibitors		
Azopt	brinzolamide	(brin-**zoh**-luh-mide)
Diamox[a]	acetazolamide	(a-**seet**-uh-**zoh**-luh-mide)
Neptazane	methazolamide	(**meth**-uh-**zole**-uh-mide)
Trusopt	dorzolamide	(dor-**zole**-uh-mide)
Cholinergics		
Miostat	carbachol	(**kar**-buh-kol)
Isopto Carpine	pilocarpine	(pye-low-**kar**-peen)
Corticosteroids		
FML	fluorometholone	(**floor**-oh-**meth**-uh-lone)
Maxidex	dexamethasone	(**dex**-uh-**meth**-uh-sone)
Pred Forte, Pred Mild	prednisolone	(pred-**niss**-uh-lone)
Zylet	loteprednol/tobramycin	(low-teh-**pred**-nol/**toe**-bruh-**my**-sin)
Prostaglandin Agonists		
Lumigan, Latisse	bimatoprost	(bye-**mat**-uh-prost)
Travatan Z	travoprost	(**trav**-uh-prost)
Xalatan, XELPROS	latanoprost	(la-**tan**-uh-prost)
Products for Conditions Affecting the Ear		
Anesthetic		
None	antipyrine/benzocaine	(an-tee-**pie**-reen/**ben**-zoe-kane)
Antiinfectives		
Moxatag	amoxicillin	(am-**ox**-ih-**sil**-in)
Augmentin	amoxicillin/clavulanate	(am-**ox**-ih-**sil**-in/**clav**-ue-lah-nate)
Ceftin[a]	cefuroxime	(**sef**-yoo-**rox**-eem)
Ocuflox	ofloxacin	(oh-**flox**-uh-sin)
None	cefdinir	(**sef**-dih-near)
Zithromax	azithromycin	(a-**zith**-row-**my**-sin)
Products for Conditions Affecting the Nose		
Flonase Allergy Relief	fluticasone	(floo-**tic**-uh-sone)
Nasonex	mometasone	(moe-**met**-uh-sone)
Neo-Synephrine, Nasal Four, 4-Way Fast Acting	phenylephrine	(feh-nill-**eh**-frin)
Rhinocort Allergy	budesonide	(byoo-**dess**-uh-nide)

[a]Brand no longer available.

Conditions of eyes, ears, nose, and throat may seem secondary or merely uncomfortable, but failure to manage these areas can result in long-term health consequences. In this chapter, we discuss the anatomy and physiology of the eyes, ears, nose, and throat, in addition to select conditions affecting these areas and common treatments.

The Eyes (Ophthalmic System)

The eyes are vital sensory organs that perceive images and translate them into nerve impulses providing visual input.

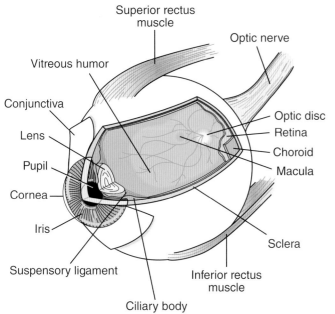

FIG. 26.1 Anatomy of the eye. (From Sorrentino SA, Remmert LN. *Mosby's Textbook for Nursing Assistants*. 9th ed. St. Louis: Mosby; 2017.)

The three different levels of health care personnel who work in eye care are opticians, optometrists, and ophthalmologists. Opticians make lenses to compensate for vision loss, but they cannot prescribe medication. Optometrists perform eye examinations and may prescribe certain eye medications. Ophthalmologists are doctors who treat major conditions affecting the eye and perform surgery.

Anatomy and Physiology of the Eye

The eye has structures that work in unison to protect it, maintain its shape, and facilitate vision. The eye sits in a bony socket called the **orbit.** The eyelids cover the eyes and have four individual layers: the outer skin, the muscles, the connective tissue, and the conjunctiva. The muscles and fibers of connective tissues are under the skin in the lid. They allow the eyelid to open and close. The **conjunctiva** is a thin, transparent mucous membrane covering the anterior eye, the eyelids, and the **sclera** (Fig. 26.1). The natural blinking reaction protects the eye from foreign objects and allows **lacrimal fluid** (tears) to cleanse the eye. The lacrimal gland, which secretes tears into the eye, has ducts that lead into the nasal cavity. Tears contain antimicrobial enzymes to protect the eye from infection.

The **cornea** is a bulging, transparent cover that allows light into the eye for visual acuity. It contains connective tissue and a thin epithelium coating. The cornea does not contain blood vessels; instead, its aqueous humor and atmospheric oxygen nourish it. The aqueous humor is in the anterior part of the eye, between the cornea and lens. Many corneal nerve fibers sense pain. The sclera attaches to the cornea but wraps around to the back of the eyeball (Fig. 26.2). The optic nerve extends from the back of the eye through the sclera. It sends images from the eye to the brain for interpretation. From the front of the eye, the sclera joins with the iris and the ciliary body. The

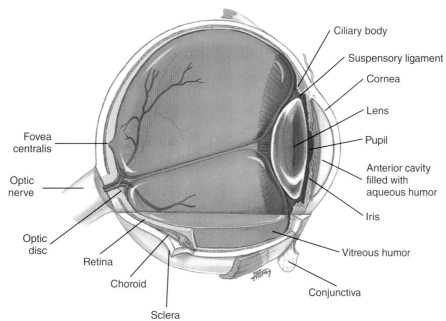

FIG. 26.2 Cross section of the eye. (From Damjanov I. *Pathology for the Health Professions*. 4th ed. Philadelphia: Saunders; 2012.)

iris is responsible for eye color and filters light. The most significant eye space is the posterior cavity, which the lens, ciliary body, and retina surround. The ciliary body forms a ring around the eye's front. The **ciliary body** holds the **lens** in place and regulates its shape to help focus vision. The area between the lens and the retina contains **vitreous humor,** a jelly-like substance that helps hold the eye's shape. The **retina** has layers of neurons, nerves, pigmented epithelium, and membranous tissues. Retinal receptor cells (known as *photoreceptors*) carry responsibility for vision, and the neurons send signals to the brain. Six major eye muscles extend from the orbit's skeletal bones. These muscles move the eye (Fig. 26.3). Other muscles close and open the eyelid and dilate and constrict the pupil.

When focusing on distant figures or in darkness, the **pupil** dilates **(mydriasis),** allowing more light inside. When exposed to excessive light, the pupil constricts **(miosis). Aqueous humor** is the watery fluid that maintains the shape of the anterior eye (ie, between the cornea and the lens) and nourishes anterior compartment structures. As the body continually synthesizes aqueous humor, it must release it to maintain proper pressure in the anterior eye chamber. Excess aqueous humor drains through small ducts, the *canals of Schlemm,* near the sclera and cornea.

> ### Tech Note!
> When we cry, the parasympathetic nervous system activates lacrimal glands directly.

Vision

As images pass through the lens, they reach the retina in the back of the eye. Retinal rods are responsible for sight in dim light and produce only black-and-white images. Retinal cones detect color. As the rods and cones synapse (connect) with nerve endings, signals pass through the optic nerve to the brain. As discussed in Chapter 17, the brain's occipital lobe interprets visuals.

Conditions That Affect the Eye

Many conditions affect the eyes. Depending on the cause, treatment can range from medication to surgery. The past decades have seen new developments in corrective lens treatment. For **myopia** (nearsightedness), laser surgery is a popular alternative to eyeglasses.

Many **ophthalmic** medications are available by prescription. Keeping eye solutions sterile is imperative because foreign objects instilled into the eyes can cause damage or infection. The pharmacist should instruct patients in the proper eye drop administration technique. This technique is essential for effective drop use and to prevent medication contamination (Box 26.1). Patients should remove contact lenses before instilling most medications. This section discusses common ophthalmic medications. Table 26.1 presents a review of nonantiinfective ophthalmic medications.

> ### BOX 26.1 Proper Administration of Eye Drops and Ointments
>
> The basic steps for administering eye drops and ointments are as follows:
> 1. Wash hands.
> 2. Tilt head back or lie down and gaze upward.
> 3. Gently pull the lower eyelid down and away from the eye to form a pouch.
> 4. Place dropper directly over the eye. Do not let dropper come in contact with the eye or any other surface (eg, fingers).
> 5. Look upward just before applying a drop.
> 6. After instilling the drop, look downward for several seconds.
> 7. Release lid slowly and close the eyes gently.
> 8. With eyes closed, use the fingertips to apply gentle pressure to the inside corner of the eye for 3 to 5 minutes (this prevents the solution from becoming part of the nasolacrimal drainage, thereby allowing the drug to enter the systemic circulation; temporary occlusion helps prevent systemic side effects and may improve drug efficacy).
> 9. Do not rub the eye or squeeze the eyelid and try not to blink.
> 10. Do not rinse the dropper.
> 11. If more than one type of eye drop is used, wait at least 5 minutes before administering the second agent.
> 12. Ointments: Follow steps 1 to 3. Then apply ointment with a sweeping motion inside the lower eyelid by squeezing the tube gently and slowly releasing the eyelid. Close the eye for 1 to 2 minutes and roll the eyeball in all directions. Remove any excess ointment from around the eye with a tissue. If using more than one kind of ointment, wait 10 minutes before applying the other ointment.

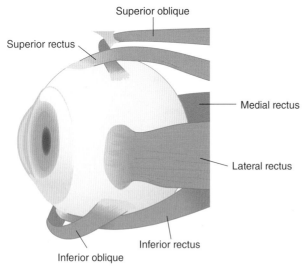

Superior oblique
Superior rectus
Medial rectus
Lateral rectus
Inferior rectus
Inferior oblique

FIG. 26.3 **Eye muscles and their direction of movement.** The superior rectus rotates upward and inward; the inferior rectus rotates downward and inward; the medial rectus rotates inward; the lateral rectus rotates outward; the superior oblique rotates downward and outward; the inferior oblique rotates upward and outward.

| | TABLE 26.1 |

Select Nonantiinfective Products for the Treatment of the Eye

Generic Name	Trade Name	Common Adult Dosage	Common Side Effects
Nonsteroidal Antiinflammatory Drugs (NSAIDs)			
ketorolac	Acular	• 1 drop 4 times daily	• Burning/stinging
flurbiprofen	Ocufen	• 1 drop every 30 min, starting 2 hr before procedure	• Crying • Increased intraocular pressure
diclofenac		• 1 drop in affected eye(s) 4 times daily, 24 hr after the procedure, and continue for 2 wk	• Keratitis • Miosis
Antihistamines: H$_1$-Antagonist (Some Mast Cell Stabilization)			
azelastine		• 1 drop in affected eye(s) twice daily	
ketotifen	Claritin Eye	• 1 drop in affected eye(s) every 8–12 hr (max 2 drops per eye per day)	• Conjunctivitis • Discharge • Dry eyes • Eyelid disorder • Pain • Photophobia
olopatadine	Patanol,[a] Pataday, Pazeo[a]	• *Patanol:* 1 drop into affected eye twice daily • *Pataday, Pazeo:* 1 drop into affected eye once daily	• Cold syndrome • Headache • Pharyngitis • Taste perversion
Mast Cell Stabilizers			
lodoxamide	Alomide	• 1–2 drops in eye(s) 4 times daily for up to 3 mo	• Blurred vision • Burning • Headache • Hyperemia • Stinging
nedocromil	Alocril	• 1–2 drops in each eye twice daily	• Headache • Photophobia • Redness • Stinging • Unpleasant taste
pemirolast	Alamast[a]	• 1–2 drops in affected eye(s) 4 times daily	• Cold/flu symptoms • Dry eyes • Headache • Rhinitis
cromolyn		• 1–2 drops in each eye 4–6 times daily	• Dryness • Itchy eyes • Puffy eyes • Redness
Anticholinergics			
cyclopentolate	Cyclogyl	• Instill 1 drop of 1% solution 3 times daily	• Blurred vision • Conjunctivitis
atropine		• 1 drop in eye(s) 40 min before procedure	• Dry eyes • Edema • Irritation • Paralysis of the ciliary eye muscle • Pupil dilation
Adrenergic Agonists			
oxymetazoline	—	• 1–2 drops in affected eye(s) every 6 hr as needed (prn); do not use longer than 3 days	• Blurred vision • Burning • Redness relief • Stinging
tetrahydrozoline	Opti-Clear[a]	• 1–2 drops in eye(s) up to 4 times daily	

Continued

TABLE 26.1

Select Nonantiinfective Products for the Treatment of the Eye—cont'd

Generic Name	Trade Name	Common Adult Dosage	Common Side Effects
brimonidine	Alphagan P	• 1 drop in affected eye(s) 3 times daily	• Conjunctivitis • Eye pain • Hyperemia • Stinging
Corticosteroids			
dexamethasone	Maxidex, Ozurdex (implant)	• 1–2 drops in conjunctival sac every hour during the day and every other hour at night (titrate down to 3–4 times daily)	• Burning • Cataract • Conjunctival hemorrhage • Hyperemia • Intraocular pressure increased • Pain
fluorometholone	FML, Flarex	• ½-inch ribbon in conjunctival sac 1–3 times daily • Suspension: 1–2 drops 2–4 times daily	
prednisolone	Omnipred,[a] Pred Forte, Pred Mild	• 1–2 drops 2–4 times daily	
loteprednol and tobramycin	Zylet	• 1–2 drops in affected eye(s) every 4–6 h	• Burning • Eyelid disorders • Headache • Increased intraocular pressure • Keratitis • Photophobia

[a]Brand no longer available.

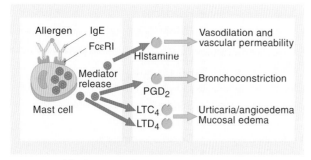

FIG. 26.4 Mechanism of a type I hypersensitivity reaction. *FceRI,* Fragment crystalline epsilon RI; *IgE,* immunoglobulin E; *PGD₂,* prostaglandin D2; *LTC₄,* leukotriene C4; *LTD₄,* leukotriene D4. (From Page C, Hoffman B, Curtis M, Walker M. *Integrated Pharmacology.* 3rd ed. St. Louis: Mosby; 2006.)

Common Conditions

Allergic Conjunctivitis

Irritants or foreign objects cause mast cells to release histamine, which causes inflammation to fight allergens (Fig. 26.4). When exposed to allergens, eyes become itchy, red, and watery, most often during allergy season. Seasonal allergies are allergic reactions to pollen from trees, grasses, and flowers. Other causes include pet dander, molds, dust mites, cigarette smoke, and exhaust fumes.

Prognosis

There is no cure for allergies. However, some patients can undergo successful desensitization. Many allergy patients can minimize symptoms with medications,

avoiding irritants, and limiting outdoor activities when allergen levels are high.

Non-Drug Treatment

Avoiding irritants, if possible, helps minimize allergic reactions. Staying indoors when pollen or other allergen levels are highest can help. Monthly allergy shots can relieve allergy symptoms associated with eyes.

Drug Treatment

Health providers use mast cell stabilizers, antihistamines, and decongestants for treatment. Mast cell stabilizers prevent mast cells from releasing chemicals that cause inflammation. They are available as ophthalmic solutions, suspensions, and systemic agents. Antihistamines inhibit histamine release, a compound responsible for itching and inflammation. Inhibition of histamine receptors diminishes seasonal allergen effects. Decongestants dry mucous secretions and relieve congestion caused by allergies and hay fever. Decongestants act on the specific receptors that cause mucous membrane constriction, lessening congestion. (See Chapters 21 and 29 for additional information on allergy treatment.) Table 26.2 provides a list of select ophthalmic decongestants, antihistamines, and mast cell stabilizer medications. Most eye drop bottles contain a preservative called benzalkonium chloride (BAK). The preservative prevents bacterial growth. Unfortunately, some patients are allergic to BAK-containing products, which can lead to eye irritation and inflammation. In this case, patients should opt for a preservative-free formulation.

TABLE 26.2
Select Ophthalmic Decongestants, Antihistamines, and Mast Cell Stabilizers

Generic Name	Trade Name	Availability
Decongestants		
naphazoline	Clear Eyes Redness Relief	Over the counter (OTC)
oxymetazoline	Afrin Original Nasal Spray	OTC
phenylephrine	Neo-Synephrine Cold + Allergy	Prescription
tetrahydrozoline	Tyzine	OTC
Antihistamines		
olopatadine	Patanol,[a] Pataday, Pazeo[a]	Prescription
azelastine	None	Prescription
epinastine	Elestat	Prescription
ketotifen	Claritin Eye, Zaditor	OTC
Mast Cell Stabilizers		
lodoxamide tromethamine	Alomide	Prescription
nedocromil	Alocril	Prescription
cromolyn sodium	Opticrom[a]	Prescription

[a]Brand no longer available.

GENERIC NAME: lodoxamide

TRADE NAME: Alomide

INDICATIONS: Conjunctivitis, vernal keratitis, vernal keratoconjunctivitis

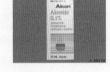

ROUTE OF ADMINISTRATION: Ophthalmic

COMMON ADULT DOSAGE: 1 or 2 drops in the affected eye(s) up to 4 times daily; not to be used for longer than 3 months

MECHANISM OF ACTION: Ophthalmic mast cell stabilizer (inhibits mast cell histamine release)

SIDE EFFECTS: Eye irritation, blurred vision, headache

AUXILIARY LABEL: For the eye

Ophthalmic Inflammation Caused by Infection or Injury

Corticosteroids relieve inflammation from infection, allergies, or injury. Doctors often prescribe them postoperatively for inflammation (Fig. 26.5). Avoid using the agents longer than necessary because they can compromise the immune system. Corticosteroid ophthalmic dosage forms include solutions, suspensions, and ointments. Side effects can consist of temporary burning sensations, blurred vision, eye pain, or headaches. Most antiinflammatory agents are solutions or suspensions. Suspensions should be shaken well before use.

GENERIC NAME: prednisolone

TRADE NAMES: Pred Forte, Omnipred, Pred Mild

INDICATIONS: Allergic conjunctivitis, postoperative ocular inflammation

ROUTE OF ADMINISTRATION: Ophthalmic

COMMON ADULT DOSAGE: 1 or 2 drops in the affected eye(s) 2–4 times daily

MECHANISM OF ACTION: Prevents or suppresses inflammation and immune responses

SIDE EFFECTS: Eye irritation, blurred vision, watery eyes

AUXILIARY LABELS:
- For the eye
- Shake well before using

Nonsteroidal antiinflammatory drugs (NSAIDs) inhibit the enzyme cyclooxygenase (COX), responsible for prostaglandin synthesis. Prostaglandins are directly related to mechanisms responsible for inflammation and pain. Ophthalmic NSAIDs are only available in solution.

GENERIC NAME: flurbiprofen

TRADE NAME: none

INDICATIONS: Miosis inhibition, postoperative ocular inflammation

ROUTE OF ADMINISTRATION: Ophthalmic

COMMON ADULT DOSAGE: *Intraoperative miosis:* Instill 1 drop every 30 minutes, beginning 2 hours before surgery for a total of 4 drops in each affected eye

MECHANISM OF ACTION: NSAID (competitively inhibits COX enzymes to reduce inflammation)

SIDE EFFECTS: Eye irritation, blurred vision, itching (pruritus)

AUXILIARY LABELS:
- For the eye
- Use as directed

GENERIC NAME: ketorolac

TRADE NAME: Acular

INDICATIONS: Allergic conjunctivitis, ocular pain, ocular pruritus, postoperative ocular inflammation

ROUTE OF ADMINISTRATION: Ophthalmic

COMMON ADULT DOSAGE: 1 drop into the affected eye(s) 4 times daily

MECHANISM OF ACTION: NSAID (competitively inhibits COX enzymes to reduce inflammation)

SIDE EFFECTS: Eye irritation, headache

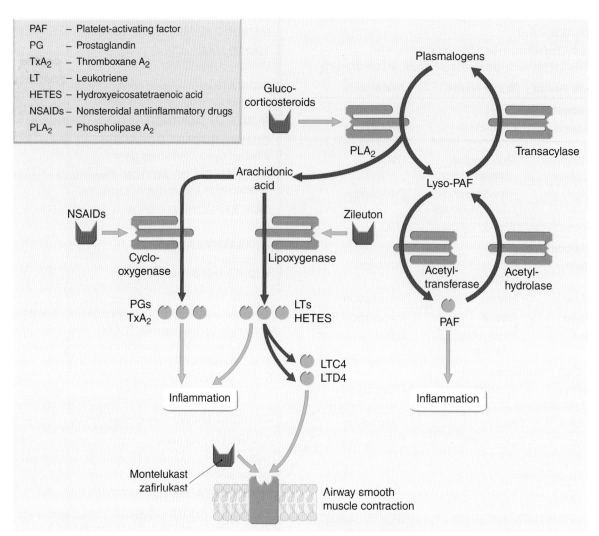

FIG. 26.5 Glucocorticosteroids reduce the production of a variety of inflammatory mediators. (From Page C, Hoffman B, Curtis M, Walker M. *Integrated Pharmacology*. 3rd ed. St. Louis: Mosby; 2006.)

COX, Cyclooxygenase; *NSAID*, nonsteroidal antiinflammatory drug.

Ophthalmic Infections

Many pathogens, including bacteria, viruses, and fungi, cause ophthalmic infections. Table 26.3 outlines select antiinfective agents for ophthalmic infections.

Bacterial ophthalmic infections Viruses, bacteria, fungi, or allergies cause conjunctivitis, an acute conjunctival inflammation (pink eye). The eye becomes red, and yellow discharge crusts over the eyelashes often after sleep. The eyes may burn and itch, causing blurred vision. Newborns can acquire a neonatal conjunctivitis form (ophthalmia neonatorum) as they pass through the birth canal. Immediate prophylaxis is crucial, or the infant may lose his or her eyesight.

Bacterial conjunctivitis is highly contagious and spread via direct contact with the eyes, secretions, or contaminated objects. Infected individuals can minimize spread by not sharing cosmetics, towels, or eye drops and avoiding touching the eyes.

Prognosis

With proper care and treatment, we can treat bacterial conjunctivitis without lasting effects. If left untreated, scarring or loss of eyesight may occur, particularly in newborns.

Non-Drug Treatment

Placing a warm compress on eyelids helps relieve pain. Patients should wash their hands frequently and avoid touching the eyes to prevent the reintroduction of bacteria. Patients should not share towels and personal care items. Patients with contact lenses should discontinue use until the infection is cleared.

Drug Treatment

Antiinfective agents combat conjunctivitis. For many bacterial infections, a broad-spectrum antibiotic, such as gentamicin or ciprofloxacin, can work well.

TABLE 26.3
Select Antiinfective Agents for the Treatment of Eye Infections

Generic Name	Trade Name	Common Dosage Range	Common Side Effects
Aminoglycoside Antibiotics			
gentamicin	Gentak	• Solution: 1–2 drops every 4 hr (2 drops/hr for severe infections) • Ointment: Instill ½-inch ribbon 2–3 times daily	• Burning • Irritation
tobramycin	Tobrex	• Solution: 1–2 drops every 4 hr until improved • Ointment: ½-inch ribbon 2–3 times daily	• Lid itching • Lid swelling • Rash
Fluoroquinolone Antibiotics			
besifloxacin	Besivance	• 1 drop in affected eye(s) 3 times daily for 7 days	• Blurred vision • Headache • Pain • Redness
ciprofloxacin	Ciloxan	• *Solution:* 1–2 drops in affected eye(s) every 2 hr while awake for the first 2 days, then 1–2 drops every 4 hr for the next 5 days • *Ointment:* ½-inch ribbon 3 times daily for the first 2 days, then twice daily for the next 5 days	• Burning • Eyelid crusting • Hyperemia • White crystalline precipitate
gatifloxacin	Zymaxid	• 1 drop in affected eye(s) every 2 hr while awake (max 8 times/day) on day 1, then 1 drop 2–4 times daily on days 2–7	• Decreased visual acuity • Dermatitis • Dry eye • Edema • Irritation
moxifloxacin	Vigamox, Moxeza	• 1 drop in affected eye(s) 2–3 times daily for 7 days	• Conjunctivitis • Decreased visual acuity • Dry eye • Hyperemia • Irritation
ofloxacin	Ocuflox	• 1–2 drops in affected eye(s) every 2–4 hr for the first 2 days, then use 4 times daily for an additional 5 days	• Blurred vision • Burning • Conjunctivitis • Photophobia • Redness • Stinging
Macrolide Antibiotics			
azithromycin	AzaSite	• 1 drop in affected eye(s) twice daily for 2 days, then 1 drop daily for 5 days	• Abnormal taste • Blurred vision • Dry eyes • Irritation • Swelling
erythromycin	—	• 1-cm ribbon up to 6 times daily	• Hypersensitivity • Irritation • Redness
Sulfonamide Antibiotics			
sulfacetamide	Bleph-10[a]	• *Solution:* 1–2 drops in lower eyelid every 2–3 hr • *Ointment:* ½-inch ribbon every 3–4 hr and at bedtime	• Burning • Conjunctivitis • Edema • Hyperemia • Ulcers
Miscellaneous Antibiotics			
bacitracin	None	• Apply 1–3 times daily	• Blurred vision • Discomfort • Stinging

Continued

■ TABLE 26.3

Select Antiinfective Agents for the Treatment of Eye Infections—cont'd

Generic Name	Trade Name	Common Dosage Range	Common Side Effects
polymyxin B/ trimethoprim	Polytrim	• 1 drop in affected eye(s) every 3 hr (max 6 doses/day) for 7–10 days	• Burning • Edema • Itching • Rash
Antifungals			
natamycin	Natacyn	• 1 drop in conjunctival sac every 1–2 h; after 3–4 days, reduce to 6–8 times daily (treat for 2–3 wk)	• Burning • Edema • Hyperemia • Paresthesia • Vision changes
Antivirals			
ganciclovir	Zirgan	• 1 drop of gel in affected eye(s) 5 times daily until ulcer heals; then 1 drop 3 times daily for 7 days	• Blurred vision • Hyperemia • Irritation • Punctate keratitis
trifluridine	Viroptic	• 1 drop in affected eye(s) every 2 hr while awake (max 9 drops/day) until ulcer heals; then 1 drop every 4 hr for 7 days	• Burning • Edema • Increased pressure • Stinging
Immunological Agent			
cyclosporine	Restasis	• 1 drop in each eye every 12 hr	• Burning • Hyperemia • Increased tear production (goal) • Itching • Pain

ªBleph-10 is only available as a solution

Ophthalmic medications come in two standard formulations: ointments and solutions. The choice of ointment or solution often depends on price, availability, and patient compliance. Ointments are thicker and can cause blurry vision due to increased viscosity and oily texture. Ointments are usually more appropriate for younger patients. On the other hand, ophthalmic solutions are better for patients who wear contacts, allowing patients to re-insert their contacts about 15 minutes after application.

SIDE EFFECT: Eye irritation

AUXILIARY LABELS:
• For the eye
• Use as directed

GENERIC NAME: sulfacetamide sodium

TRADE NAME: Bleph-10 (solution, ointment)

INDICATION: Ophthalmic bacterial infections

ROUTE OF ADMINISTRATION: Ophthalmic

COMMON ADULT DOSAGE: *Solution:* 1 or 2 drops in lower eyelid every 2–3 hours. *Ointment:* Apply ½-inch ribbon every 3–4 hours and at bedtime

MECHANISM OF ACTION: Inhibits bacterial dihydrofolate synthetase (interferes with the synthesis of folic acid, an essential component of bacterial growth and development)

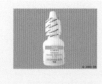

GENERIC NAME: tobramycin

TRADE NAME: Tobrex

INDICATION: Ophthalmic bacterial infections

ROUTE OF ADMINISTRATION: Ophthalmic

COMMON ADULT DOSAGE: *Solution:* Instill 1 or 2 drops every 4 hours. *Ointment:* Apply ½-inch ribbon 2–3 times a day until improvement

MECHANISM OF ACTION: Aminoglycoside antibiotic (inhibits bacterial protein synthesis, leading to bacterial cell death)

SIDE EFFECTS: Eye irritation, itching (pruritus)

AUXILIARY LABELS:
• For the eye
• Use as directed

GENERIC NAME: erythromycin

TRADE NAME: none

INDICATION: Ophthalmic bacterial infections

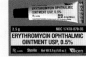

ROUTE OF ADMINISTRATION: Ophthalmic

COMMON ADULT DOSAGE: Instill an approximately 1-cm ribbon into the affected eye(s) up to 6 times daily

MECHANISM OF ACTION: Inhibits bacterial protein synthesis

SIDE EFFECTS: Eye irritation, itching, sensitivity to light

AUXILIARY LABEL: For the eye

Viral ophthalmic infections Similar to bacterial conjunctivitis, viral eye infections are contagious.

The three most common viral eye infections are herpes simplex, keratitis, and viral conjunctivitis. Viral conjunctivitis is often self-limiting, and no topical treatment exists.

Antiviral therapy means to interrupt or alter new virus synthesis at a specific replication step. Many eye viruses occur more frequently in immunocompromised patients, such as those with human immunodeficiency virus infection. Side effects of ophthalmic antiviral medications can include light sensitivity, stinging, and a mild burning sensation.

GENERIC NAME: trifluridine

TRADE NAME: Viroptic

INDICATIONS: Herpes simplex keratitis, keratoconjunctivitis, viral conjunctivitis

ROUTE OF ADMINISTRATION: Ophthalmic

COMMON ADULT DOSAGE: 1 drop in the affected eye(s) every 2 hours while awake, for a maximum of 9 drops; then treatment may decrease to 1 drop every 4 hours while awake

MECHANISM OF ACTION: Inhibits viral DNA replication

SIDE EFFECTS: Eye irritation, itching, sensitivity to light

AUXILIARY LABEL: For the eye

Fungal ophthalmic infections Fungal conjunctivitis is rare. The primary ophthalmic agent for superficial fungal eye infections is natamycin, a **fungicidal** agent. Natamycin's mechanism of action involves drug binding to the fungal cell membrane, destabilizing it, and killing the fungus.

Tech Note!

The best way to avoid conjunctivitis is by washing hands before touching eyes. Other ways of contracting infectious pathogens are from sharing towels, pillows, and even computer keyboards.

GENERIC NAME: natamycin

TRADE NAME: Natacyn

INDICATIONS: Blepharitis, fungal conjunctivitis, fungal keratitis

ROUTE OF ADMINISTRATION: Ophthalmic

COMMON ADULT DOSAGE: *Fungal conjunctivitis and blepharitis:* 1 drop in the affected eye(s) every 4–6 hours. *Fungal keratitis:* 1 drop in conjunctival sac every 1–2 hours for 3–4 days, followed by 1 drop every 6–8 hours

MECHANISM OF ACTION: Impairs fungal cell wall membranes, leading to the death of the fungus

SIDE EFFECTS: Eye irritation, itching, sensitivity to light (photophobia)

AUXILIARY LABELS:
- For the eye
- Shake well before using

Glaucoma

Glaucoma represents an ophthalmic disorder group characterized by high **intraocular pressure (IOP).** Untreated, glaucoma can lead to peripheral vision loss and blindness. Primary glaucoma has two subtypes: open-angle and closed-angle glaucoma. Open-angle glaucoma has a progressive, slow IOP increase. In this glaucoma form, the "angle" of the eye's anterior chamber through which aqueous humor is resorbed is open. In contrast, closed-angle glaucoma has a visible angle obstruction produced by the iris during contraction (Fig. 26.6). Closed-angle glaucoma often manifests suddenly, with intraocular pain, loss of vision, and redness of the eye.

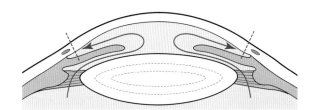

A Open-angle glaucoma

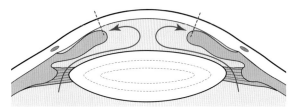

B Closed-angle glaucoma

FIG. 26.6 **Glaucoma.** (A) In open-angle glaucoma the obstruction occurs in the trabecular meshwork. (B) In closed-angle glaucoma the trabecular meshwork is covered by the root of the iris or adhesions between the iris and the cornea. (From Damjanov I. *Pathology for the Health Professions.* 4th ed. Philadelphia: Saunders; 2012.)

Prognosis

Early diagnosis and treatment can prevent irreversible vision loss. Drugs that reduce aqueous humor or intraocular pressure (IOP) help patients with glaucoma. If left untreated, glaucoma can lead to blindness. Depending on the severity, many medications and treatments can reduce IOP.

Non-Drug Treatment

A surgeon can implant drainage valves for aqueous humor outflow. Alternatively, corrective lenses may also help.

Drug Treatment

Glaucoma treatment focuses on reducing IOP by increasing drainage or reducing aqueous humor production. Ophthalmic dosage forms include drops, suspensions, and ointments. In some cases, a doctor may prescribe medicated inserts. Five drug classifications treat glaucoma: beta-adrenergic blockers, carbonic anhydrase inhibitors, cholinergic agonists (miotics), sympathomimetics, and prostaglandin analogs. In many cases, health providers use more than one medication class (Table 26.4).

Tech Note!

Several prescription combination products that include medications from several drug classes are available for glaucoma treatment.

Beta-adrenergic blockers Beta-adrenergic blockers (beta-blockers) lower the IOP in open-angle glaucoma. By blocking beta-receptors, these agents prevent the activation of the beta-adrenergic response (ie, the sympathetic, or fight-or-flight, response), which affects many body systems. In the eye, beta-blockers reduce aqueous humor production by the ciliary processes to lower IOP.

■ TABLE 26.4
Select Agents for the Treatment of Glaucoma

Generic Name	Trade Name	Common Dosage Range	Common Side Effects
Prostaglandin Analogs			
bimatoprost	Lumigan	• 1 drop in affected eye(s) every night	• Change in eye color
latanoprost	Xalatan	• 1 drop in affected eye(s) every night	• Darkening of eyelids
travoprost	Travatan Z	• 1 drop in affected eye(s) every night	• Hyperemia • Irreversible darkening of the iris • Thickening/darkening of eyelashes
Cholinergic Agonists (Miotics)			
carbachol	Miostat	• 1–2 drops up to 3 times daily	• Headaches
pilocarpine	Isopto Carpine	• 1 drop up to 3 times over a 30-min period	• Decreased night vision • Stinging • Pain • Spasm
Carbonic Anhydrase Inhibitors			
brinzolamide	Azopt	• 1 drop in affected eye(s) 3 times daily	• Blurred vision
dorzolamide	Trusopt	• 1 drop in affected eye(s) 3 times daily	• Stinging • Conjunctivitis • Keratitis
Beta-Blockers			
betaxolol	Betoptic-S	• 1–2 drop(s) in affected eye(s) twice daily	• Stinging/burning
carteolol	–	• 1 drop in affected eye(s) twice daily	• Dry eyes
levobunolol	Betagan	• 0.25%: 1–2 drop(s) in affected eye(s) twice daily • 0.5%: 1–2 drop(s) daily	• Blepharitis
metipranolol	–	• 3%: 1 drop in affected eye(s) twice daily	
timolol	Timoptic	• 1 drop in affected eye(s) 1–2 times daily	
Adrenergic Agents			
brimonidine	Alphagan P	• 1 drop in affected eye(s) 3 times daily	• Conjunctivitis • Eye pain • Stinging

GENERIC NAME: betaxolol

TRADE NAME: Betoptic-S

INDICATION: Open-angle glaucoma

ROUTE OF ADMINISTRATION: Ophthalmic

COMMON ADULT DOSAGE: 1 or 2 drops in the affected eye(s) twice daily

MECHANISM OF ACTION: Reduces the production of aqueous humor by the ciliary processes in the eye to reduce IOP

SIDE EFFECTS: Stinging, itching, dry eyes, headache

AUXILIARY LABELS:
- For the eye
- Shake well before using

IOP, Intraocular pressure.

GENERIC NAME: carteolol

TRADE NAME: none

INDICATION: Open-angle glaucoma

ROUTE OF ADMINISTRATION: Ophthalmic

COMMON ADULT DOSAGE: 1 drop in the affected eye(s) twice daily

MECHANISM OF ACTION: Reduces the production of aqueous humor by the ciliary processes in the eye to reduce intraocular pressure

SIDE EFFECTS: Burning, stinging, headache

AUXILIARY LABEL: For the eye

GENERIC NAME: timolol

TRADE NAMES: Timoptic Ocudose, Timoptic-XE (gel-forming solution), Istalol

INDICATION: Open-angle glaucoma

ROUTE OF ADMINISTRATION: Ophthalmic

COMMON ADULT DOSAGE: 1 drop twice daily in the affected eye(s). *Timoptic-XE:* 1 drop daily in the affected eye(s). *Istalol:* 1 drop once daily

MECHANISM OF ACTION: Reduces the production of aqueous humor by the ciliary processes in the eye to reduce intraocular pressure

SIDE EFFECTS: Stinging, blurred vision, headache

AUXILIARY LABEL: For the eye

Carbonic anhydrase inhibitors Carbonic anhydrase inhibitors inhibit the **carbonic anhydrase enzyme,** thereby decreasing aqueous humor formation. Directly applying these medications to the eye reduces the IOP in patients with chronic open-angle glaucoma. Doctors also prescribe carbonic anhydrase inhibitors in closed-angle glaucoma for a short duration to lower IOP and perform surgery.

Patients can apply carbonic anhydrase inhibitors locally to the eye or use them systemically (eg, methazolamide [Neptazane]).

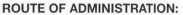

GENERIC NAME: dorzolamide

TRADE NAME: Trusopt

INDICATION: Glaucoma

ROUTE OF ADMINISTRATION: Ophthalmic

COMMON ADULT DOSAGE: 1 drop in the affected eye(s) 3 times daily

MECHANISM OF ACTION: Inhibits the carbonic anhydrase enzyme, thereby decreasing the formation of aqueous humor and lowering intraocular pressure

SIDE EFFECTS: Eye irritation, blurred vision

AUXILIARY LABEL: For the eye

Cholinergic agonists (miotics) Miotics resemble carbonic anhydrase inhibitors in their effectiveness in certain glaucoma types. The medications reduce IOP by contracting the ciliary muscle, thus increasing the outflow of aqueous humor.

GENERIC NAME: pilocarpine

TRADE NAME: Isopto Carpine

INDICATION: Glaucoma

ROUTE OF ADMINISTRATION: Ophthalmic

COMMON ADULT DOSAGE: 1 drop in the affected eye(s) up to 4 times daily

MECHANISM OF ACTION: Increases the outflow of aqueous humor from the eye by contracting the ciliary muscle

SIDE EFFECTS: Blurred vision, night blindness

AUXILIARY LABEL: For the eye

Sympathomimetics The name **sympathomimetic** refers to mimicking, or "acting like," the sympathetic system. Most agents work for patients with allergy irritation of the eyes. Sympathomimetics reduce IOP by reducing aqueous humor production and increasing its outflow. These medications treat open-angle glaucoma and in conjunction with other glaucoma medications to lower IOP.

GENERIC NAME: brimonidine

TRADE NAME: Alphagan P

INDICATION: Open-angle glaucoma

ROUTE OF ADMINISTRATION: Ophthalmic

COMMON ADULT DOSAGE: 1 drop in the affected eye(s) 3 times daily

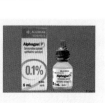

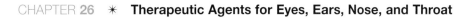

MECHANISM OF ACTION: Reduces IOP by reducing aqueous humor production and increasing its outflow

SIDE EFFECTS: Blurred vision, irritation, headache

AUXILIARY LABEL: For the eye

IOP, Intraocular pressure.

Prostaglandin analogs Several agents are prostaglandin analogs. They include latanoprost, bimatoprost, and travoprost, which reduce IOP by increasing aqueous humor outflow. Almost all prostaglandin analogs have the -prost suffix, which we derive from the word prostaglandin. Ophthalmic use of prostaglandin analogs has several unique adverse effects such as iris discoloration resulting from an increase in brown iris pigments and an increase in the length, thickness, and pigmentation of eyelashes.

GENERIC NAME: latanoprost

TRADE NAME: Xalatan

INDICATION: Open-angle glaucoma

ROUTE OF ADMINISTRATION: Ophthalmic

COMMON ADULT DOSAGE: 1 drop in the affected eye(s) once daily in the evening

MECHANISM OF ACTION: Reduces intraoperative pressure by increasing the outflow of aqueous humor

SIDE EFFECTS: Iris discoloration, eye irritation, thickening of the eyelashes

AUXILIARY LABELS:
- For the eye
- A possible permanent change in eye color, thickening and darkening of eyelashes, darkening of eyelids

Tech Note!

Xalatan should be stored in the refrigerator until opened. Once opened, it may be stored at room temperature for 6 weeks.

GENERIC NAME: bimatoprost

TRADE NAME: Lumigan

INDICATION: Open-angle glaucoma

ROUTE OF ADMINISTRATION: Ophthalmic

COMMON ADULT DOSAGE: 1 drop in the affected eye(s) once daily in the evening

MECHANISM OF ACTION: Reduces intraoperative by increasing the outflow of aqueous humor

SIDE EFFECTS: Iris discoloration, eye irritation, thickening of the eyelashes

AUXILIARY LABELS:
- For the eye
- A possible permanent change in eye color, thickening and darkening of eyelashes, darkening of eyelids

Tech Note!

A new bimatoprost formulation (Latisse) can thicken eyelashes. It is for eyelid hypotrichosis (ie, less than normal amount of hair).

Miscellaneous Ophthalmic Agents

Over-the-counter (OTC) artificial tears help dry eyes. Their ingredients include sodium chloride, buffers to adjust for pH, and other additives to prolong effects. They are all solutions with various strengths and in combination with other ingredients. A severe dry eye medication is cyclosporine (Restasis) eye drops. Restasis alleviates chronic dry eyes caused by inflammation.

Drug-Induced Ophthalmic Disorders

Due to extensive vasculature, eyes are susceptible to systemic medication toxicity through absorption. Although the body prevents most toxins from entering the eyes, some medications readily bypass the barriers resulting in localized ophthalmic injury. Injuries can range from mild (such as dry eyes) to severe symptoms (such as optic neuropathy). Common drug-induced ophthalmic disorders include dry eye disease, cataracts, retinopathy, and optic neuropathy. The severity varies on dose, duration, genetic predisposition, and the patient's natural ability to metabolize the medications. Common medications that cause ophthalmic ailments include anticholinergics, aminoquinolines, antineoplastics, corticosteroids, and retinoids.

Prognosis

In some cases, prompt medication discontinuation may lead to symptom resolution. When discontinuing the offending medication is not possible, or the benefits of continuing use outweigh the health risks, providers may recommend supportive therapies until discontinuation is appropriate. In cases of vision loss, however, the damage is irreversible.

Non-Drug Treatment

Surgery may be a viable option depending on the type of disorder and extent of the injury. For example, cataracts can be removed surgically. For drug-induced dry eye disorders, nonpharmacologic therapies include applying warm compresses, increased fluid intake, and using humidifiers.

Drug Treatment

Pharmacologic treatments for dry eye disorders include artificial tears or lubricants. Short-term ophthalmic glucocorticoids or cyclosporine can reduce inflammation.

Prevention and Monitoring

Although drug-induced ophthalmic disorders may be rare, patients must be educated on potential toxicities' signs and symptoms. They should be encouraged to seek medical help immediately with the onset symptoms. Prescribers often

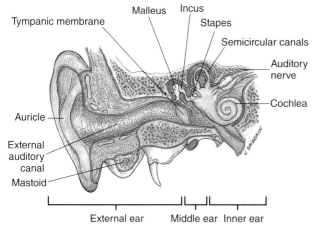

FIG. 26.7 Anatomy of the ear. (From Potter PA, Perry AG. *Fundamentals of Nursing*. 8th ed. St. Louis: Mosby; 2013.)

recommend baseline and annual vision examinations to monitor for toxicity.

The Ears (Auditory System)

The human ear is responsible for hearing, balance, and equilibrium. The ear contains three major sections: the external, middle, and inner ear (Fig. 26.7).

Anatomy and Physiology of the Ear

External Ear

The most exterior part is the **auricle.** This area has cartilage and skin and serves as an entrance for sound waves. The auricle transmits sound waves through the external **auditory canal.** This canal leads to the **tympanic membrane** (eardrum) inside the ear. This membrane has two significant functions:

- Transmission of sound waves to the middle ear
- Protection of the middle ear from foreign objects

Sound transmission happens because of vibration, much the same way a drum skin vibrates and carries sound when struck with a drumstick. Glands inside the ear produce **cerumen** (a waxy substance).

Middle Ear

Vibrations from the tympanic membrane extend into the middle ear. The middle ear has three tiny, bony structures called the **auditory ossicles:** the malleus (hammer), the incus (anvil), and the stapes (stirrup). These three small bones connect and transmit sound waves that make it to the eardrum. Another middle ear area is the **eustachian tube** that leads to the nasopharynx. When a person swallows, yawns, or moves the jaw, the eustachian tube opens and relieves pressure change between the outside and inside atmosphere.

Tech Note!

When a person in a car or plane ascends, the eustachian tube relieves the decreased pressure from the outside by causing an ear "pop." This movement equalizes the two pressure levels.

Inner Ear

After sound transmission through the ossicles, the stapes (last ossicle) continues the transfer into the third ear section, the *inner ear.* This fluid-filled area is the labyrinth and contains many components to process and transmit audible sounds via nerve impulses to the brain for interpretation (Fig. 26.8). These inner ear structures have separate, essential functions (Box 26.2).

Common Conditions Affecting the Ear

Various conditions affect hearing quality, including infections, swimmer's ear, earwax accumulation, damage to the eardrum, and congenital anatomical defects. Table 26.5 lists select products for ear condition treatment. Antibiotics are ineffective against viral ear infections. Depending on the bacterial strain, physicians can prescribe bactericidal or bacteriostatic medication. **Bactericidal** agents kill the bacteria; **bacteriostatic** agents limit bacterial growth. Bacteriostatic drugs help the body's immune system fight off bacteria.

Otitis Media

Otitis media is a middle ear infection and often occurs within the eustachian tube. Otitis media is a common ear infection treated clinically (several other ear infections are shown in Fig. 26.9). Otitis media causes changes to the eardrum that include bulging, swelling, and perforation. Antiinfectives can treat the infection. However, children with frequent, recurrent infections may need small tubes inserted through the tympanic membrane to allow drainage from the middle ear and eustachian tube. This procedure reduces reinfection. Common otitis media symptoms include fever, nausea and vomiting, earache, hearing problems, and inner ear pressure.

Tech Note!

When children tug at their ears, this is a classic sign a young child may have an ear infection.

Prognosis

Recovery from otitis media is common with proper treatment. Untreated serious infections may permanently damage the ear.

Non-Drug Treatment

Many ear infections self-limit and resolve by themselves after several days. Placing a warm compress on the ear can help relieve pain.

Drug Treatment

Antiinfectives can sometimes treat ear infections, although antibiotics are not always needed because ear infections can resolve spontaneously. Antihistamines, decongestants, and analgesics can help with otitis media symptoms (Table 26.6).

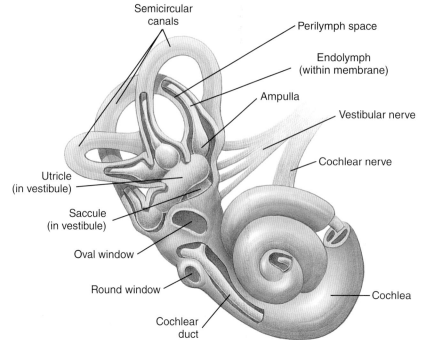

FIG. 26.8 Anatomy of the inner ear. (From Thibodeau GA, Patton KT. *Anatomy and Physiology*. 8th ed. St. Louis: Mosby; 2012.)

BOX 26.2 Three Main Areas of the Inner Ear and Their Functions

Cochlea: The cochlea is coiled and consists of three fluid-filled canals. The small, hairlike structures found here are connected to the acoustic nerve (ie, the vestibulocochlear nerve [CN VIII]) that transmits impulses to the brain. As the sound waves enter, the hairs bend and create impulses that are transmitted to the acoustic nerve.

Vestibule: The vestibule is located between the cochlea and the semicircular canals and is responsible for equilibrium and balance. Small, hairlike cells are affected by gravity, and when they move, nerve impulses are transmitted to the brain, specifically to the cerebellum and midbrain areas. Thus equilibrium is maintained. This gives humans a sense of direction and orientation.

Semicircular canals: The three semicircular canals are filled with a fluid that helps with the transfer of messages via the acoustic nerve. Small, hairlike fibers behave as sensors, moving back and forth as the person moves forward, backward, or stops. The signals sent from two of these canals provide information to the brain about the orientation of the body when at rest, whereas the third canal sends information pertaining to the body in motion.

TABLE 26.5
Select Products for the Treatment of Conditions of the Ear

Generic Name	Trade Name	Availability	Indication
carbamide peroxide, glycerin, propylene glycol, sodium stannate	Auraphene-B Gly-Oxide	OTC	Used to remove earwax

---

Cerumen Buildup

The glands near the tympanic membrane produce a waxy substance called cerumen. The cerumen acts as an infection barrier. As the amount of wax increases, it migrates out of the ear. If excessive wax accumulates, is not removed, or dries, it can impair hearing. A physician may need to remove waxy buildup to perform an examination or improve hearing quality.

Prognosis

Treating cerumen buildup appropriately improves hearing. The untreated buildup may result in partial hearing loss, tinnitus (ringing of the ears), earache, itching, or discharge.

Non-Drug Treatment

An irrigation kit with a saline solution and ear syringe removes earwax. Using warm water and the solution, it purges the ears of excessive wax. Other treatments include using a few drops of mineral oil, glycerin, or hydrogen peroxide to soften the wax. Warm water irrigation then removes earwax.

Drug Treatment

Several products help earwax removal by emulsifying it and removing it from the ear canal.

GENERIC NAME: carbamide peroxide
TRADE NAME: Debrox 6.5% Otic Drops
INDICATION: Earwax removal
ROUTE OF ADMINISTRATION: Otic
COMMON DOSAGE: Instill 5–10 drops twice daily up to 4 days
MECHANISM OF ACTION: Carbamide peroxide releases hydrogen peroxide, which serves as a source of nascent oxygen on contact with catalase; softens impacted cerumen because of its foaming action
SIDE EFFECTS: Irritation of the ear

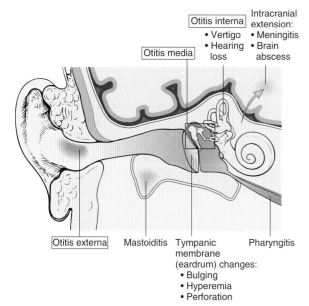

FIG. 26.9 Infections of the ear. (From Damjanov I. *Pathology for the Health Professions*. 4th ed. Philadelphia: Saunders; 2012.)

Drug-Induced Ototoxicity

Certain medications can cause temporary or permanent hearing loss, known as **ototoxicity** (Table 26.7). This injury can manifest as an ear ringing or buzzing (**tinnitus**) and can progress to permanent damage if untreated and affect balance. Aminoglycosides in high doses for extended periods are notable for ototoxicity. Health professionals assess patients who take these medications daily to ensure therapeutic outcomes without toxicity.

Prognosis

The prognosis for drug-induced ototoxicity is difficult. Although some cases reverse themselves after discontinuing drug treatment, others can be permanent. Hearing loss may not occur until after several weeks of drug treatment.

TABLE 26.6
Select Agents for the Treatment of Otitis Media in Children

Medication Class	Generic Name	Trade Name	Common Oral Dosage
Cephalosporins	ceftriaxone		• 50 mg/kg/day IM in 1–3 doses
	cefuroxime	Ceftin	• 30 mg/kg/day PO in 2 divided doses
	cefdinir		• 14 mg/kg/day PO in 1–2 doses
Macrolide	azithromycin	Zithromax	• 10 mg/kg/day PO on day 1; then 5 mg/kg/day PO on days 2–5
Penicillins	amoxicillin	Moxatag	• 90 mg/kg/day PO in 2 divided doses
	amoxicillin and clavulanate	Augmentin	• 90 mg/kg/day PO in 2 divided doses

IM, Intramuscular; *OP,* oral.

TABLE 26.7
Medications Associated With Ototoxicity or Tinnitus

Class	Specific Drugs
Aminoglycosides	gentamicin, tobramycin, amikacin
Macrolides	clarithromycin, erythromycin
Analgesics	aspirin, salicylates, nonsteroidal antiinflammatory drugs
Loop diuretics	furosemide, ethacrynic acid
Antineoplastics	cisplatin and platinum-containing agents
Antimalarial	quinine
Antiarrhythmic	quinidine
Glycopeptide antibiotic	vancomycin

Non-Drug Treatment

In most cases, no treatment is possible after hearing loss is permanent. In rare cases, amplification can help depending on the cause and drug withdrawal period.

Tech Note!

Using ophthalmic agents in the ear is acceptable because ophthalmic preparations are sterile. However, otic medicines *cannot* be used in the eyes because they are not sterile. The pH and other qualities of otic formulations may injure the eye.

Nose and Sinuses

Anatomy and Physiology of the Nose and Sinuses

As discussed in Chapter 21, the upper respiratory system contains the nose and nasal cavities, the **pharynx** (ie, the throat), and the **larynx** (ie, the voice box). The nose and sinuses play several physiological roles. The nasal septum separates the interior of the nose into two distinct cavities, lined by a mucous membrane with microscopic, hairlike cilia. The mucous membrane warms and moistens inhaled air before it passes to the lungs. The nose is also a sensory organ for smell and drains tears from the eye (Fig. 26.10). Because the nose and sinuses contact the outside world, allergens can result in allergy symptoms or infection.

Common Conditions Affecting the Nose and Sinuses

Allergic Rhinitis

Allergic rhinitis is an irritation and inflammation of the mucous membranes lining the nasal passage secondary to allergen exposure. Common allergic rhinitis symptoms include runny and itchy nose, sneezing, congestion, and postnasal drip. Postnasal drip results from the accumulation of mucus in the back of the nose and throat. OTC products help resolve these symptoms (Table 26.8). Additional symptoms include coughing, watery eyes, and headache. (See Chapter 21 for a detailed review of rhinitis and its treatment.)

GENERIC NAME: triamcinolone

TRADE NAME: Nasacort Allergy 24HR

INDICATION: Allergic rhinitis

ROUTE OF ADMINISTRATION: Intranasal

COMMON ADULT DOSAGE: 2 sprays into each nostril once daily

MECHANISM OF ACTION: Corticosteroid (has antiinflammatory and vasoconstrictive effects that help treat rhinitis symptoms)

SIDE EFFECTS: Dry mouth, nasal dryness, cough, nasal irritation

---

GENERIC NAME: fluticasone

TRADE NAME: Flonase Allergy Relief

INDICATION: Allergic rhinitis

ROUTE OF ADMINISTRATION: Intranasal

COMMON ADULT DOSAGE: 1 or 2 sprays into each nostril once daily

MECHANISM OF ACTION: Corticosteroid (has antiinflammatory and vasoconstrictive effects that help treat rhinitis symptoms)

SIDE EFFECTS: Headache, nosebleed, cough, nasal irritation

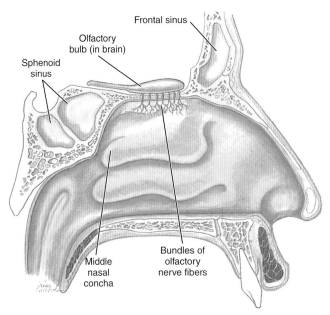

FIG. 26.10 Location and structure of the olfactory epithelium. (From Solomon EP. *Introduction to Human Anatomy and Physiology*. 3rd ed. Philadelphia: Saunders; 2009.)

TABLE 26.8
Select Over-the-Counter Products for the Treatment of Allergy Symptoms

Medication Class	Generic Name	Trade Name	Common Adult Oral Dosage
Antihistamines: Oral, nonsedating[a]	cetirizine HCl	Zyrtec Allergy	• 5–10 mg PO once daily
	fexofenadine	Allegra Allergy 12/24 hour	• 60 mg PO twice daily *or* • 180 mg PO once daily
	loratadine	Claritin	• 10 mg PO once daily
Antihistamines: Oral, sedating (first generation)	chlorpheniramine	Chlor-Trimeton	• 4 mg PO every 4–6 hr *or* • Extended-release tablets: 12 mg every 12 hr
	diphenhydramine	Benadryl Allergy	• 25–50 mg PO every 4–6 hr
Decongestant: Ophthalmic	naphazoline	Clear Eyes Redness Relief	• *0.012% or 0.03%:* 1–2 drops in eye(s) up to 4 times daily
	tetrahydrozoline	Tyzine	• 1–2 drops in each eye up to 4 times daily
Decongestants: Oral	phenylephrine	Sudafed PE Congestion	• 10 mg PO every 4–6 hr
Decongestants: Nasal[b]	cromolyn sodium	NasalCrom	• 1 spray each nostril 3–6 times daily
	oxymetazoline	Afrin Allergy Sinus	• 2–3 sprays each nostril twice daily; do not exceed 3 days' use
	phenylephrine	Neo-Synephrine Cold + Allergy	• 2–3 sprays each nostril every 4 hr as needed; do not exceed 3 days' use
Mast cell stabilizers: Ophthalmic	ketotifen	Zaditor	• 1 drop in affected eye(s) every 8–12 hr (max 2 applications/day)

[a]Medications can be available combined with pseudoephedrine 120 mg and feature a "D" after the name of the decongestant product. Dosing involves a 120-mg pseudoephedrine combination pill twice daily or a double-strength (240 mg) combination pill once daily orally.

[b]Using these nasal sprays for longer than 3 days can cause rebound nasal congestion.

PO, Oral.

Bacterial Sinusitis

Acute bacterial sinusitis is a sinus infection and corresponding inflammation of the nose and nasal passages. It can develop as a secondary infection after an upper respiratory tract viral infection. Symptoms include nasal congestion, nasal discharge, cough, sinus pressure, headache, and fever. Distinguishing between viral and bacterial sinusitis is difficult. Because viral sinusitis improves after 7 to 10 days, acute bacterial sinusitis diagnosis comes from symptoms continuing for longer than 10 days or if symptoms worsen after 5 to 7 days.

Prognosis

The prognosis for bacterial sinusitis is good with antibiotic therapy, rest, and hydration.

Non-Drug Treatment

Rest and fluids are an important aspect of recovery. Saline irrigation of the sinuses reduces the need for pain medication and improves comfort.

Drug Treatment

After a diagnosis of bacterial sinusitis, antibiotic therapy can fight the infection. Amoxicillin is a first-line therapy because of low cost and a broad antimicrobial spectrum. Amoxicillin plus clavulanate (Augmentin) works for resistant infections. Other antibiotics include doxycycline, clarithromycin, azithromycin, and trimethoprim-sulfamethoxazole. In addition to antibiotic therapy, medications for symptom management, such as analgesics, decongestants, antihistamines, mucolytics, and intranasal glucocorticoids, are widely used. See Chapter 21 for a more detailed review of these agents.

Tech Note!

Individuals who use saline irrigations to treat sinusitis should use sterile or bottled water to prepare the saline rinse. Some individuals have contracted amebic encephalitis from tap water rinses.

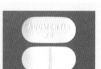

GENERIC NAME: amoxicillin plus clavulanate

TRADE NAMES: Augmentin, Augmentin XR

INDICATIONS: Sinusitis, urinary tract infection (UTI), miscellaneous bacterial infections

ROUTE OF ADMINISTRATION: Oral

COMMON ADULT DOSAGE: 250 mg every 8 hours, *or* 500 mg every 8–12 hours, *or* 875 mg every 12 hours, *or* 2000 mg every 12 hours

MECHANISMS OF ACTION: Amoxicillin is a beta-lactam antibiotic that inhibits bacterial cell wall synthesis; clavulanic acid competitively inhibits bacterial beta-lactamases to help overcome antibiotic resistance.

SIDE EFFECTS: Diarrhea, nausea, vomiting, rash

AUXILIARY LABELS:
- Take with food
- Take until gone

The Throat

The throat, composed of the pharynx and larynx (see Chapters 21 and 22), is the passageway into both the respiratory and the gastrointestinal tracts (Fig. 26.11). Many conditions can affect the throat, including viral or bacterial infections, sore throat associated with allergies, erosion of the esophagus as a result of gastric reflux, and cancers of the larynx or pharynx.

Common Conditions Affecting the Throat

Strep Throat and Tonsillitis

Streptococcal tonsillopharyngitis (or "strep throat") is a bacterial throat infection associated with an abrupt onset of throat pain, fever, and **exudate** from the tonsils (Fig. 26.12). The goals of antibiotic treatment are to reduce the following:

- Duration and severity of symptoms
- Incidence of complications (eg, rheumatic fever)
- Transmission of the bacteria to close contacts

Prognosis

With treatment, the prognosis for streptococcal infections of the throat is good. There is a risk for infrequent complications associated with such diseases, including **rheumatic fever** and **glomerulonephritis** (a form of kidney damage).

Non-Drug Treatment

As for sinusitis, adequate rest and hydration are an important component of therapy. Saltwater gargles can help with symptomatic sore throat management.

Drug Treatment

Antibiotic options include penicillin, ampicillin, amoxicillin, cephalosporins, macrolides, and clindamycin. Analgesics, lozenges, numbing sprays, and pain strips are available over the counter (OTC) for the sore throat. (See Chapter 29 for a discussion of OTC products for cough and cold symptoms including local anesthetic products for sore throat.)

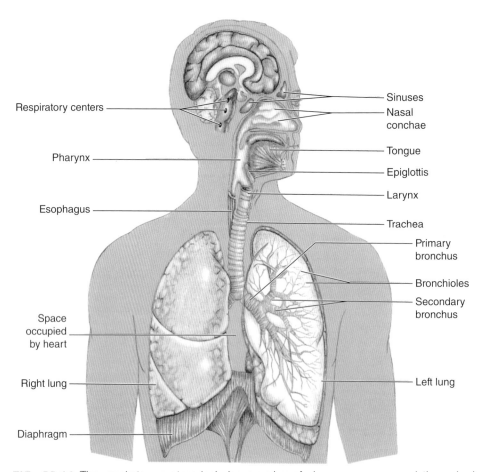

Respiratory centers — Sinuses — Nasal conchae — Pharynx — Tongue — Epiglottis — Larynx — Esophagus — Trachea — Primary bronchus — Bronchioles — Secondary bronchus — Space occupied by heart — Right lung — Left lung — Diaphragm

FIG. 26.11 The respiratory system includes a series of air passageways and the paired lungs. (From Solomon EP. *Introduction to Human Anatomy and Physiology*. 3rd ed. Philadelphia: Saunders; 2009.)

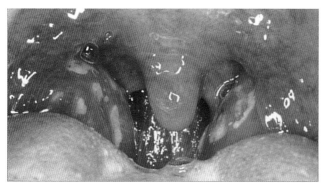

FIG. 26.12 Streptococcal tonsillitis caused by group A beta-hemolytic *Streptococcus pyogenes,* showing intense erythema of the tonsils and a creamy, yellow exudate. (From Goering R, Mims CA, et al. *Mims' Medical Microbiology*. 4th ed. St. Louis: Mosby; 2008.)

Gastroesophageal Reflux Disease

As discussed in Chapter 22, gastroesophageal reflux disease (GERD) can occur when the upper sphincter (opening) at the top of the stomach relaxes. This relaxation allows acidic stomach contents to back into the esophagus, which results in a burning sensation in the chest or throat. Risk factors for GERD include obesity, smoking, and pregnancy. If left untreated, GERD can result in significant damage to the throat. Barrett esophagus is a disorder in which the lining of the esophagus is damaged by stomach acid. Appropriate treatment of GERD helps prevent permanent damage.

Prognosis

With the use of medications and avoidance of certain aggravating foods, the outlook for GERD is good. Many people can make a full recovery from GERD symptoms.

Non-Drug Treatments

Avoiding foods that may bring about symptoms of GERD is an important treatment aspect. Another non-drug approach includes raising the head of the bed if GERD symptoms are prominent while lying down. If medication and diet are ineffective, surgery is an option but rarely necessary.

Drug Treatments

In addition to antacids, histamine-2 antagonists (H₂-antagonists) treat GERD and ulcers. Agents such as famotidine block H₂-receptors in the stomach lining. Proton pump inhibitors (PPIs) also work to treat GERD. PPIs inhibit gastric acid secretion in the stomach lining by blocking the final enzymatic reaction before acid secretion. All three classes are OTC, but some H₂-antagonists and PPIs may require a prescription.

GERD, Gastroesophageal reflux disease; *OTC,* over the counter.

GENERIC NAME: amoxicillin

TRADE NAMES: Moxatag

INDICATION: Bacterial pharyngitis, bacterial tonsillitis, miscellaneous bacterial infections

ROUTE OF ADMINISTRATION: Oral

COMMON ADULT DOSAGE: 250 mg every 8 hours *or* 500 mg every 12 hours for 7–10 days

MECHANISM OF ACTION: Beta-lactam (penicillin) antibiotic inhibits bacterial cell wall synthesis, leading to bacterial cell death

SIDE EFFECTS: Nausea, vomiting, diarrhea, allergic reactions

AUXILIARY LABELS:
- *Moxatag:* Do not chew or crush
- Take until gone

GENERIC NAME: azithromycin

TRADE NAMES: Zithromax Z-Pak, Zmax

INDICATIONS: Bacterial pharyngitis, bacterial tonsillitis, miscellaneous bacterial infections

ROUTE OF ADMINISTRATION: Oral

COMMON ADULT DOSAGE: 500 mg on day 1, followed by 250 mg daily for an additional 4 days

MECHANISM OF ACTION: Macrolide antibiotic (inhibits bacterial protein synthesis)

SIDE EFFECTS: Diarrhea, nausea, abdominal pain, anorexia

AUXILIARY LABELS:
- Take with or without food
- Take until gone

GENERIC NAME: omeprazole

TRADE NAME: Prilosec OTC (available OTC)

INDICATIONS: Gastric ulcer, duodenal ulcer, GERD, erosive esophagitis; OTC for frequent heartburn occurring 2 or more days per week for up to 2 weeks

ROUTE OF ADMINISTRATION: Oral

COMMON ADULT DOSAGES: Dosage varies, depending on the severity of the condition; a standard dose is 20 mg once daily; *OTC dosage:* 20 mg/day for up to 14 days

MECHANISM OF ACTION: Prevents gastric acid secretion from parietal cells of the stomach

SIDE EFFECTS: Diarrhea, nausea, headache, stomach pain, increased risk for fractures

AUXILIARY LABELS (Rx):
- Take before meals
- Do not crush or chew

GERD, Gastroesophageal reflux disease; *OTC,* over the counter.

GENERIC NAME: lansoprazole

TRADE NAMES: Prevacid, Prevacid 24HR (OTC)

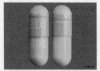

INDICATIONS: GERD, duodenal ulcer, gastric ulcer, NSAID–induced ulcer prophylaxis, erosive esophagitis

ROUTES OF ADMINISTRATION: Oral; intravenous

COMMON ADULT DOSAGE: Dosage varies, depending on the severity of the condition; standard dosage is 15–30 mg once daily

MECHANISM OF ACTION: Prevents gastric acid secretion from parietal cells of the stomach

SIDE EFFECTS: Diarrhea, nausea, headache, stomach pain, increased risk for fractures

AUXILIARY LABELS (Rx):
- Take before meals
- Do not crush or chew

GERD, Gastroesophageal reflux disease; *NSAID*, nonsteroidal antiinflammatory drug; *OTC*, over the counter.

▽ Tech Alert!

Remember the following sound-alike, look-alike drugs:
- Timoptic versus Viroptic
- Tobrex versus TobraDex
- Prednisone versus prednisolone
- Carteolol versus carvedilol

Do You Remember These Key Points?

- Names of the major anatomical components of the eyes, ears, nose, and throat and their functions
- The primary signs and symptoms of the various conditions discussed
- Medications used to treat the various conditions discussed in this chapter
- The generic and trade names for the drugs discussed in this chapter
- The appropriate auxiliary labels that should be used when filling prescriptions for drugs discussed in this chapter

Review Questions

Multiple Choice Questions

1. The cornea is responsible for:
   A. Color of the eye
   B. Lubrication of the eye
   C. Protection of the eyeball
   D. Visual acuity
2. Glaucoma is a condition of the eye that results from:
   A. Narrowing of eye blood vessels
   B. Lack of aqueous humor
   C. Increased intraocular pressure
   D. Sun exposure

3. Which medication is *not* a beta-adrenergic blocker?
   A. Timoptic
   B. Betoptic
   C. Betagan
   D. Trusopt
4. Ketorolac (Ocular) is a/an:
   A. Nonsteroidal antiinflammatory drug (NSAID)
   B. Beta-blocker
   C. Carbonic anhydrase inhibitor
   D. Prostaglandin analog
5. Miotics act by:
   A. Contraction of ciliary muscles, increasing outflow of aqueous humor
   B. Inhibition of beta sites that then relax vessels, allowing proper drainage of aqueous humor
   C. Inhibition of anhydrase, thus lessening the formation of aqueous humor
   D. The drug action is not clear
6. Natamycin is an:
   A. Antibacterial
   B. Antiviral
   C. Antifungal
   D. Antiprotozoal
7. The medical term used to describe the eardrum is:
   A. Eustachian tube
   B. Ossicle
   C. Auricle
   D. Tympanic membrane
8. The trade name of latanoprost is:
   A. Xalatan
   B. Lumigan
   C. Travatan
   D. Pilocar
9. The cavity of the middle ear contains all of the following structures *except:*
   A. Cochlea
   B. Malleus
   C. Incus
   D. Stapes
10. Cerumenex is indicated for use in the:
    A. Eye
    B. Ear
    C. Nose
    D. Throat
11. The structure in the inner ear responsible for balance is the:
    A. Semicircular canal
    B. Vestibule
    C. Cochlea
    D. A and B
12. Visine is an OTC product containing:
    A. Naphazoline
    B. Phenylephrine
    C. Tetrahydrozoline
    D. Azelastine
13. Which drug is considered first-line therapy for bacterial sinusitis?
    A. Amoxicillin
    B. Azithromycin

C. Penicillin

D. Ciprofloxacin

14. Which class of medications for glaucoma treatment has the unusual side effect of darkening of the iris?

A. Beta-blockers

B. Miotics

C. Prostaglandin agonists

D. None of the above

15. Ototoxicity can be caused by:

A. Analgesics

B. Aminoglycosides

C. Antineoplastics

D. All of the above

■ Technician's Corner

Look up the following agents in *Drug Facts and Comparisons* and list the following information on each drug: generic and trade names, normal dosage, strength(s), indication, and auxiliary labels:

- Xalatan
- Optivar
- Auralgan

Bibliography

Damjanov I. *Pathology for the Health Professions*. 4th ed. St. Louis: Saunders; 2011.

Fishback JL. *Pathology*. 3rd ed. Philadelphia: Mosby; 2005.

Goering R, Dockrell H, Zuckerman M, et al. *Mims' Medical Microbiology*. 4th ed. London: Mosby; 2008.

Huether S, McCance K. *Understanding Pathophysiology*. 5th ed. St. Louis: Mosby; 2012.

McCance KL. *Pathophysiology: The Biologic Basis for Disease in Adults and Children*. 6th ed. St. Louis: Mosby; 2010.

Page C, Hoffman B, Curtis M, Walker M. *Integrated Pharmacology*. 3rd ed. London: Mosby; 2006.

Price SA, Wilson LM. *Pathophysiology: Clinical Concepts of Disease Processes*. 6th ed. St. Louis: Mosby; 2003.

Solomon EP. *Introduction to Human Anatomy and Physiology*. 3rd ed. St. Louis: Saunders; 2009.

Thibodeau GA, Patton KT. *Anatomy and Physiology*. 8th ed. St. Louis: Mosby; 2012.

Thompson JM, Farland GK, Hirsch JE, Tucker SM. *Mosby's Clinical Nursing*. 5th ed. St. Louis: Mosby; 2001.

Websites Referenced

Clinical Pharmacology Online. Available at: https://www.clinicalkey.com/pharmacology/.

UpToDate Online. Available at: http://www.uptodate.com.

CHAPTER 27

Therapeutic Agents for the Dermatologic System

Tony Guerra

1. Describe the anatomy and physiology of the main components of the dermatologic system.
2. List the primary signs and symptoms of common conditions associated with the dermatologic system. In addition, (a) recognize prescription and over-the-counter drugs used to treat common conditions associated with the dermatologic system, (b) write the generic and trade names for the drugs discussed in this chapter, and (c) list appropriate auxiliary labels when filling prescriptions for drugs discussed in this chapter.

Acne vulgaris Commonly known as pimples, acne occurs when the skin pores clog with oil or bacteria

Alopecia Partial or complete absence of hair from body areas where it usually grows; baldness

Antiseptics Against + infection, substances that slow or stop microorganism growth on surfaces such as skin

Comedones Blackheads; plugs of keratin and sebum in hair follicles blackened at the surface

Dermis A thick layer of connective tissue that contains collagen

Eczema A condition in which patches of skin become rough and inflamed

Emollient A preparation that softens the skin

Epidermis Outer + skin, the outermost skin layer composed of the stratum corneum, or horny layer; the keratinocytes (squamous cells); and the basal layer. It also contains melanin, a pigment that contributes to skin and hair color

Eschar A slough produced by a thermal burn, by application of a corrosive agent, or by gangrene

Exfoliation The peeling off of dead skin

Head louse A louse that infests the scalp and hair of the human head

Hirsutism Abnormal growth of hair on a person's face and body

Hypodermis Below + skin, subcutaneous tissue

Keratolytics Drugs that cause shedding of the outer layer of the skin

Melanin A dark brown to black pigment found in the hair, skin, and iris of the eye

Metastasize With regard to cancer, to spread from the place of origin as a primary tumor to distant locations in the body

Nodules Small swellings or aggregations of cells in the body

Onychomycosis Nail + fungus + disease, a fungal infection of the fingernails or toenails

Papules Small, raised, solid pimples on the skin

Perspiration The process of sweating

Pruritus Itching

Pustules Small blisters or pimples on the skin containing pus

Sebaceous gland Skin glands responsible for the secretion of oil called sebum

Seborrhea Excessive discharge of sebum from the sebaceous glands

Sebum An oily/waxy substance that lubricates the skin and retains water to provide moisture

Subcutaneous layer The deepest layer of the skin, consisting of fat cells and collagen; it protects the body and conserves heat

Sweat glands Glands in the dermis that are activated by an increase in body temperature to cool the body

Urticaria Red welts that arise on the surface of the skin; they are often attributable to an allergic reaction but may have nonallergic causes; also known as hives

Xerosis Dry + condition, abnormal dryness of the skin, eyes, or mucous membranes

Common Drugs for Conditions of the Dermatologic System

Trade Name	Generic Name	Pronunciation
Antibacterials		
Bacitracin	bacitracin	(bass-ih-**tray**-sin)
Bactroban[a]	mupirocin	(myoo-**peer**-oh-sin)
Ery-Tab	erythromycin	(er-**ith**-row-**mye**-sin)
Neomycin	neomycin	(ne-oh-**mye**-sin)
Neosporin	neomycin/bacitracin/polymyxin b sulfate	(**nee**-oh-**mye**-sin/bass-ih-**tray**-sin/**pol**-ee-**mix**-in)
None	dicloxacillin	(dye-**klox**-uh-sil-in)
None	tetracycline	(**tet**-ra-**sye**-klin)
Antifungals		
Desenex	miconazole	(my-**kon**-uh-zole)
Lamisil AT	terbinafine	(**ter**-bin-uh-feen)
Lotrimin AF	clotrimazole	(kloe-**trim**-uh-zole)
Nizoral A-D	ketoconazole	(kee-tuh-**kon**-uh-zole)
Tinactin	tolnaftate	(tol-**naf**-tate)
Treatment of Eczema		
Dupixent	dipilumab	(doo-**pil**-ue-mab)
Protopic	tacrolimus	(tah-krow-**lie**-mus)
Elidel	pimecrolimus	(pih-meh-krow-**lih**-mus)
Treatment of Psoriasis		
Sotyktu	deucravacitinib	(doo-**crah**-vuh-sih-tih-nib)
Enbrel	etanercept	(eh-**tan**-er-sept)
Remicade	infliximab	(in-**flix**-ih-mab)
Stelara	ustekinumab	(**yoo**-sti-**kin**-ue-mab)
Corticosteroids		
Cordran	flurandrenolide	(flur-an-**dren**-oh-lide)
Cutivate	fluticasone propionate	(floo-**tik**-uh-sone/**pro**-pee-oh-nate)
Diprolene	betamethasone	(bay-tuh-**meth**-uh-sone)
Temovate	clobetasol propionate	(kloe-**bay**-tuh-sol/**pro**-pee-oh-nate)
Topicort	desoximetasone	(des-**ox**-ee-**met**-uh-sone)
Triderm	triamcinolone acetonide	(trye-am-**sin**-oh-lone a-**seet**-oh-nide)
Vanos	fluocinonide	(floo-oh-**sin**-oh-nide)
Immunosuppressants		
Sandimmune, Neoral	cyclosporine	(sye-kloe-**spor**-ihn)
Trexall	methotrexate	(meth-oh-**trex**-ate)

Continued

Trade Name	Generic Name	Pronunciation
Retinoids		
Retin-A, Retin-A Micro, Avita	tretinoin	(tret-**in**-oin)
Topical Vitamin D Analog		
Dovonex	calcipotriene	(cal-sih-poh-**try**-een)

ᵃBrand discontinued; now available only as generic.

The dermatologic system, in its widest sense, involves conditions affecting the skin, scalp, hair, and nails. The skin is one of the most abused organs of the body system. It withstands damage from weather, detergents, scratches, cuts, and bruises, while continually repairing itself. The skin protects the body, regulates temperature, and acts as a sensor to outside stimuli. This chapter reviews the anatomy and physiology of the skin, hair, and nails and their functions. We will discuss common conditions affecting the dermatologic system and select treatments for those conditions.

Anatomy and Physiology of the Dermatologic System

Skin

Various layers that contain nerves, glands, hair, and blood vessels form the skin, the largest body organ. The skin protects the body against heat, cold, light, dehydration, and infection. Nerve endings allow for the perception of pain, heat, and cold. The body is mostly covered with hair follicles embedded in the dermis (Fig. 27.1).

The top skin portion, the **epidermis,** further divides into three main layers: the horny outer layer, squamous cells, and basal layer. The epidermis, the outermost layer, protects the layers below. The epidermis contains melanocytes, which produce the skin pigment **melanin.** The epidermis does not

have a blood supply of its own; instead, it receives nutrition from the tissues surrounding it. Epidermis cells constantly shed, and the body replaces them. The basal layer produces new cells. The new skin cells push older cells upward, and this becomes the outer epidermis layer. Beneath the epidermis are the dermis and subcutaneous layers.

The **dermis** is a thick layer of connective tissue that contains collagen. The dermis is under the epidermis (see Fig. 27.1). Collagen, composed of interwoven, flexible fibers, helps support other structures such as dermal blood vessels, glands, and nerves. Below the dermis lies the **subcutaneous layer,** or **hypodermis,** the deepest layer. It contains fat cells for insulation. Fat also helps cushion the body against injury and serves as an energy reserve.

Hair and Nails

A protein called *keratin* is the primary component in hair. Hair has roots embedded in the dermis. The base contains melanocytes responsible for hair color. As a person ages, the melanocytes stop producing melanin, and the hair turns gray. The hair follicle is vascularized to provide nourishment to the follicle (Fig. 27.2). **Hirsutism** is an excess of hair growth, whereas **alopecia** is the loss of hair. Medications and medical conditions can cause both.

Like hair, the nails contain keratin, but they are much denser than hair. The nails cover the top surface at the end of the toes and fingers. The nail root, embedded in the epidermis, protects the surface. The lunula is the small white portion at the nail's base. The cuticle has keratin at the base and sides of the nail. The paronychium surrounds the nail and consists of softer tissue (Fig. 27.3).

Glands

The two types of glands in the skin layers are sebaceous glands and sweat glands (Fig. 27.4). The **sebaceous glands,** in the dermal skin layer, secrete an oily substance called *sebum.* **Sebum** lubricates the skin and retains water to keep the skin and hair from drying out. Ducts transport sebum to the hair follicles, where the oily substance remains. Sebaceous glands are everywhere on the skin except palms of the hands and soles of the feet.

Sweat glands are much smaller than sebaceous glands and are prevalent in hand palms and foot soles. Sweat contains mostly water and salt. When sweat glands activate, sweat escapes through skin pores. As the temperature rises, the nervous system signals the glands. **Perspiration** is the flow of sweat to the skin's surface. The subsequent evaporation cools the skin.

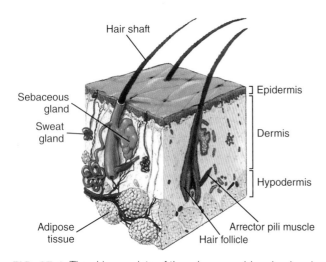

FIG. 27.1 The skin consists of three layers: epidermis, dermis, and subcutaneous tissue. (From Damjanov I. *Pathology for the Health Professions*. 4th ed. Philadelphia: Saunders; 2011.)

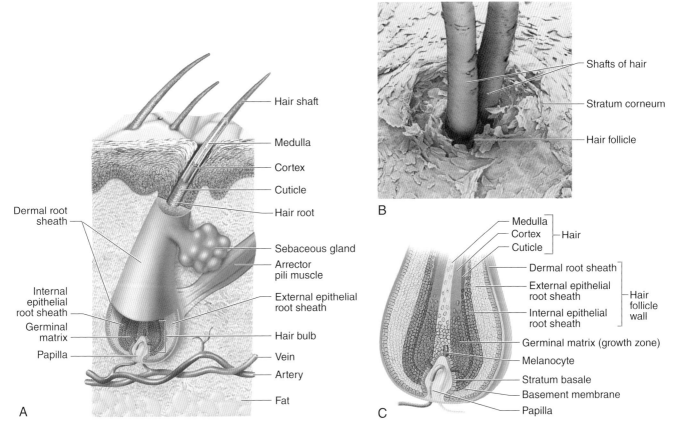

FIG. 27.2 Hair follicle. (A) Skin cross section with hair follicle. (B) Hair follicle and shaft at epidermis. (C) Hair follicle at dermis. (From Patton KT, Thibodeau GA. *Anatomy and Physiology*. 8th ed. St. Louis: Mosby; 2013.)

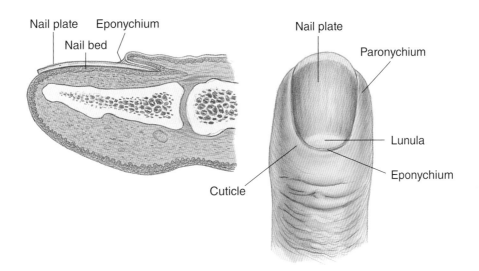

FIG. 27.3 Nail anatomy. (Redrawn from Thompson JM, McFarland GK, Hirsch JE, et al. *Mosby's Clinical Nursing*. 5th ed. St. Louis: Mosby; 2001.)

Common Conditions Affecting the Dermatologic System

This chapter outlines common conditions and treatments for the dermatologic system, starting with the skin, followed by a discussion of the hair and nails.

Dermatologic Conditions Affecting the Skin

Many conditions affect the skin. Over-the-counter (OTC) medications can relieve some issues such as acne, sunburn, and hives. Other issues, such as infection, and skin disorders, such as impetigo, require treatment by a doctor.

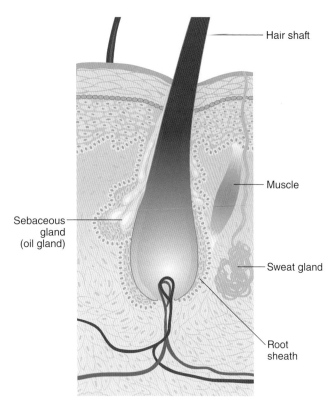

FIG. 27.4 Glands of the skin.

Labels: Hair shaft, Muscle, Sebaceous gland (oil gland), Sweat gland, Root sheath

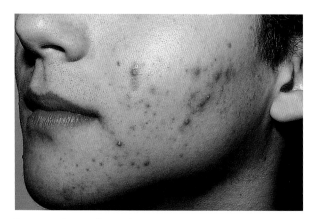

FIG. 27.5 Acne. (From Callen JP et al. *Color Atlas of Dermatology.* 2nd ed. Philadelphia: Saunders; 2000.)

Acne Vulgaris

Seborrhea, comedones, papules, pustules, nodules, and potential scarring characterize **acne vulgaris** (acne), a common skin condition. Acne most commonly affects skin with a high density of sebaceous glands, such as the face, chest, and back. Severe acne cases have inflammation. However, acne can manifest without inflammation. Because of increased testosterone levels during puberty, acne occurs most commonly during adolescence; however, it can extend into adulthood.

Hormones can enlarge and activate skin glands. Two productive glands are the sweat glands, which can become clogged, and the sebaceous glands, which produce sebum. When sebum production increases, it traps bacteria at the hair follicle's base and the likelihood of acne increases. The increased androgen production during puberty leads to increased sebum production. When this occurs, acne-causing bacteria multiply, leak from pores, and release oily chemicals onto the dermis, which can lead to inflammation (Fig. 27.5).

Prognosis

The length of time before symptoms disappear varies, depending on the acne type. Typically, as adolescents reach maturity, outbreak frequency decreases, although scarring can happen in more severe cases.

Non-Drug Treatment

The most effective non-drug acne treatment is keeping the skin clean and bacteria-free by using cleansing agents that reduce sebum production and exfoliate (ie, remove) dead skin cells. Although cleaning is essential, excessive cleansing can irritate the skin, worsening the condition. Various light therapies might improve acne; however, the efficacy of light-based therapies for the treatment of acne vulgaris remains under investigation.

Drug Treatments

Mild acne often responds to topical agents such as benzoyl peroxide, which helps dry the skin, and salicylic acid, which increases skin turnover. More severe inflammatory acne may require topical or systemic antibiotics or topical retinoids in addition to **keratolytics.** A patient may require prescription antibiotics, such as tetracycline (orally), erythromycin (orally or topically), and clindamycin (topically). Topical retinoid agents, such as tretinoin (Retin-A Micro), increase skin growth around the acne areas, which causes skin **exfoliation,** removing dead skin cells and decreasing comedone formation. With retinoid treatment, acne may seem to worsen initially but usually improves over several weeks. We reserve oral retinoids, such as isotretinoin (Amnesteem, Claravis), for severe acne. Oral retinoid therapies require that the prescriber, the pharmacy, and the patient enroll in a program called iPLEDGE. The program works to reduce fetal exposure to the medication, because systemic retinoids are known teratogens. The iPLEDGE REMS program mandates that providers dispense prescriptions no more than once every 30 days and a 7-day window in which patients must retrieve their prescription to maintain eligibility for treatment. The retrieval period is an extended 30-day window for patients who cannot become pregnant.

Table 27.1 describes select acne treatment agents.

■ Tech Note!

iPLEDGE is a program aimed to prevent pregnancy during isotretinoin product use. It educates patients and prescribers about potential side effects and risks of isotretinoin treatment. Visit *https://ipledgeprogram. com/#Main* to learn more about the program.

TABLE 27.1
Select Agents for the Treatment of Acne

Medication Class	Generic Name	Trade Name	Common Adult Dosage
Topical Treatments			
Topical skin products	benzoyl peroxide	Clearplex V, Neutrogena Clear Pore	• Apply sparingly once daily, gradually increase to 2–3 times daily
	salicylic acid	Stridex	• Apply thin layer to affected area 1–3 times daily
	adapalene	Differin	• Apply once daily at bedtime
	dapsone	Aczone	• Apply a pea-sized amount to the affected area twice daily
	azelaic acid	Azelex, Finacea	• Apply a thin film to the affected area twice daily
Lincosamide	clindamycin	Clindagel, Cleocin T, ClindaMax[a]	• Clindagel: Apply to acne once daily • Cleocin T and ClindaMax: Apply a thin film twice daily
Macrolide	erythromycin	Erygel,[a] Ery	• Apply over the affected area once or twice daily
Retinoic acid derivative	tretinoin	Retin-A Micro	• Apply once daily to acne lesions before bedtime
Oral Treatments			
Tetracyclines	doxycycline	Oracea, Vibramycin	• 50–100 mg PO twice daily
	minocycline	Minocin, Solodyn	• 50–100 mg PO twice daily
	tetracycline	—	• 1 g daily in divided doses; reduce gradually to 125–500 mg/day once improvement is noted
Macrolide	erythromycin	Ery-Tab	• 250–500 mg PO twice daily
Sulfonamide	sulfamethoxazole/trimethoprim	Bactrim	• 1 single-strength or double-strength tablet once or twice daily
Retinoic acid derivative	isotretinoin	Amnesteem, Claravis, Absorica	• 0.5–1 mg/kg/day in 2 divided doses for 15–20 wk

[a]Brand no longer available.
PO, Orally.

GENERIC NAME: tetracycline

TRADE NAME: none

INDICATION: Inflammatory acne vulgaris

ROUTE OF ADMINISTRATION: Oral

COMMON ADULT DOSAGE: 1 g/day in divided doses; reduce gradually to 125–500 mg/day on seeing improvement

SIDE EFFECTS: Nausea, vomiting, anorexia, diarrhea, photosensitivity, tooth discoloration

MECHANISM OF ACTION: Inhibits bacterial protein synthesis

AUXILIARY LABELS:
• Do not take with dairy products
• Separate from antacids or iron supplements by 4 hours
• Take on an empty stomach
• Take with a full glass of water
• Avoid exposure to sunlight or tanning beds

GENERIC NAME: tretinoin

TRADE NAMES: Retin-A, Renova

INDICATION: Acne vulgaris

ROUTE OF ADMINISTRATION: Topical

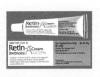

COMMON ADULT DOSAGE: Apply once daily to acne lesions in the evening or before bedtime

MECHANISMS OF ACTION: Modifies gene expression, protein synthesis, and epithelial cell growth and differentiation, leading to increased epithelial cell turnover

SIDE EFFECTS: Dry skin, itching, peeling, redness, irritation

AUXILIARY LABELS:
• For external use only
• Keep container tightly closed
• Avoid exposure to sunlight or tanning beds

GENERIC NAME: isotretinoin

TRADE NAMES: Amnesteem, Claravis, Myorisan, Absorica, Zenatane

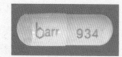

INDICATIONS: Acne (severe recalcitrant nodular)

ROUTE OF ADMINISTRATION: Oral

COMMON ADULT DOSAGE: 0.5–1 mg/kg/day given in 2 divided doses for 15–20 weeks or until the total cyst count decreases by 70%

MECHANISM OF ACTION: Inhibits sebum production through a reduction in the size of sebaceous glands and possible inhibition of follicular keratinization

SIDE EFFECTS: Inflammation of the lips, irritation, pruritus, photosensitivity, rash, congenital disabilities (pregnancy is a "Black Box Warning"), increased serum triglycerides, back pain

AUXILIARY LABELS:
- Take with food
- Swallow capsules whole with a full glass of liquid
- Avoid pregnancy (do not take this medication if you become pregnant)

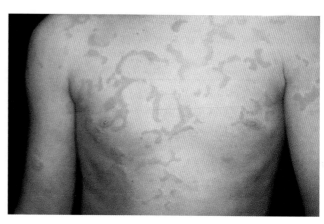

FIG. 27.6 Urticaria. (McCance KL. *Pathophysiology: The Biologic Basis for Disease in Adults and Children*. 6th ed. St. Louis: Mosby; 2010.)

■ Tech Note!

Topical diphenhydramine products are also available OTC. Health providers generally discourage topical use because of questionable efficacy and possible sensitivity reactions after prolonged or repeated use.

Urticaria

Urticaria is also known as hives. These superficial bumps range in size and are commonly associated with **pruritus** (Fig. 27.6). Hives are generally caused by hypersensitivity reactions to food, the environment, or drugs and can occur anywhere on the body. Sometimes topical agents can mitigate hives and other noninfectious inflammatory skin rashes. Some cases of urticaria are *idiopathic*, or of unknown cause. They can disappear as rapidly as they appear.

Prognosis

Hives may dissipate within several hours without treatment. However, hives resulting from allergic reactions may necessitate treatment. Removal of the allergen or cause is an important treatment component.

Non-Drug Treatment

Applying a cold, wet compress can help alleviate the pruritus that accompanies hives.

Drug Treatment

Antihistamines frequently reduce the symptoms of urticaria. Topical anesthetics can also help alleviate pruritus symptoms. If the patient needs an antihistamine, oral diphenhydramine can dramatically reduce the appearance of hives and itching. However, drowsiness is a common side effect, so patients should be cautious with sedating antihistamines. (See Chapter 29 for a review of OTC antihistamine products that can be used to treat the symptoms of urticaria.)

GENERIC NAME: diphenhydramine (OTC)

TRADE NAME: Benadryl Allergy

INDICATIONS: Hives, itching, rashes

ROUTE OF ADMINISTRATION: Oral; topical

COMMON ADULT DOSAGE: *Oral:* 25–50 mg every 4–8 hours as needed (max 300 mg/day). *Topical:* Apply 1% or 2% to affected area up to 3 or 4 times daily

MECHANISM OF ACTION: Competitively inhibits the actions of histamine at histamine-1 receptors

SIDE EFFECTS: *Oral:* Drowsiness, dry mouth, dizziness, confusion, constipation, blurred vision. *Topical:* Photosensitivity

AUXILIARY LABEL: *Oral:* May cause drowsiness

OTC, Over the counter.

GENERIC NAME: calamine 8% and pramoxine HCl 1% (OTC)

TRADE NAMES: Caladryl, Calagesic

INDICATION: Pruritus

ROUTE OF ADMINISTRATION: Topical

COMMON ADULT DOSAGE: Apply to affected area not more than 3 or 4 times daily as needed for comfort

MECHANISM OF ACTION: Calamine (a mixture of zinc and ferrous oxide) acts as a protectant against irritants; pramoxine is a local anesthetic

SIDE EFFECTS: Dryness; can aggravate contact dermatitis

AUXILIARY LABELS:
- Shake well before use
- For external use only
- Avoid contact with eyes and mucous membranes

OTC, Over the counter.

Eczema

Eczema, also known as *atopic dermatitis,* is a chronic inflammatory skin condition thought to involve a genetic defect in proteins that support the epidermal barrier (Fig. 27.7). Eczema may have a pathophysiologic immune component; therefore some of the following treatments affect the immune system. Eczema may affect 5% to 20% of children worldwide; the prevalence is approximately 11% in the United States. Eczema types include "exogenous eczema" and "endogenous eczema." Researchers believe exogenous eczema comes from environmental irritants, whereas endogenous eczema ties to systemic autoimmune disorders.

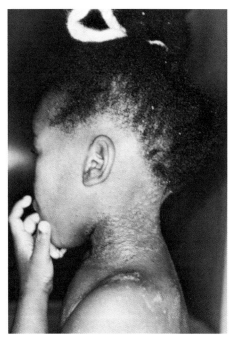

FIG. 27.7 Lichenified, thickened, scaly skin over the neck area in childhood atopic eczema. (From Price SA, Wilson LM. *Pathophysiology: Clinical Concepts of Disease Processes*. 6th ed. St. Louis: Mosby; 2003.)

Prognosis

The prognosis for eczema can vary considerably depending on the type of eczema and the person's treatment response. Approximately half of children with atopic eczema experience symptoms into adulthood.

Non-Drug Treatment

A significant management component is to eliminate exacerbating factors, such as excessive bathing, low-humidity environments, stress, dry skin, or exposure to irritants. Hydrating skin is also essential. The use of thick creams or ointments can help protect against **xerosis** (dry skin).

Drug Treatment

The pruritus associated with eczema can respond to antihistamines. Antiinflammatory agents, such as corticosteroids and topical calcineurin inhibitors (tacrolimus and pimecrolimus), can work as well. For severe cases, oral cyclosporine and methotrexate may be effective (Table 27.2). Excoriation may lead to eczema infection; therefore many patients with eczema also use antiinfective skin agents.

The injectable dupilumab (Dupixent) recently received US Food and Drug Administration (FDA) approval in patients ages 6 months to 5 years with moderate-to-severe eczema. This medicine is for patients whose symptoms do not respond to other therapies or when alternative therapies are inappropriate. Barriers to receiving dupilumab treatment include high cost and documentation of prior treatment failure(s) using other anti-eczema agents.

GENERIC NAME: dupilumab

TRADE NAME: Dupixent

INDICATIONS: Eczema, atopic dermatitis, asthma (off-label use)

ROUTE OF ADMINISTRATION: Subcutaneous injection

COMMON ADULT DOSAGE: 600 mg once, followed by 300 mg once every other week

PEDIATRIC DOSAGE: Weight- and age-based dosing (see package insert for proper dosing schedules)

MECHANISM OF ACTION: Interleukin-4 (IL-4) and interleukin-13 (IL-13) inflammatory response inhibition

SIDE EFFECTS: Injection site reactions, risk of serious hypersensitivity reactions, upper respiratory infection

AUXILIARY LABEL: For subcutaneous injection only

GENERIC NAME: tacrolimus
TRADE NAME: Protopic

INDICATIONS: Eczema, atopic dermatitis

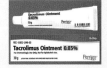

ROUTE OF ADMINISTRATION: Topical

COMMON ADULT DOSAGE: Apply a thin layer to the affected area twice daily up to 6 weeks; discontinue when symptoms have resolved

MECHANISM OF ACTION: Inhibits calcineurin, which inhibits T cell activation

TABLE 27.2

Select Agents for the Treatment of Eczema

Medication Class	Generic Name	Trade Name	Common Adult Dosage
Topical corticosteroids	betamethasone	Diprolene	• Apply to scalp/area twice daily
	clobetasol propionate	Temovate, Clobex	• Apply to scalp/area twice daily
	fluocinolone	Synalar	• Apply a thin layer to affected area 3 times daily
	fluocinonide	Vanos	• Apply a thin layer to affected area 2–4 times daily
	flurandrenolide	Cordran, Nolix[a]	• Apply a thin layer to affected area 2–3 times daily
	fluticasone propionate	Cutivate	• Apply a thin layer to affected area 1–2 times daily
	halcinonide	Halog	• Apply sparingly 2–3 times daily
	hydrocortisone	Cortizone-10	• Apply a thin layer to affected area 2–4 times daily
	triamcinolone acetonide	Triderm,[a] Kenalog	• Apply a thin layer to affected area 2–4 times daily
Topical calcineurin inhibitors	tacrolimus	Protopic	• Apply ointment twice daily
	pimecrolimus	Elidel	• Apply cream twice daily
Oral calcineurin inhibitor	cyclosporine	Sandimmune, Gengraf, Neoral	• 2.5 mg/kg PO in 2 divided doses daily
Immunosuppressants	methotrexate	Trexall	• 10–25 mg/dose PO, IM, or subcut once weekly
	mycophenolate	CellCept	• 2–3 g/day PO

[a]Brand no longer available.

IM, Intramuscularly; *PO,* orally; *subcut,* subcutaneously.

SIDE EFFECTS: Burning, irritation, increased risk for skin infections, photosensitivity

AUXILIARY LABELS:
- Increased risk of sunburn
- Use topically only
- Wash hands with soap and water before and after application

SIDE EFFECTS: Burning, irritation, increased risk of skin infections, photosensitivity

AUXILIARY LABELS:
- Increased risk for sunburn
- Use topically only
- Wash hands with soap and water before and after application

■ Tech Note!

Tacrolimus is also available orally for prophylaxis of organ transplant rejection under the trade names Prograf and Envarsus XL.

GENERIC NAME: pimecrolimus
TRADE NAME: Elidel

INDICATIONS: Eczema, atopic dermatitis

ROUTE OF ADMINISTRATION: Topical

COMMON ADULT DOSAGE: Apply a thin layer to the affected area twice daily up to 6 weeks; discontinue when symptoms have resolved

MECHANISM OF ACTION: Inhibits calcineurin, which inhibits T-cell activation

Psoriasis

Psoriasis is a common, noninfectious, painful inflammatory skin disorder that has been related to genetics, especially cases with early onset (age 40 or younger). The disease can range from mild to severe and can last a lifetime. Onset usually happens in one of two peaks, between the ages of 20 and 30 or 50 and 60. This condition is not contagious, although lesions appear inflamed. Affected areas are typically around the joints, limbs, neck, and even scalp and can appear as small or large plaques with silvery scales (Fig. 27.8).

Prognosis

Currently, psoriasis has no cure, and patients require constant treatment to prevent outbreaks. Some can develop arthritic symptoms; this happens in one-third of psoriasis patients. For these individuals, additional medications, such as nonsteroidal antiinflammatory

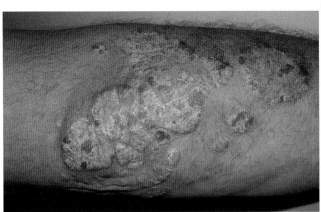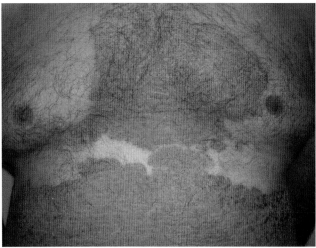

FIG. 27.8 Psoriasis. (From Lookingbill D, Marks J. *Principles of Dermatology*. 4th ed. Philadelphia: Saunders; 2006.)

drugs (NSAIDs), sulfasalazine, methotrexate, and biological response modifiers (see Chapter 25 for a detailed description of these therapies) may be effective.

Non-Drug Treatment

For mild psoriasis (covering 3%–10% of the body), the use of a high-quality moisturizer both keeps the skin moist and helps control flare-ups. **Emollients** that trap moisture work best. It may take time to determine which products are most effective.

Phototherapy (or ultraviolet [UV] exposure treatments) may be used to cause mild skin sunburn and subsequent peeling in patients with more serious disease. This treatment is based, in part, on the observation that patients often notice improvements in skin lesions during the summer months. The process is done gradually over many months with UV light. Another light therapy form involves an excimer laser to treat mild to moderate psoriasis. The UVB wavelength–only treatment requires fewer sessions. Both light therapies are thought to be antiproliferative and antiinflammatory. The American Academy of Dermatology published guidelines on UV light use for psoriasis treatment.

Drug Treatment

Treatment depends on the psoriasis type, the disease extent, and the patient's response. Although there is no cure, palliative measures (ie, care focused on pain, symptoms, and the stress of a condition) may improve the patient's quality of life. Therapy generally comes from one of three modalities: topical agents, phototherapy, and systemic agents. The application of topical agents over the affected area or areas is usually first-line treatment. Occlusion therapy uses moisturizers or topical medication applied to the skin, which is then wrapped with tape, fabric, or plastic. This therapy keeps the area moist, allowing the drug to penetrate deeply and work effectively. Dermatologists should supervise this treatment because it can lead to problems such as thinning skin. OTC bath soaks using

colloidal oatmeal (Aveeno) may reduce pruritus and skin discomfort in mild psoriasis cases. Prescribers may employ tar-based shampoos or preparations for the scalp. Calcipotriene (Dovonex) is a topical vitamin D analog commonly applied to plaques to control skin turnover.

Immunosuppressants such as topical corticosteroids may help in refractory psoriasis. Creams may be applied after bathing to facilitate absorption, and overnight occlusive dressings may help. The mechanism of action of potent corticosteroids is the suppression of T cells and other constituents that cause inflammation and an increase in cell growth; therefore patients should use caution with these agents because they impair the immune system. Etanercept (Enbrel), infliximab (Remicade), and methotrexate are for psoriatic arthritis to prevent joint damage progression. Table 27.3 presents a list of select psoriasis treatment agents.

In 2022 the FDA approved deucravacitinib (Sotyktu) for treating moderate-to-severe plaque psoriasis in adults. This oral treatment comprises a novel class of pharmacological agents called selective allosteric tyrosine kinase 2 (TYK2) inhibitors. It offers a new mechanism to target a protein that causes psoriasis.

GENERIC NAME: deucravacitinib

TRADE NAME: Sotyktu

INDICATIONS: Plaque psoriasis

ROUTE OF ADMINISTRATION: Oral

COMMON ADULT DOSAGE: 6 mg once daily

MECHANISM OF ACTION: Although the exact mechanism in psoriasis is unknown, it is thought that it inhibits tyrosine kinase 2, a protein that plays a role in causing psoriasis

SIDE EFFECTS: Increased risk of infection including pneumonia and upper respiratory tract infection

Select Agents for the Treatment of Psoriasis

Generic Name	Trade Name	Dosage Form	Common Adult Dosage
Corticosteroids			
betamethasone	Diprolene	Ointment, lotion	• Apply twice daily for up to 4 wk
clobetasol propionate	Temovate, Clobex	Ointment/cream/gel, lotion/shampoo/spray	• Apply twice daily for up to 2 wk
fluocinolone	Derma-Smoothe/ FS Scalp	Scalp oil	• Massage into wet or dampened hair/scalp; cover with a shower cap overnight, for at least 4 hr. Wash with shampoo and rinse thoroughly to remove
fluocinonide	Vanos	Cream	• Apply a thin layer to affected area 2–4 times daily
flurandrenolide	Cordran	Tape, ointment, cream, lotion	• Apply a thin layer to affected area 2–3 times daily
fluticasone propionate	Cutivate	Cream, lotion	• Apply thin layer to affected area 1–2 times daily
halcinonide	Halog	Ointment, cream	• Apply sparingly 2–3 times daily
hydrocortisone	Cortizone-10	Ointment, cream, gel	• Apply a thin layer to affected area 2–4 times daily
triamcinolone acetonide	Triderm,[a] Kenalog	Spray	• Apply a thin layer to affected area 2–4 times daily
desoximetasone	Topicort	Cream, gel, ointment, spray	• Apply a thin layer twice daily
amcinonide	Cyclocort,[a] Amcort[a]	Cream, lotion	• Apply thin layer 2–3 times daily
Vitamin D Analog			
calcipotriene	Dovonex	Cream, foam, ointment	• Apply a thin layer twice daily
Topical Retinoid			
tazarotene	Tazorac, Avage	Gel, cream	• Apply a thin layer to the affected area in the evening
Antimetabolite/Antipsoriatic Agent			
methotrexate	Trexall	Tablet	• 10–25 mg/dose PO, IM, or subcut once wkly
Coal Tar Preparation			
coal tar	DHS Tar	Shampoo, oil, ointment, cream, lotion, foam	• Body: Apply at bedtime • Scalp: Paint on scalp lesions 3–12 hr before shower/shampoo
Monoclonal Antibodies			
adalimumab	Humira	Solution for injection	• 80 mg subcut once, then 40 mg every other wk
golimumab	Simponi	Solution for injection	• 50 mg subcut once monthly
ustekinumab	Stelara	Solution for injection	• 45–90 mg subcut at wk 0 and 4, then every 12 wk
Tumor Necrosis Factor (TNF) Inhibitors			
etanercept	Enbrel	Solution for injection	• 50 mg subcut once or twice wkly
Infliximab	Remicade	Solution for injection	• 5 mg/kg IV at wk 0, 2, and 6, then every 8 wk
Calcineurin Inhibitor			
cyclosporine	Sandimmune, Neoral, Gengraf	Capsules, oral solution	• 2.5 mg/kg/day in two divided doses
Psoralens			
methoxsalen	Oxsoralen-Ultra, Uvadex	capsules, solution	• The dose depends on patient weight
Oral Retinoid			
acitretin	Soriatane	Capsule	• 25–50 mg PO once daily

[a]Brand no longer available.

IM, Intramuscularly; *IV,* intravenously; *PO,* orally; *subcut,* subcutaneously.

GENERIC NAME: calcipotriene
TRADE NAMES: Dovonex, Calcitrene, Sorilux

INDICATION: Psoriasis

ROUTE OF ADMINISTRATION: Topical

COMMON ADULT DOSAGE: Apply a thin film to the affected skin twice daily

MECHANISM OF ACTION: Synthetic analog of vitamin D_3 (inhibits cell proliferation and induction of cell differentiation in psoriatic skin)

SIDE EFFECTS: Burning, itching, redness, swelling, dryness, or peeling of the skin

AUXILIARY LABEL: For topical use only

Chickenpox and Shingles

Chickenpox is a contagious disease and may cause severe complications in young children. Typical nonserious symptoms include skin blisters, fever, and an itchy rash (Fig. 27.9). Some people can experience more severe effects, such as brain damage, pneumonia, infection, or (rarely) even death. A pregnant woman who contracts chickenpox may require hospitalization. Another disorder caused by the same virus that causes chickenpox is shingles, which may appear in adulthood in those who had childhood chickenpox. After lying dormant for several years, the virus can activate and cause acute dorsal root ganglia inflammation. Symptoms include painful lesions along the nerves. Shingles treatments include medications such as oral or intravenous valacyclovir (Valtrex). A prescriber can use acyclovir (Zovirax) over 7 days to reduce pain and promote healing. In 2006 a drug manufacturer introduced a single-dose vaccine for adults older than 60 years. The vaccine prevented shingles in about half the subjects tested and can reduce pain. Those who should not be vaccinated include pregnant women or immunocompromised

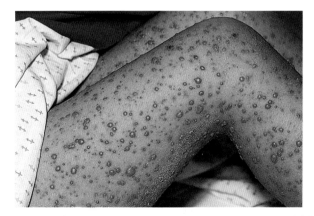

FIG. 27.9 Chickenpox. The rash begins with macules, which turn into severe papules. Symptoms can last a few days to 2 weeks. (From Callen JP et al. *Color Atlas of Dermatology*. 2nd ed. Philadelphia: Saunders; 2000.)

individuals. If the disease is contracted through immunization, only a mild form results. After the injection, the person may have soreness at the injection site and a mild fever. A vaccine was approved in 2017 for adults over 50 years of age. Shingrix is a recombinant two-dose vaccine that claims a 90% success rate. (See Chapter 25 for a more detailed description of this and other vaccines.)

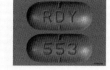

GENERIC NAME: valacyclovir
TRADE NAME: Valtrex

INDICATION: Herpes zoster (shingles)

ROUTE OF ADMINISTRATION: Oral

COMMON ADULT DOSAGE: 1 g 3 times daily for 7 days

MECHANISM OF ACTION: Inhibits viral DNA synthesis

SIDE EFFECTS: Headache, nausea, abdominal pain, fatigue

Burns

Burns range in severity from superficial to fourth-degree; fourth-degree burns are the most severe (Box 27.1). For minor wounds/burns, patients can turn to ointments such as Aquaphor to protect the skin and maintain moisture by occluding the lesion. Topical formulations include topical mupirocin, bacitracin/neomycin/polymyxin B/hydrocortisone

---

BOX 27.1   Definitions of Burn Depth and Severity

Superficial: Only the outer layer (epidermis) of the skin is burned. The skin becomes red and swells, and pain is often present. Superficial burns do not blister but are painful, dry, and red and blanch with pressure. Superficial burns commonly occur with sunburn.

Partial-thickness: The first layer of the skin (epidermis) burns through to the second layer (dermis). These burns can be further classified as superficial or deep. Superficial partial-thickness burns characteristically form blisters within 24 hours; the blisters are painful, red, and weeping and blanch with pressure. Deep partial-thickness burns extend into the deeper dermis and damage hair follicles and glands. Deep burns almost always blister, are patchy white to red, and do not blanch with pressure.

Full-thickness: The burn extends through and destroys all layers of the dermis and often injures the subcutaneous tissue. Eschar, the dead and denatured dermis, is usually intact. These burns can vary in appearance from white to leathery gray, to charred and black.

Fourth degree: The worst burns; the burn penetrates the deepest layers of the skin, including the muscles, tendons, and bones. Fourth-degree burns may be life-threatening.

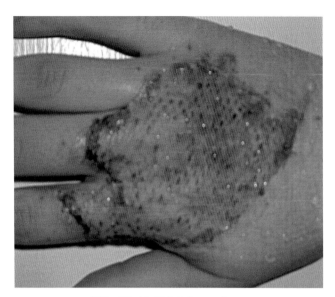

FIG. 27.10 Third-degree burn.

GENERIC NAME: silver sulfadiazine
TRADE NAMES: Silvadene

INDICATIONS: Prevention and treatment of burn wound infections

ROUTE OF ADMINISTRATION: Topical

COMMON ADULT DOSAGE: Apply to a thickness of 1/16 inch to the affected area once or twice daily

MECHANISM OF ACTION: Inhibits bacteria by damaging bacterial cell membranes and cell walls

SIDE EFFECTS: Burning, rash, skin discoloration

AUXILIARY LABEL: For topical use only; avoid contact with eyes

SPECIAL NOTE: Apply with sterile gloves

(Cortisporin) ointment, and collagenase (Santyl). If the burn degree or burn size is substantial, the patient may undergo surgery to replace the damaged skin layers (Fig. 27.10). Surgeons do this by removing and grafting healthy skin from another body part. The new skin is thinned through a rolling process and then attached to the damaged skin area. Burn hospitals require specialized solutions and medications from the pharmacy to treat patients on the burn unit. Patients can normally treat first-degree burns at home.

Prognosis

Small superficial and partial-thickness burns can often heal by themselves with simple care. Scarring is a common outcome of full-thickness and fourth-degree burns. The healing process can take a long time and may involve rehabilitation if there is damage to tissues, muscles, and tendons. A patient with severe burns over a large surface area can be at high risk for infection, sepsis, and even death.

Non-Drug Treatment

If the burn is minor, cooling it by applying a sterile, saline-soaked gauze cooled to about 55°F (13°C) can help relieve pain and limit further tissue injury. Ice should *not* be applied to the burn because this can cause additional tissue damage and pain. Any jewelry (eg, rings) close to the affected area should be removed because jewelry may become constrictive if swelling occurs. Severe burns require medical help.

Drug Treatment

Treatment can vary, depending on the burn type. For example, in addition to thermal burns, people can experience chemical and electrical burns. Topical medications may include silver cream (sulfadiazine [Silvadene]) and bacitracin ointment.

Warts

A virus causes the common wart, which is a skin growth. Verruca plana, or flat warts, commonly appear in children and may emerge on the hands, face, and neck. Plantar warts can manifest on the foot's bottom and can cause tenderness on walking. The human papillomavirus (HPV) causes common warts (Fig. 27.11A). A doctor can provide appropriate treatment, which may include drug treatment, liquid nitrogen (freezing) application, or surgical removal. Genital warts are different from common warts and come from specific strains of HPV. Genital warts are a sexually transmitted disease (see Fig. 27.11B and C; see Chapter 24 for a more detailed discussion of sexually transmitted infections).

Prognosis

Warts are contagious, although some kinds resolve on their own spontaneously within several months. Other types of warts require an evaluation and medical treatment.

Non-Drug Treatment

If no action is taken, common warts can disappear over time. No non-drug treatment is effective for common warts or genital warts. The best strategy for genital warts is sexual transmission prevention. The human papillomavirus vaccine (Gardasil) can prevent the contraction of genital warts and cervical cancer in young women.

Drug Treatment

OTC agents with salicylic acid or that freeze the wart can be effective. Topical fluorouracil (Carac, Efudex) treats warts by interfering with skin cell growth and is usually reserved for resistant plantar warts. Fluorouracil must be applied topically while wearing gloves or using nonmetal applicators.

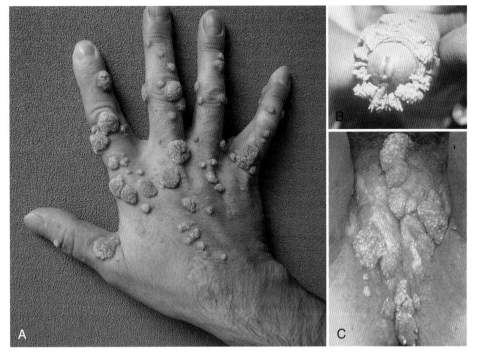

FIG. 27.11 (A) Human papillomavirus (common warts). (B) Genital warts, male patient. (C) Genital warts, female patient. (A, From Lookingbill D, Marks J. *Principles of Dermatology*. 4th ed. Philadelphia: Saunders; 2006; B and C, Courtesy New York City Health Department.)

GENERIC NAME: salicylic acid (OTC)

TRADE NAME: Compound W

INDICATIONS: Common warts, plantar warts

ROUTE OF ADMINISTRATION: Topical

COMMON ADULT DOSAGE: Soak the wart in warm water for 5 minutes; dry thoroughly; apply to the entire wart surface, allow to dry, and then apply again. Apply once or twice daily for 4–6 weeks

MECHANISM OF ACTION: Removes warts by acting as a topical keratolytic agent

SIDE EFFECT: Skin irritation

SPECIAL NOTE: Wash hands after application

Tech Note!

Dermatophytosis is defined as any infection of the skin, hair, or nails caused by a dermatophyte (fungus) and is characterized by redness of the skin, small papular vesicles, fissures, and scaling. Fungal transmission can occur through direct contact with infected lesions or with infections present on the skin of cats and dogs, soiled or contaminated clothing, or articles such as shoes, towels, or shower stalls. Tinea pedis (athlete's foot) is a common condition affecting the toes and soles of the feet.

Athlete's Foot

Athlete's foot, medically known as *tinea pedis*, is most commonly caused by the fungus *Trichophyton rubrum*. The name of a tinea infection depends on the site. Tinea pedis causes scaling and blisters between the toes. Severe infection can cause inflammation of the skin on the entire sole and may include relentless pruritus and pain when walking. The infection can spread by contact with shower floor surfaces or clothing; for example, by sharing socks. Direct contact is required for the transfer of the fungal infection (Fig. 27.12).

Other types of tinea infections include:

- Tinea barbae (bearded skin)
- Tinea capitis (hair of the head)
- Tinea corporis (ringworm of the skin)
- Tinea cruris (groin, also known as "jock itch")
- Tinea manuum (hands)
- Tinea unguium (nails)

Prognosis

In most cases, the prognosis for a tinea infection is good with the use of antifungals and if the feet are kept clean and dry. Most people can avoid this infection through education on proper foot care.

Non-Drug Treatment

Good hygienic practices help prevent infection. Keeping the feet dry and in clean, comfortable socks and shoes helps prevent athlete's foot. Exposing the feet to air whenever possible is also helpful. Walking barefoot in community showers or other places where transmission is possible should be avoided.

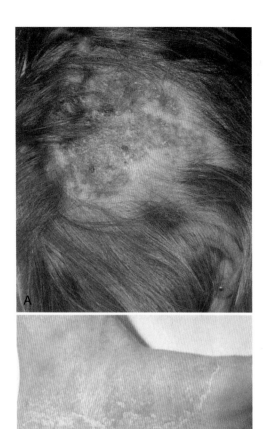

GENERIC NAME: clotrimazole (OTC)
TRADE NAME: Lotrimin AF

INDICATIONS: Tinea pedis and other fungal infections of the skin

ROUTE OF ADMINISTRATION: Topical

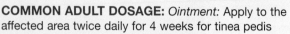

COMMON ADULT DOSAGE: *Ointment:* Apply to the affected area twice daily for 4 weeks for tinea pedis

MECHANISM OF ACTION: Azole antifungal (inhibits the proper functioning of fungal cell membranes)

SIDE EFFECTS: Erythema, skin irritation, peeling, pruritus

OTC, Over the counter.

GENERIC NAME: tolnaftate (OTC)
TRADE NAME: Tinactin

INDICATIONS: Tinea pedis and other fungal infections of the skin

ROUTE OF ADMINISTRATION: Topical

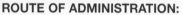

COMMON ADULT DOSAGE: Apply twice daily for 2–4 weeks

MECHANISM OF ACTION: Inhibits fungal cell growth in susceptible fungi

SIDE EFFECTS: Erythema, pruritus, inflammation, skin irritation

OTC, Over the counter.

FIG. 27.12 (A) Tinea capitis (head). (B) Tinea pedis (athlete's foot).

Drug Treatment

Most treatments involve topical agents available either over the counter (OTC) or by prescription. Antifungals kill fungus and treat athlete's foot. OTC products can come in powder or spray form. More severe infections can involve chronic thickening of the skin; those refractory to topical treatments often require treatment with oral antifungals. If the infection affects the nails, systemic therapy may be needed to clear the nail infection completely. Table 27.4 lists select topical antifungal agents for athlete's foot and other dermatologic fungal infections.

Impetigo

A comprehensive review of bacterial skin infections is beyond the scope of this chapter; however, we associate numerous bacteria with many skin infections. Impetigo is one such infection. Impetigo is a highly contagious condition caused by streptococcal organisms or *Staphylococcus aureus.* The bacteria can enter the body through broken skin caused by animal bites, injuries, trauma, or insect bites, although impetigo may appear without a skin break. Potentially affected areas include the face, limbs, and abdomen. A thick, yellow crust

▪ TABLE 27.4
Select Topical Agents for the Treatment of Dermatologic Fungal Infections

Medication Class	Generic Name	Trade Name	Common Adult Oral Dosage
Topical antifungals	miconazole	Desenex	• Apply twice daily for 4 wk
	terbinafine	Lamisil AT	• Apply to affected area once daily for at least 1 wk
	clotrimazole	Lotrimin AF	• Apply to skin twice daily for 2 wk
	ketoconazole	Nizoral A-D	• *Shampoo:* Apply once to damp skin, lather, leave on for 5 min, rinse off
	nystatin	Nystop	• Apply to the affected area 2–3 times daily

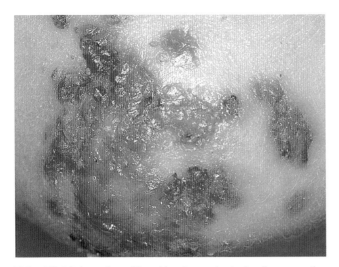

FIG. 27.13 Impetigo. The skin shows typical yellow, crusting blisters containing pus. (From Damjanov I. *Pathology for the Health Professions*. 4th ed. Philadelphia: Saunders; 2012.)

characteristically forms. Sores are often itchy and oozing, and blistering is common (Fig. 27.13). The infection is contagious because of the lesions' discharge.

Prognosis

The sores of impetigo heal slowly, although they rarely cause scarring. Children may have recurrences.

Non-Drug Treatment

Keeping the skin clean by washing several times daily with an antibacterial soap can remove crusted skin and oozing discharge. The condition is very contagious, so patients should wash sheets, towels, and clothing frequently to help prevent the spread of infection. A health provider may advise isolation to reduce bacterial transfer to others.

Drug Treatment

Treatment includes topical antibiotics, such as mupirocin 2% ointment (Bactroban, Centany) or retapamulin 1% ointment (Altabax); these are effective for limited areas and have the advantage of having no systemic side effects. Table 27.5 lists select topical antibacterial agents for impetigo and other bacterial skin infections. Oral antibiotics are for extensive cases of impetigo or for patients who have concurrent systemic symptoms. Prescribed antibiotics can include penicillins (eg, dicloxacillin or amoxicillin/clavulanate) or cephalosporins (eg, cephalexin or cefuroxime) as first choices. Erythromycin is typically a second-line antibiotic.

GENERIC NAME: retapamulin
TRADE NAME: Altabax
INDICATION: Impetigo
ROUTE OF ADMINISTRATION: Topical

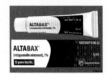

COMMON ADULT DOSAGE: Apply a thin layer to the affected area(s) twice daily for 5 days

MECHANISM OF ACTION: Inhibits bacterial protein synthesis

SIDE EFFECTS: Skin irritation, headache, diarrhea, nausea

AUXILIARY LABEL: For topical use only

SPECIAL NOTE: Wash hands after application

■ Tech Note!

Prolonged retapamulin (Altabax) use may cause a possible overgrowth of resistant organisms. This overgrowth may lead to severe resistant infections.

Diaper Rash

Diaper rash is a common form of dermatitis in babies. Although it is not life-threatening, it can be painful. These rashes occur more frequently in babies due to the nature of their thin and sensitive skin. When a baby's skin maintains exposure to urine or stools for extended periods of time, the moist environment irritates the skin leading to a tender, inflamed rash.

■ TABLE 27.5
Select Topical Antibacterial Products

Product	Trade Names	Dosage Forms
bacitracin (OTC)	Bacitracin	Ointment
mupirocin 2% (Rx)	Bactroban, Centany	Ointment, cream
polymyxin B sulfate, neomycin, bacitracin (OTC)	Neosporin Original Formula	Ointment, cream
retapamulin 1% (Rx)	Altabax	Ointment

OTC, Over the counter; *Rx,* prescription.

Prognosis

Treatment can ease the pain and discomfort and minimize the risk of infection.

Non-Drug Treatment

Caregivers should change diapers often, allowing the skin to air-dry when possible, being sure to wipe the entire area well with water or unscented wipes. Skin protectants such as petrolatum, lanolin, or zinc oxide can prevent diaper rash and should be part of every diaper change.

Drug Treatment

Should a yeast infection be suspected, topical formulations may treat and prevent further infection or complications. Dermal yeast infection treatment includes topical clotrimazole, topical miconazole, and topical nystatin. Topical corticosteroids may be appropriate for children ages two and older in minimal quantities for concise terms. Avoid topical steroids for several consecutive days to avoid increasing infection risk. As with the initiation of any new medication, parents, guardians, or caregivers should be directed to the child's pediatrician for proper evaluation of infections and appropriateness of therapy.

Skin Cancer

Any abnormal growth of new skin tissue that results in malignancy is known as skin cancer. Melanomas are cancerous skin growths emanating from moles and areas of the skin that may have been sunburned. The three main types of skin cancer are melanoma, squamous cell cancer, and basal cell cancer (nonmelanomas) (Fig. 27.14). The most aggressive and severe type of cancer is melanoma. Melanomas typically appear as an irregular shape, elevated off the skin; they are discolored and change in size. These can occur anywhere on the body (Box 27.2). Melanomas start in the lower part of the epidermis, in the melanocytes (cells that color the skin). Individuals with light-colored or freckled skin, red- and blond-haired people, and white people aged 20 or older are at higher risk. The usual treatment course depends on the cancer stage or severity. Basal cell cancer grows very slowly, occurs on the skin's surface, and often comes from sun damage. This cancer type usually first appears on the face and rarely spreads to other areas. Squamous cell skin cancer occurs typically on parts of the body other than the face that have been overexposed to the sun. This cancer type can spread to lymph nodes and **metastasize** to other organs.

Prognosis

The cancer prognosis depends on several factors, such as early detection, effective treatment, and a strong support system. With skin cancers, the outcome is good if detected early. Constant vigilance can help catch new skin areas changing in a suspicious way. Regularly scheduled visits to the physician can play an important role in early detection.

Non-Drug Treatment

Prevention is the best treatment, including protection from harmful sun rays. The first line of treatment is

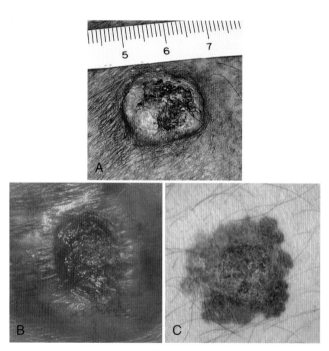

FIG. 27.14 Types of skin cancer. (A) Squamous cell. (B) Basal cell. (C) Malignant melanoma. (A, From Noble J. *Textbook of Primary Care Medicine*. 3rd ed. Philadelphia: Mosby; 2001; B, From Goldman L, Ausiello D. *Cecil Textbook of Medicine*. 23rd ed. Philadelphia: Saunders; 2003; C, From Townsend C et al. *Sabiston Textbook of Surgery*. 18th ed. Philadelphia: Saunders; 2008.)

BOX 27.2 **Instructions for Detecting Possible Skin Cancers**

Check yourself regularly for skin cancer using the ABCD method. This examination takes only a few minutes and may allow you to catch skin cancer in the early stages. Stand in front of a mirror and examine your entire body for any moles. Remember, not all moles look the same on every person; they can be different colors (red, black, brown), flat, raised, round, oval, or even irregularly shaped from the beginning. By examining yourself, you can determine whether any suspicious changes have taken place. A sudden or continuous change in the appearance of a mole is a sign that you should see your doctor. If you note such changes, see your dermatologist right away.

A—Asymmetry

Moles should appear symmetrical; this means that the two halves of the mole should look alike or be a mirror image of one another.

B—Border

The border of moles should be well defined and clear. It should not be fuzzy, blotchy, or irregular in any way.

C—Color

The color of moles must be monitored to note whether any changes occur, such as a change from light to dark in color.

D—Diameter

Melanomas are usually larger in diameter than the size of the eraser on a pencil. Anything over 6 mm should be examined by your doctor.

---

removal surgery. Treatments include photodynamic therapy or radiation therapy. Both squamous and basal cell carcinomas are less severe and respond to various therapies.

Drug Treatment

If cancer penetrates deep in the skin tissue, topical chemotherapy can be appropriate for large cancer areas inappropriate for surgical removal. Topical fluorouracil, an antimetabolite that inhibits cancer cells from synthesizing DNA, can treat basal cell and squamous cell cancers on the surface of the skin.

GENERIC NAME: fluorouracil
TRADE NAMES: Efudex, Fluoroplex,[a] Carac,[a] Tolak[a]
INDICATION: Basal cell carcinoma

ROUTE OF ADMINISTRATION: Topical

COMMON ADULT DOSAGE: Apply to affected lesions twice daily for 3–6 weeks

MECHANISM OF ACTION: Antimetabolite (inhibits cancer cells' synthesis of DNA)

SIDE EFFECTS: Skin irritation, dryness, photosensitivity, burning, erythema, pruritus

AUXILIARY LABELS:
• For topical use only
• Avoid contact with eyes, nose, and mouth
• Do not use if pregnant or breastfeeding
• Avoid sunlight
• Apply using gloves

SPECIAL NOTE: Must be applied using gloves or with a nonmetal applicator; thoroughly wash hands after application.

[a]Brand no longer available.

Common Dermatologic Conditions Affecting the Scalp and Hair

Head Lice

The parasite *Pediculus humanus capitis*, or the **head louse,** causes head lice. Many children come home from school with head lice. Lice transfer easily with hairbrushes and hats. Other ways to transmit lice include sleeping next to or sharing clothes with someone with lice. Symptoms include itching, head sores, and a feeling of something moving in the hair. Several products treat this infestation. Treatment of the whole family is essential, even if the infestation appears to affect only one child (Fig. 27.15A).

Another type of lice, spread through sexual contact, affects the pubic area. It is commonly called *crabs*. Lice can live on leg hair, armpits, mustaches, beards, eyebrows, and adult eyelashes. If lice are on children's eyelashes or eyebrows, it is considered head lice. Symptoms include pruritus and visible nits (lice eggs) or crawling lice in the genital area (see Fig. 27.15B).

Prognosis

Treatments can eliminate lice, although resistance is sometimes an issue.

Non-Drug Treatment

Patients should clean all brushes, combs, and hats in hot, soapy water or alcohol, and they should not be shared. All bed linen should be washed in hot water and dried for at least 20 minutes on the hottest setting. Nonwashable items should be dry-cleaned. Affected families should place all stuffed animals and blankets in a sealed plastic bag for at least 2 weeks to kill the lice. They should thoroughly clean and vacuum carpets and furniture. In adults, if genital lice also are present in the eyebrows or eyelashes, the lice should be removed with the fingers. Do not use medicated treatments on or around the eyes. With genital lice, avoid sexual contact

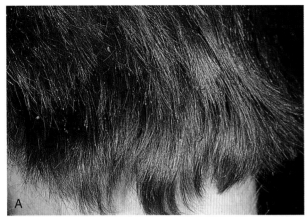

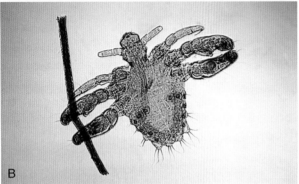

FIG. 27.15 (A) Head lice. (B) Crab louse. (A, From Callen JP et al. *Color Atlas of Dermatology*. 2nd ed. Philadelphia: Saunders; 2000; B, From Auerbach PS. *Wilderness Medicine*. 5th ed. St. Louis: Mosby; 2007.)

until the infestation is gone. Physical removal of all nits is essential to adequately treat a lice infestation.

Drug Treatment

OTC agents are available, such as permethrin (Nix Lice Killing Creme Rinse) topical cream rinse and pyrethrins and piperonyl butoxide as shampoos. Prescription treatments include malathion (Ovide 5% Topical Lotion) topical; these are reserved for resistant cases. Lindane may cause neurotoxicity and seizures if improperly used; patient counseling on its proper use is essential for safety.

A pediculicide (eg, permethrin or pyrethrin) is used to treat pubic lice infestations; prescription therapies are reserved for resistant cases.

OTC, Over the counter.

GENERIC NAME: permethrin (OTC)
TRADE NAME: Nix Lice Killing Creme Rinse

INDICATION: Lice

ROUTE OF ADMINISTRATION: Topical

COMMON ADULT DOSAGE: Before application, wash hair with conditioner-free shampoo, rinse with water, and towel dry. Apply a sufficient amount of

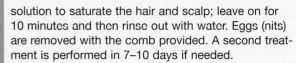

solution to saturate the hair and scalp; leave on for 10 minutes and then rinse out with water. Eggs (nits) are removed with the comb provided. A second treatment is performed in 7–10 days if needed.

MECHANISM OF ACTION: Disrupts sodium channels on the nerve cell membrane of lice, leading to paralysis and death of the parasite

SIDE EFFECTS: Itching, burning, stinging, redness, swelling

AUXILIARY LABEL: For topical use only

OTC, Over the counter.

Common Dermatologic Conditions Affecting the Nails

Onychomycosis

Nails on both the hands and feet endure daily abuse and can become damaged. Bacterial and fungal infections or trauma can occur that may discolor, deform, or cause detachment of the nail. **Onychomycosis,** a fungal infection of the nails, is the most common nail disease. The infection starts typically at the tip of one or more toenails. It produces thickening, discoloration, and nail crumbling, possibly affecting the entire nail. Infections attributable to candidal organisms are referred to as *onychomycosis.* Most nail infections are superficial and rarely become systemic. Therefore they are typically treated with topical agents. If a fungal infection becomes systemic, a doctor may prescribe oral agents, such as ketoconazole or fluconazole.

Prognosis

With proper treatment, the prognosis for onychomycosis is good. Although nails may require removal in severe cases, they typically grow back, and their absence does not hinder normal daily activities.

Non-Drug Treatment

Health providers should educate people about avoiding direct contact with high-risk areas in public places (eg, locker room floors) to prevent subsequent infections. Good hand hygiene is paramount in keeping the nails in good condition. In some instances, a combination of oral and topical agents, along with surgical removal of the affected nails, may be necessary.

Drug Treatment

Onychomycosis treatment depends on the infection severity and the number of affected nails. The severity also determines the dosage form and treatment length. We can treat certain infections with topical antifungals, such as ciclopirox olamine 8% lacquer solution. Oral therapy may be used either alone or in combination with topical treatments. Oral antifungals (eg, terbinafine) provide higher cure rates than previous agents, such as itraconazole and griseofulvin. In severe cases, the treatment duration can be lengthy to allow for the eradication of the causative infection and outgrowth of healthy nails. Although this chapter focuses on onychomycosis, other fungal and viral infections also can occur on the skin.

GENERIC NAME: terbinafine
TRADE NAME: Lamisil

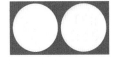

INDICATION: Onychomycosis

ROUTE OF ADMINISTRATION: Oral

COMMON ADULT DOSAGE: 250 mg once daily for 6 weeks (fingernails) or for 12 weeks (toenails)

MECHANISM OF ACTION: Interferes with the cell membrane strength of sensitive fungi

SIDE EFFECTS: Diarrhea, abdominal pain, headache, rash

AUXILIARY LABEL: Take as directed

■ Tech Note!

Soap and water have always been an excellent way to remove bacteria from the skin; however, they do not necessarily kill all bacteria. **Antiseptics** are necessary for the health care worker because they do kill and/or inhibit the growth of germs. Unfortunately, both good and bad germs are killed when these agents are used. It is wise not to overuse antiseptics because bacteria can mutate into strains that become resistant to them. Using gloves can reduce the necessity of constant hand hygiene and also help the skin stay hydrated.

Do You Remember These Key Points?

- The names of the major components of the dermatologic system and their functions
- The primary signs and symptoms of the various dermatologic conditions discussed
- Medications used to treat the different dermatologic conditions discussed
- The generic and trade names for the drugs discussed
- The appropriate auxiliary labels that should be used when filling prescriptions for medicines discussed

Review Questions

Multiple Choice Questions

1. The skin has many functions. Which of the following is *not* one of its main functions?
   A. Regulates body temperature
   B. Acts as a sensor to a stimulus
   C. Protects the internal organs from the elements
   D. All of the above are the main functions of the skin

2. _____ lubricate(s) the skin and retains water to keep the skin and hair from drying out.
   A. Sweat
   B. Sebum
   C. Pustules
   D. Retinoids

3. Which condition is associated with the development of comedones?
   A. Eczema
   B. Acne
   C. Psoriasis
   D. Tinea pedis

4. Which type of burn is the most severe?
   A. Partial-thickness
   B. Superficial
   C. Fourth-degree
   D. Full-thickness

5. Which product requires the patient and pharmacy to enroll in the iPLEDGE program because of the risk for teratogenicity?
   A. Isotretinoin
   B. Doxycycline
   C. Pimecrolimus
   D. Mycophenolate

6. The vitamin D analog calcipotriene (Dovonex) is indicated for the treatment of:
   A. Psoriasis
   B. Acne
   C. Human papillomavirus
   D. Thermal burns

7. Retapamulin (Altabax) is a topical:
   A. Antibacterial agent
   B. Antifungal agent
   C. Antiviral agent
   D. Keratolytic

8. Topical salicylic acid products are used to treat:
   A. Warts
   B. Acne
   C. Psoriasis
   D. A and B

9. Which medication could be used to treat pruritus of the skin?
   A. Tolnaftate
   B. Salicylic acid
   C. Bacitracin
   D. Caladryl

10. Impetigo can be treated with all of the following methods *except*:
    A. Keeping the skin clean and dry
    B. Using both oral and topical bacterial antibiotics
    C. Using a topical antiviral
    D. Washing with antibacterial soap

■ Technician's Corner

Using a comprehensive drug reference (eg, *Drug Facts and Comparisons*), look up the oral medications listed in Table 27.1 for the treatment of acne and determine what side effects are common with these medications and what warning labels, if any, should be placed on these prescriptions before they are dispensed.

Bibliography

Damjanov I. *Pathology for the Health Professions*. 4th ed. St. Louis: Saunders; 2011.

Fishback JL. *Pathology*. 3rd ed. Philadelphia: Mosby; 2005.

Lookingbill D, Marks J. *Principles of Dermatology*. 4th ed. Philadelphia: Saunders; 2006.

McCance KL. *Pathophysiology: The Biologic Basis for Disease in Adults and Children*. 6th ed. St. Louis: Mosby; 2010.

Patton KT, Thibodeau GA. *Mosby's Handbook of Anatomy and Physiology*. St. Louis: Mosby; 2000.

Potter PA, Perry AG. *Fundamentals of Nursing*. 8th ed. St. Louis: Mosby; 2013.

Price SA, Wilson LM. *Pathophysiology: Clinical Concepts of Disease Processes*. 6th ed. St. Louis: Mosby; 2003.

Solomon EP. *Introduction to Human Anatomy and Physiology*. 3rd ed. St. Louis: Mosby; 2009.

Thompson JM, McFarland GK, Hirsch JE, et al. *Mosby's Clinical Nursing*. 5th ed. St. Louis: Mosby; 2001.

Websites Referenced

Clinical Pharmacology Online. Available at: https://www.clinicalkey.com/pharmacology/.

UpToDate Online. Available at: http://www.uptodate.com.

CHAPTER 28

Therapeutic Agents for the Hematologic System

Tony Guerra

OBJECTIVES

1. Describe the major components of the hematologic system.
2. List the primary symptoms of conditions associated with the hematologic system. In addition, (a) recognize drugs used to treat the conditions associated with the hematologic system, (b) write the generic and trade names for the drugs discussed in this chapter, and (c) list appropriate auxiliary labels when filling prescriptions for drugs discussed in this chapter.

TERMS AND DEFINITIONS

Absolute neutrophil count (ANC) The number of white blood cells that are neutrophils

Albumin The major protein found in plasma

Anemia Without + blood condition, a decrease in the number of red blood cells or hemoglobin, which impairs the blood's ability to carry oxygen to the tissues

Bone marrow The tissue that fills the cavities in long bones, the source of red blood cells and many white blood cells

Colony-stimulating factor (CSF) A hormone that stimulates the bone marrow to synthesize hematopoietic cells

Cryoprecipitate Cold + precipitate, any precipitate that results from cooling; sometimes explicitly used to describe a precipitate rich in coagulation factor VIII obtained from the cooling of blood plasma

Erythrocyte Red + cell, a cell that contains hemoglobin and can carry oxygen to the body; also known as a red blood cell

Erythropoiesis The formation of erythrocytes

Erythropoietin A hormone secreted by the kidney that stimulates the production of red blood cells by stem cells in bone marrow

Granulocytopenia A reduction in granulocyte number, which encompasses specific types of white blood cells that contain "granules"; these white blood cells include neutrophils, eosinophils, and basophils, which are all known as granulocytes. These contrast to lymphocytes, white blood cells devoid of granules

Hemoglobin The oxygen-carrying component of red blood cells

Hemophilia A hereditary coagulation disorder that leads to a decreased ability to clot normally

Hydrostatic pressure The pressure exerted by a fluid because of the force of gravity

Hypoxia Low + oxygen, an oxygen supply reduction to a tissue despite adequate tissue perfusion

Idiopathic A term meaning "of unknown cause"

Leukemia White + blood condition, a progressive, malignant disease of the blood-forming organs, marked by distorted proliferation and development of leukocytes and their precursors in blood and bone marrow

Leukocyte White + cell, a white blood cell

Leukopenia White + reduction, a reduction in the number of leukocytes (white blood cells) in the blood

Lymphoid organ A component of the system of interconnected tissues and organs by which lymph circulates throughout the body

Lymphoma Cancer of the lymphatic system

Neutropenia Abnormally low level of neutrophils in the blood

Osmosis Diffusion of fluid through a semipermeable membrane from a solution with a low solute concentration to a solution with a higher solute concentration to achieve equilibrium

Osmotic pressure The pressure exerted by water flowing through a semipermeable membrane separating two solutions with different concentrations of solutes

Pallor A deficiency in color, particularly of the face

Phlebotomy The act or practice of opening a vein by incision or puncture to remove blood

Plasma The transparent, yellowish fluid portion of the blood

Plasma protein Any of the dissolved proteins of blood plasma

Polycythemia Many + cell + blood condition, an increase in the total cell mass of the blood

Serum The clear, yellowish fluid obtained by separating whole blood into its solid and liquid components after it has been allowed to clot; plasma minus clotting factors

Solute A substance dissolved in another substance; usually the component of a solution present in less amount

Splenectomy Surgical removal of the spleen

Thrombocyte A platelet

Thrombocytopenia Platelet + cell + reduction, a decrease in the number of platelets in the blood

von Willebrand disease The most common inherited bleeding disorder, associated with a deficiency in the clotting protein von Willebrand factor

Whole blood Blood drawn from the body from which no constituent, such as plasma or platelets, has been removed

Common Drugs for Conditions of the Hematologic System

Trade Name	Generic Name	Pronunciation
Iron Deficiency Anemia Medications		
FerrouSul[a]	ferrous sulfate	(**fare**-us **sul**-fate)
Ferate[a]	ferric gluconate	(**fer**-ik **gloo**-koe-nate)
Colony-Stimulating Factors		
Aranesp[a]	darbepoetin alfa	(**dar**-be-**poe**-ee-tin **al**-fuh)
Epogen	epoetin alfa	(e-**poe**-ee-tin **al**-fuh)
Leukine	sargramostim	(sar-**gra**-moe-stim)
Neulasta	pegfilgrastim	(peg-fil-**gras**-tim)
Neupogen	filgrastim	(fil-**gras**-tim)
Chemotherapeutic Agents for the Treatment of Leukemia		
None	cytarabine	(sye-**tar**-uh-bean)
None	cyclophosphamide	(sye-kloe-**foss**-fuh-mide)
Gleevec	imatinib	(im-**ma**-tuh-nib)
Trexall	methotrexate	(meth-oh-**trex**-ate)
Rituxan	rituximab	(ri-**tux**-ih-mab)

[a]Brand discontinued; now available only as generic.

Anatomy and Physiology of the Hematologic System

As discussed in Chapter 20, adequate blood flow is critical to delivering oxygen and nutrients to the body's tissues and organs. Not only does the blood carry oxygen and nutrients throughout the body, it also carries wastes from the tissues and organs that it supports to organs such as the kidneys and liver for elimination. The blood also transports immune system cells (see Chapter 25) to sites of infection and injury. The following is a brief review of the components that make up whole blood and a description of the functions these components serve in the body. (See Chapter 25 for a refresher on the structure and function of the major **lymphoid organs;** ie, thymus, spleen, and lymph nodes.)

Major Components of Blood

Plasma

Whole blood includes plasma and cellular components (Fig. 28.1). **Plasma** is the fluid component of whole blood that includes water, plasma proteins, and other solutes such as electrolytes and nutrients. Plasma accounts for approximately 50% of whole blood volume in a normal, healthy adult. **Serum,** used for some laboratory tests, is plasma that has been allowed to clot in the laboratory to remove clotting factors that can interfere with some blood tests.

Plasma Proteins

Various **plasma proteins** are present in the blood, such as albumin, globulins, fibrinogen, and prothrombin (see Fig. 28.1). **Albumin** is critical for maintaining water and solute balance in the blood. Albumin is a large protein that cannot diffuse across the vascular epithelium, as do water and electrolytes. Thus albumin helps maintain blood volume and the transport of **solutes** between the blood and tissues (see the discussion of osmotic pressure later in the chapter). Another important albumin function is to serve as a carrier molecule for blood components and drugs. Drug interactions between agents that bind to albumin are relatively common. Phenytoin is an example of a drug that is highly bound to albumin. Its use with other drugs that bind to albumin can lead to phenytoin toxicity. We can use intravenous albumin to increase plasma volume or to increase albumin levels in people with low serum albumin levels.

Two primary forces regulate the movement of fluids and solutes into and out of the vasculature: hydrostatic pressure and osmosis. Blood pressure generated by heart contraction drives **hydrostatic pressure.** The hydrostatic pressure in the arterial capillaries pushes water and solutes out of the

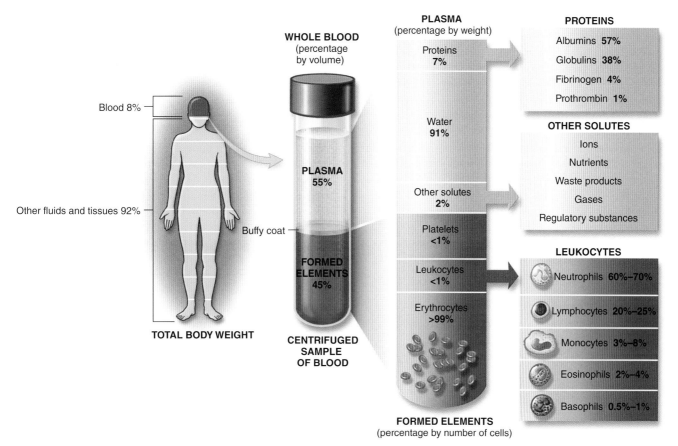

FIG. 28.1 Composition of whole blood. Approximate values for the components of blood in a healthy adult. (From Patton KT, Thibodeau GA. *Anatomy and Physiology*. 8th ed. St. Louis: Mosby; 2013.)

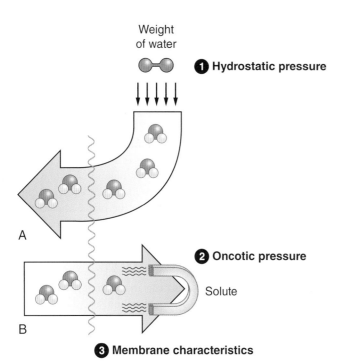

Weight
of water

1 Hydrostatic pressure

A

2 Oncotic pressure

Solute

B

3 Membrane characteristics

FIG. 28.2 (A) Hydrostatic pressure and (B) osmotic (oncotic) pressure in plasma. (From McCance KL, Huether SE. *Pathophysiology: The Biologic Basis for Disease in Adults and Children.* 7th ed. St. Louis: Elsevier; 2014.)

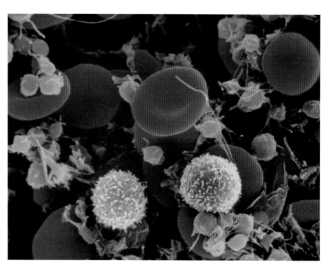

FIG. 28.3 Blood cells. (From Huether S, McCance K. *Understanding Pathophysiology.* 5th ed. St. Louis: Mosby; 2012.)

arterioles into the tissues. **Osmosis** is the movement of water down a concentration gradient. Once the blood has passed through the arterioles and returns to the venous system, **osmotic pressure** (also known as *oncotic pressure*) becomes greater than the hydrostatic pressure. Therefore water and solutes move out of tissues and back into the venous system. Albumin is the major blood protein that maintains osmotic pressure in the vascular system. In certain cases, people can produce less albumin (eg, individuals with liver disease or malnutrition) or lose albumin from the bloodstream (eg, in certain types of kidney disease). When this happens, osmotic pressure decreases, leading to fluid accumulation and edema (Fig. 28.2).

Other plasma proteins contribute to clotting (eg, fibrinogen), immune function (antibodies), transport proteins, and lipoproteins (eg, low-density lipoprotein [LDL] and high-density lipoprotein [HDL], discussed in Chapter 20).

Platelets

Platelets (also known as **thrombocytes**) are blood components essential to coagulation. Because platelets are vital to clotting, low platelet levels (**thrombocytopenia**) can increase bleeding risk. A platelet's life span is approximately 10 days.

Cellular Components of the Blood

We can divide the cell types found primarily in the blood into two main groups, leukocytes and erythrocytes (Fig. 28.3). These cells (and platelets) form through hematopoiesis (Fig. 28.4). **Leukocytes,** or white blood cells (WBCs), are immune system cells that help defend the body against infection.

Leukocyte examples are lymphocytes, neutrophils, and monocytes. (See Chapter 25 for a review of leukocytes and their immune system functions.)

Erythrocytes, or red blood cells (RBCs), are the most prevalent cells in the blood. The main RBC function is to carry oxygen to the tissues and organs. RBC production, or **erythropoiesis,** takes place in the **bone marrow,** and the hormone **erythropoietin** (produced by the kidneys) largely drives it (Fig. 28.5). Health professionals can use erythropoietin for people with low RBC counts because of kidney disease or other medical conditions.

RBCs can effectively transport oxygen because they contain **hemoglobin.** Hemoglobin is an oxygen-carrying RBC protein that binds to oxygen as blood passes through the lungs. The heart then pumps blood throughout the body, allowing RBCs to deliver oxygen to tissues. Iron is essential for hemoglobin production. Various other building blocks, also required for hemoglobin and erythrocyte formation, can be deficient and lead to anemia.

Conditions Affecting the Hematologic System

Based on the anatomy and physiology of the hematologic system, it is easy to see that conditions affecting the hematologic system have significant overlap with organ systems and conditions discussed in other chapters. For example, in the renal system discussion (Chapter 23), we saw that because the kidneys produce erythropoietin, patients with kidney disease can have reduced RBC production. Another example is the discussion of thromboembolic diseases in Chapter 20. Thrombus formation resulting in myocardial infarction, stroke (also known as a *cerebrovascular accident*), and deep vein thrombosis is due to a complex interplay between atherosclerotic plaques, platelets, and immune system cells. This chapter focuses on hematologic conditions,

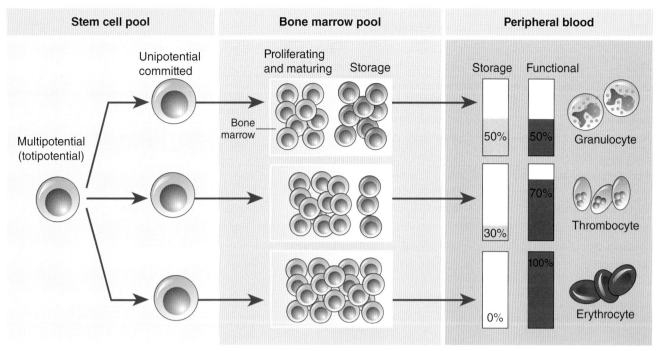

FIG. 28.4 Hematopoiesis. (From Huether S, McCance K. *Understanding Pathophysiology*. 5th ed. St. Louis: Mosby; 2012.)

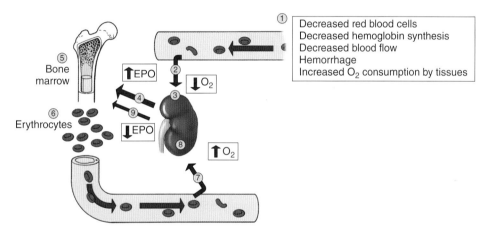

① Decreased red blood cells
Decreased hemoglobin synthesis
Decreased blood flow
Hemorrhage
Increased O₂ consumption by tissues

FIG. 28.5 Role of erythropoietin (EPO) in the regulation of erythropoiesis. (From Huether S, McCance K. *Understanding Pathophysiology*. 5th ed. St. Louis: Mosby; 2012.)

such as anemia, low cell counts (thrombocytopenia, leukopenia, and neutropenia), and hematologic cancers. It also provides a brief review of bleeding disorders and their treatment.

Common Conditions

Anemia

In general, a reduction in the total RBC number available to carry oxygen or a deficiency in the quality or quantity of hemoglobin present in RBCs is **anemia.** This chapter does not provide an exhaustive review of all forms of anemia. Rather, it presents a brief overview of iron deficiency anemia, the most common form of anemia worldwide. There are many types of anemia, and not all forms require iron supplementation (Table 28.1).

Iron deficiency anemia Iron deficiency anemia is the most common form worldwide. People at particular risk for the development of iron deficiency anemia include children, women of childbearing age, and people living in poverty. A common cause of iron deficiency anemia is continuous blood loss, such as gastrointestinal bleeding. Symptoms of iron deficiency anemia include fatigue, weakness, shortness of breath, and **pallor** (Fig. 28.6).

> **Tech Note!**
>
> Gastrointestinal bleeding, such as that from a nonsteroidal antiinflammatory drug–induced ulcer, can lead to iron deficiency anemia. When individuals present with iron deficiency anemia, it is important for the doctor to rule out hidden (ie, occult) bleeding.

TABLE 28.1
Classification of Anemia

Name	Cause and/or Contributing Factors
Anemia of chronic inflammation	Increased demand for erythrocyte production resulting from chronic inflammation, infection, and/or malignancy
Aplastic anemia	Depressed stem cell proliferation
Folate deficiency anemia	Dietary folate deficiency
Hemolytic anemia	Destruction of mature erythrocytes because of cell lysis
Iron deficiency anemia	Lack of sufficient iron to produce hemoglobin as a result of chronic blood loss, dietary iron deficiency, or disruption of iron metabolism
Pernicious anemia	Vitamin B_{12} deficiency resulting from congenital or acquired deficiency of intrinsic factor
Sickle cell anemia	Abnormal hemoglobin synthesis and abnormal red blood cell shape
Sideroblastic anemia	Dysfunctional iron uptake by erythroblasts and heme synthesis
Thalassemia	Impaired synthesis of the hemoglobin molecule

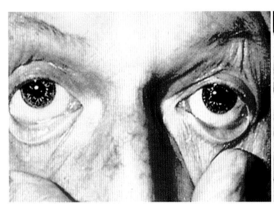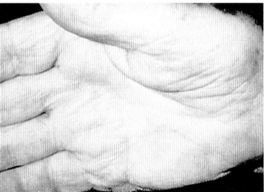

FIG. 28.6 Pallor and iron deficiency. (From Huether S, McCance K. *Understanding Pathophysiology*. 5th ed. St. Louis: Mosby; 2012.)

Prognosis
Iron deficiency anemia responds well to current treatments.

Non-Drug Treatment
Iron deficiency anemia may indicate bleeding or another metabolic contributor. The first step in managing iron deficiency anemia should be identifying and/or ruling out blood loss. Unless bleeding, if present, is resolved, iron replacement therapy proves ineffective. Patients can treat mild anemia with dietary changes, including an increase in iron-rich foods (eg, spinach, beef, broccoli, liver).

Drug Treatment
Iron replacement therapy is the primary treatment for iron deficiency anemia (Table 28.2). With adequate supplementation, the resolution of symptoms can occur within 4 weeks. Supplementation duration depends on the extent of the deficiency and the causative factors.

GENERIC NAME: ferrous sulfate (over the counter)

TRADE NAMES: Slow Fe,[a] FerrouSul[a]

INDICATION: Iron deficiency anemia

ROUTE OF ADMINISTRATION: Oral

COMMON ADULT DOSAGE: 250–325 mg 2–3 times daily

MECHANISMS OF ACTION: Iron supplement to increase iron stores and support erythropoiesis

SIDE EFFECTS: Constipation, abdominal pain, dyspepsia, stool discoloration

AUXILIARY LABEL: Administer with meals to minimize gastrointestinal side effects

[a]Brand discontinued; now available only as generic.

■ Tech Note!

Doctors sometimes prescribe oral iron supplements in combination with ascorbic acid (vitamin C). Vitamin C's acidity helps iron absorb from the gastrointestinal tract. Having the patient take oral iron with a glass of orange juice is another strategy.

GENERIC NAME: sodium ferric gluconate complex

TRADE NAME: Ferrlecit

INDICATION: Iron deficiency anemia in people on hemodialysis

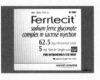

TABLE 28.2
Iron Preparations for the Treatment of Iron Deficiency Anemia

Generic Name	Trade Name	Common Dosage Range	Elemental Iron Content	Common Side Effects
Oral Iron Salts				
ferrous sulfate	Slow Fe,[a] FerrouSul[a]	• 250–325 mg 2–3 times daily	*Slow Fe:* 50 mg/156 mg tab *FerrouSul:* 65 mg/325 mg tab	• Dark stools • Nausea • Vomiting • Constipation
ferrous gluconate	Ferate[a]	• 240 mg PO 2–3 times daily	27 mg/tab	
Parenteral Iron				
iron dextran	INFeD	• Max daily dose: 100 mg	50 mg/mL	• Chills • Dizziness • Injection site reactions • Nausea • Hypotension
sodium ferric gluconate complex	Ferrlecit	• 125 mg in 100 mL NS IV over 1 hr	12.5 mg/mL	
iron sucrose	Venofer	• 100–300 mg IV	20 mg/mL	

[a]Brand discontinued; now available only as generic.
IV, Intravenously; *NS,* normal saline; *PO,* orally; *tab,* tablet.

ROUTE OF ADMINISTRATION: Intravenous (IV)

COMMON ADULT DOSAGE: 125 mg elemental IV during each dialysis session

MECHANISM OF ACTION: Iron supplement to increase iron stores and support erythropoiesis

SIDE EFFECTS: Injection site reaction, headache, anaphylaxis

Sickle Cell Disease

Sickle cell disease, an anemia most commonly found in African Americans, can lead to many complications. Normal red blood cells are donut-like shaped and move readily through different sized blood vessels. Sickle cells are curved and somewhat rigid. Consequently, patients may develop pain from ischemia, as well as other chronic complications.

Prognosis
Curing the disease requires bone marrow transplantation.

Non-Drug Treatment
Blood transfusions provide healthy red blood cells to increase the oxygen-carrying capacity of blood. Bone marrow transplantation is costly and risks infection.

Drug Treatment
Therapy can minimize pain, relieve symptoms, and prevent complications. Analgesics, such as NSAIDs, acetaminophen (Tylenol), or opioids, can alleviate pain. Hydroxyurea

can stimulate hemoglobin F (HbF) to help prevent red blood cell collapse into the sickled shape.

An amino acid, L-glutamine powder (Endari), can reduce disease complications. In 2019 the US Food and Drug Administration (FDA) approved Voxelotor (Oxbryta), a hemoglobin S (HbS) polymerization inhibitor, for patients 4 years and older with or without hydroxyurea.

GENERIC NAME: voxelotor

TRADE NAME: Oxbryta

INDICATIONS: Sickle cell disease

ROUTE OF ADMINISTRATION: Oral

COMMON ADULT DOSAGE: 1.5 g once daily

MECHANISM OF ACTION: Works by inhibiting hemoglobin S (HbS) polymerization to allow increased hemoglobin binding to oxygen to improve anemia

SIDE EFFECTS: Skin rash, abdominal pain, diarrhea, headache, fever

AUXILIARY LABEL: Swallow whole. Do not cut, crush, or chew the tablets

Polycythemia

Although many conditions of the hematologic system involve a deficiency in a specific cell type (eg, thrombocytopenia, leukopenia, and neutropenia, discussed later), some forms of hematologic dysfunction involve the *overproduction* of hematopoietic cells. **Polycythemia** is excessive RBC production. People can develop either primary or secondary polycythemia. Secondary polycythemia, the most common form, occurs as a result of a physiological response to **hypoxia.** This polycythemia form occurs when the body has difficulty oxygenating blood. For example, people living at high altitudes, those who smoke tobacco, and those with chronic obstructive pulmonary disease (COPD) struggle to oxygenate the blood. Primary polycythemia, also known as *polycythemia vera,* is a chronic condition of RBC overproduction. This overproduction is due to an increased sensitivity of stem cells in the bone marrow to the effects of erythropoietin.

Prognosis

For people with secondary polycythemia, proper treatment of the underlying condition can result in a good prognosis. For those with polycythemia vera, the prognosis can be poor if the person does not receive appropriate treatment. However, with proper treatment, survival of 10 to 15 years is common.

Non-Drug Treatment

The treatment of contributing factors is a critical management component. Health professionals recommend smoking cessation for smokers and medical intervention for chronic obstructive pulmonary disease and heart failure to minimize hypoxia. For individuals with polycythemia vera, **phlebotomy** can reduce blood volume and RBC numbers.

Drug Treatment

Drug therapy in polycythemia vera involves treatments aimed at minimizing thrombosis risk with myelosuppressive agents (eg, hydroxyurea as the first choice and interferon alpha or busulfan as alternatives). In 2021 Besremi (ropeginterferon-alfa-2b-njft) was granted FDA approval for the treatment of polycythemia vera in adults. Besremi, a long-acting subcutaneous injection administered every 2 weeks, is the first interferon therapy approved for use in this disease.

GENERIC NAME: hydroxyurea

Trade Name: Droxia

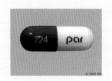

INDICATIONS: Polycythemia vera (off-label use), sickle cell disease, chronic myelogenous leukemia, head and neck cancers

ROUTE OF ADMINISTRATION: Oral

COMMON ADULT DOSAGE: 15–20 mg/kg/day

MECHANISM OF ACTION: Inhibits DNA synthesis

SIDE EFFECTS: Leukopenia, neutropenia, anemia, diarrhea, rash, fever

AUXILIARY LABELS:
- Wear gloves when handling capsules
- Wash hands before and after contact with bottle or capsules

Low Cell and Platelet Counts

A variety of conditions and secondary factors can contribute to impaired hematopoiesis, resulting in conditions such as thrombocytopenia, leukopenia, and neutropenia. Agents known broadly as **colony-stimulating factors (CSFs)** can stimulate hematopoiesis and treat such conditions (Table 28.3).

Thrombocytopenia *Thrombocytopenia* is a term that describes low platelet count. Thrombocytopenia has many causes. Some of the most common causes are pregnancy (gestational thrombocytopenia), drug side effects (drug-induced thrombocytopenia) (Box 28.1), and **idiopathic** thrombocytopenia. The principal treatment goal is bleeding prevention.

Prognosis

The prognosis for thrombocytopenia varies widely, depending on thrombocytopenia severity and the underlying cause.

Non-Drug Treatment

We should pursue resolution of contributing factors when the underlying cause can be corrected. Individuals with particularly low platelet counts may need transfusions to increase platelet levels. Severe thrombocytopenia may necessitate activity restrictions, such as limiting contact sports.

Drug Treatment

In immune-mediated thrombocytopenia, glucocorticoid medications (eg, prednisone, dexamethasone, hydrocortisone, and methylprednisolone) can suppress the immune response. Eltrombopag (Promacta) is available for patients whose condition does not respond to corticosteroids, immunoglobulins, or **splenectomy.**

GENERIC NAME: eltrombopag

TRADE NAME: Promacta

INDICATIONS: Thrombocytopenia, idiopathic thrombocytopenic purpura (ITP), severe aplastic anemia

ROUTE OF ADMINISTRATION: Oral

COMMON ADULT DOSAGE: 25–50 mg once daily adjusted based on platelet response

MECHANISM OF ACTION: Thrombopoietin receptor agonist (increases platelet production)

SIDE EFFECTS:
Thrombosis, nausea, vomiting, dyspepsia

AUXILIARY LABELS:
- Take on an empty stomach
- Take at least 1 hour before or 2 hours after meals
- Do not crush tablets

TABLE 28.3
Select Colony-Stimulating Factors for the Treatment of Low Hematologic Cell Counts

Generic Name	Trade Name	Common Dosage Range	Common Side Effects
Erythropoiesis (Red Blood Cell [RBC]–Stimulating Agents)			
darbepoetin alfa	Aranesp[a]	• 0.45–2.25 mcg/kg subcut once wkly *or* • 500 mcg every 3 wk or 0.75 mcg/kg every 2 wk	• Abdominal pain • Cough • Edema • Hypertension • Shortness of breath
epoetin alfa	Epogen, Procrit	• 50–300 units/kg IV or subcut 3 times wkly	• Cough • Fever • Headache • Itching • Nausea • Pain • Vomiting
White Blood Cell–Stimulating Agents			
filgrastim	Neupogen, Granix, Zarxio	• 5–10 mcg/kg/day subcut or IV	• Bone pain • Fever • Nose bleeds • Rash • Splenomegaly
pegfilgrastim	Neulasta	• 6 mg subcut once per chemotherapy cycle	• Bone pain • Limb pain
sargramostim	Leukine	• 250 mcg/m^2/day subcut or IV	• Diarrhea • Edema • Fever • Headache • Hyperglycemia • Hypertension • Rash

[a]Brand discontinued; now available only as generic.

IV, Intravenous; *subcut,* subcutaneous.

BOX 28.1 Select Drugs Frequently Associated With Drug-Induced Thrombocytopenia

- abciximab
- carbamazepine
- eptifibatide
- heparin
- linezolid
- measles-mumps-rubella (MMR) vaccine
- phenytoin
- piperacillin
- quinidine
- quinine
- rifampin
- sulfamethoxazole/trimethoprim
- tirofiban
- valproic acid
- vancomycin

- **Leukopenia:** A low total WBC count (granulocytes and lymphocytes); almost all people with leukopenia also have neutropenia.
- **Granulocytopenia:** A reduced number of circulating granulocytes (neutrophils, eosinophils, and basophils). Because neutrophils are the predominant granulocyte cell type, people with granulocytopenia almost always have neutropenia.

The primary concern in a patient with neutropenia is increased infection risk. However, neutropenia can be a symptom of an underlying condition that requires identification and treatment.

Neutropenia **Neutropenia** can occur in conjunction with other conditions (eg, aplastic anemia, leukemia, vitamin B$_{12}$ deficiency, folate deficiency), during chemotherapy treatment, and as an isolated condition. To assess a patient for neutropenia, the **absolute neutrophil count** (**ANC**) classifies the neutropenia as mild, moderate, or severe.

Health professionals sometimes use other terms interchangeably with *neutropenia,* but these are slightly different conditions:

Prognosis

Recurrent infection is the primary risk associated with neutropenia. The prognosis depends largely on the degree of neutropenia and the cause.

Non-Drug Treatment

Non-drug treatment for patients with chronic neutropenia includes infection avoidance. A critical component of care involves regular dental care to prevent gingivitis and associated infection.

Drug Treatment

The primary drugs used to treat neutropenia are recombinant growth factors or colony-stimulating factors (CSFs). Doctors can prescribe these agents prophylactically for chemotherapy-induced neutropenia and therapeutic use in people with preexisting neutropenia. Current therapies are either granulocyte colony-stimulating factors (G-CSFs) or granulocyte-macrophage colony-stimulating factors (GM-CSFs; see Table 28.3). Fig. 28.7 shows where these growth factors act in the differentiation of hematopoietic cells.

GENERIC NAME: filgrastim

TRADE NAME: Neupogen

INDICATIONS: Neutropenia resulting from chemotherapy, bone marrow transplantation, hematopoietic radiation injury

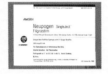

ROUTE OF ADMINISTRATION: Subcutaneous injection

COMMON ADULT DOSAGE: 5–10 mcg/kg once daily

MECHANISM OF ACTION: Recombinant granulocyte colony-stimulating factor (stimulates the production of neutrophils in the bone marrow)

SIDE EFFECTS: Bone pain, hypotension, hyperuricemia

AUXILIARY LABEL: Avoid eye contact

GENERIC NAME: sargramostim

TRADE NAME: Leukine

INDICATIONS: Neutropenia resulting from chemotherapy, bone marrow transplantation

ROUTES OF ADMINISTRATION: Intravenous; subcutaneous

COMMON ADULT DOSAGE: 250 mcg/m^2/day infused over 2 hours

MECHANISM OF ACTION: Recombinant granulocyte-macrophage colony-stimulating factor (stimulates the production of neutrophils, eosinophils, and monocytes within the bone marrow)

SIDE EFFECTS: Bone pain, hypotension, peripheral edema, nausea, vomiting, skin rash

Hematologic Cancers

Several cancers are associated with the lymphatic organs and cells of the hematologic system. This chapter briefly reviews the epidemiology, prognosis, and treatment of leukemia and lymphoma.

Leukemia Leukemia is a cancer characterized by cancerous hematopoietic stem cell production that replaces normal WBCs in the bone marrow. Forms of leukemia include acute lymphoblastic leukemia (ALL), acute myeloblastic leukemia (AML), chronic myelogenous leukemia (CML), and chronic lymphocytic leukemia (CLL), among others. Both men and women can develop leukemia. It can arise at any age. Both genetics and environmental factors

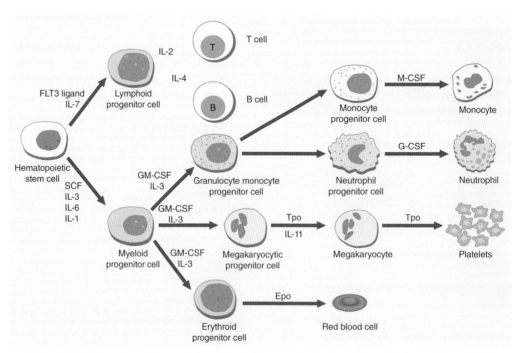

FIG. 28.7 Hematopoiesis and hematopoietic growth factors. *Epo,* Erythropoietin; *FLT3,* FMS-related tyrosine kinase 3; *G-CSF,* granulocyte colony-stimulating factors; *GM-CSF,* granulocyte-macrophage colony-stimulating factors; *IL,* interleukin; *M-CSF,* macrophage colony-stimulating factor; *SCF,* stem cell factor; *Tpo,* thrombopoietin. (From Page C, Hoffman B, Curtis M, et al: *Integrated Pharmacology.* 3rd ed. St. Louis: Mosby; 2006.)

can contribute to its development. Environmental factors can include exposure to radiation and chemicals, including radiation and chemotherapeutic agents used to treat other cancers.

Prognosis

Statistics show approximately 65% of patients with leukemia who resume normal hematopoiesis after treatment achieve remission. Because treatment results in bone marrow suppression, infection is the leading cause of death in patients with leukemia.

Non-Drug Treatment

Infection morbidity and mortality can cause death in patients treated for leukemia. Essential elements of non-drug therapy include precautions against infectious disease transmission. In line with bone marrow suppression, individuals receiving chemotherapy for leukemia have an increased bleeding risk. Sometimes blood products (eg, red blood cells, platelets) are required to treat or prevent bleeding events.

Drug Treatment

Drug therapy works to eliminate cancerous hematopoietic cells in the bone marrow. Table 28.4 presents select chemotherapeutic agents for leukemia (and other hematologic cancers). Although this chapter focuses on hematologic cancers, the doctors use the same chemotherapeutic agents for different cancers. Several key categories of chemotherapeutic agents and how they work are described briefly.

Antimetabolite agents. Individual nucleotides form DNA and RNA nucleic acids. Nucleotides contain purine or pyrimidine bases. These bases are part of nucleotides used in DNA synthesis. The antimetabolite's structure resembles these bases. Because they are not identical, antimetabolites prevent cell division completion, or mitosis. Antimetabolites are for leukemia. Common side effects include nausea, vomiting, fever, anorexia, bone marrow suppression, and jaundice. Examples of antimetabolites include the following:
- cytarabine
- fludarabine
- 5-fluorouracil (5-FU)
- 6-mercaptopurine
- methotrexate

Antibiotics. The antibiotics for cancer are in different categories than those for infection. These chemotherapeutic antibiotics bind directly to cancer cell DNA and prevent new cancer cell development. We do not use these agents for infections because of toxic side effects. Because they also destroy healthy cells with cancer cells, they produce side effects that include severe emesis (vomiting), nausea, diarrhea, and hair loss. Some examples include the following:
- bleomycin
- daunorubicin
- doxorubicin
- idarubicin
- mitomycin-C

Mitotic inhibitors. Mitotic inhibitors prevent mitosis at the metaphase stage. Mitosis is the process of cell division that all cells must perform (Fig. 28.8). The agents that prevent this cellular reproduction are a group of plant-derived alkaloids. Hodgkin disease and various cancers that may not respond to other medications often require treatment with mitotic inhibitors. Side effects may include appetite loss, back pain, diarrhea, hair loss, increased sweating, nausea, vomiting, voice changes, and discoloration of the skin. These agents include the following:
- etoposide
- vinblastine
- vincristine
- vinorelbine

Alkylating agents. The two major types of alkylating agents are nitrogen mustards and nitrosoureas. Although similar in structure, their modes of action and side effects differ. Because alkylation is a normal reaction that takes place in DNA between chemical compounds, these agents can bind to specific DNA bases. New bonds (created by alkylation) form between components. This bonding damages the rapidly dividing cancer cells, which cannot proliferate further. Doctors most often use alkylating agents with Hodgkin disease, retinoblastoma, lymphocytic leukemia, and inoperable cancers.

Nitrogen mustards. Nitrogen mustards represent some of the first chemotherapeutic cancer agents. World War I saw their use in chemical warfare. Soldiers exposed to these agents had a reduced number of WBCs. Because of this effect on WBCs, they were used to treat leukemia, which is marked by a high WBC count. Although effective, the first nitrogen mustards had severe side effects. They have been replaced with agents derived from the same chemical structure but better tolerated. Side effects may include low blood counts, nausea, vomiting, mouth sores, hair loss, darkening of veins used for infusion, and fertility loss. Examples of nitrogen mustard agents include the following:
- chlorambucil
- cyclophosphamide
- ifosfamide

■ Tech Note!

When preparing chemotherapeutic agents, the technician must wear special chemotherapy gloves or double-glove to protect the skin. Gowns and masks are essential when preparing agents that must be compounded, reconstituted, or admixed. Technicians prepare such agents in a special laminar flow hood to prevent unwanted exposure. If a chemotherapeutic agent spills on the gloves, the top gloves can be removed and discarded into an appropriate hazardous waste container. New gloves can then replace the old. Always follow proper procedures for the chemotherapeutic agent type.

TABLE 28.4

Select Chemotherapeutic Agents Used in the Treatment of Hematologic Cancers

Generic Name	Trade Name	Common Dosage Range[a]	Select Common Side Effects
Alkylating Agents			
chlorambucil	Leukeran	• 0.1–0.2 mg/kg/day for 3–6 wk	• Amenorrhea • Edema • Fever • Neutropenia • Rash • Sterility
cyclophosphamide		• 650 mg/m^2 on day 1 every 3 wk as a part of BEACOPP for 8 cycles	• Alopecia • Hemorrhagic cystitis • Nausea • Sterility • Urinary fibrosis • Vomiting
carboplatin		• Target AUC 5 (max 800 mg) for 2 cycles (in combination with ifosfamide and etoposide)	• Electrolyte imbalance • Myelosuppression • Pain • Renal complications • Vomiting
Purine Nucleoside Analogs			
fludarabine		• 25 mg/m^2/day IV on specific cycle days	• Anorexia • Bleeding • Cough • Edema • Fever • Nausea • Rash
pentostatin	Nipent	• 4 mg/m^2/dose IV every 2 wk	• Anemia • Fever • Nausea • Rash • Weakness
cladribine		• 0.09 mg/kg/day continuous IV infusion for 7 days	• Flulike symptoms • Infection • Injection site reactions • Rash
mercaptopurine	Purixan	• 1.5–2.5 mg/kg/day PO	• Anemia • Anorexia • Bleeding • Hepatotoxicity
Pyrimidine Analog			
cytarabine		• 100–2000 mg/m^2/dose IV depending on indication and regimen	• Fever • Nausea • Rash
Monoclonal Antibodies			
rituximab	Rituxan	• 375–500 mg/m^2/dose IV once wkly	• Fatigue • Fever • Infusion reaction • Nausea • Neuropathy • Rash • Tumor lysis syndrome

Generic Name	Trade Name	Common Dosage Range[a]	Select Common Side Effects
alemtuzumab	Campath, Lemtrada	• 30 mg/dose IV infusion 3 times wkly	• Fever • Hypotension • Injection site reaction • Nausea • Rash • Vomiting
Anthracyclines			
daunorubicin		• 30–60 mg/m²/day IV	• Alopecia • Cardiac toxicity • Injection site reaction • Nausea • Urine discoloration • Vomiting
idarubicin	Idamycin	• 12 mg/m²/day or infuse over 3 days	• Alopecia • Vomiting
Topoisomerase II Inhibitor			
etoposide	Etopophos	• 50–100 mg/m²/day IV for 5 days	• Alopecia • Anorexia • Nausea • Neuropathy
Vinca Alkaloids			
vindesine		• 3–4 mg/m²/wk IV	• Flulike symptoms • Loss of reflexes • Nausea
vincristine	Vincasar PFS[b]	• 2 mg/dose IV at specified cycle days	• Alopecia • Constipation • Hearing loss • Pain • Peripheral neuropathy
Tyrosine Kinase Inhibitors			
dasatinib	Sprycel	• 100–180 mg PO once daily for cycle	• Anemia • Arthralgia • Headache • Nausea • Rash
imatinib	Gleevec	• 400–800 mg PO once daily for cycle	
nilotinib	Tasigna	• 300–400 mg PO twice daily for cycle	
Retinoic Acid Derivative			
tretinoin	Vesanoid[b]	• 45 mg/m²/day PO in 2 divided doses	• Chest discomfort • Edema • Fever • Headache • Liver toxicity
Antimetabolites			
methotrexate	Trexall	• 12 mg/dose intrathecally	• Headache • Infections • Rigidity
hydroxyurea	Hydrea, Droxia	• 50–100 mg/kg/day PO until WBC <100,000/mm³	• Drowsiness • Edema • Fever • Nausea

[a]Doses can vary by patient and indication for use.
[b]Brand discontinued; now available only as generic.

AUC, Area under the curve; *BEACOPP*, *b*leomycin + *e*toposide + *A*driamycin (doxorubicin) + *c*yclophosphamide + *O*ncovin (vincristine) + *p*rocarbazine + *p*rednisone; *IV*, intravenously; *PO*, orally; *WBC*, white blood cell.

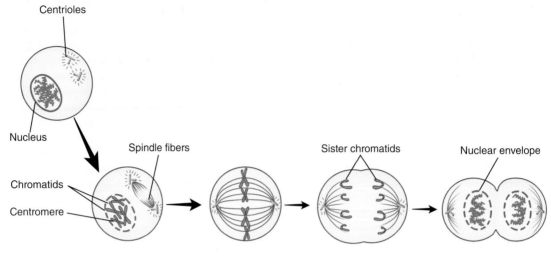

FIG. 28.8 Mitosis.

Nitrosoureas. These agents can cross the blood-brain barrier that surrounds the central nervous system; thus they can affect brain cancers. Side effects may include nausea, vomiting, intense skin flushing, red eyes, headache, and rash. The following drugs are nitrosoureas:

• carmustine
• lomustine

Other antineoplastic agents. Antiandrogens, for example, are part of prostate cancer treatment. Also known as *immunotherapy*, biological therapy is a type of cancer treatment that uses natural or laboratory substances. Some of these substances stimulate the body's immune system to resist cancer. In addition, they can stop or slow cancer cell growth and prevent cancer spread. This therapy type affects certain cancers. Prescribers often pair these drugs with other chemotherapy and radiation therapy. Biological therapy can treat diseases other than cancer. For example, rituximab can improve rheumatoid arthritis.

Lymphoma **Lymphomas,** as the name suggests, are cancers of the lymphatic system. Lymphomas initially develop in the lymph nodes or spleen. (For a review of the anatomy and physiology of the lymphatic system, see Chapter 25.) Inflammation-associated lymphoma development often leads to enlarged lymph nodes, which can be an early cancer symptom (Fig. 28.9). A major risk factor, lymphoma development is the presence of an immunodeficiency disorder (eg, acquired immunodeficiency syndrome [AIDS]). Another risk factor includes exposure to herbicides, pesticides, and organic solvents. Viruses, such as Epstein-Barr, also have been tied to certain lymphomas. The two broad categories of lymphoma are Hodgkin disease and non-Hodgkin lymphoma. Although the signs and symptoms of these two lymphomas overlap, they have different treatments and prognoses.

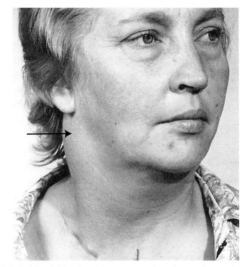

FIG. 28.9 Hodgkin lymphoma and enlarged cervical lymph node. (From Huether S, McCance K. *Understanding Pathophysiology*. 5th ed. St. Louis: Mosby; 2012.)

Prognosis

The prognosis for lymphoma varies widely based on the type and stage (Table 28.5).

Non-Drug Treatment

As with leukemia, supportive measures for lymphoma, such as prevention and aggressive infection treatment, are important. Radiation therapy can accompany other methods depending on the lymphoma type and stage.

Drug Treatment

Hematologic cancers respond to various chemotherapeutic agents depending on the cancer type and stage (see Table 28.4). Combination therapies are common.

TABLE 28.5
Stages of Cancer

Stage	Description
Stage I	Defined by small tumors located in one part of the body. Many cancers of this type are very treatable because the cancer is small and localized. This type of cancer may be cured by surgery and a small dose of radiation therapy.
Stage II	Slightly more severe than stage I cancer. Stage II tumors are more substantial but have not spread to the surrounding tissues and lymph nodes. The tumor can still be extracted surgically, and radiation can help ensure that the cancer does not return.
Stage III	The cancer has begun to move from the local organ to the surrounding lymph nodes. After this occurs, treatment and cure become more difficult. Treatment typically involves surgery to remove the tumor and radiation and chemotherapy to kill the cancer cells that have moved to the lymph nodes and surrounding tissues.
Stage IV	Metastatic cancer, the most advanced form of cancer. This type of cancer is characterized by large tumors that have spread to surrounding organs. After cancer has metastasized, it generally cannot be completely removed by surgery.

For example, a Hodgkin disease treatment includes the standard combination ABVD (*A*driamycin [doxorubicin] + *b*leomycin + *v*inblastine + *d*acarbazine) or, alternatively, BEACOPP (*b*leomycin + *e*toposide + *A*driamycin [doxorubicin] + *c*yclophosphamide + *O*ncovin [vincristine] + *p*rocarbazine + *p*rednisone) or Stanford V (doxorubicin + vinblastine + mechlorethamine + vincristine + bleomycin + etoposide + prednisone).

Bleeding Disorders

A defect in one or more clotting factors involved in the coagulation process can lead to bleeding disorders (Fig. 28.10). Bleeding disorders can be drug induced, genetic (hemophilia, von Willebrand disease), or the result of other disease processes (eg, liver disease or vasculitis). Drug-induced bleeding is relatively common with antiplatelet agents (eg, aspirin and clopidogrel), anticoagulants (eg, warfarin), and NSAIDs.

Hemophilia is a hereditary coagulation disorder associated with intermittent bleeding episodes. Hemophilia ties to either a deficiency or lack of either antihemophilic factor VIII (known as *hemophilia A*) or factor IX (Fig. 28.11). Hemophilia treatment involves prophylactic blood infusions or the use of recombinant factor VIII or factor IX products.

Von Willebrand disease is the most common inherited coagulation disorder and is associated with decreased activity of von Willebrand factor. Von Willebrand factor facilitates platelet binding in the vasculature. Treatment involves strategies to increase the availability of von Willebrand factor and include the use of **cryoprecipitate,** factor VIII concentrates, desmopressin (DDAVP), fresh frozen plasma, and estrogen therapy.

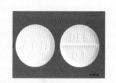

GENERIC NAME: desmopressin

TRADE NAME: DDAVP, Stimate

INDICATIONS: Bleeding prophylaxis, hemophilia A, hemorrhage, surgical bleeding, von Willebrand disease, diabetes insipidus, nocturia

ROUTES OF ADMINISTRATION: Intravenous (IV); subcutaneous (subcut); intranasal; oral

COMMON ADULT DOSAGE: *IV/subcut:* 0.3 mcg/kg. *Intranasal:* <50 kg: 150 mcg (1 spray in a single nostril); 50 kg: 300 mcg (1 spray each nostril)

MECHANISM OF ACTION: Synthetic analog of the antidiuretic hormone arginine vasopressin that increases plasma factor VIII and von Willebrand factor

SIDE EFFECTS: Facial flushing, headache, hyponatremia

I. Subendothelial exposure

- Occurs after endothelial sloughing
- Platelets begin to fill endothelial gaps
- Promoted by thromboxane A$_2$ (TXA$_2$)
- Inhibited by prostacyclin I$_2$ (PGI$_2$)
- Platelet function depends on many factors, especially calcium

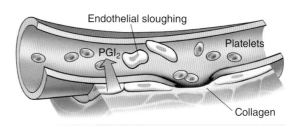

II. Adhesion

- Adhesion is initiated by loss of endothelial cells (or rupture or erosion of atherosclerotic plaque), which exposes adhesive glycoproteins such as collagen and von Willebrand factor (vWF) in the subendothelium. vWF and, perhaps, other adhesive glycoproteins in the plasma deposit on the damaged area. Platelets adhere to the subendothelium through receptors that bind to the adhesive glycoproteins (GPIb, GPIa/IIa, GPIIb/IIIa).

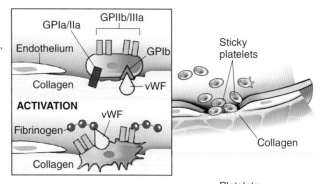

III. Activation

- After platelets adhere they undergo an activation process that leads to a conformational change in GPIIb/IIIa receptors, resulting in their ability to bind adhesive proteins, including fibrinogen and von Willebrand factor
- Changes in platelet shape
- Formation of pseudopods
- Activation of arachidonic pathway

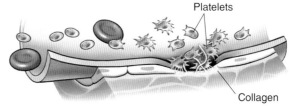

IV. Aggregation

- Induced by release of TXA$_2$
- Adhesive glycoproteins bind simultaneously to GPIIb/IIIa on two different platelets
- Stabilization of the platelet plug (blood clot) occurs by activation of coagulation factors, thrombin, and fibrin
- Heparin neutralizing factor enhances clot formation

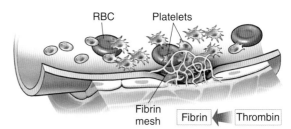

V. Platelet plug formation

- Red blood cells and platelets enmeshed in fibrin

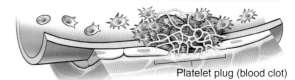

VI. Clot retraction and clot dissolution

- Clot retraction, using large number of platelets, joins the edges of the injured vessel
- Clot dissolution is regulated by thrombin and plasminogen activators

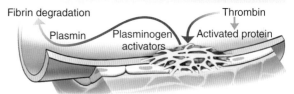

FIG. 28.10 Blood vessel damage, blood clot, and clot dissolution. *RBC,* Red blood cell.(From Huether S, McCance K. *Understanding Pathophysiology*. 5th ed. St. Louis: Mosby; 2012.)

Do You Remember These Key Points?

- Names of the major components of the hematologic system and their functions
- The primary symptoms of the various hematologic conditions discussed
- Medications used to treat the various hematologic conditions discussed
- The generic and trade names for the drugs discussed in this chapter
- The appropriate auxiliary labels that should be used when filling prescriptions for drugs discussed in this chapter

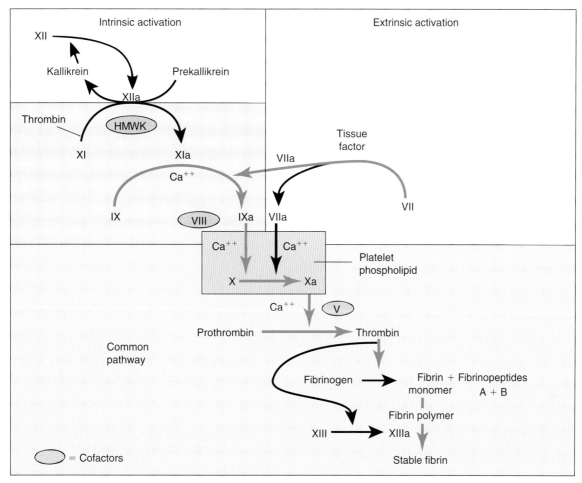

FIG. 28.11 Activation of factor X by the steps in the extrinsic and intrinsic coagulation pathways. *HMWK,* High-molecular-weight kininogen. (*From Price SA, Wilson LM. Pathophysiology: Clinical Concepts of Disease Processes.* 6th ed. St. Louis; Mosby; 2003.)

Review Questions

Multiple Choice Questions

1. _____ is the movement of water down a concentration gradient.
   A. Hydrostatic pressure
   B. Osmosis
   C. Diuresis
   D. Plasmolysis

2. Plasma that has been allowed to clot in the laboratory to remove clotting factors that can interfere with some blood tests is known as _____.
   A. Serum
   B. Whole blood
   C. Erythrocytes
   D. Fibrinogen

3. A condition associated with abnormally low platelets in the blood is known as:
   A. Leukocytosis
   B. Leukopenia
   C. Thrombocytopenia
   D. Neutropenia

4. Which hormone is produced in the kidney and stimulates the bone marrow to produce red blood cells?
   A. Prothrombin
   B. Fibrinogen
   C. Leukine
   D. Erythropoietin

5. What is the trade name for sodium ferric gluconate complex?
   A. Epogen
   B. Neulasta
   C. Ferrlecit
   D. Feosol

6. _____ is defined as excessive red blood cell production.
   A. Polycythemia
   B. Thrombocytopenia
   C. Anemia
   D. None of the above

7. Which medication is approved for the treatment of polycythemia vera?
   A. Epoetin alfa
   B. Darbepoetin alfa
   C. Anagrelide
   D. Sargramostim

8. Which condition(s) is/are associated with the development of neutropenia?
   A. Aplastic anemia
   B. Leukemia
   C. Vitamin B_{12} deficiency
   D. All of the above

9. ABVD is a combination therapy for the treatment of:
   A. Hodgkin disease
   B. Leukemia
   C. Non-Hodgkin lymphoma
   D. Hemophilia

10. Which drug is *not* thought to contribute to drug-induced bleeding?
    A. Ibuprofen
    B. Warfarin
    C. Clopidogrel
    D. Acetaminophen

11. Which condition is associated with a deficiency or a lack of either factor VIII or factor IX?
    A. Hemophilia
    B. von Willebrand disease
    C. Thrombocytopenia
    D. Hodgkin disease

12. _____ is associated with the destruction of mature erythrocytes because of cell lysis.
    A. Aplastic anemia
    B. Pernicious anemia
    C. Hemolytic anemia
    D. Iron deficiency anemia

13. The trade name for pegfilgrastim is:
    A. Aranesp
    B. Leukine
    C. Neulasta
    D. Neupogen

14. Eltrombopag (Promacta) is indicated for the treatment of:
    A. Thrombocytopenia
    B. Hemophilia
    C. Neutropenia
    D. Leukopenia

15. Which medication(s) is/are *not* associated with drug-induced thrombocytopenia?
    A. Heparin
    B. Quinine
    C. Vancomycin
    D. All of the above are associated with drug-induced thrombocytopenia.

■ Technician's Corner

Using an online drug information reference, perform a search of medications associated with the development of anemia as a drug side effect. If a person were picking up a refill for one of these medications and also was purchasing an over-the-counter (OTC) iron supplement, what (if anything) would you do?

Bibliography

Damjanov I. *Pathology for the Health Professions.* 4th ed. St. Louis: Saunders; 2011.

Fishback JL. *Pathology.* 3rd ed. Philadelphia: Mosby; 2005.

Huether S, McCance K. *Understanding Pathophysiology.* 5th ed. St. Louis: Mosby; 2012.

McCance KL. *Pathophysiology: The Biologic Basis for Disease in Adults and Children.* 6th ed. St. Louis: Mosby; 2010.

Page C, Hoffman B, Curtis, M, Walker M. *Integrated Pharmacology.* 3rd ed. St. Louis: Mosby; 2006.

Price SA, Wilson LM. *Pathophysiology: Clinical Concepts of Disease Processes.* 6th ed. St. Louis: Mosby; 2003.

Solomon EP. *Introduction to Human Anatomy and Physiology.* 3rd ed. St. Louis: Mosby; 2009.

Thibodeau GA, Patton KT. *Anatomy and Physiology.* 8th ed. St. Louis: Mosby; 2012.

Thompson JM, McFarland GK, Hirsch JE, et al. *Mosby's Clinical Nursing.* 5th ed. St. Louis: Mosby; 2001.

Websites Referenced

Clinical Pharmacology Online. Available at: https://www.clinicalkey.com/pharmacology.

UpToDate Online. Available at: http://www.uptodate.com.

CHAPTER 29

Over-the-Counter Medications

Tony Guerra

OBJECTIVES

1. Discuss important considerations that consumers should address before buying and using over-the-counter (OTC) medications.
2. Discuss how US Food and Drug Administration regulations affect OTC products and describe the process of how a prescription drug becomes an OTC drug.
3. Describe the most common conditions treated with OTC products. In addition, (a) recognize OTC drugs used to treat the conditions discussed in this chapter, (b) write the generic and trade names for the OTC drugs in this chapter, and (c) recognize common dosage forms and safety considerations for OTC products.
4. Describe scenarios in which special populations need to consider whether OTC drugs are appropriate for their use. In addition, discuss restricted OTC products.

TERMS AND DEFINITIONS

Analgesics Not + pain, drugs that relieve pain

Antiinflammatory A drug that reduces swelling

Antipyretics Not + fire, drugs that reduce fever

Antitussive Not + cough, a drug that can decrease the coughing reflex

Behind-the-counter drug A nonprescription medication kept "behind the [prescription] counter" that patients must buy at a pharmacy

Circadian rhythms The 24-hour cycles of regular biological changes. In pharmacology, this often involves medications affecting sleep/wake cycles

Expectorants Chemicals that loosen and thin sputum and bronchial secretions

Legend drugs Medications that need a prescription

Nutraceutical A food or supplement with added health benefits

Over-the-counter (OTC) drugs Nonprescription medicines generally found outside the secure part of the pharmacy

Pruritus An itch

Unlike in other countries, retail pharmacies in the United States make **over-the-counter (OTC) drugs** readily available to allow students to explore and work with medicines early in the program. Customers often request that pharmacy technicians help them find medications. Although only pharmacists can provide therapeutic advice, pharmacy technicians can guide patients to the correct section. Technicians need a comprehensive understanding of how pharmacies group medications in the aisle.

Different pharmacies use different signage as markers. For example, one pharmacy might place antacids under "Antacids," and another might place these products under "Digestive." Some smaller pharmacies might forgo signage, depending on significant conversations with pharmacy staff instead. Pharmacy technicians who familiarize themselves with the different ways pharmacies group or refer to OTC medications can better help patients.

Customers can buy OTC products without a prescription. Patients often buy these products without advice from the pharmacy staff about their correct use. Just as people keep food staples in the kitchen, certain nonprescription medications are home medicine cabinet staples. An essential shopping list might include food items such as flour, sugar, eggs, and analgesics, such as acetaminophen (Tylenol) or ibuprofen (Advil, Motrin).

Consumer access to OTC drugs has increased sharply since the mid-1980s. The Consumer Healthcare Products Association offers useful data on OTC sales, possible health care cost reductions, and the future of these products. The Association cites four broad reasons that patients use OTC drugs: accessibility, affordability, trust, and empowerment.

- *Accessibility:* Pharmacies remain open well before and after the physician's office hours, providing round-the-clock access to care.
- *Affordability:* OTC drug costs may exceed copays, but they can save the time and expense of meeting with health care providers.
- *Trust:* Most health care providers and consumers think OTC medications are safe and effective.
- *Empowerment:* Patients can involve pharmacists as advisers to make their own decisions about care.

In this chapter, we explore recommended OTC medications and present common dose forms and dosages. This chapter also includes a review of the US Food and Drug Administration (FDA) rules.

Federal law dictates that pharmacists counsel patients with Medicaid receiving new prescriptions. Individual states have added counseling expectations. Unless the prescriber writes a script for nonprescription items, they do not fall under these categories. During patient counseling for prescription items, pharmacists ask about OTC medication use because these items can interact with prescription drugs and medical conditions. The ready availability of OTC drugs can provide cost savings, but it can pose risks if excluded from the patient profile.

What should consumers consider in choosing OTC medicines? Correctly identifying the cause of the disease is the first step. If the diagnosis is wrong, the nonprescription medicine may aggravate an underlying condition. For example, patients who employ antidiarrheals to treat bacterial intestinal infections trap microbes. This action relieves the symptoms but worsens the condition. Therefore patient education is critical to providing the correct recommendation.

Many OTCs list specific age groups that should not take the medication. Parents should consult with their child's pediatrician before giving these medications, especially to children younger than 4 years of age. In addition, children with colds may develop ear infections and other conditions that warrant a visit to the pediatrician. Consumers should address these considerations before buying and using OTC medications.

- Various OTCs have identical ingredients; however, consumers often buy a more expensive name brand, not realizing that they are getting the same medication as the less costly generic form.
- Manufacturers may swap "like ingredients." The label shows the ingredient change or reformulation. Consumers often overlook this if they do not read labels carefully. Thus consumers may be unaware that they are using a formula different from what they used previously.
- Patients on special diets or with allergies, diabetes, or interacting medications should use caution in selecting an OTC.
- Parents should check with the pharmacist when buying nonprescription medications for infants or young children.
- When trying a new agent, individuals should watch for any adverse reactions that may occur.
- Pregnant or breastfeeding women cannot take many prescription and nonprescription medications. Pregnant or breastfeeding women should always seek professional advice before taking an OTC product.

US Food and Drug Administration Regulations

The FDA regulates OTC and prescription medications differently. New drugs must undergo a new drug application (NDA) before approval. Drugs judged "generally recognized as safe and effective" (GRASE) are exempt. Historically, some drug products, such as aspirin, were available OTC before the NDA. To handle these products, the FDA set up the OTC monograph system. This method allows expert panels to review OTCs for the GRASE label. To handle the more than 300,000 marketed nonprescription products, the FDA evaluates active ingredients and labeling expectations of drug classes rather than individual products. The *Federal Register* houses published OTC drug monographs and outlines acceptable ingredients, dosages, formulas, and labeling. Products not covered by a monograph because of an active ingredient or ingredients and labeling expectations need approval by the traditional NDA. Manufacturers can market new products that conform to a final monograph without further FDA review.

How a Prescription Drug Becomes an Over-the-Counter Drug

The process of transferring a drug from prescription (Rx) to nonprescription, or an "Rx-to-OTC switch," takes place through one of two methods: (1) under the OTC drug review or (2) through manufacturer submission of added information to the original product NDA. The FDA's primary concern is whether patients can safely use the medication without a health care provider's oversight. The manufacturer must also show that consumers can independently read, understand, and follow the product's labeling. Significant research precedes a new OTC release as the FDA works to approve drugs meeting its strict guidelines (as discussed in Chapter 2). OTC drug approval has similar safety and effectiveness standards as those placed **on legend drugs** (those needing a prescription). A prospective nonprescription formula may have a lower dosage than its prescription counterpart. Studies must confirm its effectiveness at the new dosage. If the agent meets the standards, the FDA will likely approve the medication. If the agent has previous prescription drug approval and the manufacturer wants an OTC version, it does not need further testing.

Some medications have an OTC *and* legend drug approval. Often the dose form or dosage strength separates them. Topical low-dosage lidocaine, an anesthetic, is nonprescription; injectable lidocaine (Xylocaine) for dental procedures is Rx. Ibuprofen in 200-mg strength is available OTC, whereas 400-, 600-, or 800-mg doses need a prescription. Notable agents making the Rx-to-OTC switch include the following:

- *Nonsedating antihistamines:* Loratadine (Claritin), fexofenadine (Allegra Allergy 12/24 Hour), and cetirizine (Zyrtec Allergy)
- *Proton pump inhibitors:* Omeprazole (Prilosec OTC), esomeprazole (Nexium 24HR), and lansoprazole (Prevacid 24HR)
- *Laxative:* Polyethylene glycol (MiraLAX)
- *Allergic rhinitis medications:* Budesonide (Rhinocort Allergy Spray), fluticasone (Flonase Allergy Relief), and triamcinolone (Nasacort Allergy 24HR)
- *Patch for overactive bladder:* Oxybutynin (Oxytrol For Women)

Patient Perceptions and Safety of OTC Medications and Herbal Supplements

It is not uncommon for patients to perceive OTC medications and herbal supplements as risk free. All OTC medications and herbal supplements come with the risk of side effects or adverse drug interactions. For example, acetaminophen causes liver toxicity at high doses, and St. John's wort can reduce the effectiveness of warfarin. Just because a drug is available without a prescription does not indicate that it comes without risk—a medication, by prescription or over the counter, is only safe and effective when used to treat intended conditions and administered appropriately.

Common Routes of Administration for Over-the-Counter Drugs

Table 29.1 lists some of the most common OTC medications, the symptoms they treat, and popular routes of administration. For example, a patient may try a topical formula to treat acne, and if that proves unsuccessful, ask a prescriber for an oral medication. As new medicines enter the OTC market, consumers can have more choices.

Over-the-Counter Pain Relievers and Antipyretics

Analgesics relieve pain. **Antipyretics** reduce fever. Acetaminophen (Tylenol) is both an analgesic and an antipyretic. Aspirin (acetylsalicylic acid) is an analgesic, antipyretic, and **antiinflammatory** agent at higher doses. As noted in Chapter 19, aspirin, in a low dosage, can prevent platelet clotting to help avoid heart attack and stroke. However, because of the bleeding risk with aspirin, patients are advised to consult their providers before starting therapy.

TABLE 29.1
Common OTC Product Categories

Drug Type	Symptom Treated	Route of Administration
Acne products	Pimples	Topical
Analgesics	Pain	Oral, topical, rectal
Antacids	Indigestion	Oral
Antibiotics	Topical infection treatment/prophylaxis	Topical
Antidiarrheals	Diarrhea	Oral
Antifungals	Dry, flaking skin and pain caused by fungus	Topical
Antihistamines	Allergies	Oral, intranasal
Antiinflammatories	Inflammation/arthritis pain	Oral, topical
Antipyretics	Fever	Oral, rectal
Cold sore preparations	Painful canker sores	Topical
Cough suppressants	Dry cough	Oral
Decongestants	Congestion	Oral, intranasal
Expectorants	Productive cough	Oral
Headache products	Pain	Oral
Laxatives	Constipation	Oral, rectal
Sleep aids	Insomnia	Oral
Sore throat products	Pain	Oral
Sunburn products	Pain/inflammation	Topical
Sunscreens	Sunburn prophylaxis	Topical
Wart removal products	Wart growth	Topical

> ### ■ Tech Note!
>
> Reye syndrome is a rare condition that can affect children and teenagers with an active case of certain viral illnesses (eg, chickenpox or influenza) who take products containing aspirin. The symptoms include vomiting, drowsiness, delirium, and coma. Permanent brain damage can occur, and the condition can be fatal. Proper aspirin and other salicylate use can prevent such adverse effects.

Patients widely use pain relievers for arthritis, headaches, and other aches and pains. Nonsteroidal antiinflammatory drugs (NSAIDs), such as ibuprofen and naproxen, are staples of most medicine cabinets in the United States and are effective analgesics, antipyretics, and antiinflammatory agents. Acetaminophen (Tylenol) is another widely used OTC product that acts as both an analgesic and an antipyretic. Table 29.2 lists select OTCs to treat pain and fever.

> ### ■ Tech Note!
>
> A potential and common side effect of NSAIDs is an increase in blood pressure. Alert the pharmacist if the patient is taking blood pressure medications and OTC NSAIDs.

> ### ■ Tech Note!
>
> Acetaminophen is a common ingredient of many OTC products, such as Tylenol, combination cough and cold preparations, and prescription pain relievers. Patients may not realize that many products contain acetaminophen. Excessive daily use puts them at risk for liver toxicity.

Over-the-Counter Allergy Treatments

Various OTC products treat allergy symptoms (Table 29.3). These products can contain several agents, such as antihistamines and decongestants. (See Chapter 21 for a detailed discussion of allergy treatments.) Antihistamines block histamine (H_1) receptors, which cause allergic symptoms. Customers use antihistamines to reduce symptoms of **pruritus** (itching), hives, sneezing, and itchy, runny eyes. First-generation sedating agents include diphenhydramine (Benadryl Allergy) and chlorpheniramine (Chlor-Trimeton). Cetirizine (Zyrtec Allergy) is a weakly sedating antihistamine that causes less drowsiness than first-generation agents. Loratadine (Claritin) does not typically cause drowsiness. OTC antihistamines usually relieve mild symptoms of allergy, but people with severe allergies may need a prescription. Decongestants relieve sinus congestion through vasoconstriction. Nasal corticosteroid sprays such as budesonide, fluticasone, and triamcinolone work to improve allergic rhinitis. It may take a few weeks to see their effects.

Over-the-Counter Products to Treat Cough and Cold Symptoms

The pharmacy cold and flu section is expansive. Many manufacturers offer similar ingredients in different combinations (Table 29.4). For congested coughs, **expectorants** can help break up phlegm. Use an **antitussive** (anticough) medicine for dry, nonproductive coughs.

Sore, scratchy, and dry throats often arise from a cold or flu. Nonprescription agents regularly provide symptomatic relief. A prescriber should evaluate symptoms that persist for more than a few days. A sore throat can hallmark a streptococcal bacterial infection, strep throat. Nonprescription syrups, sprays, and analgesics again manage the associated discomfort. Product ingredients include menthol, alcohol, and a topical anesthetic such as benzocaine, or a combination of these ingredients.

Over-the-Counter Products for Insomnia

Many customers treat insomnia with nonprescription products first. Effective first-generation sedating antihistamines include diphenhydramine and doxylamine (Table 29.5). Some combination products also contain a pain reliever such as acetaminophen to help with nighttime aches. These sleep aids handle transient insomnia and are not for extended use.

■ TABLE 29.2
Select OTC Pain Medications

Medication Class	Generic Name	Trade Name	Common Adult Dosage
Nonnarcotic analgesic	acetaminophen	Tylenol	• 325–650 mg PO or PR every 4–6 hr as needed; max 4 g/day[a]
Nonsteroidal antiinflammatory drugs (NSAIDs)	aspirin	Ecotrin	• 325–650 mg PO or PR every 4–6 hr as needed (max 4 g/day)
	ibuprofen	Advil, Motrin	• 200–400 mg PO every 4–6 hr as needed (max 1200 mg/day)
	naproxen	Aleve	• 200–440 mg PO once, then 200 mg PO every 8–12 hr (max 600 mg/day)

[a]Makers of Tylenol Extra Strength recommend a limit of 3 g/day, but the US Food and Drug Administration upholds a 4 g/day maximum. *https://www.fda.gov/drugs/drug-safety-and-availability/fda-drug-safety-communication-prescription-acetaminophen-products-be-limited-325-mg-dosage-unit*
PO, Orally; *PR,* rectally.

TABLE 29.3
Select OTC Products for Allergy Symptoms

Medication Class	Generic Name	Trade Name	Common Adult Dosage
Antihistamines: Oral nonsedating[a]	cetirizine HCl	Zyrtec Allergy	• 5–10 mg PO once daily
	fexofenadine	Allegra	• 60 mg PO twice daily *or* • 180 mg PO once daily
	loratadine	Claritin	• 10 mg PO once daily *or* • 5 mg twice daily
Antihistamines: Oral sedating	chlorpheniramine	Chlor-Trimeton	• 4 mg PO every 4–6 hr *or* • *ER:* 12 mg twice daily
	diphenhydramine	Benadryl Allergy	• 25–50 mg PO every 4–6 hr
Decongestant: Oral	pseudoephedrine	Sudafed 12 hr	• *IR:* 60 mg PO every 4–6 hr • *ER:* 120 mg every 12 h or 240 mg every 24 h
Decongestants: Nasal[b]	oxymetazoline	Afrin	• 2–3 sprays in each nostril twice daily (max 3 days)
	phenylephrine	Neo-Synephrine Cold and Allergy Spray	• 2–3 sprays in each nostril every 4 hr as needed (max 3 days)
Mast cell stabilizer: Nasal	cromolyn sodium	NasalCrom	• 1 spray in each nostril 3–6 times daily
Antihistamine/mast cell stabilizer: Ophthalmic	ketotifen	Zaditor	• 1 drop into the affected eye(s) every 8–12 hr
Antihistamine/decongestant: Ophthalmic	naphazoline	Clear Eyes[c]	• 1–2 drops into the eye(s) up to 4 times daily as needed
	tetrahydrozoline	Opti-Clear	• 1–2 drops in the affected eye(s) up to 4 times daily
Nasal corticosteroids	budesonide	Rhinocort Allergy Spray	• 2 sprays in each nostril once daily (max 4 sprays/nostril daily)
	fluticasone	Flonase Allergy Relief	• Begin with 2 sprays in each nostril; once symptoms improve, reduce to 1 spray in each nostril daily
	triamcinolone	Nasacort Allergy 24HR	• Begin with 2 sprays in each nostril; once symptoms improve, reduce to 1 spray in each nostril daily

[a]Combination pseudoephedrine products may feature a "D" after the name of the other ingredient; for example, "Loratadine-D" for a medication containing loratadine (an antihistamine) and pseudoephedrine (a decongestant).
[b]Using these nasal sprays longer than 3 days can cause rebound nasal congestion.
[c]Brand discontinued; now available only as generic.
ER, Extended-release; *IR,* immediate-release; *PO,* orally.

Melatonin is a **nutraceutical** widely used for sleep issues. The pineal gland secretes this endogenous hormone that plays a role in **circadian rhythms**.

Customers should discuss the correct use of these products with their pharmacist, physician, or other health care provider, because other conditions often underlie insomnia. The recommended duration for nonprescription sleep aids is 2 weeks maximum. People with lengthy sleep trouble should make an appointment with their physician. Non-drug approaches may help treat sleeplessness. These methods include a regular sleep schedule, exercise, stress reduction, and avoiding caffeine and long daytime naps.

Tech Note!

Diphenhydramine regularly causes next-day drowsiness in older adults. Drowsiness and confusion may increase the risk for falls in older individuals, so sedating antihistamines warrant caution in these patients.

Gastroesophageal Reflux Disease and Indigestion

Acid reducers relieve indigestion and gastroesophageal reflux disease (GERD) symptoms (Table 29.6). Antacids such as calcium carbonate and magnesium hydroxide increase the

Select OTC Products for Cough and Cold Symptoms[a]

Medication Class	Generic Name	Trade Name	Common Adult Dosage
Antipyretic (fever) and analgesics	acetaminophen	Tylenol	• 325–650 mg PO or PR every 4–6 hr as needed; max 4 g/day[b]
	ibuprofen	Advil	• 200–400 mg PO every 4–6 hr as needed (max 1200 mg/day)
Cough suppressant (antitussive)	dextromethorphan	Delsym	• *IR:* 10–20 mg PO every 4 hr as needed *or* • 20–30 mg every 6–8 h as needed • *ER:* 60 mg every 12 hr as needed
Expectorant	guaifenesin	Mucinex	• *IR:* 200–400 mg PO every 4 hr • *ER:* 600–1200 mg twice daily (max 2400 mg/day)
Systemic decongestant	pseudoephedrine	Sudafed 12 Hr	• *IR:* 60 mg PO every 4–6 hr • *ER:* 120 mg every 12 h or 240 mg every 24 h
	phenylephrine	Sudafed PE	• 10 mg PO every 4–6 hr
Local anesthetics	benzocaine	Chloraseptic Sore Throat Lozenges	• 1 lozenge (10–15 mg) dissolved slowly in the mouth; may repeat every 2 hr
	menthol	Halls Lozenges	• 1–2 lozenges dissolved in the mouth over time; may repeat every 2 hr
	phenol	Chloraseptic Sore Throat Spray	• Up to 5 sprays to the affected area, keep in place for 15 seconds, then spit; may repeat every 2 hr
	benzocaine, glycerin	Cepacol Extra Strength Sore Throat	• 1 spray to the affected area, wait longer than 1 min and spit; may repeat 4 times daily
Antihistamine, sedating	diphenhydramine	Benadryl Allergy	• 25–50 mg PO every 4–8 hr

[a]Refer to other sections and tables for additional options and more information on antihistamines, decongestants, sleep medications, and pain/analgesia medications. Many cough and cold products are available in a combination form.

[b]Makers of Tylenol Extra Strength recommend a limit of 3 g per day, but the US Food and Drug Administration maintains 4 g per day maximum. *https://www.fda.gov/drugs/drug-safety-and-availability/fda-drug-safety-communication-prescription-acetaminophen-products-be-limited-325-mg-dosage-unit*

ER, Extended-release; *IR,* immediate-release; *PO,* orally; *PR,* rectally; *prn,* as needed.

■ TABLE 29.5

Select OTC Products for Insomnia[a]

Medication Class	Generic Name	Trade Name	Common Adult Dosage
Hormone/nutritional supplement	melatonin	n/a	• 3–5 mg PO daily
Histamine antagonist (first generation)	doxylamine	Unisom SleepTabs	• 25 mg PO once daily before bedtime
	diphenhydramine	Benadryl (as the "PM" in Tylenol PM)	• 50 mg PO at bedtime

[a]The US Food and Drug Administration recommends developing healthy sleep habits before trying medications.

n/a, Not available; *PO,* orally.

stomach's pH level in a few minutes to reduce heartburn. H_2 antagonists such as famotidine and ranitidine block the H_2 receptor, reduce gastric acid, and improve hyperacidic states. Proton pump inhibitors (PPIs) also decrease acid but may take a few days for maximum effect. (See Chapter 22 to review these medication classes.) Note that all forms of ranitidine were removed from shelves in the United States in April 2020.

■ **Tech Note!**

Ulcers may cause chronic stomach pain. *Helicobacter pylori,* a bacterium associated with stomach and intestinal ulcers, can cause this discomfort. If the condition lasts more than 2 weeks, patients should contact their physician.

TABLE 29.6
Select OTC Products for Gastroesophageal Reflux Disease and Indigestion

Generic Name	Trade Name	Common Dosage Range
Antacids		
Neutralize Existing Stomach Acid		
calcium carbonate	Tums	• 1–4 tablets as symptoms occur (max 8 g/day for 2 wk)
magnesium hydroxide	Phillips' Milk of Magnesia	• 2–4 tablets or 5–15 mL PO prn every 4 h up to 4 times daily
sodium bicarbonate		• 325 mg to 2 g PO 1–4 times daily
Histamine-2 Blockers		
Block the Action of Histamine That Causes Secretion of Stomach Acid		
cimetidine	Tagamet HB 200	• 200 mg PO once or twice daily 30 min before ingesting heartburn-causing agents (max 400 mg/day)
famotidine	Pepcid AC	• 10–20 mg PO every 12 h (max 40 mg/day)
Proton Pump Inhibitors		
Inactivate the Acid Pumps Throughout Cells in the Stomach		
esomeprazole	Nexium 24HR	• 20 mg PO once daily for up to 14 days
omeprazole	Prilosec OTC	• 20 mg PO once daily for up to 14 days
lansoprazole	Prevacid 24HR	• 15 mg PO once daily for up to 14 days

OTC, Over the counter; *PO,* orally; *prn,* as needed.

Antacids work best for short-term heartburn relief. H_2-receptor antagonists and PPIs provide maintenance therapy or work as part of triple ulcer therapy. Triple therapy commonly includes one acid reducer and two antibiotics. Antacids can cause varying side effects, such as constipation, diarrhea, stomach cramps, and drug-drug interactions. Antacids containing calcium, magnesium, and aluminum may chelate (bind with) tetracycline and quinolone antibiotics. Antacids also affect thyroid hormone absorption. Antacids, H_2-receptor antagonists, and PPIs also interact with drugs that need an acidic environment for proper absorption.

Tech Note!

Calcium absorption is acid dependent. Researchers linked long-term proton pump inhibitor use and increased stomach alkalinity to an increased bone fracture risk.

Over-the-Counter Products for Nausea and Vomiting

Antiemetics can prevent nausea and vomiting. Emetrol and Pepto-Bismol provide relief from nausea and upset stomach. Although Emetrol is appropriate for children ages 2 and older, Pepto-Bismol is not recommended for children under age 12 because bismuth subsalicylate, its active ingredient, can cause Reye syndrome, a life-threatening disorder. Emetrol's brand name alludes to "emesis control," or control of vomiting.

With severe vomiting, fluid replacement may be appropriate. Children who need fluid replacement can use rehydration fluids such as Enfalyte or Pedialyte. Children must be 2 years old to use Enfalyte, but Pedialyte is safe for infants younger than 1 year with a physician's care.

First-generation antihistamines such as dimenhydrinate (Dramamine) and meclizine (Bonine) can relieve motion sickness and nausea. They block acetylcholine and histamine-1 receptors, inhibiting the vestibular system. First-generation antihistamines may cause drowsiness and dry mouth, although meclizine can cause less sedation than dimenhydrinate. Table 29.7 includes these medications.

Over-the-Counter Agents for Other Gastrointestinal Conditions

Table 29.8 presents medicines for intestinal discomfort and pain resulting from constipation, diarrhea, or gas (flatulence). (See Chapter 22 for a review of constipation and diarrhea treatments.) Simethicone (Gas-X Extra Strength) is the most common agent for gas. Beano, with the alpha-galactosidase enzyme, works to counter foods with gas-producing carbohydrates. Beano neutralizes gas produced as a bacterial by-product.

Tech Note!

Psyllium, a bulk-forming agent, treats constipation *and* diarrhea. This dual effect earns psyllium the label "bowel stabilizer" because some patients cycle between constipation and diarrhea episodes.

Miscellaneous Over-the-Counter Products for Skin-Related Conditions

Table 29.9 highlights drugs for minor cuts, scrapes, and other skin conditions. Neosporin kills topical bacteria in superficial

■ TABLE 29.7
Select Medications for Management of Nausea and Vomiting

Medication Class	Generic Name	Trade Name	Common Dosage
Antiemetics	fructose, dextrose, and phosphoric acid	Emetrol	15 to 30 mL; repeat dose every 15 min until distress subsides. No more than 5 doses in an hr
	bismuth subsalicylate	Pepto-Bismol	1 dose every 30–60 min as needed. No more than 8 doses in a 24-hr period Refer to the Drug Facts label for specific instructions as dosing varies by formula and form.
Rehydration fluids	oral electrolyte therapy	Enfamil Enfalyte	Children 2 years of age and older: small, frequent sips every 15–30 min Children 1–10 years: up to 32 fluid oz in 24 hr Children 10 years to adults: up to 64 fluid oz in 24 hr
	oral electrolyte therapy	Pedialyte	Children 1 year of age and older: 1–2 L/day
Antihistamines	meclizine	Bonine, Antivert, Motion-Time	12.5 to 25 mg every 6–8 hr as needed
	dimenhydrinate	Dramamine	50 to 100 mg every 4–6 hr

■ TABLE 29.8
Select OTC Products for Gastrointestinal Conditions Such as Constipation and Diarrhea

Medication Class	Generic Name	Trade Name	Common Dosage Range	Onset
Fiber/bulk laxative	psyllium	Metamucil	• 2.5–30 g/day in divided doses	12–72 hr
Stool softener	docusate sodium	Colace	• 50–360 mg/day PO once daily or in divided doses	12–72 hr
Hyperosmolar agent	sorbitol	None	• 30–45 mL/day PO	1–2 days
Stimulants	bisacodyl	Dulcolax Laxative	• 5–15 mg PO once daily	6 hr
	sennosides	Senokot	• 2 tabs PO once daily (max 4 tabs)	6–12 hr
Saline laxatives	magnesium citrate	Citroma[a]	• 195–300 mL PO once or divided doses	0.5–3 hr
	magnesium hydroxide	Milk of Magnesia	• 2–4 tablets or 5–15 mL PO as needed every 4 h up to 4 times daily	0.5–6 hr
Lubricant laxative	mineral oil	Kondremul	• *Plain mineral oil:* 15–45 mL PO once daily • *Kondremul:* 30–90 mL/day in a single dose or divided doses	6–8 hr
Suppositories	glycerin	Fleet Glycerin Suppository	• 1 supp PR prn once daily	15–60 min
	bisacodyl	Dulcolax	• 1 supp PR prn once daily	15–60 min
Enemas	sodium phosphate	Fleet Saline Enema	• 1 unit PR as a single dose	5–15 min
	mineral oil	Fleet Mineral Oil Enema	• 118 mL PR as a single dose	6–8 hr
Antidiarrheals	loperamide	Imodium A-D	• 4 mg PO initially, then 2 mg after each loose stool (max 16 mg/day)	1 hr
	bismuth subsalicylate	Pepto-Bismol	• 524 mg PO every 30–60 min prn, up to 8 doses daily	1 hr

[a]Brand discontinued; now available only as generic.
PO, Orally; *PR,* rectally; *prn,* as needed; *supp,* suppository.

TABLE 29.9
Select Miscellaneous Topical OTC Products for a Variety of Skin Conditions

Skin Condition	Generic Name	Trade Name	Dosage Form
Acne	benzoyl peroxide	Clearskin	Cream
		Clearplex-X	Gel
		Acne Medication	Lotion
		Zaclir Cleansing	Lotion
Athlete's foot	clotrimazole	Lotrimin-AF	Cream
	miconazole	Zeasorb-AF	Powder
	tolnaftate	Tinactin	Liquid, powder, aerosol, cream
	terbinafine	Lamisil AT	Cream, topical solution
Cuts/scrapes	bacitracin	Bacitracin	Ointment
	neomycin	None	Ointment
	polymyxin B sulfate, neomycin, bacitracin	Neosporin Original Formula	Ointment, cream
Hives, inflammation	diphenhydramine	Benadryl	Lotion, cream
	hydrocortisone	Cortizone-10	Cream, ointment
Warts	salicylic acid	DuoFilm	Liquid
		Compound W	Gel, liquid
		Salisol	Solution

wounds. Benzoyl peroxide clears acne, which is common among teenagers. Systemic antihistamines, such as diphenhydramine, and topical corticosteroids, such as hydrocortisone, provide relief from hives, which is an allergic reaction. Topical antifungals resolve athlete's foot (tinea pedis) and jock itch (tinea cruris). Topical salicylic acid removes common warts.

Considerations for Special Populations

Elderly patients may have multiple conditions that make self-treatment risky. Apart from chronic conditions such as hypertension, diabetes, and arthritis, they may have degenerating eyesight or hearing problems. Often, taking extra time to listen and make them comfortable provides an avenue to a full medication history. Some patients worry about asking too many questions. Reassure them that their questions are welcome.

Another high-risk group for medication errors includes infants and young children. Most pediatric products carry age- and/or weight-based dosage calculations. The parent may have trouble measuring the proper dose or assume that a child's dose is simply a smaller version of an adult's dose. For example, diphenhydramine works as a sleep aid in adults, but its primary purpose in children is allergy relief. The FDA recommends that parents only use nonprescription drugs in children 2 years and older. For this age group, the FDA provides several recommendations.

- Check the Drug Facts label's "active ingredients" section to ensure the product ingredients match the child's symptoms.

- With multiple cough and cold children's medicines, look carefully for repeat ingredients.
- Carefully follow the Drug Facts label directions.
- Use measuring spoons or cups included with the medicines or those properly marked for measuring drugs.
- Choose cough and cold medicines with childproof safety caps, when available. Store out of reach of children.
- Understand that cough and cold medicines only treat the child's symptoms.
- Do not use OTC cough and cold medicines to sedate a child.
- If questions arise about the correct cough or cold medicine to use in children aged 2 or older, call a physician, pharmacist, or other health care professional.

Restricted Over-the-Counter Products

Table 29.10 lists drugs kept behind the counter to regulate access. Although we refer to them as **behind-the-counter drugs**, they do not belong to a specific OTC "class" of drugs under FDA rules, unlike in England and Canada. Also, under the 2005 Combat Methamphetamine Epidemic Act (see Chapter 2), pharmacies must keep pseudoephedrine products behind the pharmacy counter and log and keep information about the people who buy them.

Most pharmacies stock insulin vials behind the counter for safety, because insulin can lead to serious harm if not used appropriately. Some insulins can be purchased without insurance or a prescription, but they still require needles and syringes, which are available separately.

TABLE 29.10
Current Medications Available Behind the Counter in the United States

Trade Name	Generic Name	Conditions
Sudafed 12 Hr	pseudoephedrine	Log book or electronic record containing customer's name, address, identification, and signature; date and time of sale; and name and quantity of product sold. Keep records for at least 2 years. Limited purchase amounts for 1-day and 1-month intervals
ReliOn Novolog	Insulin aspart, vial	Requires needles for use
ReliOn Novolin NPH	Insulin NPH, vial	
ReliOn Novolin 70/30 mix	Insulin regular and NPH, vial	

◼ Tech Note!

If a patient has not used insulin before or has yet to be educated on self-administration using needles, encourage a discussion with the pharmacist to address any concerns or questions regarding safety and administration.

Urinary Incontinence (Overactive Bladder)

Oxybutynin (Oxytrol For Women) is an anticholinergic patch to treat overactive bladder. The patch duration of action is 4 days. Although anticholinergic side effects such as dry mouth or constipation might be expected, these side effects were comparable to placebo. The patient may experience drowsiness, dizziness, or blurry vision. The patient should avoid alcohol during treatment. After removing the patch, the user may experience site-specific itching, rash, or redness.

Do You Remember These Key Points?

- The most common conditions treated with OTC products
- Trade (brand) and generic names of common OTC drugs used to treat the conditions discussed in this chapter
- Regulations concerning the manufacture of OTC products as established by the FDA
- Common dose forms and safety considerations for the OTC products discussed in this chapter

Review Questions

Multiple Choice Questions

1. Drugs available over the counter (OTC) are 100% safe and effective for all patients.
   A. True
   B. False

2. Which medication *does not* block histamine-2 receptors?
   A. Cimetidine (Tagamet HB 200)
   B. Famotidine (Pepcid AC)
   C. Loperamide (Imodium AD)
   D. Ranitidine

3. Which drug class does not affect stomach acid?
   A. Proton pump inhibitors (PPIs)
   B. H_2-receptor antagonists
   C. Antidiarrheals
   D. Antacids

4. The US Food and Drug Administration (FDA) recommends that children under the age of _____ should *not* use OTC cough and cold products.
   A. 1 year
   B. 2 years
   C. 4 years
   D. 5 years

5. Which analgesic works to prevent heart attacks?
   A. Acetaminophen
   B. Aspirin
   C. Ibuprofen
   D. Naproxen

6. Which drug does *not* have antiinflammatory properties?
   A. Aspirin
   B. Ibuprofen (Advil)
   C. Acetaminophen (Tylenol)
   D. Naproxen (Aleve)

7. Which agent treats both constipation and diarrhea?
   A. Psyllium
   B. Loperamide
   C. Calcium carbonate
   D. Docusate

8. Which drug class has an association with increased blood pressure?
   A. NSAIDs
   B. Stimulant laxatives
   C. Topical corticosteroid creams
   D. Allergic rhinitis nasal inhalers

9. What is the generic name for the active ingredient of Prilosec OTC?
   A. Clotrimazole
   B. Omeprazole
   C. Esomeprazole
   D. Lansoprazole
10. The OTC product most commonly used as an antihistamine is:
   A. Aspirin
   B. Ibuprofen
   C. Diphenhydramine
   D. Polyethylene glycol
11. Advil and Motrin carry the generic name:
   A. Ibuprofen
   B. Doxylamine
   C. Acetaminophen
   D. Diphenhydramine
12. Melatonin:
   A. Stops diarrhea
   B. Is an endogenous hormone
   C. Comes as a topical agent
   D. Effectively treats athlete's foot
13. OTC agents such as Tums and Milk of Magnesia can reduce the effectiveness of:
   A. Quinolones
   B. Tetracyclines
   C. Insulin
   D. A and B
14. Ibuprofen can reduce:
   A. Fever
   B. Inflammation
   C. Pain
   D. All of the above
15. An expectorant such as ___ thins mucus.
   A. Guaifenesin
   B. Diphenhydramine
   C. Naphazoline
   D. Cetirizine

Bibliography

Consumer Healthcare Products Association. Available at: http://www.chpa.org.

US Food and Drug Administration. Drug applications for nonprescription drugs. Available at: https://www.fda.gov/drugs/types-applications/drug-application-process-nonprescription-drugs.

US Food and Drug Administration. Now available without a prescription. Available at: https://www.fda.gov/drugs/information-consumers-and-patients-drugs/now-available-without-prescription.

US Food and Drug Administration, Public Health Advisory. Should you give medicine to kids for coughs and colds https://www.fda.gov/consumers/consumer-updates/should-you-give-kids-medicine-coughs-and-colds.

Websites Referenced

Clinical Pharmacology Online. Available at: https://www.clinicalkey.com/pharmacology/.

UpToDate Online. Available at: http://www.uptodate.com.

CHAPTER 30

Complementary and Alternative Medicine

Tony Guerra

OBJECTIVES

OBJECTIVES

1. Define complementary and alternative medicine (CAM) and list the three primary goals of the National Center for Complementary and Integrative Health (NCCIH).
2. Recognize the most common herbal products used in the United States and recognize conditions they are used to treat. In addition, (a) understand potential risks, such as side effects and drug-herbal interactions, that can occur with herbal product use, and (b) write the common and scientific names for the herbal products discussed in this chapter.
3. Recognize other CAM practices, including those pertaining to mind and body medicine and manipulative practices.

TERMS AND DEFINITIONS

Alternative medicine Any range of medical therapies not regarded as orthodox by Western medicine

Ayurveda A holistic traditional medical system originating in India that emphasizes disease prevention

Biofeedback The use of electronic monitoring of an automatic bodily function to train someone to acquire voluntary control of that function

Chiropractic medicine Manual manipulation of the joints and muscles

Complementary medicine A range of medical therapies that fall beyond the scope of Western medicine. They are complementary to traditional medicine

Diagnosis A physician's recognition of a condition or disease based on its outward signs and symptoms and/or confirming tests or procedures

Herb Any plant that is valued for its aromatic, medicinal, flavorful, or other properties

Homeopath A practitioner of homeopathy

Homeopathy A therapeutic belief that dilutions of medicinal substances that cause a specific symptom can treat an illness that yields the same symptoms. The US Food and Drug Administration (FDA) under the Food, Drug, and Cosmetic Act regulates homeopathic medications

Prophylaxis Treatment or measure to prevent disease

Synthetic medicine A medication made in a laboratory from chemical processes

Traditional Chinese medicine Complementary and alternative medicine whole medical system that includes a range of traditional medicine practices originating in China

Select Common Herbal Products

Common Name	Scientific Name	Select Common Uses
Garlic	*Allium sativum*	Hypertension, hypercholesterolemia, antimicrobial
Echinacea	*Echinacea angustifolia, Echinacea pallida, Echinacea purpurea*	Immunostimulant, treatment of common cold and other respiratory infections
Saw palmetto	*Serenoa repens*	Benign prostatic hyperplasia
Ginkgo	*Ginkgo biloba*	Dementia, peripheral vascular disease, intermittent claudication
Soy	*Glycine max*	Hyperlipidemia, menopausal symptoms, osteoporosis prevention, cardiovascular disease prevention
Cranberry	*Vaccinium macrocarpon*	Urinary tract infections
Ginseng	*Panax quinquefolius*	Stimulant, diabetes, digestive aid
Black cohosh	*Actaea racemosa*	Menopausal symptoms, premenstrual syndrome
St. John's wort	*Hypericum perforatum*	Depression, anxiety
Milk thistle	*Silybum marianum*	Antioxidant, toxin-induced liver damage

This chapter presents information on complementary and alternative medicine (CAM), including the origins of various nontraditional therapies from Eastern and Western cultures. Many people use CAM to pursue better health. The 2007 National Health Interview Survey (NHIS) reported that approximately 38% of adults use CAM. Because CAM use is prevalent, it is vital to have a general understanding of these practices. The chapter presents a review of herbal remedies with monographs for 10 select top-selling herbal products and explains common uses and known herb interactions.

What Is Complementary and Alternative Medicine?

Defining CAM is difficult. The field is vast and continually evolving. It is easier to contrast CAM with traditional medicine. Traditional medical treatment often includes prescription medication after physician visits, possibly with radiographic examinations and/or laboratory tests for a proper **diagnosis**. Conventional medicine includes legend (prescription) and over-the-counter (OTC) medications. Follow-up visits ensure treatment success, and regular visits monitor the patient's condition.

The alternative approach may consist of visits to a practitioner of **chiropractic medicine** (chiropractor), a homeopathic physician (**homeopath**), or other practitioners, followed by treatments in those specific areas (Table 30.1). Treatments may include herbs, acupuncture, acupressure, yoga, and tai chi. Many alternative approaches have been around for thousands of years, whereas traditional medicine has a history of only a few hundred years. Nevertheless, conventional medicine is the Western world standard.

CAM, by definition, is complementary and alternative medicine. **Alternative medicine** includes a range of medical therapies not regarded as orthodox by Western medicine that are used in place of conventional medicine. **Complementary medicine** refers to these same alternative therapies along with traditional medicine. Acupressure or acupuncture with prescription pain medication is a complementary strategy for pain.

CAM therapies, including herbal remedies, have high sales, reflecting their extensive use. Because CAM use is prevalent, a division of the National Institutes of Health (NIH) is dedicated to the study of CAM. The National Center for Complementary and Integrative Health (NCCIH) (formerly known as the National Center for Complementary and Alternative Medicine) was formed in the early 1990s with three primary goals: (1) to perform research on alternative treatments, (2) to train individuals interested in learning CAM techniques, and (3) to provide the consumer with information on various CAM therapies. More than half of US medical schools offer classes on CAM, which can include dietary supplement therapy (eg, vitamins and minerals), herbal medicine, acupuncture, and homeopathy.

FDA Regulation of Dietary Supplements

The Dietary Supplement Health and Education Act (DSHEA) of 1994 regulates supplement use. DSHEA requires manufacturers of herbal and dietary supplements to produce a backed statement that an herbal or dietary supplement is "reasonably expected to be safe" before it can be legally marketed. Unlike manufacturers of drug-containing products, manufacturers of herbal or dietary supplements do not need to provide proprietary experimental and effectiveness data as proof of a product's effectiveness. The US Food and Drug Administration (FDA) is responsible for ensuring evidence of safety and effectiveness only for drug-containing products utilizing rigorous clinical trials and safety analyses. Nevertheless, herbal and dietary supplements are still subject to FDA labeling standards. Mislabeling herbal or dietary supplements breaches adulteration regulations. When a product is mislabeled or adulterated, whether OTC medication, herbal remedy product, or dietary supplement, the FDA can remove the product from the shelves and ban its sale.

Regarding patient safety data, all manufacturers are responsible for investigating and reporting serious adverse events to the FDA. Adverse events associated with dietary supplements can be reported to the FDA's Safety Reporting

TABLE 30.1
Select Examples of Complementary and Alternative Medicine Treatments

Type of Treatment	Description
Acupressure	Acupressure is based on the same principles as acupuncture. Instead of using needles to unblock pathways carrying energy, the practitioner uses his or her hands to apply pressure to specific points on the body.
Acupuncture	Acupuncture is based on the meridians in the body. These lines are thought to carry energy to particular parts of the body. When they become blocked, illness or pain can occur. The practitioner relieves blocked pathways with the use of needles.
Aromatherapy	Through the sense of smell, various blends of fragrances result in relief of certain ailments. Aromatic herbs, perfumes, and oils are frequently used.
Ayurveda	Ayurveda is based on the spiritual side of the body and all that affects the body, including the environment, emotional stability, and physical health. Practitioners find ways to change what is necessary to enable the patient to be more in tune with the outside world. This mode includes various postures, meditation, and massage. Changing habits is a large part of this treatment.
Biofeedback	Biofeedback is a learned technique that enables the self-control of various physiological responses of the body. This technique includes voluntary systems and involuntary systems of the body. A practitioner teaches it only until the patient is proficient in using the technique on his or her own.
Chiropractic medicine	Chiropractic treatment is based on the belief that the realignment of the body, specifically the spine, can remedy certain conditions. Periodic adjustments usually are required to align the spine and various joints throughout the body. In this way, pressure or pain is relieved.
Herbal remedies	The medicinal purposes of herbs have been learned through historical literature and by word of mouth. Herbal therapies are available for the treatment of a variety of ailments and are frequently sold in pharmacies and health food stores. Physicians and other health care providers often recommend herbal therapies; herbals are a common component of complementary medicine.
Homeopathy	Homeopathy is the traditional belief that "like cures like." Various types of toxins are mixed in extreme dilutions to the point at which they are often undetectable by scientific means. This minute amount of "toxin" from which the patient is suffering allows the patient's body to fight the illness.
Traditional Chinese medicine	Chinese medicine is based on the body spirits of the yin and yang, which are acknowledged as having similar elements yet are different in order. Therefore each is treated differently. Diagnosis is based on the person's dreams, tastes, sensations, smell, and other senses. Various types of treatments are used, including herbal remedies and acupuncture.

Portal. Once the product is deemed unsafe, the FDA has the authority to remove the product from the market. Before using dietary supplements or herbal products, consumers should be aware of a product's active and inactive ingredients to discuss their concerns with their doctor, pharmacist, or other health care professional.

The FDA requires the manufacture of a dietary supplement to include the following information on the label:
1. Product name
2. A clear statement that it is a "dietary supplement"
3. Name and place of the manufacturer
4. Supplement Facts (including serving size, number of servings per container, dietary ingredients, and the amount of dietary ingredients per serving)
5. Net quantity of contents
6. A domestic address or phone number for patients to report adverse events to the manufacturer

Marketing a dietary supplement with claims to treat or cure a disease is illegal. For example, it is unlawful for a manufacturer of an herbal product to claim that it is a cure for bone cancer. Instead, health claims of dietary supplements or herbal products must be limited to generalized claims and supplemented by the statement that the product is "not intended to treat, cure, or prevent any disease."

When manufacturers of dietary and herbal supplements make structure/function claims (claims that demonstrate how a product affects or maintains typical body structure or function), the label must also include a statement claiming that the FDA has not evaluated the claim or product for validity or safety.

Medical Food

Medical foods are neither medication nor supplements. They are specially formulated compounds that patients with specific nutritional needs use. Per the FDA, medical food is a food that is:
Administered enterally
Taken under the supervision of a physician, although not all require a prescription

Intended to treat a condition or disease with distinctive nutritional requirements

The FDA does not regulate medical foods the same way as drugs; instead, the regulation is like that for food and subject to following requirements for food labeling. However, a medical food with a false or misleading claim is subject to removal by the FDA based on misbranding. Like dietary supplements, the FDA does not maintain an updated list of medical foods. The FDA mandates that all ingredients added to medical food be proven to be safe. Common medical foods include Lofenalac (infant powder formula), Ketonex-2 (amino acid–modified medical food), and GlutarAde (lysine-free powdered formula).

Tech Note!

When performing medication reconciliation, ask the patient about past or current use of over-the-counter medications, dietary supplements, and medical food. Dietary supplements and herbal remedies are easy to overlook when gathering patient information, and patients often need to be made aware of the need to report the use of these products. There is always a risk for drug-dietary interactions, drug-drug interactions, or other potential adverse reactions associated with OTC or supplement use. You may also encounter patients who prefer to self-treat a condition using OTC products rather than prescription drugs. These patients may be more likely to have relevant information missing from an electronic health record, such as past medication history or diagnosis. Therefore it is best to use open-ended questions that allow patients to share such information openly.

Types of Complementary and Alternative Medicine

CAM is continuously changing and adapting; as a result, many types of CAM have become available. The NCCAM website is a great resource for researching these therapies. This chapter briefly reviews the more common CAM practices, but it is not a comprehensive review. Although there are no formal CAM categories, many resources, including NCCAM, group CAM practices into broad categories. In this chapter we discuss CAM practices that fall in the general categories of natural products, mind and body medicine, and manipulative practices. Although these categories are not formally defined (and some CAM practices may fit into more than one category), they help in discussions about the various types of CAM.

Natural Products

Natural products constitute a broad category of CAM that includes the use of **herbs** (herbal remedies), vitamins, minerals, and other natural products, such as probiotics. By this definition, vitamin use is considered CAM, but daily multivitamins are not usually considered CAM. Herbal products are the most common forms of CAM. According to the 2007 NHIS, nearly 18% of US adults take a nonvitamin and

nonmineral natural product. Accordingly, this section focuses on herbal remedies and 10 common herbal products.

Tech Note!

Herbal medicines account for some of the first attempts to improve human health. The mummified prehistoric "iceman" discovered in the Italian Alps in 1991 had medicinal herbs with him.

Herbal Products

Although herbal remedies have existed for thousands of years, herbal therapies have gained increasing popularity. The herbal remedy market continues to grow with an aging population and the rising cost of traditional health care. Because pharmacies sell many herbals products, technicians should familiarize themselves with the most popular ones (Table 30.2). Many people do not report herbal use to health care providers. Some patients think that because herbal products are "natural," they are not harmful. However, dangerous interactions exist between natural products, legend drugs, and OTC medications (Table 30.3).

Many traditional medicines came from plant sources. Chemicals that have undergone efficacy and safety testing for certain medical conditions or ailments are often manufactured as **synthetic medicines**. For this reason, most Western medicine discovered from plants does not incorporate the whole or even part of the plant. Although herbs and herbal supplements are subjected to regulations enforced by the FDA, they are not regulated in the same way as drugs because they are considered dietary supplements. (See Chapter 29 for a discussion of OTC and dietary supplement regulation.)

Because many cultures have used herbs for thousands of years, they may have different names. For example, *Echinacea* is also known as black sampson, sampson root, narrow-leafed purple coneflower, and red sunflower. An herb's family name is essential in case of unwanted interactions. For instance, if someone is allergic to an herb, then an herb from the same family may cause an allergic response. Species can vary even if they are closely related. Studies may have focused only on one species used to prepare the supplement. Several herbal textbooks help one determine the herb's family. Another excellent reference for herbal product information is the Natural Medicines Comprehensive Database.

Garlic Oral garlic (Fig. 30.1) has antihyperlipidemic, antihypertensive, and antifungal effects. However, the evidence supporting garlic for the conditions varies. Garlic is considered safe when used orally at appropriate doses. It was used safely in clinical studies lasting up to 7 years without reports of significant toxicity.

Scientific name. *Allium sativum*

Also known as. Ail, ajo, Da Suan, Lasuna, Rason, stinking rose

Possibly effective to treat. Atherosclerosis, hyperlipidemia, hypertension, ringworm (garlic gel), athlete's foot (garlic gel), jock itch (garlic gel), reduce the number of tick bites

TABLE 30.2
Common Uses and Cautionary Notes for Select Herbal Products

Herb	Scientific Name	Uses	Cautions
Black cohosh	Cimicifuga racemosa[a]	Menopause, premenstrual syndrome	• Should not be used if pregnant • May cause liver toxicity
Chamomile	Matricaria recutita[a]	Gastrointestinal upset, skin conditions	• Should not be used if pregnant • Safe if used in small quantities and short term
Garlic	Allium sativum	Antihypertensive, antihyperlipidemic	• Safe if used in small quantities
Ginkgo	Ginkgo biloba	Increases circulation	• Should not be used if pregnant
Ginseng	Panax quinquefolius	Antidiabetic, estrogenic effects, improve memory	• Safe if used in small quantities
Milk thistle	Silybum marianum	Dyspepsia	• Studies are not complete because of the many different species and parts of herbaceous plant used
St. John's wort	Hypericum perforatum	Antidepressant	• Safe if used in small quantities

[a]Various species are used; some side effects may differ, depending on the species.

TABLE 30.3
Select Examples of Herb-Drug Interactions

Herb	Drug	Potential Interaction
Black cohosh	Cisplatin	May decrease cytotoxic effect on breast cancer
Echinacea	Caffeine	May increase caffeine levels by 30%
	Tacrolimus	May decrease effects of tacrolimus
Garlic	Isoniazid	May decrease isoniazid levels by 65%
	Nimodipine	May increase antihypertensive effect
	Quinapril	May increase antihypertensive effect
	Reserpine	May increase antihypertensive effect
	Warfarin	May increase risk for bleeding
Ginkgo biloba	NSAIDs	May increase risk for bleeding
	Chlorothiazide	May increase blood pressure
	Clopidogrel	May increase risk for bleeding
	Atorvastatin	May decrease effectiveness of atorvastatin
	Carbamazepine	May decrease seizure threshold
	Warfarin	May increase risk for bleeding
Ginseng	Glimepiride	May increase risk for hypoglycemia
	Cyclosporine	May decrease effectiveness of cyclosporine
	Phenelzine	May cause insomnia, headache, and tremors
	Warfarin	May decrease effectiveness of warfarin
St. John's wort	Alprazolam	May decrease effect of alprazolam
	Clopidogrel	May increase risk for bleeding
	Contraception	May decrease contraceptive effectiveness
	Dapsone	May decrease dapsone blood concentration
	Desipramine	May increase desipramine's pharmacological effects and risk for toxicity
	Digoxin	May reduce effectiveness of digoxin
	Estrogen, esterified	May decrease levels of esterified estrogens
	Fluoxetine	May increase fluoxetine's pharmacological effects and risk of toxicity

◼ TABLE 30.3
Select Examples of Herb-Drug Interactions—cont'd

Herb	Drug	Potential Interaction
	Ketamine	May decrease serum levels of ketamine
	Lamivudine and many antiviral drugs for HIV	May decrease blood concentration and effectiveness in treating HIV
	Methocarbamol	May increase CNS depression
	Oxytetracycline	May increase risk for photosensitivity
	Paroxetine	May increase paroxetine's pharmacological effects and risk for toxicity
	Piroxicam	May increase risk for phototoxicity
	Quinine	May decrease quinine levels
	Reserpine	May increase CNS depression
	Sulfisoxazole	May cause photosensitization
	Theophylline	May decrease metabolism of theophylline
	Venlafaxine	May increase sedative effect of venlafaxine
	Warfarin	May decrease the effects of warfarin

CNS, Central nervous system; *HIV*, human immunodeficiency virus; *NSAID*, nonsteroidal antiinflammatory drug.

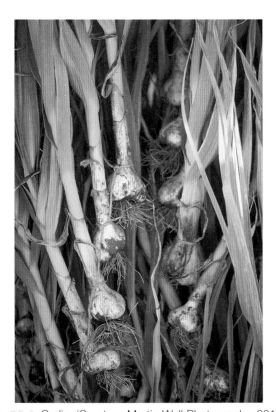

FIG. 30.1 Garlic. (Courtesy Martin Wall Photography, 2011.)

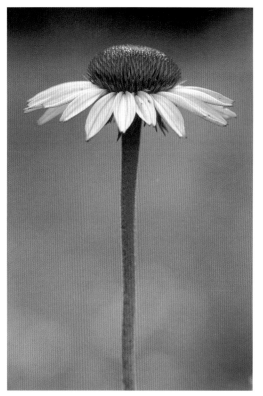

FIG. 30.2 Purple coneflower. (Courtesy Martin Wall Photography, 2011.)

Potential side effects. Gastrointestinal (GI) irritation, heartburn, flatulence, nausea, vomiting, breath and body odor

Echinacea *Echinacea*, often also referred to as purple coneflower (Fig. 30.2), is used orally for treating and preventing the common cold and other upper respiratory tract conditions. *Echinacea* is characterized as an immunostimulant. This herb is considered safe when used orally at appropriate doses in the short term. Although studies lasting

up to 6 months have demonstrated safety with several formulations of *Echinacea*, safety data for long-term use are lacking.

Scientific names. *Echinacea angustifolia*, *Echinacea pallida*, *Echinacea purpurea*

Also known as. Purple coneflower, American coneflower, comb flower, red sunflower, snakeroot

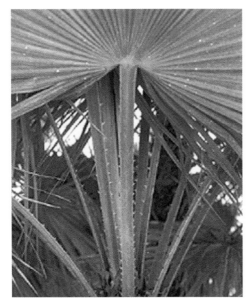

FIG. 30.3 Saw palmetto. (From Freeman LW. *Mosby's Complementary and Alternative Medicine: A Research-Based Approach.* 3rd ed. St. Louis: Mosby; 2009.)

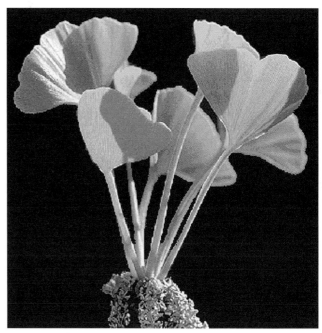

FIG. 30.4 *Ginkgo biloba.* (From Freeman LW. *Mosby's Complementary and Alternative Medicine: A Research-Based Approach.* 3rd ed. St. Louis: Mosby; 2009.)

Possibly effective to treat. Common cold

Potential side effects. Nausea, diarrhea, heartburn, headache, dizziness

Saw palmetto Saw palmetto (Fig. 30.3) is widely used as an herbal treatment for benign prostatic hyperplasia (BPH) but is also used orally as a mild diuretic, sedative, antiseptic, and antiinflammatory agent. The ripe fruit of the plant is used medicinally. Saw palmetto has been used safely in clinical studies lasting up to 3 years, but it is considered unsafe to use during pregnancy because of its hormonal activity.

Scientific names. *Serenoa repens, Serenoa serrulata, Sabal serrulata*

Also known as. American dwarf palm tree, cabbage palm, Ju-Zhong, Sabal, Sabal fructus, saw palmetto berry

Possibly effective to treat. Transurethral resection of the prostate

Potential side effects. Dizziness, headache, nausea, constipation, diarrhea

Ginkgo biloba *Ginkgo biloba*, also known as ginkgo, is widely used for conditions of memory, such as Alzheimer disease and vascular dementia (Fig. 30.4). The applicable parts of ginkgo are the leaf and the seed; an extract made from the ginkgo leaf is the most commonly used form. Standardized extracts have been used safely in clinical trials lasting several weeks to 6 years.

Scientific name. *Ginkgo biloba*

Also known as. Fossil tree, ginkgo folium, Japanese silver apricot, kew tree, maidenhair tree, Yinhsing

Possibly effective to treat. Anxiety, cognitive function, dementia, diabetic retinopathy, glaucoma, peripheral vascular disease, premenstrual syndrome, schizophrenia, tardive dyskinesia, vertigo

Potential side effects. Headache, dizziness, palpitations, constipation, rash

Soy Soy is widely used as a milk substitute in food products for individuals with lactose intolerance and in infant feeding formulas. As an oral herbal product, soy is used for many conditions, from high cholesterol to cardiovascular disease prevention. Soy products in doses up to 60 g/day have been safely used in studies lasting up to 16 weeks.

Scientific name. *Glycine max*

Also known as. Isoflavones, isolated soy protein, plant estrogen, soybean, soy isoflavone, soy fiber, soy protein isolate, texturized vegetable protein

Possibly effective to treat. Diabetes, diarrhea, galactosemia, hyperlipidemia, kidney disease, lactose intolerance, menopausal symptoms, osteoporosis

Potential side effects. Constipation, diarrhea, bloating, nausea

Cranberry The cranberry fruit (Fig. 30.5) is most widely used for the treatment and/or prevention of urinary tract infections (UTIs). Patients can drink a cranberry juice product (eg, Ocean Spray cranberry juice cocktail) or take as cranberry capsules. Cranberry is considered quite safe.

Scientific name. *Vaccinium macrocarpon*

Also known as. Agrio, craneberry, Da Guo Yue Jie, Tsuru-Kokemomo

Possibly effective to treat. UTIs

Potential side effects. GI upset and diarrhea with substantial doses (3–4 L of juice per day)

Ginseng (American) Ginseng root is used for a variety of conditions, such as diabetes, respiratory tract infections, and attention-deficit/hyperactivity disorder (ADHD). Also, ginseng often is used for overall wellness and as an antiinflammatory agent. American ginseng 100 to 3000 mg has been safely used for up to 12 weeks but should not be used in pregnancy.

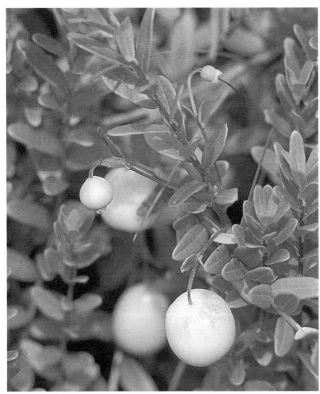

FIG. 30.5 Cranberry. (From Freeman LW. *Mosby's Complementary and Alternative Medicine: A Research-Based Approach*. 3rd ed. St. Louis: Mosby; 2009.)

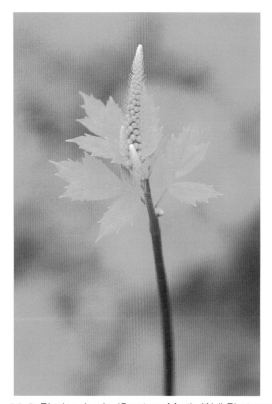

FIG. 30.6 Black cohosh. (Courtesy Martin Wall Photography, 2011.)

Scientific name. *Panax quinquefolius*

Also known as. Red berry, Ren Shen, Sang, Shang, Shi Yang Seng, Xi Yang Shen

Possibly effective to treat. Diabetes, respiratory tract infections

Potential side effects. Headache, insomnia, GI discomfort

Black cohosh Black cohosh (Fig. 30.6) is primarily for hot flashes associated with menopause. Although short-term studies lasting up to a year have concluded that black cohosh is safe, some studies have shown that liver toxicity may occur. Therefore a cautionary statement must be included on the label of this agent. Black cohosh must not be confused with herbs with similar-sounding names, such as blue and white cohosh. These are not used for the same purpose and have different interactions with other medications.

Scientific name. *Actaea racemosa*

Also known as. Black snakeroot, bugbane, bugwort, cohosh negro, phytoestrogen, rattle root, rattle weed, Sheng Ma, squaw root

Possibly effective to treat. Menopausal symptoms

Potential side effects. GI upset, rash, headache, dizziness, weight gain, breast tenderness

St. John's wort St. John's wort (Fig. 30.7) is frequently used for neuropsychiatric conditions such as depression and anxiety. The parts of the plant that are used are the flowers and leaves. Interestingly, several active constituents have been isolated from St. John's wort, including melatonin. Scientists think St. John's wort has serotonergic effects, which may account for its beneficial effects for depression

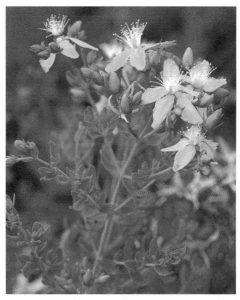

FIG. 30.7 St. John's wort. (From Freeman LW. *Mosby's Complementary and Alternative Medicine: A Research-Based Approach*. 3rd ed. St. Louis: Mosby; 2009.)

and anxiety. St. John's wort extract is safe when used appropriately for up to 12 weeks.

Scientific name. *Hypericum perforatum*

Also known as. Goatweed, hard hay, *Hypericum*, Klamath weed, Saynt Johannes wort, Tipton weed

Likely effective to treat. Depression

Possibly effective to treat. Menopausal symptoms, wound healing

Potential side effects. Insomnia, vivid dreams, restlessness, GI discomfort, dizziness, headache

Milk thistle The milk thistle seed is the most commonly used part of the plant. One of the most common reasons people take milk thistle is for toxic liver damage caused by chemicals. It also has been used intravenously for the treatment of mushroom poisoning. Preliminary clinical research suggests that milk thistle may be beneficial in improving liver function in people with alcoholic liver disease; however, this has yet to be proven.

Scientific name. *Silybum marianum*

Also known as. Holy thistle, lady's thistle, Marian thistle, silibinin, *Silybum*, silymarin, St. Mary thistle

Possibly effective to treat. Diabetes, dyspepsia

Potential side effects. Diarrhea, nausea, flatulence, bloating, anorexia

Herbal Preparations

How companies prepare herbs determines the active ingredient strength. Herbs brewed for teas are usually more potent than a capsule form. Providers and patients can prepare teas in different ways. Pouring hot water on herbs and letting them steep for several minutes is an *infusion*. Simmering herbs in water for 15 to 20 minutes creates a decoction. Allowing herbs to soak in cold water over many hours is a *cold infusion*. The various methods depend on the herb type (Table 30.4). Some medical schools include herbal remedies and their preparation in courses because of their prevalence and possible benefits to complement traditional medicine.

> **Tech Note!**
>
> As alternative therapy popularity increases, the medical community must stay up to date. Increased herbal use may have a significant impact on medication interactions because of their effect on prescribed or over-the-counter drugs. The pharmacy technician should know the most common interactions between herbal remedies and legend drugs. In this way, the technician can help the pharmacist identify patients who may want or need counseling.

Mind and Body Medicine

Mind and body CAM practices are based on the interactions among the brain, mind, body, and behavior. The intent of these CAM practices is to use the power of the mind to affect physical function and health positively. A variety of forms of CAM fall into this category; specific information on meditation, yoga, acupuncture, and acupressure is presented in the following sections.

> **Tech Note!**
>
> Hippocrates, referred to as the father of Western medicine, noted the moral and spiritual aspects of healing. He thought that attitude, environmental factors, and natural remedies were all integral components of medical treatment.

Meditation

Meditation is a popular mind-body form of CAM that has many variations. Most meditation forms began in ancient religious and spiritual traditions. To practice meditation, individuals learn to focus attention on achieving greater calmness, psychological balance, and physical relaxation.

Yoga

Yoga is a form of mind-body practice that originated in ancient Indian philosophy (Fig. 30.8). Yoga can maintain physical health and flexibility, and it incorporates elements of physical posturing, breathing techniques, and meditation. The 2007 NHIS identified yoga as one of the top 10 complementary health practices used by adults in the United States; approximately 6% of respondents reported using yoga for health purposes in the previous 12 months. Hatha yoga is the most commonly practiced form of yoga in the United States and Europe. Hatha yoga incorporates the use of postures *(asanas)* and breathing exercises *(pranayama)*. Because yoga helps maintain flexibility, posture, and balance, older adults use it for aging-associated conditions.

◾ TABLE 30.4
Examples of Various Herbal Preparations

Dosage Form	Route of Administration	Ingredients	Use, Strength, Onset of Action
Syrups, diluted; tinctures	Internal	Alcohol, glycerin	Usually a potent form
Tablets, capsules	Internal	Powdered	Slower to act; broken down in the stomach
Teas	Internal	Syrups, sweeteners	May be better tasting with sweeteners added; teas may be stronger than tablets or capsules
Aromatic solutions, baths	External	Scented water	Used to treat skin conditions and burns
Oils	External	Extracted oil from herbs	Used for sore muscles and skin conditions
Compresses, salves	External	Compresses made from teas, salves from herbal oils	For compresses, a cloth soaked in herbal tea is applied to skin site; used for conditions such as bruises and cramps

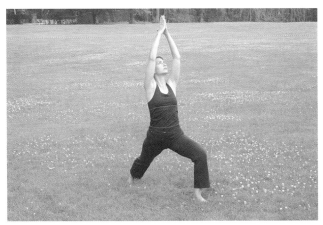

FIG. 30.8 Standing pose for alignment and balance. (From Deutsch JE, Anderson EZ. *Complementary Therapies for Physical Therapy: A Clinical Decision-Making Approach*. Philadelphia: Saunders; 2008.)

Acupuncture

Acupuncture has been used for thousands of years. Extensive studies have been done in the Eastern and Western worlds. Acupuncture is a complementary treatment for conditions such as chronic pain, depression, and addiction. It is based on the Chinese belief that the body contains energy channels. When the energy channels are blocked, sickness may result. Needles inserted at specific points throughout the body are thought to release channels, bringing the body into harmony (Fig. 30.9).

Acupressure

Acupressure is closely related to acupuncture because it also uses specific energy points across the body. Instead of using needles, practitioners apply pressure to a specific point to unblock channels (Fig. 30.10). Insurance companies are beginning to pay for acupuncture and acupressure treatment if a physician recommends it for pain. Acupressure classes are available in which a person can learn to perform the technique on himself or herself.

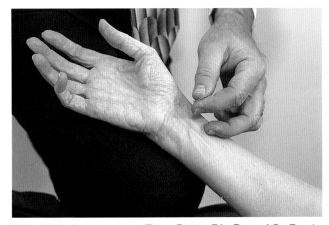

FIG. 30.9 Acupuncture. (From Potter PA, Perry AG. *Fundamentals of Nursing*. 8th ed. St. Louis: Mosby; 2013.)

Manipulative and Body-Based Practices

Manipulative and body-based CAM practices focus on alignment and proper functioning of various structures and body systems. Structures and systems that may be the focus of these forms of CAM are the bones and joints, soft tissue, circulatory system, and lymphatic system. The two most common types of CAM in this category include spinal manipulation and massage therapy.

■ Tech Note!

Spinal manipulation dates back to the ancient Greeks. Massage therapy dates back thousands of years and is referenced in ancient writings from China, Japan, India, Egypt, Greece, and Rome.

Spinal Manipulation

Chiropractic therapy is an orthopedic approach to treating pain resulting from misalignment of bones and joints. Chiropractors think that skeletal structure changes interfere with the nervous system and other organ systems. The treatment is *manipulation*. Treatment can include hands-on adjustments of the spine or joints and the application of massage and heat therapy. Research has proved that some forms of manipulation can be helpful, specifically manipulation of the lower back. Although chiropractic therapy use is increasing, various treatment forms are controversial. Some physicians promote the use of manipulation of certain parts of the skeletal structure, whereas other doctors think it may be harmful. Skepticism about the ability of manipulation to treat many common illnesses abounds, and studies will determine exactly which therapy works and why it is effective. Practitioners must attend an accredited school to attain the degree Doctor of Chiropractic (DC). Many insurance companies cover chiropractic treatment.

Massage Therapy

Massage therapy encompasses many different techniques. It generally involves the use of the hands and fingers, but practitioners may use their forearms, elbows, or feet (Fig. 30.11). Massage can manipulate muscles and soft body tissues. It is used for many health-related purposes such as to relieve pain, rehabilitate physical injuries, induce relaxation, and reduce anxiety and stress. As with spinal manipulation, insurance plans may cover massage therapy, particularly for musculoskeletal conditions, with a proper medical referral.

Other Complementary and Alternative Medicine Practices

In addition to the small sample of CAM practices briefly described in this chapter, a multitude of CAM therapies are available. Whole medical systems, which are complete systems of medical theory and practice, such as **traditional Chinese medicine** and **Ayurveda**, are also considered CAM. Traditional Chinese medicine has been a well-known art based on more than 4000 years of trial and error. Although herbal remedies might come to mind readily when

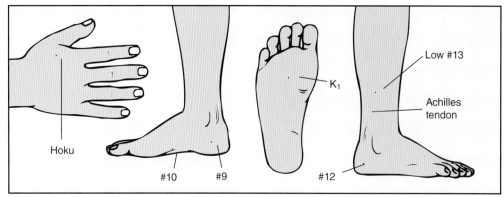

FIG. 30.10 Acupressure points. (From Potter PA, Perry AG. *Fundamentals of Nursing*. 8th ed. St. Louis: Mosby; 2013.)

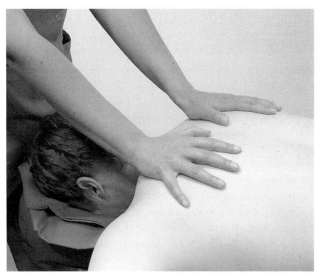

FIG. 30.11 Massage is most typically delivered with the hands, although the forearms, elbows, or feet also may be used. (From Freeman LW. *Mosby's Complementary and Alternative Medicine: A Research-Based Approach*. 3rd ed. St. Louis: Mosby; 2009.)

the topic of Chinese medicine is discussed, it involves much more than the use of herbs. The heart of Chinese practice is yin and yang, which represent male and female entities, respectively. The ancient Chinese belief contends that although men and women are made of the same substances, their spirits are different; therefore appropriate treatment is different. Practitioners conduct examinations by asking the patient about dreams, strange tastes, or smells experienced. Also, a visual examination of the skin and voice tone is performed. After the diagnosis is complete, the practitioner may prescribe the necessary treatment, which could include a variety of herbs, minerals, and/or vegetables. Herbs and other remedies are used in Chinese medicine to cure the body of the original illness and for disease **prophylaxis**. Chinese medicine is currently still in use; many health care providers, including pharmacists, take classes based on Chinese knowledge of herbs and their medicinal uses.

Ayurveda is an ancient Indian approach to medicine that is currently still practiced. Dating back thousands of years, Ayurveda is based on the person knowing and understanding the spiritual self. This knowledge encompasses the body and all that affects it. With insight into the various effects of outside influences on the body's spirit, it is possible to make assumptions. A person can predict whether something will have a positive effect or a negative effect on the body. For example, certain colors, sounds, clothing, and other environmental stimuli are taken into consideration. The types of foods and herbs patients consume also play a role in overall health. These assumptions are then applied to physical and spiritual activities. Based on the individual's personality type, practitioners suggest ways to alter the diet and/or lifestyle to cure and prevent illnesses. This treatment is currently practiced in many parts of the world. Medical schools teaching this approach are in India. Courses in Indian medicine are also offered in various medical schools in the United States.

Biofeedback is another form of CAM that is used for stress, hypertension, and other conditions. Biofeedback uses the patient's mental ability to alter his or her vital signs, such as blood pressure, heart rate, and even GI activity. The body has two movement types, voluntary and involuntary. Voluntary movements include the musculoskeletal system and involve purposeful actions such as walking, sitting, standing, and bending. People have control over these functions daily; therefore adjusting behavior does not take much conscious effort. With biofeedback, a person is taught how to mentally access and alter involuntary body functions such as heartbeat, breathing, and digestion. These functions do not normally require conscious thought. Biofeedback usually is taught by an instructor who uses electrical leads that provide a readout of data. Patients are connected to monitors that allow them to see what their bodies are experiencing (Fig. 30.12). For example, the instructor might have the patient alter the heart rate to a certain level through concentration. Gradually, the person is able to adjust body functions as needed without the monitor. Biofeedback connects the mind to the body. Patients need to practice these techniques frequently to achieve full benefit. Biofeedback can be used as an alternative to or in addition to medication for conditions such as anxiety, low back pain, neuromuscular dysfunction, and tension headaches. Biofeedback therapy is partially reimbursed by many insurance companies, with a physician's approval. After the technique of biofeedback has been perfected, it can be done at any time without supervision.

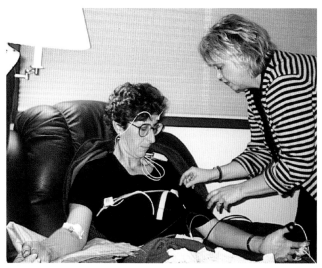

FIG. 30.12 Example of electrode placement for biofeedback. (From Potter PA, Perry AG. *Fundamentals of Nursing*. 8th ed. St. Louis: Mosby; 2013.)

The term *homeopathy*, translated from Greek, simply means "like suffering." The premise of **homeopathy** is the belief that "like cures like." Homeopathy is also sometimes referred to as the law of similars. The idea is that consuming a small amount of the substance that caused a person's disease or condition enables the body to fight the disease. Homeopathy became well known in the late 1700s through the efforts of Samuel Hahnemann, a German physician. After ingesting a small amount of quinine, he exhibited symptoms of malaria, the disease that quinine cured. Over time he perfected the necessary minute amount of quinine that was needed to instigate a cure rather than illness. Homeopathy was first used in the United States in the 1800s and became a popular treatment. Although homeopathy has remained a well-accepted form of treatment in parts of Europe, it is generally considered an alternative treatment in the United States.

Thousands of homeopathic remedies are available, but only one remedy is correct for each illness; therefore homeopathic physicians must know what will work for the patient. Unlike with herbs and other alternative treatments, the FDA oversees the manufacture of homeopathic drugs. Under FDA guidelines, a homeopathic drug must meet standards for strength, quality, purity, and other parameters established in the *Homeopathic Pharmacopeia*, which contains monographs on ingredients used in homeopathic medicine. All homeopathic agents must be manufactured using good manufacturing practices (GMPs). In addition, if the homeopathic drug is a prescription, it must contain the same label as that indicated for prescription drugs. If it is sold over the counter, the agent must comply with the general labeling provisions for OTC products (eg, indications for use, warnings, and directions for use). Although more medical schools are offering classes on homeopathic medicine, it is still somewhat controversial in the traditional medical community.

Do You Remember These Key Points?

- The definition of complementary and alternative medicine (CAM) and examples of CAM therapies currently in use
- The most common herbal products used in the United States and the conditions they are most commonly used to treat
- The potential risks of herbal use
- The common and scientific names for the herbal products discussed in this chapter

Review Questions

Multiple Choice Questions

1. Homeopathy is known as the law of similars, which can be best described as:
   A. Taking a similar drug that works but at a much-reduced cost
   B. Taking a drug that is similar to legend drugs but does not require a prescription
   C. Taking a drug that causes the same illness as the one you are trying to cure
   D. Taking a drug that causes a reaction similar to that of traditional agents

2. *Silybum marianum* is known commonly as _____ and is used most commonly to treat _____.
   A. Ginger, motion sickness
   B. St. John's wort, depression
   C. Milk thistle, liver conditions
   D. Garlic, infections

3. Which herbal product is commonly used to treat depression?
   A. *Echinacea*
   B. *Ginkgo biloba*
   C. St. John's wort
   D. Milk thistle

4. Which herbal product is used to treat menopausal symptoms?
   A. Saw palmetto
   B. *Ginkgo biloba*
   C. St. John's wort
   D. Black cohosh

5. Which herbal product is used to treat conditions associated with impaired memory?
   A. Saw palmetto
   B. *Ginkgo biloba*
   C. Soy
   D. Black cohosh

6. Which herbal product is commonly used to treat the symptoms of benign prostatic hyperplasia?
   A. Saw palmetto
   B. *Ginkgo biloba*
   C. Soy
   D. Milk thistle

7. Which herbal product is commonly taken to help treat and prevent urinary tract infections?
   A. *Ginkgo biloba*
   B. St. John's wort

C. Cranberry

D. Garlic

8. Which herbal product is commonly used as an immunostimulant to prevent the common cold?

    A. Echinacea

    B. *Ginkgo biloba*

    C. Black cohosh

    D. Milk thistle

9. _____ is closely related to acupuncture but uses pressure instead of needles to unblock energy channels.

    A. Massage therapy

    B. Acupressure

    C. Biofeedback

    D. Yoga

10. The one drug classification that has unwanted interactions with many herbal drugs is:

    A. Antiulcer agents

    B. Anticoagulants

    C. Vitamins

    D. Analgesics

■ Technician's Corner

Using an appropriate drug/herbal medication reference, research the typical uses, preparations, and potential side effects of the following herbal products not specifically discussed in this chapter:

- Melatonin
- Valerian
- Kava kava

Bibliography

Deutsch JE, Anderson EZ. *Complementary Therapies for Physical Therapy: A Clinical Decision-Making Approach*. Philadelphia: Saunders; 2008.

Freeman LW. *Mosby's Complementary and Alternative Medicine: A Research-Based Approach*. 3rd ed. St. Louis: Mosby; 2009.

National Institutes of Health. National Center for Complementary and Integrative Health (NCCAM). National Institutes of Health. Available at: https://www.nccih.nih.gov/.

Natural Medicines Comprehensive Database. Available at: https://naturalmedicines.therapeuticresearch.com/.

Potter P, Perry A. *Fundamentals of Nursing*. 8th ed. St. Louis: Mosby; 2013.

Skidmore L. *Mosby's Handbook of Herbs and Natural Supplements*. 4th ed. Philadelphia: Elsevier; 2010.

Websites Referenced

Clinical Pharmacology Online. Available at: https://www.clinicalkey.com/pharmacology/.

UpToDate Online. Available at: http://www.uptodate.com.

Top 200 Prescription Drugs

	Brand Name	Generic Name	Drug Classification[a]	Indication or Use
1	Abilify	aripiprazole	Antipsychotic	Schizophrenia
2	Accupril	quinapril	ACE inhibitor	Hypertension
3	Actonel	risedronate	Bone strengthener	Osteoporosis
4	Actos	pioglitazone hydrochloride	Thiazolidinedione	Type 2 diabetes mellitus
5	Adderall XR	amphetamine/ dextroamphetamine	CNS stimulant	ADHD
6	Adipex	phentermine	CNS stimulant	Obesity
7	Advair Diskus	fluticasone propionate/ salmeterol xinafoate	Beta-2 agonist/corticosteroid	Asthma, COPD
8	Aldactone	spironolactone	Potassium-sparing diuretic	Hypertension, edema, hypokalemia
9	Altace	ramipril	ACE inhibitor	Hypertension
10	Amaryl	glimepiride	Sulfonylurea	Type 2 diabetes mellitus
11	Ambien	zolpidem tartrate	Gamma-aminobutyric acid agonist	Insomnia
12	Amoxil	amoxicillin	Penicillin antibiotic	Bacterial infection
13	Androgel	testosterone topical	Androgen	Hypogonadism
14	Antivert	meclizine	H1 antagonist	Antivertigo
15	Apresoline	hydralazine hydrochloride	Vasodilator	Hypertension
16	Aricept	donepezil hydrochloride	Acetylcholinesterase inhibitor	Alzheimer disease
17	Armour Thyroid	thyroid	Thyroid hormone	Hypothyroidism
18	Aspir-Low, Ecotrin	aspirin	NSAID	Analgesic, stroke prevention
19	Ativan	lorazepam	Benzodiazepine	Anxiety
20	Augmentin	amoxicillin/clavulanate potassium	Penicillin/beta-lactamase combination antibiotic	Bacterial infection
21	Avelox	moxifloxacin	Antibiotic	Bacterial infections
22	Avodart	dutasteride	5-Alpha-reductase inhibitor	Reduces enlarged prostate (BPH)
23	Bactrim or Septra	sulfamethoxazole/trimethoprim	Sulfa antibiotic	Bacterial infection
24	Bactroban	mupirocin	Antibiotic	Topical infections
25	Benadryl	diphenhydramine hydrochloride	H_1 antagonist	Allergies
26	Benicar	olmesartan medoxomil	ARB	Hypertension
27	Buspar	buspirone hydrochloride	$5\text{-}HT_{1a}$ receptor partial antagonist	Anxiety
28	Bystolic	nebivolol hydrochloride	Beta-blocker	Hypertension
29	Calan	verapamil hydrochloride	Nondihydropyridine CCB	Hypertension
30	Calcium	calcium	Vitamin	Calcium deficiency
31	Cardizem	diltiazem hydrochloride	Nondihydropyridine CCB	Hypertension

Continued

Drugs by Brand, Generic, Classification, Indication—cont'd

	Brand Name	Generic Name	Drug Classification[a]	Indication or Use
32	Cardura	doxazosin mesylate	Alpha-1 blocker	Hypertension
33	Catapres-TTS	clonidine	Alpha-agonist	Hypertension
34	Celebrex	celecoxib	NSAID, COX-2 inhibitor	Inflammation
35	Celexa	citalopram	SSRI	Depression
36	Cipro	ciprofloxacin	Quinolone antibiotic	Bacterial infection
37	Claritin	loratadine	H_1 antagonist	Allergies
38	Cleocin	clindamycin	Lincosamide antibiotic	Bacterial infection
39	Cogentin	benztropine mesylate	Anti-Parkinson	Parkinson disease
40	Combivent	albuterol/ipratropium	Anticholinergic/beta-2 agonist	Asthma
41	Concerta	methylphenidate	Central nervous system stimulant	ADHD
42	Coreg	carvedilol	Beta-blocker	Hypertension
43	Cortef	hydrocortisone	Corticosteroid	Inflammatory disorders
44	Coumadin	warfarin	Vitamin K antagonist	Anticoagulation
45	Cozaar	losartan potassium	ARB	Hypertension
46	Crestor	rosuvastatin calcium	HMG-CoA reductase inhibitor	Hyperlipidemia
47	Cymbalta	duloxetine	SNRI	Depression
48	Deltasone	prednisone	Corticosteroid	Inflammation
49	Depakote ER	divalproex sodium	Neurologic	Bipolar disorder, migraine headache, seizure disorder
50	Desyrel	trazodone hydrochloride	Serotonin reuptake inhibitor	Insomnia, depression
51	Diflucan	fluconazole	Antifungal	Fungal infection
52	Dilantin	phenytoin	Hydantoin	Status epilepticus
53	Diovan	valsartan	ARB	Hypertension
54	Diovan HCT	hydrochlorothiazide/valsartan	ARB/thiazide combination	Hypertension
55	Ditropan	oxybutynin	Antispasmotic	Overactive bladder
56	Dramamine	meclizine hydrochloride	H_1 antagonist	Motion sickness
57	Duragesic	fentanyl transdermal patch	Analgesic	Pain
58	Dyazide	triamterene/HCTZ	Diuretic combo	Hypertension
59	Edarbi	azilsartan	Angiotensin II receptor blocker	Hypertension
60	Effexor	venlafaxine hydrochloride	SNRI	Depression
61	Elavil	amitriptyline	TCA	Depression
62	Eliquis	apixaban	Anticoagulant	Anticoagulant
63	Evista	raloxifene	Estrogen modulator	Osteoporosis
64	Flexeril	cyclobenzaprine hydrochloride	Muscle relaxant	Skeletal muscle relaxant
65	Flomax	tamsulosin hydrochloride	Alpha-blocker	BPH
66	Flonase	fluticasone	Corticosteroid	Allergic rhinitis
67	Focalin XR	dexmethylphenidate hydrochloride	CNS stimulant	ADHD
68	Folic Acid	folic acid	Vitamin	Dietary supplement
69	Fosamax	alendronate	Bisphosphonate	Osteoporosis
70	Furadantin	nitrofurantoin	Antibiotic	UTI
71	Gianvi	drospirenone/ethinyl estradiol	Monophasic oral contraceptive	Oral contraceptive
72	Glucophage	metformin hydrochloride	Biguanide	Type 2 diabetes mellitus
73	Glucotrol	glipizide	Sulfonylurea	Type 2 diabetes mellitus
74	Haldol	haloperidol	Antipsychotic	Schizophrenia
75	Humalog	insulin lispro	Insulin	Diabetes mellitus
76	Humulin N	insulin NPH	Insulin	Diabetes mellitus

	Brand Name	Generic Name	Drug Classification[a]	Indication or Use
77	Hytrin	terazosin	Alpha-1 blocker	BPH
78	Hyzaar	hydrochlorothiazide/losartan potassium	ARB/thiazide combination	Hypertension
79	Imdur	isosorbide mononitrate	Vasodilator	Angina
80	Imitrex	sumatriptan	Serotonin 5-HT$_1$ receptor agonist	Migraine headache
81	Inderal	propranolol hydrochloride	Beta-blocker	Hypertension
82	Iron	ferrous sulfate	Supplement	Iron-deficiency anemia
83	Janumet	metformin hydrochloride/sitagliptin phosphate	Biguanide/DPP-4 inhibitor	Type 2 diabetes mellitus
84	Januvia	sitagliptin phosphate	DPP-4 inhibitor	Type 2 diabetes mellitus
85	Jardiance	empagliflozin	Antidiabetic	Diabetes
86	K-Dur, Klor-Con, Klor-Con M, Micro K	potassium chloride	Electrolyte	Potassium supplement
87	Kariva	desogestrel/ethinyl estradiol	Monophasic oral contraceptive	Oral contraceptive
88	Keflex	cephalexin	Cephalosporin antibiotic	Bacterial infection
89	Keppra	levetiracetam	Antiepileptic	Seizure
90	Klonopin	clonazepam	Benzodiazepine	Seizure
91	Lamictal	lamotrigine	Antiepileptic	Bipolar disorder
92	Lanoxin	digoxin	Cardiac glycoside	Arrhythmia, myocardial infarction
93	Lantus	insulin glargine	Insulin	Diabetes mellitus
94	Lasix	furosemide	Loop diuretic	Hypertension
95	Levaquin	levofloxacin	Quinolone antibiotic	Bacterial infection
96	Levemir	insulin detemir	Insulin	Diabetes mellitus
97	Lexapro	escitalopram oxalate	SSRI	Depression
98	Lioresal	baclofen	Muscle relaxer	Muscle spasms
99	Lipitor	atorvastatin	HMG-CoA reductase inhibitor	Hyperlipidemia
100	Lithobid	lithium	Antimanic	Bipolar disorder
101	Lopid	gemfibrozil	Antilipemic agent	Hyperlipidemia
102	Lopressor	metoprolol tartrate	Beta-blocker	Hypertension
103	Loratadine	cetirizine hydrochloride	H$_1$ antagonist	Allergies
104	Lotensin	benazepril hydrochloride	ACE inhibitor	Hypertension
105	Lotrel	amlodipine besylate/benazepril hydrochloride	ACE inhibitor/CCB combination	Hypertension
106	Lyrica	pregabalin	GABA analogue	Neuropathic pain
107	Maxzide or Dyazide	hydrochlorothiazide/triamterene	Potassium-sparing/thiazide diuretic	Hypertension
108	Medrol	methylprednisolone	Corticosteroid	Inflammation
109	Mevacor	lovastatin	HMG-CoA reductase inhibitor	Hyperlipidemia
110	Micronase or DiaBeta	glyburide	Sulfonylurea	Type 2 diabetes mellitus
111	Mobic	meloxicam	NSAID	Osteoarthritis
112	Motrin[b]	ibuprofen	NSAID	Inflammation
113	Namenda	memantine hydrochloride	NMDA receptor agonist	Alzheimer disease
114	Nasacort AQ	triamcinolone	Corticosteroid	Allergic rhinitis
115	Neurontin	gabapentin	Neurologic	Seizure
116	Nexium[b]	esomeprazole	PPI	GERD

Continued

	Brand Name	Generic Name	Drug Classification[a]	Indication or Use
117	Nitrostat	nitroglycerin	Vasodilator	Angina
118	Norvasc	amlodipine besylate	CCB	Hypertension
119	Novolog	insulin aspart	Insulin	Diabetes mellitus
120	Ortho-Tri-Cyclen Lo	ethinyl estradiol/norgestimate	Triphasic oral contraceptive	Oral contraceptive
121	Oxycontin	oxycodone	Opioid	Analgesic
122	Ozempic[b]	semaglutide	H_2 blocker	GERD
123	Pamelor	nortriptyline hydrochloride	TCA	Depression
124	Paxil	paroxetine	SSRI	Depression
125	Pen VK -brand	penicillin VK	Penicillin antibiotic	Bacterial infection
126	Pepcid[b]	famotidine	H_2 blocker	GERD
127	Phenergan	promethazine hydrochloride	Antihistamine	Antiemetic
128	Plaquenil	hydroxychloroquine sulfate	Aminoquinoline	Antimalarial
129	Plavix	clopidogrel bisulfate	Antiplatelet	Thrombotic event prevention
130	Pravachol	pravastatin	HMG-CoA reductase inhibitor	Hyperlipidemia
131	Premarin	estrogens conjugated	Estrogen	Vasomotor symptoms
132	Prevacid[b]	lansoprazole	PPI	GERD
133	Prilosec[b]	omeprazole	PPI	GERD
134	Pristiq	desvenlafaxine	SNRI	Depression
135	ProAir HFA, Proventil HFA, Ventolin HFA	albuterol	Bronchodilator	Asthma
136	Procardia	nifedipine	Dihydropyridine CCB	Hypertension
137	Proscar	finasteride	5 Alpha-reductase inhibitor	BPH
138	Protonix	pantoprazole sodium	PPI	GERD
139	Prozac	fluoxetine hydrochloride	SSRI	Depression
140	Pyridium	phenazopyridine	Urinary analgesic	UTI
141	Relafen	nabumetone	Dopamine antagonist	antiinflammatory
142	Remeron	mirtazapine	Antidepressant	Depression
143	Requip	ropinirole hydrochloride	Dopamine agonist	Parkinson disease
144	Restoril	temazepam	Benzodiazepine	Insomnia
145	Risperdal	risperidone	Antipsychotic	Schizophrenia
146	Robaxin	methocarbamol	Skeletal muscle relaxant	Spasticity
147	Robitussin	guaifenesin	Expectorant	Congestion
148	Seroquel	quetiapine fumarate	Antipsychotic	Schizophrenia
149	Singulair	montelukast	Leukotriene receptor antagonist	Asthma
150	Soma	carisoprodol	Muscle relaxant	Skeletal muscle relaxant
151	Spiriva HandiHaler	tiotropium	Anticholinergic	COPD
	Sterapred	prednisone	Corticosteroid	Inflammation
152	Stool softener	docusate	Laxative	Constipation
153	Strattera	atomoxetine	Antistimulant	ADHD
154	Suboxone	buprenorphine	Opioid	Opioid recovery
155	Symbicort	budesonide/formoterol	Corticosteroid/beta-2 agonist	Asthma
156	Synthroid	levothyroxine sodium	Thyroid hormone	Hypothyroidism
157	Tamiflu	oseltamivir	Antiviral	Pneumonia
158	Tapazole	methimazole	Anti thyroid hormone	Hyperthyroidism
159	Tegretol	carbamazepine	Anticonvulsant	Seizures

	Brand Name	Generic Name	Drug Classification[a]	Indication or Use
160	Tenex	guanfacine	Antihypertensive	Hypertension
161	Tenormin	atenolol	Beta-blocker	Hypertension
162	Tessalon Perles	benzonatate	Antitussive	Cough
163	Topamax	topiramate	Antiepileptic	Seizures
164	Trandate	labetalol	Antihypertensive	Hypertension
165	Tresiba	insulin degludec	Insulin (long acting)	Diabetes
166	Tricor	fenofibrate	Fibrate	Hyperlipidemia
167	Trileptal	oxcarbazepine	Antiepileptic	Partial seizures
168	Trulicity	dulaglutide	Antidiabetic	Diabetes
169	Tylenol	acetaminophen	Nonopioid analgesic	Analgesic
170	Ultram	tramadol hydrochloride	Opioid	Analgesic
171	Valium	diazepam	Benzodiazepine	Anxiety
172	Valtrex	valacyclovir	Antiviral	Viral infection
173	Vasotec	enalapril maleate	ACE inhibitor	Hypertension
174	Vibramycin	doxycycline hyclate	Tetracycline antibiotic	Bacterial infection
175	Vicodin	acetaminophen/hydrocodone bitartrate	Opioid combination	Analgesic
176	Victoza	liraglutide	GLP-1 receptor agonist	Type 2 diabetes mellitus
177	Vistaril	hydroxyzine	H_1 antagonist	Allergies
178	Vitamin B$_{12}$	cyanocobalamin	Vitamin	Vitamin B$_{12}$ deficiency
179	Vitamin D 50,000[b]	ergocalciferol	Vitamin	Vitamin D deficiency
180	Vitamin D$_3$	cholecalciferol/alpha-tocopherol	Vitamin	Vitamin D deficiency
181	Vyvanse	lisdexamfetamine	CNS stimulant	ADHD
182	Wellbutrin XL	bupropion	Antidepressant	Depression
183	Xalatan	latanoprost	Prostaglandin analogue	Glaucoma
184	Xanax	alprazolam	Benzodiazepine	Anxiety
185	Xarelto	rivaroxaban	DOAC	Anticoagulant
186	Xyzal	levocetirizine dihydrochloride	H_1 antagonist	Allergies
187	Yaz	ethinyl estradiol/drospirenone	Oral contraceptive	Oral contraceptive
188	Zanaflex	tizanidine	Alpha-2 agonist	Muscle relaxant
189	Zestoretic	hydrochlorothiazide/lisinopril	ACE inhibitor/thiazide combination	Hypertension
190	Zestril or Prinivil	lisinopril	ACE inhibitor	Hypertension
191	Zetia	ezetimibe	Cholesterol absorption inhibitor	Hyperlipidemia
192	Zithromax	azithromycin	Macrolide antibiotic	Bacterial infection
193	Zocor	simvastatin	HMG-CoA reductase inhibitor	Hyperlipidemia
194	Zofran	ondansetron	5-HT$_3$ receptor antagonist	Antiemetic
195	Zoloft	sertraline hydrochloride	SSRI	Depression
196	Zovirax	acyclovir	Antiviral	Viral infection
197	Zyloprim	allopurinol	Xanthine oxidase inhibitor	Gout

[a] According to Epocrates.

[b] Prescription.

ACE, Angiotensin-converting enzyme; ADHD, attention deficit/hyperactivity disorder; ARB, angiotensin II–receptor blocker; BPH, benign prostatic hypertrophy; CCB, calcium channel blocker; CNS, central nervous system; COPD, chronic obstructive pulmonary disease; COX, cyclooxygenase; DPP-4, dipeptidyl peptidase 4; DOAC, direct-acting oral anticoagulant; DVT, deep vein thrombosis; GERD, gastroesophageal reflux disease; GLP, glucagon-like peptide; GU, genitourinary; HMG-CoA, 3-hydroxy-3-methylglutaryl/coenzyme A; NMDA, N-methyl-D-aspartate; NSAID, nonsteroidal antiinflammatory drug; PDE-5, phosphodiesterase type 5; PPI, proton pump inhibitor; SERM, selective estrogen receptor modulator; SNRI, serotonin-norepinephrine reuptake inhibitor; SSRI, selective serotonin reuptake inhibitor; TCA, tricyclic antidepressant.

Modified from Mizner JJ. *Mosby's Review for the Pharmacy Technician Certification Examination.* 3rd ed. St. Louis: Mosby, 2014.

Top Herbal Remedies

Drugs by Brand, Generic, Classification, Indication

Common Name	Scientific Name	Common Reported Uses
Aloe vera (leaf)	*Aloe* spp.	Wound and burn healing
Bilberry (berry)	*Vaccinium myrtillus*	Eye and vascular support
Black cohosh (root)	*Cimicifuga racemosa*	Menopause, premenstrual syndrome (PMS)
Cascara sagrada (aged bark)	*Rhamnus purshiana*	Laxative
Cat's claw (root, bark)	*Uncaria tomentosa*	Antiinflammatory, immune system support
Chondroitin	Chondroitin 4- and 6-sulfate	Osteoarthritis
Dong quai (root)	*Angelica sinensis*	Energy (females), menopause, dysmenorrhea, PMS
Echinacea (flower, root)	*Echinacea purpurea, Echinacea angustifolia*	Support of common cold, immunostimulant
Evening primrose (seed oil)	*Oenothera biennis*	PMS, menopause
Feverfew (leaf)	*Tanacetum parthenium*	Antiinflammatory, migraine prevention
Fish oils	Nutraceutical	Lower triglycerides, heart health
Garlic (bulb)	*Allium sativum*	Lower blood pressure, lower cholesterol
Ginger (root)	*Zingiber officinale*	Antiemetic, gastrointestinal distress, dyspepsia
Ginkgo (root)	*Ginkgo biloba*	Support of memory, increased blood flow to brain, prevention of dementia
Ginseng (American)	*Panax quinquefolius*	Increase physical endurance and concentration, lessen fatigue, support energy, stress, immune system
Glucosamine	3-Amino-6-(hydroxymethyl) oxane-2,4, 5-triol sulfate or (3R,4R,5S,6R)-3-amino-6-(hydroxymethyl)oxane-2,4,5-triol hydrochloride	Osteoarthritis
Goldenseal (root)	*Hydrastis canadensis*	Chest congestion
Grape seed (seed, skin)	*Vitis vinifera*	Support circulation
Green tea (leaf)	*Camellia sinensis*	Improve cognitive performance and mental alertness
Kava (root)	*Piper methysticum*	Anxiety, sedation
Melatonin	N-acetyl-5-methoxytryptamine	Insomnia, jet lag
Milk thistle (seed)	*Silybum marianum*	Antioxidant, liver support
Saw palmetto (berry)	*Serenoa repens*	Diuretic
Siberian ginseng (root)	*Eleutherococcus senticosus*	Athletic performance, stress, immune system builder
St. John's wort (flowering buds)	*Hypericum perforatum*	Depression, anxiety
Valerian (root)	*Valeriana officinalis*	Sedative, muscle spasms, insomnia
Wild yam (tuber)	*Dioscorea villosa*	PMS, infertility

A

Abortifacient Any treatment that causes abortion of a fetus

Absolute neutrophil count (ANC) The number of white blood cells that are neutrophils

Absorption Movement of nutrients, fluids, and medications from the gastrointestinal tract into the bloodstream

Accreditation Council for Pharmacy Education (ACPE) A national agency for the accreditation of professional degree programs in pharmacy and providers of continuing pharmacy education

Acidification (urinary) The conversion of urine to a more acidic content

Acidosis Increase in the blood's acidity, resulting from the accumulation of acid or loss of bicarbonate; the blood's pH is lower

Acne vulgaris Commonly known as pimples, acne occurs when the skin pores clog with oil or bacteria

Acromegaly A condition caused by excessive growth hormone production during adulthood

Act A statutory proposal passed by Congress or any legislature that is a "bill" until it is enacted and becomes law

Addison disease A condition resulting in decreased levels of adrenocortical hormones (eg, mineralocorticoids and glucocorticoids), which causes symptoms such as muscle weakness and weight loss

Adjudication The process by which a prescription is submitted electronically to a third-party payer to obtain reimbursement for the pharmacy for the medication dispensed

Adrenal cortex A portion of the adrenal gland that secretes steroids, including mineralocorticoids, glucocorticoids, and sex steroids

Adrenal medulla A portion of the adrenal gland that synthesizes and secretes the catecholamines norepinephrine and epinephrine

Adulteration The mishandling of medication that can lead to contamination or impurity, falsification of contents, or loss of drug quality or potency; adulteration may cause injury or illness to the consumer

Albumin The major protein found in plasma

Aldosterone A steroid hormone secreted by the adrenal cortex that regulates the salt and water balance in the body; the principal mineralocorticoid in the body that maintains sodium and potassium homeostasis by stimulating the kidneys to conserve sodium and excrete potassium

Alkalosis Increase in the blood's alkalinity, resulting from the accumulation of alkali or reduction of acid content; the blood's pH is higher

Allergen A substance that causes an allergic reaction

Alligation A mathematical method of solving problems that involves the mixing of two solutions or two solids of different percentages to achieve a desired third strength

Alopecia Partial or complete absence of hair from body areas where it usually grows; baldness

Alternative medicine Any range of medical therapies not regarded as orthodox by Western medicine

Alveoli Tiny air sacs in the lungs where oxygen and carbon dioxide exchange takes place

Alzheimer disease (AD) A progressive form of dementia that affects memory, thinking, and behavior

Amendment A change in an original act or law

American Association of Pharmacy Technicians (AAPT) The first pharmacy technician association: founded in 1979

American Pharmacists Association (APhA) The oldest pharmacy association: founded in 1852

American Society of Health-System Pharmacists (ASHP) An association of pharmacists, pharmacy students, and technicians practicing in hospitals and health care systems including home health care; the ASHP has a long history of advocating patient safety and establishing best practices to improve medication use; it was founded in 1942

American Society of Health-System Pharmacists (ASHP) Model Curriculum for Pharmacy Technician Education and Training A model that provides details on how to meet the ASHP

goals for pharmacy technician training programs

Amino acids Molecules that are the building blocks of proteins

Analgesic A drug that relieves pain

Anaphylaxis An extreme, potentially life-threatening allergic reaction

Androgen Male sex hormone

Anemia A decrease in the number of red blood cells or hemoglobin, which impairs the blood's ability to carry oxygen to the tissues

Aneurysm A balloon-like bulge or dilation of an artery resulting from weakening of the arterial wall

Angina Chest pain due to an inadequate supply of oxygen to the heart muscle

Angiotensin II A peptide hormone that causes vasoconstriction and a subsequent increase in blood pressure

Anion A negatively charged ion

Antibodies Complex molecules (immunoglobulins) made in response an antigen's presence (eg, a protein of bacteria or other infecting organism) that neutralize a foreign substance's effect

Anticholinergic An agent that inhibits the physiologic action of acetylcholine

Anticoagulant An agent used to prevent the formation of blood clots

Antiemetics A drug that prevents or treats nausea and vomiting

Antigen A substance that prompts antibody production, resulting in an immune response

Antigen-presenting cell (APC) An immune system cell that presents antigens to lymphocytes to activate an immune response

Antihistamine A drug or other compound that inhibits the effects of histamine; often used to treat allergies

Antihyperlipidemics A diverse group of pharmaceuticals used in the treatment of hyperlipidemia

Antiinflammatory A drug that reduces swelling

Antipyretic A drug that prevents or reduces fever

Antiseptics Substances that slow or stop microorganism growth on surfaces such as skin

Antitussive A drug that can decrease the central nervous system coughing reflex

Aorta The great arterial trunk that carries blood from the heart to be distributed to tissues of the body

Aphasia A communication disorder that results from damage or injury to the language parts of the brain; it is more common in older adults, particularly those who have had a stroke

Apothecary The Latin term for pharmacist; also, a place where drugs are sold

Apothecary system A system of measurement once used in the practice of pharmacy to measure both volume and weight; it has been mostly replaced by the metric system

Aqueous humor The fluid found in the anterior chamber of the eye, in front of the lens

Arrhythmias Abnormal or irregular heart rhythms

Arteriosclerosis A condition characterized by thickening, loss of elasticity (hardening), and calcification of the arterial walls

Artery A vessel that carries oxygenated blood from the heart to the tissues of the body

Arthroplasty Surgical reconstruction or replacement of a joint

ASAP order As soon as possible but not an emergency

Aseptic technique A technique used in the sterile compounding of hazardous and nonhazardous materials to minimize the introduction of microbes or unwanted debris that could cause contamination of the preparation; the procedures used to eliminate the possibility of a drug becoming contaminated with microbes or particles

Aspiration To draw a foreign substance into the respiratory tract during inhalation

Atherosclerosis A process of progressive thickening and hardening of the walls of medium-sized and large arteries as a result of fat deposits on their inner lining

Atrium The entry chamber on both sides of the heart

Attention-deficit/hyperactivity disorder (ADHD) A physiologic brain disorder that affects the ability to engage in quiet, passive activities or to focus one's attention; attributable to a neurotransmitter imbalance

Attenuated A term that describes an altered or weakened live vaccine made from the disease organism against which the vaccine protects

Auditory canal A 1-inch segment of tube that extends from the external ear to the middle ear

Auditory ossicles Small bones (ossicles) of the middle ear that transmit sound from the eardrum to the inner ear

Auricle The outer projecting portion of the ear

Automated dispensing system (ADS) Computerized cabinets that control inventory on nursing floors, in emergency departments, and in surgical suites and other patient care areas; electronic systems used to dispense medications

Autonomic nervous system (ANS) The nervous system branch that carries out "automatic" bodily functions. It includes the sympathetic and parasympathetic systems

Auxiliary label A label that provides supplementary information about proper and safe administration, use, or storage of a medication

Average wholesale price (AWP) The average price at which a drug is sold; the data are compiled from information provided by manufacturers, distributors, and pharmacies; the AWP is often used in calculations related to medication reimbursement

Avoirdupois system A system of measurement previously used in pharmacy for the determination of weight in ounces and pounds; this system has been mostly replaced by the metric system

Ayurveda A holistic traditional medical system originating in India that emphasizes disease prevention

B

Bactericidal Causes bacterial cell death

Bacteriostatic Inhibits bacterial cell growth

Bank Identification Number (BIN) A six-digit number on a prescription drug card that is used for routing and identification to process a prescription claim

Barbiturate A drug derived from barbituric acid; a barbiturate acts as a central nervous system depressant; barbiturates are often used in the treatment of seizures and as sedative and hypnotic agents

Behind-the-counter drug A nonprescription medication kept "behind the [prescription] counter" that patients must buy at a pharmacy

Benign A condition, tumor, or growth that is not cancerous and therefore will not metastasize (spread)

Benign prostatic hyperplasia (BPH) Enlargement of the prostate

Beyond-use date (BUD) Defined by USP Chapter <797> as the date or time after which a compounded sterile preparation (CSP) shall not be administered, stored, or transported; the BUD is determined from the date the preparation is compounded

Bioavailability The degree to which a drug or other substance becomes available to the target tissue after administration

Bioequivalence The relationship between two drugs that have the same dosage and dosage form and that have similar bioavailability; generic versions of a medication must show bioequivalence to the original approved brand product as a requirement of drug approval

Biofeedback The use of electronic monitoring of an automatic bodily function to train someone to acquire voluntary control of that function

Biological response modifier (BRM) An agent used to modify the body's immune response

Biological safety cabinet (BSC) A hood that should be used for hazardous sterile preparations in the clean room

Blister pack See *bubble pack*

Blood-brain barrier (BBB) A brain barrier that results from special permeability characteristics of capillaries that supply brain cells; the capillaries prevent certain solutes or chemicals from passing from the blood to the brain

Bloodletting The practice of draining blood; it was believed to release illness

Blood pressure The pressure of the blood within the arteries

Board of Pharmacy (BOP) A state-managed agency (board) that licenses pharmacists and may either register or license pharmacy technicians to work in a pharmacy

Body mass index (BMI) A measure of body fat based on height and weight of a patient.

Bone fracture A break or rupture of a bone

Bone marrow A fatty network of connective tissue that fills the cavities in long bones, the source of red blood cells and many white blood cells

Boxed warning A drug warning that is placed in the prescribing information or package insert of a product and indicates a significant risk for potentially dangerous side effects. It is the strongest warning the US Food and Drug Administration (FDA) can give. It is common in the pharmacy profession to call these warnings "Black Box Warnings" because of their appearance on a drug label; the warning is often enclosed in a black outlined box to draw attention to the content

Bradykinesia Slowed movement

Brainstem A section of the brain consisting of the medulla oblongata, pons, and midbrain, which connect the forebrain and cerebrum to the spinal cord

Brand name The name a company assigns to a commercial drug product for marketing and identification purposes. Most proprietary names are trademarked and belong to originator products. The named products are often protected, for a time, by patents; also known as the *proprietary name* or *trade name*

Bronchi The major lung air passages that diverge from the windpipe

Bronchioles Small branches that divide from the bronchus in the lungs

Bubble pack A preformed card with 28-, 30-, and 31-day depressions that can hold medications; they are sealed with a foil card backboard and usually used for long-term care medications

Bulk repackaging The process by which the pharmacy transfers a medication manually or by means of an automated system from a manufacturer's original container to another type of container unrelated to dispensing a prescriber's order

C

Caduceus Often confused as the symbol of the medical field; it is a staff with two entwined snakes and two wings at the top

Calcitonin A thyroid hormone that helps to regulate blood concentrations of calcium and phosphate and promotes the formation of bone

Calibration The markings on a measuring device

Cancellous bone A meshwork of spongy bone typically found at the core of vertebral bones in the spine and the ends of long bones; also called spongy bone

Capillary A tiny vessel that connects the ends of the smallest arteries (arterioles) to the smallest veins (venules), where exchange of nutrients, waste products, oxygen (O_2), and carbon dioxide (CO_2) occurs

Carbohydrates Chemical compounds that contain carbon, hydrogen, and oxygen; examples include sugars, glycogen, starches, and cellulose

Carbonic anhydrase An enzyme that converts carbonic acid into carbon dioxide and water

Cardiac muscle A type of muscle tissue found in the heart

Cardiac output (CO) The amount of blood the heart pumps through the circulatory system in a minute

Catecholamines Hormones produced in the brainstem, nervous system, and adrenal glands that help the body respond to stress and prepare the body for the "fight-or-flight" response; they are important in regulating heart rate, blood pressure, and nervous system functions

Cation A positively charged ion

Central nervous system (CNS) Consists of the brain and spinal cord; it coordinates sensory and motor body function control

Cerebellum A structure posterior to the pons and medulla oblongata responsible for posture, balance, and voluntary muscle movement

Cerebrospinal fluid (CSF) A continually produced and absorbed clear, watery fluid that flows in the ventricles around the brain surface and spinal cord

Certified pharmacy technician (CPhT) A technician who has passed the national certification examination; the technician can use the abbreviation CPhT after his or her name

Cerumen Earwax

Chain pharmacy A corporate-owned group of pharmacies that share a brand name and central management and usually have standardized business methods and practices

Channel In communications, a written message, spoken words, or body language

Chemical structure The makeup of a chemical, including factors such as the elements, shape, bonding types, and molecular configurations; the nature of a chemical's structure has much to do with the chemical's stability, reactivity, and physical and chemical properties

Chiropractic medicine Manual manipulation of the joints and muscles

Chloasma Hyperpigmentation of the skin that is limited or confined to a certain area

Chronic kidney disease (CKD) A condition that reduces the kidneys' ability to function properly

Chyme The resulting soupy mixture (semifluid) after food mixes with stomach acids and digestive enzymes

Cilia Short, microscopic, hairlike structures

Ciliary body The part of the eye that connects the iris to the choroid

Circadian rhythms 24-hour cycles of regular biological changes. In pharmacology, this often involves medications affecting sleep/wake cycles

Civilian Health and Medical Program of the Department of Veterans Affairs (CHAMPVA) A program for veterans with permanent service-related disabilities and their dependents and for the spouses and children of veterans who died from service-connected disability; also known as the Veterans Health Administration (VHA)

Clean room A contained and controlled environment in the pharmacy that has a low level of environmental pollutants such as dust, airborne microbes, aerosol particles, and chemical vapors; the clean room is used for preparing sterile medication products

Closed-door pharmacy A pharmacy to which medications are called in from institutions, such as long-term care facilities, and the medications are then delivered; closed door pharmacies are not open to the public

Closed formulary A system in which medication use is tightly restricted to medications provided on the formulary list; medications that are not listed as preapproved drugs per the health plan provider or pharmacy benefits manager are not reimbursed except under extenuating circumstances and with proper documentation

Coagulation Solidification or change from a fluid state to a solid state, as in the formation of a blood clot

Coinsurance A type of insurance in which the policyholder pays a share of the payment made against a claim

Collecting duct A series of tubules in the kidneys that connect the nephrons to the ureter

Colony-stimulating factor (CSF) A hormone that stimulates bone marrow to synthesize hematopoietic cells

Comedones Blackheads; plugs of keratin and sebum in hair follicles blackened at the surface

Communication The ability to express oneself in such a way that one is readily and clearly understood

Community pharmacy Pharmacies that serve patients in their communities; consumers can walk in and purchase a prescription or OTC drug; also known as *outpatient pharmacies* or retail pharmacies

Comorbidity A concomitant, but not necessarily related, medical condition existing simultaneously with another condition

Compact bone Rigid bone, which makes up most of the skeleton; also known as cortical bone

Compassion A feeling of wanting to help someone who is sick or in trouble

Competency The capability or proficiency to perform a function

Complementary medicine A range of medical therapies that fall beyond the scope of Western medicine. They are complementary to traditional medicine

Compounded sterile preparations (CSPs) Substances prepared in a sterile environment with nonsterile ingredients or devices that must be sterilized before they are used

Compounding The act of mixing, reconstituting, and packaging a drug

Compounding record (CR) Documentation of nonsterile compounding

Computerized physician order entry (CPOE) A computerized order entry

Confidentiality The practice of keeping privileged customer information from being disclosed without the customer's consent

Conjunctiva The transparent protective mucous membrane that lines the underside of the eyelid

Continuing education (CE) Courses taken beyond the basic technical education, usually required for license or certification renewal

Controlled substance Any drug or other substance categorized as Schedule I through V and regulated by the Drug Enforcement Administration

Conversion factor A fraction used to convert one unit into another without changing the value of the number

Copayment The portion of the prescription bill that the patient is responsible for paying

Cornea The transparent tissue covering the anterior portion of the eye

Coronary artery Either of two arteries that arise from the aorta (one from the left side and one from the right side) and supply the tissues of the heart itself

Crash carts Moveable carts containing trays of medications, administration sets, oxygen, and other materials that are used in life-threatening situations such as cardiac arrest; also known as *code carts*

Cream A hydrophilic base

Cretinism A condition in which the development of the brain and body is inhibited by a congenital lack of thyroid hormone secretion

Cryoprecipitate Any precipitate that results from cooling; sometimes explicitly used to describe a precipitate rich in coagulation factor VIII obtained from cooling of blood plasma

Cyclooxygenase (COX) Either of two related enzymes that control prostaglandin production

Cytokine A protein that signals cells of the immune system

D

Decongestant A drug that shrinks the swollen membranes in the nasal cavity, making it easier to breathe

Deductible The amount paid by a policyholder out of pocket before the insurance company pays a claim

Depot An area of the body where a substance can accumulate or be stored for later distribution

Dermis A thick layer of connective tissue that contains collagen

Diagnosis A physician's recognition of a condition or disease based on its outward signs and symptoms and/or confirming tests or procedures

Dialysate The fluid into which material passes by way of the membrane in dialysis

Dialysis The passage of a solute through a semipermeable membrane to remove toxic materials and to maintain fluid, electrolyte, and pH levels when the kidneys malfunction

Diaphragm A dome-shaped, muscular partition separating the thorax from the abdomen that plays a major role in breathing

Diastole The period when the heart is in a state of relaxation and dilation

Digestion The mechanical, chemical, and enzymatic action of breaking food into molecules for metabolism

Diluent/solvent An inert product, either liquid or solid, that is added to a preparation to reduce the strength of the original product

Dilution The process of adding a diluent or solvent to a compound, resulting in a product of increased volume or weight and lower concentration

Diplomacy The skill of dealing with others without causing bad feelings

Direct manufacturer ordering A process in which pharmacies may join a group purchasing organization (GPO) and contract directly with the manufacturer to obtain better pricing

Dispense as written (DAW) codes A numerical set of codes, created by the National Council for Prescription Drug Programs (NCPDP), that is used when filling prescriptions; the code can affect reimbursement amounts from insurance companies

Distribution The movement of a medication throughout the blood, organs, and tissues after administration

Diuretic An agent that increases urine output and excretion of water

Dogma A principle or set of principles laid down by an authority as incontrovertibly true

Drip rate/drop rate The number of drops (gtt) administered over a specific time by an intravenous infusion (eg, gtt/min)

Drop factor The size of the drops produced by tubing used to administer a medication; the size is measured in gtt/mL, and the drop factor is indicated on the tubing package

Drug classification Categorization of a drug based on its various characteristics, including chemical structure, action, and/or therapeutic or anatomical use

Drug diversion The intentional misuse of a drug intended for medical purposes; the Drug Enforcement Administration usually defines diversion as the recreational use of a prescription or scheduled drug; diversion also can refer to the channeling of the prescription drug supply away from legal distribution and to the illegal street market

Drug Enforcement Administration (DEA) The agency of the US

Department of Justice that enforces US laws and regulations related to controlled substances

Drug Enforcement Administration (DEA) number An alphanumeric number consisting of two letters and seven numbers that is assigned to prescribers authorized by the DEA to prescribe controlled substances

Drug Facts and Comparisons A reference book found in pharmacies that contains detailed information on medications

Drug Topics Red Book A reference book listing National Drug Code (NDC) numbers, manufacturers, and average wholesale pricing of drug products; pharmacies often include this type of product and pricing information on their online database systems, which are provided by companies such as First DataBank and Gold Standard

Drug utilization evaluation (DUE) A program for ensuring that prescribed drugs are used appropriately; an authorized, structured, ongoing review of health care provider prescribing, pharmacist dispensing, and patient use of medication; the primary goal of any DUE program is an increase in medication-related efficacy and safety; formerly known as *drug utilization review*

Dwarfism A condition characterized by a growth hormone deficiency during adolescence, resulting in short stature and decreased organ size

Dyspnea Difficult or labored breathing

E

Eczema A condition in which patches of skin become rough and inflamed

Edema An excess of watery fluid in the cavities or tissues of the body

Electronic medication administration record (E-MAR) Technology that automatically documents the administration of medication into certified electronic health record (EHR) systems; the report serves as a legal record of medications administered to a patient at a facility by a health care professional

Elimination The final evacuation of a drug or other substance from the body by normal body processes, such as kidney elimination (urine), biliary excretion (bile to stool), sweat, respiration, or saliva

Elixir A base solution that is a mixture of alcohol and water

Embolus A clump of material, often a blood clot, that travels from one part of the body to another and obstructs a blood vessel; an embolus can consist of any material, including bacteria or air

Emesis A medical term for vomiting

Emollient A preparation that softens the skin

Emulsion A mixture of two or more liquids that do not usually blend together, which are mixed using a stabilizing agent; the process of making an emulsion is called *emulsification*

Endocardium The thin membrane that lines the interior of the heart; the inner layer of the heart wall

Endocrine glands Glands that produce hormones that enter the bloodstream to reach their target or act at target sites near the area of hormone release

Endocrinologist A physician who specializes in treating endocrine system conditions

Endometrium The mucous membrane lining the inner wall or layer of the uterus

Enteral A route of administration by way of the intestine, such as orally, rectally, or sublingually

Enzyme A protein that accelerates a reaction by reducing the amount of energy required to initiate the reaction

Epicardium The outer layer of the heart wall; the inner layer of the pericardium

Epidermis The outermost skin layer composed of the stratum corneum, or horny layer, the keratinocytes (squamous cells), and the basal layer. It also contains melanin, a pigment that contributes to skin and hair color

Epilepsy A brain disorder marked by repeated seizures over time

e-Prescribing The computer-to-computer transfer of prescription data between pharmacies, prescribers, and payers

Erectile dysfunction (ED) Inability of a man to maintain an erection sufficient for satisfying sexual activity

Erythrocyte A cell that contains hemoglobin and can carry oxygen to the body; also known as a red blood cell

Erythropoiesis The formation of erythrocytes

Erythropoietin A hormone secreted by the kidney that stimulates the production of red blood cells by stem cells in bone marrow

Eschar A slough produced by a thermal burn, by application of a corrosive, or by gangrene

Essential hypertension The most common form of hypertension; it occurs in the absence of any evident cause

Estrogen Any of a group of anabolic sex hormones that promote the development and maintenance of female sexual characteristics

Ethics The values and morals used within a profession

Etiquette An unwritten guideline or rule of behavior

Euphoria A feeling or state of intense excitement and happiness

Eustachian tube A structure in the middle ear that connects with the nasopharynx (throat); it equalizes pressure between the outside air and middle ear and drains mucus

Excipient An inert substance added to a drug to form a suitable consistency for dosing

Excretion Elimination of waste products mainly through stools and urine

Exfoliation The peeling off of dead skin

Exocrine glands Glands that produce hormones sent to the target organ or tissue via a tube or duct outside the body

Exophthalmos Eyeball prominence (protrusion) from the orbit; increased thyroid hormone is a common cause of bilateral presentation

Expectorant A drug that helps remove mucous secretions from the respiratory system; it loosens and thins sputum and bronchial secretions for ease of expectoration

Expiration The act of breathing out; exhalation

Extrapyramidal symptoms (EPS) Often result from taking antipsychotic medications and include Parkinsonism, dystonia, and tremors

Exudate A mass of cells and fluid that has seeped out of blood vessels as a result of inflammation

F

Fallopian tube A narrow tube that connects the ovary to the uterus

Fascicles A bundle such as muscle fibers

FDA See *Food and Drug Administration (FDA)*

Federal legend The statement found on the labeling of all prescription medications: "Federal law prohibits the dispensing of this *drug* without a prescription"

Fertilization The process by which a sperm unites with an ovum

Fibrates An antihyperlipidemic drug class that primarily lowers triglycerides

First-pass effect The process by which a portion of the dose is metabolized before the drug has a chance to be distributed systemically

Fistulae Permanent abnormal passageways between two organs or between an organ and the outside

Floor stock Drugs that are not labeled for a specific patient and maintained at a nursing station or other department of the institution (excluding the pharmacy) for the purpose of administration to a patient of the facility

Flow rate/infusion rate The amount of intravenous solution administered over a specified period (eg, mL/min, mL/hr, gtt/min); volume/time

Food and Drug Administration (FDA) The agency in the US Department of Health and Human Services responsible for ensuring the safety, efficacy, and security of human and veterinary drugs, biological products, medical devices, the national food supply, cosmetics, and radioactive products

Formulary A list of drugs that have been approved for use in hospitals by the pharmacy and therapeutics committee of the institution and are the standard stock carried by the pharmacy and other departments; also, a list of drugs covered by an insurance company

Formulation record A document similar to a recipe used in preparation of nonsterile compounds

Franchise A form of business organization in which a firm that already has a successful product or service (the franchisor) enters into a continuing contractual relationship with other businesses (franchisees) operating under the franchisor's trade name and usually with the franchisor's guidance, in exchange for a fee

Fungicidal Able to destroy or inhibit the growth of fungi

G

Gametes Sex cells, or ova and sperm

Gastroparesis Delayed gastric emptying

Gauge The size of a needle opening

Generic name The name assigned to a medication; the nonproprietary name of a drug

Gigantism A condition of excessive growth hormone production during childhood or adolescence that results in excessive height and body tissue growth

Glomerulonephritis Acute inflammation of the kidney, typically caused by an immune response

Glucometer A device used to test blood sugar levels in patients with diabetes mellitus (DM)

Goiter A condition in which the thyroid gland is enlarged because of a lack of iodine; it can be either a simple goiter or a toxic goiter (ie, resulting from a tumor)

Good Manufacturing Practices (GMPs) Federal guidelines that must be followed by all entities that prepare and package medication or medical devices

Gout A painful form of arthritis characterized by defective metabolism of uric acid

Granulocytopenia A reduction in granulocyte number, which encompasses specific types of white blood cells that contain "granules"; these white blood cells include neutrophils, eosinophils, and basophils, which are all known as granulocytes. These contrast to lymphocytes, white blood cells devoid of granules

Graves disease A condition caused by thyroid hormone hypersecretion; symptoms include diffuse goiter, exophthalmos, and skin changes

H

Half-life (1) The amount of time it takes a chemical to be decreased by one half; (2) the time required for half the amount of a substance, such as a drug in a living system, to be eliminated or disintegrated by natural processes; (3) the time required for the concentration of a substance in a body fluid (blood plasma) to decrease by half

Hashimoto thyroiditis An autoimmune disease leading to hypothyroidism

Hazardous drug Any drug that has been proven to have dangerous effects during animal or human testing; it may cause cancer or may harm to certain organs or pregnant women

Hazardous waste Any waste that meets the Resource Conservation and Recovery Act (RCRA) definition of ignitability, corrosiveness, reactivity, or toxicity

Head louse A louse that infests the scalp and hair of the human head

Health care–associated infection (HAI) An infection that patients acquire during the course of receiving treatments for other conditions in an institutional setting

Health Insurance Portability and Accountability Act of 1996 (HIPAA) A federal law that protects patients' rights, establishes national standards for electronic health care communication, and ensures the security and privacy of health data

Health maintenance organization (HMO) An insurance plan that that allows coverage for in-network only physicians and services and uses the primary care physician (or provider) as the "gatekeeper" for the patient's health care; patients often have copays to defray the costs of medical care and prescription drugs

Heart failure (HF) A condition in which the heart cannot keep up with demand; failure of the heart to pump blood with normal efficiency

Help desk A 24/7 toll-free hotline to an insurance company that pharmacists can use to ask specific questions about insurance claims and coverage, in addition to pharmacy-specific inquiries

Hematopoiesis The formation of blood cells

Hemoglobin The oxygen-carrying component of red blood cells

Hemophilia A hereditary coagulation disorder that leads to a decreased ability to clot normally

Hemorrhagic stroke A stroke caused by a brain blood vessel rupture

Herb Any plant that is valued for its aromatic, medicinal, flavorful, or other properties

Herbals A substance made from or using herbs

Heterozygous familial hypercholesterolemia (HeFH) A genetic disorder based on a gene that encodes LDLR. Very high LDL levels in the blood characterize this disorder

High-density lipoprotein (HDL) A blood plasma lipoprotein composed of a high proportion of protein with little triglyceride and cholesterol and associated with a decreased probability of developing atherosclerosis

Hippocratic oath An oath taken by physicians concerning the ethics and practice of medicine

Hirsutism Abnormal growth of hair on a person's face and body

Homeopathy A therapeutic belief that dilutions of medicinal substances that cause a specific symptom can treat an illness that yields the same symptoms. The US Food and Drug Administration (FDA) under the Food, Drug, and Cosmetic Act regulates homeopathic medications.

Homeostasis The body's tendency to maintain stability, as with body temperature; the equilibrium pertaining to the balance of fluid levels, pH level, osmotic pressures, and concentrations of various substances

Horizontal laminar flow hood An environment for the preparation of compounded sterile preparations in which air originating from the back of the hood moves forward across the hood and into the room

Hormones Chemical substances produced and secreted by an endocrine duct into the bloodstream that result in a physiologic response at a specific target tissue

Household system A system of measurement commonly used in the United States; volumes are measured using household utensils

Humoral immunity The immune response mediated by antibodies

Hydrophilic Water loving; any substance that easily mixes in water

Hydrophobic Water hating; any substance that does not mix or dissolve in water

Hydrostatic pressure The pressure exerted by a fluid because of the force of gravity

Hyperalimentation Parenteral (intravenous) nutrition for patients who are unable to eat solids or liquids; also known as *total parenteral nutrition* (TPN)

Hyperglycemia Elevated concentration of glucose in the blood

Hyperlipidemia Also known as hypercholesterolemia—a condition marked by an increase in bloodstream cholesterol that can lead to atherosclerosis, or artery hardening

Hypertension Elevated blood pressure

Hyperthyroidism Excessive secretion of thyroid hormone

Hypocalcemia Low concentration of calcium in the blood

Hypodermis Subcutaneous tissue

Hypoglycemia Excessively low concentration of glucose in the blood

Hypokalemia Low concentration of potassium in the blood

Hypopituitary dwarfism Short stature caused by a deficiency in growth hormone during childhood

Hypotension Low blood pressure

Hypoxia An oxygen supply reduction to a tissue despite adequate tissue perfusion

I

Idiopathic A term meaning "of unknown cause"

Immunity An infection resistance type caused by the body's immune response after exposure to antigens or vaccine administration

Immunization The act of conferring immunity, such as with vaccination

Immunoglobulin An antibody

Inert ingredient An ingredient that has little or no effect on body functions

Infection control Policies and procedures put in place to minimize the risk of spreading infections in hospitals or other health care facilities

Infix A meaningful stem in a generic name in the middle of the word (eg, methylprednisolone)

Inflammation A localized physical condition associated with red, swollen, hot, and often painful tissue

Influenza A respiratory tract infection caused by an influenza virus

Ingestion Taking in food, liquid, or other substances (eg, medications)

INN International nonproprietary name, a generic name

Innate immunity Natural immunity

Inpatient pharmacy A pharmacy in a hospital or institutional setting

Inscription The name, dosage form, strength, and quantity of the medication prescribed

Insomnia Difficulty falling or staying asleep

Inspiration The act of breathing in; inhalation

Instill To place into; instillation instructions are commonly used for ophthalmic or otic drugs

Institute for Healthcare Improvement (IHI) A nonprofit organization committed to the improvement of health care by promoting promising concepts through safety, efficiency, and other patient-centered goals

Institute for Safe Medication Practices (ISMP) A nonprofit organization devoted entirely to promoting safe medication use and preventing medication errors; the organization gathers information on drug errors and suggests new, safer standards to prevent such errors

Institute of Medicine (IOM) Established under the National Academies and a part of the National Academy of Sciences, this nonprofit organization provides scientifically informed analysis and guidance regarding health and health policy; projects include studies of drug safety systems within the United States and recommendations for patient safety

Institutional pharmacy A pharmacy in which patients receive care on site, such as in hospitals, extended-living homes, long-term care, and hospice facilities; institutional pharmacies are also found in government-supported hospitals run by the Veterans Health Administration, Indian Health Service, and the Bureau of Prisons

Insulin resistance Resistance of body tissues (skeletal muscle and fat) to insulin effects; insulin resistance is associated with the development of type 2 diabetes mellitus

International System of Units (SI) A system of measurement based on seven base units with prefixes that change units by multiples of 10; the prefixes for the modern metric system are taken from the French Système International d'Unités and were adopted to provide a single worldwide system of weights and measures

International time A 24-hour method of keeping time in which hours are not distinguished between am and pm, but rather are counted continuously throughout the day

Interstitial space Small, narrow spaces between tissues

Intraocular pressure (IOP) The pressure exerted by the fluids inside the eyeball

Inventory The amount of product a pharmacy has for sale

Investigational drug A drug that has not been approved by the FDA for marketing but is in clinical trials; the term can also pertain to an FDA-approved drug for which the manufacturers are seeking approval of a new indication for use

Ions Atoms or molecules with a net electrical charge (positive or negative)

Iris The colored part of the eye seen through the cornea; it consists of smooth muscles that regulate pupil size

Ischemic stroke A stroke caused by a brain blood vessel blockage

J

Just-in-time ordering A system in which a product is ordered just before it is used

Juvenile rheumatoid arthritis (JRA) Rheumatoid arthritis that affects children

K

Keratolytics Drugs that cause shedding of the outer layer of the skin

L

Lacrimal fluid The fluid in the eye that cleans and lubricates the eyes

Laminar flow hood An environment for the preparation of sterile products

Larynx A hollow muscular organ that forms an air passage to the lungs and holds the vocal cords

Laudanum A mixture of opium and alcohol used to treat dozens of illnesses through the 1800s

Leech A type of segmented worm with suckers that attaches to the skin of a host; leeches engorge themselves on the host's blood

Legend drugs Medications that need a prescription

Lens Flexible, clear tissue that focuses images

Leukemia A progressive, malignant disease of the blood-forming organs, marked by distorted proliferation and development of leukocytes and their precursors in blood and bone marrow

Leukocyte A white blood cell (WBC)

Leukopenia A reduction in the number of leukocytes (white blood cells) in the blood

Licensed pharmacy technician A pharmacy technician who is licensed by the state board; licensing ensures that an individual has at least the minimum level of competency required by the profession

Ligament A fibrous connective tissue that connects to bones

Lithotripsy Treatment with ultrasound shock waves to break kidney stones into small particles

Low-density lipoprotein (LDL) A lipid (fat) and protein combined molecule. It is associated with an increased probability of developing atherosclerosis

Low-density lipoprotein receptor (LDLR) A protein found mainly on liver cells that binds to and removes blood LDL

Lumen A channel within a tube (eg, a blood vessel)

Lymph node A structure that consists of many small, oval nodules that filter lymphatic fluid and fight infection; the site of lymphocyte, monocyte, and plasma cell production

Lymphocyte A mononuclear leukocyte found in the blood, lymph, and lymphoid tissues

Lymphoid organ A component of the system of interconnected tissues and organs by which lymph circulates throughout the body

Lymphoma Cancer of the lymphatic system

M

Maggots Fly larvae that feed on dead tissue; they are used in medicine to clean wounds that do not respond to routine antibiotics

Mammary gland The milk-producing gland of women

Managed care An organized health care delivery system designed to improve both the quality and the accessibility of health care, including pharmaceutical care, while containing costs

Markup The amount (usually a percentage) added to a wholesale price to make a profit

Medicaid A federal- and state-operated insurance program that covers health care costs and prescription drugs for low-income children, adults, and elderly and those with disabilities

Medicare A government-managed insurance program composed of several coverage plans for health care services and supplies; it is funded by both federal and state entities, and individuals must meet specific requirements to be eligible; individuals must be 65 years or older, or younger than 65 with long-term disabilities, or suffer from end-stage renal disease

Medicare Modernization Act (MMA) A law that provides for prescription drug coverage for those covered by Medicare

Medication error Any preventable event that may cause or lead to inappropriate medication use or patient harm

Medication error prevention Methods used by pharmacy, medicine, nursing, and other allied health professionals to prevent medication errors

Medication order A prescription written for administration in a hospital or institutional setting

Medication reconciliation The process of comparing a patient's medication orders with all the medications the patient was taking before admission to the hospital

Medicine The science and art dealing with the maintenance of health and the prevention, alleviation, or cure of disease

Medigap plan Supplemental insurance provided through private insurance companies to help cover costs not reimbursed by the Medicare plan, such as coinsurance, copays, and deductibles

MedMARx A national, Internet-accessible database that hospitals and health care systems use to track adverse drug reactions and medication errors

MedWatch A program established by the FDA for reporting drug and medical product safety alerts and label changes; the program also provides a voluntary adverse event reporting system for medications, medical products, and devices

Melanin A dark brown to black pigment found in the hair, skin, and iris of the eye

Menopause Cessation of menstruation; a natural phenomenon in which a woman passes from a reproductive state to a nonreproductive state

Menses The time of menstruation

Metabolism The processes by which the body breaks down or converts

Metastasize With regard to cancer, to spread from the place of origin as a primary tumor to distant locations in the body

Metric system The approved system of measurement for pharmacy in the United States based on multiples of 10; the basic units of measurement are the gram (g) for weight, the liter (L) for volume, and the meter (m) for length

Micturition Urination

Miosis Constriction of the pupil of the eye

Misbranding Labeling of a product that is false or misleading; label information must include the directions for use; safe and/or unsafe dosages; manufacturer, packer, or distributor; quantity; and weight

Monocyte A phagocytic leukocyte

Monograph Comprehensive information on a medication's actions within that class of drugs; it also lists generic and trade names, ingredients, dosages, side effects, adverse effects, how the patient should take the medication, and foods or other drugs (eg, OTC medications, herbals) to avoid while taking the medication

Morals Beliefs concerning or relating to what is right or wrong in human behavior

Mortar and pestle A bowl and tool with a rounded knob used to grind substances into fine powder or to mix liquids

Motor nerve A nerve carrying impulses from the brain or spinal cord to a muscle or gland

Multiple sclerosis (MS) An autoimmune disorder that affects CNS nerves; it leads to hindered motor function

Muscle fiber Muscle cell

Myasthenia gravis A neuromuscular disorder leading to skeletal muscle weakness

Mydriasis Dilation of the pupil

Myocardial infarction (MI) Myocardial tissue death due to sudden deprivation of oxygenated blood flow, often a result of a blood clot plugging a coronary artery; also known as a *heart attack*

Myocardium The middle muscular layer of the heart wall; it consists of cardiac muscle tissue

Myopia Nearsightedness

Myxedema A condition associated with a decrease in overall adult thyroid function; also known as hypothyroidism

N

Narcotic A nonspecific term used to describe a drug (eg, opium) that in moderate doses dulls the senses, relieves pain, and induces profound sleep but that in excessive doses causes stupor, coma, .or convulsions and may lead to addiction; from the standpoint of US law, opium, opiates (derivatives of opium), and opioids, in addition to cocaine and coca leaves, are "narcotics"

National Association of Boards of Pharmacy (NABP) A national organization for members of state boards of pharmacy

National Coordinating Council for Medication Error Reporting and Prevention (NCC MERP) An independent council of more than 25 organizations, founded by the United States Pharmacopeia (USP), that addresses interdisciplinary causes of medication errors and strategies for prevention

National Drug Code (NDC) number A unique 10- or 11-digit number given to all drugs for identification purposes; in health and drug databases, the NDC has three segments (the first four digits identify the drug manufacturer, the next four identify specifics about the product, and the last two identify the drug packaging); placeholder zeros are inserted in the proper order in the code to standardize data transmissions

National Healthcareer Association (NHA) A certifying organization for a variety of health care careers, including the National Board for Certification of Pharmacy Technicians (NBCPT) and the Institute for the Certification of Pharmacy Technicians (ICPT)

National Pharmacy Technician Association (NPTA) A pharmacy association primarily for technicians: founded in 1999

National Provider Identifier (NPI) A unique, 10-digit identification number for covered health care providers that is issued by the Centers for Medicare and Medicaid Services (CMS) to standardize health data transmissions

Negative feedback A self-regulating mechanism in which the output of a system has input or control on the process; in this case, the stimulus results in reactions that reduce the effects of the stimulus

Negligence A legal concept that describes an action taken without the forethought that should have been used by a reasonable person of similar competency

Nephron The filtering unit of the kidneys

Neuromuscular junction The junction between a nerve fiber and the muscle it supplies

Neuron The nervous system's basic building block and cell

Neutropenia Abnormally low level of neutrophils in the blood

Nicotinic acid A member of the vitamin B complex; also known as niacin

Nitrates A class of drugs used to treat heart conditions, such as angina

NKA No known allergies

NKDA No known drug allergy

Nocturia Urination at night

Nodules Small swellings or aggregations of cells in the body

Nonformulary drugs A list of drugs that are not included in the list of preferred medications that a committee of pharmacists and physicians deems to be the safest, most effective, and most economical; they are drugs not included in the drug list approved for reimbursement by the health care plans unless specific exceptions are filed and accepted by the institutional protocols

Nonproprietary (generic) name A short name coined for a drug or chemical that is not subject to proprietary (trademark) rights and recommended or recognized by an official body

Nonsterile compounding A process of compounding two or more medications in a nonsterile environment (no clean room or hood required)

Nonverbal communication The act of giving or exchanging information without using any spoken words

Nosocomial infection An infection that originates in the hospital or institutional setting

NSAID Nonsteroidal antiinflammatory drug, such as ibuprofen

Nutraceutical A food or supplement with added health benefits

O

Occupational Safety and Health Administration (OSHA) A federal agency that oversees safety in the workplace; OSHA is responsible for establishing the Safety Data Sheet (SDS) requirements

Ointment A hydrophobic product, such as petroleum jelly

Oleaginous base An ingredient used in compounding that does not dissolve in water

Omnibus Budget Reconciliation Act of 1990 (OBRA '90) A law that changed reimbursement limits and mandated drug utilization evaluation, pharmacy patient consultation, and educational outreach programs

Onychomycosis A fungal infection of the fingernails or toenails

Oocyte (ovum) The female reproductive germ cell, more commonly known as an egg

Oogenesis Production or development of an egg

Open formulary A formulary list that is essentially unrestricted in the types of drugs offered or that can be prescribed and reimbursed under the health provider plan or pharmacy benefit plan

Ophthalmic Pertaining to the eye

Opioid analgesic An analgesic medication that activates opioid receptors

Opium An analgesic that is made from the poppy plant

Orbit The eye socket

Orthostatic hypotension A temporary, often rapid lowering of blood pressure, usually related to standing up suddenly

Osmosis Diffusion of fluid through a semipermeable membrane from a solution with a low solute concentration to a solution with a higher solute concentration in an effort to achieve equilibrium

Osmotic pressure The pressure exerted by water flowing through a semipermeable membrane separating two solutions with different concentrations of solutes

Osteoarthritis (OA) Degeneration of joint cartilage and the underlying bone

Osteoporosis A medical condition in which the bones become brittle and fragile from loss of bone density and poor microarchitecture

Otic Pertaining to the ear

Ototoxicity Toxic effects on the organs of hearing or balance or on the auditory nerve

Outpatient pharmacies Pharmacies that serve patients in community or ambulatory settings

Ovaries The female reproductive organs in which ova, or eggs, are produced

Over-the-counter (OTC) medication A nonprescription medicine generally found outside the secure part of the pharmacy

Ovulation Release of an egg from the ovary

P

Package insert The official prescribing information for a prescription drug; the medication information sheet provided by the manufacturer that includes side effects, dosage forms, indications, and other important information

Palliative Something that brings relief but does not cure

Pallor A deficiency in color, particularly of the face

Pancreas An endocrine gland that produces both insulin and glucagon

Papules Small, raised, solid pimples on the skin

PAR See *periodic automatic replacement (PAR) level*

Parasympathetic nervous system (PSNS) An autonomic nervous system division that functions during rest

Parenteral A term indicating administration of a substance by a route other than by mouth

Parenteral medication A medication that bypasses the digestive system but is intended for systemic action; the term most commonly describes medications given by injection, such as intravenously or intramuscularly

Parkinson disease (PD) A movement disorder with the classic symptoms of tremor, rigidity, bradykinesia, and postural instability

Patient profile An electronic or written record listing important patient personal and health information, including comprehensive information on the medications the patient takes, disease states, and any food or drug allergies the patient may have

Pelvic inflammatory disease (PID) Inflammation of the female genital tract, accompanied by fever and lower abdominal pain

Perception The way a person thinks about or understands someone or something

Pericardium A fluid-filled membrane that surrounds the heart; also called the pericardial sac

Periodic automatic replacement (PAR) level A minimum set amount of stock that must be kept on hand

Peripheral nervous system (PNS) The nervous system division outside the brain and spinal cord

Peripheral neuropathy Damage to nerves of the peripheral nervous system

Peripheral parenteral administration Injection of a medication into the veins on the periphery of the body rather than a central vein or artery

Peripheral parenteral nutrition (PPN) Intravenous nutrition administered through the veins on the periphery of the body rather than through a central vein or artery

Peripheral resistance Vascular resistance to the flow of blood in peripheral arterial vessels

Peristalsis Tubular muscle contraction and relaxation of the esophagus, stomach, and intestines to move substances through the gastrointestinal tract

Peritonitis Inflammation of the peritoneum, typically caused by bacterial infection

Perspiration The process of sweating

Phagocyte A cell of the immune system that engulfs cells, debris, and antigens

Pharmacist A health care professional who dispenses drugs and counsels patients on the use of medications and any interactions the drugs may have with food or other drugs

Pharmacokinetics The study of the absorption, metabolism, distribution, and elimination of drugs

Pharmacy A place where drugs are sold

Pharmacy and therapeutics committee (P&T committee) A medical staff composed of physicians, pharmacists, pharmacy technicians, nurses, and dieticians, who provide necessary information and advice to the institution or insurer on whether a drug should be added to a formulary

Pharmacy benefit management (PBM) The development and management of broad and cost-efficient prescription drug benefits for a large group of patient populations

Pharmacy clerk A person who assists the pharmacist at the front counter of the pharmacy; the person who accepts payment for medications

Pharmacy technician A person who assists a pharmacist by filling prescriptions and performing other nondiscretionary tasks

Pharmacy Technician Certification Board (PTCB) A national board for the certification of pharmacy technicians; the PTCB provides a national exam for pharmacy technicians

Pharmacy Technician Educators Council (PTEC) A US organization that promotes teachers' strategies and instructions for pharmacy technician education

Pharynx The membrane-lined cavity behind the nose and mouth that connects them to the esophagus

Phlebotomy The act or practice of opening a vein by incision or puncture to remove blood

Physicians' Desk Reference **(PDR)** One of the many reference books on medications; it compiles and publishes select manufacturer-provided package inserts and prescribing information useful for health professionals

Plasma The clear, yellowish fluid portion of blood

Plasma cell A cell of the immune system that secretes antibodies

Plasma protein Any of the dissolved proteins of blood plasma

Pleural cavity The cavity in the thorax that contains the lungs and heart

Point of sale (POS) A system that allows inventory to be tracked as it is used

Polycythemia An increase in the total cell mass of the blood

Polyneuropathy A neurologic disorder that occurs when many nerves malfunction; it may include painful neuropathy

Precipitate To separate from solution or suspension; a solid that emerges from a liquid solution

Preferred provider organization (PPO) An insurance plan in which patients choose a provider from a specified list, resulting in reduced costs for medical services

Prefix A meaningful stem in a generic name in the beginning of the word (eg, *cef*dinir)

Pregnancy Category A system used by the FDA to describe five levels of assessment of the fetal effects caused by a drug; a required section of current prescription drug labeling; introduced in 1979, the system is currently under reevaluation for usefulness and inclusion on the prescription label

Prescription An order for medication issued by a physician, dentist, or other properly licensed practitioner, such as a physician assistant or nurse practitioner

Prime vendor A large distributor of medications and retail products that contracts with the pharmacy to deliver the bulk of the pharmacy's medications in exchange for lower prices (eg, McKesson, Cardinal Health, and AmerisourceBergen)

Prior authorization Insurance-required approval for a restricted, non-formulary, or noncovered medication before a prescription medication can be filled

PRN An abbreviation for a Latin term *(pro re nata)* meaning "as needed"

Prodrug An inactive substance that is converted to a drug in the body by the action of enzymes or other chemicals

Professionalism Conforming to the right principles of conduct (work ethics) as accepted by others in the profession

Progesterone An anabolic sex hormone that stimulates the uterus to prepare for pregnancy

Prophylactic Treatment given before an event or exposure to prevent the condition or symptom

Prophylaxis Treatment or measure to prevent disease

Proprotein convertase subtilisin/kexin type 9 (PCSK9) An enzyme that binds to and breaks down LDLR

Prostaglandin A mediator responsible for the features of inflammation, such as swelling, pain, stiffness, redness, and warmth

Prostate A gland surrounding the neck of the bladder in males that produces a fluid component of semen

Protected health information (PHI) A patient's personal health data; under HIPAA, this information is protected from sharing or distribution without permission

Protocol A set of standards and guidelines by which a facility operates

Pruritus Itching

Psychosis A mental illness characterized by loss of contact with reality. Psychosis may be a genuine mental illness due to an underlying medical condition (eg, dementia, drug withdrawal syndromes) or induced by medications, recreational drugs, or poisons

Pulmonary artery One of two vessels formed as terminal branches of the pulmonary trunk; conveys unaerated blood to the lungs

Punch method Manual filling of capsules with powdered medication that has been premixed

Pupil The circular opening in the iris that allows light to enter

Pustules Small blisters or pimples on the skin containing pus

Pyxis An automated dispensing system

R

RAAS Renin-angiotensin-aldosterone system, helps regulate blood pressure

Reconstitute To add a diluent (eg, saline or sterile water) to a powder to form a suspension or solution

Refill Permission by a prescriber to replenish a prescription

Registered pharmacy technician (RPhT) A pharmacy technician who is registered through the state board of pharmacy; the registration process helps maintain a list of those working in pharmacies

Renal artery One of the pair of arteries that branch from the abdominal aorta; each kidney has one renal artery

Renal osteodystrophy A condition resulting from chronic kidney disease (CKD) and renal failure; it is marked by elevated serum phosphorus levels, low or normal serum calcium levels, and stimulation of parathyroid function, resulting in bone disease

Renal vein The vein in which filtered blood from the kidneys is sent back into the body's circulatory system; each kidney has one renal vein

Renin An enzyme secreted by and stored in the kidneys that promotes the production of the protein angiotensin; it is released by the kidney in response to low sodium levels or blood volume

Repackaging The act of reducing the amount of medication taken from a bulk bottle

Resorption The process or action by which something is reabsorbed (eg, bone resorption in the development of osteoporosis)

Resorption (bone) Removal of osseous tissue by osteoclasts

Retail price The wholesale price plus markup

Retina The innermost layer of the eye; a complex structure considered part of the central nervous system (CNS); the retina contains photoreceptors (rods and cones) that transmit impulses to the optic nerve, in addition to the macula lutea (a yellow spot in the center of the retina)

Reye syndrome A life-threatening metabolic disorder of uncertain cause in young children; aspirin use may precipitate the syndrome

Rheumatic fever A noncontagious acute fever marked by inflammation and pain in the joints

Rheumatoid arthritis (RA) A progressive degenerative and crippling autoimmune joint disease

Risk evaluation and mitigation strategy (REMS) A strategy to manage a known or potential serious risk associated with a drug or biological product

S

Safety Data Sheets (SDSs) Documents that provide chemical product information; an SDS includes the product name, composition (chemicals in the product), hazards, toxicology, and other information regarding the proper steps to take with spills, accidental exposure, handling, and storage of the product; filing of an SDS in the pharmacy or workplace is usually a requirement to meet Occupational Safety and Health Administration (OSHA) standards; formerly known as Material Safety Data Sheets

Satellite pharmacy A specialty pharmacy located away from the central pharmacy, such as with an operating room (OR), emergency department (ED), or a neonatal pharmacy; it typically is staffed by a pharmacist and a pharmacy technician

Schizophrenia A disorder characterized by inappropriate emotions and unrealistic thinking

Sclera The white of the eyes

Sebaceous glands Skin glands responsible for the secretion of oil called sebum

Seborrhea Excessive discharge of sebum from the sebaceous glands

Sebum An oily/waxy substance that lubricates the skin and retains water to provide moisture

Secondary hypertension Hypertension that results from an underlying identifiable cause

Serum The clear, yellowish fluid obtained by separating whole blood into its solid and liquid components after it has been allowed to clot; plasma minus clotting factors

Shaman A person who holds a high place of honor in a tribe as a healer and spiritual mediator

Signatura (signa or sig) The directions on a prescription that explain how the patient is to take the prescribed medication; a Latin expression meaning to "write on label"

Skeletal muscle Muscle that is connected to the skeleton to form part of the mechanical system that moves the limbs and other parts of the body

Skeletal system The hard structure (bones and cartilages) that provides a frame for the body

Society for the Education of Pharmacy Technicians (SEPhT) A national pharmacy technician organization that promotes the education and training of pharmacy technicians; it provides links to medication safety and quality practices for technicians

Sole proprietorship An unincorporated business owned by one person

Solute A substance dissolved in another substance; usually the component of a solution present in less amount

Solution A water base in which the ingredient or ingredients are dissolved completely

Solvent The greater part of a solution that dissolves a solute

Somatic nervous system The motor neurons of the peripheral nervous system that control voluntary actions of the skeletal muscles and provide sensory input (touch, hearing, sight)

Sperm (plural, spermatozoa) The male reproductive germ cell

Spermatogenesis The development of sperm in the testes

Spermicide An agent that kills sperm

Spleen A lymphatic organ involved in blood cell production and removal as well as lymphocyte storage

Splenectomy Surgical removal of the spleen

Spongy bone Meshwork of spongy bone typically found at the core of vertebral bones in the spine and the ends of long bones, also known as cancellous bone

Sputum Fluid (mucus) expectorated from the lungs and bronchial tissues

Staff of Asclepius The symbol of the medical profession; it is a wingless staff with one snake wrapped around it

Standard operating procedures (SOPs) Written guidelines and criteria that list specific steps for various competencies

Standard Precautions (Universal Precautions) A set of standards that reduces the possibility of contamination and the risk of transmission of infectious disease; Standard Precautions are used throughout a health care facility, including to prepare medications

Standing order Written protocols for drugs or treatment that is to be used in a specific situation

Statin An informal term for HMG-CoA reductase inhibitors referring to the last six letters in the name of each medication name in the class, for example, atorvastatin, simvastatin. Used for the treatment of hyperlipidemia, primarily to lower LDL cholesterol

Stat order A medication order that must be filled immediately; that is, as quickly as is safely possible to prepare the dose, usually within 5 to 15 minutes

Stem A meaningful group of letters in a generic name that allows one to classify the medication by those letters

Stent A tube designed inserted into a vessel or passageway to keep it open

Sterile preparation A preparation that contains no living microorganisms

Stress incontinence Involuntary emission of urine when pressure in the abdomen suddenly increases

Strip pack A strip of heat-sealed packets, each holding one tablet or capsule, that is used in the bulk repackaging process

Stroke The sudden death of brain cells due to oxygen deprivation when brain blood flow is impaired by blockage (ischemic stroke) or rupture (hemorrhagic stroke) of an artery to the brain

Subchondral bone Bone located below the cartilage, particularly within a joint

Subcutaneous layer The deepest layer of the skin, consisting of fat cells and collagen; it protects the body and conserves heat

Subscription The part of the prescription that provides specific instructions to the pharmacist on how to compound the prescription

Superscription The heading of a prescription, represented by the Latin symbol Rx, meaning "take thou" or "you take"; the symbol has come to represent prescription or pharmacy

SureMed An automated dispensing system often used in hospitals

Surface area Extent of an object's surface in contact with its surroundings

Suspension A solution in which the powder does not dissolve into the base; the solution must be shaken before use

Sweat glands Glands in the dermis that are activated by an increase in body temperature to cool the body

Sympathetic nervous system (SNS) An autonomic nervous system division that activates during stress; the "fight-or-flight" response

Sympathomimetic Producing physiologic effects resembling those caused by the sympathetic nervous system

Syndrome A set of conditions that occur together

Synovium A thin membrane in synovial (freely moving) joints that lines the joint capsule and secretes synovial fluid

Synthetic medicine A medication made in a laboratory from chemical processes

Syrup A sugar-based liquid

Systemic Pertaining to the entire organism; "widespread" in contrast to "local"

Systemic lupus erythematosus (SLE) An autoimmune inflammatory disease of connective tissue with variable features, including fever, weakness, fatigue, and other systemic manifestations

Systole The period when the heart is contracting, specifically when the left ventricle of the heart contracts

T

Tachycardia A rapid heart rate, usually defined as greater than 100 beats per minute

Tact The ability to do or say things without offending or upsetting other people

Tardive dyskinesia (TD) A type of dyskinesia (unwanted, involuntary rhythmic movements) recognized as a potential side effect of dopamine antagonists (eg, phenothiazines, metoclopramide); the symptoms may continue even after the offending drug is discontinued

Telepharmacy The provision of pharmaceutical care through the use of telecommunications and information technologies to patients at a distance

Tendon A flexible but inelastic cord of strong fibrous collagen tissue that attaches a muscle to a bone

Teratogen Any agent that causes abnormal embryonic or fetal development

Testes The male reproductive organs that produce sperm

Testosterone An anabolic sex hormone produced in the testes that stimulates the development of male sexual characteristics

The Joint Commission (TJC) An independent, nonprofit organization that accredits hospitals and other health care organizations in the United States; accreditation is required to accept Medicare and Medicaid payments

Therapeutic alliance A trust relationship between a health care professional and a patient that incorporates the patient's perceptions of the acceptability of interventions and mutually agreed upon goals for treatment

Thrombin A blood coagulation enzyme from prothrombin; thrombin reacts with fibrinogen and converts it to fibrin, which is essential in the formation of blood clots; thrombin levels are tested by performing a prothrombin time or partial thromboplastin time blood test

Thrombocyte A platelet

Thrombocytopenia A decrease in the number of platelets in the blood

Thrombolytic A medication used to break up a thrombus or blood clot

Thrombosis The formation or presence of a blood clot in a blood vessel

Thyroxine (T$_4$) A thyroid hormone derived from tyrosine (amino acid) that influences the metabolic rate

Tinnitus Ringing or buzzing in the ears

Tort An act that causes harm or injury to a person intentionally or because of negligence

Total parenteral nutrition (TPN) Large-volume intravenous nutrition administered through the central vein (eg, subclavian vein), which allows for a higher concentration of solutions

Toxoid A vaccine type in which a toxin has been rendered harmless but still invokes an antigenic response, improving immunity against the active toxin at some future date

Traditional Chinese medicine Complementary and alternative medicine whole medical system that includes a range of traditional medicine practices originating in China

Transient ischemic attack (TIA) A neurologic event in which the signs and symptoms of a stroke appear but resolve within a short time

Transplant rejection An immune response after tissue or organ transplantation

Treatment authorization request (TAR) The process used by Medicare and Medicaid for authorization of assistive technology devices costing more than $100; durable medical equipment (eg, wheelchairs, walkers) also requires a TAR; similar to a preauthorization form

Trephining The practice of making an opening in the head to allow disease to leave the body

TRICARE A health benefit program for active-duty and retired personnel in all seven US uniformed services. It also covers dependents of military personnel who were killed while on active duty; formerly CHAMPUS

Triglyceride The dominant form of body-stored fat consisting of three fatty acid molecules and a molecule of the alcohol glycerol

Triiodothyronine (T$_3$) A thyroid hormone that helps regulate growth and development and controls metabolism and body temperature; it is mainly produced through the metabolism of thyroxine

Triturate To grind or crush powder (eg, a tablet) into fine particles

Troche A flat, disklike tablet that dissolves between the gum and cheek

Tubular reabsorption The conservation of protein, glucose, bicarbonate, and water from the glomerular filtrate by the tubules

Tubular secretion A function of the nephron in which ions, toxins, and water are secreted into the collecting duct to be excreted

Tympanic membrane A thin membrane that separates the external ear from the middle ear; also known as the eardrum

Type 1 diabetes mellitus (T1DM) A form of diabetes mellitus associated with an absolute deficiency of insulin production by the pancreas; people with T1DM require insulin therapy

Type 2 diabetes mellitus (T2DM) A form of diabetes mellitus associated with insulin resistance and a relative deficiency of insulin; people with T2DM can be treated with oral therapies, noninsulin injectable medications, and insulin

U

Unit dose A single dose of a drug; individualized packaged doses used in institutional practice settings

United States Pharmacopeia (USP) An independent, nonprofit organization that establishes documentation on product quality standards, drug quality and information, and health care information on medications, over-the-counter products, dietary supplements, and food ingredients to ensure the appropriate purity, quality, and strength; Chapter 797 (Pharmaceutical Compounding—Sterile Preparations) in the USP-NF is a set of enforceable sterile compounding standards and describes the guidelines, procedures, and compliance requirements for compounding sterile preparations; it also establishes the standards that apply to all settings in which sterile preparations are compounded

United States Pharmacopeia–National Formulary (USP-NF) A publication of the USP that contains standards for medications, dosage forms, drug substances, excipients, medical devices, and dietary supplements

Ureteroscopy Examination of the upper urinary tract, usually performed with an endoscope passed through the urethra

Urethritis Inflammation of the urethra

Urge incontinence Urinary incontinence because of involuntary bladder contractions that result in an urgent need to urinate

Uric acid The water-insoluble end product of purine metabolism; deposition of uric acid as crystals in the joints and kidneys causes gout

Urinary acidification The conversion of urine to a more acidic content

Urolithiasis Solid mineral deposits that form stones in the urinary tract

Urticaria Red welts that arise on the surface of the skin; they are often attributable to an allergic reaction but may have nonallergic causes; also known as *hives*

USANC United States Adopted Names Council, the body that makes decisions on drug names

Uterus The organ in the lower abdomen of a woman where gestation of a fetus occurs

V

Vaccine A biological preparation that improves immunity to a particular disease by invoking an immune response and a "memory" of the response for future use

Vasoconstriction Blood vessel narrowing resulting from contraction of the vessel muscular walls

Vasodilation Widening of blood vessel, relaxation of muscular vessel wall, leading to increased blood flow

Vasopressin Another term used for antidiuretic hormone (ADH)

Vein A vessel that carries deoxygenated blood to or toward the heart

Vena cava One of the two large veins that carry deoxygenated blood from the upper (superior vena cava) and lower (inferior vena cava) parts of the body to the right atrium of the heart

Ventricle One of the two lower chambers of the heart

Verbal communication The sharing of information by individuals through the use of speech

Vertical laminar flow hood An environment for the preparation of chemotherapeutic and other hazardous agents in which air originating from the roof of the hood moves downward (over the agent) and is captured in a vent on the floor of the hood

Virion A virus particle

Virus A microscopic, nonliving organism that replicates exclusively inside the host's cell using parts of the host cell, including DNA, ribosomes, and proteins

Vitreous humor A gel-like substance that fills the posterior cavity of the eye between the lens and retina; it helps maintain the shape of the eye

Volume The amount of liquid in a container

von Willebrand disease The most common inherited bleeding disorder, associated with a deficiency in the clotting protein von Willebrand factor

W

Whole blood Blood drawn from the body from which no constituent, such as plasma or platelets, has been removed

Wholesale cost The purchase price of a product (eg, medicine) that is then marked up for resale

Wholesalers Companies that stock a variety of drug manufacturers' medications and normally have a "just-in-time" turnaround for ordered drugs; this means that drugs ordered today will arrive tomorrow

Workers' compensation Government-required and government-enforced medical coverage for workers injured on the job, paid for by the employer. The programs are managed by each state in accordance with the state's workers' compensation laws

X

Xerosis Abnormal dryness of the skin, eyes, or mucous membranes

INDEX

A

AAPT. *see* American Association of Pharmacy Technicians
Abacavir, for human immunodeficiency virus infection and acquired immunodeficiency syndrome, 570t
Abatacept, 585–587t, 589, 589–590b
Abbreviations, 167–168t, 265t
  for allergies, 194b
  "Do Not Use List" of, 96, 97–102t
  for dosage forms, 96, 112t
  for dosing schedules, 137b
  for drops, 141b
  in *Drug Topics Red Book*, 152
  for IV supplies, 257, 258t
  for medical field, 121t
  origins of, 96
  primary units and areas, 208b
  for routes of administration, 96, 112–114, 112t
Abducens nerve, 373t
Abilify. *see* Aripiprazole
Abortifacient, 558
Absinthe, 9
Absorica. *see* Isotretinoin
Absorption, 116, 116f, 506, 507f, 527
  bases, 244b
ACA. *see* Affordable Care Act
Academy of Managed Care Pharmacy (AMCP), 315
ACAM2000, 592–593t
Acarbose, 398–400t, 421–422t
Accessibility, of over-the-counter medications, 662
Accolate. *see* Zafirlukast
Accreditation Council for Pharmacy Education (ACPE), 59
Acebutolol, 458t
Acetadote. *see* Acetylcysteine
Acetaminophen, 357, 430b, 430f
  caplets, 106
  common adult dosage of, 664t
  for cough and cold symptoms, 666t
  for osteoarthritis, 429–430, 429b, 434t
  in over-the-counter medications, 663, 664b
Acetaminophen/codeine, 426–427t
Acetazolamide, 537t
Acetylcholine, 372
Acetylcholinesterase, 372, 379t
Acetylcysteine, 492t
Acidosis, 527–528
Aciphex. *see* Rabeprazole
Acitretin, 632t
Aclidinium, 495b, 495f
Acne Medication. *see* Benzoyl peroxide

Acne vulgaris, 626–628, 626b, 626f, 627t
ACPE. *see* Accreditation Council for Pharmacy Education
Acquired immunodeficiency syndrome, treatment for, 570t
Acromegaly, 398–400t, 411, 411f
Act, 23
Actemra. *see* Tocilizumab
ACTH. *see* Adrenocorticotropic hormone
ActHIB, 592–593t
Actin, 427
Activase. *see* Alteplase
Active acquired immunity, 594
Active pharmaceutical ingredient (API), 229–230
Active transport, 529
Actonel. *see* Risedronate
Actos. *see* Pioglitazone
Acular. *see* Ketorolac
Acupressure, 674t, 681, 682f
Acupuncture, 674t, 681, 681f
Acute inflammation, 583–584, 584f
Acute lymphoblastic leukemia (ALL), 652–656
Acute myeloblastic leukemia (AML), 652–656
Acyclovir, 569t, 633
Aczone. *see* Dapsone
AD. *see* Alzheimer disease
Adacel, 592–593t
Adalat. *see* Nifedipine
Adalimumab, 514t, 585–587t, 589b, 589f, 632t
Adamantane antivirals, for influenza, 490t
Adapalene, 627t
Adaptability, 79
Adaptive immunity, 583f
Adderall. *see* Amphetamine/dextroamphetamine
Adderall XR. *see* Amphetamine/dextroamphetamine
Addison disease, 398–400t, 409t, 416–417, 416–417b
  therapeutic agents for, 357
Additives, 118–119, 119t, 236, 237t
  parenteral, 280, 280t
  for taste, 237t
ADD-Vantage system, 276, 276f
Adefovir, for hepatitis B, 571t
Adenovirus vaccine, 592–593t
ADEs. *see* Adverse drug events
ADH. *see* Antidiuretic hormone
ADHD. *see* Attention-deficit/hyperactivity disorder
Adipose tissue, 624f
Adjudication, 171–172, 172t, 290
Administration, medication error in, 317t
Adrenal cortex, 404–405, 406f, 531

Adrenal glands, 404–405, 405f
  conditions of, 409t, 415–418
    Addison disease, 416–417
    Cushing disease, 415–416, 416f
    hyperaldosteronism, 416
  functions of, 402t
Adrenal medulla, 404–405, 406f
  conditions affecting, 418
Adrenergic agents, 610t
Adrenergic agonist, 475–476t
  for conditions affecting the eye, 599–600t,
    603–604t
Adrenocorticotropic hormone (ACTH), 402t
ADS. see Automated dispensing system
Adulteration, 21–22, 23
Advair Diskus. see Fluticasone/salmeterol
Advair HFA. see Fluticasone/salmeterol
Adverse drug events (ADEs), 215
Adverse effect, medication errors and, 318
Adverse reactions, 44
  reporting of, 31, 31b, 32f
Advil. see Ibuprofen
Aerosols, 109–110
Affordability, of over-the-counter medications, 662
Affordable Care Act (ACA), 292, 292b
Afinitor. see Everolimus
Afluria Quadrivalent, 592–593t
Afrezza, 109–110
Afrin. see Oxymetazoline
Afrin Allergy Sinus. see Oxymetazoline
Aggrastat. see Tirofiban
Aggrenox. see Aspirin/dipyridamole
AHFS DI. see American Hospital Formulary Service Drug
    Information
Air lock, 267b
Air pressure, 267b
Airflow, 267–269
Akinetic seizure, 376t
Alamast. see Pemirolast
Albumin, 645
Albuterol, 109–110, 354, 492t, 495b, 495f
Albuterol sulfate, 109–110
Albuterol/ipratropium, 492t
Alcohol, 9, 9b
Aldactone. see Spironolactone
Alderton, Charles, 13t
Aldomet. see Methyldopa
Aldosterone, 402t, 416, 453–457
Aldosterone antagonists, 537t
Aldosterone inhibitors, 475–476t
Alemtuzumab, 585–587t, 654–655t
Alendronate, 426–427t, 440b, 440f, 441t
Aleve. see Naproxen
Alfuzosin, 565t
Alirocumab, 463t, 466b
Aliskiren, 456b, 456f, 459–460t
Alkalosis, 527–528

Alka-Seltzer. see Sodium bicarbonate/citric acid/potassium
    bicarbonate
Alka-Seltzer Gold. see Sodium bicarbonate/citric acid/
    potassium bicarbonate
Alkylating agents, 653, 654–655t
ALL. see Acute lymphoblastic leukemia
Allegra. see Fexofenadine
Allegra Allergy 12/24 hour. see Fexofenadine
Allergens, 488
Allergic conjunctivitis, 604–605, 604b, 604f
Allergic rhinitis, 616
  therapeutic agents for, 360
Allergies, 486t, 488–489, 488b, 488t
  anaphylaxis and, 584
  medication error and, 324–325
  therapeutic agent for, 358
  treatment of, over-the-counter medications for, 664, 665t
Alli. see Orlistat
Alligation alternate, 144, 145b
Allopurinol, 426–427t, 443t, 536b, 536f
Almacone. see AlOH, MgOH, and simethicone
Almotriptan, 364–366t
Alocril. see Nedocromil
Alogliptin, 398–400t, 421–422t
AlOH, MgOH, and simethicone, 510t
AlOH and magnesium carbonate, 510t
AlOH and MgOH, 510t
Alomide. see Lodoxamide
Alopecia, 624
Alosetron, 516b, 516f
Alpha-2 adrenergic agonists, 459–460t
Alpha-adrenergic blockers, 566
Alpha-blockers, 449–451t
Alpha-1 blockers, 565b, 565t
Alpha-glucosidase inhibitors, 398–400t
Alpha-4 integrin antagonist, 514t
Alpha-1 receptor blockers, 459–460t
Alphagan P. see Brimonidine
5-Alpha-reductase inhibitors, 546–547t, 565b, 565t
  birth defects and, 566b
  for conditions affecting the male and female reproductive
    systems, 546–547t, 565–566
Alprazolam, 364–366t, 388b, 388f
Alprostadil, 568t
Altabax. see Retapamulin
Altace. see Ramipril
Alteplase (t-PA), 470t, 472t
Alternative medicine. see Complementary and alternative
    medicine
Altoprev. see Lovastatin
Aluminum hydroxide, 509t
Alveolar sacs, 480, 481f
Alveoli, 481
Alzheimer disease (AD), 378, 378b
  stages associated with, 379t
  treatment of, 364–366t, 379t
AMA. see American Medical Association

Amantadine, 364–366t, 381t, 490t
Amaryl. *see* Glimepiride
Ambien. *see* Zolpidem
Amcinonide, 632t
Amcort. *see* Amcinonide
Amendment, 23
Amenorrhea, 553b
American Association of Pharmacy Technicians (AAPT), 77t, 78
American Drug Index, 155
American Hospital Formulary Service Drug Information (AHFS DI), 152–153, 157t
American Medical Association (AMA), 183, 217
American Pharmacists Association (APhA), 13, 59, 77, 77t
American Recovery and Reinvestment Act (2009), 197–198
American Sign Language (ASL), 91, 91b
American Society of Health-System Pharmacists (ASHP), 13, 58–59, 77t, 78, 316, 338
  certification from, 216–217
  institutional technicians and, 200b
  on medication errors, 318, 319b
  Model Curriculum for Pharmacy Technician Education and Training, 68–70, 68–70b
  Pharmacy Practice Model Initiative, 210–211
Amiloride, 537t
Amino acids, 280, 506
Aminoglycosides, 607–608t
5-Aminosalicylates, 514t
Amiodarone, 281t, 322t, 474t
Amitiza. *see* Lubiprostone
Amitriptyline, 364–366t, 385b, 385f, 386–387t
AML. *see* Acute myeloblastic leukemia
Amlodipine, 457b, 457f, 459–460t
Amnesteem. *see* Isotretinoin
Amoxicillin, 615t
  for bacterial sinusitis, 619b, 619f
Amoxicillin plus clavulanate, 615t, 617–618b, 617f
Amoxicillin/clavulanate suspension, 111
Amphetamine/dextroamphetamine, 364–366t, 394t
Ampicillin, 277t
Ampicillin/sulbactam, 560t
Ampule breaker, 259t
Ampules, 261f
  medication preparation, aseptic technique in, 274–276
  proper manipulation of, 275f
Ampyra. *see* Dalfampridine
Amrix. *see* Cyclobenzaprine
Anabolic Steroids Control Act, 30t
Anakinra, 585–587t
Analgesics, 663, 666t
  delivery systems for
    cassette system, patient-controlled, 263, 264f
    continuous, 263
    syringe system, patient-controlled, 263
  opioid, 426–427t
  for otitis media, 615t
Anaphylaxis, 584, 584b

Ancef. *see* Cefazolin
Ancient beliefs, medicine and, 4
AndroGel. *see* Testosterone
Androgen, 563b
  functions of, 548t
  for male and female reproductive system conditions, 546–547t, 551, 552–553t
  supplements for, 563t
Anemia, 647–649
  classification of, 648t
  iron deficiency, 644t, 647–649, 647b, 648f, 649t
Anesthetics
  for conditions affecting the ear, 599–600t
  for cough and cold symptoms, 666t
Aneurysm, 472–473
Angina, 466
Angina pectoris, 466–468, 467f
Angiomax. *see* Bivalirudin
Angioplasty, 467–468b
Angiotensin I, 531
Angiotensin II, 453, 531
Angiotensin receptor blockers (ARBs), 449–451t, 459–460t
Angiotensin II receptor antagonists, 455, 455b
  for cardiovascular system, 358
Angiotensin-converting enzyme (ACE) inhibitors, 322t
  for cardiac conditions, 449–451t, 453–454, 454b, 458t, 459–460t, 475–476t
  for cardiovascular system, 358
Anions, 531
Anoro Ellipta. *see* Umeclidinium/vilanterol
Anovulation, 555
ANS. *see* Autonomic nervous system
Antacids, 508
  for GERD, 509, 509t, 510t
    and indigestion, 667t
  interactions, 508b
Ante area, 265t
Anteroom, 267, 267b
Anthracenedione, 585–587t
Anthracyclines, 654–655t
Anthrax, 592–593t
Antiandrogens, 568t
Antianginal agents, 472t
Antiarrhythmics, 449–451t
Antibacterials, 623–624t, 637t
Antibiotics, 237t
  for colds, 490b
  for impetigo, 637b
  for leukemia, 653
  parenteral, 277, 277b, 277t
  for urinary tract infections, 526–527t
Antibodies, 579
Antibody-mediated immunity, 580–582
Anticholinergics, 372, 379t, 381t, 479t, 603–604t
  for asthma and COPD, 492t, 495
  for urinary incontinence, 540b, 541t
Anticoagulant technician, 64

Anticoagulants, 449–451t, 469, 470, 470t

Anticonvulsants, 377t

Antidepressants, liothyronine and, 414b

Antidiarrheals, for gastrointestinal conditions, 668t

Antidiuretic hormone (ADH), 402t, 403–404

Antiemetics, 521b, 668t

Antifungals, 607–608t
  for dermatological conditions, 623–624t
  for fungal infections, 635–636b, 636t
  for onychomycosis, 640–641b

Antigen, 579

Antigen-presenting cell (APC), 579

Antihistamine/decongestant, for allergy, 665t

Antihistamine/mast cell stabilizer, for allergy, 665t

Antihistamines, 237t, 479t
  for allergies, 488t
  for allergy symptoms, 617t
  for colds, 486, 666t
  for conditions affecting the eye, 599–600t, 603–604t, 605t
  for cough, 666t
  for hypertension, 457b
  for insomnia, 392t
  for nausea and vomiting, 668t
  topical, 628b
  for urticaria, 628b

Antihyperlipidemics, 449–451t

Anti-IgE antibody, for asthma and COPD, 492t

Antiinfectives
  for conditions affecting the ear, 599–600t, 607–608t
  for conditions affecting the eye, 599–600t

Antiinflammatory drugs, 663
  for asthma, 358

Antimetabolite agents, 585–587t, 653, 654–655t

Antimuscarinic medications, for urinary incontinence, 541t

Antineoplastic agents, 656

Antiplatelet agents, 449–451t, 458t, 470t, 471, 472t

Antipyretics, 663–664, 666t

Antiseptics, for onychomycosis, 641b

Antitoxins, 576–577t, 596, 596b

Antitussives, 486–487, 664, 666t

Antivenins, 596, 596b

Antivirals, 607–608t
  for hepatitis C, 571t
  therapeutic agents for, 359

Anxiety, therapeutic agents for, 356

Anxiety disorders, 364–366t, 387–388, 387b

Aorta, 451–452

APC. see Antigen-presenting cell

APhA. see American Pharmacists Association

Aphasia, 182–183

API. see Active pharmaceutical ingredient

Apidra. see Insulin glulisine

Apixaban, 470t

Aplastic anemia, 648t

Apnea, 484t

Apothecary system, 8, 135, 135b, 135f

Apresoline. see Hydralazine

Apriso. see Mesalamine

Aqueous humor, 601–602

Arabic numerals, 127, 127t

Aranesp. see Darbepoetin alfa

ARBs. see Angiotensin receptor blockers

Arformoterol, 492t

Argatroban, 470t

Aricept. see Donepezil

Aripiprazole, 364–366t, 390b, 390f

Aristotle, 5–6

Arixtra. see Fondaparinux

Armour Thyroid. see Desiccated thyroid; Thyroid

Army Medical Corps, 4, 5f

Aromatherapy, 674t

Aromatic spirits of ammonia, 108

Arrector pili muscle, 624f, 625f

Arrhythmias, 474t

ART. see Assisted reproductive technology

Artane. see Trihexyphenidyl

Arteriosclerosis, 466

Artery, 451, 625f

Arthritis
  gouty, 440–441b, 442f
  psoriatic, 630–631b
  rheumatoid, 427, 588–590, 588f, 589b

Arthroplasty, 427–428, 428–429b

Asacol. see Mesalamine

Asacol HD. see Mesalamine

ASAP order, 197

Asclepius, 4

Aseptic technique, 204, 271–272, 274f
  donning of gloves and gown, 272
  hand hygiene in, 273b
  hand placement in, 273, 273b, 275f
  personnel cleansing and garbing order in, 274b
  in use of ampules to prepare medications, 274–276
  vials and, 276, 276b

ASHP. see American Society of Health-System Pharmacists

ASL. see American Sign Language

Aspiration, 481b

Aspiration pneumonia, 481b, 498

Aspirin, 357, 426–427t, 431b, 431f, 434t, 458t, 470t
  common adult dosage of, 664t
  inhibition of prostaglandins, 583
  niacin and, 465b
  for osteoarthritis, 430–431

Aspirin/dipyridamole, 470t

Assisted reproductive technology (ART), for infertility, 555b

Associations, for pharmacy technicians, 77, 77t

Astagraf XL. see Tacrolimus

Asthma, 490–495, 491b, 491f, 492t, 493f, 494b
  therapeutic agent for, 358

Atacand. see Candesartan

Atazanavir, for human immunodeficiency virus infection and acquired immunodeficiency syndrome, 570t

Atenolol, 456b, 456f, 459–460t

Atherosclerosis, 461–464, 462f, 466

Athlete's foot, 635–636, 635b, 636f, 636t
Ativan. *see* Lorazepam
Atomoxetine, 356, 364–366t, 394t
Atorvastatin, 358, 458t, 463t, 464b, 464f
Atracurium, 426–427t, 445t
Atrioventricular (AV) node, 452
Atrium, 451–452
Atropine, 603–604t
Atropine/diphenoxylate (C-V), 517b, 517f
Atrovent. *see* Ipratropium
Atrovent HFA. *see* Ipratropium
Attention-deficit/hyperactivity disorder (ADHD), 364–366t, 393–394b, 393–395, 394t
Attenuated, definition of, 594
Attitude, 91
Auditory canal, 613
Auditory nerve, 613f
Auditory ossicles, 613
Auditory system, 613–616
Augmentin. *see* Amoxicillin plus clavulanate
Augmentin XR. *see* Amoxicillin plus clavulanate
Auraphene-B. *see* Carbamide peroxide
Auricle, 613, 613f
Autocrine hormones, 401
Autoimmune disorders, 584–591
    biological response modifiers and immunomodulators for, 585, 585–587t
    Graves disease, 590, 590b, 590f
    Hashimoto thyroiditis, 591, 591b
    immunosuppressive agents for transplant rejection and, 577t
    myasthenia gravis, 372–374, 375f
    rheumatoid arthritis, 588–590, 588f, 589b
    systemic lupus erythematosus (SLE), 587–588, 588b
    type 1 diabetes mellitus, 584–585
Automated dispensing system (ADS), 194, 201–202, 202b, 305, 305b, 306f
    in community pharmacy, 339, 339f
    in institutional pharmacy, 343, 344b, 344f
    medication safety and
        in community pharmacy, 329–330, 330b, 330f
        in hospital pharmacy, 329, 329f
Automated return companies, 308–310
Autonomic nervous system (ANS), 367, 368f, 371–372, 371b
    heart rate and, 453
Auxiliary labels, 173, 173f, 173t
    for nonsterile compounding, 240, 240t
Average wholesale price (AWP), 299–300, 303
Avoirdupois system, 136, 136t
Avonex. *see* Interferon beta-1a
AWP. *see* Average wholesale price
Axert. *see* Almotriptan
Axon, 367
Ayurveda, 674t, 681–682
Azasan. *see* Azathioprine
AzaSite. *see* Azithromycin

Azathioprine, 364–366t, 374b, 374f, 585–587t, 588b, 588f
Azelaic acid, 627t
Azelastine, 603–604t
Azelex. *see* Azelaic acid
Azilect. *see* Rasagiline
Azithromycin, 498b, 498f, 569t, 607–608t, 615t, 619b, 619f
Azmacort. *see* Triamcinolone acetonide
Azopt. *see* Brinzolamide
Azulfidine. *see* Sulfasalazine

B

B lymphocytes (B cells), 579
Bacitracin, 607–608t, 637t, 669t
Bacitracin/neomycin/polymyxin ointment, 111
Baclofen, 426–427t, 444t
Bacon, Roger, 6
Bacterial infection, ophthalmic, 606–609, 606b
Bacterial sinusitis, 617–618, 617b
Bacterial vaccines, 576–577t, 595, 595b
Bacterial vaginitis, 569t
Bactericidal agents, 613
Bacteriostatic agents, 613
Bactrim. *see* Sulfamethoxazole/trimethoprim
Bactroban. *see* Mupirocin
Baker Cell systems, 305, 329
Balance
    Class A, 235, 238b
    for compounding, 235, 236f
    electronic, 235
Balsalazide, 514t
Bank identification number (BIN), 171
Banks, Janelle, 318
Bar coding, 305
Barbiturates, 22, 237t
Barcode point of entry (BPOE), 198, 198f
Barcodes, 198, 198f
    medication safety and, 326, 326f, 328
Barrier method, of contraception, 556–558
Basal cell cancer, 638–639, 638f
Basal ganglia, 378–380
Basiliximab, 585–587t
Baur, Jacob, 12
Baxa's Repeater pump, 258–259
Bayer. *see* Aspirin
Bayer Company, 430
BBB. *see* Blood-brain barrier
Beclomethasone, 488t, 492t
Beconase AQ. *see* Beclomethasone
Behind-the-counter (BTC) medications, 102–103, 166, 669
Belatacept, 585–587t, 591–592b
Belimumab, 585–587t, 588b
Belsomra. *see* Suvorexant
Benadryl. *see* Diphenhydramine
Benadryl Allergy. *see* Diphenhydramine
Benazepril, 454b, 154f, 458t, 459–460t, 475–476t
Benicar. *see* Olmesartan
Benign, defined, 564–565

Benign prostatic hyperplasia, 359
Benign prostatic hypertrophy, 564–565b, 564–566, 564f, 565t
Benlysta. *see* Belimumab
Bentyl. *see* Dicyclomine
Benuryl. *see* Probenecid
Benzathine, 569t
Benzocaine, 111
 for cough and cold symptoms
  glycerin, 666t
  menthol, 666t
 menthol lozenge and, 106
Benzodiazepines, 388b, 391b, 392t
Benzoyl peroxide, 627t, 669t
Benztropine, 381t
Besifloxacin, 607–608t
Besivance. *see* Besifloxacin
Beta-blockers, 449–451t, 456–457, 457b, 458t, 459–460t, 472t, 475–476t
 for cardiovascular system, 358
 for conditions affecting the eye, 599–600t, 610–611, 610t
Betagan. *see* Levobunolol
Betamethasone, 630t, 632t
 cream, 111
Betapace. *see* Sotalol
Betapace AF. *see* Sotalol
Betaseron. *see* Interferon beta-1b
Betaxolol, 610t, 611b, 611f
Betoptic-S. *see* Betaxolol
Bevacizumab, 522b, 522f
Bexsero, 592–593t
Beyond-use date (BUD), 179–180, 261–262, 265t
 for bulk repackaging, 228, 228b
 for nonsterile compounding, 229–230, 230t
Beyond-use dating, 207
Bicarbonate, 531
Biguanide, 398–400t, 421–422t
Bile acid sequestrants, 458t, 463t, 464, 464b
Billing
 pharmacy, 312
 third-party, 297–299, 297t
  claim problems in, 300, 301f
  coverage expiration policy for drugs and, 300–301
  filling prescription too soon, 302
  handling nonformulary drugs or noncovered National Drug Codes, 302
  limitation of plan exceeded and, 301–302, 302b
  nonidentification match in, 302
  patient profiles and, 299–300, 300f
  plan limitations in, 303, 303b
  point of sale billing and, 297, 297b
  prior authorization and, 297–299, 298f, 299b
  processing claims in, 300, 301f
  resubmitting rejected claims in, 303
Bimatoprost, 610t, 612b, 612f
BIN. *see* Bank identification number
Bioavailability, 118
Bioequivalence, 118

Biofeedback, 674t, 682, 683f
Biological response modifiers (BRMs), 585, 585–587t
Biological safety cabinet (BSC), 204–205, 206f, 265t, 267, 267b
 cleaning, 272b
 spills in, 282
Biological therapy, 656
Biomaterials, 106
BioThrax, 592–593t
Bipolar disorder, 364–366t, 388–389, 388b
Bisacodyl, 519b, 519f, 519t
 for gastrointestinal conditions, 668t
 suppositories, 112
Bismuth subsalicylate, 517t, 518b, 518f
 for gastrointestinal conditions, 668t
Bisoprolol, 458t
Bisphosphonates, 440b, 441t
 for musculoskeletal system, 357
Bivalirudin, 470t
Black Box Warning, 44
Black cohosh, 673t, 676t, 679, 679f
Bladder, 527, 528f
 overactive, 526–527t
Bleeding disorders, 659f
Bleph-10. *see* Sulfacetamide
Blister card, 224, 228
Blister pack containers, 225f
Blister package cards, 342, 342b, 342f
Blood. *see also* Hematologic system
 major components of, 645–646, 658f
  cellular components of blood, 646, 646f, 647f
  plasma, 645
  plasma proteins, 645–646, 646f
  platelets, 646
Blood glucose meters, 423
Blood oxygenation, 451–452, 452f, 453f
Blood pressure, 453
 classification of, 455t
 high. *see* Hypertension
 hormones and, 453
 low. *see* Hypotension
Blood-brain barrier (BBB), 369
 propranolol and, 457b
Bloodletting, 7
BMI. *see* Body mass index
Board of pharmacy (BOP), 58, 60–61, 61b
 controlled substances and, 39
Boceprevir, for hepatitis C, 571t
Body mass index (BMI), 419–422b
Body surface area, calculating, 138
Body systems, classifications of medications and, 102, 103t, 122–123t
Body weight, calculating, 137, 138b
Bolus, 263
Bone fracture, 438
Bone marrow, 427, 429f, 578, 578f, 579f
 erythropoiesis in, 646, 647f
Bone remodeling, 439f

Bones, 427
    anatomy of, 429f
    microscopic structure of, 430f
Boniva. *see* Ibandronate
Boostrix, 592–593t
BOP. *see* Board of pharmacy; State Board of Pharmacy
Bore sizes, 260
Botox, 290
Bowman capsule, 528
Boxed warning, 44, 46b
BPH. *see* Benign prostatic hyperplasia
BPOE. *see* Barcode point of entry
Bradham, Caleb, 13t
Bradykinesia, 378–380
Bradypnea, 484t
Brain, 369, 370b, 371f
Brainstem, 369, 371f
Brand names, 150b, 289–290. *see also* Trade names
    generic names *vs.*, 352
    Medicare insurance in, 294
Breasts, 550, 551f
Breo Ellipta. *see* Fluticasone/vilanterol
Brexpiprazole, 390b, 390f
Brick-and-mortar pharmacies, 51–52
Brimonidine, 603–604t, 610t, 611–612b, 611f
Brinzolamide, 610t
BRMs. *see* Biological response modifiers
Brompheniramine/phenylephrine elixir, 108
Bronchi, 480, 480f
Bronchioles, 480, 481f
Bronchodilators, 479t
    for asthma, 358
Brovana. *see* Arformoterol
BSC. *see* Biological safety cabinet
BTC medications. *see* Behind-the-counter (BTC)
        medications
Bubble pack, 224, 228
Buccal agents, 113, 113f
BUD. *see* Beyond-use date
Budesonide, 488t, 491b, 492t, 665t
Budesonide/formoterol, 492t
Buffer room, 265t, 267b
Buffers, 239
Bulk repackaging, 224–226
    beyond-use date and, 228
    containers for, 224, 224b, 225f, 225t
    documentation of, 226, 226t, 227f
    equipment for, 224–225, 225f
    expiration dates and, 228
    gloves and, 228b
    good manufacturing practices in, 224, 224t
    labeling and checking, 226–228
    long-term care packaging in, 228, 229f
    regulatory and quality control of, 250
    storage and stability in, 228
    techniques for, 225–226, 226b
Bulk vials, 276
Bulk-forming laxatives, 518, 519t

Bumetanide, 458t, 459–460t, 537t
Bumex. *see* Bumetanide
Buprenorphine, 50, 437t
Bupropion, 364–366t, 386–387t, 387b
Burns, 633–634, 633b, 634b, 634f
Business calculations, 145–147
BuSpar. *see* Buspirone
Buspirone, 364–366t, 388b, 388f
Bydureon. *see* Exenatide
Byetta. *see* Exenatide
Bypass surgery, 461b

C

CABG. *see* Coronary artery bypass graft
CACI. *see* Compounding aseptic containment isolator
CADM. *see* Computerized adverse drug event monitoring
Caduceus, 4, 5f
Caffeine, 12
CAI. *see* Compounding aseptic isolator
Caladryl. *see* Calamine
Calagesic. *see* Calamine
Calamine, 628–629b, 628f
Calan. *see* Verapamil
Calcijex. *see* Calcitriol
Calcineurin inhibitors, 585–587t
    for eczema, 630t
Calcipotriene, 630–631b, 632t, 633b, 633f
Calcitonin, 401, 402t, 441t
Calcitonin hormone analog, 441t
Calcitrene. *see* Calcipotriene
Calcitriol, 398–400t, 415b, 415f, 534b, 534f
Calcium, 405f, 427, 441t, 531
    absorption, 667b
Calcium acetate, 534b, 534f
Calcium carbonate, 509t, 534b, 534f
    for gastroesophageal reflux disease and indigestion, 667t
Calcium channel blockers (CCBs), 449–451t, 457, 457b,
        458t, 459–460t
Calcium gluconate, 280t
Calculate with Confidence, 160t
Calculations, 126b, 148
    apothecary system and, 135, 135b, 135f
    avoirdupois system and, 136, 136t
    basic math skills and, 129–132, 129t
    compounding, 251–253
    differences among systems, 136, 137b
    dilution, 143, 144b
    household system and, 132, 134, 134b, 135b
    international time and, 128, 128b, 128f
    with liquid medication, 137–140
        alligation alternate in, 144, 145b
        body surface area in, 138, 138b
        body weight in, 137, 138b
        dilution and, 143
        dimensional analysis, 137, 142b
        intramuscular injections, 140
        intravenous medications, 140–141, 141f
        involving units and milliequivalents, 139–140, 140b

Calculations (Continued)
    oral and injectable syringes and, 138, 139f
    in pediatric and geriatric dosing, 138, 139b
    percentage and ratio strengths in, 142, 142b
    single-step proportion problem, 137
    subcutaneous injections, 140
    total parenteral nutrition, 144
  metric system and, 126–127, 132–134, 133t
  of percentages of quantities, 145–146
  pharmacy, history of, 126–127
  Roman numerals and, 127–128, 127t
Calibration, 230
  of molds, 240, 241b
CAM. see Complementary and alternative medicine
Campath. see Alemtuzumab
Camphor, 108
Camptosar. see Irinotecan
Canagliflozin, 398–400t, 421–422t
Canals of Schlemm, 602
Canasa. see Mesalamine
Cancellous bone, 427, 438–439
Cancer
  colorectal, 522, 522b
  hematologic, 652–657, 654–655t, 657t
    leukemia, 652–656, 653b, 654–655t
    lymphoma, 656–657, 656f
  lung, 500, 500b
  prostate, 567–568, 567–568b, 568f, 568t, 656
  skin, 637b, 638–639, 638 639b, 638f, 639b
Candesartan, 459–460t
Candida albicans, 569t
Candidiasis, vaginal, 569t
Cannabidiol, 37
Cannabis legality, 37
Capillary, 451
Capillary action, 238
Capitation, 290
Caplets, 104–105, 105b, 105t
Capoten. see Captopril
Capsaicin, 364–366t, 376b, 376f
Capsules, 105–106, 105f
  compounding, 241, 242f
  repackaging of, containers for, 224, 225f
  sizes of, 105–106, 106f, 242t
  types of, 105f
Captopril, 458t, 459–460t, 475–476t
Carac. see Fluorouracil
Carbachol, 610t
Carbamazepine, 356, 364–366t, 377b, 377f, 377t
Carbamide peroxide, 614t, 615b, 615f
Carbohydrates, 507–508
Carbon dioxide, oxygen and, gas exchange of, 481, 485f
Carbonic anhydrase, 610b
Carbonic anhydrase inhibitors, 537t
  for conditions affecting the eye, 599–600t, 610t, 611
Carboplatin, 654–655t
Carcinogenic effects, of drugs, 356
Cardene. see Nicardipine

Cardiac conduction system, 452, 453f
Cardiac cycle, 452, 454f
Cardiac glycoside, 475–476t
Cardiac muscle, 451
Cardiac notch, 481
Cardiac output (CO), 453
Cardiovascular system, 477
  anatomy of, 451–452, 452f
    cardiac conduction system and, 452, 453f
    cardiac cycle, 452, 454f
    oxygenation and, 451–452, 452f, 453f
  conditions affecting, 457–476
    arrhythmias, 474t
    common drugs for, 449–451t
    common medication classes used to treat, 453–457, 454b,
      455b, 457b, 458t
    coronary artery disease, 465b, 466–468, 466f, 467f,
      468b, 468f, 468t
    dysrhythmia, 473, 473b, 474t
    heart failure, 473–476, 473b, 474b, 475–476t
    hyperlipidemia, 461–465, 462f, 463t, 464b
    hypertension, 455t, 457–459, 457b, 459–460t
    hypotension, 460–461, 461b
    thrombotic events, 468–473, 469b, 470t
      myocardial infarction, 471–472, 472t
      transient ischemic attacks and strokes, 472–473
  regulation of, 453, 453b, 455f
  therapeutic agents for, 357–358
Cardizem. see Diltiazem
Cardura. see Doxazosin
Cardura XL. see Doxazosin
Caregivers, for elderly patients, 183–184
Cariprazine, 388b, 388f
Carisoprodol, 426–427t, 443b, 443f, 444t
Carpuject cartridge, 259–260, 260f
Carteolol, 610t, 611b, 611f
Cartridge systems, 259–260
Carvedilol, 459–460t, 475–476t
Cassette system, patient-controlled analgesia, 263, 264f
Catapres. see Clonidine
Catapres-TTS. see Clonidine
Catecholamines, 404–405
Catechol-*O*-methyltransferase (COMT) inhibitors, 381t
Cations, 531
CCBs. see Calcium channel blockers
CCR5 blocker, for human immunodeficiency virus infection
  and acquired immunodeficiency syndrome, 570t
Cefazolin, 277t
Cefdinir, 615t
Cefixime, 569t
Cefotaxime, 277t
Cefotetan, 560t
Ceftazidime, 277t, 280b
Ceftin. see Cefuroxime
Ceftizoxime, 560t
Ceftriaxone, 277t, 560t, 569t, 615t
Cefuroxime, 615t
Celebrex. see Celecoxib

Celecoxib, 426–427t, 434t, 435f

Celexa. *see* Citalopram

Cell phone etiquette, 88–89, 88b, 88f

CellCept. *see* Mycophenolate

Celsius, temperature conversion between Fahrenheit and, 129

Centany. *see* Mupirocin

Centers for Medicare and Medicaid Services (CMS), 195, 292b

Central nervous system (CNS), 367, 367b, 369–371
  brain and, 369, 371f
  diseases and conditions of, 376–384
    Alzheimer disease, 364–366t, 378, 379t
    epilepsy, 364–366t, 376–378
    migraine headaches, 364–366t, 383–384
    multiple sclerosis, 364–366t, 380–383, 382f, 382t
    Parkinson disease, 364–366t, 380f, 381t
    stroke, 384
  spinal cord and, 369–370, 371f

Central supply, 210

Cephalexin, 540b, 540f

Cephalosporins, 539t
  for otitis media, 615t

Cerebellum, 369, 371f

Cerebral cortex, 369

Cerebrospinal fluid (CSF), 369–370

Certification
  of pharmacists, 15
  of pharmacy technicians, 15, 70–78, 71b, 72–73t, 73–74b, 74b

Certified pharmacy technician, 60, 70

Certolizumab pegol, 514t, 585–587t

Cerumen, 613
  buildup of, 614–615, 614–615b

Cervarix, 592–593t

Cervical caps, 558

Cetirizine HCl, 617t, 665t

Cetylev. *see* Acetylcysteine

CFCs. *see* Chlorofluorocarbons

Chain pharmacy, 165

Chamomile, 676t

CHAMPUS. *see* TRICARE

CHAMPVA. *see* Civilian Health and Medical Program of the Department of Veterans Affairs

Channel, definition of, 84

Chemical structure, 150

Chemokines, 582f

Chemotherapeutic agents, 281–282, 282f
  airflow in, 268
  for leukemia, 644t, 654–655t
    preparation of, 653b

Chemotherapy
  medication, counting trays for, 226b
  preparing for, 205
  technician responsibilities on, 199t

Chemotherapy technician, 64

Chewable lozenges, 243

Chickenpox, 633, 633f

Childhood immunizations, 594b

Children
  breathing rates in, 481, 481b
  dosing of liquid medications, 138
    calculating, 138, 139b

Children's Health Insurance Program (CHIP), 195

Child-resistant containers, 175

Child-resistant packaging, 50

Chinese medicine, 674t, 681–682

CHIP. *see* Children's Health Insurance Program

Chiropractic medicine, 673, 674t

Chlamydia, 569, 569t

Chlamydia trachomatis, 569, 569t

Chlorambucil, 654–655t

Chloraseptic Sore Throat Lozenges. *see* Benzocaine

Chloraseptic Spray. *see* Phenol

Chloride, 531

Chlorofluorocarbons (CFCs), inhalers and, 494b

Chlorothiazide, 458t, 459–460t

Chlorpheniramine, 617t, 665t

Chlorthalidone, 537t

Chlor-Trimeton. *see* Chlorpheniramine

Cholesterol absorption inhibitors, 463t

Cholestyramine, 458t, 463t, 464, 464b, 464f

Cholinergic agonists, 610t, 611

Cholinergics, for conditions affecting the eye, 599–600t

Choriogonadotropin alfa, 552–553t

Choroid, 601f

Chronic inflammation, 583–584

Chronic kidney disease, 531–535, 532t, 533f
  agents for, 526–527t

Chronic lymphocytic leukemia, 652–656

Chronic obstructive pulmonary disease (COPD), 491f, 492t, 495–498, 496f, 497b

Chronic venous insufficiency, 536b

Chyme, 506

Cilia, 480, 616

Ciliary body, 601–602, 601f

Cilostazol, 470t

Ciloxan. *see* Ciprofloxacin

Cimetidine, 280, 280t, 511t
  for gastroesophageal reflux disease and indigestion, 667t

Cimzia. *see* Certolizumab pegol

Cinacalcet, 398–400t, 415b, 415f, 534–535b, 535b

Cinchona bark, 8

Ciprofloxacin, 281t, 322t, 607–608t

Circadian rhythms, 664–665

Cirrhosis, 536b

Cisatracurium, 426–427t, 445t

Cisplatin, 500b, 500f

Citalopram, 364–366t, 386–387t

Citroma. *see* Magnesium citrate

Citrucel. *see* Methylcellulose

Civil War, 9, 9b

Civilian Health and Medical Program of the Department of Veterans Affairs (CHAMPVA), 295–296, 296f

Cladribine, 654–655t

Claforan. *see* Cefotaxime

Claravis. *see* Isotretinoin
Clarinex. *see* Desloratadine
Claritin. *see* Loratadine
Claritin Eye. *see* Ketotifen
Clark's Rule, 139
Clean room, 258–259, 265t, 267b
Clear Eyes. *see* Naphazoline
Clear Eyes Redness Relief. *see* Naphazoline
Clearplex. *see* Benzoyl peroxide
Clearskin. *see* Benzoyl peroxide
Cleocin. *see* Clindamycin
Cleocin T. *see* Clindamycin
Clindagel. *see* Clindamycin
ClindaMax. *see* Clindamycin
Clindamycin, 560t, 569t, 627t
Clinical Pharmacology, 153, 154f
Clinical technician, 13, 64
Clinical trials, 200
Clobetasol propionate, 630t, 632t
Clobex. *see* Clobetasol propionate
Clomiphene, 552–553t, 555b, 555f
    for male infertility, 555b
Clonidine, 459–460t
Clopidogrel, 458t, 470t, 471b, 471f, 472t
Closed formulary, 288
Closed-angle glaucoma, 609–610, 609f
Closed-door pharmacy, 66–67, 67b, 67f
Clotrimazole, 106, 569t, 636b, 636f, 636t, 669t
Clozapine, 390b, 390f
CMS. *see* Centers for Medicare and Medicaid Services
CNS. *see* Central nervous system
Coagulation, 468–469
Coal tar, 632t
Coatings, 237t
Coca-Cola, 12
Cocaine, 12
Cochlea, 613f, 614b, 614f
Cogentin. *see* Benztropine
Colace. *see* Docusate; Docusate sodium
Colazal. *see* Balsalazide
Colchicine, 426–427t, 443t
Colcrys. *see* Colchicine
Cold
    symptoms, over-the-counter medications for, 664, 666t
    therapeutic agent for, 358
Colesevelam, 463t, 464b
Colestid. *see* Colestipol
Colestipol, 458t, 463t
Collaboration, 79
Collecting duct, 529
College of Pharmacy and Sciences in Philadelphia, 12
Colony-stimulating factor, 578, 644t, 650
Colorectal cancer, 522, 522b
Colostomy, 513
Combat Methamphetamine Epidemic Act, 28–29, 29b, 29f, 30t, 166
Combivent. *see* Albuterol/ipratropium
Combivent Respimat. *see* Albuterol/ipratropium

Comedones, 626
Common cold, 485–486b, 485–488, 486t
Communication, 79, 84–87, 84f, 181–182
    barriers, eliminating, 91, 91b
    cycle of, 84, 84f
    with the health care team, 91, 91f
    with hearing-impaired patients, 91, 91b
    listening skills and, 84
    medication errors and, 333
    with non-English-speaking patients, 90, 90b
    nonverbal, 84–85, 85b, 85f
    of nursing staff, institutional pharmacy and, 195f, 198
    optimizing, 86–87, 87b
    outpatient pharmacies and, 65
    scenario, 84, 91
    with special patient groups, 90–91
    telephone etiquette, 87–89, 88b, 88f
    with terminally ill patients, 90
    verbal, 85–86, 86b, 87b
    written, 89–90, 89b, 90b
Community pharmacy, 163–189, 338–343
    automated counters in, 339, 339f
    automated dispensing system and, 329–330, 330b, 330f
    checking area in, 340, 340b
    communication and, 181–182
    consultation area at, 180, 180f
    drive-through window at, 180–181, 181f
    durable and nondurable supplies and equipment in, 186–187, 186f, 187b
    for elderly patients, 182–185, 182f
        with caregivers, 183–184
        with health literacy issues, 183
        with mental health problems, 183
        terminally ill, 183
    "fast-moving" items in, 339, 339f
    front counter area in, 338, 339b, 339f, 346f
    immunizations in, 185, 185b
    layout of, 177–181, 338, 338f, 346f
    long-term care services in, 187, 187f
    medication therapy management in, 185–186
    patient bins at, 180, 180f
    patient counseling and, 176, 176f
    prescription in, 166–170
        calculating day's supply, 171
        checking, 175
        data input, 170–172
        date of, 168–169, 169b
        directions for use, 171
        drug benefit, 170–171, 170f
        filing, 175–176
        information, 166–167, 167–168t
        intake, 170
        intake window, 177
        labeling, 172–173
        packaging, 175
        patient information in, 168
        payment, 176
        pick-up window, 180

Community pharmacy *(Continued)*
    preparation, 173–176, 174f
    prescriber information in, 168, 169f
    processing of, 170–173
    scanning, 172
  records in, 180
  repackaging area of, 179–180, 179t
  role of pharmacy technician in, 165–166, 165f
    interacting with, 181–182
    interacting with patient, 182, 182b
    prescription refilling by, 176
    requesting prescription refill authorization by, 176
    transferring prescription by, 176–177
  setting requirements in, 64b, 65–66, 65b, 66b, 66f
  synchronization of medications in, 186, 186b, 186f
  wellness and disease prevention in, 187–188
Compact bone(s), 427
Compassion, 84
Competencies, 60–61, 61b
  closed-door pharmacy requirements, 66–67, 67b, 67f
  community (outpatient) setting requirements, 65–66, 65b, 66b, 66f
  for compounding, 238b, 282
  definition of, 60–61
  inpatient setting requirements, 63–64, 64b, 64f, 65b
  levels of pharmacy technicians, 70
  medical terminology, 123
  nondiscretionary duties, 61–64, 63b
  state and national boards of pharmacy, 60–61, 61b
  training programs for pharmacy technician student, 68–70, 68–70b
Complementary and alternative medicine (CAM), 681–683, 684
  types of, 674t, 675–683
    acupressure, 674t, 681, 682f
    acupuncture, 674t, 681, 681f
    ayurveda, 674t, 681–682
    biofeedback, 674t, 682, 683f
    Chinese medicine, 674t, 681–682
    chiropractic medicine, 673, 674t
    herbal products. *see* Herbal products
    homeopathy, 674t, 683
    massage therapy, 681, 682f
    meditation, 680
    spinal manipulation, 681
    yoga, 680, 681f
Compliance error, 317t
Compound W. *see* Salicylic acid
Compounded nonsterile preparation (CNSP), 247–249
Compounded sterile preparations (CSPs), 257
  of chemotherapeutic agents, 281–282, 282f
  education and training in, 282, 283b, 283f
  routes of administration and, 262
  supplies for, 258–262, 259t
    filters, 260–261, 261f
    needles, 260, 260b, 260f
    stock levels, 261–262
    syringes, 259–260, 260f

Compounded sterile preparations *(Continued)*
  United States Pharmacopeia 797 (USP 797), 263–271
    history of, 263–264, 264t
    intravenous environment in, 266–267, 266f, 267b, 268f
    requirements for compounding in, 266, 267t
    risk levels in, 265–266, 265f, 266f, 267t
    sections of, 264–265, 265t
    stock levels in, 261
Compounding, 223–224
  nonsterile, 254
    additional supplies for, 235–236
    area for, 230, 230b
    beyond-use dating for, 229–230, 230t
    calculations in, 251–253
    competencies for, 238b
    documentation in, 247–249, 248f, 250b
    equipment for, 230–235, 230f, 231t, 232–233f
    excipients and, 236, 237t
    flavorings in, 236, 237t
    history of, 228–229, 229b
    measuring liquids in, 239, 239f
    mold forms and, 235–236
    nasal preparations in, 246–247, 247b
    packaging in, 247, 247b, 247t
    personal preparation for, 236–238
    preparing solutions in, 239
    professionalism in, 250
    reconstituting premade suspensions in, 240, 240t
    safety in, 250
    semisolids in, 243–244, 244b
    solids in, 240–243
    stability in, 247
    use of, 229, 230b
    weighing techniques for, 237–238, 238b
  non-sterile, area for, 178–179, 178f
  personnel training on, 250–251b, 251
  reasons for, 229, 229b
  regulatory and quality control of, 250
  sterile, 284
  sterile, area for, 179
  veterinary medications and, 250–251, 251b, 251t
Compounding areas, 340–341, 340f, 341b, 341f
Compounding aseptic containment isolator (CACI), 205, 267, 267b
Compounding aseptic isolator (CAI), 265t, 267b
Compounding Quality Act, 30
Compounding record (CR), 247–249
Comprehensive Drug Abuse Prevention and Control Act 1970, 24
Compressed tablets and lozenges, 240–243
Compro. *see* Prochlorperazine
Computer skills, 63, 65
Computer support technician, 76
Computerized adverse drug event monitoring (CADM), 198
Computerized physician order entry (CPOE), 197–198
  area, 343
  medication errors and, 325–326, 326b, 326f
Computers on wheels (COWs), 197

Comtan. *see* Entacapone
Concerta. *see* Methylphenidate
Confidentiality, 65b
  breaching, 27b
  patient, 26, 27b
  of patient, coverage expiration policy for drugs and, 300–301
Conflict resolution skills, 79
Conjugated estrogens, 552–553t, 559b, 559f
Conjunctiva, 601, 601f
Conjunctivitis
  allergic, 604–605, 604b, 604f
  prevention of, 609b
Connective tissue, 431f
Constipation, 504t, 518–520, 518b, 519t
  bowel evacuants and, 518b
Consultation area, 180, 180f
Consumer Product Safety Commission (CPSC), 22
Containers, 175
  amber-colored, 224b
  blister pack, 225f
  for bulk repackaging, 224, 225t
  disposal of, 281, 281b
  in filling ointment jars, 244
  for measuring liquids, in nonsterile compounding, 239
  in medication delivery systems, 262
    patient-controlled analgesia, 263
    piggyback, 262, 262f
  for nonsterile compounding, 230f, 247t
  requirements for medications, 24
  sharp, 281, 281b, 310
Containment ventilated enclosure (CVE), for nonsterile compounding, 230, 234f
Continuing education (CE)
  for national certification, 74–76, 75b
  websites for, 75t
Continuous analgesic delivery systems, 263
Contraception, 556–558
Contraceptives, types of, 556f, 557t
  barrier method, 556–558, 556f
  emergency form of, 557t, 558
  implantable device, 557t
  injection, 557t
  intrauterine, progestin, 557t
  long-acting, 546–547t
  oral, 546–547t, 556–558, 556b, 557b, 557t
  spermicides, 558
  transdermal, 557b, 557t
Contraindications, 43
Controlled Substance Act, 24, 175
Controlled substances, 31–41, 36f, 202–203
  DEA's stair-step schedule of, 24
  dispensing, without prescriptions, 42
  disposal of, 310
  documentation of, 262b
  lending/transferring to another pharmacy, 42–43
  mailing, 43
  narcotic inventory, 40
  ordering, 39–40, 39f, 40b

Controlled substances *(Continued)*
  prescriptions for
    cannabidiol, 37
    cannabis legality, 37
    filling, 41–43
      DEA verification, 49–50, 49b
      emergency, 41–42
      original, 41–43
      partial, 42
    refilling, 39, 42
    tamper-proof, 37, 38b, 38f
    transferring, 42
  ratings of scheduled, 36–41, 36b, 37t
  record keeping of, 40, 40t, 41f
  return of (reverse distributor), 40–41
  technician responsibilities and, 199t
Controlled-release infusion system (CRIS), 276–277
Controls, in drug trials, 353
Conversion factor, 133
Conversions, 126b, 148
  apothecary system, 135, 135b, 135f
  avoirdupois system, 136, 136t
  differences among systems, 136, 137b
  of fractions, 129–130
  household to metric volume, 134, 134t
  metric system, 132–134
  of percentages, 130
  of ratios, 131
  temperature, between Fahrenheit and Celsius, 129
Copaxone. *see* Glatiramer
Copay, 290, 300
Copayment, 289
COPD. *see* Chronic obstructive pulmonary disease
Cordarone. *see* Amiodarone
Cordran. *see* Flurandrenolide
Coreg. *see* Carvedilol
Corgard. *see* Nadolol
Cornea, 601–602, 601f
Coronary artery, 451–452
Coronary artery bypass graft (CABG), 467–468b, 467f
Coronary artery disease, 465b, 466–468, 466f, 467–468b, 467f, 468f, 468t
Corporate pharmacy analyst, 76
Corpus Hippocraticum, 5
Cortef. *see* Hydrocortisone
Cortex, 625f
Cortical bone, 427, 438–439
Corticosteroids
  for allergies, 479t
  for asthma, 491–494
  for conditions affecting the eye, 599–600t, 603–604t, 605
  for dermatological conditions, 623–624t
  for diaper rash, 638b
  for eczema, 630t
  for gout, 443t
  inhaled, 479t
  nasal, 479t
  for psoriasis, 632t

Corticotropin, 410

Cortisol, 402t, 415–416

Cortizone-10. *see* Hydrocortisone

Cough
  over-the-counter medications for, 664, 666t
  therapeutic agent for, 358

Coumadin. *see* Warfarin

Counseling, patient, 176, 176f

Counseling area, 341

Counterfeit drugs, 67

Counting trays, 174f

Coverage expiration policy, for drugs, 300–301

COWs. *see* Computers on wheels

COX-2 inhibitors. *see* Cyclooxygenase-2 inhibitors

Cozaar. *see* Losartan

CPE Monitor, 74–75

CPOE. *see* Computerized physician order entry

CPSC. *see* Consumer Product Safety Commission

CR. *see* Compounding record

Crab louse, 639–640, 640f

Cranberry, 673t, 678, 679f

Cranial nerves, 371, 372f, 373t

Crash carts, 208–210, 208b, 209b, 209f, 209t

Creams, 111, 111f, 243

CREST Initiative, 60, 70

Crestor. *see* Rosuvastatin

Cretinism, 413

Crick, Francis, 10

CRIS. *see* Controlled-release infusion system

Critical observation skills, 79

Critical site, 265t

Crohn disease, 513–515, 514f, 515f

Cromolyn sodium, 487–488, 487–488b, 487f, 492t,
    603–604t, 617t, 665t

Cryoprecipitate, 657

CSF. *see* Cerebrospinal fluid

CSPs. *see* Compounded sterile preparations

Cushing disease, 409t, 415–416, 416b, 416f

Cushing syndrome, 398–400t

Customer service, 184–185, 185b

Cuticle, 624, 625f

Cutivate. *see* Fluticasone propionate

CVS, 165

Cyanosis, 484t

Cyclobenzaprine, 426–427t, 443b, 443f, 444t

Cyclogyl. *see* Cyclopentolate

Cyclooxygenase (COX), 431, 583

Cyclooxygenase-2 inhibitors (COX-2 inhibitors), 426–427t,
    431, 434t

Cyclopentolate, 603–604t

Cyclophosphamide, 654–655t

Cyclosporine, 607–608t

Cyclosporine A, 585–587t

Cyclosporine ophthalmic emulsion, 110

Cymbalta. *see* Duloxetine

Cystic fibrosis, 500–501, 500–501b, 501b

Cystitis, 539

Cytarabine, 654–655t

Cytokines, 579–580, 582f

Cytomel. *see* Liothyronine sodium

Cytotoxic agents, 308, 311

D

DA. *see* Dimensional analysis

Dabigatran, 470, 470b, 470f, 470t

Dalfampridine, 364–366t

Daliresp. *see* Roflumilast

Dalmane. *see* Flurazepam

Dalteparin, 470t

Damaged stock, 308

Danazol, 552–553t

Dapagliflozin, 398–400t, 421–422t

Dapsone, 627t

Daptacel, 592–593t

Darbepoetin alfa, 534b, 534f, 651t

Darifenacin, 541t, 542b, 542f

Darunavir, for human immunodeficiency virus infection and
    acquired immunodeficiency syndrome, 570t

Dasabuvir, 572b, 572f
    for hepatitis C, 571t

Dasatinib, 654–655t

Data entry area, 339

Date of birth (DOB), 299b

Daunorubicin, 654–655t

DAW codes. *see* Dispense as Written (DAW) codes

Daytrana. *see* Methylphenidate

DCA. *see* Direct compounding area

DDAVP. *see* Desmopressin; Desmopressin acetate

DEA. *see* Drug Enforcement Administration

Debrox. *see* Carbamide peroxide

Declomycin. *see* Demeclocycline

Decoction, 680

Decongestants, 237t
    for allergy, 617t, 665t
    for colds, 487, 487b, 666t
    for cough, 666t
    for hypertension, 457b
    ophthalmic, 605t
    pseudoephedrine, 28, 29f
    rebound congestion and, 487b

Deductible, 291

DEERS. *see* Defense Enrollment Eligibility Reporting
    System

Defense Enrollment Eligibility Reporting System (DEERS),
    295

Delsym. *see* Dextromethorphan

Deltasone. *see* Prednisone

Demeclocycline, 398–400t, 410b, 410f

Demerol. *see* Meperidine

Denosumab, 426–427t, 440b, 440f, 441t

Depakote. *see* Divalproex sodium; Valproic acid

Depakote ER. *see* Divalproex sodium

Department of Health and Human Services (DHHS), 195

Department of Public Health (DPH), 195

Depolarization, 367–369, 370f

Depot, 551

Depression, 385–387, 385b
    therapeutic agents for, 357
    treatment for, 364–366t, 386–387t
Dermal root sheath, 625f
Dermatologic system, 641
    anatomy and physiology of, 624
        glands, 624, 626f
        hair and nails, 624, 625f
        skin, 624, 624f
    conditions of, 625–641
        acne vulgaris, 626b, 626f, 627t
        athlete's foot, 635–636, 635b, 636f, 636t
        burns, 633–634, 633b, 634b, 634f
        cancer, 637b, 638–639, 638–639b, 638f, 639b
        chickenpox and shingles, 633, 633f
        common drugs for, 623–624t
        eczema, 629–630, 629f, 630t
        head lice, 639–640, 640f
        impetigo, 636–637, 637f, 637t
        onychomycosis, 640–641, 641b
        psoriasis, 623–624t
        urticaria, 628–629, 628b, 628f
        warts, 634–635, 635f
    therapeutic agents for, 360
Dermatophytosis, 635b
Dermis, 624, 624f
Desenex. see Miconazole
Desiccated thyroid, 398–400t
Desloratadine, 488t, 489b, 489f
Desmopressin, 657f
Desmopressin acetate, 398–400t
Desogestrel, 557t
Desoximetasone, 632t
Desvenlafaxine, 364–366t, 386–387t
Desyrel. see Trazodone
Deteriorated drug error, 317t
Deucravacitinib, 631b
Dexamethasone, 585–587t
    for conditions affecting the eye, 603–604t
Dexilant. see Dexlansoprazole
Dexlansoprazole, 511t
Dexmethylphenidate, 364–366t, 394t
DexPak. see Dexamethasone
Dextroamphetamine, 364–366t, 394t
Dextromethorphan, 486b, 486f
    for cough and cold symptoms, 666t
    syrup, 107
Dextrose, 280
DHS Tar. see Coal tar
DiaBeta. see Glyburide
Diabetes insipidus, 409t, 410b
Diabetes mellitus, 418–419, 418–419b
    gestational, 409t, 418–419
    therapeutic agents for, 357
    treatment of, 398–400t, 421–422t, 464b
    type 1, 409t, 418, 584–585
    type 2, 409t, 418
        treatment of, 422t

Diagnosis, 673
Dialysate, 532–533, 532–533b
Dialysis, 532, 532–533b
Diaper rash, 637–638
Diaphragm, 481
Diarrhea, 504t, 516–518, 517b, 517t
Diastole, 452
Diazepam, 364–366t, 378f
Diclegis. see Doxylamine succinate and pyridoxine
        hydrochloride
Diclofenac, 426–427t, 434t, 603–604t
Dicyclomine, 516b, 516f
Didanosine, for human immunodeficiency virus infection
        and acquired immunodeficiency syndrome,
        570t
Dietary Supplement Health and Education Act, 30t
Dietary supplements, 675b
    FDA regulation of, 673–674
Differin. see Adapalene
Diflucan. see Fluconazole
Digestion, 505, 508f
Digoxin, 322t, 473b, 473f, 474t, 475–476t
    overdose, 474b
Dilantin. see Phenytoin
Dilatrate-SR. see Isosorbide dinitrate
Dilaudid. see Hydromorphone
Diltiazem, 457b, 457f, 458t, 459–460t
Diluent, 276b, 277b, 280b
Diluent/solvents, 143
Dilution, 143, 144b
Dimensional analysis (DA), 132, 132b, 142b
Diovan. see Valsartan
Dipeptidyl peptidase-4 (DPP-4) inhibitor, 398–400t,
        421–422t
Diphenhydramine, 364–366t, 486b, 486f, 617t, 665b, 665t,
        669t
    for cough and cold symptoms, 666t
    for insomnia, 392t, 666t
    for skin conditions, 669t
    topical, 628b
    for urticaria, 628b, 628f
Diplomacy, 84
Diprolene. see Betamethasone
Direct compounding area (DCA), 265t
Direct manufacturer ordering, 310
Direct renin inhibitor, 459–460t
Direct thrombin inhibitor, 449–451t, 470, 470t
Disaster medications, 345
Discharge pharmacies, 193–194, 199t
Disease-modifying antirheumatic drugs (DMARDs),
        585–587t, 588–590
Disintegrants, 237t
Disopyramide, 474t
Dispense as Written (DAW) codes, 171, 172b, 289
Disposal, of containers, 281, 281b
Distal convoluted tubule, 529
Distribution, 117, 117b, 527
Ditropan. see Oxybutynin

Diuretics, 449–451t, 458t, 459–460t, 473b, 475–476t, 537, 537t
  for renal system, 359
  side effects of, 538b
Diuril. *see* Chlorothiazide
Divalproex sodium, 364–366t
  for epilepsy, 377t
Division (math), 129
DLA. *see* Drug Listing Act
DMARDs. *see* Disease-modifying antirheumatic drugs
DOB. *see* Date of birth
Dobutamine, 475–476t
Dobutrex. *see* Dobutamine
Documentation
  of bulk repackaging, 226, 227f, 227t
  of controlled substances, 262b
  of nonsterile compounding, 247–249, 248f, 250b
Docusate, 518–519b, 518f, 519t
Docusate sodium, for gastrointestinal conditions, 668t
Dofetilide, 474t
Dogma, 4
Domagk, Gerhard, 9–10
Donepezil, 364–366t, 379t
Dopamine agonists, 381t
Dorzolamide, 610t, 611b, 611f
Dosage and administration, 43
Dosage forms, 103–111, 103f, 104b, 104t
  abbreviations for, 96
  additives and, 118–119, 119t
  approval of manufactured types of, 120t
  categories of, 103
    liquids, 103, 107–111, 107f
    semisolids, 103, 111–112
    solids, 103, 104–107
  of controlled substances, 262b
  manufactured products of, 119
  medication error in, 317t
  of nitroglycerin, 467–468b
  pet, 251t
  routes of administration and, 94–124, 97t
    inhalants, 114
    injectables, 114–115, 115f
    instructions of, 102
    miscellaneous, 115
    ophthalmic, otic, nasal agents, 114
    oral agents, 113
    parenteral agents, 114
    rectal, 113
    topical agents, 113–114
  and strengths, 43
Dosing schedules, abbreviations for, 137b
Double-blinded trials, 353
Dovonex. *see* Calcipotriene
Doxazosin, 459–460t, 565t
Doxepin, 386–387t
Doxercalciferol, 398–400t, 415b, 415f
Doxycycline, 277t, 560t, 569t, 627t

Doxylamine, 364–366t, 392t
  for insomnia, 666t
Doxylamine succinate and pyridoxine hydrochloride, 521b, 521f
DPP-4 inhibitor. *see* Dipeptidyl peptidase-4 (DPP-4) inhibitor
Dramamine Less Drowsy. *see* Meclizine
Dress, professional, 79–80, 80f
Drip rate/drop rate, 141
Drips, 262
Drive-through window, 180–181, 181f
Dronabinol, 36–37
Dronedarone, 474t
Drop factor, 141
Drops, 141b
  eye, administration of, 602, 602b
Drospirenone, 557t
Droxia. *see* Hydroxyurea
Drug abuse
  dependence and, 44
  monitoring programs and, 51, 51b
Drug Abuse Control Amendments, 22
Drug Addiction Treatment Act of 2000, 28
Drug allergy, drug intolerance *vs.*, 584
Drug classifications, 150, 361, 455b
  by Drug Enforcement Agency (DEA), 360
Drug coupon cards, 303
Drug discount card, 303
Drug diversion, 40
Drug Enforcement Administration (DEA), 22, 31
  drug classifications by, 360
  number, 168
  verification process for, 49–50, 49b
Drug Facts and Comparisons, 152, 157t
Drug information references, 149–162, 150f, 160t
  American Drug Index, 155
  American Hospital Formulary Service Drug Information (AHDS DI), 152–153, 157t
  Clinical Pharmacology, 153, 154f
  considerations when choosing, 161, 161b
  Drug Facts and Comparisons, 152, 157t
  Drug Topics Red Book, 152, 157t
  electronic referencing, 156–157
  Geriatric Dosage Handbook, 156, 157t
  Goodman & Gilman's The Pharmacological Basis of Therapeutics, 155, 157t
  Handbook of Nonprescription Drugs, 155
  Handbook on Injectable Drugs, 154, 157t
  Ident-A-Drug, 153, 155f, 157t
  Internet, 158, 158t
  journals and news magazines, 159, 159t
  Martindale's The Complete Drug Reference, 156
  Micromedex Healthcare Series, 154
  Orange Book, 152, 157t
  Pediatric and Neonatal Dosage Handbook, 156, 157t
  Physicians' Desk Reference, 152, 157t
  pocket-sized reference books, 156
  Purple Book, 152

Drug information references *(Continued)*
  Remington's Pharmaceutical Sciences: The Science and Practice of Pharmacy, 156, 157t
  through pharmacy associations, 160b
  United States Pharmacists' Pharmacopeia, 153
  United States Pharmacopoeia-National Formulary (USP-NF), 153, 157t
  used in pharmacy, 151–153, 157t
Drug interactions, 44
  medication errors and, 321–322, 322t
Drug intolerance, drug allergy *vs.,* 584
Drug Listing Act (DLA), 24, 30t
Drug monographs, 43–46, 45f
Drug preparation, medication error in, 317t
Drug Quality and Security Act, 30–31
Drug research, 150–151, 150b
Drug sales, classifications of, 102–103
Drug Supply Chain Security Act (DSCSA), 215
Drug Topics Red Book, 152, 157t
  average wholesale price in, 299–300
Drug utilization, 288–289, 289b
Drug utilization evaluation (DUE), 25–26, 166–167, 172, 288–289
Drug utilization review (DUR), 288–289
DRUGDEX, 154
Drug-induced ototoxicity, 615–616, 615t
Drugs
  agonists and antagonists, 355
  brand name of, 352
  chemical name of, 352
  effectiveness of, 353
  effects of, 356
  generic name of, 352
  interactions, 356
  medication characteristics of, 353
  pharmacodynamics of, 354–355
  pharmacokinetics of, 354, 355f
  and receptors, 355
  safety of, 353
  selectivity of, 353
  tall man lettering in, 352–353, 353t
  testing of, four phases of, 353
  therapeutic index, 355–356
  trials of, 353
DSCSA. *see* Drug Supply Chain Security Act
Dual orexin receptor antagonist, 392t
DUE. *see* Drug utilization evaluation
Dulcolax. *see* Bisacodyl
Dulera. *see* Formoterol/mometasone
Duloxetine, 356, 364–366t, 375b, 375f, 386–387t
Duodenum, 506
DuoNeb. *see* Albuterol/ipratropium
Dupilumab, 629–630, 629b
Dupixent. *see* Dupilumab
DUR. *see* Drug utilization review
Duragesic. *see* Fentanyl
Durham-Humphrey Amendment, 24
Dutasteride, 565t, 566b, 566f

Dwarfism, 411
Dyrenium. *see* Triamterene
Dysarthria, 182
Dysmenorrhea, 551, 553b
Dyspnea, 484t, 490–491
Dysrhythmia, 473, 473b, 474t

E

Ears, 613–616, 621
  anatomy and physiology of, 613
    external, 613, 613f
    inner, 613, 613f, 614b, 614f
    middle, 613, 613f
  conditions of, 613–616
    cerumen buildup as, 614–615, 614–615b
    drug-induced ototoxicity as, 615–616, 615–616b, 615t
    drugs for, 599–600t, 614t, 616b
    medications for, 114
    otitis media as, 613, 613b, 615f, 615t
  therapeutic agents for, 360
Echinacea, 673t, 677, 677f
Ecotrin. *see* Aspirin
Ectopic pregnancy, 559
Eczema, 629–630, 629f, 630t
Edema, 536–539
  causes of, 536b
  drug treatment for, 536–537b, 537t
  heart failure and, 473–474, 473b
  non-drug treatment for, 536–537b
  pitting, 536–537, 536f
Edluar. *see* Zolpidem
Education
  on compounded sterile preparations, 282, 283b, 283f
  on medication error prevention, 334
  training programs for pharmacy technician student, 68–70, 68–70b
Efavirenz, for human immunodeficiency virus infection and acquired immunodeficiency syndrome, 570t
Effexor. *see* Venlafaxine
Effient. *see* Prasugrel
Efudex. *see* Fluorouracil
Ejaculatory duct, 561–562, 561f
Elavil. *see* Amitriptyline
Elbow, 427
Eldepryl. *see* Selegiline
Elderly patients, 182–185, 182f
  caregivers for, 183–184
  with health literacy issues, 183
  medication errors and, 323
  with mental health problems, 183
  terminally ill, 183
Electrolytes, 237t, 280, 280t, 529b
  importance of, 531
Electronic Medicaid Eligibility Verification System (EMEVS), 295
Electronic medication administration record (E-MAR), 198, 198b
Electronic prescription records, 175, 175b

Electronic prior authorization modules, 297b
Electronic referencing, 156–157
Eletriptan, 364–366t, 384b, 384f
Elexacaftor/tezacaftor/ivacaftor and ivacaftor, 501b
Elidel. *see* Pimecrolimus
Elimination, of drugs, 118
Eliquis. *see* Apixaban
Elixir, 107–108, 108f, 239
Elixophyllin. *see* Theophylline
Eltrombopag, 650b
E-MAR. *see* Electronic medication administration record
Embolus, 468–469
Emergency carts, 208–210
Emergency contraceptive, for conditions affecting the male
    and female reproductive systems, 546–547t, 558
Emergency medication box, 210, 210f
Emergency medications, 345
Emesis, 520–521
EMEVS. *see* Electronic Medicaid Eligibility Verification
    System
Emily's Law, 318
Emollient laxatives (stool softeners), 518–519
Emollients, 630–631b
Empagliflozin, 421–422t
Empowerment, in over-the-counter medications, 662
Emtricitabine, for human immunodeficiency virus infection
    and acquired immunodeficiency syndrome, 570t
Emulsifying agents, 237t
Emulsion, 110, 110b, 239
    bases, 244b
E-Mycin. *see* Erythromycin
Enalapril, 459–460t, 475–476t
Enbrel. *see* Etanercept
Endocardium, 451
Endocrine glands, function of, 403–409
    hypothalamus, 403
    ovaries, 406–408
    pancreas, 405–406
    parathyroid glands, 404, 404f
    pineal gland, 404
    pituitary gland, 403–404, 403f
    testes, 408–409, 408f
    thyroid gland, 404, 404f
Endocrine system
    anatomy of, 400–401, 400f
    conditions of, 409–423, 409t
        adrenal glands, 415–418
            Addison disease, 416–417
            Cushing disease, 415–416, 416f
            hyperaldosteronism, 416
        common drugs for, 398–400t
        pancreas, 418–423
        parathyroid glands, 409t, 414–415
            hyperparathyroidism, 398–400t, 409t, 414–415
            hypoparathyroidism, 415
        pituitary gland and hypothalamus, 409–411
            diabetes insipidus, 410
            hypersecretion of growth hormone, 409t

Endocrine system *(Continued)*
            hypopituitarism, 409t, 410–411
            syndrome of inappropriate antidiuretic hormone
                secretion (SIADH), 398–400t, 409–410
        mechanism of action of, 401–403, 403f
        structure and function of hormones, 401, 401f, 402t
        therapeutic agents for, 357, 424
        thyroid gland, 409t, 412–414
            conditions of, 412–414
                hyperthyroidism, 412, 412b, 412f
                hypothyroidism, 413–414, 413b, 413f
Endocrinologists, 400
Endometriosis
    agents for, 546–547t
    hormonal therapies for, 552–553t
Endometrium, 550
Endomysium, 431f
End-stage renal disease (ESRD), 532
    Medicare and, 291
Enemas, 111
    for gastrointestinal conditions, 668t
Enfuvirtide, for human immunodeficiency virus infection
    and acquired immunodeficiency syndrome, 570t
Engerix-B, 592–593t
Enoxaparin, 470t
Entacapone, 364–366t, 381t
Entecavir, for hepatitis B, 571t
Enteral route, of administration, 104
Entresto, 456
Envarsus XR. *see* Tacrolimus
Enzyme, 453
Eosinophils, 578, 581f
e-pharmacy, 51–52, 67
Epicardium, 451
Epidermis, 624, 624f
Epididymis, 561–562, 561f
Epididymitis, 569
Epiglottis, 480
Epilepsy, 364–366t, 376–377b, 376–378, 376t
    therapeutic agents for, 356
Epimysium, 431f
Epinephrine, 402t
    autoinjector, 584
    in refilling of crash carts, 208
Epithelial cells, 506
Eplerenone, 475–476t, 537t
Epocrates, 156
Epoetin alfa, 533–534b, 533f, 651t
Epogen. *see* Epoetin alfa
Eponychium, 625f
e-prescribing, 166, 316
EPS. *see* Extrapyramidal symptoms
Eptifibatide, 470t, 472t
Erectile dysfunction, 566–567, 567b, 567t
    agents for, 546–547t
Error, 316
Ery. *see* Erythromycin
Erygel. *see* Erythromycin

Ery-Tab. *see* Erythromycin
Ery-tab. *see* Erythromycin
Erythrocyte, 646
Erythromycin, 569t, 607–608t, 609b, 609f
  for acne vulgaris, 627t
  dosage forms of, 103–104, 104t
  dosing times, solutions, and appropriate volumes for, 277t
  reconstituting, 280b
Erythropoiesis, 646, 647f
Erythropoiesis stimulating agents, 651t
Erythropoietin, 532–533, 646, 647f
Eschar, 633b
Escherichia coli, 539
Escitalopram, 364–366t, 386–387t
Esidrex. *see* Hydrochlorothiazide
Eskalith. *see* Lithium
Esomeprazole, 510b, 510f, 511t
  for gastroesophageal reflux disease and indigestion, 667t
Esophagitis, 359
Esophagus, 505f, 507f, 508f
ESRD. *see* End-stage renal disease
Essential hypertension, 457
Esterified estrogen, 552–553t, 559b, 559f
Estradiol, 551, 552–553t, 559b, 559f
Estradiol and levonorgestrel, 552–553t
Estrogen, 359, 402t, 546–547t, 547–549
  for conditions affecting the male and female reproductive systems, 546–547t, 551
  function of, 547–549
  secretion of, 558
  therapy with, 556
Estropipate, 559b, 559f
Eszopiclone, 364–366t, 392t, 393b, 393f
Etanercept, 585–587t, 589b, 589f, 630–631b, 632t
Ethacrynic acid, 537t
Ethambutol, 499t
Ethics
  professional, 54
  in workplace, 54, 54b
Ethinyl estradiol, 556, 557b, 557f
Ethionamide, 499t
Ethosuximide, 377–378b, 377f
  for epilepsy, 377t
Ethynodiol diacetate, 557t
Etiquette
  telephone, 87–89, 88b, 88f
  virtual communication, 89
Etodolac, 426–427t, 434t
Etonogestrel, 359, 556, 557t
Etoposide, 654–655t
Etravirine, for human immunodeficiency virus infection and acquired immunodeficiency syndrome, 570t
Euphoria, 435–436
Eustachian tube, 613, 613b
Everolimus, 585–587t
Evista. *see* Raloxifene
Evolocumab, 463t, 466b

Exam for the Certification of Pharmacy Technicians (ExCPT), 71, 72–73t
Excessive workload, medication errors and, 321
Excipients, 118–119, 236
Excretion, 505, 527
Exelon. *see* Rivastigmine
Exempt controlled substances, 36
Exenatide, 398–400t, 421–422t
Exfoliation, in acne vulgaris, 626b
Exocrine glands, 401
Exophthalmos, 412
Expectorants, 237t, 487, 664, 666t
Expiration, 481, 484f
Expiration dates, repackaged medications, 228
Expired stock, 308, 308b
Extavia. *see* Interferon beta-1b
External auditory canal, 613f
External ear, 613, 613f
External epithelial root sheath, 625f
Extrapyramidal symptoms (EPSs), 388b
Exudate, 618–619
Eyelids, 601
Eyes, 601–602
  anatomy and physiology of, 601–602, 601f, 602f
  conditions of, 602–613
    allergic conjunctivitis, 604–605, 604b, 604f
    drugs for, 599–600t, 603–604t
    glaucoma as, 609–612, 609f, 610b, 610t
    infections as, 606–609, 607–608t
    medications for, 114
    ophthalmic inflammation caused by infection or injury as, 605–606, 606f
  therapeutic agents for, 360
  vision and, 602
Ezetimibe, 463t, 465b, 465f

F

Facial expression, 85f
Facial nerve, 373t
Factor Xa inhibitors, 470t
Fahrenheit, temperature conversion between Celsius and, 129
Fair Packaging and Labeling Act, 30t
Fallopian tubes, 406–408, 547–549, 550
Famciclovir, 569t
Family Smoking and Tobacco Control Act, 30t
Famotidine, 280, 280t, 509b, 509f, 511t
  for gastroesophageal reflux disease and indigestion, 667t
Fanapt. *see* Iloperidone
Farxiga. *see* Dapagliflozin
Fascicles, 427, 431f
Fast movers, 306, 339, 339f
Fat, in hair, 625f
FDA. *see* Food and Drug Administration
Febuxostat, 426–427t, 443t
Federal Food, Drug, and Cosmetic Act, 23, 31
Federal Legend, 166

Female reproductive system, 547–550, 550f
  conditions of, 550–560
    common drugs for, 546–547t
    contraception and, 556–558, 556f, 557b, 557t
    hormones affecting, 548t
    hypogonadism as, 554–555, 554f
    infertility as, 546–547t, 552–553t, 555–556
    menopause as, 558–559
    menstrual disorders as, 551, 553b
    pelvic inflammatory disease as, 559–560, 560b, 560t
  menstrual cycle in, 549f
  pelvic organs of, 547–549, 548f
Fenofibrate, 463t
Fentanyl, 426–427t, 437t, 438b, 438f
  patch, 107
Ferrous sulfate, 360, 533b, 533f, 648b
FerrouSul. see Ferrous sulfate
Fertilization, 550
Fesoterodine, 541t, 542b, 542f
Fexofenadine, 488t, 489b, 489f, 617t, 665t
Fiber/bulk laxative, for gastrointestinal conditions, 668t
Fibrates, 463t, 464–465
Filgrastim, 651t, 652b, 652f
Filter needles, 259t, 274–275
Filter straws, 259t, 260–261
Filters, 259t, 260–261, 261f
Fimbriae, 550
Finacea. see Azelaic acid
Finasteride, 565–566b, 565f, 565t, 566b
Fingertip Formulary, 157
Fingolimod, 364–366t
First air, 265t, 268
First-pass effect, 117–118
Fish oil, 463t, 465
Fistulae, 513–515
Flarex. see Fluorometholone
Flat warts, 634–635
Flatulence, 504t, 520, 520b
Flavoring additives, for taste, 236, 237t
Flecainide, 474t
Fleet. see Sodium phosphate
Fleet Mineral Oil Enema. see Mineral oil
Fleming, Alexander, 9–10
Flexeril. see Cyclobenzaprine
Flexible spending account, 303
Flomax. see Tamsulosin
Flonase. see Fluticasone
Flonase Allergy Relief. see Fluticasone
Floor stock, 192–193, 207–208
Florinef. see Fludrocortisone acetate
Flovent Diskus. see Fluticasone
Flovent HFA. see Fluticasone
Flow hood, laminar, when preparing chemotherapeutic
  agents, 653b
Fluad, 592–593t
Fluarix, 592–593t
Flublok, 592–593t
Flucelvax, 592–593t

Fluconazole, 569t
Fludarabine, 654–655t
Fludrocortisone, 461b, 461f
Fludrocortisone acetate, 398–400t, 417b, 417f
Flulaval, 592–593t
Flumadine. see Rimantadine
FluMist Quadrivalent, 592–593t
Flunisolide, 488t
Fluocinolone, 630t, 632t
Fluocinonide, 630t
Fluorometholone, for conditions affecting the eye, 603–604t
Fluoroplex. see Fluorouracil
Fluoroquinolone, 539t, 607–608t
Fluoroquinolone antibiotics, 498b
Fluorouracil
  for basal cell carcinoma, 639b, 639f
  for skin cancer, 639b, 639f
  for warts, 634b
Fluoxetine, 356, 364–366t, 386–387t
Fluoxymesterone, 563t
Flurandrenolide, 630t, 632t
Flurazepam, 392t
Flurbiprofen, 603–604t, 605b, 605f
Flutamide, 568t
Fluticasone, 488t, 489b, 489f, 492t, 616b, 616f, 665t
Fluticasone propionate, 494b, 494f, 630t, 632t
Fluticasone/salmeterol, 492t, 497b, 497f
Fluticasone/vilanterol, 497b, 497f
Fluvastatin, 463t
Fluvirin, 592–593t
Fluzone, 592–593t
Fluzone high-dose, 592–593t
Fluzone Intradermal, 592–593t
FML. see Fluorometholone
Focalin. see Dexmethylphenidate
Folate deficiency anemia, 648t
Follicle-stimulating hormone (FSH), 402t, 406–408
  functions of, 548t
  secretion of, 558
  testosterone and, 562f
Fondaparinux, 470t
Food and Drug Administration (FDA), 21, 31
  drug recalls and, 308, 309b, 309t
  good manufacturing practices, 224
  history of, 21–23
  recalled drugs and, 31, 35–36b
  reporting process and adverse reactions, 31, 31b, 32f
Food and Drug Administration Amendments Act of 2007,
  51
Food and Drug Administration Modernization Act, 30t
Forceps, 259t
Formoterol, 492t, 494b
Formoterol/budesonide, 497b, 497f
Formoterol/mometasone, 492t
Formulary, 280–289, 289b, 306
  definition, 154
  medications, 194
Formulation record (FR), 247–249, 248f

Fortaz. *see* Ceftazidime

Fosamax. *see* Alendronate

Fosamprenavir, for human immunodeficiency virus infection and acquired immunodeficiency syndrome, 570t

Fosinopril, 458t

Fourth-degree burns, 633–634, 633b, 634b

Fovea centralis, 601f

FR. *see* Formulation record

Fragmin. *see* Dalteparin

Franchise, 164–165

Front counter area, 338, 339b, 339f, 346f

Frontal lobe, 369

Frova. *see* Frovatriptan

Frovatriptan, 364–366t

FSH. *see* Follicle-stimulating hormone

Full-thickness burns, 633b, 634b

Fundamentals of Nursing, 160t

Fungal infections
    athlete's foot, 635–636, 635b, 636f, 636t
    ophthalmic, 609
    vaginal, agents for, 546–547t

Fungicidal, 609

Furosemide, 458t, 459–460t, 475–476t, 537t, 538b, 538f

Fusion inhibitor, for human immunodeficiency virus infection and acquired immunodeficiency syndrome, 570t

G

Gabapentin, 356, 364–366t, 375f

Gabitril. *see* Tiagabine

GAD. *see* Generalized anxiety disorder

Galantamine, 364–366t, 379t

Galen, Claudius, 6

Gallbladder, 506, 508f

Gametes, 547–549

Ganciclovir, 607–608t

Garamycin. *see* Gentamicin

Gardasil 9, 592–593t

Gardnerella vaginalis, 569t

Garlic, 7, 673t, 675–677, 676t, 677f

Gas, 472t

Gas exchange, 481–484, 485f

Gastric juice, 505–506

Gastrocrom. *see* Cromolyn sodium

Gastroesophageal reflux disease (GERD), 504t, 509–511, 509b, 510t, 511t, 619–620
    over-the-counter medications for, 665–667, 667t

Gastrointestinal system, 524
    anatomy and physiology of, 505–508, 505f
        absorption, 506, 507f
        auxiliary organs, 507–508, 508f
        excretion, 506–507
        ingestion, 505–506, 505b, 505f, 506f, 507f
    conditions affecting, 508–523
        colorectal cancer, 522
        common drugs for, 504t
        intestines, 513–520
            constipation, 504t, 518–520, 518b, 519t

Gastrointestinal system *(Continued)*
        diarrhea, 504t, 516–518, 517b, 517t
        flatulence, 504t, 520
        inflammatory bowel disease (IBD), 513–515, 513f, 514–515b, 514f, 514t
        irritable bowel syndrome (IBS), 504t, 516, 516b
    nausea and vomiting, 520–522
    stomach, 508–512, 509b, 511b
        gastroesophageal reflux disease (GERD), 504t, 509–511, 509b, 510t, 511t
        peptic ulcer disease (PUD), 511–512, 511f, 512f, 512t
    form and role of, 505
    therapeutic agents for, 359

Gastroparesis, 418–419b

Gas-X. *see* Simethicone

Gatifloxacin, 607–608t

Gauges, 260

Gaviscon Extra Strength. *see* AlOH and magnesium carbonate

Gels, 111
    preparing, 247

Gemcitabine, 523b

Gemfibrozil, 463t, 465b, 465f

Generalized anxiety disorder (GAD), 387

Generalized seizures, 376–377, 376t

Generic drugs
    as formulary drugs, 289
    insurance in, 289
    Medicare insurance in, 294
    in multiple dosage forms, 103–104, 104t
    substitution, 171
    trade name drugs *vs.*, 289–290

Generic name, 150–151, 150b, 151b
    brand names *vs.*, 352
    drug classification and, 455b
    tall man lettering and, 352, 353t

Genetics, 7

Gengraf. *see* Cyclosporine; Cyclosporine A

Genital herpes, 569, 569t

Genital warts, 634–635, 635f

Gentak. *see* Gentamicin

Gentamicin, 277t, 560t, 607–608t

Geodon. *see* Ziprasidone

George, Homer, 24

GERD. *see* Gastroesophageal reflux disease

Geriatric Dosage Handbook, 156, 157t

Geriatric patients, 139
    liquid medications and, 138

Geriatrics, 237t

Germinal matrix, 625f

Gestational diabetes mellitus, 409t, 418–419

Gigantism, 411

Gilenya. *see* Fingolimod

Ginkgo biloba, 673t, 676t, 678, 678f, 679f

Ginseng, 673t, 676t, 678–679

Glass syringes, 259

Glatiramer, 364–366t, 383b, 383f, 585–587t

Glaucoma, 609–612, 609f, 610b, 610t

Gleevec. *see* Imatinib

Gliadel Wafer, 106–107

Glimepiride, 398–400t, 421–422t

Glipizide, 398–400t, 421–422t

Global Initiative for Chronic Obstructive Lung Disease (GOLD), 495–498

Glomerulonephritis, 618b

Glomerulus, 528

Glossopharyngeal nerve, 373t

Glove boxes, 205, 206b, 206f, 268

Gloves

  for bulk repackaging, 228b

  donning of, in aseptic technique, 272

  labeling, 207b

  when preparing chemotherapeutic agents, 653b

Glucagon, 402t, 407f

Glucocorticoids, 417b

  for Addison disease, 417–418

  therapeutic use of, 585–587t

Glucometer, 423

Glucophage. *see* Metformin

Glucotrol. *see* Glipizide

Glyburide, 398–400t, 421–422t

Glycerin, for gastrointestinal conditions, 668t

Glycerinated gelatins, 245

Glycoprotein IIb/IIIa inhibitors, 470t, 472t

Gly-Oxide. *see* Carbamide peroxide

Glyset. *see* Miglitol

GMP. *see* Good Manufacturing Practices

GnRH. *see* Gonadotropin-releasing hormone

Goiter, 412

GOLD. *see* Global Initiative for Chronic Obstructive Lung Disease

Gold Standard/ Elsevier products, 153

Golimumab, 585–587t, 632t

Gonadotropin, 563t

Gonadotropin-ovulation stimulator, 552–553t

Gonadotropin-releasing hormone (GnRH), 550, 552–553t, 558

  functions of, 548t

  male sex hormones and, 562f

  release of, 558, 562

Gonorrhea, 569, 569t

Good Manufacturing Practices (GMP), 24, 224, 224t, 683

Goodman & Gilman's The Pharmacological Basis of Therapeutics, 155, 157t

Goserelin, 552–553t, 568t

Gout, 426–427t, 440–441, 440–441b, 442f, 443t

Government-managed insurance programs, 291–292

  CHAMPVA, 295–296, 296f

  Medicaid. *see* Medicaid

  Medicare. *see* Medicare

  TRICARE, 295, 296f

  workers' compensation in, 296–297, 297b

Gown

  chemotherapy, 281–282

  donning of, in aseptic technique, 272

  when preparing chemotherapeutic agents, 653b

Graduated cylinders, 231–234, 234f, 234t, 238, 239f

Grand mal seizures, 376–377

Granix. *see* Filgrastim

Granulocytopenia, 651

Graves disease, 412, 590, 590b, 590f

Gray matter, 369

Group purchasing organization, 310

Growth hormone, irregular secretion of, 411, 411b

Guaifenesin, 487b, 487f

  for cough and cold symptoms, 666t

Gums, 237t

Gyne-Lotrimin. *see* Clotrimazole

H

Hahnemann, Samuel, 683

HAI. *see* Health care-associated infection

Hair

  anatomy and physiology of, 624, 625f

  head lice, 639–640, 640f

Hair bulb, 625f

Hair follicle, 624f, 625f

Hair root, 625f

Hair shaft, 624f, 625f, 626f

Halcinonide, 630t, 632t

Halcion. *see* Triazolam

Haldol. *see* Haloperidol

Half-life, 118

Halls Lozenges. *see* Menthol

Halog. *see* Halcinonide

Haloperidol, 357, 364–366t, 389b, 389f

Hand hygiene, proper, 273b, 273f

Hand placement, aseptic technique in, 273, 273b, 275f

Handbook of Nonprescription Drugs, 155

Handbook on Injectable Drugs, 154, 157t

Hand-rolling method, in preparing suppositories, 246

Hard lozenges, 242–243

  formula for, 243

Hard sticks, 245

Harrison Narcotics Act of 1914, 12, 23

Hashimoto thyroiditis, 591, 591b

Hatha yoga, 680

Havrix, 592–593t

Hayhurst, Susan, 13t

Hazardous chemicals, 250

Hazardous drugs (HD), 265t, 268, 281–282

Hazardous Substances Labeling Act of 1960, 24

Hazardous waste, 282b

HCTZ. *see* Hydrochlorothiazide

HDL. *see* High-density lipoprotein

Head lice, 639–640, 640f

Health care team, communication with, 91, 91f

Health care-associated infection (HAI), 263–264

  medication errors and, 323

  urinary tract and, 540b

Health Careers Today, 160t

Health Information Technology for Economic and Clinical Health (HITECH) Act, 197–198

Health Insurance Portability and Accountability Act (HIPAA), 26
   Medicare and, 291–292
Health literacy, definition of, 183
Health maintenance organization (HMO), 216, 290
Health Maintenance Organization Act (1973), 216
Health savings account, 303
Hearing impairments, in elderly patients, 182
Hearing-impaired patients, communication with, 91, 91b
Heart. *see also* Cardiovascular system
   anatomy of, 451–452, 452f
      cardiac conduction system and, 452, 453f
      cardiac cycle, 452, 454f
      oxygenation and, 451–452, 452f, 453f
   regulation of, 453, 453b, 455f
Heart failure (HF), 473–476, 473b, 474b, 475–476t, 536b
Heartburn, 511b
Hectorol. *see* Doxercalciferol
HeFH. *see* Heterozygous familial hypercholesterolemia
Helicobacter pylori infection, 666b
   treatment of, 512t
Help Desk, 172
Hematologic system, 660
   anatomy and physiology of, 645–646
      cellular components of blood, 646, 646f, 647f
      plasma, 645, 645f
      plasma proteins, 645–646, 645f, 646f
   conditions of, 646–657
      anemia, 647–649, 618t
      bleeding disorders, 657, 657b
      cancer, 652–657, 654–655t, 657t
      common drugs for, 644t
      low cell and platelet counts, 650–652, 651t
      polycythemia, 649–650
      sickle cell disease, 649
   therapeutic agents for, 360
Hematopoiesis, 578, 579f, 647f, 652f
Hematopoietic agents, 526–527t
Hematopoietic growth factors, 652f
Hemochromatosis, 11
Hemodialysis, 532, 533f
Hemoglobin, 646
Hemolytic anemia, 648t
Hemophilia, 657
Hemorrhagic strokes, 384
HEPA filters. *see* High-efficiency particulate air (HEPA) filters
Heparin, 103, 469b, 470t, 472t
   measurement of, 139, 140b
   overdose, 325
Heparin-lock solutions, 325
Hepatitis, 569
Hepatitis A vaccine, 592–593t
Hepatitis B
   treatment for, 571t
   vaccine, 592–593t
Hepatitis C, 572
   treatment for, 571t

Herbal products, 673t, 674t, 675–680, 675b
   common uses and cautionary notes for, 676t
   drug interactions with, 676–677t
   popularity of, 680b
   preparations for, 680, 680t
Herbal remedies, ancient treatments using, 7
Hermes, 4
Herpes simplex, 569t
Herpes zoster, 592–593t
Heterozygous familial hypercholesterolemia (HeFH), 465–466
HFA. *see* Hydrofluoroalkane
Hiberix, 592–593t
High alert medications, 139
High-density lipoprotein (HDL), 461–464
High-efficiency particulate air (HEPA) filters, 205, 267
   airflow and, 268
Hilus, 527
HIPAA. *see* Health Insurance Portability and Accountability Act
Hippely, Beth, 318
Hippocrates, 5, 680b
Hippocratic oath, 5, 5b
Hires, Charles Elmer, 13t
Hirsutism, 624
Histamine antagonist, for insomnia, 666t
Histamine-₂ antagonists (H₂-antagonists), 509, 509b, 511t
   for gastroesophageal reflux disease and indigestion, 667, 667t
   for gastrointestinal system, 359
   for GERD, 619b
Histex. *see* Triprolidine
HITECH Act. *see* Health Information Technology for Economic and Clinical Health (HITECH) Act
HIV. *see* Human immunodeficiency virus
HMO. *see* Health Maintenance Organization
Home health care, medication errors in, 323
Home health pharmacies, 66, 67f
Home infusion pharmacy technician, 76
Homeopathic Pharmacopeia, 683
Homeopathy, 674t, 683
Homeostasis, 366–367, 401, 531
Honey, 11
Hood
   cleaning and maintaining, 269, 269–270b, 271b
   hand placement and, 273
   horizontal laminar flow, 204–205, 205f, 263, 269–270b
   vertical flow, 204–205, 206f
   vertical laminar flow, 267, 271b
Horizontal laminar flow hood, 205, 205f, 263
   cleaning, 269–270b, 269f, 270f
   spills in, 282
Hormone replacement therapy, 554–555b
   for female hypogonadism, 552–553t, 554–555
   for menopause, 558–559, 558–559b
Hormone/nutritional supplement, for insomnia, 666t

Hormones, 400, 401–403
  adrenocorticotropic, 402t
  autocrine, 401
  blood pressure and, 453
  calcitonin, 401, 402t
  gonadotropin-releasing, 550, 558, 562
  growth, 402t
  luteinizing, 402t, 548t, 558, 562
  oxytocin, 402t
  parathyroid, 401, 402t
  pineal gland, 402t
  pituitary gland, 402t
  of pituitary gland, 547–549
  structure and function of, 401
  thyroid, 402t
Hospital
  burn, 633–634
  orders, 195 198
  pharmacies. see Institutional pharmacy
  Standard Precautions and, 257
  types of, 192–194, 192f, 193t
Household measurements, 127
Household system, 132, 134, 134b, 135b
Humalog. see Insulin lispro
Human chorionic gonadotropin, 563t
Human immunodeficiency virus (HIV)
  symptoms of, 569
  treatment for, 570t
  vaccines for, 570–572
Human papillomavirus, 635f
Human papillomavirus vaccine, 634–635
Humatrope. see Somatropin
Humira. see Adalimumab
Humoral immunity, 580–582
Humors, of body system, 5, 5b
Humulin N. see Isophane insulin
Hydralazine, 475–476t
Hydrea. see Hydroxyurea
Hydrochloric acid, 505–506
Hydrochlorothiazide (HCTZ), 458t, 459–460t, 475–476t,
    537t, 538b, 538f
Hydrocodone and chlorpheniramine syrup, 107
Hydrocodone/acetaminophen, 426–427t, 436b, 436f
Hydrocortisone, 111, 398–400t, 417b, 417f, 630t, 632t, 669t
  cream, 111
  lotion, 111
Hydrofluoroalkane (HFA), inhalers and, 494b
Hydromorphone, 426–427t, 437t
Hydrophilic solution, 240
Hydrophobic solution, 240
Hydrostatic pressure, 645–646, 646f
Hydroxychloroquine, 588b
Hydroxyurea, 650f, 654–655t
Hydroxyzine pamoate capsules, 106
Hyperaldosteronism, 409t, 416, 416b
Hyperalimentation, 277–278, 278b, 278f, 279f
  preparation of, 63
Hypercholesterolemia, 358

Hyperglycemia, 418
Hyperlipidemia, 461–465, 461b, 462f, 463t, 464b
Hyperosmolar agent, for gastrointestinal conditions, 668t
Hyperparathyroidism, 398–400t, 409t, 414–415, 414b
Hyperplasia, benign prostatic, therapeutic agents for, 359
Hypersecretion of growth hormone, 409t
Hypertension, 358, 455t, 457–459, 457b, 458–459b,
    459–460t
  essential, 457
  hyperaldosteronism and, 416
  medications used for, treatment of, 459–460t
  during pregnancy, 459
  secondary, 457
Hyperthyroidism, 398–400t, 409t, 412, 412b, 412f, 590f
Hyperventilation, 484t
Hypocalcemia, 414–415
Hypodermis, 624, 624f
Hypoglossal nerve, 373t
Hypoglycemia, 410
Hypogonadism
  female, 554–555, 554f
  male, 562–564, 563t
Hypokalemia, 416
Hypomenorrhea, 553b
Hypoparathyroidism, 409t, 415, 415b
Hypopituitarism, 409t, 410–411, 410–411b
Hypopituitary dwarfism, 410
Hypopnea, 484t
Hypotension, 460–461, 461b
Hypothalamus
  conditions of, 409–411
    diabetes insipidus, 410
    syndrome of inappropriate antidiuretic hormone
        secretion (SIADH), 398–400t, 409–410
  functions of, 403, 403f
Hypothyroidism, 398–400t, 409t, 413–414, 413f
Hypoxia, 649–650
Hytrin. see Terazosin

I

Iatrogenic effects, of drugs, 356
Ibandronate, 426–427t, 441t
IBD. see Inflammatory bowel disease
IBM Micromedex Drug Information, 157
IBS. see Irritable bowel syndrome
Ibuprofen, 352, 426–427t, 435b, 435f
  common adult dosage of, 664t
  for cough and cold symptoms, 666t
  for gout, 443t
  suspension, 111
ICHP. see Illinois Council of Health-System Pharmacists
Icosapent ethyl, 465b
Idamycin. see Idarubicin
Idarubicin, 654–655t
Idarucizumab, 471b
Ident-A-Drug, 153, 155f, 157t
IDENTIDEX, 154
Identification number (ID #), 299b

Idiopathic thrombocytopenia, 650
IHI. *see* Institute for Healthcare Improvement
Ileostomy, 513
Illinois Council of Health-System Pharmacists (ICHP), 71
Iloperidone, 364–366t
Imatinib, 654–655t
Imdur. *see* Isosorbide mononitrate
Imipenem-cilastatin, 277t
Imipramine, 364–366t
Imitrex. *see* Sumatriptan
Immune globulins, 576–577t
Immune system
    anatomy and physiology of, 577–584, 578f
        bone marrow, 578, 578f, 579f
        cells and mediators, 578–582, 581f, 582f
        inflammation, 583–584, 584f
        spleen, 578, 578f, 580f
        thymus, 578, 578f
        types of immunity, 580–582, 583f
    autoimmune disorders, 584–591
        biological response modifiers and immunomodulators for, 585, 585–587t
        Graves disease, 412, 590, 590b, 590f
        Hashimoto thyroiditis, 591, 591b
        immunosuppressive agents for transplant rejection and, 577t
        rheumatoid arthritis, 588–590, 588f, 589b
        systemic lupus erythematosus (SLE), 587–588, 588b
        type 1 diabetes mellitus, 418, 584–585
    therapeutic agents for, 359–360, 597
    transplant rejection and, 577t, 585–587t, 591–592, 591b, 591f
    vaccines that affect, 576–577t
Immunity, 578
    types of, 580–582, 583f
Immunizations, 592–596, 594b, 594t. *see also* Vaccines
    for adult, 595t
    childhood, 594b
    in community pharmacy, 185, 185b
Immunoglobulins, 580–582
Immunological agent, 607–608t
Immunomodulators, 479t
    for autoimmune disorders and transplant rejection prophylaxis, 585–587t
Immunosuppressants, 577t, 623–624t, 630t
Immunotherapy, 656
Imodium. *see* Loperamide
Imodium A-D. *see* Loperamide
Imovax Rabies, 592–593t
Impetigo, 636–637, 637f, 637t
Implants, 106–107
Impotence, 566–567
Improper dose error, 317t
Imuran. *see* Azathioprine
Incentive programs, for employees, 76–77
Incretin mimetics, 398–400t
Incus, 613f
Independent pharmacy, 164

Independent physician association (IPA), 290
Inderal. *see* Propranolol
Indications and usage, 43
Indigestion, over-the-counter medications for, 665–667, 667t
Indinavir, for human immunodeficiency virus infection and acquired immunodeficiency syndrome, 570t
Indocin. *see* Indomethacin
Indomethacin, 426–427t, 434t, 443t
Infanrix, 592–593t
Infant, breathing rates in, 481b
Infection control, 257
Infections
    athlete's foot, 635–636, 635b, 636f, 636t
    ophthalmic, 606–609, 607–608t
        bacterial, 606–609, 606b
        fungal, 609
        viral, 609
    ophthalmic inflammation caused by, 605–606, 606f
Inferior rectus muscle, 601f
Infertility, 555–556
    medications for, 546–547t, 552–553t
Infix, term, 352
Inflammation, 583–584, 584f
    ophthalmic, by infection or injury, 605–606, 606f
Inflammatory bowel disease (IBD), 513–515, 513f, 514–515b, 514f, 514t, 516b
Inflectra. *see* Infliximab
Infliximab, 514t, 515b, 515f, 585–587t, 630–631b, 632t
Influenza, 486t, 489–490, 490b, 490f, 490t
    vaccines, 592–593t
Infusion, herbal, 680
Ingestion, 505–506, 505b, 505f, 506f, 507f
INH. *see* Isoniazid
Inhalant, cross-contamination of, 247b
Inhalers, 109–110, 109f, 110b, 110f, 491–494, 493f, 494b
    metered dose, 109
INN. *see* International Nonproprietary Names
Innate immunity, 580, 583f
Inner ear, 613, 613f, 614b, 614f
Innovator product, 289
Inpatient pharmacy, 15
    setting requirements in, 63–64, 64b, 64f, 65b
Inscription, 169
Insomnia, 364–366t, 391–393, 391b, 392t, 404b
    over-the-counter medications for, 664–665, 666t
Inspiration, 481, 484f
Inspra. *see* Eplerenone
Instillation, 114
Institute for Healthcare Improvement (IHI), 331
Institute for Safe Medication Practices (ISMP), 315
    list of error-prone abbreviations, symbols, and dose designations, 96, 97–102t
    on tall man lettering, 320–321
Institute of Medicine (IOM), on point-of-entry system, 197
Institutional pharmacy, 191–192, 343–345
    automated dispensing system and, 201–202, 202b, 329, 329f, 343, 344b, 344f

Institutional pharmacy *(Continued)*
  communication between nurses and, 198, 198b
  discharge pharmacies, 193–194
  flow of orders in, 195–197, 196f
  point-of-entry systems in, 197–198
  policies and standard operating procedures, 194, 194b
  protocol of, 194
  regulatory agencies and, 195
  satellite pharmacies, 192–193
  settings, 192–194, 193f
  stat, ASAP, and standing orders in, 197
  technician, 199–200, 199t
    automated dispensing systems and, 201–202, 202b
    counting, dispensing, and tracking controlled substances
        and, 202
    future for, 210–211, 211b
    intravenous preparations, 203–204
    labeling, 207–210, 207b, 207f
    maintaining stock and supplying specialty areas,
        207–208, 208b
    nonhazardous intravenous preparation, 204–206, 204b
    patient cassette drawers and/or Pyxis machine, 200–201
    refilling of crash carts, 208, 208b, 209b, 209f, 209t
    specialty tasks, 199–200, 200b
    supplying nonclinical areas, 210, 210b
    unit dose medications, 201f, 202, 224
  types of hospitals and, 192–194, 192f, 193t
Institutional pharmacy practice, 212
Insulin, 280t, 402t, 670b
  for diabetes mellitus, 418, 420t
  measurement of, 139–140, 140b
  overdose, 325
Insulin aspart, 398–400t
Insulin detemir, 398–400t
Insulin glargine, 398–400t
Insulin glulisine, 398–400t
Insulin lispro, 398–400t
Insulin resistance, 418
Insurance
  DAW codes in, 289, 289b
  formularies and, 288
  in generic drugs, 289
  types of, 289–290
    CHAMPVA, 295–296, 296f
    health maintenance organization, 290
    Medicaid. *see* Medicaid
    Medicare. *see* Medicare
    preferred provider organization, 291, 291f
    respect, 297b
    TRICARE, 295, 296f
    workers' compensation in, 296–297
Insurance billing technician, 65–66
Integrase inhibitor, for human immunodeficiency virus
        infection and acquired immunodeficiency syndrome, 570t
Integrilin. *see* Eptifibatide
Interdisciplinary team, 214
Interferon alfa-2a, for hepatitis C, 571t
Interferon alfa-2a pegylated, for hepatitis B and C, 571t

Interferon alfa-2b, for hepatitis B and C, 571t
Interferon beta-1a, 364–366t, 382b, 382f, 383b, 383f, 585–587t
Interferon beta-1b, 364–366t, 383b, 383f, 585–587t
Interferons, 585–587t
  for hepatitis B and C, 571t
Interleukin antagonists, 585–587t
Interleukin-1 (IL-1), 579–580, 582f
Intermezzo. *see* Zolpidem
Internal epithelial root sheath, 625f
International Nonproprietary Names (INN), 352
International System of Units (SI), 132–133
International time, 128, 128b, 128f
Internet
  e-pharmacies and, 51–52
  as reference source, 158, 158t
Interstitial cell-stimulating hormone, 562
Interstitial space, 536–537
Intestines, 505–506, 505f
  conditions affecting, 513–520
    constipation, 504t, 518–520, 518b, 519t
    diarrhea, 504t, 516–518, 517b, 517t
    flatulence, 504t, 520
    inflammatory bowel disease (IBD), 513–515, 513f,
        514–515b, 514f, 514t
    irritable bowel syndrome (IBS), 504t, 516, 516b
Intramuscular agents, 114
Intraocular pressure (IOP), 609–610
Intrauterine devices, 557t
Intravenous infusion rates/flow rates, 141, 141b, 142b
Intravenous medications, 114, 116f
  calculating, 140–141, 141f
  label for, 280–281, 280b, 281f
  preparation of, 63, 64f, 203–204
Intravenous room, 199t, 203, 344–345
  supplies used in, 259t
Invega. *see* Paliperidone
Inventory, 288
  technician responsibilities and, 199t
Inventory control technician, 304–305, 304f, 306b
Inventory management, 63, 303–311, 312
  automated return companies in, 308–310
  damaged stock in, 308
  drug recall in, 307–308, 309b, 309t
  expired stock in, 308, 308b
  inventory control technician in, 304–305, 304f
  new stock in, 306, 307b
  nonreturnable drugs and, 310
  ordering process in, 305
    automated dispensing systems and, 305, 305b, 306f
    bar coding and, 305
    manual, 305–306, 306b
    special considerations in, 311
    special orders, 305
    suppliers in, 310–311, 311t
  pharmacy stock in, 303–304
  proper storage in, 306–307
  returns in, 307–310, 310b
    patient medications not picked up, 310

Inventory technician, 64
Inventory/stock technician, 66
Investigational drugs, 192, 200, 311
Invokana. *see* Canagliflozin
Iodine, 404
IOM. *see* Institute of Medicine
Ions, 527
IPA. *see* Independent physician association
iPLEDGE program, 51, 626b
IPOL, 592–593t
Ipratropium, 492t, 495b, 495f
Ipratropium bromide, 109–110
Ipratropium/albuterol, 497–498b, 497f
Irinotecan, 522b
Iris, 601–602, 601f
Iron. *see* Ferrous sulfate
Iron deficiency anemia, 647–649, 647b, 648f
    treatment for, 644t, 649t
Iron supplement, 526–527t
Irritable bowel syndrome (IBS), 504t, 516, 516b
Ischemic stroke, 384
"Islets of Langerhans," 401
ISMP. *see* Institute for Safe Medication Practices
Isolator hoods, 268
Isoniazid (INH), 499b, 499f, 499t
Isophane insulin, 398–400t
Isopropyl alcohol, 259t
Isoptin. *see* Verapamil
Isopto Carpine. *see* Pilocarpine
Isordil. *see* Isosorbide dinitrate
Isosorbide dinitrate, 458t, 472t, 475–476t
Isosorbide mononitrate, 472t
Isotretinoin, 51, 302, 627t, 628b, 628f
    iPLEDGE program, 51, 626b
IV technician, 64, 204
Ivacaftor, 501b
Ixiaro, 592–593t

J

Januvia. *see* Sitagliptin
Japanese encephalitis vaccine, 592–593t
JCAHO. *see* Joint Commission on Accreditation of
    Healthcare Organizations
Jenner, Edward, 10–11t
Job search, approaches to, 80–81, 80b
Joint Commission on Accreditation of Healthcare
    Organizations (JCAHO), 52
Joints, 427
Journals, 159, 159t
JRA. *see* Juvenile rheumatoid arthritis
Just-in-time ordering, 288
Juvenile rheumatoid arthritis (JRA), 588–590

K

Kariva. *see* Desogestrel
Kefauver-Harris Amendments, 24
Keflex. *see* Cephalexin
Kefzol. *see* Cefazolin

Kenalog. *see* Triamcinolone acetonide
Keppra. *see* Levetiracetam
Keratin, 624
Keratolytics, for acne vulgaris, 626b
Ketoconazole, 636t
Ketoprofen, 352
Ketorolac, 426–427t, 603–604t, 605–606b, 605f
Ketotifen, 603–604t, 617t, 665t
Kidney disease, 536b
Kidney stones, 535–536, 535f
Kidneys
    anatomy and physiology of, 527–531, 528f, 529f
    conditions of
        chronic kidney disease as, 531–535, 532t, 533f
        kidney stones as, 535–536, 535f
    function of, 527–528
Kineret. *see* Anakinra
Kinrix, 592–593t
KL20, 329, 330f
Knee joint, 428f
Koch, Robert, 10–11t
Kondremul. *see* Mineral oil
Kübler-Ross, Elisabeth, 183
Kyphosis, 439f

L

Labeling
    in institutional pharmacy, 207–210, 207f
    medication errors and, 321
    for nonsterile compounding, 240, 240t
    repackaged medications, 226–228
    for veterinary medications, 251b
Labels
    for intravenous medication, 280–281, 280b, 281f
    for prescriptions, 47, 48f
    for repackaged medications, 47
Labetalol, 459–460t
Lacosamide, for epilepsy, 377t
Lacrimal fluid, 601
LAFH. *see* Laminar air flow hood
Lamictal. *see* Lamotrigine
Laminar air flow hood, 266–267, 267b
    horizontal, 204–205, 205f, 263, 269–270b
    vertical, 204–205, 206f, 267, 271b
Laminar air flow workbench (LAFW), 266–267
Lamisil. *see* Terbinafine
Lamisil AT. *see* Terbinafine
Lamivudine
    for hepatitis B, 571t
    for human immunodeficiency virus infection and acquired
        immunodeficiency syndrome, 570t
Lamotrigine, 364–366t
    for epilepsy, 377t
Lanoxin. *see* Digoxin
Lansoprazole, 510b, 510f, 511t, 620b, 620f
    for gastroesophageal reflux disease and indigestion,
        667t
Lantus. *see* Insulin glargine

Large-volume drips, in medication delivery systems, 262, 262b
Larynx, 480, 482f, 616
LASA drugs. *see* Look-alike, sound-alike (LASA) drugs
Lasix. *see* Furosemide
Latanoprost, 610t, 612b, 612f
  storage of, 612b
LaTourette, Steve, 318
Latuda. *see* Lurasidone
Laudanum, 9, 9b
Laws, pharmacy, 21
  FDA history and, 21–23
  federal, 22–23, 23t
  liabilities, 53, 53b
  scenario checkup, 21, 26–31, 41–43, 53–54
  state, 53
LDL. *see* Low-density lipoprotein
Ledipasvir, for hepatitis C, 571t, 572b, 572f
Leeches, 7, 11
Legend drugs, 24, 47, 102–103, 662–663
Lemtrada. *see* Alemtuzumab
Lens, 601f
Leroux, Henri, 430
Lescol. *see* Fluvastatin
Letrozole, 555b
Leukemia, 644t, 652–656, 654–655t
Leukeran. *see* Chlorambucil
Leukine. *see* Sargramostim
Leukocytes, 578–579, 646, 647f
Leukopenia, 651
Leukotriene inhibitors, 479t, 488t, 494–495
Leukotriene receptor antagonists, for asthma and COPD, 492t, 494–495
Leuprolide, 552–553t, 556b, 568t
Levalbuterol, 492t
Levaquin. *see* Levofloxacin
Levemir. *see* Insulin detemir
Levetiracetam, 364–366t
  for epilepsy, 377t
Levobunolol, 610t
Levocetirizine, 488t
Levodopa/carbidopa, 364–366t, 380b, 380f, 381t
Levofloxacin, 498b, 498f, 569t
Levonorgestrel, 557, 557t, 558, 558b
Levothroid. *see* Levothyroxine sodium
Levothyroxine, 398–400t
Levothyroxine sodium, 414b, 414f
Levoxyl. *see* Levothyroxine sodium
Lexapro. *see* Escitalopram
Lexicomp, 152
LH. *see* Luteinizing hormone
LHRH. *see* Luteinizing hormone-releasing hormone
Liabilities, 53, 53b
Lice, 639–640, 640t
Licensed pharmacy technician, 70
Lidocaine, 474t
Ligaments, 427
Limitation of plan exceeded, 301–302, 302b

Linagliptin, 398–400t, 421–422t
Lincosamide, 627t
Lioresal. *see* Baclofen
Liothyronine, 398–400t
Liothyronine sodium, 414b, 414f
Lipids, 280
Lipitor. *see* Atorvastatin
Liquid medications, 103, 107–111, 107f
  calculations with, 137–140
    alligation alternate in, 144, 145b
    body surface area in, 138, 138b
    body weight in, 137, 138b
    dilution and, 143
    dimensional analysis, 137, 142b
    intramuscular injections, 140
    intravenous medications, 140–141, 141f
    involving units and milliequivalents, 139–140, 140b
    oral and injectable syringes and, 138, 139f
    in pediatric and geriatric dosing, 138, 139b
    percentage and ratio strengths in, 142, 142b
    single-step proportion problem, 137
    subcutaneous injections, 140
    total parenteral nutrition, 144
  unit dose, 202
Liquids, repackaging of, containers for, 224
Liraglutide, 398–400t, 421–422t
Lisdexamfetamine, 364–366t, 394t
Lisinopril, 358, 454b, 454f, 458t, 459–460t, 475–476t
Listening skills, 84
Lithium, 364–366t, 388b, 388f, 389b
Lithotripsy, 535–536b
Liverwort, 7
LMWHs. *see* Low-molecular-weight heparins
Lock-and-key mechanism, 370f
Lodine. *see* Etodolac
Lodoxamide, 603–604t, 605b, 605f
Lomotil. *see* Atropine/diphenoxylate
Long-acting beta-agonists, for asthma, 491–494, 492t
Long-acting contraceptives, for conditions affecting the male and female reproductive systems, 546–547t
Long-term care packaging, 228, 341–342, 341f, 342b, 342f
Long-term care services, 187, 187f
Look-alike, sound-alike (LASA) drugs, medication errors and, 320
Loop diuretics
  in cardiovascular conditions, 459–460t, 473b
  for conditions of the renal and urinary systems, 526–527t, 537t, 538
Loop of Henle, 529
Loperamide, 517b, 517f, 517t
  for gastrointestinal conditions, 668t
Lopid. *see* Gemfibrozil
Lopinavir and ritonavir, for human immunodeficiency virus infection and acquired immunodeficiency syndrome, 570t
Lopressor. *see* Metoprolol
Loratadine, 617t, 665t. *see also* Cetirizine HCl
Lorazepam, 281t, 364–366t

Lortab. *see* Hydrocodone/acetaminophen

Losartan, 358, 455b, 455f, 459–460t

Lot numbers, 308

Lotensin. *see* Benazepril

Loteprednol and tobramycin, for conditions affecting the eye, 603–604t

Lotions, 111

Lotrimin. *see* Clotrimazole

Lotrimin AF. *see* Clotrimazole

Lovastatin, 358, 458t, 463t, 464b, 464f

Lovaza. *see* Fish oil

Lovenox. *see* Enoxaparin

Low cell and platelet counts, 650b, 651–652b, 651b

Low-density lipoprotein (LDL), 461–464

Low-density lipoprotein receptor (LDLR), 465–466

Lower respiratory system
  disorders and conditions of, 490–500
    asthma, 490–495, 491b, 491f, 492t, 493f, 494b
    chronic obstructive pulmonary disease (COPD), 495–498, 496f, 497b
    pneumonia, 498, 498b
    tuberculosis, 498–500, 499b, 499f, 499t
  structure and function of, 481, 481f

Low-molecular-weight heparins (LMWHs), 449–451t, 469, 470t

Lozenges, 106

Lozenges, compressed tablets and, 240–243

Lubiprostone, 516b, 516f, 519t

Lubricant laxative, for gastrointestinal conditions, 668t

Lubricants, 237t

Luer-Lok syringe, 259, 260f

Lumen, 467, 506

Lumigan. *see* Bimatoprost

Lunesta. *see* Eszopiclone

Lung cancer, 500, 500b

Lungs, 480, 482f, 483f

Lunula, 624, 625f

Lurasidone, 364–366t

Luteinizing hormone (LH), 402t
  functions of, 548t
  secretion of, 558, 562

Luteinizing hormone-releasing hormone (LHRH), 568t

Lutropin alfa, 552–553t

Lymph nodes, 577–578, 578f

Lymphatic vessels, 578f

Lymphocytes, 466, 577–578

Lymphocyte-specific agents, 585–587t

Lymphoma, 656–657, 656–657b, 656f

Lysodren. *see* Mitotane

M

Maalox Advanced Maximum Strength. *see* AlOH, MgOH, and simethicone

Macrolides, 607–608t, 627t
  for otitis media, 615t

Macrophages, 466, 579, 581f

Macula, 601f

Mag-Al. *see* AlOH and MgOH

Maggots, 11

Magnesium, 531

Magnesium citrate, for gastrointestinal conditions, 668t

Magnesium hydroxide, 509t
  for gastroesophageal reflux disease and indigestion, 667t
  for gastrointestinal conditions, 668t

Magnesium sulfate, 280t

Mailing controlled substances, 43

Mail-order pharmacy, 51–52, 67

Mainstreaming Addiction Act, 30t

Malaria, 8

Male reproductive system, 560–562, 561f
  conditions of, 562–568
    benign prostatic hypertrophy as, 564–566, 564f, 565t
    common drugs for, 546–547t
    erectile dysfunction as, 546–547t, 566–567, 567t
    hypogonadism as, 562–564, 563t
    prostate cancer as, 567–568, 568f, 568t
  hormones affecting, 548t

Male/female adapter, 259t

Malleus, 613f

Malpractice insurance, 53

Mammary gland, 550, 551f

Managed care, 216

Managed care pharmacy technician, 216

Manipulative and body-based practices, 681, 681b, 682f

Mannitol, 539b

Manufacturer's bottle, scanning, 175, 175b

Manuka honey, 11

MAO. *see* Monoamine oxidase

MAO$_B$-I. *see* Monoamine oxidase-B inhibitors

MAOIs. *see* Monoamine oxidase inhibitors

Maraviroc, for human immunodeficiency virus infection and acquired immunodeficiency syndrome, 570t

Marinol. *see* Dronabinol

Markup, 146

Martindale's The Complete Drug Reference, 156

Massage therapy, 681, 682f

Mast cell stabilizers, 479t, 492t
  for allergy, 617t, 665t
  for conditions affecting the eye, 599–600t, 603–604t, 604b, 605t

Mast cells, 579, 581f

Master formulation record (MFR), 247–249

Mastoid, 613f

Math skills, basic, 129–132, 129t

Maxalt. *see* Rizatriptan

Maxidex. *see* Dexamethasone

MDVs. *see* Multidose vials

Measles, mumps, and rubella (MMR) vaccine, 592–593t

Measurements
  apothecary system, 135
  avoirdupois system, 136
  basic math skills and, 129–132, 129t
  household system, 132, 134, 134b, 135b
  international time and, 128, 128b, 128f

Measurements *(Continued)*
  metric system, 126–127, 132–134, 133t
  systems, 132–136
Meclizine, 522b, 522f
MedCarousel, 329, 329f
MedGuides, 44–46, 320
Media-fill tests, 265t, 283b
Medicaid, 25–26
  chronological changes in, 293t
  current use of, 294–295
  history of, 291–292, 292b
  institutional pharmacies and, 195
  TAR form and, 297–298, 298f
Medical Device Amendments, 22–23
Medical equipment area, durable and nondurable, 342–343,
    343f
Medical food, 674–675
Medical staff, 4, 5f
Medical terminology, 119–123, 121b, 121t, 123b
Medicare, 28
  chronological changes in, 293t
  current use of, 292–294, 292b
  history of, 291–292, 292b
  institutional pharmacies and, 195
  Medigap plan and, 294, 294b
  parts of, 292–294, 292b, 295f
  supplies covered by, 295b
  TAR form and, 297–298, 298f
Medicare Modernization Act (MMA), 28, 292
Medication, 171
  administration, 'five rights' of, 184
  change in, request of, 302b
  classifications of
    by availability to consumers, 102–103
    by body systems, 102, 103t
    packaging and storage requirements for, 119, 120t
  delivery systems, 262–263
  disposal of, 310
  respiratory rates and, 481b
  synchronization of, 186, 186b, 186f
Medication error, 341
  age-related, 323–324
  allergies and, 324–325
  causes of, 319–320
  drug interactions as, 321–322, 322t
  elderly and, 323
  health care-associated infections and, 322t
  "high alert" in connection with, 315, 316b
  home health care, 323
  parenteral, 325, 325f
  patient care and, 323
  pediatric patients and, 323–324, 324f
  pharmacy and, 322–323
  reporting, 326–328, 326b, 327b
  responsibility for, 318
  settings for, 318, 319b
  sustained-released dosage form, 325
  types of, 316–318, 317t

Medication error prevention, 327, 334b, 335
  computerized prescription order entry and, 325–326,
      326b, 326f
  MERP on, 326–327
  strategies for, 328
  training and education for, 334
Medication orders, 192–193, 195–196
  flow of, 195–196, 196f
Medication reconciliation, 331–333, 331b, 332f
  definition of, 215
  job descriptions for institutional pharmacy technicians,
      199t
Medication reconciliation technicians, 215–216, 215f
Medication safety, 335
  automated dispensing system and
    in community pharmacy, 329–330, 330b, 330f
    in hospital pharmacy, 329, 329f
  barcodes for, 328
  medication reconciliation, 331–333, 331b, 332f
  patient dose-specific orders and, 330
  rights of, 315–316
  Robot-Rx machines for, 328, 329f
  USP 797 regulations and, 330–331
Medication sticks, 243
Medication therapy management, 185–186
Medicine
  advances in drug therapy and vaccinations in, 10–11t,
      10–11
  ancient beliefs and treatments in, 4
  eighteenth- and nineteenth-century, 7–9, 8b, 8t, 9b
  evolution of, 4–7, 5b, 6–7t
  history of, 4–7
  in North America, 8–9, 8b, 9t
  twentieth-century, 9–10
Medigap plan, 294, 294b
Meditation, 680
MedMARx, 327
Medrol. *see* Methylprednisolone
Medroxyprogesterone, 554b, 554f
Medroxyprogesterone acetate, 557t
Medscape Mobile, 157
Medulla, 625f
Medulla oblongata, 484
MedWatch, 31, 31b, 32f, 323
Meglitinides, 398–400t
Melanin, 624
Melanocyte, 625f
Melanomas, 638–639, 638f
Melatonin, 392t, 402t, 404
  for insomnia, 666t
Melatonin receptor agonists, 392t
Meloxicam, 426–427t, 434t, 435b, 435f
Memantine, 364–366t, 379t
Menactra, 592–593t
Mendel, Gregor, 8
Meningitis
  in New England Compounding Center, 264
  outbreak in fall of 2012, 30–31

Meningococcal vaccine, 592–593t
Meniscus, 238, 239f
Menopause, 551, 558–559
  premature, 553b
Menorrhagia, 553b
Menotropins, 552–553t, 555b, 555f
  for male infertility, 555b
Menses, 550
Menstrual disorders, 551, 553b
Menstruation, 401
Mental health problems, elderly patients with, 183
Menthol, for cough and cold symptoms, 666t
Menveo, 592–593t
Meperidine, 426–427t, 437t
Mercaptopurine, 654–655t
Mercury, 8
Mesalamine (5-ASA), 514t, 515b, 515f
Mesalamine enema, 111
Message-taking, 89
Mestinon. see Pyridostigmine
Metabolism, 117–118, 117f, 118t, 527
Metadate. see Methylphenidate
Metamucil. see Psyllium
Metastasis, of skin, 638–639
Metaxalone, 444t
Metformin, 398–400t, 421–422t
Methadone, 437t
  maintenance treatment, 50
Methimazole, 398–400t, 412b, 412f, 590b, 590f
Methocarbamol, 426–427t, 444t
Methotrexate, 585–587t, 589b, 589f
  for eczema, 630t
  for hematologic cancer, 654–655t
  for psoriasis, 630–631b, 632t
Methoxsalen, 632t
Methylcellulose, 519t
Methyldopa, 459–460t
Methylin. see Methylphenidate
Methylnaltrexone, 438b
Methylphenidate, 364–366t, 394–395b, 394f, 394t
Methylprednisolone, 417b, 417f, 443t
Methylprednisolone sodium succinate, 398–400t, 417b, 417f
Methyltestosterone, 563b, 563f
Methylxanthines, for asthma and COPD, 492t
Metipranolol, 610t
Metoclopramide, 521b, 521f
Metolazone, 458t, 459–460t, 475–476t, 537t, 538b, 538f
Metopirone. see Metyrapone
Metoprolol, 456b, 456f, 458t, 459–460t, 472t, 475–476t
Metric system, 126–127, 132–134, 133t
  conversions, 133–134
  measurements of, 133, 133b
  prefixes, 133t
Metric-household conversions, 168t
Metronidazole, 560t, 569t
Metyrapone, 398–400t

MI. see Myocardial infarction
Michigan Pharmacists Association (MPA), 13, 71
Miconazole, 569t, 636t, 669t
Miconazole powder, 112
Miconazole vaginal suppositories, 112
Micromedex, 152
Micromedex Healthcare Series, 154
Micronase. see Glyburide
Microzide. see Hydrochlorothiazide
Micturition, 540–542
Middle ear, 613, 613f
Midodrine, 461b, 461f
Mifeprex, 558
Mifepristone, 558
Miglitol, 398–400t, 421–422t
Migraine
  propranolol and, 457b
  therapeutic agents for, 356–357
Migraine headaches, 364–366t, 383–384, 383–384b
Military time, 128, 128b, 128f
Milk of Magnesia. see Magnesium hydroxide
Milk thistle, 673t, 676t, 680
Millard, Rick, 184
Milliequivalent (mEq), 140
Milrinone, 475–476t
Mind and body medicine, 680–681, 681b, 681f, 682f
Mineral oil, for gastrointestinal conditions, 668t
Mineralocorticoids, 405
  for Addison disease, 417
Minipress. see Prazosin
Minispike, 259t
Minocin. see Minocycline
Minocycline, 627t
Mintox Plus. see AlOH, MgOH, and simethicone
Miosis, 435–436, 602
Miostat. see Carbachol
Miotics, for glaucoma, 610t, 611
Mirabegron, 542b, 542f
MiraLax. see Polyethylene glycol
Mirapex. see Pramipexole
Misbranding, 21–22, 23
Miscellaneous analgesics, 426–427t
Miscellaneous vaccines, 595–596, 595b
Missed dose, medication errors and, 318
Mitosis, 653, 656f
Mitotane, 398–400t
Mitotic inhibitors, 653
Mitoxantrone, 364–366t, 585–587t
MMA. see Medicare Modernization Act
MMR vaccine. see Measles, mumps, and rubella (MMR) vaccine
Mobic. see Meloxicam
Mobile PDR, 157
Moexipril, 458t
Mold forms, 235–236
Molded tablets, 240, 240b
  compounding procedure for, 242b
Molds, in preparing suppositories, 245–246, 246f

Mometasone, 488t

Monitoring error, 317t

Monoamine oxidase (MAO), 385–387

Monoamine oxidase inhibitors (MAOIs), 386–387t

Monoamine oxidase-$_B$ inhibitors (MAO$_B$-I), 381t

Monoclonal antibodies

    for gastrointestinal system, 359

    for hematologic cancer, 654–655t

    for osteoporosis, 441t

    for psoriasis, 632t

Monocytes, 579

Monographs, 43–46, 45f, 150, 154f

Monopril. *see* Fosinopril

Montelukast, 488t, 492t, 495b, 495f

Morals, in workplace, 54

Morning-after pill, 558

Morphine, 437t, 472t

Mortars and pestles, 228, 234–235, 234f, 234t, 235f

Mosby's Dictionary of Medicine, Nursing and Health Professions,
    160t

Motor nerve, 427

Motrin. *see* Ibuprofen

Mounjaro, 423b

Mouth, 505, 505f, 508f

Movantik. *see* Naloxegol

Moxatag. *see* Amoxicillin

Moxeza. *see* Moxifloxacin

Moxifloxacin, 607–608t

MPA. *see* Michigan Pharmacists Association

MS. *see* Multiple sclerosis

MS-Contin. *see* Morphine

Mucinex. *see* Guaifenesin

Mucolytics, 479t, 492t

Mucomyst. *see* Acetylcysteine

Multaq. *see* Dronedarone

Multidose vials (MDVs), 265t, 276

Multiple sclerosis (MS), 364–366t, 380–383, 382b, 382f, 382t

Multiple trace elements, 280t

Multiplication, 129, 129t

Multitasking, medication errors and, 320

Multivitamin, 280t

Mupirocin, 637t

Muscle contraction, 432f

Muscle fibers, 427, 431f, 433f

Muscle relaxants, skeletal, 426–427t, 441–444, 444t

Muscles

    of eye, 602f

    structure of, 431f

Musculoskeletal system

    anatomy and physiology of, skeletal system, 427, 428f

    conditions of, 427–441

        common drugs for, 426–427t, 427–441

        gout, 440–441, 440–441b, 442f

        osteoporosis, 438–440, 439b, 439f

    medication classes that affect, 441–444

        neuromuscular blockers, 444, 444b, 445t

        skeletal muscle relaxants, 426–427t, 441–444, 444t

    therapeutic agents for, 357, 446

Myambutol. *see* Ethambutol

Myasthenia gravis, 364–366t, 372–374, 373b, 375f

    therapeutic agents for, 356

Mycobutin. *see* Rifabutin

Mycophenolate, 585–587t, 630t

Mydriasis, 602

Myelin sheath, 367, 369f

Myfortic. *see* Mycophenolate

Mylanta. *see* AlOH and MgOH

Mylanta Classic Maximum Strength. *see* AlOH,
    MgOH, and simethicone

Myocardial infarction (MI), 471–472, 471–472b,
    472t

Myocardium, 451

Myofibrils, 427, 431f

Myopia, 602

Myosin filaments, 427, 431f

Myxedema, 413–414, 413f

N

NABP. *see* National Association of Boards of Pharmacy

Nabumetone, 434t

NACDS. *see* National Association of Chain Drug Stores

Nadolol, 458t, 459–460t

Nafarelin, 552–553t

Naftifine gel, 111

Nail, anatomy and physiology of, 624, 625f

Nail bed, 625f

Nail plate, 625f

Nalbuphine, 437t

Naloxegol, 519t, 520b, 520f

Naloxone, 437t

Naltrexone, 437t

Namenda. *see* Memantine

Naphazoline, 617t, 665t

Naprosyn. *see* Naproxen

Naproxen, 435b

    common adult dosage of, 664t

    for gout, 443t

Naproxen sodium, 426–427t, 434t

Narcotics. *see also* Controlled substances

    inventory of, 40

    registration requirements for maintaining, 38–39

Narcotics area, 344

Nasacort Allergy 24HR. *see* Triamcinolone

Nasacort AQ. *see* Triamcinolone

Nasal corticosteroids, for allergy, 665t

Nasal preparations

    compounding in, 246–247

    cross-contamination of, 247b

Nasal wall, 482f

NasalCrom. *see* Cromolyn sodium

Nasarel. *see* Flunisolide

Nasonex. *see* Mometasone

Natacyn. *see* Natamycin

Natalizumab, 364–366t, 514t, 585–587t

Natamycin, 607–608t, 609

Nateglinide, 398–400t, 421–422t

National Association of Boards of Pharmacy (NABP), 51, 59, 60–61
  Model Pharmacy Act of, 218
  USP 797, 263–264
National Association of Chain Drug Stores (NACDS), 74
National Center for Complementary and Integrative Health (NCCIH), 673
National Commission for Certifying Agencies (NCCA), 74
National Community Pharmacists Association (NCPA), 77t, 78
National Coordinating Committee on Large Volume Parenterals (NCCLVP), 263–264
National Coordinating Council for Medication Error Reporting and Prevention (NCCMERP), 316
National Council for Prescription Drug Programs (NCPDP), 170–171
National Drug Code (NDC), 24, 25b, 25f, 197, 296, 300, 301f
  number, 173
National Formulary (NF), 21–22
National Healthcareer Association (NHA), 58–59, 74
National Institute of Mental Health (NIMH), 183
National Institute on Drug Abuse (NIDA), 51
National Institutes of Health (NIH), 673
National Patient Safety Foundation (NPSF), 183
National Patient Safety Goal, 52–53
National Pharmacy Technician Association (NPTA), 74, 77t, 78
National Poison Prevention Week, 24
National Precursor Log Exchange (NPLEx), 28
National Provider Identifier (NPI), 294
  number, 168
National Vaccine Error Reporting Program (VERP), 327
Natural killer (NK) cells, 579, 581f
Nausea, 504t, 520–522
NCCA. see National Commission for Certifying Agencies
NCCIH. see National Center for Complementary and Integrative Health
NCCLVP. see National Coordinating Committee on Large Volume Parenterals
NCCMERP. see National Coordinating Council for Medication Error Reporting and Prevention
NCPA. see National Community Pharmacists Association
NCPDP. see National Council for Prescription Drug Programs
NDC. see National Drug Code
Nebulizers, 109, 109b
Nedocromil, 603–604t
Needles
  disposal of, 281
  in parenteral medications, 260, 260b, 260f
Negative feedback, 550
Negative pressure room, 265t
Negligence, 53
Neisseria gonorrhoeae, 569, 569t
Nelfinavir, for human immunodeficiency virus infection and acquired immunodeficiency syndrome, 570t

Neomycin, 669t
Neomycin/bacitracin/polymyxin b sulfate, 637t
Neoral. see Cyclosporine
Neosporin. see Polymyxin B sulfate, neomycin, bacitracin
Neosporin Original Formula. see Neomycin/bacitracin/polymyxin b sulfate
Neo-Synephrine. see Phenylephrine
Neo-Synephrine Cold + Allergy. see Phenylephrine
Nephrogenic diabetes insipidus, 410
Nephrons, 528–529, 529f
  function of, 528–531
Nephropathy, 358
Nerve transmission, 367–369, 370f
Nervous system, 366–369, 367b, 367f
  central, 367, 367b, 369–371, 376–384
    brain, 369, 371f
    spinal cord and, 369–370, 371f
  diseases and conditions of, 364–366t, 376–384
    Alzheimer disease, 364–366t, 378, 379t
    anxiety disorders, 364–366t, 387–388
    attention-deficit/hyperactivity disorder, 364–366t, 393–395, 394t
    bipolar disorder, 364–366t, 388–389
    depression, 385–387, 386–387t
    epilepsy, 364–366t, 376–378
    insomnia, 364–366t, 391–393, 392t
    migraine headache, 364–366t, 383–384
    migraine headaches, 364–366t, 383–384
    multiple sclerosis, 364–366t, 380–383, 382f, 382t
    myasthenia gravis, 364–366t, 372–374, 373b, 375f
    Parkinson disease, 364–366t, 378–380, 380f, 381t
    schizophrenia, 364–366t, 389–395
    stroke, 384
    treatment for, 372–395
  nerve transmission, 367–369, 370f
  neurons, 367, 369f
  peripheral, 371–372
    autonomic system, 368f, 371–372, 374f
      heart rate and, 453
    parasympathetic system, 372, 374f
    somatic system, 368f, 372
    sympathetic system, 371, 374f, 374t
  spinal cord, 369–370, 371f
  therapeutic agents for, 356–357, 396
Nesina. see Alogliptin
Neulasta. see Pegfilgrastim
Neupogen. see Filgrastim
Neupro. see Rotigotine
Neuraminidase inhibitors, for influenza, 490t
Neuromuscular blockers, 426–427t, 444, 444b, 445t
Neuromuscular junction, 427, 433f
Neurons, 367, 369f
Neurontin. see Gabapentin
Neurotransmitters, 369, 369f
Neut. see Sodium bicarbonate
Neutrogena Clear Pore. see Benzoyl peroxide
Neutropenia, 650
Neutrophils, 578, 581f

Nevirapine, for human immunodeficiency virus infection and acquired immunodeficiency syndrome, 570t

News magazines, 159, 159t

Nexium. *see* Esomeprazole

Nexium 24HR. *see* Esomeprazole

NHA. *see* National Healthcareer Association

Niacin, 463t, 465b

Niacor. *see* Niacin

Niaspan ER. *see* Niacin

Nicardipine, 459–460t

Nicotinic acid, 463t, 465, 465b, 465f

NIDA. *see* National Institute on Drug Abuse

Nifedipine, 458t, 459–460t

Nightingale, Florence, 8

NIH. *see* National Institutes of Health

Nilutamide, 568t

Nimbex. *see* Cisatracurium

NIMH. *see* National Institute of Mental Health

Nipent. *see* Pentostatin

Nitrates, 449–451t, 458t, 467–468b, 468t

Nitro-Dur. *see* Nitroglycerin

Nitrofuran antibacterial, 539t

Nitrofurantoin, 540b, 540f

Nitrogen mustards, 653

Nitroglycerin, 281t, 458t, 472t
   for angina, 467–468b
   dosage forms, 467–468b
   for heart failure, 475–476t
   for myocardial infarction, 472t
   patches, 107
   sublingual tablets, 468b, 468f

Nitroglycerin SL spray, 108

Nitropress. *see* Nitroprusside

Nitroprusside, 475–476t

Nitrosoureas, 656

Nitrostat. *see* Nitroglycerin

Nix. *see* Permethrin

Nizatidine, 511t

Nizoral A-D. *see* Ketoconazole

N-methyl-D-aspartate receptor antagonist, 379t

NNRTI. *see* Non-nucleoside reverse transcriptase inhibitor

No known allergies (NKA), 194b

No known drug allergy (NKDA), 194b

Nocturia, 564–565

Nocturnal hemodialysis, 533

Nodules, 626

Noise, medication errors and, 319–320

Nolix. *see* Flurandrenolide

Nonbenzodiazepine hypnotics, 392t

Non-child-resistant bottles, 50t

Noncompliance, medication errors and, 318

Nondiscretionary duties, 61–64, 63b

Nonformulary agents, 153

Nonformulary medications, 194
   handling, in third-party billing, 302

Nonhazardous intravenous preparation, 204–206, 204b

Nonidentification match, in third-party billing, 302

Nonnarcotic analgesic, 664t

Non-nucleoside reverse transcriptase inhibitor (NNRTI), for human immunodeficiency virus infection and acquired immunodeficiency syndrome, 570t

Nonopioid analgesic, for musculoskeletal system, 357

Nonproprietary (generic) name, 173

Nonreturnable drugs, 310

Nonsedating antihistamines, for allergy, 665t

Nonsterile compounding, 254
   additional supplies for, 235–236
   area for, 178–179, 178f, 230, 230b
   beyond-use dating for, 229–230, 230t
   calculations in, 251–253
   competencies for, 238b
   documentation in, 247–249, 248f, 250b
   equipment for, 230–235, 230f, 231t, 232–233f
   excipients and, 236, 237t
   flavorings in, 236, 237t
   history of, 228–229, 229b
   measuring liquids in, 239, 239f
   mold forms and, 235–236
   nasal preparations in, 246–247, 247b
   packaging in, 247, 247b, 247t
   personal preparation for, 236–238
   personnel training in, 250–251b, 251
   preparing solutions in, 239
   professionalism in, 250
   reconstituting premade suspensions in, 240, 240t
   regulatory and quality control of, 250
   safety in, 250
   semisolids in, 243–244, 244b
   solids in, 240–243
   stability in, 247
   use of, 229, 230b
   weighing techniques for, 237–238, 238b

Nonsteroidal antiinflammatory drugs (NSAIDs), 426–427t, 431–435, 434t, 664, 664b, 664t
   for conditions affecting the eye, 599–600t, 603–604t, 605–606
   for hypertension, 457b
   for musculoskeletal system, 357

Nonverbal communication, 84–85, 85b, 85f, 181

Norco (C-II). *see* Hydrocodone/acetaminophen

Norcuron. *see* Vecuronium

Norelgestromin, 557–558, 557t

Norepinephrine, 402t, 405b

Norethindrone, 557t

Norethindrone acetate, 557t

Norgestimate, 557t

Norgestrel, 557t

Norpace. *see* Disopyramide

Nortriptyline, 364–366t, 386–387t

Norvasc. *see* Amlodipine

Nose, 480, 616–618, 621
   anatomy and physiology of, 616
   conditions of, 616–618
      allergic rhinitis as, 616
      bacterial sinusitis as, 617–618, 617b
   conditions of, drugs for, 599–600t
   therapeutic agents for, 360

Nosocomial infection, 540b
Notices of privacy practices (NPPs), 26
Notifiable Infectious Diseases, 568–569
Novantrone. *see* Mitoxantrone
Novel drug agents, 419
Novolin N. *see* Isophane insulin
NovoLog. *see* Insulin aspart
NPI. *see* National Provider Identifier
NPLEx. *see* National Precursor Log Exchange
NPPs. *see* Notices of privacy practices
NPSF. *see* National Patient Safety Foundation
NPTA. *see* National Pharmacy Technician Association
NRTI. *see* Nucleoside reverse transcriptase inhibitor
NSAIDs. *see* Nonsteroidal antiinflammatory drugs
NTRTI. *see* Nucleotide reverse transcriptase inhibitor
Nuclear pharmacy, 217
Nuclear pharmacy technician, 76, 217–218, 218b
Nucleoside reverse transcriptase inhibitor (NRTI)
    for hepatitis B, 571t
    for human immunodeficiency virus infection
        and acquired immunodeficiency syndrome,
        570t
Nucleotide reverse transcriptase inhibitor (NTRTI)
    for hepatitis B, 571t
    for human immunodeficiency virus infection and
        acquired immunodeficiency syndrome,
        570t
Nucynta. *see* Tapentadol
Nulojix. *see* Belatacept
Numoisyn lozenge, 106
Nursing Interventions & Clinical Skills, 160t
Nursing staff
    communication between, institutional pharmacy and,
        195f, 198, 198b
    pharmacy and, relationship between, 194–195
Nutraceutical, 664–665
Nutrition Labeling and Education Act, 30t
Nystatin, 636t
    powder, 112
Nystop. *see* Nystatin

O

OA. *see* Osteoarthritis
Obesity, 419–422b, 419–423, 422b
OBRA. *see* Omnibus Budget Reconciliation Act
Obsessive-compulsive disorder (OCD), 387–388
Occipital lobe, 369
Occlusion therapy, 630–631b
Occupational Safety and Health Administration (OSHA),
    52, 52b
OCD. *see* Obsessive-compulsive disorder
Octreotide, 398–400t, 411b, 411f
Ocufen. *see* Flurbiprofen
Ocuflox. *see* Ofloxacin
Oculomotor nerve, 373t
ODA. *see* Orphan Drug Act
Ofloxacin, 569t, 607–608t
Ointment mill, 234–235, 235f

Ointments, 111, 243
    bases of, classification of, 244b
    eye, administration of, 602, 602b
    jars, filling of, 244
    preparing, 247
    tubes, filling of, 244
Olanzapine, 364–366t, 390b, 390f
Oleaginous bases, 244b, 245
Olfactory nerve, 373t
Oligomenorrhea, 553b
Oligospermia, 555b
Olmesartan, 459–460t
Olopatadine, 488t, 603–604t
Omalizumab, 492t
Ombitasvir, 572b, 572f
    for hepatitis C, 571t
Omega-3 acid ethyl esters, 465b
Omega-3 fatty acids, 463t
Omeprazole, 511b, 511f, 511t, 619b, 619f
    for gastroesophageal reflux disease and indigestion, 667t
Omeprazole + sodium bicarbonate, 511t
Omission error, 317t
Omnibus Budget Reconciliation Act (OBRA), 15–16,
    25–26, 166–167
Omnipen. *see* Ampicillin
Omnipred. *see* Prednisolone
OmniRx, 305, 306f
On Death and Dying, 183
OnabotulinumtoxinA, 542b, 542f
Ondansetron, 521–522b, 521f
Onglyza. *see* Saxagliptin
Online pharmacies, 51–52
Oocyte, 550
Oogenesis, 406–408
Open formulary, 288
Open-angle glaucoma, 609–610, 609f
Open-ended questions, 86–87
Ophthalmic preparations, therapeutic agents for, 360
Ophthalmic system. *see* Eyes
Ophthalmologists, 601
Opioid analgesics, 426–427t
    for musculoskeletal system, 357
Opioid antagonists, 437t, 519t
Opioid-induced constipation, 438
Opioids, 9, 31–36, 41b, 472t
    addiction to, treatment of, 50, 51f
Opium, 9, 9b
Optic disc, 601f
Optic nerve, 373t, 601f
Opticians, 601
Opti-Clear. *see* Tetrahydrozoline
Opticrom. *see* Cromolyn sodium
Optometrists, 601
Oracea. *see* Doxycycline
Oral administration, of drugs, 113
Oral contraceptives, for conditions affecting the male
    and female reproductive systems, 546–547t, 556–558,
    556b

Orange Book, 152, 157t
Orapred. *see* Prednisolone; Prednisone
Orbit, 601
Orchidectomy, 567–568b
Orencia. *see* Abatacept
Orlistat, 422b, 422f
Orphan Drug Act (ODA), 23, 24
Orthopnea, 484t
Orthostatic hypotension, 418–419b, 460–461
Oseltamivir, 490t
OSHA. *see* Occupational Safety and Health Administration
Osmosis, 529, 530f, 645–646
Osmotic diuretic, 526–527t, 539
Osmotic laxatives, 519t, 520
Osmotic pressure, 645–646, 646f
Osteoarthritis (OA), 357, 427–438, 433f
  drug treatment of, 428–429b
    acetaminophen for, 429–130, 429b
    aspirin, 430–431
    cyclooxygenase-2 inhibitors for, 435
    NSAIDs, 431–435
    opioid analgesics for, 435–438, 436f, 437t
  non-drug treatment of, 427–428
  pain route, 433f
Osteoblasts, 427, 438
Osteoclasts, 438
Osteoporosis, 357, 438–440
  medications of, 426–427t
  treatment of, 441t
OTC medications. *see* Over-the-counter (OTC) medications
Otic medicines, 616b
Otic preparations, cross-contamination of, 247b
Otitis media, 613, 613b, 615f, 615t
Ototoxicity, drug-induced, 615–616, 615–616b, 615t, 616b
Otrexup. *see* Methotrexate
Outdated medications, 207–208
Outpatient pharmacy, 65
Ovaries, 402t, 406–408, 408f
  functions of, 547–549, 550f
Overactive bladder, agents for, 526–527t
Overdosage, 44
Over-the-counter area, 340, 340f
Over-the-counter (OTC) medications, 22f, 102–103, 166, 671
  acetaminophen in, 663, 664b
  for allergy treatment, 617t, 664, 665t
  considerations for special populations, 669
  for cough and cold symptoms, 664, 666t
  for eyes, 612
  FDA regulations on, 24, 662
  FDA reporting process and adverse reactions, 31, 31b, 32f
  for gastroesophageal reflux disease and indigestion, 665–667, 667t
  for gastrointestinal conditions, 667, 668t
  for insomnia, 664–665, 666t
  nausea and vomiting, 667
  pain relievers, 435
    antipyretics and, 663–664, 663t, 664t
  perception to, 663

Over-the-counter (OTC) medications *(Continued)*
  prescription drug to, 662–663
  restricted, 669–670, 670t
  routes of administration for, 663–669, 663t
  for skin-related conditions, 667–669, 669t
  in United States, 670t
  for urinary incontinence, 670
  for warts, 634b
Ovulation, 406–408, 547–549, 549f
Ovum, 550
Oxaliplatin, 522b, 522f
Oxaprozin, 434t
Oxazepam, 364–366t
Oxcarbazepine, 364–366t
  for epilepsy, 377t
Oxybutynin, 540–541b, 540f, 541t
Oxycodone, 436f, 437t
Oxycodone/acetaminophen, 426–427t
OxyContin. *see* Oxycodone
Oxygen, 472t
  carbon dioxide and, gas exchange of, 484, 485f
Oxygenation, 451–452, 452f, 453f
Oxymetazoline, 603–604t, 617t, 665t
Oxymetazoline nasal spray, 108
Oxymorphone, 437t
Oxytocin, 402t
Ozurdex. *see* Dexamethasone

P

Pacerone. *see* Amiodarone
Package code, 24
Package inserts, 43, 152
Packaging
  compounding and, 247, 247b, 247t
  suppositories, 246
Pain relievers, over-the-counter, 435, 663–664, 663t, 664t
Paliperidone, 364–366t
Palliative, defined, 563b
Pallor, 647–649, 648f
Pamelor. *see* Nortriptyline
Pancreas, 402t, 405–406, 407f, 409t
  conditions of, 418–423
Pancreatic cancer, 522–523, 522–523b, 523b
Pancuronium, 426–427t, 445t
Panic disorders, 387
Pantoprazole, 511b, 511f, 511t
Papilla, 625f
Papules, 626
PAR levels. *see* Periodic automatic replacement (PAR) levels
Paracelsus, 6, 9
Parasites, 639, 640f
Parasympathetic nervous system (PNS), 371–372, 374f, 602b
  heart rate and, 453
Parasympathomimetics, 372
Parathyroid glands, 404, 404f
  conditions of, 402t, 409t, 414–415
    hyperparathyroidism, 398–400t, 409t, 414–415

Parathyroid glands (Continued)
    hypoparathyroidism, 415
    hormones, 401, 402t
Parathyroid hormone analog, 441t
Parenteral administration, 114
Parenteral medications, 64, 114, 204, 257, 259t
    abbreviations for, 258t
    administration of, errors in, 325, 325f
    antibiotics in, 277, 277b, 277t
    compatibility considerations of, 280, 281t
    delivery systems of, 262–263
        continuous analgesic, 263
        patient-controlled analgesia, 263, 264f
        piggyback containers in, 262, 262f
    electrolytes and additives in, 280, 280t
    hyperalimentation in, 277–278, 278b, 278f, 279f
    label for, 280, 281f
    preparations of, 205f
    routes of administration for, 262
    supplies for, 258–262, 259t
        filters, 260–261, 261f
        needles, 260, 260b, 260f
        stock levels, 261–262
        syringes, 259–260, 260f
Paricalcitol, 398–400t, 415b, 415f
Parietal lobe, 369
Paritaprevir, 572b, 572f
    for hepatitis C, 571t
Parkinson disease (PD), 378–380, 378–380b, 380b, 380f
    hypotension and, 461b
    metoclopramide for, 521b
    swallowing and, 481b
    therapeutic agents for, 356
    treatment of, 364–366t, 381t
Paronychium, 624, 625f
Parotid gland, 505, 505f
Paroxetine, 364–366t, 386–387t
Partial seizures, 376–377, 376t
Partial-thickness burns, 633b, 634b
Pastes, 111–112, 243
Pasteur, Louis, 10, 10–11t
Pataday. see Olopatadine
Patanase. see Olopatadine
Patanol. see Olopatadine
Patient bins, 180, 180f
Patient cassette drawers, 200–201
Patient confidentiality, 26, 27b
    coverage expiration policy for drugs and, 300–301
Patient counseling, 176, 176f
    information, 44
Patient dose-specific orders, 330
Patient information, 168, 170
Patient package inserts, 48
Patient product information, 173
Patient profiles, third-party billing and, 299–300, 300f
Patient Protection and Affordable Care Act, 29–30
Patient-centered care, 182

Patient-controlled analgesia (PCA)
    cassette system, 263, 264f
    syringe system, 263
Patient's medical record, 50
Pavulon. see Pancuronium
Paxil. see Paroxetine
Pazeo. see Olopatadine
PBM. see Pharmacy benefit management
PCA. see Patient-controlled analgesia
PCAT. see Pharmacy College Admissions Test
PCN. see Pharmacy Benefit Processor Control Number
PCP. see Primary care physician
PCSK9 inhibitors, 463t, 465–466, 466b
    for cardiovascular system, 358
PD. see Parkinson disease
PDMA. see Prescription Drug Marketing Act
PDR. see Physicians' Desk Reference
PEC. see Primary engineering control
Pediarix, 592–593t
Pediatric and Neonatal Dosage Handbook, 156, 157t
Pediatric dosing, 138
    calculating, 138, 139b
Pediatrics, 208
    medication errors and, 323–324, 324f
Pediculus humanus capitis, 639
PedvaxHIB, 592–593t
PEG polymers, 245
Pegfilgrastim, 651t
Pelvic inflammatory disease (PID), 559–560, 560b
    select treatment regimens for, 560t
Pelvic muscle (Kegel) exercises, 540b
Pemberton, John, 12, 13t
Pemirolast, 603–604t
Penicillin, 539t
    discovery of, 9–10
    for otitis media, 615t
Penicillin and aminoglycoside, 539t
Penicillin G, 569t
Pentacel, 592–593t
Pentasa. see Mesalamine
Pentostatin, 654–655t
Pepcid. see Famotidine
Pepcid AC. see Famotidine
Peppermint spirit, 108
Peptic ulcer disease (PUD), 511–512, 511f, 512f
Pepto-Bismol. see Bismuth subsalicylate
Percentages, 130
    of liquid medications, calculating, 142, 142b
    of quantities, 145–146
Perception, definition of, 84
Percocet. see Oxycodone/acetaminophen
Perforomist. see Formoterol
Pericardium, 451
Perimysium, 431f
Periodic automatic replacement (PAR) levels, 226–227, 228b
Periodic automatic replenishment (PAR), 201–202, 304

Peripheral nervous system (PNS), 371–372
  autonomic system, 368f, 371–372, 374f
  diseases and conditions of, 372–376
    myasthenia gravis, 372–374, 375f
    polyneuropathy, 375–376, 375b
  parasympathetic system, 372, 374f
  somatic system, 368f, 372
  sympathetic system, 371, 374f, 374t
Peripheral neuropathy, 364–366t, 418–419b
Peripheral parenteral nutrition (PPN), 278
Peripheral resistance, 453
Peristalsis, 505
Peritoneal dialysis, 532–533, 533f
Peritonitis, 532–533b
Permethrin, 639–640b, 640b, 640f
Pernicious anemia, 648t
Person code, 299b
Personal protective equipment, for nonsterile compounding, 231
Perspiration, 624
Pertussis vaccine, 592–593t
Petit mal seizures, 376t
pH scale, 506f
Phagocytes, 577–578
Phagocytic cells, 580
Pharmaceutical elegance, 250
Pharmaceutical sales representatives, 217, 217f
Pharmacists
  certification of, 15
  daily routine of, 325
  history of, 12, 12f
  role of, changes in, 59
  trust in, 15–16
Pharmacodynamics, 116, 354–355
Pharmacokinetics, 116, 354, 355f
Pharmacy
  changing requirements in, 15–16
  in early America, 12–14
  history of, 12–16
  laws, 21
    FDA history and, 21–23
    federal, 22–23, 23t
    liabilities, 53, 53b
    state, 53
  medication errors and, 322–323
  terminology used in, 257, 258t
Pharmacy and therapeutics committee (P&T committee), 194, 288
Pharmacy bench, 177, 177f
Pharmacy Benefit International Identification number (RxBIN), 299b
Pharmacy benefit management (PBM), 216
Pharmacy Benefit Processor Control Number (PCN), 299b
Pharmacy billing, 312
Pharmacy business management operators, 76
Pharmacy calculations, 126–127
Pharmacy clerks, 12–13

Pharmacy College Admissions Test (PCAT), 15
Pharmacy informatics, 219
Pharmacy informatics analyst, 64, 65b
Pharmacy operations management, 347
  efficiency techniques in, 345
Pharmacy order check-in area, 179
Pharmacy Practice Model Initiative, 338
Pharmacy purchasing agents, 214–215, 214f
Pharmacy sites, 51–52
Pharmacy stock, 303–304
Pharmacy stock area, 177–178, 178f
Pharmacy Technician Accreditation Commission (PTAC), 60
Pharmacy Technician Certification Board (PTCB), 13, 21, 53, 334, 338
  continuing education and, 74
  CREST Initiative of, 60, 70
  examination, 145
    math problems using percentages on, 145–146
  history of, 58–59
Pharmacy Technician Certification Exam (PTCE), 71–73, 72–73t
Pharmacy technician coordinator, 76
Pharmacy technician director/instructor, 76
Pharmacy technician educator or trainer, 216–217, 216f
Pharmacy technician student, training programs for, 68–70, 68–70b
Pharmacy technicians, 15f, 50b, 70, 220b
  advanced roles for, 221
    as inventory and purchasing agent, 214–215, 214f
    as lead pharmacy technician, 219
    as managed care pharmacy technicians, 216
    as medication adherence or compliance technician, 219
    as medication reconciliation technician, 215–216, 215f
    as nuclear pharmacy technician, 217–218, 218b
    as pharmaceutical sales representatives, 217, 217f
    as pharmacy technician educator or trainer, 216–217, 216f
    as prior approval or investigational drug coordinator, 216
    as remote/telepharmacy technician, 218, 218f
  associations for, 77, 77t
  career, 60
  certification for, 15, 70–78, 71b, 72–73t, 73–74b, 74b
  closed-door facility, 67b
  code of ethics of, 54b
  common job duties and requirements for, 75b
  communication skills for. see Communication
  competencies required of. see Competencies
  employment growth rate for, 214
  future of, 81, 219–220, 220b
  historical data for, 59–60, 59b
  history of, 13–14t, 13–14
  levels of, 70
  liability for actions of, 53, 53b
  opportunities for, 76, 76t
    advanced or specialized, 214–216, 214b
  role of, 214

Pharmacy technicians (*Continued*)
  scenario, 58–59, 61, 64–70
  state requirements, 62–63b
  trust in, 15–16, 16b
  of twenty-first century and beyond, 16
PharmacyChecker.com, 67
Pharynx, 480, 482f, 616
Phazyme. *see* Simethicone
Phenazopyridine, 540b
Phenelzine, 386–387t
Phenergan with Codeine (C-V). *see* Promethazine/codeine
Phenol, 306–307
  for cough and cold symptoms, 666t
Phentermine/topiramate, 423b
Phenylephrine, 487b, 487f, 617t, 665t
Phenytoin, 356, 364–366t, 377b, 377f
  albumin and, 645
  for epilepsy, 377t
Pheochromocytomas, 418
PHI. *see* Protected health information
Phlebotomy, 8, 650b
Phobias, 387–388
Phone calls, institutional pharmacy and, 194, 195b
Phosphate, 531
Phosphodiesterase enzyme inhibitor, 475–476t
Phosphodiesterase-4 inhibitor, for asthma and COPD, 492t, 495
Phosphodiesterase-5 inhibitors, 565t, 568t
Phosphorus, 438
Phosphorus-binding agents, 526–527t
Photoreceptors, 601–602
Phototherapy, 630–631b
Physicians' Desk Reference (PDR), 43, 152, 157t
Physician's handwriting, 316
Physician's Labeling Rule, 30t
Pickup areas, 341
Pictograms, 323–324, 324f
PID. *see* Pelvic inflammatory disease
Piggyback containers, delivery systems for, 262, 262f
Pill counters, 329, 330f
Pill counting trays, 226b, 228b
Pilocarpine, 610t, 611b, 611f
Pimecrolimus, 630b, 630f, 630t
Pindolol, 458t
Pineal gland, 402t, 404
  hormones, 402t
Pioglitazone, 398–400t, 421–422t
Pipettes, 231–234
Pitressin. *see* Vasopressin
Pituitary gland, 403–404, 403f, 409t
  conditions of, 409–411
    hypersecretion of growth hormone, 409t
    hypopituitarism, 409t, 410–411
    syndrome of inappropriate antidiuretic hormone secretion (SIADH), 398–400t, 409–410
  hormones of, 402t, 547–549
Plan limitations, in third-party billing, 303, 303b
Plantar warts, 634–635

Plaquenil. *see* Hydroxychloroquine
Plasma, 528–529, 645
Plasma cells, 579
Plasma proteins, 645–646, 645f, 646f
Plasticizers, 237t
Platelets, 646
Plavix. *see* Clopidogrel
Pneumatic tube area, 344
Pneumatic tube system, 196, 196f
Pneumococcal vaccine, 592–593t
Pneumonia, 498, 498b
  aspiration, 481b, 498
  therapeutic agents for, 358–359
Pneumovax 23, 592–593t
PNS. *see* Parasympathetic nervous system; Peripheral nervous system
Pocket-sized reference books, 156
Point of sale (POS) billing, 297, 297b
Point-of-entry systems, 197–198
Poison control call center operator, 76
Poison Prevention Packaging Act (PPPA), 24, 25b, 175
Polarization, 367, 370f
Policies and procedures (P&P), 194, 194b
Polio vaccine, 592–593t
Polycythemia, 649–650, 650b
Polyethylene glycol, 519t, 520b, 520f
Polymenorrhea, 553b
Polymyxin B sulfate, neomycin, bacitracin, 669t
Polymyxin B/trimethoprim, 607–608t
Polyneuropathy, 375–376, 375b
  therapeutic agents for, 356
Polytrim. *see* Polymyxin B/trimethoprim
Positive pressure room, 265t
Post-traumatic stress disorder (PTSD), 387
Potassium, 531
Potassium acetate, 280t
Potassium chloride (KCl), 280t, 325
Potassium citrate, 536b, 536f
Potassium phosphate, 280t
Potassium-sparing diuretics, 459–460t, 526–527t, 537t, 538
Powder hood, for nonsterile compounding, 230, 234f
Powders, 112
P&P. *see* Policies and procedures
PPD skin test, 498–500, 499f
PPIs. *see* Proton pump inhibitors
PPN. *see* Peripheral parenteral nutrition
PPO. *see* Preferred provider organization
PPPA. *see* Poison Prevention Packaging Act
Pradaxa. *see* Dabigatran
Praluent. *see* Alirocumab
Pramipexole, 364–366t, 380b, 380f, 381t
Pramlintide, 421–422t
Pramoxine, 628–629b, 628f
Prandin. *see* Repaglinide
Prasugrel, 470t, 472t
Pravachol. *see* Pravastatin
Pravastatin, 458t, 463t
Prazosin, 459–460t

Precipitate, in chemicals, 278b
Precose. *see* Acarbose
Pred Forte. *see* Prednisolone
Pred Mild. *see* Prednisolone
Prednisolone, 417b, 417f, 585–587t
   for conditions affecting the eye, 603–604t, 605b, 605f
   ophthalmic suspension, 111
Prednisone, 398–400t, 418, 418b, 418f, 443t, 585–587t
Preferred provider organization (PPO), 291, 291f
Prefix
   metric, 133t
   term, 352
Pregnancy, category, 46, 47b
Premarin. *see* Conjugated estrogens
Premenstrual syndrome, 553b
Prescriber information, 168, 169f, 171
Prescribing error, 317t
Prescription, 166–170
   calculating day's supply, 171
   checking, 175
   data input, 170–172
   date of, 168–169, 169b
   directions for use, 171
   drug benefit, 170–171, 170f
   filing of, 175–176
   filling of, controlled substances, 41–43
   information, 166–167, 167–168t
   intake, 170
   intake window, 177
   labeling, 172–173
   labels in
      repackaging, 48–49
      requirements for, 49t
      special, 48, 48b
   limitation of plan exceeded and, 301–302
   packaging, 175
   patient information in, 168
   payment, 176
   pick-up window, 180
   preparation, 173–176, 174f
   prescriber information in, 168, 169f
   processing of, 170–173
   refilling, 39, 42
   regulations on, 47–50
      DEA verification, 49–50, 49b
      mailing medications, 43
      non-child-resistant bottles, 50t
      who can prescribe, 47, 47b
      who can receive, 47, 47b
   risk management programs for, 51
   scanning, 172
   tamper-proof, 37, 38b, 38f
   transferring, for controlled substances, 42
   veterinary medications, 48
Prescription Drug Marketing Act (PDMA), 25
Prescription group number (Rx Grp #), 299b
Prescription information, 166–167, 167–168t
Prevacid. *see* Lansoprazole

Prevacid 24HR. *see* Lansoprazole
Prevalite. *see* Cholestyramine
Prevnar 13, 592–593t
Priftin. *see* Rifapentine
Prilosec. *see* Omeprazole
Primacor. *see* Milrinone
Primary care physician (PCP), 290
Primary engineering control (PEC), 265t, 267–271, 267b,
      268b, 268f
   airflow in, 267–269, 268b, 268f
   cleaning and maintaining, 269–270b, 269–271, 271b, 272b
Primaxin. *see* Imipenem-cilastatin
Prime vendors, 310
Prinivil. *see* Lisinopril
Prior authorization, 290, 297–299, 298f, 299b
Pristiq. *see* Desvenlafaxine
Private plans, 303
prn, 197
ProAir HFA. *see* Albuterol
Probenecid, 426–427t, 443t
Problem-solving, 79
Procainamide, 474t
Procanbid. *see* Procainamide
Procardia. *see* Nifedipine
ProCentra Solution. *see* Dextroamphetamine
Prochlorperazine, 521b, 521f
Procrit. *see* Epoetin alfa
Proctor, William, Jr, 13t
Prodrugs, 117
Product code, 24
Professionalism
   compounding, 250
   in workplace, 78–81, 79f, 80b
Progesterone, 402t, 551–554, 552–553t, 553–554b, 553f
   functions of, 548t
   secretion of, 547–549, 558
Progestins, 552–553t
   for conditions affecting the male and female reproductive
      systems, 546–547t
   for reproductive system, 359
Prograf. *see* Tacrolimus
Prolia. *see* Denosumab
Promacta. *see* Eltrombopag
Promethazine suppositories, 112
Promethazine/codeine, 486–487b, 486f
Pronestyl. *see* Procainamide
Propafenone, 474t
Prophylactic agent, 487–488
Prophylaxis, 681–682
Propofol, 110
Proportions, 131, 131b
Propranolol, 456–457b, 456f, 457b, 459–460t
Proprietary (brand or trade) name, 173, 289
Propylthiouracil (PTU), 398–400t, 412b, 412f, 590b, 590f
ProQuad, 592–593t
Proscar. *see* Finasteride
Prostaglandin agonists, for conditions affecting the eye, 599–600t
Prostaglandin analogs, 610t, 612, 612b

Prostaglandins, 431, 568t, 583

Prostate, 562

Prostate cancer, 567–568, 568f, 568t, 656

Prostatic hyperplasia, benign, 359

Protease inhibitors (PIs)
    for hepatitis B and C, 571t
    for human immunodeficiency virus infection and acquired
        immunodeficiency syndrome, 570t

Protected health information (PHI), 26

Protocol, 194

Proton pump inhibitors (PPIs), 508
    for gastroesophageal reflux disease and indigestion, 667t
    for gastrointestinal system, 359
    for GERD, 510–511, 511t, 619b

Protonix. see Pantoprazole

Protopic. see Tacrolimus; tacrolimus

Proventil HFA. see Albuterol

Proximal convoluted tubule, 529

Prozac. see Fluoxetine

Pruritus, 628, 664

Pseudoephedrine, 28, 29b, 29f, 487b, 487f, 665t, 670t
    for cough and cold symptoms, 666t

Psoralens, 632t

Psoriasis, 623–624t, 630–633, 631f

Psychosis, 389

Psychotherapy, for depression, 385b

Psyllium, 517t, 518b, 518f, 519t, 667b
    for gastrointestinal conditions, 668t

PTAC. see Pharmacy Technician Accreditation Commission

PTCB. see Pharmacy Technician Certification Board

PTCE. see Pharmacy Technician Certification Exam

PTSD. see Post-traumatic stress disorder

PTU. see Propylthiouracil

Puberty, 408–409
    in females, 547–549
    in males, 560–561

PUD. see Peptic ulcer disease

Pulmicort Flexhaler. see Budesonide

Pulmicort Respules. see Budesonide

Pulmonary artery, 451–452

Punch method, 241

Pupil, 601f

Pure Food and Drug Act of 1906, 21, 23

Purine nucleoside analogs, 654–655t

Purixan. see Mercaptopurine

Purple Book, 152

Purple coneflower, 677f

Pustules, 626

Pyelonephritis, 539

Pyridostigmine, 356, 364–366t, 373b

Pyxis, 191–192, 201

PZA, 499t

Q

Qnasl. see Beclomethasone

Qsymia. see Phentermine/topiramate

Quadracel, 592–593t

Quality assurance (QA), 345
    medication errors and, 333, 333b

Quality control (QC), 345

Quantity sufficient (qs), 239b

Questran. see Cholestyramine

Quetiapine, 364–366t

Quinidex. see Quinidine

Quinidine, 474t

Quinine, 8, 473b

Quinolones, 322t

Qvar Redihaler. see Beclomethasone

R

RA. see Rheumatoid arthritis

RAAS. see Renin-angiotensin-aldosterone system

RabAvert, 592–593t

Rabeprazole, 511t

Rabies vaccine, 592–593t

Radical prostatectomy, 567–568b

"Radiopharmaceuticals," 217–218

Raloxifene, 426–427t, 440b, 440f, 441t

Raltegravir, for human immunodeficiency virus infection
    and acquired immunodeficiency syndrome, 570t

Ramelteon, 364–366t, 392t, 393b

Ramipril, 458t, 459–460t, 475–476t

Randomization, in drug trials, 353

Ranitidine, for gastroesophageal reflux disease and
    indigestion, 667t

Rapamune. see Sirolimus

Rapamycin inhibitors, 585–587t

Rapidly disintegrating oral tablets, 113

Rasagiline, 364–366t, 381t

Rasuvo. see Methotrexate

Ratio strengths, of liquid medications, 142, 142b

Ratios, 131

Razadyne. see Galantamine

Rebif. see Interferon beta-1a

Recalled drugs, 31, 35–36b

Receptors, drugs and, 355

Recombivax HB, 592–593t

Reconstituted medication, 262

Reconstituted vial, 276b

Reconstituting premade suspensions, 240, 240t

Reconstitution, 240

Reconstitution area, 179, 340–341

Record keeping, for controlled substances, 40, 40t, 41f

Red pulp, 578, 580f

Reference books, 160t
    American Drug Index, 155
    American Hospital Formulary Service Drug Information (AHDS DI),
        152–153, 157t
    Clinical Pharmacology, 153, 154f
    Drug Facts and Comparisons, 152, 157t
    Drug Topics Red Book, 152, 157t
    Geriatric Dosage Handbook, 156, 157t
    Goodman & Gilman's The Pharmacological Basis of
        Therapeutics, 155, 157t
    Handbook of Nonprescription Drugs, 155
    Handbook on Injectable Drugs, 154, 157t
    Ident-A-Drug, 153, 155f, 157t
    Martindale's The Complete Drug Reference, 156

Reference books *(Continued)*
  Micromedex Healthcare Series, 154
  Orange Book, 152, 157t
  Pediatric and Neonatal Dosage Handbook, 156, 157t
  Physicians' Desk Reference, 152, 157t
  Purple Book, 152
  Remington's Pharmaceutical Sciences: The Science and Practice of Pharmacy, 156, 157t
  United States Pharmacists' Pharmacopeia, 153
  United States Pharmacopoeia-National Formulary (USP-NF), 153, 157t
Refilling prescriptions, controlled substances, 39, 42
Refills, 171
Registered pharmacy technician, 70
Reglan. *see* Metoclopramide
Rehydration fluids, for nausea and vomiting, 668t
Relenza. *see* Zanamivir
Relpax. *see* Eletriptan
Remicade. *see* Infliximab
Remington's Pharmaceutical Sciences: The Science and Practice of Pharmacy, 156, 157t
REMS. *see* Risk Evaluation and Mitigation Strategy
Renal artery, 527
Renal failure, 532–533
Renal system
  anatomy and physiology of, 527–531, 528f, 529f
    function of the kidneys, 527–528
    importance of electrolytes in, 531
    nephron function in, 528–531, 529f
  conditions of, 531–542
    chronic kidney disease, 531–535, 532t, 533f
    common drugs for, 526–527t
    edema as, 536–539, 536b, 536f, 537t
    kidney stones as, 535–536, 535f
    urinary incontinence as, 540–542
    urinary tract infections as, 539–540, 539b, 539t
  therapeutic agents for, 359, 543
Renal vein, 527
Renflexis. *see* Infliximab
Renin, 453, 455f, 531
Renin inhibitors, 456, 459–460t
Renin-angiotensin-aldosterone system (RAAS), 357–358, 453, 455f, 531f
Repackaging medications. *see also* Bulk repackaging
  area for, 179–180, 179t, 344
  reasons for, 61
Repaglinide, 398–400t, 421–422t
Repatha. *see* Evolocumab
Repolarization, 367–369, 370f
Reports, preparation of, 63
Reproductive system
  female, 547–550, 550f
    conditions of, 550–560
      common drugs for, 546–547t
      contraception and, 556–558, 556f, 557b, 557t
      hypogonadism as, 554–555, 554f
      infertility as, 546–547t, 552–553t, 555–556
      menopause as, 558–559
      menstrual disorders as, 551

Reproductive system *(Continued)*
      pelvic inflammatory disease as, 559–560, 560b, 560t
    hormones affecting, 548t
    menstrual cycle in, 549f
  male, 560–562, 561f
    conditions of, 562–568
      benign prostatic hypertrophy as, 564–566, 564f, 565t
      common drugs for, 546–547t
      erectile dysfunction as, 546–547t, 566–567, 567t
      hypogonadism as, 562–564, 563t
      prostate cancer as, 567–568, 568f, 568t
    hormones affecting, 548t
  therapeutic agents for, 359, 573
Requip. *see* Ropinirole
Requisitions, filling, technician responsibilities and, 199t
Resorption, 438
Respiration, 481, 481b, 484f, 484t
  dysfunction, 484t
  rate of, 481, 481b
Respiratory system, 502
  common drugs for, 479t
  disorders and conditions of, 485–501
    lower respiratory system, 490–500
      asthma, 490–495, 491b, 491f, 492t, 493f, 494b
      chronic obstructive pulmonary disease (COPD), 495–498, 496f, 497b
      pneumonia, 498, 498b
      tuberculosis, 498–500, 499b, 499f, 499t
      lung cancer, 500, 500b
    upper respiratory system, 485–490, 486t
      allergies, 486t, 488–489, 488b, 488t
      common cold, 485–488, 487b
      influenza, 486t, 489–490, 490b, 490f, 490t
      rhinitis, 486t, 489, 489b
  structure and function of, 480–484, 480f, 481f
    gas exchange, 481–484, 485f
    lower respiratory system, 481, 482f
    respiration, 481, 481b, 484f, 484t
    upper respiratory system, 480–481, 481b, 482f
  therapeutic agent for, 358–359
Restasis. *see* Cyclosporine
Restoril. *see* Temazepam
Resume, 80, 80b
Retail price, 146
Retail technician, 66
Retapamulin, 637b, 637f, 637t
Retavase. *see* Reteplase
Reteplase, 470t
Retina, 601–602, 601f
Retin-A Micro. *see* Tretinoin
Retinoic acid, 627t
Retinoids, 623–624t, 626b, 632t
Returns, of medication, 307–310
Reverse distributor, 40–41
Reye syndrome, 430, 664b
Rheumatic fever, 618b
Rheumatoid arthritis (RA), 427, 588–590, 588f, 589b
  therapeutic agents for, 359–360
Rhinitis, 486t, 489, 489b

Rhinitis, allergic, therapeutic agents for, 360
Rhinocort Allergy. *see* Budesonide
Rhinocort Allergy Spray. *see* Budesonide
Ribavirin, for hepatitis C, 571t
Rifabutin, 499t
Rifadin. *see* Rifampin
Rifampin, 499t, 500b, 500f
Rifapentine, 499t
Rimantadine, 490t
Risedronate, 426–427t, 441t
Risk Evaluation and Mitigation Strategy (REMS), 51, 320–321
Risk management, medication errors and, 333, 333b
Risperdal. *see* Risperidone
Risperidone, 364–366t, 390b, 390f
Ritalin. *see* Methylphenidate
Ritonavir, 572b, 572f
  for hepatitis C, 571t
  for human immunodeficiency virus infection and acquired immunodeficiency syndrome, 570t
Rituxan. *see* Rituximab
Rituximab, 585–587t, 654–655t
Rivaroxaban, 470t
Rivastigmine, 364–366t, 379t
Rizatriptan, 364–366t
ROA. *see* Routes of administration
Robaxin. *see* Methocarbamol
Robitussin. *see* Dextromethorphan
Robot filler, 64
Robot technology, 329–330
Robot-Rx machines, 328, 329f
Rocaltrol. *see* Calcitriol
Rocephin. *see* Ceftriaxone
Rocuronium, 445t
Roflumilast, 492t, 495b, 495f
Roman numerals, 127–128, 127t
  determining, rules for, 127–128
Roosevelt, Franklin D., 22
Roosevelt, Theodore, 21–22
Ropinirole, 364–366t, 381t
Rosuvastatin, 463t
Rotarix, 592–593t
RotaTeq, 592–593t
Rotavirus vaccine, 592–593t
Rotigotine, 364–366t, 380b, 380f, 381t
Routes of administration (ROA), 112–114, 112t
  dosage forms and, 94–124, 97t
    inhalants, 114
    injectables, 114–115, 115f
    instructions of, 102
    ophthalmic, otic, nasal agents, 114
    oral agents, 113
    parenteral agents, 114, 262
    rectal, 113
    topical agents, 113–114
  miscellaneous, 115
Rowasa. *see* Mesalamine
Roxicodone. *see* Oxycodone
Rozerem. *see* Ramelteon

RU-486. *see* Mifepristone
Ryan Haight Online Consumer Protection Act, 67
Rythmol. *see* Propafenone

S

Sabin, Albert, 10–11t
Sabril. *see* Vigabatrin
Sacubitril, 456b, 456f
Safe Medical Devices Act (SMDA), 30t
Safety
  medication. *see* Medication safety
  in nonsterile compounding, 250
Safety Data Sheet (SDS), 52, 311
Salicin, 430
Salicylic acid, 669t
  for acne vulgaris, 627t
  for warts, 635b, 635f
Saline irrigations, 617b
Saline laxatives, for gastrointestinal conditions, 668t
Salisol. *see* Salicylic acid
Saliva, 505
Salivary glands, 505, 508f
Salk, Jonas, 10–11t
Salmeterol, 492t, 494f, 497b, 497f
Salmeterol Multicenter Asthma Research Trial (SMART), 491–494
Salt intake, high, 536b
Salt-restricted diets, 453b
Sandimmune. *see* Cyclosporine; Cyclosporine A
Sandostatin. *see* Octreotide
Sani-supp. *see* Glycerin
Saquinavir, for human immunodeficiency virus infection and acquired immunodeficiency syndrome, 570t
Sargramostim, 651t
Satellite pharmacies, 192–193, 199t
Saw palmetto, 673t, 678, 678f
Saxagliptin, 398–400t, 421–422t
Scalp, 639–640, 640f
Schizophrenia, 364–366t, 389–395, 389b
  therapeutic agents for, 357
Sclera, 601, 601f
Scopolamine transdermal patches, 107
Scrotum, 408–409, 560–561
SDS. *see* Safety Data Sheet
Sebaceous glands, 624, 624f, 625f, 626f
Seborrhea, 626
Sebum, 624
Secondary hypertension, 457
Sectral. *see* Acebutolol
Sedating antihistamines, for allergy, 665t
Seizures, 376t
Selective estrogen receptor modulator (SERM), 441t
Selective estrogen receptor modulator (SERM)-ovulation simulator, 552–553t
Selective serotonin reuptake inhibitors (SSRIs), 385b, 386–387t
Selegiline, 364–366t, 381t
Selenium, 280t
Self-pay, 303

Semicircular canals, 613f, 614b, 614f
Semisolids, 103, 111–112
 compounding, 243–244, 244b
Senna, 519–520b, 519f, 519t
 for gastrointestinal conditions, 668t
Senokot. *see* Senna
Sensipar. *see* Cinacalcet
SEPhT. *see* Society for Education of Pharmacy Technicians
Serax. *see* Oxazepam
SERM. *see* Selective estrogen receptor modulator
Seroquel. *see* Quetiapine
Serotonin norepinephrine reuptake inhibitors (SNRIs), 386–387t
Sertraline, 357, 364–366t, 385b, 385f, 386–387t
Serum, 645
Service level agreements (SLAs), 290
Sevelamer, 534b, 534f
Sex code, 299b
Sexually transmitted diseases, 568–572, 569t, 634–635
 agents for, 546–547t
 causes of, 568–569
 genital herpes, 569
 HIV as, 569
 oral contraceptives and, 556b
 pelvic inflammatory disease and, 560
 symptoms of, 569
SGLT2 inhibitors. *see* Sodium-glucose co-transporter 2 (SGLT2) inhibitors
Shaman, 4
Sharps container, 310
 disposal of, 281, 281b
Shingles, 633
Shingrix, 592–593t
Short-acting beta-agonists, for asthma and COPD, 492t, 495
Show globes, 12, 12f
SIADH. *see* Syndrome of inappropriate antidiuretic hormone secretion
Sickle cell anemia, 648t
Sickle cell disease, 649, 649b
Sideroblastic anemia, 648t
Signatura *(signa* or *sig)*, 170
Sildenafil, 567b, 568t
Silvadene. *see* Silver sulfadiazine
Silver sulfadiazine, 634b, 634f
Simethicone, 520b, 520f
Simponi. *see* Golimumab
Simulect. *see* Basiliximab
Simvastatin, 294, 458t, 463t, 464b, 464f
Sinemet. *see* Levodopa/carbidopa
Single-dose vials (SDVs), 265t, 276
Singulair. *see* Montelukast
Sinoatrial (SA) node, 452
Sinuses, 616–618
 anatomy and physiology of, 616
 conditions of, 616–618
  allergic rhinitis as, 616
  bacterial sinusitis as, 617–618, 617b
Sinusitis, bacterial, 617–618, 617b

Sirolimus, 585–587t, 591b, 591f
Sitagliptin, 398–400t, 421–422t
Skeletal muscle relaxants, 426–427t, 441–444, 444t
Skeletal muscles, 426–427t
 anatomy and physiology of, 427
Skeletal system, 427
Skin
 anatomy and physiology of, 624, 624f
 conditions of
  acne vulgaris, 626–628, 626b, 626f, 627t
  athlete's foot, 635–636, 635b, 636f, 636t
  burns, 633–634, 633b, 634b, 634f
  cancer, 637b, 638–639, 638–639b, 638f, 639b
  chickenpox and shingles, 633, 633f
  diaper rash, 637–638
  eczema, 629–630, 629f, 630t
  head lice, 639–640, 640f
  impetigo, 636–637, 637f, 637t
  psoriasis, 623–624t, 630–633, 631f
  urticaria, 628–629, 628f
  warts, 634–635, 635f
Skin cancer, 637b, 638–639, 638–639b, 638f, 639b
Skull, 427
SLAs. *see* Service level agreements
SLE. *see* Systemic lupus erythematosus
Slow Fe. *see* Ferrous sulfate
Slow mover, 306
Small intestine, 506, 507f, 508f
Smallpox vaccine, 592–593t
Small-volume drips, in medication delivery systems, 262, 262b
SMART. *see* Salmeterol Multicenter Asthma Research Trial
Smart BMI, 422b
SMDA. *see* Safe Medical Devices Act
Smoking cessation, 395, 395b
SNRIs. *see* Serotonin norepinephrine reuptake inhibitors
SNS. *see* Sympathetic nervous system
Social anxiety disorder, 387
Social Security Administration, 291
Society for Education of Pharmacy Technicians (SEPhT), 77t, 78
Society for the Education of Pharmacy Technicians (SEPhT), 334
Soda fountain pharmacy, 12
Sodium, 529b, 531
Sodium acetate, 280t
Sodium bicarbonate, for gastroesophageal reflux disease and indigestion, 667t
Sodium bicarbonate/aspirin/citric acid, 510t
Sodium bicarbonate/citric acid/potassium bicarbonate, 510t
Sodium chloride, 280t
Sodium ferric gluconate complex, 648–649b, 648f
Sodium phosphate, 280t
 for gastrointestinal conditions, 668t
Sodium phosphate enema, 111
Sodium-glucose cotransporter 2 (SGLT2) inhibitors, 398–400t, 421–422t
Sofosbuvir, for hepatitis C, 571t, 572b, 572f

Soft lozenges, 243
Soft sticks, 244
Software writer, 76
Sole proprietorship, 164
Solid medications, 103, 104–107
  compounding, 240–243
Solifenacin, 541t, 542b, 542f
Solodyn. *see* Minocycline
Solubility, 239, 239b, 239f
Solu-Medrol. *see* Methylprednisolone sodium succinate
Solutes, 239
  albumin and, 645
Solutions, 239
  parenteral, 277, 277b, 277t
  preparing, 246
Solvent, 239, 276b, 277b, 280b
Soma. *see* Carisoprodol
Somatic nervous system, 368f, 372
Somatropin, 411, 411b, 411f
Sonata. *see* Zaleplon
SOPs. *see* Standard operating procedures
Sorbitol, for gastrointestinal conditions, 668t
Soriatane. *see* Acitretin
Sorilux. *see* Calcipotriene
Sotalol, 474t
Sotyktu. *see* Deucravacitinib
Sound-alike, look-alike drugs, 657b
  for eyes, ears, nose and throat, 620b
  in heart failure, 476b
  for renal system, 542b
  for reproductive system, 572b
Soy, 673t, 678
Spacers, 491b
Spansules, 105
Spatula, 234–235, 234t
Special orders, 306
Specialty Sterile Pharmaceutical Society (SSPS), 264
Speech impairments, 182
Sperm, 408–409, 547–549, 560–561
Spermatogenesis, 560–561
Spermicide, 558
Spinal accessory nerve, 373t
Spinal cord, 369–370, 371f, 435–436
Spinal manipulation, 681, 681b
Spirits, 108, 108f
Spiriva. *see* Tiotropium
Spironolactone, 322t, 458t, 459–460t, 475–476t, 537t, 538b, 538f
Spleen, 578, 578f, 580f
Splenectomy, 650b
Spongy bone, 427
Sprays, 108, 108f
Sprycel. *see* Dasatinib
Sputum, 499b
Squamous cell cancer, 638–639, 638f
SSPS. *see* Specialty Sterile Pharmaceutical Society
SSRIs. *see* Selective serotonin reuptake inhibitors
St. John's wort, 673t, 676t, 679–680, 679f

Stability
  in bulk repackaging, 228
  in nonsterile compounding, 247
Staff of Asclepius, 4
Standard operating procedures (SOPs), 264
Standard Precautions, 271–272, 273
Standing orders, 197
Stapes, 613f
Staphylococcus aureus, 636–637
Starlix. *see* Nateglinide
Stat order, 64, 197
State Board of Pharmacy (BOP), 195
State laws, pharmacy, 53
Statins, 458t, 461, 461b, 463t, 464b
  for cardiovascular system, 358
Status epilepticus, 376t
Stavudine, for human immunodeficiency virus infection and acquired immunodeficiency syndrome, 570t
Stelara. *see* Ustekinumab
Stent, 467–468b
Sterile 70% alcohol pads, 259t
Sterile compounding, 284
  area for, 179
  personnel cleansing and garbing order for, 204b
Sterile preparation, 281
Steroids, for asthma and COPD, 492t
Stewart, Ella Phillips, 13t
Sticks, medication, 243
  hard, 245
  soft, 244
  veterinary, 250–251
Stimate. *see* Desmopressin
Stimulant laxatives, 519–520, 519t
  for gastrointestinal conditions, 668t
Stock
  area, pharmacy, 177–178, 178f
  damage, 308
  expired, 308, 308b
  floor, 192–193
  levels of, in intravenous room, 261–262
  maintaining, 207–208, 208b
  new, 306, 307b
  ordering of, 63
  PAR levels and, 226–227, 228b
  pharmacy, 303–304
    abbreviations of, 258t
Stocking area, 339
  nonclinical, 345
Stomach, 505f
  acidity, 505b
  anatomy and physiology of, 505–508, 507f
  conditions affecting, 508–512, 509b, 511b
    gastroesophageal reflux disease (GERD), 504t, 509–511, 509b, 510t, 511t
    peptic ulcer disease (PUD), 511–512, 512f
Stool softener (emollient laxative), 519t
  for gastrointestinal conditions, 668t

Storage
  of medications, 119, 120t, 228, 306–307
  of vaccines, 596, 596b
Storefront, 340, 340f
Strattera. *see* Atomoxetine
Stratum basale, 625f
Stratum corneum, 625f
Strep throat, 618–619, 619f
Streptomycin, 499t
Stress, medication errors and, 319
Stress incontinence, 540–542
Stridex. *see* Salicylic acid
Strip packaging process, 341–342, 341f
Strip packs, 224
Stroke, 384, 384b, 461–464, 472–473
Subchondral bone, 427–428
Subcutaneous agents, 114
Subcutaneous layer, 624, 624f
Sublingual agents, 113, 113f
Sublingual gland, 505, 505f
Submandibular gland, 505, 505f
Suboxone, 50
Subscription, 169–170
Succinylcholine, 445t
Sudafed. *see* Pseudoephedrine
Suffix, term, 352
Sulfacetamide, 607–608t, 608b, 608f
Sulfamethoxazole/trimethoprim, 103, 627t
Sulfasalazine, 514t, 585–587t
Sulfonamides, 9–10, 539t, 607–608t
  for acne vulgaris, 627t
Sulfonylureas, 398–400t
Sumatriptan, 356–357, 364–366t, 384b, 384f
Superficial burns, 633b, 634b
Superior rectus muscle, 601f
Superior vena cava, 451–452
Superscription, 169
Supervisory technician, 64–65
Supplementation, 441t
Suppositories, 112, 112f, 245–246
  for gastrointestinal conditions, 668t
SureMed, 201
Surface area, 506
Suspending agents, 237t
Suspensions, 110–111, 110f, 111b, 239
  preparing, 246
  reconstituting premade, 240, 240t
Suspensory ligament, 601f
Sustained-released dosage form errors, 325
Suvorexant, 392t, 393b, 393f
Swallowing, 481b
Sweat glands, 624, 624f, 626f
Symbicort. *see* Budesonide/formoterol
Sympathetic nervous system (SNS), 371, 374f, 374t
  heart rate and, 453
Sympatholytics, 371
Sympathomimetics, 371, 611–612
Synalar. *see* Fluocinolone

Synapses, 367
Syncope, 460–461
Syndrome, definition of, 466
Syndrome of inappropriate antidiuretic hormone secretion
  (SIADH), 398–400t, 409–410
Synovium, 427–428
Synthetic amylin analog, 421–422t
Synthetic medicine, 675
Synthetic opioid fentanyl, 50
Synthroid. *see* Levothyroxine sodium
Syphilis, 8, 569t
Syringe caps, 259t
Syringe needles, 259t
Syringe system, patient-controlled analgesia, 263
Syringes, 231–234, 259t
  in measuring liquid medications, 138, 139f
  in parenteral medications, 259–260, 259f
Syrup, 107, 108f, 239
Systemic, definition of, 583–584
Systemic lupus erythematosus (SLE), 587–588, 588b
Systole, 452

T

T lymphocytes, 466, 579
Tablet molds, 240
Tablets, 104–105, 105b, 105t
  compounding
    compressed, 240–243
    molded, 240, 240b, 242b
  repackaging of, containers for, 224, 225f
  types of, 103, 103f
Tachycardia, 456
Tachyphylaxis, 356
Tachypnea, 484t
Tacrolimus, 585–587t, 629–630b, 629f, 630b, 630t
  ointment, 111
Tact, 84
Tadalafil, 565t, 568t
Tagamet HB 200. *see* Cimetidine
Tall man lettering, 320–321, 352–353, 353t
Tambocor. *see* Flecainide
Tamiflu. *see* Oseltamivir
Tamper-proof prescriptions, 37, 38b, 38f
Tamsulosin, 565t, 566b, 566f
Tapazole. *see* Methimazole
Tapentadol, 426–427t
TAR. *see* Treatment authorization request
Tardive dyskinesia, 389b
Tasmar. *see* Tolcapone
Taste, flavoring additives for, 236, 237t
Tazarotene, 632t
Tazorac. *see* Tazarotene
TCAs. *see* Tricyclic antidepressants
TD. *see* Tardive dyskinesia
Tea, herbal, 680
Teamwork, 79
Tears, 601
  artificial, 612

Technician manager, 66
Technician recruiter, 66
Technician trainer, 66
Technician verifiers, 64
Tegretol. *see* Carbamazepine
Tekturna. *see* Aliskiren
Telaprevir, for hepatitis C, 571t
Telepharmacy, 218, 218f
Telephone etiquette, 87–89, 88b, 88f
Temazepam, 364–366t, 392b, 392f, 392t
Temovate. *see* Clobetasol propionate
Temperature conversion, between Fahrenheit and Celsius, 129
Temporal lobe, 369
Tendons, 427
Tenecteplase, 470t
Tenivac, 592–593t
Tenofovir
  for hepatitis B, 571t
  for human immunodeficiency virus infection and acquired immunodeficiency syndrome, 570t
Tenormin. *see* Atenolol
TENS. *see* Transcutaneous electrical nerve
Teratogen, 558–559b
Teratogenic effects, of drugs, 356
Teratogenicity, 302
Terazosin, 459–460t, 565t, 566b, 566f
Terbinafine, 636t, 641b, 641f, 669t
Terconazole, 569t
Teriparatide, 440f, 441t
Terminally ill patients, communication with, 90, 90t
Terminology
  environment, 267b
  medical, 119–123, 121b, 121t, 123b
Testes, 402t, 408–409, 408f, 560–561, 561f, 562f
Testosterone, 402t, 547–549, 560–561, 562, 563t, 564, 564f
  functions of, 408–409, 548t, 560–561, 562f
  for male hypogonadism, 564b
  secondary exposure of children to, 564b
Tetanus vaccine, 592–593t
Tetracyclines, for acne vulgaris, 627b, 627f, 627t
Tetrahydrozoline, 603–604t, 617t, 665t
Thalassemia, 648t
Thalidomide, 22, 24
Thalitone. *see* Chlorthalidone
The Joint Commission (TJC), 52–53
  "Do Not Use List" of abbreviations, 96, 97t
  on medication error prevention, 327–328
  survey, of hospitals, 195
  on tall man lettering, 320–321
  USP 797 and, 264
Theo-24. *see* Theophylline
Theochron. *see* Theophylline
Theophylline, 322t, 492t
Theophylline elixir, 108
Therapeutic alliance, 182
Therapeutic alternatives, 288
Therapeutic index, 355–356

Thiazide
  for cardiac conditions, 459–460t, 475–476t
  for renal and urologic system conditions, 526–527t, 538
Thiazide-like diuretics, 526–527t, 537t, 538
Thiazolidinedione, 398–400t
Third-degree burn, 634f
Third-party billing, 297–299, 297t
  claim problems in, 300, 301f
  coverage expiration policy for drugs and, 300–301
  filling prescription too soon, 302
  handling nonformulary drugs or noncovered National Drug Codes, 302
  limitation of plan exceeded and, 301–302, 302b
  nonidentification match in, 302
  patient profiles and, 299–300, 300f
  plan limitations in, 303, 303b
  point of sale billing and, 297, 297b
  prior authorization and, 297–299, 298f, 299b
  processing claims in, 300, 301f
  resubmitting rejected claims in, 303
Thorax, 481
Throat, 618–620, 618f, 621
  conditions of, 618–620
    drugs for, 599–600t
    gastroesophageal reflux disease as, 619–620
    strep throat and tonsillitis as, 618–619, 618f
  therapeutic agents for, 360
Thrombin, 468–469
Thrombocytes, 646
Thrombocytopenia, 646, 650, 651b
Thrombolytics, 449–451t, 470t, 472t
Thrombophlebitis, 536b
Thrombosis, 468–469
Thrombotic events, 468–473, 469b, 470t
Thumb, metric rule of, 134
Thymus, 401, 578, 578f
Thyroid gland, 402t, 404, 404f, 409t
  conditions of, 412–414
    hyperthyroidism, 412, 412b, 412f
    hypothyroidism, 413–414, 413f
  desiccated, 414b, 414f
Thyroiditis, 413
Thyroid-stimulating hormone (TSH), 402t
Thyrotoxicosis, 412, 412f
Thyroxine (T_4), 401
TIA. *see* Transient ischemic attack
Tiagabine, 364–366t
  for epilepsy, 377t
Ticagrelor, 470t, 472t
Tikosyn. *see* Dofetilide
Time, international, 128, 128b, 128f
Time error, medication error in, 317t
Timolol, 610t, 611b, 611f
Timoptic. *see* Timolol
Tinactin. *see* Tolnaftate
Tinea capitis, 636f
Tinea pedis, 635, 636f
Tinidazole, 569t

Tinnitus, 615–616
Tiotropium, 492t
Tipranavir, for human immunodeficiency virus infection and acquired immunodeficiency syndrome, 570t
Tirofiban, 470t, 472t
Tirosint. see Levothyroxine sodium
Tirzepatide, 423b
Tissue mast cells, 581f
Tizanidine, 444b, 444f
TJC. see The Joint Commission
TNF. see Tumor necrosis factor
TNF inhibitors. see Tumor necrosis factor (TNF) inhibitors
TNF-alpha inhibitors. see Tumor necrosis factor (TNF)-alpha inhibitors
TNKase. see Tenecteplase
Tobramycin, 607–608t, 608b, 608f
Tobrex. see Tobramycin
Tocilizumab, 585–587t
Tofranil. see Imipramine
Tolak. see Fluorouracil
Tolcapone, 381t
Tolnaftate, 636b, 636f, 636t, 669t
Tolterodine, 541b, 541f, 541t
Tongue, 505, 505f
Tonsillitis, 618–619, 618f
Tonsils, 480, 578f
Topamax. see Topiramate
Topamax Sprinkles, 105–106
Topicort. see Desoximetasone
Topiramate, 364–366t
  for epilepsy, 377t
Toprol-XL. see Metoprolol
Toradol. see Ketorolac
Torsemide, 537t
Tort, 53
Total parenteral nutrition (TPN), 64, 278, 278f, 279f
  calculations in, 144
Toxoids, 595
TPN. see Total parenteral nutrition
Trabeculae, 427
Trabecular bone, 438–439
Trachea, 480, 480f, 481b
Tracrium. see Atracurium
Trade names, 150–151, 151b
  generic name vs., 289–290
Traditional Chinese medicine, 674t, 681–682
Tradjenta. see Linagliptin
Training
  in compounded sterile preparations, 282, 283b, 283f
  programs for pharmacy technician student, 68–70, 68–70b
Tramadol, 426–427t
Trandate. see Labetalol
Transcutaneous electrical nerve (TENS), 375b
Transdermal patches, 107, 107b, 107f
  contraceptive, 557b, 557t
Transfer needles, 259t
Transfer of prescriptions, for controlled substances, 42

Transient ischemic attack (TIA), 472–473, 472–473b
Transplant rejection, 577t, 585–587t, 591–592, 591b, 591f
  tacrolimus, 630b
Travatan. see Travoprost
Travel Sickness. see Meclizine
Travoprost, 610t
Trazodone, 386–387t
Treatment authorization request (TAR), 297–298, 298f
Trecator. see Ethionamide
Trephining, 4
Treponema pallidum, 569t
Tretinoin
  for acne vulgaris, 627b, 627f
  for hematologic cancer, 654–655t
Trexall. see Methotrexate
Triamcinolone, 443t, 488t, 489b, 489f, 616b, 616f, 665t
Triamcinolone acetonide
  for eczema, 630t, 632t
  for psoriasis, 632t
Triamterene, 458t, 459–460t, 537t, 538b, 538f
Triazolam, 364–366t
TRICARE, 295, 296f
Trichomonas vaginalis, 569t
Trichomoniasis vaginalis, 569t
Trichophyton rubrum, 635
Tricor. see Fenofibrate
Tricyclic antidepressants (TCAs), 386–387t
Triderm. see Triamcinolone acetonide
Trifluridine, 607–608t, 609b, 609f
Trigeminal nerve, 373t
Triglycerides (TGs), 461–464
Trihexyphenidyl, 381t
Triiodothyronine (T$_3$), 401
Trileptal. see Oxcarbazepine
Triostat. see Liothyronine sodium
Triprolidine, 488t
Triptans, 356–357
Trissel, Lawrence, 154
Triturate, 240
Troches, 106, 241–242, 243f
Trochlear nerve, 373t
Trospium, 541b, 541f, 541t
Trumenba, 592–593t
Trusopt. see Dorzolamide
Trust, in over-the-counter medications, 662
TSH. see Thyroid-stimulating hormone
Tuberculin skin test, 498–500, 499f
Tuberculosis, 498–500, 499b, 499f, 499t
  in employee, of hospitals, 257
  treatment of, 479t
  vaccine, 595b
Tubex cartridge, 259–260, 260f
Tubing, for pumps, 259t
Tubing transfer sets, 259t
Tubular reabsorption, 529, 530f
Tubular secretion, 529–531
Tudorza Pressair. see Aclidinium
Tumor necrosis factor (TNF), 579–580, 582f

Tumor necrosis factor (TNF)-alpha inhibitors, 514t, 585–587t
Tumor necrosis factor (TNF) inhibitors, 632t
Tumor treatment, propranolol and, 457b
Tums. *see* Calcium carbonate
Turner syndrome, 554–555, 554f
21st Century Cures Act, 30t
Twinrix, 592–593t
Tylenol. *see* Acetaminophen
Tylenol w/ Codeine. *see* Acetaminophen/codeine
Tympanic membrane, 613, 613f
Type 1 diabetes mellitus (T1DM), 409t, 418
Type 2 diabetes mellitus (T2DM), 409t, 418
Typhim Vi, 592–593t
Typhoid vaccine, 592–593t
Typing skills, 63
Tyrosine kinase inhibitors, 654–655t
Tysabri. *see* Natalizumab
Tyzine. *see* Tetrahydrozoline

U

Ubrogepant, 384b
UCFs. *see* Universal claim forms
Ulcerative colitis, 515, 515b, 515f
Ulcers, 666b
Uloric. *see* Febuxostat
Ultram. *see* Tramadol
Umeclidinium/vilanterol, 497b, 497f
Unauthorized drug error, 317t
Unisom. *see* Doxylamine
Unit dose (UD), 224, 344
    medications, 202
    packs, 224
    record, 226, 226t, 227f
United States Adopted Names Council (USANC), 352
United States Pharmacists' Pharmacopeia, 153
United States Pharmacopeia (USP), 126–127, 195, 263–264
United States Pharmacopeia 795 (USP 795), 229–230
United States Pharmacopeia 797 (USP 797), 263–271
    in chemotherapeutic agents, 281–282
    history of, 263–264, 264t
    intravenous environment in, 266–267, 266f, 267b, 268f
    regulations, 330–331
    requirements for compounding in, 266, 267t
    risk levels in, 265–266, 265f, 266f, 267t
    sections of, 264–265, 265t
    stock levels in, 261
United States Pharmacopeia 800 (USP 800), in chemotherapeutic agents, 281–282
United States Pharmacopeial (USP) Convention, 330
United States Pharmacopoeia-National Formulary (USP-NF), 153, 157t, 177
Unithroid. *see* Levothyroxine sodium
Units
    calculations with liquid medication, 139
    definition of, 139
Univasc. *see* Moexipril
Universal claim forms (UCFs), 300, 301f
Universal Precautions, 271–272, 273
Upper respiratory system
    disorders and conditions of, 485–490, 486t
        allergies, 488–489, 488b, 488t
        common cold, 485–488, 487b
        influenza, 489–490, 490b, 490f, 490t
        rhinitis, 489, 489b
    structure and function of, 480–481, 481b, 482f
Upset stomach, 511b
Ureteroscopy, 535–536b
Ureters, 527
Urethra, 562
Urethritis, 539
Urge incontinence, 540–542
Uric acid, 440
Uricosuric agent, 443t
Urinary acidification, 529
Urinary analgesic, 539t
Urinary antispasmodic, 539t
Urinary incontinence, 540–542
Urinary system
    anatomy and physiology of, 527–531, 528f, 529f
        function of the kidneys, 527–528
        importance of electrolytes in, 531
        in males, 561–562, 561f
        nephron function in, 528–531, 529f
    conditions of, 531–542
        chronic kidney disease, 531–535, 532t, 533f
        common drugs for, 526–527t
        edema as, 536–539, 536b, 536f, 537t
        kidney stones as, 535–536, 535f
        urinary incontinence as, 540–542
        urinary tract infections as, 539–540, 539b, 539t
Urinary tract, 528f
Urinary tract infections, 526–527t, 539–540, 539b, 539t
Urine, 529
Urofollitropin, 552–553t
Urolithiasis, 535–536
Urticaria, 628–629, 628f
US Adopted Names Council, 151
US Department of Agriculture, 21
USANC. *see* United States Adopted Names Council
Use in specific populations, 44
USP. *see United States Pharmacopeia*
USP-NF. *see United States Pharmacopoeia-National Formulary*
Ustekinumab, 632t
Uterus, 547–549

V

Vaccine Information Statement, 594b
Vaccines, 592, 592–593t
    acellular, 595b
    adenovirus, 592–593t
    adult immunizations, 595t
    advances in, 10–11t, 10–11
    affecting immune system, 576–577t
    anthrax, 592–593t
    antiidiotypic, 595b

Vaccines *(Continued)*
  bacterial, 576–577t, 595, 595b
  childhood immunizations, 594b
  conjugated, 595b
  diphtheria, 592–593t
  hepatitis A, 592–593t
  hepatitis B, 592–593t
  herpes zoster, 592–593t
  human papillomavirus, 592–593t, 634–635
  for immune system, 360
  influenza, 592–593t
  Japanese encephalitis, 592–593t
  live, 594
  measles, 592–593t
  miscellaneous, 595–596, 595b
  mumps, 592–593t
  pertussis, 592–593t
  pneumococcal, 592–593t
  polio, 592–593t
  rabies, 592–593t
  rotavirus, 592–593t
  for shingles, 633
  storage of, 596, 596b
  subunit, 595b
  tetanus, 592–593t
  typhoid, 592–593t
  varicella, 592–593t
  viral, 576–577t, 594–595
  yellow fever, 592–593t
Vagifem. *see* Estradiol
Vaginal candidiasis, 569t
Vaginal fungal infections, agents for, 546–547t
Vaginal suppositories, 112
Vagus nerve, 373t
Valacyclovir, 572b, 572f, 633b, 633f
Valium. *see* Diazepam
Valproic acid, 364–366t
Valsartan, 358, 455b, 455f, 459–460t
Valtrex. *see* Valacyclovir
Vanos. *see* Fluocinonide
Vaporizers, 109
Vaqta, 592–593t
Vardenafil, 568t
Varenicline, 395b, 395f
Varicella vaccine, 592–593t
Varivax, 592–593t
Vas deferens, 561–562
Vasoconstriction, 453
Vasodilation, 453, 583
Vasodilators, 472t, 475–476t, 568t
Vasopressin, 398–400t, 403–404
Vasotec. *see* Enalapril
Vecuronium, 426–427t, 445t
Vein, 451–452
  in hair, 625f
Vena cava, 451–452
Venesection, 8
Venlafaxine, 357, 364–366t, 385b, 385f, 386–387t

Ventolin HFA. *see* Albuterol
Ventricle, 451–452
Verapamil, 322t, 458t, 459–460t
Verbal communication, 85–86, 86b, 87b
Verbal skills, 86
Verified Internet Pharmacy Practice Sites (VIPPS), 51–52, 67
Vernor, James, 13t
VERP. *see* National Vaccine Error Reporting Program
Vertical airflow hoods, 204–205, 206, 206f
Vertical laminar flow hood, cleaning, 267, 271b
Vesanoid. *see* Tretinoin
Vestibule, 614b, 614f
Vestibulocochlear nerve, 373t
Veterinary medications, 48, 250–251, 251b, 251t
Viaflex bags, 207, 262
Vials
  aseptic technique and, 276, 276b
  for parenteral medications, 261f
Vibegron, 542b
Vibramycin. *see* Doxycycline
Vicodin. *see* Hydrocodone/acetaminophen
Victoza. *see* Liraglutide
Vigabatrin, for epilepsy, 377t
Vigamox. *see* Moxifloxacin
Vilazodone, 386–387t
Villus, 506
Viloxazine, 395b
Vimpat. *see* Lacosamide
Vinca alkaloids, 654–655t
Vindesine, 654–655t
Vinorelbine, 500b
VIPPS. *see* Verified Internet Pharmacy Practice Sites
Viral infections, ophthalmic, 609
Viral vaccines, 576–577t, 594–595
Virion, 594–595
Viroptic. *see* Trifluridine
Virtual communication etiquette, 89
Viruses, 594–595
Vision, 602
Visken. *see* Pindolol
Vitamin D, 441t
Vitamin D analog, 526–527t
Vitamin K antagonist (VKA), 470t
Vitreous humor, 601–602, 601f
Vivotif Berna, 592–593t
VKA. *see* Vitamin K antagonist
Vocal cords, 480
Vocal skills, 86
Voltaren. *see* Diclofenac
Volume, 132–133
  in avoirdupois system, 136
  household measurements of, 134, 134t
  in nonsterile compounding, 238, 239f
Vomiting, 504t, 520–522
von Behring, Emil, 10–11t
Von Willebrand disease, 657
VoSpire ER. *see* Albuterol

Voxelotor, 649b
Vyvanse. *see* Lisdexamfetamine

W

Walgreens, 165, 318
Warfarin, 469b, 469f, 470t
    adverse drug events and, 657b
    interactions, medication errors and, 322, 322t
Warnings and precautions, 44
Warts, 634–635, 635f
Washington, George, 7
Water-soluble bases, 244b, 245
Watson, James, 10
Wearable devices, 423
Weighing, in nonsterile compounding, 235, 235b, 236f
    techniques for, 237–238, 238b
Weight
    in apothecary system, 135, 135b
    in avoirdupois system, 136, 136t
    in household system, 134
    in metric system, 132–133
WelChol. *see* Colesevelam
Wellbutrin. *see* Bupropion
Wellbutrin XL. *see* Bupropion
White matter, 369
White Paper on Pharmacy Technicians 2002, 59, 59b
White pulp, 578, 580f
Whitney, Harvey A.K., 13t
Whole blood, 645, 645f
Wholesale cost, 146
Wholesalers, 310
Wiley, Harvey, 21
Wiley Act, 21–22
Wilkins, Maurice, 10
Window pickup area, 344
Winsley, William, 318
Word problems, 131–132
Workers' compensation, 296–297, 297b
World Health Organization, 385
Written communication skills, 89–90, 89b, 90b

X

Xalatan. *see* Latanoprost
Xanax. *see* Alprazolam
Xanthine, 479t
Xanthine oxidase inhibitor, 443t
Xarelto. *see* Rivaroxaban
Xatmep. *see* Methotrexate
Xenical. *see* Orlistat
Xerosis, 629b
Xolair. *see* Omalizumab
Xopenex. *see* Levalbuterol
Xopenex HFA. *see* Levalbuterol
Xylocaine. *see* Lidocaine
Xyzal. *see* Levocetirizine

Y

Yellow fever vaccine, 592–593t
YF-Vax, 592–593t
Yoga, 680, 681f
Young's Rule, for pediatric dosing, 139

Z

Zaclir Cleansing. *see* Benzoyl peroxide
Zaditor. *see* Ketotifen
Zafirlukast, 492t
Zaleplon, 364–366t
Zanaflex. *see* Tizanidine
Zanamivir, 490t
Zantac. *see* Ranitidine
Zantac 150. *see* Ranitidine
Zarontin. *see* Ethosuximide
Zaroxolyn. *see* Metolazone
Zarxio. *see* Filgrastim
Zeasorb-AF. *see* Miconazole
Zebeta. *see* Bisoprolol
Zegerid. *see* Omeprazole + sodium bicarbonate
Zelapar. *see* Selegiline
Zemplar. *see* Paricalcitol
Zenatane. *see* Isotretinoin
Zestril. *see* Lisinopril
Zetia. *see* Ezetimibe
Zidovudine, for human immunodeficiency virus infection and acquired immunodeficiency syndrome, 570t
Zinc, 280t
Zinc oxide paste, 112
Ziprasidone, 364–366t, 391b, 391f
Zirgan. *see* Ganciclovir
Zithromax. *see* Azithromycin
Zocor. *see* Simvastatin
Zofran. *see* Ondansetron
Zofran ODT. *see* Ondansetron
Zoladex, 106–107
Zoledronic acid, 441t
Zolmitriptan, 364–366t
Zoloft. *see* Sertraline
Zolpidem, 364–366t, 392t, 393b, 393f
Zolpimist. *see* Zolpidem
Zomig. *see* Zolmitriptan
ZonaCort. *see* Dexamethasone
Zonegran. *see* Zonisamide
Zonisamide, for epilepsy, 377t
Zortress. *see* Everolimus
Zostavax, 592–593t
Zostrix. *see* Capsaicin
Zovirax. *see* Acyclovir
Zuplenz. *see* Ondansetron
Zylet. *see* Loteprednol and tobramycin
Zyloprim. *see* Allopurinol
Zymaxid. *see* Gatifloxacin
Zyprexa. *see* Olanzapine
Zyrtec. *see* Cetirizine HCl